WOMEN'S HEALTH ACROSS THE LIFESPAN

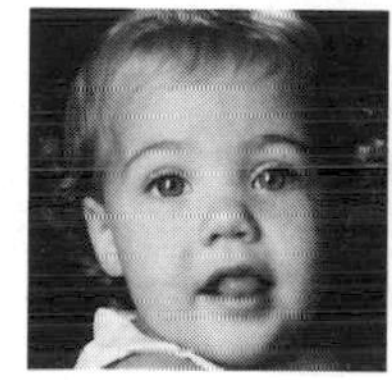
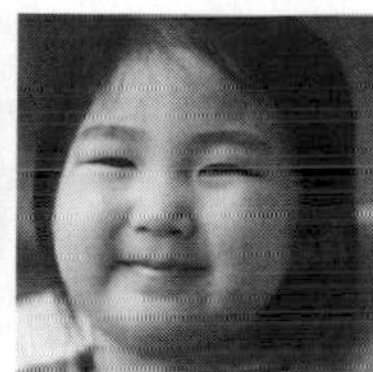
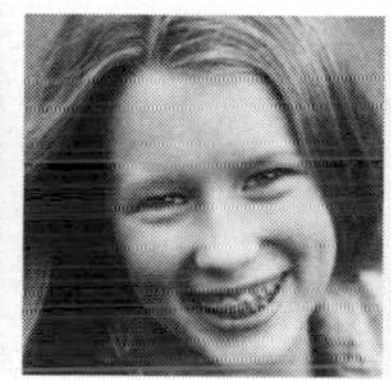
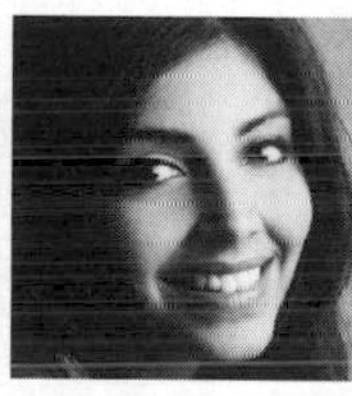
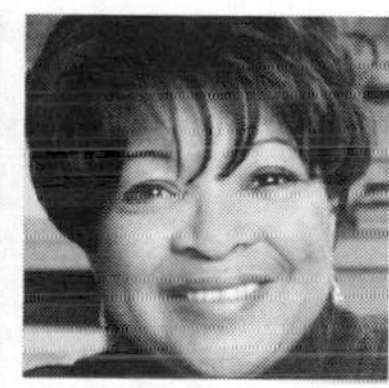
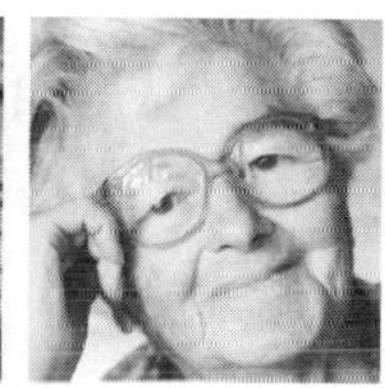

A PHARMACOTHERAPEUTIC APPROACH

Laura Marie Borgelt, Pharm.D., BCPS, FCCP

Mary Beth O'Connell, Pharm.D., BCPS, FASHP, FCCP

Judith Ann Smith, Pharm.D., BCOP, FCCP, FISOPP

Karim Anton Calis, Pharm.D., MPH, FASHP, FCCP

Disclaimer: *Dr. Calis contributed to this textbook in his personal capacity. The views expressed are his own and do not necessarily represent the views or policies of the Food and Drug Administration, the National Institutes of Health, or the United States Government.*

American Society of Health-System Pharmacists®

BETHESDA, MARYLAND

Any correspondence regarding this publication should be sent to the publisher, American Society of Health-System Pharmacists, 7272 Wisconsin Avenue, Bethesda, MD 20814, attention: Special Publishing.

Director, Special Publishing: Jack Bruggeman
Acquisitions Editor: Rebecca Olson
Senior Editorial Project Manager: Dana Battaglia
Production Editor: Kristin Eckles
Editorial assistance: Moyo Myers
Cover and page design: DeVall Advertising
Original art: Holly Fischer, MFA

Library of Congress Cataloging-in-Publication Data

Women's health across the lifespan : a pharmacotherapeutic approach / [edited by] Laura Marie Borgelt ... [et al.].
p. ; cm.
Includes bibliographical references and index.
ISBN 978-1-58528-194-7
1. Women's health services. 2. Women--Diseases--Chemotherapy. I. Borgelt, Laura Marie. II. American Society of Health-System Pharmacists.
[DNLM: 1. Women's Health. 2. Drug Therapy. 3. Sex Factors. WA 309.1 W87263 2010]
RA564.85.W666522 2010
613′.04244--dc22

2010003646

ISBN 978-1-58528-194-7

DEDICATION

I dedicate this book to my three wonderful boys—Thor, Leif, and Lars—who remind me to cherish every moment and create lasting memories; and to my amazing mom Ellen, who has been an inspiring role model in becoming an independent, loving, and confident woman.

—Laura Marie Borgelt

I would like to thank my Mom and Aunt Dolores; the nurses in my upbringing who paved the way for a healthcare profession; my Dad; my Grandma Guelig; my brother and his family; my sister and her family; and all my great relatives, friends, teachers, and colleagues who consistently provide support, encouragement, happiness, and especially love along the way of my professional endeavors.

—Mary Beth O'Connell

I dedicate this book to my wonderful son, Lance, whose arrival has been a blessing and source of endless happiness in my life and to my husband, Heath, for all his love and endless support....steady as we go.

—Judith Ann Smith

This book is dedicated to my loving wife and our precious little girls; to my devoted mom, sisters, and brother; and to my beloved dad who left us too soon—with special thanks to our Blessed Mother for her guidance and inspiration.

—Karim Anton Calis

December 2009

Contents

FOREWORD

Women's bodies are different from those of men! This seems such an obvious statement—even children recognize the differences at an early age. Yet, it has been only recently that the scientific and healthcare communities have begun to give due attention to the fact that these differences exist beyond just body shape and reproductive systems and organs, and that they are very important in the full understanding of the health and well-being of women and men, and how we can best prevent, diagnose, or treat all conditions and diseases. Important causes of mortality and morbidity such as osteoporosis, cardiovascular disease, chronic pain, addiction, and mental health, among many others, may differ in various aspects between women and men. Almost all organ systems have shown sex and gender variations from differences in anatomy, physiology, and pathophysiology to the response to medications. Even more attention is needed in consideration of pharmacotherapeutic approaches to women, with the appreciation of sex differences that can and do influence their effectiveness or effects. This new text, *Women's Health Across the Lifespan: A Pharmacotherapeutic Approach,* goes beyond the reproductive healthcare issues that are unique to women and examines the issues of chronic illness that have a higher prevalence in women and warrant sex/gender differences in treatment regimens. Its publication is not only timely but provides a needed comprehensive source of valuable information.

Healthcare providers must integrate the biopsychosocial aspects of sex/gender specific care in confronting treatment adherence problems and disparities in health status and health outcomes. Women's health research is a model for expanding the study of the many important factors that affect the health of girls and women. This holistic approach, reaching beyond biomedical and biobehavioral contributors, includes poverty; culture and ethnicity; geographic location and environmental influences; access to healthcare; education; gender differences in provider-patient interaction; communications; sexual orientation; occupational stresses; and the unique demands of disabilities as potential contributing factors to the health of women. Furthermore, women can be considered as the portal to family and community health—often as motivators or caregivers for their families and those around them and as givers of life through whom their own preconception and pregnancy bodily health can affect future generations. So, considerations of how healthcare is delivered to women have far reaching implications. The editors have applied the holistic approach in the development of this text to assist healthcare professionals and others to identify and effectively consider all of these issues when treating their female patients.

Since the establishment of the NIH Office of Research on Women's Health, the concept of women's health has expanded to embrace the entire lifespan, from in utero to infancy and childhood, adolescence, reproductive years, menopause, and the elderly years. Additionally, this concept has extended further to include the totality of physical, mental, behavioral, and sociocultural factors that contribute to the total body health of women. This text helps respond to many of these concerns through its chapters that detail not only the historical, biological, and behavioral facets of women's health across the lifespan as we understand it today, but also by informing through narrative and case studies the challenges for principles of pharmacotherapeutics in the care of women. This book provides an interdisciplinary and multidisciplinary resource for the future care of girls and women through its incredible wealth of information, especially as one of the first to place emphasis on sex and gender differences in regards to medication protocols.

I hope that *Women's Health Across the Lifespan* will stimulate change in some practice paradigms, especially shifting from lack of consideration of sex/gender differences to algorithms and practices specific to a more individualized treatment of disease and promotion of healthy lifestyle behaviors including known sex/gender differences. Medications are important to the care of girls and women, but adherence to these therapies may not always be optimal due to many reasons in the lives of women. By understanding the concept of the totality of girls and women, providers can help improve individual female wellness and disease prevention and control. With a sex/gender approach, we are learning more about the health of women, their families, and their communities.

This book will be a valuable resource for new and established healthcare practitioners. The reader will be able to incorporate a better understanding of sex/gender influences into the delivery of care and his or her own standards of approach to patient issues. The reader should also be able to individualize medication therapy and maximize the resultant health outcomes from preconception to the end of life for girls and women. The cases and bioethical challenges help the reader identify sex and gender differences and then individualize care based on sex/gender principles. And, hopefully, readers will gain an appreciation of the importance of new scientific advances related to evolving technologies, therapies, and practices that can unravel the continuing and emerging gaps in knowledge about women's health, spurring them to become advocates for women's health and the study of sex/gender factors.

Vivian W. Pinn, MD
Associate Director for Research on Women's Health
Director, Office of Research on Women's Health
National Institutes of Health
U.S. Department of Health and Human Services
November 2009

Preface

That men and women are different seems obvious. The sexes are different physically, physiologically, emotionally, and socially. They are also potentially different in their pharmacokinetics, pharmacodynamics, and response to drug therapy. But historically, the same approach has been applied to the medical care of both sexes. In fact, until now, no one comprehensive resource existed that addressed the complex pharmacotherapeutic and health needs of women. As a result, there has been a significant gap in knowledge that we believe has limited the ability of medical professionals to provide optimal healthcare for girls and women. Healthcare providers need to have an appreciation for the potential influences of sex and gender on medication disposition, response, and quality of life as these can profoundly affect wellness and disease.

To illustrate this point, imagine your next clinical encounter with a girl, woman, mother-to-be, or grandmother. Providing your patient with the best care will mean individualizing her medication therapy to fit her unique medical needs while balancing the complex psychosocial influences of her everyday life. Physiologic and hormonal stresses, social pressures, psychologic issues, emotional challenges, and economic strains are among the factors that must be considered along with sex-related clinical differences.

We developed *Women's Health Across the Lifespan: A Pharmacotherapeutic Approach* to be a comprehensive primary reference for healthcare professionals and students who work or interact with female patients. Several goals guided us as we planned the book. First, we wanted to ensure that in discussing pharmacotherapy issues, we addressed not only sex- and gender-specific medication response, but also the social, economic, physiologic, spiritual, emotional, and ethical issues that directly or indirectly affect medication use. In order to present a well-balanced approach for each topic, we enlisted the assistance of a diverse group of healthcare professionals and content experts from around the world to serve as contributors and reviewers. We also strongly believed that the information presented in this book should further enhance and augment the information already available in primary care resources. Finally, we made every effort to ensure that the content is comprehensive, authoritative, objective, up-to-date, and evidenced based. All of these principles informed our goal of making this book a necessary resource that complements other references by providing a greater depth of coverage on sex and gender issues, which are vitally important to health.

We chose not to present the book in a chronological order so we could more comprehensively address broader social and ethical issues that affect girls and women at various stages in their lifespan. To achieve this goal, the book is organized into eight sections:

1. The historical and social context of women's health
2. The biology, physiology, and wellness of girls and women
3. Menstrual health
4. Contraceptive methods
5. Preconception, pregnancy, and postpartum care
6. Selected conditions that affect women differently or disproportionately compared to men
7. Cancers that affect women
8. Ethical issues in women's healthcare

In order to provide a logical, orderly presentation for readers, we created a standard template for our clinical chapters. The clinical presentation and pathophysiology sections will be helpful for readers to fully understand the rationale for medication therapy. Guidelines and preventive therapy are discussed where applicable. The treatment sections include the overall treatment goals along with a discussion of nonpharmacologic and pharmacologic therapies, monitoring, and patient education. Information regarding complementary and alternative therapies is provided where appropriate based on available evidence.

We felt strongly that some special features within each chapter would make the information more relevant to users, particularly students. As a result, specific pedagogy was incorporated to enhance learning in the classroom. Each chapter in this book includes measurable learning objectives that can be used to assess learning. All chapters include a patient case, typically presented in a "book end" fashion, where subjective and objective information appears at the beginning of the chapter and the assessment and plan close the chapter. This allows the case to complement the chapter content and highlight critical concepts in therapeutics and clinical practice. Chapters also include a feature called "therapeutic challenges." The therapeutic challenges present difficult or unresolved issues in women's health pharmacotherapy that can be debated and further studied. They are intended to spur critical thinking and further exploration of a topic, and may be particularly suitable for in-class and group discussions. Tables and figures highlight the most relevant content. For many chapters, additional textbook content—including more patient cases, tables, and figures—can be found online at www.ashp.org/womenshealth. The added content is noted in the book with the following text and computer screen icon:

Additional content available at
www.ashp.org/womenshealth

An important and innovative feature of the book is that full reference lists for each chapter can be found online. Where possible, these references are hyperlinked to their corresponding PubMed citations or other relevant sources of additional information.

Our goal was to create a book that would help healthcare professionals, educators, and students to

- discover the unique facets of girls' and women's healthcare;
- address healthcare needs across the female lifespan;
- describe rational, evidence-based pharmacotherapeutic interventions based on sex and gender differences;
- foster lively discussions about controversies and challenges in the care of girls and women; and
- stimulate research that leads to advances in women's healthcare.

We are confident that this comprehensive resource will help to advance educational endeavors in girls' and women's health, and ultimately improve the care provided to these patients. We are sincerely grateful for the contributions of the chapter authors and reviewers who generously shared their knowledge, experience, and time to enhance the scope, depth, and accuracy of this resource. We greatly appreciate the support, guidance, and assistance of the staff at the American Society of Health-System Pharmacists. The expertise, insight, and positive encouragement of Dana Battaglia and Rebecca Olson were especially valuable. Our greatest hope is that you, the reader, will find that this resource helps you in caring for and treating your patients in a way that considers all the unique, complex, and dynamic aspects of girls and women during their lifetime.

Laura Marie Borgelt
Mary Beth O'Connell
Judith Ann Smith
Karim Anton Calis

October 2009

EDITORS

Laura Marie Borgelt, Pharm.D., BCPS, FCCP
Associate Professor
Schools of Pharmacy and Medicine
Anschutz Medical Campus
University of Colorado Denver
Aurora, Colorado

Mary Beth O'Connell, Pharm.D., BCPS, FASHP, FCCP
Associate Professor
Pharmacy Practice Department
Eugene Applebaum College of Pharmacy and Health Sciences
Wayne State University
Detroit, Michigan

Judith Ann Smith, Pharm.D., BCOP, FCCP, FISOPP
Associate Professor and Director, Pharmacology Research
Department of Gynecologic Oncology, Division of Surgery
Director, Oncology Translational Research Fellowship
Division of Pharmacy
The University of Texas M. D. Anderson Cancer Center
Houston, Texas

Karim Anton Calis, Pharm.D., MPH, FASHP, FCCP
Clinical Reviewer
Division of Metabolism and Endocrinology Products
U.S. Food and Drug Administration
Silver Spring, Maryland
Clinical Investigator
Eunice Kennedy Shriver National Institute of Child Health and Human Development and National Institute of Diabetes and Digestive and Kidney Diseases
National Institutes of Health
Bethesda, Maryland
Clinical Professor
University of Maryland School of Pharmacy
Baltimore, Maryland
Professor
Medical College of Virginia
Virginia Commonwealth University School of Pharmacy
Richmond, Virginia

Contributors

Jean Abbott, MD, MH
Professor Emeritus
Emergency Medicine Faculty
Center for Bioethics and Humanities
University of Colorado Denver—Health Sciences Center
Aurora, Colorado

Kyle Anderson, MD
Research Assistant
Department of Dermatology
Northwestern University
Chicago, Illinois

Alicia Armstrong MD, MHSCR
Associate Fellowship Director
Reproductive Endocrinology and Infertility
Program in Reproductive and Adult Endocrinology
NICHD
National Institutes of Health
Bethesda, Maryland

Margaret B. Artz, Ph.D., R.Ph.
Senior Researcher
Clinical Informatics
Ingenix
Eden Prairie, Minnesota

Teresa M. Bailey, Pharm.D., BCPS, FCCP
Professor
Ferris State University College of Pharmacy
Big Rapids, Michigan

Jacquelyn L. Bainbridge, B.S.Pharm., Pharm.D.
Professor
Department of Clinical Pharmacy/Department of Neurology
University of Colorado Denver
Aurora, Colorado

Tiki Bakhshi, MD
MAJ, US Army, MC
Staff, Maternal—Fetal Medicine
Tripler Army Medical Center
Honolulu, Hawaii

Chad Barnett, Pharm.D, BCOP
Clinical Pharmacy Specialist—Breast Oncology
The University of Texas M. D. Anderson Cancer Center
Houston, Texas

Sneha Baxi, Pharm.D.
Clinical Assistant Professor
Chicago State University
Chicago, Illinois

Evelyn S. Becker, Pharm.D, MA
Professor of Biology
St. Louis College of Pharmacy
St. Louis, Missouri

James A. Berch, AB, MA
Permanent Deacon
Archdiocese of Detroit
St. Clair Shores, Michigan

Pamela D. Berens, MD
Professor
Department of Obstetrics, Gynecology & Reproductive Sciences
University of Texas Medical School—Houston
Houston, Texas

Laura Marie Borgelt, Pharm.D., BCPS, FCCP
Associate Professor
Schools of Pharmacy and Medicine
Anschutz Medical Campus
University of Colorado Denver
Aurora, Colorado

Wendy B. Bostwick, Ph.D., MPH
Assistant Professor
Public Health and Health Education Programs
Northern Illinois University
School of Nursing and Health Studies
De Kalb, Illinois

Susan K. Bowles, B.Sc.Pharm., Pharm.D., M.Sc.
Associate Professor of Clinical Pharmacy and Geriatric Medicine
Dalhousie University
Halifax, Nova Scotia, Canada

Jennie Broders, Pharm.D.
PGY2 Ambulatory Care Pharmacy Resident
Duke University Medical Center
Clinical Instructor
Eshelman School of Pharmacy
University of North Carolina at Chapel Hill
Durham, North Carolina

Candace S. Brown, Pharm.D., MSN
Professor
Departments of Clinical Pharmacy, Ob/Gyn, and Psychiatry
University of Tennessee Health Science Center
Memphis, Tennessee

Jubilee Brown, MD
Associate Professor
Department of Gynecologic Oncology
The University of Texas M. D. Anderson Cancer Center
Houston, Texas

Kimberley C. Brown, Pharm.D., AAHIVE
Science and Research Liaison
Tibotec Therapeutics
Jacksonville, Florida

Karim Anton Calis, Pharm.D., MPH, FASHP, FCCP
Clinical Reviewer
Division of Metabolism and Endocrinology Products
U.S. Food and Drug Administration
Silver Spring, Maryland
Clinical Investigator
Eunice Kennedy Shriver National Institute of Child Health and Human Development and National Institute of Diabetes and Digestive and Kidney Diseases
National Institutes of Health
Bethesda, Maryland
Clinical Professor
University of Maryland School of Pharmacy
Baltimore, Maryland
Professor
Medical College of Virginia
Virginia Commonwealth University School of Pharmacy
Richmond, Virginia

Raymond Cha, Pharm.D.
Assistant Clinical Professor
Pharmacy Practice Department
Eugene Applebaum College of Pharmacy and Health Sciences
Wayne State University
Detroit, Michigan

Mary L. Chavez, B.S.Pharm., Pharm.D., FAACP
Professor and Chair of Pharmacy Practice
Texas A&M HSC Rangel College of Pharmacy
Kingsville, Texas

Kai I. Cheang, Pharm.D., M.Sc., BCPS, FCCP
Associate Professor of Pharmacy
Virginia Commonwealth University
Richmond, Virginia

Judy T. Chen, Pharm.D, BCPS, CDE
Clinical Assistant Professor of Pharmacy Practice
Wishard Health Services
Purdue University School of Pharmacy and Pharmaceutical Sciences
Indianapolis, Indiana

Lynn M. Cloutier RN, MSN, ACNP, AOCN
Inpatient Nurse Practitioner
Department of Gynecologic Oncology
M. D. Anderson Cancer Center
Houston, Texas

Andrea L. Coffee, Pharm.D., BCPS, MBA
Pharmacy Clinical Specialist
Scott & White Healthcare
Temple, Texas

Lisa B. Cohen, Pharm.D., CDE
Assistant Professor
University of Rhode Island
Kingston, Rhode Island

Nicole S. Culhane, Pharm.D., BCPS, FCCP
Director of Experiential Education
Associate Professor
Clinical and Administrative Sciences
College of Notre Dame of Maryland School of Pharmacy
Baltimore, Maryland

Devra K. Dang, Pharm.D., BCPS, CDE
Associate Clinical Professor
University of Connecticut School of Pharmacy
Storrs, Connecticut

Susan R. Davis, MBBS, Ph.D., FRACP
Professor of Women's Health
Women's Health Program
Department of Medicine
Central Clinical School
Monash University
Prahran, Victoria, Australia

Heather E. Dillaway, Ph.D.
Associate Professor
Director of Undergraduate Studies
Department of Sociology
Wayne State University
Detroit, Michigan

Bethany A. DiPaula, Pharm.D., BCPP
Assistant Professor
Director of Pharmacy
University of Maryland School of Pharmacy
Baltimore, Maryland

Don Downing, R.Ph.
Clinical Professor
Department of Pharmacy
University of Washington
Seattle, Washington

Shareen Y. El-Ibiary, Pharm.D., BCPS
Associate Professor of Pharmacy Practice
Department of Pharmacy Practice
Midwestern University College of Pharmacy—Glendale
Glendale, Arizona

Janet L. Espirito, Pharm.D., BCOP
Clinical Coordinator
US Oncology
The Woodlands, Texas

Joslyn W. Fisher, MD, MPH, FACP
Associate Professor of Medicine and Medical Ethics
Baylor College of Medicine
Houston, Texas

Alicia B. Forinash, Pharm.D., BCPS, CCD
Associate Professor of Pharmacy Practice
St. Louis College of Pharmacy
St. Louis, Missouri

Jaclyn Michelle Graham, Pharm.D.
Clinical Pharmacist
Bay Pines VA
St. Petersburg, Florida

Philip J. Gregory, Pharm.D.
Editor, Natural Medicines Comprehensive Database
Assistant Professor, Pharmacy Practice
Center for Drug Information and Evidence-Based Practice

School of Pharmacy and Health Professions
Creighton University
Omaha, Nebraska

Amy M. Haddad, Ph.D.
Director
Center for Health Policy and Ethics
Dr. C.C. and Mabel L. Criss Endowed Chair in the Health Sciences
Creighton University
Omaha, Nebraska

Thomas W. Hale, R.Ph., Ph.D.
Professor
Department of Pediatrics
Texas Tech University School of Medicine
Amarillo, Texas

Sharon L. Hame, MD
Associate Clinical Professor
Department of Orthopaedic Surgery
David Geffen UCLA School of Medicine
Los Angeles, California

Brian A. Hemstreet, Pharm.D., BCPS
Associate Professor
Director, Pharmaceutical Care Learning Center
University of Colorado Denver School of Pharmacy
Aurora, Colorado

Jaou-Chen Huang, MD, FACOG
Associate Professor
Division of Reproductive Endocrinology and Infertility
Department of Obstetrics, Gynecology, and Reproductive Sciences
University of Texas Medical School at Houston
Houston, Texas

Andrea K. Hubbard, Ph.D.
Associate Dean
University of Connecticut School of Pharmacy
Storrs, Connecticut

Anne L. Hume, Pharm.D., FCCP, BCPS
Professor of Pharmacy
University of Rhode Island
Kingston, Rhode Island
Adjunct Professor of Family Medicine
Warren Alpert School of Medicine
Brown University
Providence, Rhode Island

Mary E. S. Indritz, Ph.D., R.Ph., FASHP
President
Compass Healthcare Consulting, LLC
St. Paul, Minnesota

Lisa D. Inge, Pharm.D. BCPS, AAHIVE
Jacksonville Assistant Campus Director
Assistant Professor of Pharmacotherapy and Translational Research
University of Florida College of Pharmacy
Jacksonville, Florida

Fiona Jane, MBBS
Research Fellow
Women's Health Program
Department of Medicine
Monash University
Prahran, Victoria, Australia

Sarah L. Johnson, Pharm.D.
Investigator Initiated Clinical Trials Manager
Rocky Mountain Multiple Sclerosis Center at the Anschutz Medical Campus
Department of Neurology
University of Colorado Denver
Aurora, Colorado

Sophia N. Kalantaridou, MD, Ph.D.
Associate Professor of Obstetrics and Gynecology
Division of Reproductive Endocrinology
Department of Obstetrics and Gynecology
University of Ioannina Medical School
Ioannina, Greece

Julie J. Kelsey, Pharm.D.
Clinical Pharmacy Specialist—Women's Health
University of Virginia Health System
Charlottesville, Virginia

Charlie C. Kilpatrick, MD
Assistant Professor
Department of Obstetrics, Gynecology, and Reproductive Sciences
University of Texas Houston Medical School
Houston, Texas

Karissa Y. Kim, Pharm.D., CACP, BCPS
Associate Clinical Professor
Division of Pharmacy Practice and Administrative Sciences
James L. Winkle College of Pharmacy
University of Cincinnati
Cincinnati, Ohio

Connie Kraus, Pharm.D., BCPS
Clinical Professor
University of Wisconsin School of Pharmacy
Madison, Wisconsin

Trisha LaPointe, Pharm.D., BCPS
Assistant Professor of Pharmacy Practice
Department of Pharmacy of Practice, School of Pharmacy
Massachusetts College of Pharmacy and Health Sciences—Boston
Boston, Massachusetts

Lazaros G. Lavasidis, MD
Division of Reproductive Endocrinology
Department of Obstetrics and Gynecology
University of Ioannina Medical School
Ioannina, Greece

Jennifer J. Lee, Pharm.D., BCPS, CDE
Assistant Clinical Professor
University of Connecticut School of Pharmacy
Storrs, Connecticut

Sandra R. Leiblum, Ph.D.
Sex Therapist
Bridgewater, New Jersey

Kimberly Braxton Lloyd, Pharm.D.
Assistant Dean for Pharmacy Health Services
Associate Professor
Auburn University's Harrison School of Pharmacy
Auburn University, Alabama

Catherine L. Lysack, Ph.D., OT(C)
Deputy Director, Institute of Gerontology
Professor of Gerontology and Occupational Therapy
Wayne State University
Detroit, Michigan

Claire M. Mach, Pharm.D.
Assistant Professor
University of Houston College of Pharmacy
Houston, Texas

Somjate Manipalviratn, MD
Obstetrician and Gynecologist
Reproductive Endocrinology and Infertility Specialist
Jetanin Hospital
Bangkok, Thailand

Carla Ann Martinez, MD
Assistant Professor
Maternal Fetal Medicine
Department of Obstetrics and Gynecology
Texas Tech University Health Sciences Center
El Paso, Texas

Joan M. Mastrobattista, MD
Professor
Department of Obstetrics, Gynecology, and Reproductive Sciences
Director, Prenatal Diagnosis
University of Texas Medical School Houston
Houston, Texas

Kelly L. Matson, BSN, Pharm.D.
Clinical Associate Professor
Department of Pharmacy Practice
University of Rhode Island
Kingston, Rhode Island

Desireé McCarthy-Keith, MD, MPH
National Institutes of Health
Bethesda, Maryland

Jennifer A. McIntosh, Pharm.D., MHS
Assistant Clinical Professor
Bouvé College of Health Sciences School of Pharmacy
Northeastern University
Boston, Massachusetts

Marisa Navo Mendoza, Pharm.D.
Quality Assurance Specialist
Pharmacy Academic Programs
University of Texas M. D. Anderson Cancer Center
Houston, Texas

Ginat W. Mirowski, DMD, MD
Professor
Department of Dermatology
Indiana University
Indianapolis, Indiana

Manju Monga, MD
Berel Held Professor and Division Director
Maternal Fetal Medicine
Department of Obstetrics, Gynecology, and Reproductive Sciences
University of Texas Houston Medical School
Houston, Texas

Edna Elise Moore, MSN, ARNP, WHNP-C
Nurse Practitioner
Atlanta Geriatrics and Extended Care—Incontinence Clinic
Nurse Researcher
Birmingham/Atlanta GRECC
Veterans Administration Medical Center
Atlanta, Georgia

Baochau (Lisa) Nguyen, Pharm.D.
Clinical Pharmacist
Exempla St. Joseph Hospital
Denver, Colorado

Mary Beth O'Connell, Pharm.D., BCPS, FASHP, FCCP
Associate Professor
Pharmacy Practice Department
Eugene Applebaum College of Pharmacy and Health Sciences
Wayne State University
Detroit, Michigan

Carol M. Odell, MSN, FNP
Senior Clinical Instructor
Department of Family Medicine
University of Colorado at Denver School of Medicine
University Family Medicine—A.F. Williams Clinic
Denver, Colorado

Katherine A. O'Hanlan, MD, FACOG, FACS, SGO
Director
Laparoscopic Institute for Gynecologic Oncology
Portola Valley, California

Nancy D. Ordonez, Pharm.D., BCPS
Clinical Assistant Professor
University of Houston College of Pharmacy
Houston, Texas

Norma J. Owens, Pharm.D., BCPS, FCCP
Professor and Chair
University of Rhode Island College of Pharmacy
Kingston, Rhode Island

Makala Pace, Pharm.D., BCOP
Clinical Pharmacy Specialist
The University of Texas M. D. Anderson Cancer Center
Houston, Texas

Dennis Parker Jr., Pharm.D.
Assistant Clinical Professor
Pharmacy Practice Department
Eugene Applebaum College of Pharmacy and Health Sciences
Wayne State University
Clinical Specialist Neuroscience
Detroit Receiving Hospital
Detroit, Michigan

Nima M. Patel, Pharm.D., BCPS
Associate Professor
Temple University School of Pharmacy
Philadelphia, Pennsylvania

Kathryn E. Peek, MS, MA, Ph.D.
Assistant Vice President for University Health Initiatives
University of Houston
Houston, Texas

Kirk D. Ramin, MD
Professor
Department of Obstetrics, Gynecology, and Women's Health
University of Minnesota
Minneapolis, Minnesota

Mildred M. Ramirez, MD
Professor
Department of Obstetrics, Gynecology, and Reproductive Sciences
Division of Maternal Fetal Medicine
University of Texas Medical School Houston
Houston, Texas

Charmaine D. Rochester, Pharm.D., CDE, BCPS
Associate Professor
Department of Pharmacy Practice and Science
University of Maryland School of Pharmacy
Baltimore, Maryland

Debbie Rodriquez, RN, Pharm.D.
Kaiser Permanente
Denver, Colorado

Melody Ryan, Pharm.D., MPH
Associate Professor
Departments of Pharmacy Practice & Science and Neurology
University of Kentucky
Lexington, Kentucky

Claire Saadeh, Pharm.D, BCOP
Associate Professor
College of Pharmacy
Ferris State University
Big Rapids, Michigan

Rosalie Sagraves, Pharm.D., F.A.Ph.A., FCCP
Dean Emerita and Professor Emerita
University of Illinois at Chicago
Chicago, Illinois

Imam Achmat Salie, DBA, AFK, MBA
Oakland University
American Muslim Diversity Association
Rochester Hills, Michigan

Bethanee J. Schlosser, MD, Ph.D.
Assistant Professor
Department of Dermatology
Northwestern University
Chicago, Illinois

Arthur A. Schuna, MS, FASHP
Clinical Coordinator
William S. Middleton VA Medical Center
Clinical Professor
University of Wisconsin School of Pharmacy
Madison, Wisconsin

Neha Shah, MD
Research Assistant
Department of Dermatology
Northwestern University
Chicago, Illinois

Amy Heck Sheehan, Pharm.D.
Associate Professor of Pharmacy Practice
Purdue University School of Pharmacy and Pharmaceutical Sciences
Indianapolis, Indiana

Sheetal Sheth, Pharm.D., BCOP
Clinical Coordinator
US Oncology, Inc.
The Woodlands, Texas

Leslie A. Shimp, Pharm.D., MS
Professor of Pharmacy
University of Michigan College of Pharmacy
Ann Arbor, Michigan

Jeri J. Sias, Pharm.D., MPH
Clinical Associate Professor
UTEP/UT Austin Cooperative Pharmacy Program
El Paso, Texas

Perry Silverschanz, Ph.D., MSW
Lecturer
University of Michigan
Eastern Michigan University
Ann Arbor, Michigan

Tracy L. Skaer, Pharm.D., FABFE, FASCP, FASHP
Professor of Pharmacotherapy
Professor of Health Policy and Administration
Pharmacoeconomics and Pharmacoepidemiology Research Unit
Washington State University College of Pharmacy
Pullman, Washington

Judith Ann Smith, Pharm.D., BCOP, FCCP, FISOPP
Associate Professor and Director, Pharmacology Research

Department of Gynecologic Oncology, Division of Surgery
Director, Oncology Translational Research Fellowship
Division of Pharmacy
The University of Texas M. D. Anderson Cancer Center
Houston, Texas

Gail Goodman Snitkoff, Ph.D.
Associate Professor
Albany College of Pharmacy and Health Sciences
Albany, New York

Martha Stassinos, Pharm.D.
Women's Health Clinical Pharmacist Specialist
Veterans Administration of Northern California Health Care System
Berkeley, California

Julie L. Strickland, MD, MPH
Associate Professor
Department of Obstetrics and Gynecology
University of Missouri Kansas City
Kansas City, Missouri

Deborah A. Sturpe, Pharm.D., BCPS
Associate Professor
University of Maryland School of Pharmacy
Baltimore, Maryland

Robert Taylor
Author
Priest in the Vaishnava Hindu tradition
Grosse Pointe, Michigan

Tracy E. Thomason, Pharm.D.
Adjunct Assistant Professor
UNC Eshelman School of Pharmacy
University of North Carolina at Chapel Hill
Chapel Hill, North Carolina

Kimberly Thrasher, Pharm.D., BCPS, FCCP, CPP
Associate Director of Pharmacotherapy
South East Area Health Education Center (SEAHEC)
Wilmington, NC
Clinical Associate Professor, UNC Eshelman School of Pharmacy
Clinical Assistant Professor, UNC School of Medicine
University of North Carolina
Chapel Hill, North Carolina

Peter V. Tortorice, Pharm.D., BCOP
Senior Manager, Pharmaceutical Services
US Oncology, Inc.
Schaumburg, Illinois

Timothy S. Tracy, Ph.D.
Professor and Department Head
Department of Experimental and Clinical Pharmacology
University of Minnesota
Minneapolis, Minnesota

Jeanne Hawkins VanTyle, Pharm.D., MS
Professor of Pharmacy Practice
College of Pharmacy and Health Sciences
Butler University
Indianapolis, Indiana

Fei Wang, M.Sc., Pharm.D., BCPS, FASHP
Associate Clinical Professor
Department of Pharmacy Practice
University of Connecticut School of Pharmacy
Storrs, Connecticut

Dennis P. West, Ph.D., FCCP, CIP
Professor in Dermatology and Pediatrics
Vincent W. Foglia Family Research Professor of Dermatology
Director Dermatopharmacology Program
Director Dermatology Translational Core
Department of Dermatology
Feinberg School of Medicine, Northwestern University
Chicago, Illinois

Lee E. West, B.S.Pharm.
Clinical Pharmacist
Northwestern Memorial Hospital
Chicago, Illinois

Jessica L. White, Pharm.D., BCPS
Clinical Assistant Professor
University of Houston College of Pharmacy
Houston, Texas

Patricia Rozek Wigle, Pharm.D., BCPS
Associate Clinical Professor
Division of Pharmacy Practice and Administrative Sciences
James L. Winkle College of Pharmacy
University of Cincinnati
Cincinnati, Ohio

Jacki S. Witt, JD, MSN, WHNP, CNM
Project Director
Clinical Training Center for Family Planning
Clinical Associate Professor
Kansas City, Missouri

Yasuko Yamamura, MD
Assistant Professor
Department of Obstetrics, Gynecology, and Women's Health
University of Minnesota
Minneapolis, Minnesota

Barbara W. K. Yee, Ph.D.
Professor and Chair
Family and Consumer Sciences/ CTAHR
University of Hawaii at Manoa
Honolulu, Hawaii

Reviewers

Julie Wright Banderas, Pharm.D., BCPS, FCCP
Assistant Dean for Graduate Studies
University of Missouri-Kansas City School of Medicine
Kansas City, Missouri

David W. Bartels, Pharm.D., CDE, FCCP
Clinical Professor and Vice Dean
University of Illinois College of Pharmacy at Rockford
Rockford, Illinois

Judith L. Beizer, Pharm.D., CGP, FASCP
Clinical Professor
College of Pharmacy and Allied Health Professions
St. John's University
Jamaica, New York

Kathleen Hill Besinque, Pharm.D., M.S.Ed., FASHP
Associate Professor of Clinical Pharmacy
University of Southern California School of Pharmacy
Los Angeles, California

Nancy L. Borja-Hart, Pharm.D., BCPS
Assistant Professor of Pharmacy Practice
Nova Southeastern University College of Pharmacy
Ft. Lauderdale, Florida

Thomas E. R. Brown, Pharm.D.
Associate Professor and Director of the Doctor of Pharmacy Program
Leslie Dan Faculty of Pharmacy
University of Toronto
Toronto, Ontario, Canada

Robert A. Buerki, Ph.D., R.Ph.
Professor
Division of Pharmacy Practice and Administration
The Ohio State University College of Pharmacy
Columbus, Ohio

Joanna Cain, MD
Chair of Obstetrics and Gynecology
Alpert Medical School
Brown University
Providence, Rhode Island

Deborah Stier Carson, Pharm.D., FCCP
Associate Program Director for Education
South Carolina Area Health Education Consortium
Charleston, South Carolina

Philip E. Empey, Pharm.D., Ph.D., BCPS
Assistant Professor, Department of Pharmacy and Therapeutics
Center for Clinical Pharmacy Research
University of Pittsburgh School of Pharmacy
Pittsburgh, Pennsylvania

Mary H. H. Ensom, Pharm.D., FASHP, FCCP, FCSHP, FCAHS
Professor and Director, Doctor of Pharmacy Program
Faculty of Pharmaceutical Sciences
Distinguished University Scholar
The University of British Columbia
Clinical Pharmacy Specialist
Children's and Women's Health Centre of British Columbia
Vancouver, British Columbia, Canada

Ema Ferreira, B.Pharm., M.Sc., Pharm.D., FCSHP
Pharmacist in Obstetrics and Gynecology at CHU Ste-Justine
Clinical Associate Professor
Faculté de Pharmacie, Université de Montréal
Montréal, Québec, Canada

David R. Foster, Pharm.D.
Associate Professor of Pharmacy Practice
Purdue University
Adjunct Associate Professor of Medicine
Indiana University
Indianapolis, Indiana

Carla B. Frye, Pharm.D., BCPS, FASHP
Senior Clinical Research Scientist
EPI-Q, Inc.
Oak Brook, Illinois

Barry R. Goldspiel, Pharm.D., BCOP, FASHP
Deputy Chief
NIH Clinical Center Pharmacy Department
Bethesda, Maryland

Tawara D. Goode, MA
Assistant Professor
Georgetown University Center for Child and Human Development
Director
National Center for Cultural Competence
Washington, District of Columbia

Susan Goodin, Pharm.D., FCCP, BCOP
Associate Director, Clinical Trials and Therapeutics
The Cancer Institute of New Jersey
Professor of Medicine
UMDNJ-Robert Wood Johnson Medical School
New Brunswick, New Jersey

Jennifer L. Hardman, Pharm.D.
Clinical Pharmacist
Froedtert Hospital
Milwaukee, Wisconsin

Ila M. Harris, Pharm.D., FCCP, BCPS
Associate Professor
Department of Family Medicine and Community Health
University of Minnesota Medical School
Adjunct Associate Professor
Department of Pharmaceutical Care and Health Systems
University of Minnesota College of Pharmacy
Minneapolis, Minnesota

Thomas K. Hazlet, Pharm.D., Dr.P.H.
Pharmaceutical Outcomes Research and Policy Program
Associate Professor
University of Washington School of Pharmacy
Seattle, Washington

Cheryl Horlen, Pharm.D., BCPS
Associate Professor of Pharmacy Practice
Feik School of Pharmacy
University of the Incarnate Word
San Antonio, Texas

Paul R. Hutson, Pharm.D.
Associate Professor
UW School of Pharmacy
Madison, Wisconsin

Robert Ignoffo, Pharm.D., FASHP, FCSHP
Clinical Professor Emeritus
University of California, San Francisco
Professor of Pharmacy
College of Pharmacy, Touro University—California
Vallejo, California

Amir Anthony Jazaeri, MD, FACS, FACOG
Assistant Professor
Division of Gynecologic Oncology
Department of Obstetrics and Gynecology
University of Virginia Health System
Charlottesville, Virginia

Kellie L. Jones, Pharm.D., BCOP
Clinical Associate Professor
Department of Pharmacy Practice
Purdue University School of Pharmacy and Pharmaceutical Sciences
Indianapolis, Indiana

Barbara F. Kelly, MD
Associate Professor
Department of Family Medicine
University of Colorado Denver
Aurora, Colorado

David C. Knoppert, B.S.Pharm., M.Sc.Pharm., FCCP, FCSHP
Liaison Neonatology
St Joseph's Health Care
London, Ontario, Canada

Howard S. Kurtzman, Ph.D.
Deputy Executive Director for Science
American Psychological Association
Washington, District of Columbia

Knoll Larkin, MPH
Research Associate
Bioethics Program—Internal Medicine/General Medicine
The University of Michigan
Ann Arbor, Michigan

Gary M. Levin, Pharm.D., BCPP, FCCP
Dean and Professor
LECOM School of Pharmacy—Bradenton
Bradenton, Florida

Nicole M. Lodise, Pharm.D.
Associate Professor of Pharmacy Practice
Albany College of Pharmacy and Health Sciences
Albany, New York

Judette Louis, MD, MPH
Assistant Professor
Reproductive Biology
MetroHealth Medical Center
Case Western Reserve University
Cleveland, Ohio

David L. Lourwood, Pharm.D., BCPS, FCCP
Clinical Pharmacy Specialist
Department of Pharmacy Services
Poplar Bluff Regional Medical Center
Poplar Bluff, Missouri

Kirsten J. Lund, MD
Associate Professor, OB-GYN
Denver Health Medical Center
Denver, Colorado

Eric J. MacLaughlin, Pharm.D., FCCP, BCPS
Associate Professor and Head of Adult Medicine
Texas Tech University Health Sciences Center School of Pharmacy
Amarillo, Texas

Linda Gore Martin, Pharm.D., MBA, BCPS
Associate Professor
Social and Administrative Pharmacy
University of Wyoming School of Pharmacy
Laramie, Wyoming

Cydney E. McQueen, Pharm.D.
Clinical Associate Professor
Pharmacy Practice and Administration
UMKC School of Pharmacy
Kansas City, Missouri

Mary G. Mihalyo, BS, Pharm.D.
Assistant Professor Pharmacy Practice
Mylan School of Pharmacy
Duquesne University
Pittsburgh, Pennsylvania

Julie Moldenhauer, MD

Lawrence M. Nelson, MD
Captain, United States Public Health Service
Integrative Reproductive Medicine Unit
Intramural Research Program on Reproductive and Adult Endocrinology
National Institute of Child Health and Human Development
National Institutes of Health
Bethesda, Maryland

John E. Nestler, MD
Vice Chairman
William G. Blackard Professor of Medicine
Chair, Division of Endocrinology and Metabolism
Vice Chair, Department of Internal Medicine
Virginia Commonwealth University
Richmond, Virginia

Melinda M. Neuhauser, Pharm.D., MPH
Clinical Pharmacy Specialist, Infectious Diseases
Department of Veterans Affairs
Pharmacy Benefits Management Services
Hines, Illinois

Anuradha Paranjape, MD, MPH, FACP
Associate Professor of Medicine and Public Health
Section of General Internal Medicine
Temple University School of Medicine
Philadelphia, Pennsylvania

Amy L. Pittenger, Pharm.D., MS
Associate Director, Office of Cyber Learning and Outreach
Assistant Professor, Pharmaceutical Care and Health-Systems
University of Minnesota College of Pharmacy
Minneapolis, Minnesota

Charles D. Ponte, Pharm.D., BC-ADM, BCPS, CDE, CPE, F.A.Ph.A., FASHP, FCCP
Professor of Clinical Pharmacy and Family Medicine
Robert C. Byrd Health Sciences Center
West Virginia University Schools of Pharmacy and Medicine
Morgantown, West Virginia

Vaishali Popat, MD, MPH
Endocrinologist
National Institutes of Health
Bethesda, Maryland

Frank Pucino, Jr., Pharm.D., BCPS, FASHP, FDPGEC
Clinical Investigator
National Institute of Arthritis and Musculoskeletal and Skin Diseases
National Institutes of Health
Bethesda, Maryland

Julie L. Puotinen, Pharm.D., BCPS
System Drug Policy Coordinator
Aurora Health Care
Milwaukee, Wisconsin

Erin C. Raney, Pharm.D., BCPS
Associate Professor of Pharmacy Practice
Midwestern University College of Pharmacy—Glendale
Glendale, Arizona

Jerrie S. Refuerzo, MD
Assistant Professor, Division of Maternal Fetal Medicine
Department of Obstetrics, Gynecology, and Reproductive Sciences
University of Texas Health Science Center at Houston
Houston, Texas

Denise Rhoney, Pharm.D., FCCP, FCCM
Associate Professor
Pharmacy Practice Department
Eugene Applebaum College of Pharmacy and Health Sciences
Wayne State University
Detroit, Michigan

Jane L. Rogan, B.S.Pharm., MA
Curator, Pharmuseum
Eugene Applebaum College of Pharmacy and Health Sciences
Wayne State University
Detroit, Michigan

Ronald J. Ruggiero, BS, Pharm.D.
Clinical Professor Emeritus
Departments of Clinical Pharmacy and Obstetrics
Gynecology and Reproductive Sciences
The University of California San Francisco Schools of Pharmacy and Medicine
San Francisco, California

O. J. Rustad, MD, FAAD
Mohs Surgeon
Medical Director
Medical and Surgical Divisions of Advanced Dermatology Care
Adjunct Clinical Professor
University of Minnesota Medical School
Minneapolis, Minnesota

Ruth A. Rustad, MD
Medical Director of Advanced Esthetics
Division of Advanced Dermatology Care
Clinical Instructor
University of Minnesota Medical School
Minneapolis, Minnesota

Joseph Saseen, Pharm.D., FCCP, BCPS
Professor
Schools of Pharmacy and Medicine
Anschutz Medical Campus
University of Colorado Denver
Aurora, Colorado

Terry L. Seaton, Pharm.D., FCCP, BCPS
Professor and Associate Director

Division of Pharmacy Practice
St. Louis College of Pharmacy
St. Louis, Missouri

James Segars, MD
Head, Unit on Reproductive Endocrinology and Infertility
Eunice Kennedy Shriver National Institute of Child Health and Human Development
National Institutes of Health
Bethesda, Maryland

Susan M. Sirmans, BS, Pharm.D., BCPS
Associate Professor
University of Louisiana at Monroe College of Pharmacy
Monroe, Louisiana

Rebecca B. Sleeper, Pharm.D., FASCP, BCPS
Associate Professor and Division Head
Geriatrics Division
TTUHSC School of Pharmacy
Lubbock, Texas

Leon Speroff, MD
Professor Emeritus of Obstetrics and Gynecology
Oregon Health & Science University
Portland, Oregon

Sarah A. Spinler, Pharm.D., BCPS (AQ Cardiology), FAHA, FCCP
Professor of Clinical Pharmacy
Residency and Fellowship Program Coordinator
Philadelphia College of Pharmacy
University of the Sciences in Philadelphia
Philadelphia, Pennsylvania

Scott K. Stolte, Pharm.D.
Associate Dean of Academic Affairs
Bernard J. Dunn School of Pharmacy
Shenandoah University
Winchester, Virginia

Pamela Stratton, MD
Chief, Gynecology Consult Service
Program in Reproductive and Adult Endocrinology
National Institutes of Health
Bethesda, Maryland

Marie Boyle Struble, Ph.D., RD
Adjunct Professor
College of Saint Elizabeth
Morristown, New Jersey
Adjunct Professor
University of Massachusetts
Amherst, Massachusetts

Stephanie B. Teal, MD, MPH
Associate Professor of Obstetrics and Gynecology
Director, Fellowship in Family Planning
Denver School of Medicine
University of Colorado
Aurora, Colorado

Candy Tsourounis, Pharm.D.
Professor of Clinical Pharmacy
San Francisco School of Pharmacy
University of California
San Francisco, California

Elena M. Umland, Pharm.D.
Associate Dean for Academic Affairs
Jefferson School of Pharmacy
Thomas Jefferson University
Philadelphia, Pennsylvania

Sheryl F. Vondracek, Pharm.D., BCPS, FCCP
Associate Professor
Department of Clinical Pharmacy
University of Colorado Denver
Aurora, Colorado

Mitzi Wasik, Pharm.D., BCPS
Clinical Assistant Professor
Center for Women's Health
University of Illinois at Chicago College of Pharmacy
Chicago, Illinois

Emily Weidman-Evans, Pharm.D., AE-C, CPE
Associate Professor
Department of Clinical and Administrative Sciences
University of Louisiana College of Pharmacy
Clinical Pharmacist, Department of Family Medicine
Louisiana State University Health Sciences Center
Shreveport, Louisiana

Frank R. Witter, MD
Professor of Gynecology and Obstetrics
Johns Hopkins University School of Medicine
Baltimore, Maryland

Patrick T. Wong, Pharm.D., BCOP, BCPS
Health Sciences Assistant Clinical Professor
San Francisco School of Pharmacy
University of California
San Francisco, California

Gary C. Yee, Pharm.D., FCCP, BCOP
Professor of Pharmacy Practice
Associate Dean for Academic Affairs
University of Nebraska Medical Center College of Pharmacy
Omaha, Nebraska

Rosa F. Yeh, Pharm.D., BCPS, AAHIVE
Research Assistant Professor
University of Houston College of Pharmacy
Houston, Texas

ABBREVIATIONS

17P	17-alpha hydroxyprogesterone caproate
Ab	antibody
ACCP	American College of Chest Physicians
ACEI	angiotensin-converting enzyme inhibitors
ACG	American College of Gastroenterology
ACOG	American College of Obstetricians and Gynecologists
ACS	American Cancer Society
ACSs	acute coronary syndromes
AEDs	antiepileptic drugs
AGA	American Gastroenterological Association
AGC	atypical glandular cells of uncertain significance
AIs	aromatase inhibitors
AIS	adenocarcinoma in situ
ALLHAT	Antihypertensive and Lipid-Lowering Treatment to Prevent Heart Attack Trial
ALND	axillary lymph node dissection
ANA	antinuclear antibodies
ANC	acid-neutralizing capacity
Anti-CCP	anticyclic citrullinated peptide
APs	antipsychotics
aPTT	activated partial thrombin time
ARBs	angiotensin receptor blockers
ART	assisted reproductive technology
ASC	atypical squamous cells
ASC-US	atypical squamous cells–unspecified
ASRM	American Society for Reproductive Medicine
AUC	area under the curve
BAP	British Association for Psychopharmacology
BBT	basal body temperature
BCT	breast-conserving therapy
BDD	body dysmorphic disorder
BED	binge-eating disorder
BIA	bioelectrical impedance analysis
BI-RADS	Breast Imaging Reporting and Data System
BMD	bone mineral density
BMI	body mass index
BMR	basal metabolic rate
BNP	B-type natriuretic peptide
BSE	breast self-evaluation
BSO	bilateral salpingo-oophorectomy
cAMP	cyclic adenosine monophosphate
CBE	clinical breast evaluation
CBT	cognitive behavioral therapy
CCBs	calcium channel blockers
CCRs	chemokine coreceptor antagonists
CD	Crohn's disease
CHCs	combined hormonal contraceptives
CHD	coronary heart disease
CI	confidence interval
CIN	cervical intraepithelial neoplasia
CLAS	culturally and linguistically appropriate services
CMF	cyclophosphamide, methotrexate, and fluorouracil
CMV	cytomegalovirus
CNS	central nervous system
COC	combined oral contraceptive
COX	cyclo-oxygenase
CR	complete response
CRP	C-reactive protein
CT	computed tomography
CXR	chest x-ray
D&C	dilatation and curettage
DASH	Dietary Approaches to Stop Hypertension
DCIS	ductal carcinoma in situ
DFS	disease-free survival
DHEA	dehydroepiandrosterone
DHHS	Department of Health and Human Services
DHT	dihydrotestosterone
DIG	Digitalis Investigation Group
DMARDs	disease-modifying antirheumatic drugs
DMPA	depot medroxyprogesterone acetate
DMSO	dimethyl sulfoxide
DNA	deoxyribonucleic acid
DSM-IV	Diagnostic and Statistical Manual of Mental Disorders, fourth edition
DUB	dysfunctional uterine bleeding
DVT	deep vein thrombosis
EASI	extra-amniotic saline infusions
EBAF	endometrial bleeding associated factor
EBRT	external beam radiotherapy

EBV	Epstein-Barr virus
ED	emergency department
EDNOS	eating disorders not otherwise specified
EE	esterified estrogens
EE	ethinyl estradiol
EEG	electroencephalogram
EGFR	epidermal growth factor receptor
EIC	endometrial intraepithelial carcinoma
EMB	endometrial biopsy
EPDS	Edinburgh Postnatal Depression Score
EPL	early pregnancy loss
EPS	extrapyramidal symptoms
ER	estrogen receptor
ESBC	early-stage breast cancer
ESR	erythrocyte sedimentation rate
ET	estrogen therapy
FAMs	fertility awareness methods
FDA	U.S. Food and Drug Administration
FEV1	forced expiratory volume in 1 second
FIGO	International Federation of Gynecology and Obstetrics
FOD	female orgasmic disorder
FSAD	female sexual arousal disorder
FSH	follicle stimulating hormone
GABA	gamma-aminobutyric acid
GAD	general anxiety disorder
GD	gestational diabetes
GERD	gastroesophageal reflux disease
GFR	glomerular filtration rate
GI	gastrointestinal
GIFT	gamete intrafallopian transfer
GMT	geometric mean titer
GnRH	gonadotropin releasing hormone
GOG	Gynecologic Oncology Group
H_2RA	histamine-2 receptor antagonists
HAART	highly active antiretroviral therapy
HBOC	hereditary breast/ovarian cancer
HCG	human chorionic hormone
HDL-C	high-density lipoprotein cholesterol
HER2	human epidermal growth factor 2
HELLP	hemolysis, elevated liver enzymes, low platelet count
HERS	Heart and Estrogen/progestin Replacement Study
HIV	human immunodeficiency virus
HLA	human leukocyte antigen
hMG	human menopausal gonadotropin
HNPCC	hereditary nonpolyposis colorectal cancer
HPA	hypothalamic-pituitary-adrenal
HPO	hypothalamic-pituitary-ovarian
hPTH	human parathyroid hormone
HPV	human papillomavirus
HSDD	hypoactive sexual desire disorder
HSG	hysterosalpingogram
HSV	herpes simplex virus
HT	hormone therapy
IBC	inflammatory breast cancer
IBD	inflammatory bowel disease
IBS	irritable bowel syndrome
IBS-C	irritable bowel syndrome with constipation
IBS-D	irritable bowel syndrome with diarrhea
IBS-M	mixed IBS
IBS-U	unsubtyped IBS
ICD	International Classification of Diseases
ICSI	intracytoplasmic sperm injection
ICSs	inhaled corticosteroids
IGT	impaired glucose tolerance
IL	interleukin
IMS	International Menopause Society
IND	investigational new drug
INR	international normalized ratio
IP	intraperitoneal
ISMP	Institute of Safe Medication Practices
IUC	intrauterine contraceptive
IUI	intrauterine insemination
IVF	in vitro fertilization
IVF-ET	in vitro fertilization–embryo transfer
IVF-ICSI	in vitro fertilization–intracytoplasmic sperm injection
JNC	Joint National Committee
LABA	long-acting beta-2 agonist
LABC	locally advanced breast cancer
LCD	low-calorie diet
LCIS	lobular carcinoma in situ
LDL-C	low-density lipoprotein cholesterol
LEEP	loop electrosurgical excision procedure
LES	lower esophageal sphincter
LGSIL	low-grade squamous intraepithelial lesion
LH	luteinizing hormone
LHRH	luteinizing hormone–releasing hormone
LMP	last menstrual period
LMWH	low molecular weight heparin
LND	lymph node dissection
LNG	levonorgestrel
LNG-IUD	levonorgestrel intrauterine device
LNG-IUS	levonorgestrel-releasing intrauterine system
LPS	lipopolysaccharides
LUNA	laparoscopic uterosacral nerve ablation
LVEF	left ventricular ejection fraction

MAOIs	monoamine oxidase inhibitors
MBC	metastatic breast cancer
MDD	major depressive disorder
MHC	major histocompatibility complex
MI	myocardial infarctions
MMPs	matrix metalloproteinases
MMSE	mini-mental state exam
MOMPs	major outer-membrane proteins
MPA	medroxyprogesterone acetate
MRM	modified radical mastectomy
MS	multiple sclerosis
mT	methyltestosterone therapy
MTCT	mother-to-child transmission
N-9	nonoxynol-9
NAAT	nucleic acid amplification tests
NAMS	The North American Menopause Society
NAS	neonatal abstinence syndrome
NCCN	National Comprehensive Cancer Network
NCEP	National Cholesterol Education Program
NFP	natural family planning
NHLBI	National Heart, Lung, and Blood Institute
NIH	National Institutes of Health
NK	neurokinin
NNRTIs	non-nucleoside reverse transcriptase inhibitors
NO	nitric oxide
nPEP	nonoccupational exposure prophylaxis
NRT	nicotine replacement therapy
NRTIs	nucleoside reverse transcriptase inhibitors
NSAIDs	nonsteroidal anti-inflammatory drugs
NSTEMI	non-ST-elevation myocardial infarction
NTDs	neural tube defects
NVP	nausea and/or vomiting during pregnancy
OB/GYN	obstetrics and gynecology
OCs	oral contraceptives
OCD	obsessive-compulsive disorder
OCPs	oral contraceptive pills
OGTT	oral glucose tolerance test
OHSS	ovarian hyperstimulation syndrome
OMH	Office of Minority Health
OR	odds ratio
ORT	oral replacement therapy
OS	overall survival
PCOS	polycystic ovary syndrome
PCR	polymerase chain reaction
PE	pulmonary embolism
PEG	polyethylene glycol
PEFR	peak expiratory flow rate
PET	positron-emission tomography
PFMT	pelvic floor muscle training
PFS	progression-free survival
PGE_2	prostaglandin E_2
$PGF_{2\alpha}$	prostaglandin $F_{2\alpha}$
PIs	protease inhibitors
PID	pelvic inflammatory disease
PMDD	premenstrual dysphoric disorder
PMS	premenstrual syndrome
POI	primary ovarian insufficiency
POP	progestogen-only pill
PPA	phenylpropanolamine
PPIs	proton-pump inhibitors
PPPH	persistent primary pulmonary hypertension
PR	progesterone receptor
PSN	presacral neurectomy
PT	prothrombin time
PTSD	post-traumatic stress disorder
PTU	propylthiouracil
RA	rheumatoid arthritis
RCTs	randomized controlled trials
REM	rapid eye movement
RF	rheumatoid factor
RID	relative infant dose
ROC	risk of ovarian cancer
RPR	rapid plasma reagin
RR	response rate
RR	relative risk
RT	radiation therapy
SAD	seasonal affective disorder
SEER	Surveillance and Epidemiology and End Results
SERMs	selective estrogen receptor modulators
SGO	Society of Gynecologic Oncologists
SGOT	serum glutamic oxaloacetic transaminase
SGPT	serum glutamatic pyruvate transaminase
SHBG	sex-hormone binding globulin
SIL	squamous intraepithelial lesions
SIR	standardized incidence ratio
SLE	systemic lupus erythematosus
SNB	sentinel node biopsy
SNRIs	serotonin-norepinephrine reuptake inhibitors
sono-HSG	sonohysterography
SR	sustained release
SREs	skeletal related events
SS	Sjögren's syndrome
SSRIs	selective serotonin reuptake inhibitors
STDs	sexually transmitted diseases

STEMI	ST-elevation myocardial infarction
STIs	sexually transmitted infections
SWOG	Southwest Oncology Group
TAH/BSO	total abdominal hysterectomy with bilateral salpingo-oophorectomy
TCAs	tricyclic antidepressants
Tdap	tetanus toxoid, reduced diphtheria toxoid, and acellular pertussis
TENS	transcutaneous electrical nerve stimulation
TNF	tumor necrosis factor
TNF-α	tumor necrosis factor alpha
TNM	tumor-node-metastasis
TPMT	thiopurine-methyl transferase
TRAb	TSH receptor antibodies
TSH	thyroid-stimulating hormone
TSI	thyroid-stimulating immunoglobulin
TSS	toxic shock syndrome
TTTS	twin-to-twin transfusion syndrome
TVUS	transvaginal ultrasound
TWEL	transepidermal water loss
TZDs	thiazolidinediones
UC	ulcerative colitis
UFH	unfractionated heparin
UI	urinary incontinence
UKCTOCS	United Kingdom Collaborative Trial of Ovarian Cancer Screening
U.S.	United States
USPSTF	U.S. Preventive Services Task Force
UV	ultraviolet
VDRL	venereal disease research laboratory
VEGF	vascular endothelial growth factor
VLPs	virus-like particles
VTE	venous thromboembolism
WBC	white blood cell
WHI	Women's Health Initiative
WHO	World Health Organization
WISDOM	Women's International Study of Long Duration after Menopause
WISE	Women's Ischemia Syndrome Evaluation
XRT	external radiation therapy
ZIFT	zygote intrafallopian transfer

List of Web Resources

SECTION ONE

Historical and Social Issues

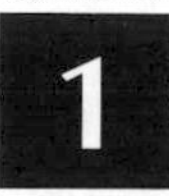

1 History of Women's Healthcare and Research

Rosalie Sagraves, Pharm.D., F.A.Ph.A., FCCP; Jennifer A. McIntosh, Pharm.D., MHS

Learning Objectives

1. Describe how government funded social welfare programs and medical education have influenced the definition of women's health.
2. Outline changes in society that have altered women's roles at home and in the workplace, education and careers, and sexuality and explain their impact on women's health and healthcare delivery.
3. Explain changing trends and significant healthcare and research advancements leading to decreased morbidity and mortality of women.
4. Evaluate the impact of actions taken by federal agencies, legislators, and pharmacy associations/organizations on women's healthcare and research.

The history of modern women's health is a complex story that involves significantly more than the advancement of medical theory. Improvements in women's health are intimately linked to changing social and political norms that have laid the foundation for the current U.S. women's health movement. Without equal access to higher education, the right to vote and be elected to public office or the ability to work outside the home, women would not be in a position to demand things like prescription coverage for contraception or adequate funding for breast cancer screening and treatment. To understand the significance of more recent developments, it is imperative to briefly examine key events that laid the groundwork for what is now known as women's health.

Women's health has no founding mothers like the U.S. had founding fathers. Instead, the efforts of generations of women represent the collective "mothers" of women's health, and women of the Revolutionary War era (1775–1783) were critical in laying the foundation for this movement. While their husbands, fathers, and brothers crafted arguments for independence, women called for their inclusion in government and better education of their sex. Although it would be nearly 150 years until women would obtain the right to vote, gains in education were achieved more rapidly, thanks to the reform efforts of both men and women. After the Revolutionary War, an educated citizenry was deemed critical to the success of the new nation, resulting in the establishment of new academies and seminaries for women. Although women were barred from attending traditional male colleges until Oberlin College opened its doors to women in 1837, the new all female academies were the beginnings of the education women from the Revolutionary War era had demanded.[1]

Many of the women who benefited from these improvements in education played pivotal roles in the abolitionist and suffrage movements of the 18th and 19th centuries with the latter continuing into the early part of the 20th century. These movements, which ultimately led to the 13th Amendment to the U.S. Constitution (ratified in 1865) banning slavery and the 19th Amendment (ratified in 1920) giving women the right to vote, enabled women to more actively participate in government, but by no means guaranteed equality. For example, women's participation in the work force increased only modestly between 1900 and 1940, due to considerable stigma and even legal restrictions against married women working outside the home.[2] Women typically left the work force permanently once they were married or had children. Not until World War II (1941–1945) did a significant number of married women enter the work force, gaining the economic and social benefits of employment. Unfortunately many of these benefits lasted only as long as the war.[3]

Case Presentation

Patient Case: Part 1

In 1910, M.E. was a 25-year-old mother of four living children who worked in one of the many sweatshops in New York City to subsidize the family income. Although some women of her generation had access to higher education, M.E. immigrated to the U.S. with her parents when she was 15-years-old and did not have the finances or formal training necessary for higher education. In theory, labor laws of the early 1900s limited the number of hours women could work, but many factory owners violated these laws. M.E. considered joining a union to protest the harsh working conditions at the factory but feared she might lose her job. M.E. felt lucky that she had survived the birth of her last child—the delivery was difficult. A neighbor had attended the birth, as M.E. could not afford the services of a trained midwife. The infant died a few months later when an outbreak of measles swept through the neighborhood. M.E. worried about having additional children and wanted to learn more about contraceptive options, but it was illegal for anyone to distribute information on contraception. So like many of her friends, M.E. relied on her husband to withdraw during intercourse.

In 1982, J.S., M.E.'s great-granddaughter, was 18-years-old and has graduated from high school. A star basketball player, she secured a full scholarship to the state university and was excited for fall to arrive. She would be the first in her family to attend college, and was grateful for the new opportunities in sports and education for women of her generation. Although her mother (M.C.) was intelligent and enjoyed being physically active, there had been few organized women's sports and no athletic scholarships offered to women in the late 1960s and early 1970s. Because M.C.'s family could not afford a college education, M.C. opted to be a career homemaker. J.S. did not want to do anything to jeopardize her scholarship, so although she was sexually active, she used contraception to avoid an unplanned pregnancy. It was easy for her to obtain low cost birth control pills from the clinic located in her neighborhood, and she appreciated the extra counseling and confidentiality the staff provided. Many of J.S.'s friends used drugs like marijuana, and a few got high on cocaine at parties. J.S. had experimented with pot when she was a sophomore, but with her scholarship depending on her athletic ability, she no longer used illicit drugs.

The fight for women's rights continued throughout the 20th century, and eventually played out in the medical arena. Where women once demanded improved access to education, they would later call for increased numbers of female scientists, healthcare providers, and gender specific health curricula. Women who fought for a voice in their own government would eventually oversee government programs dedicated to their own health. The fact that modern women's health has its foundations in social and political movements illustrates that women's health is achieved not merely by treating disease, but through action at individual, community, and national levels. In addition to discussing historical trends in morbidity and mortality, this chapter will describe social and political events that have shaped women's health and women's health research, providing a context for later chapters.

Definition of Women's Health

The definition of women's health has been evolving over time, from a biomedical model focusing on reproductive health to a biopsychosocial model taking into account the biological and social influences on women's health across the lifespan. Historically, women's health has been linked to reproduction and a woman's role as mother—a notion that has been reinforced socially, as well as through government sponsored programs and medical education.[4] Today multiple definitions of women's health exist (Table 1-1).[5-7] The National Institutes of Health's (NIH) research goals to improve women's health emphasize an integrated model incorporating social and behavioral factors with the biomedical model. The more recent definition by the Fourth World Conference on Women in Beijing also takes a biopsychosocial approach, addressing health from a wellness perspective and acknowledging the role of the social and economic environment on women's health. Only by understanding the factors influencing women's health, can a more comprehensive healthcare system encompassing the whole woman be developed.

The Woman as Mother: Women's Healthcare and Reproductive Health

GOVERNMENT PROGRAMS FOR WOMEN

The modern U.S. welfare system has its roots in protecting laborers, but instead of covering all workers, early U.S. public assistance programs targeted

Table 1-1. Definitions of Women's Health[5-7]

Organization	Year	Definition
Public Health Service and National Institutes of Health	1985 1987	Diseases or conditions unique to women or some subgroup of women; diseases or conditions more prevalent in women; diseases or conditions more serious among women or some subgroup of women; diseases or conditions for which the risk factors are different for women or some subgroup of women; or diseases or conditions for which the interventions are different for women or some subgroup of women. An additional distinction was made between diseases or conditions whose effect on women (or some women) is medically, physiologically, or sociologically different than those diseases or conditions that affect women differently because of access, resource, or delivery mode considerations.
Public Health Service	1991	Women's health is devoted to the preservation of wellness and prevention of illness in women, and includes screening, diagnosis and management of conditions which are unique to women, are more common in women, are more serious in women, and/or have manifestations, risk factors or interventions which are different in women
Fourth World Conference on Women in Beijing	1995	Health is a state of complete physical, mental and social well-being and not merely the absence of disease or infirmity; women's health involves their emotional, social and physical well-being and is determined by the social, political and economic context of their lives, as well as by biology

women. This was justified by their role, or potential role, as mothers. As early as the 1890s laws limiting work hours for women were enacted, and between 1911 and 1920, 40 states adopted "mother's pensions" to enable widows to care for their children.[8]

In 1912 the Federal Children's Bureau was established with a mission to "investigate and report...upon all matters pertaining to the welfare of children."[9] It was specifically charged with investigating infant mortality, which led to some of the first improvements in prenatal care.[9] Based on reports from the Children's Bureau, the Sheppard-Towner Act (officially the Federal Act for the Promotion of Welfare and Hygiene of Maternity and Infancy of 1921) established grants to states for maternal and child health services. Although allowed to lapse in 1929, activities initiated under the Sheppard-Towner Act laid the foundation for Title V of the Social Security Act.[10] Established as part of the Social Security Act of 1935, Title V provides funds for states to expand "services for promoting the health of mothers and children."[11] Funding from this act provided the foundation for many state health department activities, and it continues to be one of the major sources of funding for today's maternal and child health activities.

Programs enacted in the 1960s and 1970s, including Medicaid and Title X, also link access to healthcare and social services to reproduction. Signed into law in 1965, Medicaid is the largest federal assistance program for the poor. To qualify under the original rules, a woman needed to either be the mother of a child eligible for Aid to Families with Dependent Children (AFDC or welfare), be disabled, or indigent. In 1984 Medicaid eligibility was expanded to include pregnant women up to 133% of the federal poverty level.[12] In 1970 Title X of the Public Health Service (PHS) Act became the first and only federal program dedicated to providing family planning services. Available to low income women for free and to all women on a sliding scale, services provided by Title X funds are limited to those relating to reproductive health but do not currently include abortion.[13]

In all of the examples cited, access to government-sponsored healthcare is linked to motherhood and/or reproductive health. By linking a woman's access to healthcare to motherhood, these programs have institutionalized the notion that women's health is synonymous with reproductive health.

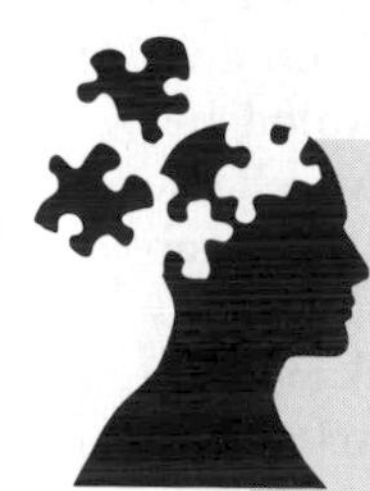

Therapeutic Challenge:

What health reform related to women's health is currently being explored via federal legislation?

MEDICAL EDUCATION

Although women's health content in medical education has progressed over the years, it has been slow to adopt a comprehensive view of women's health. In 1993 a report from the Department of Health and Human Services (DHHS) Committee on Appropriations concluded, "To date, there is no medical specialty which provides comprehensive primary healthcare to women."[14] Based on this observation, a national survey of medical school curricula on women's health was conducted. Although this study represents a single point in time and cannot be interpreted to represent all medical education, results indicated that many chronic conditions primarily affecting women were not consistently covered, while sexual and reproductive health topics were almost universally taught, reinforcing the link between women's health and reproduction.[14]

Effects of Various Societal Changes on Women's Lives and Health

WOMEN IN THE WORK FORCE

Prior to the 1940s, married women primarily managed the home and cared for children while single women who worked outside the home typically

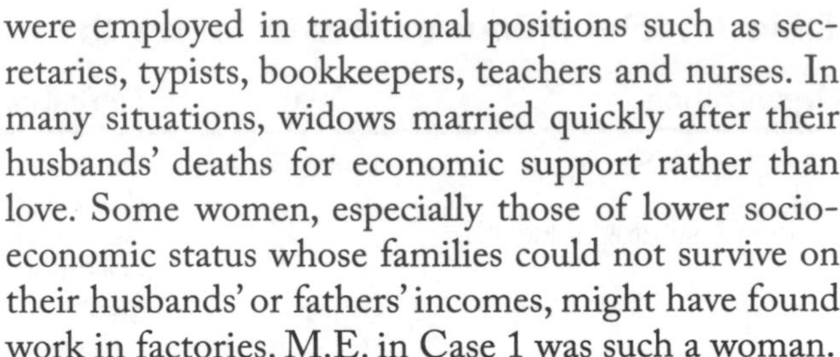

were employed in traditional positions such as secretaries, typists, bookkeepers, teachers and nurses. In many situations, widows married quickly after their husbands' deaths for economic support rather than love. Some women, especially those of lower socioeconomic status whose families could not survive on their husbands' or fathers' incomes, might have found work in factories. M.E. in Case 1 was such a woman.

Women's lives in the U.S. changed dramatically during WWII as women entered the work force in large numbers while men were involved in military actions around the globe. The country's war support efforts on the home front were undertaken to a great extent by women. After WWII ended and men returned home, many women left outside employment to again become fulltime housewives to free up jobs for returning veterans and to start families. Some of these jobs disappeared because certain manufactured products were no longer needed after the war. Some women supported their husbands as they went to college in large numbers on the GI education bill. Many other women yearned to return to employment outside the home.

From the 1940s to the 1960s, the number of women working outside the home doubled and the number of working mothers increased by 4 times so that families could afford a better life style.[17] For many women, it was not just the increased standard of living that appealed to them but the social interactions that occurred in the workplace.[17] Betty Friedan said there was a problem for women in the U.S.—"the problem that has no name"—which arose from "the boredom and dissatisfaction experienced by young wives and mothers across the country."[17] By 1960, 30% of all married women were working outside of the home, and of those with children, the figure was 39%.[17] To better expand their horizons, women in the 1950s began asking for a better birth control method to space their children and/or control the number of children they wanted. They sought a contraceptive method they could control because they were the ones who got pregnant. So the desires

MARGARET SANGER (1879–1966)[15,16]

Margaret Sanger was a pioneer in the field of family planning, and devoted her life to the cause. Trained as a nurse, she initially practiced on the Lower East Side of New York City where she cared for poor immigrant women suffering from failed illegal abortions. Based on this experience she focused her efforts on improving access to contraception. In 1916 she opened the first birth control clinic in the country, and in 1921 helped establish the American Birth Control League, the precursor to the Planned Parenthood Federation (name used beginning in 1942). Sanger was arrested twice and finally jailed on charges of obscenity for distributing information on contraceptives.[15] In later years, Sanger devoted her energy to finding an easier and more reliable method of contraception. Her dream was realized in 1951 when she paired scientist Gregory Pincus and heiress Katharine McCormick in a collaboration that ultimately led to the development of the first oral contraceptive.[16]

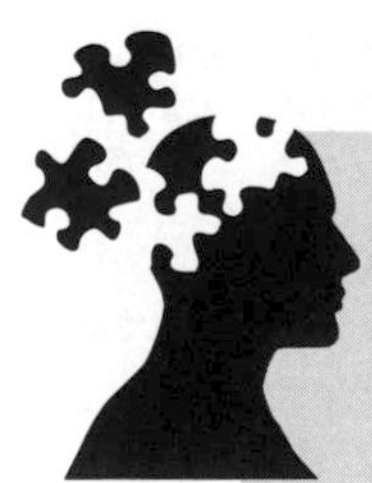

Therapeutic Challenge:

How have advances in healthcare contributed to gender equity in the work place?

of women and the sexual revolution began to intertwine in the 1960s.

After the sexual revolution of the 1960s, the number of women in the work force continued to increase in the U.S. and is predicted to continue to do so until at least 2014 when 51% of new workers will be women.[18] In 2006, a record number of women (67 million) were employed in the U.S. with 75% of these individuals being employed on a fulltime basis.[18]

SEXUAL ACTIVITY CHANGES

Presexual Revolution

Although women's lives began changing during the 1940s, sexual norms changed at a slow pace. For example, before the sexual revolution of the 1960s, girls and women who became pregnant out of wedlock went to homes for unwed mothers and typically gave their offspring up for adoption. Abortions were illegal and women who decided to have abortions did so at the risk of dying or having fertility problems thereafter. For women who went to college in increasing numbers after WWII, universities served as parents as young women transitioned from their family's home to the ones they would share with their husbands. Student dormitories were separated by gender and women had "hours." Women had to be in their rooms by a specified time nightly under the eyes of their dorm mothers.

Sexual Revolution

The availability of the birth control pill influenced the early 1960s while the mid-to-late 1960s were also influenced by the hippie movement as the oldest of the baby-boomer generation (post-WWII babies born between 1946 and 1964) became young adults who enrolled in college and/or went to war in Vietnam. *Cosmopolitan* and other publications for women revealed a "freer" life style. The feminist movement was growing. This time frame is also known as the sexual revolution. Debate is ongoing as to the origins of the sexual revolution. Some say it occurred secondarily to the availability of the "pill" while others say that this was partially true, but not totally responsible for the enormous social changes that occurred in the 1960s, a time of social upheaval on many fronts.[17] However, the pill probably helped expand the sexual freedom that women desired. During this same time, the Boston Women's Health Book Collective organized and began their publication of *Our Bodies, Ourselves* in response to women's needs to have information about their bodies and how to use the healthcare system to help meet their health needs. (See Web Resources for The Boston Women's Health Book Collective and *Our Bodies, Ourselves*.)[19] This book has undergone subsequent revisions and the group has published additional books on other women's health topics.

Additional content available at
www.ashp.org/womenshealth

The Pill

In the 1950s and 1960s, population control and economic development together helped change the U.S. In 1960, Searle's Enovid® was approved by the U.S. Food and Drug Administration (FDA) and other oral contraceptives followed. By 1965, 6.5 million married women and unknown numbers of unmarried women obtained prescriptions for the pill (data only for married women, numbers for unmarried women were not included; see *Griswold vs. Connecticut* later in this chapter).[17] Statistics from Planned Parenthood Clinics in 1961 showed that 14% of new clinic patients wanted an oral contraceptive; by 1963 these numbers increased to 42%, and by 1966 it rose to 70%.[17] Some have said that the numbers rose quickly because of advertisements for the pill, and financial incentives for physicians to be involved with contraception via more office visits to write prescriptions and for additional patient follow-up.

Divorce Rates and Cohabitation

The U.S. divorce rates increased during the 20th century with a peak of 23 divorces/1,000 married women occurring in 1978.[20] This likely occurred in industrialized countries such as the U.S. because women were increasingly working outside the home and thus had a lesser need for spousal financial support, and better birth control methods enabled couples to separate having children from having sex.[20] This is reflected by a divorce rate of only 5/1,000 married women in 1950 prior to the previously mentioned changes.

Since the late 1970s, a slow decline or leveling off of divorces has occurred in the U.S. (e.g., in 2005 there were 17.7 divorces/1,000 married women).[21] This has resulted from a variety of factors including a decrease in those getting married, an increase in the rate of cohabitation, and the aging of the population with older individuals typically remaining married. With heterosexual cohabitation (8.1% of coupled U.S. households in 2005), it is believed that there is increased instability in families because "cohabiting couples have twice the breakup rate of married couples," and ... "in the U.S., 40% bring [children] into these often shaky live-in relationships."[21]

Roe vs. Wade, The Family Leave Act (FLA), and the Equal Rights Amendment (ERA)

The U.S. Supreme Court decision, *Roe vs. Wade* (1973), gave women the right to have an abortion legally. This decision along with others such as The Family and Medical Leave Act of 1993 gave women more freedom and decision-making powers for her own health and for others.[22] For example, this latter act is a labor law that allows employees to take an unpaid leave for a serious health condition, which makes the employee unable to perform his/her job, care for an ill family member, or care for a newborn child (including by birth, adoption, or foster care).

The ERA was proposed as a new amendment to the U.S. Constitution that would guarantee that equal rights could not be denied because of sex under any federal, state, or local law. It passed the U.S. House of Representatives in 1971 and the Senate in 1972.[23] Thereafter, it was sent to state legislatures for ratification, which required a positive vote by three-quarters of legislatures within a 7-year time period. This did not occur before the deadline, and since 1982, the ERA or new resolutions entitled Women's Equality Amendment have been introduced in the U.S. House and Senate without passage.[23] The ERA, although never enacted, placed a spotlight on the feminist movement and helped advance women's rights in the workplace.

TITLE IX

Title IX of the Education Amendments of 1972 prohibits discrimination against women in education programs receiving federal funds. Although Title IX pertains to all aspects of education including employment, salary, and promotion, its most emotional and controversial application is to athletics.[24] This has also been its greatest impact, exemplified by the staggering increase of women athletes since its inception. In 1971 only 294,015 girls played high school sports, accounting for less than 8% of all participants.[25] By 2006 there were nearly 3 million female high school athletes, representing 41% of all participants.[26] Similar gains have been seen at the collegiate level, with over 155,000 women participating in competitive athletics in 2004—up almost fivefold from 1971.[27] Title IX has also opened doors to educational opportunities, including funding for female athletic scholarships, which were virtually nonexistent prior to 1972. Other groups, including pharmacy organizations, were also affected by Title IX. After its passage, gender segregated professional fraternities were forced to open their membership to both genders, creating modern coeducational organizations.

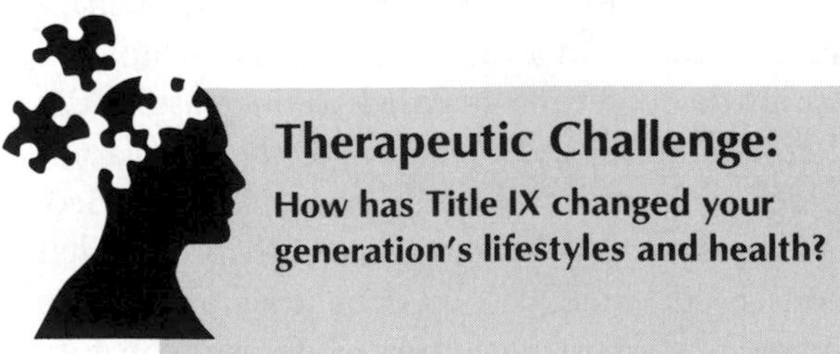

Therapeutic Challenge:
How has Title IX changed your generation's lifestyles and health?

Health Insurance and Women's Health

Changes in government programs, the aging of the population, and shifting work patterns have all influenced health insurance coverage for women. As previously discussed, government sponsored health programs such as Medicaid and Title X have improved access to healthcare for women. In addition to the expansion of Medicaid in the 1980s to include pregnancy, Medicaid has also been broadened to include screening and treatment for breast and cervical cancer. Building on the Breast and Cervical Cancer Mortality Prevention Act of 1990, which only provided screening services, the Breast and Cervical Cancer Prevention and Treatment Act of 2000 gives states the option of expanding Medicaid to provide qualifying women treatment for breast and cervical cancer.[28] Since the inception of the program, the number of women over 40 years of age reporting having a mammogram in the last 2 years has increased from 51.7% in 1990 to 69.5% in 2003.[29]

Because so many women are living into older age, Medicare can also be thought of as a health program to improve women's health. Instituted in 1965, Medicare provides hospital coverage for eligible people age 65 years and older, with the option to buy into additional outpatient and prescription drug coverage. In 1960, 9.1 million (10%) of all women were age 65 years and over, but this number is expected to expand to 42.2 million (19%) in 2040 making Medicare a primary source of health insurance for U.S. women.[30]

As more women have entered the workplace, employer-sponsored insurance (ESI) has become an important source of coverage for women. Women still face barriers to ESI, as women are less likely to be employed and more likely to work part time than men. Women are also more likely to obtain coverage through their spouse than are men, which places women at risk for becoming uninsured as employers scale back benefits for dependents.[31] Lesbians are one group of women who have seen a substantial increase in access to ESI over the last 25 years. In 1982 the *Village Voice* newspaper became the first company to offer domestic partner benefits to same sex partners, and the number of Fortune 500 companies offering domestic partner benefits increased from three in 1992 to 249 in 2006.[32,33] Another growing source of government healthcare for women is the Veteran's Health Care System. Historically women's participation in the military was restricted, but in 1967 the 2% cap on women enlisting in the military was lifted. The end of the male draft in 1973 and the opening of military academies to women in 1976 also contributed to an increasing number of women joining the military.[34] Women now make up 20% of new military recruits, and by 2036 the Veterans Administration expects there to be over 2.1 million female veterans, forcing a system that has historically been thought of as male healthcare to adapt to the needs of its female patients.[35,36]

In the future women will likely see significant changes in health insurance options as both state and federal legislators move to reform the healthcare system. How these reform efforts play out will dramatically influence the type of care women are able to receive, and ultimately their health outcomes. Issues such as the inclusion of reproductive health and preventative care; continuity of coverage regardless of employment, marital status, or health condition; adequate coverage of prescription drugs, and ensuring affordability for women and families will all be important elements of new insurance programs.

Advancement of Women's Healthcare

All the major political, social, scientific, product, and educational advancements influencing women's health, healthcare, and research cannot be discussed within this chapter. Some additional noteworthy changes are delineated in the Web Resources (see Advances in Women's Healthcare and Research Not Covered in the Text and Historical Timeline of Selected Events, Policies, and Key Decisions Related to Women, Women's Health, and the Role of Pharmacy in Women's Health). The historical timeline is also on the inside book cover.

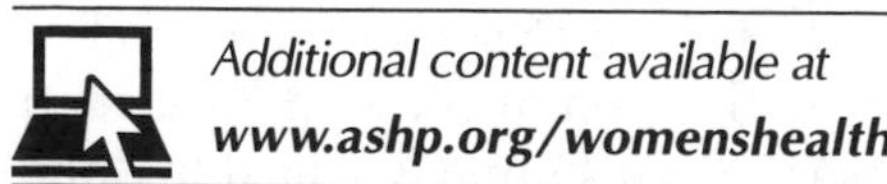
Additional content available at
www.ashp.org/womenshealth

ADVANCES IN REPRODUCTIVE HEALTH

The following areas are snapshots of advances made in women's reproductive health primarily since 1900 and certainly is not inclusive.

Maternal Mortality

The decline in maternal mortality by almost 99% between 1900 and 1997 is one of the great achievements in women's health in the 20th century. The period between 1935 and 1956 saw one of the steepest declines in maternal mortality rates going from 582 deaths per 100,000 live births to 40.[37] This overall decline is attributed to multiple factors, including improvements in nutrition and living standards, use of aseptic technique, introduction of antibiotics, improvements in access to care, improved surveillance, and the legalization of induced abortion.[37,38]

Availability and Use of Family Planning

For much of the first half of the 20th century distribution of information on contraception was illegal, even for married women. Not until 1965 in *Griswold vs. Connecticut* when the U.S. Supreme Court struck down Connecticut's law prohibiting contraceptive use by married couples was contraception made truly legal in the U.S.[39] Oral contraceptives have consistently been one of the most popular methods of birth control since first approved by the FDA in 1960, with approximately 16% to 18% of reproductive aged women reporting it as their current contraceptive method between 1982 and 2002.[40,41] Among married couples, sterilization is the most frequently used contraceptive method with its use increasing significantly since 1973 when the first survey of family planning methods was conducted. Use of sterilization increased from 24% in 1973 to a peak of 44% in 1988 decreasing slightly to 37% in 2002.[40,41]

Of note, many initiatives in the 1970s that expanded access to or improved surveillance of family planning were not initiated as women's health programs. The National Survey of Family Growth

(NSFG), which measures contraception use, was initiated as a reaction to concerns about population growth and its negative impact on the environment, the economy, and quality of life. In response to these concerns, President Richard Nixon in 1969 called for the formation of The Commission on Population Growth and The American Future. Chaired by John D. Rockefeller III, the Commission recommended that legal restrictions on contraception be lifted, state laws on abortion be liberalized, and that the NSFG be initiated.[42] Likewise, Title X was established as part of Nixon's war on poverty, aimed at curbing the negative economic and social effects of unintended pregnancy.[13]

Papanicolaou (Pap) Smear and Cervical Cancer

The introduction of the Pap smear in 1943 dramatically altered cervical cancer mortality in the U.S. Between 1950 and 2003, mortality due to cervical cancer in the U.S. decreased by 81.6% and the 5-year relative survival rate increased from 59% to 74.3%, making cervical cancer one of the least deadly cancers affecting women in the developed world.[43] The development of the vaccine for human papillomavirus, the virus necessary for cervical cancer, promises to reduce cervical cancer rates even more, although the long-term impact of the vaccine on actual mortality rates has yet to be measured.[44]

TRENDS IN MORBIDITY AND MORTALITY

Shift to Chronic Conditions

One of the most significant changes in women's health over the last century has been the increase in life expectancy and the shift in the leading cause of mortality away from infectious diseases to chronic conditions. Between 1900 and 2004 life expectancy at birth for all U.S. women increased by over 31 years, from 48.3 to 80.1 years.[29] More significant is the proportion of women living into older age. In 1950 only about 10% of women and 5% of men reaching age 50 years lived to age 90, but in 1990 this proportion jumped to 23% for women and 10% for men.[30]

In 1900 the leading three causes of death in the U.S. were due to infections, whereas in 2004 chronic diseases and cancer were the leading causes of mortality.[29,45] Gender specific data on leading causes of death are only available from 1971 onward, in part reflecting the lack of attention paid to gender specific healthcare during a significant portion of the 20th century.[45] Between 1971 and 2004, suicide, congenital anomalies, and conditions originating in early infancy have been replaced by Alzheimer's disease, septicemia, and renal disease as leading causes of death among women in recent years. (See Web Resources for Leading Causes of Death in the U.S. from 1900–2004.)

Additional content available at ***www.ashp.org/womenshealth***

The shift toward chronic disease is of particular importance to women as the probability of having multiple chronic conditions increases with age, and many diseases common in women, such as osteoporosis and arthritis, contribute to disability.[46] As women continue living longer and the baby-boomer generation ages, there will be an even greater proportion of women living with one or more chronic conditions. Table 1-2 highlights trends in selected chronic conditions over time.[29] Of note is the decline of women reporting high cholesterol and hypertension. This decline, along with a decrease in cigarette smoking and improved medical care, has contributed to the decline in mortality from heart disease and stroke, although the increasing prevalence of women who are overweight and obese threatens this success as seen by the rise in diabetes. (See Chapter 32: Overweight and Obesity.)[47]

Table 1-2. Selected Chronic Conditions in U.S. Women[29]

Condition	1960–1962	1988–1994	2001–2004
	(% of Population)		
Hypertension[a,b]	33.7	20.8	26.2
High serum cholesterol[a]	35.6	20.5	16.2
Overweight[a,c]	40.2	51.2	61.4
Obesity[a,d]	15.7	26.0	34.0
Diabetes[e]	--	5.4	7.1

[a]Aged 20–74 years, age adjusted to 2000 standard population.
[b]Excludes pregnant women.
[c]Body mass index (BMI) ≥25.
[d]BMI ≥30.
[e]Aged 20 years or older; physician-diagnosed; excludes diabetes during pregnancy.

Re-emergence of Infectious Diseases: Human Immunodeficiency Virus (HIV)/Acquired Immune Deficiency Syndrome (AIDS)

Although chronic conditions and cancer are the leading cause of mortality among women, infections again are playing a major role in women's health. Since the emergence of HIV/AIDS in 1981, women, and especially African-American women, are bearing an increasing burden of the disease. (See Chapter 38: Sexually Transmitted and Infectious Diseases.) Between 1990 and 1999 rates of AIDS diagnosis decreased among men by over 40% (42.9% vs. 29.3%) but increased among women (5.8% vs. 8.8%).[48] Likewise, between 1986 and 2005 the cumulative percentage of AIDS cases among women increased from 6.7% to 19% and the percentage of new AIDS cases in women increased from 7% to 26%.[49-51] In 2004, AIDS was the fifth leading cause of death among women aged 25–44 years and the third leading cause of death for African-American women of this age group.[29]

LESBIAN, BISEXUAL, AND TRANSGENDERED WOMEN

Significant changes have developed for women who are lesbian, bisexual, or transgendered; however, significant stereotypes, prejudices, and health disparities still exist. For information about the social welfare and healthcare of lesbian, bisexual, and transgendered women and men refer to Chapter 5: Issues in Lesbian, Bisexual, and Transgender Healthcare.

TRENDS IN SUBSTANCE USE

The feminist movement of the 20th century opened multiple political, economic, and social opportunities for women. Ironically, it also allowed them to more freely engage in some of the same negative health behaviors that many men practiced. (See Chapter 36: Substance-Use Disorders.) Advertisements marketing cigarettes to women utilized the women's liberation movement by referring to cigarettes as a "torch of freedom."[52] Women exercised their equality in the 1960s and 1970s by smoking marijuana in record numbers.[53] Body image also played a significant role in the use of tobacco and other drugs. Early cigarette ads promoted smoking as a diet suppressant by warning women, "you can't hide fat clumsy ankles," and amphetamines were over prescribed to women in the 1960s mainly as appetite suppressants.[54]

Cigarette Smoking

Early in the 20th century smoking cigarettes was considered taboo for women, and in 1908 in New York it was actually illegal for women to smoke in public, but this began changing in the 1920s.[54] Although there are no reliable national estimations of smoking prevalence prior to 1955, estimates based on early industry data suggested that approximately 6% of women smoked in 1924, increasing to 12% in 1929.[55] During WWII smoking among both men and women increased, with 36% of women and 48% of men identifying as smokers in a 1944 Gallup pole.[56] Smoking was included in the National Health Interview Survey (NHIS) for the first time in 1965, and since that time current smoking status among women has declined from 34% to 19%, while for men the rate decreased from 52% to 23%.[29] During this period of overall decline, there have been spikes in youth smoking rates. Initiation of smoking among girls aged 14–17 increased between 1966 and 1979 in parallel with sales of niche brands targeting young women, whereas during the same time period initiation rates among boys aged 16–17 declined.[55] Ads for theses brands echoed earlier themes of freedom and liberation with tag lines such as, "You've come a long way, baby" or "Find your voice." Another increase was seen in the 1990s with the percentage of high school senior girls who reported smoking increasing from 26% in 1992 to 35% in 1997 while smoking rates for high school boys went from 29% to 37%.[57] This change follows the debut of the Joe Camel character in 1988. Although Marlboro continued to be the most popular teen brand, it is possible the Joe Camel campaign affected the overall popularity of smoking.[55] Cigarette ads targeting women, and some critics claim young women, continue into the 21st century with the introduction of Camel No. 9, a repackaged new "Light and Lushes" version of the original product.[58]

Alcohol Use

Women began consuming alcohol more openly in the 1920s, even though some still considered women who opposed prohibition to be "immoral." As women continued gaining their social and economic independence, alcohol consumption increased.[54] The percentage of women who drank alcohol went from 45% in 1939 to a peak of 66% in 1981 but has declined in recent years to 46%.[56,59] Men have had consistently higher rates of alcohol use over the same time period but followed a similar pattern with 70%, 75%, and 57% reporting drinking during the same years. Another factor influencing women and drinking is the increased awareness of the effects of

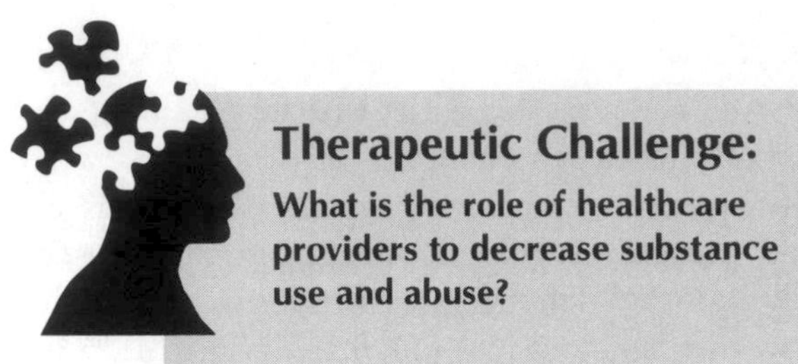

Therapeutic Challenge:

What is the role of healthcare providers to decrease substance use and abuse?

alcohol during pregnancy, highlighted by the U.S. Surgeon General's first report on the topic in 1981 and required warning labels on alcoholic beverages beginning in 1989.[60,61]

Drugs of Abuse

Drug abuse has been common among women since the 1800s, and in the early 20th century women made up the majority of people addicted to opiates. Women have been consistently over prescribed certain classes of medications including sedatives and amphetamines, leading to addiction among women, which sometimes has been classified as iatrogenic. In 1914 the use of opiates for nonmedicinal use was made illegal, dramatically decreasing the number of female users. Use of prescription medications again surged from the 1950s through the early 1980s. Between 1969 and 1982, an estimated 1–2 million women were addicted to prescription drugs and in 1978 approximately 20% of women were taking diazepam (Valium®).[54]

In addition to prescription medications, illicit drugs have also been a source of abuse by women. Between 1960 and 1970, the proportion of women with addictions doubled from 14% to 30%, and the proportion with heroin addiction increased from 18% to 30% in 1970.[54,62] With the introduction of crack cocaine in the 1980s, cocaine use among women also increased; between 1983 and 1989 approximately one-third to two-fifths of callers to a national cocaine help line were women.[63]

FDA AND THE FDA OFFICE OF WOMEN'S HEALTH (OWH)

There have been numerous ways by which the FDA, and specifically the FDA OWH, has advanced women's healthcare since the early 1990s. Prior to that time, many FDA policies and guidelines prohibited wide participation of women in clinical trials, but after the 1993 *Guideline for the Study and Evaluation of Gender Differences in the Clinical Evaluation of Drugs* was released, and the OWH was established, there has been an increased acknowledgement of women's health needs through policy changes and decisions on medications to be used by women, some of which can be found in the timeline.[64]

The OWH has worked with pharmacy organizations such as the American Pharmacists Association (APhA) and the National Association of Chain Drug Stores (NACDS) to advance women's health (Table 1-3).

DHHS AND THE DHHS OWH

This department has advanced women's health in a variety of ways via establishing general health policies that affect all people (e.g., Healthy People 2000, 2010, and the upcoming 2020 reports), but also by specifically addressing women's health under the direction of its OWH, which established Centers of Excellence in Women's Health (CoE) and other related organizations (see the timeline).[65,66] The CoEs have for many years helped advance education, research, care, and outreach in the area of women's health through selected academic institutions. Although many of these CoEs still exist by generating their own funding, federal funds no longer support their efforts.

PHARMACY PROFESSIONAL ORGANIZATIONS

In the 1990s and early 2000s, pharmacy organizations such as the American Association of Colleges of Pharmacy (AACP), APhA, and NACDS began increasing their support of women's health through journal publications, special programming, and partnering with federal agencies (e.g., FDA OWH and NACDS combined their efforts on the Women's Health "Take Time to Care" campaign). The AACP received support from NIH Office of Research on Women's Health (ORWH), FDA OWH, and DHHS OWH to establish a women's health database to supplement resources of colleges/schools of pharmacy. In addition, U.S. pharmacists have been advancing women's health globally through their participation in international pharmacy organizations such as the International Pharmaceutical Federation (FIP) (Table 1-3).

Table 1-3. Pharmacy Professional Organizations—Additional Involvement in Women's Health and Research Not Covered in the Text

Organization	Activity, Program, and/or Report	Date	Comments
American Association of Colleges of Pharmacy (AACP)	Women Faculty Special Interest Group (includes women educator luncheons at the AACP Annual Meetings)	1994	Established
American College of Clinical Pharmacy (ACCP)	Task Force on Women's Health Research	1991	Established
	Policy statement on women as research subjects	1992	Issued
	NIH ORWH public policy sessions on women's health research	1992, 1993, and 1996	Member testified
	White paper *Women as Research Subjects*	1993	Published
	Women's Health Practice and Research Network (WH-PRN)	1994	Established
	Grant for women's health research	1995–2002	Funded by Wyeth
	Programming on women's health	Began in 1995	Presented annually by the WH-PRN and periodically as ACCP special programming
	Research in Women and Special Populations; revised white paper on women's health research	2008	Published
American Pharmacists Association (APhA)	Passes policy *Use of Representative Populations in Clinical Studies*	1990	Policy revised in 2005
	Members testified at NIH ORWH public policy sessions on women's health research	1993 and 1996	
	Programming on women's health held during annual meetings	Began in early 1990s	
	Articles on women's health in APhA publications	Began in early 1990s	
	FDA has booths at APhA Annual Meetings	Began in late 1990s	
American Society of Health-System Pharmacists (ASHP)	*Women's Health Across the Lifespan: A Pharmacotherapeutic Approach*	2010	First pharmacy textbook on women's health
International Pharmaceutical Federation (FIP)	International women's leadership symposium	1987	*Proceedings of the International Leadership Symposium: The Role of Women in Pharmacy*
	Women in Pharmacy International luncheons	1989–2006	
	International Forum of Women for Pharmacy (name changed various times)	1989–1998	Presentations on women in pharmacy
National Association of Chain Drug Stores (NACDS) and/or the NACDS Foundation	Partnered with FDA's Office of Women's Health (OWH) to advance "Take Time to Care" (TTTC) campaign. The campaign was held to advance women's health and improve medication safety.	1999 and 2000	Also involved pharmacies nationwide and some colleges/schools of pharmacy
	FDA has booths at NACDS meetings	Began in late 1990s	

Policy Decisions That Have Impacted Women's Healthcare and Research in the U.S.

Research that today is defined as medical or clinical began in the 20th century after methods to conduct clinical trials were first established in the 1930s and 1940s.[67] At approximately this same time, Congress passed a series of acts to increase the quality and purity of drugs (e.g., Food, Drug, and Cosmetic Act enacted in 1938 that required safety testing of drugs prior to their being marketed).[67] Even with the government's requirement for clinical trials, women's participation in these trials is relatively new, typically going back less than two decades. Prior to the end of this past century, Caucasian men were the norm for human participation in clinical trials. Many policy decisions slowed the inclusion of women in the clinical trials process, which might have negatively affected women's health. The remainder of this section presents an overview of policies, guidelines, statements and events that have had the greatest impact, both positive and negative, on women's healthcare research in the U.S. Related information can also be found in a table in the Web Resources (see Advances in Women's Healthcare and Research Not Covered in the Text and Historical Timeline of Selected Events, Policies, and Key Decisions Related to Women, Women's Health, and the Role of Pharmacy in Women's Health). The historical timeline is also on the inside book cover.

Additional content available at ***www.ashp.org/womenshealth***

NUREMBERG CODE OF ETHICS

The Nuremberg Code of Ethics is considered one of the most important documents in biomedical ethics because it laid the foundation for the protection of human subjects participating in research.[68,69] It stemmed from the war crimes trials of Nazi Germany that were held in Nuremberg, Germany following WWII and established research ethics beyond the Hippocratic oath so that nations and scientists would not in the future conduct unethical research involving human subjects. Thereafter, significant components of the code were adopted by U.S. government agencies involved in human research. These included the concept of informed consent—a need for scientifically valid research designs that would produce results for the good of society while subjects enrolled in clinical trails had the right to end their participation at any time. In the Nuremberg Code of Ethics, patient autonomy was equal to that of the researcher (i.e., the rights of the patient were as important as those of the researcher). This code, written to especially protect populations believed vulnerable (e.g., children, pregnant women, and their fetuses), became the landmark document that U.S. government officials cited when writing policies such as the *PHS Policy on the Protection of Human Subjects* (issued in 1966 and rewritten many times) that essentially excluded women from research studies.[69] Therefore, the autonomy in healthcare included in the Nuremberg Code of Ethics was something that U.S. women did not gain along with men. Women began to demand these rights in the 1960s and finally received them in the 1990s after changes were made in the conduct of clinical trials funded by the NIH, and via policy changes at the FDA that allowed women to participate in all phases of clinical trials.

U.S. FEDERAL GUIDELINES FOR THE CONDUCT OF HUMAN SUBJECTS RESEARCH

In the early years of clinical research, studies conducted involving human subjects were not regulated and some abuses occurred. Examples of such unethical practices included the PHS Syphilis Study (begun in 1932), the testing of oral contraceptives in women without some participants being totally informed about the study, and alleged abuses in the healthcare of children and prisoners. Hearings were held about abuses and thereafter, Congress enacted the National Research Act of 1974, formed the National Commission for the Protection of Human Subjects of Biomedical and Behavioral Research, and placed a moratorium on federally funded research involving live human fetuses.[67,69] Among the Commission's reports (1974–1978) were those involving research conducted in vulnerable populations (e.g., pregnant women, live human fetuses, children, prisoners, mentally disabled). These reports further decreased women's participation in clinical trials because of childbearing potential even if the women were not pregnant, were using birth control, were sterile, and/or did not have a male sex partner. Postmenopausal women were typically not thought of for clinical trail participation because of their longevity compared to men. Thus they were thought to require less medical research aimed at their needs when exploring therapy for diseases that affected both men and women. The assumption was drugs that benefited and were safe in men would also benefit and be safe in women at the same doses. Prior to congressional hearings, federal funding for clinical research had been expanded in the 1960s. As a result, NIH developed the first *PHS Policy on the Protection of Human Subjects* in 1966.[69] This policy was expanded to cover all Department of Health, Education, and Welfare (later called the Department of Health and Human Services, DHHS) supported human research, and thereafter has been revised many times.

WOMEN AS VULNERABLE SUBJECTS

Other events that also led to women being considered a vulnerable research group included the effects of diethylstilbestrol (DES) and thalidomide on fetuses secondary to maternal use during pregnancy. The consequences were the enactment of policy decisions that in the past led to women being excluded from clinical trials for decades, the result of which was a lack of knowledge about medications and their specific effects in women.

DES Use During Pregnancy

While the Nuremberg Code of Ethics provided an underpinning for research that involved humans, the use of certain medications by pregnant women for which research had not been carried out prior to its general use led to outcomes that further blocked women from participating in clinical trails.[70] DES was prescribed for pregnant women in the U.S. from the 1940s until the early 1970s to prevent threatened, spontaneous abortions, and preterm births. Even though a study undertaken in 1953 demonstrated that DES was no more effective than placebo in preventing miscarriages or preterm deliveries, the drug was used until the early 1970s when a report linked DES to cases of vaginal clear cell adenocarcinoma (CCAC) in daughters exposed in utero when their mothers took DES.[71,72] These daughters were also noted to have an increased risk of cervical CCAC, vaginal epithelial changes, reproductive tract abnormalities, ectopic pregnancies, miscarriages, etc., while their mothers were at an increased risk for developing breast cancer.[70] Sons of DES mothers were noted to have increased reproductive tract abnormalities.[70] Adverse health effects associated with DES have been noted in some DES grandchildren (e.g., preterm labor and deliveries). Therefore, three generations are being followed in large cohort studies to evaluate DES adverse effects.[70]

Thalidomide Tragedy

Thalidomide had not been approved for use in the U.S. when over 10,000 children worldwide (1957–1962) were noted to have various birth defects (e.g., defects of the limbs including **phocomelia,** axial skeleton, head, eyes, and ears as well as cardiovascular, central nervous, gastrointestinal, genitourinary, and respiratory systems) resulting from their mothers' use of this drug during pregnancy.[67,73] Of these children, 17 born in the U.S. had malformations because their mothers received drug samples from physicians before the FDA acted on the drug.[73] The impact in the U.S. was minimal because the FDA had not yet approved the use of this medication. This wide-scale tragedy facilitated the U.S. Congress passing the Kefauver-Harris Amendments (1962) that modified the Federal Food, Drug, and Cosmetic Act of 1938, which gave the FDA increased control over drug experimentation in humans and the regulation of new drugs.[73] Thereafter, drug manufacturers had to demonstrate that drugs were safe and effective.

FDA Guideline of 1977

An FDA guideline entitled, *General Consideration for the Clinical Evaluation of Drugs,* issued in 1977 contained a section "Women of Childbearing Potential" that essentially prohibited women from participating in clinical studies.[74] This guideline was not revised until 1993 to include both sexes in drug development trials. The revised statement denoted a need for comparing trial data between the sexes. Thus, the FDA now notes that women and men might respond differently to drugs.

PHS TASK FORCE ON WOMEN'S HEALTH ISSUES (1985) AND NIH ADVISORY COMMITTEE ON WOMEN'S HEALTH (1986)

In 1985, the PHS Task Force on Women's Health Issues under the guidance of Edward N. Brandt, Jr., MD, Ph.D., then Assistant Secretary of DHHS, released a report in which members recommended that "biomedical and behavioral research should be expanded to insure emphasis on those conditions and diseases unique to, or more prevalent in, women in all age groups as well as those conditions for which the interventions were different, or the health risks greater, for women than for men."[75-77] For his leadership and political clout, Dr. Brandt is considered the godfather of women's health.[75] This report was a landmark government report, which emphasized the need for women to be research participants. This report was followed by the recommendations of the 1986 NIH Advisory Committee on Women's Health that concluded women should be included in clinical trials and researchers should evaluate study data for gender differences.[76,78]

EDWARD N. BRANDT, JR., MD, Ph.D. (1933–2007)

This chapter is dedicated to Edward N. Brandt, Jr., MD, Ph.D., for his lifelong support of women's health and women's health research. From a successful academic career in obstetrics and gynecology at the University of Oklahoma Health Sciences Center, Dr. Brandt became the Assistant Secretary, U.S. Department of Health and Human Services. He established the Public Health Service Task Force on Women's Health Issues that was the first to bring to the forefront the need to have women included in clinical research trials. This landmark report started individuals at the NIH and some members of the U.S. Congress to think about the great need to increase support of women's health research. For his ongoing leadership and support of women's health and women's health research, Dr. Vivian Pinn, Director of the NIH ORWH, recognized Dr. Brandt as the "godfather" of women's health. She also stated that he was "instrumental in promoting the careers of many people, especially women in science and women's health."[75] Later in his career after holding many distinguished positions in academic administration, he returned to the University of Oklahoma as Professor Emeritus, where he continued his passions, such as serving as a member of the NIH ORWH Advisory Committee. There he shared his knowledge and imparted his wisdom, especially on how to push forth a women's health agenda in a political environment.

While DHHS Assistant Secretary, Dr. Brandt not only advanced women's health research, but he provided the initial federal response to the AIDS epidemic and worked to establish requirements for tamper-proof drug packaging following the Tylenol® poisonings.[75]

U.S. GENERAL ACCOUNTING OFFICE (GAO) REPORT OF 1990

By the late 1980s, women were clamoring for greater federal government support of women's health and research. Activists, some with ties to the NIH and the Congressional Caucus for Women's Issues (CCWI), became interested in what the NIH had accomplished since putting forth its 1986 policy to increase women's participation in clinical trails. At about this same time, results from a large NIH-funded study were released that explored aspirin use to reduce heart attacks among 22,000 male physicians.[79] This and other issues resulted in the CCWI asking Congressman Henry Waxman (Chair, Energy and Commerce Subcommittee on Health and the Environment) to request a GAO investigation of how the NIH was fulfilling its policy to include women and minorities in federally funded research.[80] Thereafter, the GAO stated in its landmark report that the NIH was slow to implement its policy on including women and minorities in clinical trials, and that the evaluation of sex/gender differences had not been required in studies.[80,81] It was also noted that only 13.5% of the $778 million that NIH was spending on research was funding women's health research.[76]

WOMEN'S HEALTH EQUITY ACT OF 1990 AND ESTABLISHMENT OF THE NIH ORWH

The CCWI drafted the Women's Health Equity Act in 1990.[76,78] Out of this process came the establishment of the NIH ORWH within the Office of the NIH Director. Shortly thereafter, Dr. Ruth Kirschstein was appointed its acting director. (See Web Resources for Key Women in the Advancement of Women's Health Research at the National Institutes of Health.)[82] The ORWH was given three main objectives by Congress:

1. "to ensure that issues pertaining to women are adequately addressed, including diseases, disorders, and conditions that are unique to, more prevalent among, or far more serious in women, or for which there are different risk factors or interventions for women than for men;
2. to ensure appropriate participation in clinical research, especially clinical trials; and
3. to foster increased involvement of women in biomedical research, especially in decision-making roles in clinical medicine and research environments."[76,83] In addition, starting in February 1991, no PHS clinical research grant applications (including those supported by NIH) were accepted for funding unless women were adequately represented, except in cases where exclusion was justified.[76]

Additional content available at
www.ashp.org/womenshealth

ESTABLISHMENT OF WOMEN'S HEALTH OFFICES IN VARIOUS DHHS AGENCIES

After the establishment of the NIH ORWH, offices addressing women's health were founded within other DHHS agencies. These included the appointment of the Special Assistant for Women's Health at FDA (1990, now the Office of Women's Health [OWH] that Congress mandated in 1994), DHHS Office on Women's Health (1991), and Centers for Disease Control and Prevention (CDC) OWH (1994). Today these offices work closely together to advance women's health and research on a national basis.

NIH REVITALIZATION ACT OF 1993

As part of the NIH Revitalization Act of 1993, the ORWH was authorized by statute. The NIH was also directed by Congress to establish guidelines for the inclusion of women and minorities in clinical research. The NIH Director was to ensure that women and minorities are included as subjects in each research project.[84] In addition, if differences among various subpopulations (e.g., women, minorities, seniors) were identified, additional analyses and studies were to be conducted. A data system for the collection, storage, analysis, retrieval and dissemination of information regarding NIH sponsored research on women's health was to be established. In 1994 NIH issued new guidelines for the inclusion of women in medical research in accordance with the 1993 guideline.[78]

GAO REPORT OF 2000

In 2000 the GAO released a report entitled, *NIH Has Increased Its Efforts to Include Women in Research*, in response to a request by Congress about the status of women's health research. This report assessed "NIH's progress in conducting research on women's health in the past decade" after a previous GAO report (1990) found NIH slow to do so.[81] Overall, according to the report, the NIH had made significant progress toward achieving its goals. This was accomplished by establishing "guidelines to implement the NIH Revitalization Act of 1993 and conduct(ing) extensive training for scientists and (grant) reviewers."[81,84]

The NIH ORWH was complimented by the GAO for developing a women's health research agenda for the 21st century, and for wisely leveraging their funds by working with various NIH institutes and centers to increase funding for women's health research. Between fiscal years 1993 and 1999, funding for women's health research at NIH grew by 39% vs. 23% for men's health and 27% for research that affected both men and women.[81]

FDA STATEMENTS AND POLICIES THAT HAVE AFFECTED WOMEN IN RESEARCH STUDIES

DHHS revised *Title 45 Code of Federal Regulations Part 46, Protection of Human Subjects* (45 CFR 46) in 1991 concerning pregnant women's participation in clinical studies (45 CFR 46.207).[85] Thereafter, when the GAO released a report in 1992 that investigated the under-representation of women in drug trials, the FDA issued the *Guideline for the Study and Evaluation of Gender Differences in the Clinical Evaluation of Drugs* (1993).[64] This guideline called for the inclusion of both genders in drug development and the section "Women of Childbearing Potential" included in the 1977 FDA guideline *General Consideration for the Clinical Evaluation of Drugs* was revised. It also gave more authority to institutional review boards, investigators, and research subjects to ensure that women of childbearing potential could participate in clinical trials.

In 1998, the FDA published a final ruling for Investigational New Drug Applications and New Drug Applications that modified previous language including "the requirement to present effectiveness and safety data for important demographic subgroups, specifically gender, age, and racial subgroups."[86] It was also stated that the FDA declined "to define subpopulations of women because it is not necessary. Usually, pregnant women would only participate in clinical trials intended specifically to study drug effects during pregnancy. The data generated from such trials would, therefore, reflect use in this subpopulation of women."[86] Thus, the FDA let companies that required their approval to market drugs, devices, etc. have more leeway in the inclusion of women as subjects in clinical trails than did the NIH. Differences between the two agencies could be due to their different roles. The NIH directly funds clinical research while the FDA is a regulatory agency that ensures that drugs and medical devices are safe and effective.

Advancement of Women's Health Research

NURSES' HEALTH STUDY AND ASSOCIATED STUDIES

Prior to the 1990s, the Nurses' Health Study was the only major research study in the U.S. that addressed women's health. The study design was a prospective epidemiology trial. It was launched in the mid-1970s, about 10 years after oral contraceptives were marketed in the U.S., after a group of Harvard School of Medicine faculty asked the question, "Do birth control pills have long-term health effects?"[87] This question "sparked the beginning of what has since become one of the largest and most comprehensive studies of women's health."[87] These Harvard researchers received NIH support for a pilot study for which recruitment began in 1976. Thereafter, over 120,000 married nurses between the ages of 30 and 55 years responded to a survey, which contained questions about contraception and other health issues. Questionnaires have been modified over time to reflect health issues and conditions that affect participants as they age. In addition to answering questionnaires, these nurses have periodically been asked to provide various biological samples (e.g., blood and nail clippings). Today this is the longest running and largest women's health study worldwide.[87]

Additional women's prospective epidemiology trials have developed from this study. In 1989 the Nurses' Health Study II was initiated because women in the original study could no longer respond to certain reproductive health questions such as those concerning the use of low-dose oral contraceptives. Over 116,000 nurses (ages 25–42 years) initially enrolled in this second study with up to 90% responding to questionnaires concerning their reproductive history, overall health status, lifestyle choices, medication use, etc.[87] An observational study, Growing Up Today Study, enrolled over 17,000 children of women who were participants in the Nurses' Health Study II.[87] Since 1995 these children, now adolescents and young adults, have annually filled out questionnaires about health issues, diet, exercise, weight gain, etc.

LACK OF WOMEN'S HEALTH RESEARCH STUDIES

Except for the Nurses' Health Study, little research was undertaken before the 1990s in the area of women's health compared to advances made in men's health via federally funded clinical research trials. This was primarily the result of policies and guidelines that were previously discussed. A new era in women's health research began with changes at the NIH and FDA in the early- to mid-1990s. For example, Dr. Bernadine Healy, then director (and first woman director, see Web Resources for Key Women in the Advancement of Women's Health Research at the National Institutes of Health) of the NIH, launched a major women's health research project, the Women's Health Initiative (WHI), in April 1991 shortly after the establishment of the NIH ORWH.[88] Thereafter, the WHI advanced via the efforts of the ORWH and the National Heart, Lung, and Blood Institute (NHLBI), sponsor of the WHI within the NIH community.[89]

Additional content available at **www.ashp.org/womenshealth**

WHI

WHI was a major 15-year, multimillion dollar research program that eventually enrolled 161,808 postmenopausal women (ages 50–79 years) in a series of randomized controlled clinical trials and/or an observational study.[89] It addressed the effects of postmenopausal hormone therapy, diet modification, calcium and vitamin D supplements on cardiovascular disease, osteoporosis, and breast and colorectal cancer. The hormone trial had two studies: the estrogen-plus-progestin study of women with a uterus and the estrogen-alone study of women without a uterus.[89] These two studies were stopped early, but many study participants were enrolled in a "follow-up phase" that is to finish in 2010. In addition, a 5-year prevention study in partnership with the CDC studied strategies to increase healthy behaviors in women 40 years of age and older via community-based public health intervention models.[89] Overall, WHI enrollment cut across geographical, ethnic, race, and socioeconomic circumstances.

NIH AND THE NIH ORWH

In 1999 NIH ORWH under the leadership of Dr. Vivian Pinn (see Web Resources for Key Women in the Advancement of Women's Health Research at the National Institutes of Health), and with the help and support of others at NIH and external partners, published the *Agenda for Research on Women's Health for the 21st Century* that is currently used to guide funding priorities.[90,91] The ORWH also works closely with various NIH institutes and centers to plan conferences on women's health, develop research initiatives that cut across NIH boundaries, and cofund meritorious research, which advances women's health among its many other responsibilities.[92]

Additional content available at **www.ashp.org/womenshealth**

Beyond its initial mandates, ORWH today 1) "coordinates and serves as a focal point for women's health research funded by the NIH; 2) promotes, stimulates, and supports efforts to improve the health of women through biomedical and behavioral research on the roles of sex (biological characteristics of being female or male) and gender (social influences based on sex) in health and disease; 3) works in partnership with the NIH institutes and centers to ensure that women's health research is part of the scientific framework at NIH and throughout the scientific community; 4) advises the NIH Director and staff on matters relating to research on women's health; 5) strengthens and enhances research related to diseases, disorders, and conditions that affect women; 6) ensures that research conducted and supported by NIH adequately addresses issues regarding women's health; 7) ensures that women are appropriately represented in biomedical and biobehavioral research studies supported by NIH; 8) develops opportunities for and supports recruitment, retention, re-entry, and advancement of women in biomedical careers; and 9) supports research on women's health issues."[92] For further information about ORWH and its accomplishments, see Web Resources for Advances in Women's Healthcare and Research Not Covered in the Text and Historical Timeline of Selected Events, Policies, and Key Decisions Related to Women, Women's Health, and the Role of Pharmacy in Women's Health or go to the ORWH website at http://orwh.od.nih.gov/.

Additional content available at
www.ashp.org/womenshealth

Without the guidance of Drs. Bernadine Healy, Ruth Kirschstein, and Vivian Pinn, the NIH ORWH might not have accomplished all it has thus far for women's health and research at the NIH. These individuals were the right people in the right place to make a difference that will affect women's lives for years to come. (See Web Resources for Key Women in the Advancement of Women's Health Research at the National Institutes of Health.)

Additional content available at
www.ashp.org/womenshealth

CHALLENGES OF RECRUITING WOMEN FOR CLINICAL TRIALS, ESPECIALLY FROM SOME MINORITY GROUPS

Although progress has been made concerning the inclusion of women in clinical trials, recruitment of women from some minority groups is still difficult. One of the first actions of the NIH ORWH as part of its mandate was "to ensure appropriate participation (of women) in clinical research, especially clinical trials."[73,80] Thus in 1993, ORWH held public hearings and a meeting entitled, *Recruitment and Retention of Women in Clinical Studies.* Information gained was published as a chapter entitled, "Selected Issues in Research Design: Sex and Gender Differences" in *The Agenda for Research on Women's Health in the 21st Century.* This chapter addressed issues of not only recruiting and retaining women as a whole but also of specific minority groups who have low levels of clinical study involvement. This chapter served as the foundation for some WHI recruitment and other NIH endeavors.[93]

FDA AND THE FDA OWH

In 1994 Congress mandated the establishment of the FDA OWH to advise the commissioner and other FDA officials on "scientific, ethical, and policy issues relating to women's health."[94] Thereafter, the OWH "began its work by establishing a science program to address the gaps in scientific knowledge about women's health."[94] As its mission, OWH "serves as a champion for women's health both within and outside the agency." In addition it 1) "ensures that FDA functions, both regulatory and oversight, remain gender sensitive and responsive; 2) works to correct any identified gender disparities in drug, device and biologics testing, and regulation policy; 3) monitors progress of priority women's health initiatives within FDA; 4) promotes an integrative and interactive approach regarding women's health issues across all the organizational components of the FDA; and 5) forms partnerships with government and nongovernment entities, including consumer groups, health advocates, professional organizations, and industry, to promote FDA's women's health objectives."[94] To accomplish its mission, the OWH has supported "many key scientific research initiatives on behalf of women, (has) provided unbiased science-based information and worked with partners in the private sector, nonprofit and government agencies to advance women's health and well-being."[94] The OWH continues to advance women's health in policy, science, outreach and education. Other information not included in this chapter about OWH may be found at http://www.fda.gov/womens/, in Table 1-3, and the Historical Timeline of Selected Events, Policies, and Key Decisions Related to Women, Women's Health, and the Role of Pharmacy in Women's Health appearing in the Web Resources and on the inside book cover.

Additional content available at
www.ashp.org/womenshealth

PHARMACY PROFESSIONAL ORGANIZATIONS

In the 1990s, the American College of Clinical Pharmacy (ACCP) and the APhA began actively supporting research in women's health (see Table 1-3 for

CASE PRESENTATION

Patient Case: Part 2

Social factors of the time greatly influenced M.E.'s health, healthcare, and healthcare decisions. M.E.'s low socioeconomic status and lack of education contributed significantly to her health. They influenced her unhealthy job selection while limiting her access to skilled medical care and more reliable contraception. Societal views on sex also affected her health—sexuality was not accepted as a healthy part of life or marriage. The association between sex and obscenity formed the basis for laws that criminalized contraception.

M.E.'s primary health concerns were access to contraception, the complications of childbirth, and healthcare for her children. During M.E.'s lifetime, healthcare changed secondary to government programs and laws such as the Children's Bureau, Sheppard-Towner Act, and Title V of the Social Security Act and key social movements such as those lead by Margaret Sanger.[15,16]

The political, social, and medical changes described above and in the Web Resources have greatly influenced J.S.'s health, activities, and career options (i.e., increased contraceptive options and access, the ability to participate in more organized sports, and a greater number of career options for women in her generation compared with those of previous generations). Title IX of the Education Amendments of 1972, Title X of the PHS Act of 1970, and birth control pills are some examples of these major factors influencing her life options. The relatively common use of drugs and alcohol during this time could potentially have had negative effects on her health, education, and career.

some of their initiatives). This occurred in response to the NIH ORWH opening channels of communication with professional health and grassroots organizations and some key pharmacy leaders. The first textbook on women's health for pharmacy, this book, was published by the American Society of Health-System Pharmacists (ASHP).

OTHER GROUPS AND ORGANIZATIONS

Various groups and organizations have been involved in advancing research in women's health and the need for more women scientists who would have a significant interest in women's health research. For example, the Society for Women's Health Research was founded in 1990 to specifically increase the importance of women's health research. The Institute of Medicine (IOM, one of the National Academies) and the National Academies as an organization have published reports and books as well as establishing committees to address research that affects women's health. (See Web Resources for Advances in Women's Healthcare and Research Not Covered in the Text and Historical Timeline of Selected Events, Policies, and Key Decisions Related to Women, Women's Health, and the Role of Pharmacy in Women's Health.) Medical journals outside the realm of obstetrics and gynecology (e.g., *Journal of the American Medical Association* and the *New England Journal of Medicine*) increased coverage of women's health research in the 1990s as have various pharmacy journals including the *Journal of the American Pharmacists Association* and *Pharmacotherapy*.

Additional content available at
www.ashp.org/womenshealth

Summary

Although great strides have been made over the last century in expanding the definition of women's health and creating federal agencies and regulations to address quality healthcare for women, reproductive and maternal health still play a central role in the field. Issues such as access to planned pregnancy terminations, emergency contraception, and coverage of prescription contraceptives remain controversial and receive widespread coverage in the popular press. The role that chronic diseases play in the lives of women has received increased attention, but many women still face barriers to receiving regular preventive healthcare and treatment. Reproductive health is and will always be an important component of women's health, but the rise in chronic conditions, the aging of the population, and changing societal norms will bring significant needs and changes in the future. Providers need to be cognizant of the history that has brought women's healthcare and research to this point and vigilant in ensuring that future research and policy initiatives protect and promote all aspects of women's health.

References

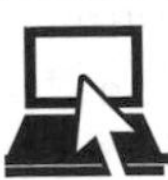

Additional content available at
www.ashp.org/womenshealth

2 Race, Ethnic, and Religious Issues

Jeri J. Sias, Pharm.D., MPH; Mary Beth O'Connell, Pharm.D., BCPS, FASHP, FCCP; James A. Berch, AB, MA; Imam Achmat Salie, DBA, AFK, MBA; Robert Taylor

Learning Objectives

1. Explore definitions related to culture and women's health.
2. Identify cultural issues that might affect women's health and healthcare delivery.
3. Discuss race, ethnic and religious issues influencing women's healthcare and decisions from conception to end-of-life.
4. Compare and contrast healthcare beliefs and practices of women from selected race, ethnic and religious groups.
5. Recognize opportunities to improve pharmaceutical care for women from various cultural backgrounds.

The face of the U.S. population is becoming culturally and linguistically more diverse.[1-3] With at least 106 **ethnic** groups, over 500 American Indian Nations, and over 300 languages spoken in the U.S., these changing demographics increase the complexity of healthcare for women.[4,5]

Women from specific **race** and ethnic groups experience differences in mortality rates and healthcare services.[6] Although heart **disease** and cancer mortality are common for women from all race/ethnic groups, differences in the rest of the top 10 causes of mortality exist. For example, diabetes related mortality is number 4 for Native American women and number 5–7 for women of other race/ethnicities. The framework for the *Healthy People 2020* goals for the U.S. include seeking to "achieve health equity, eliminate disparities, and improve the health of all groups" with many of the developing objectives related to women's health.[7] All healthcare providers should be able to navigate across **cultures** to provide patient-centered, effective, safe, and equitable care to everyone.[8] (See Web Resources for Leading Causes of Death Among Women by Race and Hispanic Origin: United States, 2004.)

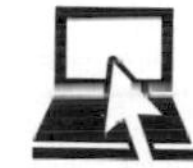

Additional content available at ***www.ashp.org/womenshealth***

Women from various cultural backgrounds bring different beliefs about wellness, **illness,** self-image, divine/spiritual intervention, and treatment preferences to the healthcare setting.[9] Recognizing that these variations exist can help healthcare providers adapt their approach and improve care of women from different cultures and improve patient and family trust. However, understanding the cultural identity of a person is not an easy process. If a provider ignores the subtleties of culture, lack of trust in the healthcare system[10] and increased medication errors can result. Although knowing about all of the cultural nuances influencing women's health is not a realistic expectation, healthcare providers can better prepare themselves for working with women of diverse backgrounds by learning key definitions, concepts, and frameworks. Recognizing the importance of beliefs, values, communication, **health literacy,** and **acculturation** in working with women of different cultures is also helpful. The purpose of this chapter is to help healthcare providers better understand the important role that culture—especially race, ethnicity, and **religion**—can play in the healthcare of women. Not every culture can be discussed in this chapter; however, the cultural examples included will help healthcare providers cultivate their attitude and develop a framework to respect and utilize a woman's cultural beliefs to improve her healthcare.

CASE PRESENTATION

Patient Case: Part 1

J.B. is an 18-year-old female high school senior whose family has just moved into a new urban community. She will be starting at a public school that has a high pregnancy rate. The school district has a new policy that allows for the school clinic to provide pregnancy prevention counseling and contraception. Prior to the start of the academic year, the school has an open clinic to ensure students are current with vaccination requirements and physicals. Parents give consent for all of these health services to be provided. The pharmacist administers immunizations and helps with any medication related needs. After the provider evaluates the patient, the pharmacist administers vaccines for tetanus-diphtheria toxoid, hepatitis B, and human papillomavirus (HPV) as needed. Following protocol, the pharmacist then starts to counsel the patient on how to use birth control. During the counseling session, J.B. begins to turn red, bows her head down, and shakes her head in apparent disbelief and embarrassment.

Cultural Influences on Women's Health

CULTURAL DEFINITIONS

Many definitions of culture exist. Culture can be described as "the learned and shared knowledge that specific groups use to generate their behavior and interpret their experience of the world."[11] Culture can encompass a set of beliefs, customs, values, experiences and behaviors, as well as manners of communication, and concepts of identity, relationships, roles in society, health, wellness, illness, and death.[4,11-14] These traits affect how people define their reality and interact with the world. Culture is often passed on to future generations through families, religious institutions, and social infrastructures.[4] **Subcultures**—which include age, race, ethnicity, sex, gender expression, sexual orientation, religion, socioeconomic status, chronic illness, and other characteristics for identifying oneself—also have unique characteristics that add variation to one's primary culture. Based on cultures and subcultures, women and men often develop behaviors and beliefs that affect, for example, their roles in society, the way they dress, patterns of communication, responsibilities in the family, and participation in healthcare.[11]

Race and ethnicity are important cultural terms that are often used together but are not interchangeable. While there is just one human race with very little genetic variation, race is often used to broadly describe a group of people throughout the world by their physical traits that can be genetically transferred to offspring.[11] Race is also a term that can be based on social, political, and/or biological definitions and connotations, which sometimes creates stratification and discrimination. When a group of people has a unique set of characteristics that they share based on culture or national origin, they are often referred to as an ethnic group.[11,15] Ethnicity has also been defined by self-perception and how a person is seen by others.[11] For example, when using U.S. Census classifications, Black or White people would be considered races whereas Hispanic would be considered an ethnic group because a Hispanic woman could also identify as being from the White, Black, or Asian race.[16]

Religion is a set of common beliefs and values based on the teachings of or reverence to a divine being(s).[17] Some people can be spiritual and believe in a superior being or force but do not embrace or affiliate with a formal religion. Others have chosen to not adopt religious or spiritual beliefs.

STEREOTYPE VS. GENERALIZATION

When discussing cultures, the differences between stereotyping and making a **generalization** must be recognized.[18] A **stereotype** may be viewed as an endpoint—a final analysis made about a person or culture that fits a preconceived idea or definition. On the other hand, a generalization might be viewed as a starting point. Generalizations acknowledge common links, understanding, or practices among a group of people while recognizing that individual differences exist. For example, a stereotype might lead a healthcare provider to counsel a Latina woman with diabetes to say "You can help keep your blood sugar under control by not eating so much rice and beans." However, a generalization might lead the healthcare provider to reflect, "This patient identifies herself as Latina. Many of the Latino patients in this community eat rice and beans. I will need to keep this in mind as I determine her specific dietary habits and help her control her diabetes better." The healthcare provider can actually follow-up with the Latina patient by asking the open-ended question, "What types of food do you eat throughout the day?" Learning about some of the common traits of different cultures can be helpful to have a context for understanding behaviors and providing care. Ultimately, at the individual patient or family level, the healthcare provider must evaluate the unique cultural beliefs and experiences to make a therapeutic recommendation.

ACCULTURATION

One factor influencing the subtleties of culture is acculturation or the adaptation to a dominant host culture. Four areas of acculturation have been described: integration, assimilation, marginalization, and separation.[19] A person with high acculturation can integrate or assimilate into the dominant culture. A person who integrates into a dominant culture (e.g., a young girl raised in a bilingual or bicultural home) can navigate in her home culture and in the dominant host culture at the same time. Someone who has assimilated has been willing to take on the dominant host culture often at the expense of losing the home culture. One example of assimilation might be of a woman who lets go of her home culture of being Protestant and takes on the culture of her spouse who is Catholic. Those persons who have been exposed to both cultures but never fully adopt or understand either culture may be considered to be marginalized. Those persons who experience separation have not been able to adapt to the dominant host culture. They may hold on to their home culture while trying to function and live in the new host culture. Separation might be more pronounced for example, in an elderly woman who has moved to the U.S. with her family and has a hard time adjusting to the new culture and learning a new language. New immigrants may have more difficulty adapting to the U.S. culture and feel marginalized or separated.

HEALTH AND ILLNESS VS. DISEASE

Understanding terminology related to health and illness compared to disease is an important concept in working with culturally diverse patients. Concepts of health are based on culture or individual beliefs and can be defined as the state of being well or being balanced emotionally, physically, mentally, socially, and spiritually.[4] Illness can be described as how an individual experiences symptoms and disability, the state of "not being well" or the state of imbalance (e.g., hot/cold or yin/yang).[4,20,21] In the **biomedical model,**[22] the term *disease* refers to a biological mechanism for an illness (e.g., germ, DNA damage) and does not generally include psychological and social explanations. Within the biomedical model, drug mechanisms are usually related to a physiologic process. However, cultural beliefs can affect behaviors and attitudes about adhering to a recommended treatment including prescription, over-the-counter, and herbal medications, which can influence medication outcomes.

BELIEFS, VALUES, AND COMMUNICATION

Other factors influencing healthcare decisions and delivery include culturally-based values and beliefs about social organization, understanding of time, and communication styles (Table 2-1).[4, 23-26] To provide culturally competent care, healthcare providers need to understand their own cultures and beliefs about the role of women and medication therapies related to women's health and also be aware of conflicts with other cultural beliefs as learned or confronted. Cultural self-assessment tools for healthcare providers and systems exist.[27]

An important example of social organization is the decision-making capacity between individuals and within nuclear (immediate), extended (relatives), or fictive (nontraditional, such as godparents) families.[28] Decision making within social organizations can be based on hierarchy or equality within and outside the nuclear family structure as well as legal rules. For example, pharmacists who are working with a female patient who is accustomed to deferring to her husband for decisions might have better success in convincing their patient to receive immunizations or adhere to a medication regimen if the husband also understands the need and importance. Or, a patient who is lesbian and has a terminal cancer might wish for her partner to make her healthcare decisions as opposed to her parents.

If a female patient values the family, but the healthcare provider makes recommendations that focus on individual health, the patient might not see the importance of the health intervention unless it affects the family. For example, a healthcare provider might try to influence a woman to quit smoking by focusing on the patient's individual health and potential future complications. However, if the woman is family-oriented, the healthcare provider might have greater influence on helping the patient to quit by acknowledging that the woman has a child with asthma and then explaining how second-hand smoke poses risks to her family in general.

Some cultures view concepts of time in relationship to valuing the past, the present, or the future. A culture that is future-oriented might place more value on preventive measures, whereas a culture that is present-oriented might focus on immediate health needs.[4] For some cultures, time is not regimented and thus patients may arrive for scheduled clinic visits at a different time than originally scheduled.

Table 2-1. Generalized Communication and Family Characteristics of Various Race and Ethnic Groups[4,23-26]

	Communication[a]	Family[a]
American Indian and Alaska Native	Format: Use of silence and body language; may not ask questions; may not disagree with provider; some distrust of healthcare system; may appreciate storytelling, humor, or talking about family and community first Eye contact: Indirect Physical contact: Respect space; may appreciate handshake Time: Present-oriented	Extended family and tribe/Nation orientation may be found Sometimes medicine woman/man and/or tribal leader is decision maker Community might gather to heal an individual patient
Arab American	Format: Indirect; may provide a story unrelated to questions asked; some prefer same gender provider Eye contact: Indirect Physical contact: Limited opposite gender contact; frequently avoid handshakes especially with opposite gender; chest to knee area covered for women	Extended family-centered Sometimes male decision makers Family may withhold serious or terminal health issues from elders May include imam (spiritual leader) as a decision maker
Asian American	Format: Use of silence, nonverbal Eye contact: Indirect Physical contact: Noncontact Time: Present-oriented	Extended family and/or clan-centered Hierarchy within family Sometimes shaman or ethnic leader is decision maker
Black and African American	Format: Listen, storytellers, some distrust of healthcare system Salutation: Use last name Eye contact: Essential Physical contact: Close proximity Time: Present-oriented	Extended family and fictive kin (e.g., friends) centered Affiliations strong with church and community May be in female single-parent homes
Hispanic/Latino/Latina American	Format: Listen Salutation: Use last name (check with patient preference) Eye contact: Expected from provider; might avoid with provider (out of respect) Physical contact: Acceptable (hand shake, hug) Time: Present-oriented	Extended family centered Involvement of godparents Affiliations strong with church
Non-Hispanic White American	Format: Willing to discuss; verbalize Salutation: First or last name (check with patient preference) Eye contact: Direct; expected Physical contact: Noncontact-distant; some Southern states contact more accepted Time: Future-oriented	Nuclear family centered

[a]This information provides generalizations, which can be helpful to identify differences in communication and family structure in cultures. However, each person within a culture is an individual who may or may not have the same beliefs or behaviors. Thus, each person should be evaluated and provided care based on her/his own culture, experience, and needs.

Taboo numbers or times exist in some cultures. For example, in the Mexican culture, *martes trece* (Tuesday the 13th) is considered by some to be unlucky. Having an appointment on Tuesday the 13th might cause some Mexican-American patients to skip an appointment on that day for fear of hearing bad news about their health. In some Asian cultures, the number four sounds like the word *death* and is considered unlucky.

Communication styles vary greatly across cultures and can be influenced by perceptions of personal space, eye contact, volume, and rate of speaking and the ability to listen, among other factors. Being aware of the potential for building or breaking down trust based on one's communication style with another person is important for making health connections. For example, depending on her specific cultural background, an older woman who self-identifies as American Indian might not say very much when communicating with the healthcare provider.[4] Rather, she might expect the healthcare provider to listen carefully, read her body language, and instinctively understand her health situation. The patient might not volunteer that she does not understand a concept or medication instructions unless asked. She might not appreciate having lots of questions asked and feel that note-taking is disruptive.[4]

HEALTH LITERACY

Health literacy can be defined as the "degree to which individuals have the capacity to obtain, process, and understand basic health information and services needed to make appropriate health decisions."[7,29] Health literacy includes **prose literacy, document literacy,** and **quantitative literacy.**[30] Health literacy can be influenced by factors such as primary language or language spoken at home, education level, age, and emotion, among other factors. For example, a well-educated woman with diabetes might not understand medical terms when she receives a prescription for insulin and education about using syringes and a glucometer.

Within the U.S., about 47 million people (or 17%) do not speak English at home.[31,32] About 11 million of these persons live in a household with no one over the age of 14 years who speaks English at least very well (defined as linguistic isolation). Healthcare providers should be prepared to provide assistance to a woman, who due to differences in language, age, or other cultural issues, might have difficulty navigating through the healthcare system and understanding medication information.

MEDICAL EDUCATION TRANSLATIONS

While internet and pharmacy dispensing software can provide translations of English into Spanish, healthcare providers should still be careful when using these tools. Notice what happens to the following medication instructions "Give 1½ teaspoonfuls by mouth every 8 hours with food as needed for pain" when translated by an online translator. The Spanish translation becomes *"Dé uno y una medias cucharaditas por boca cada ocho horas con alimento necesitaron como para el dolor."* Several errors occur. In Spanish "1½ teaspoons" would be "one teaspoon and a half" or *"una cucharadita y media."* Also, *"necesitaron"* is plural for "needed" and loses meaning in the way it is translated. These errors are not caught in translation and might be confusing to patients.

Cultural Competency

In order to provide the best possible care, healthcare providers need to consider multiple factors to provide culturally competent care. Cultural competency can be defined as a process by which individuals and organizations value and can "demonstrate behaviors, attitudes, policies and structures that enable them to work effectively" across cultures.[33,34] Providers and organizational leaders should value diversity and understand their own cultural identity, biases, and beliefs in order to better appreciate and work with other cultures. To provide culturally competent care, it is important to understand the patient's and family's cultural beliefs and practices related to health, illness, and treatment. Governmental, health system, and accreditation/regulatory policies and guidelines related to cultural competency also exist to inform decisions about care and improve the process of caring for persons from diverse backgrounds.[33,34]

CULTURAL COMPETENCY MODEL

While several models exist for describing cultural competency, one example of a cultural competency continuum is well cited and easy to use to evaluate one's own behaviors and attitudes.[33] When applying this model to religious and other cultural considerations in women, *cultural destructiveness* can occur when the status of women and their religious, race, and or ethnic backgrounds are devalued. For example, perhaps healthcare is denied to a pregnant woman because she is a minority patient with no health insurance. *Cultural incapacity* exists when stereotypes are perpetuated. *Cultural blindness* occurs when assumptions are made about treating everyone equally regardless of gender, sexual orientation, gender identity, religion, race, ethnicity, age, or other cultural influences. For example, certain religions might find the use of contraception unacceptable and not embrace public or broad education about contraception use. (See Web Resources for Cultural Competency Continuum and Cultural Competency Patient Case.)

Additional content available at
www.ashp.org/womenshealth

In *cultural precompetency*, the healthcare provider might understand the inherent values and differences of unique cultures, but might think that making one or two changes in the practice setting will suffice. For example, a community pharmacy might hire technicians who speak Spanish or the predominant non-English languages in their community. However, subtleties in language related to health or medication use might not be known by untrained (in language) pharmacy technicians and errors can still occur. *Culturally competent* healthcare providers respect diversity, accept and incorporate a patient's cultural beliefs, work to improve their cultural competency skills, make practice and setting changes to increase outcomes secondary to cultural competency issues, and engage in cultural events in the community (e.g., community health fairs, cultural art fairs). *Cultural proficiency* extends beyond the boundaries of cultural competency to foster continued growth and excellence. Organizations that are moving toward culturally proficiency increase leadership capacity, implement policies, make organizational change, develop community partnerships, conduct research, develop and disseminate new knowledge, and promote advocacy in the area of culturally competent care on an ongoing basis. Some consider cultural proficiency a continuous process vs. an achievable endpoint. At this stage, healthcare providers and organizations continue to strive to deepen their knowledge and skills to address cultural dynamics in healthcare.

PATIENT'S EXPLANATORY MODEL

In the 1980s Arthur Kleinman, a medical anthropologist, provided some tools to evaluate patients' explanation of their illness. He described a common disconnect between the biomedical model and individual, family, and even cultural beliefs of health. By eliciting the patient's and sometimes family's understanding of illness, healthcare providers can gain insight and further trust in working with their patients. The following questions constitute the patient explanatory model[21]:

1. What do you call the problem? (patient/family view of illness)
2. What do you think has caused the problem? (etiology)
3. Why do you think it started when it did? (time of onset of symptoms)
4. What do you think the sickness does? How does it work? (pathophysiology)
5. How severe is the sickness? Will it have a short or long course? (course of illness)
6. What kind of treatment do you think you should receive? What are the most important results you hope to receive from this treatment? (appropriate therapy)
7. What are the chief problems the sickness has caused? (quality of life)
8. What do you fear most about the sickness? (significance of illness to self and family).

Five of these questions coincide with the biomedical model because they evaluate etiology, onset of disease, pathophysiology, course of disease, and appropriate therapy. However, when healthcare providers give patients the opportunity to explain their understanding of disease etiology, their answer might be very different from the biomedical model explanation. A patient's explanation of an infection might be due to a divine intervention or perhaps an imbalance between hot and cold. The patients' understanding of illness can affect how seriously they accept the recommended medication therapy. The final three questions allow healthcare providers to understand the significance of the health problem or illness to the patient.

PRACTICE MODEL

One model for working with patients from different cultures is RESPECT (**R**apport, **E**mpathy, **S**upport, **P**artnership, **E**xplanations, **C**ultural Competence, and **T**rust).[35] Healthcare providers should work to develop a *rapport* with the female patient without casting judgment or making assumptions. They should have *empathy* for the patient as she has come to the healthcare provider for help and should try to understand her views and beliefs about disease and illness. The healthcare provider should *support* the woman and, when appropriate, involve family members to overcome barriers (e.g., language, financial barriers, literacy). A *partnership* should be developed with the patient that is consistent with her belief system. Being open to how the woman *explains* her understanding of her medical situation, as well as verifying her medication use, would be incorporated into the visit. Healthcare providers should understand their own beliefs, values, and biases in relationship to the patient and her family by working toward *cultural competence*. Sometimes being culturally competent may mean having the patient work with a different pharmacist. Recognizing that *trust* can take time but will provide great insight into the patient's pharmaceutical and medical care is another key factor.

Health-system accreditation bodies now require assessment of issues related to culture to help give the healthcare provider valuable information about the patient beliefs.[36-39] Sometimes people can not use certain medications or eat certain foods. Some patients want to include their family when they make decisions about their health. To gather this information when working with a new patient, the healthcare provider could ask "Do you have any health beliefs or concerns that I should know about?" If the answer is yes, open-ended questions or statements should be used to identify the cultural issues. For example, "Tell me what cultural or religious issues we should consider to make you confident and comfortable in the care that we provide to you." Some health systems and pharmacies already have categories in their charts and computer documentation systems to collect and record patient cultural issues that need to be utilized by all healthcare providers.[37]

ORGANIZATIONAL POLICY CONSIDERATIONS

To optimize care for the patient, healthcare providers and the organizations they work for should embrace cultural and linguistic competency. The Joint Commission on Accreditation of Healthcare Organizations (The Joint Commission) and the Health Resource Services Administration (HRSA) have guidelines for cultural and linguistic competency in healthcare organizations.[38,39] Further according to the CLAS (Culturally and Linguistically Appropriate Services) standards in Title VI under the Civil Rights Act of 1964, organizations receiving federal funding (e.g., Medicare) must provide language-appropriate services.[39-41] To provide culturally competent care, healthcare providers and their employers should be willing to undergo individual and organizational self-assessments of beliefs and values as well as actively participate in adapting and developing attitudes, knowledge, and skills respectful and inclusive of diverse cultural beliefs.[34,38] (See Web Resources for Organizational and Individual Provider Requirements for Culturally Competent Care and Culturally and Linguistically Appropriate Service Standards.)

> **ADDITIONAL CULTURE AND HEALTHCARE INFORMATION**
>
> **The U.S. government has been responsive to creating more resources and research to help healthcare providers be more culturally competent. The U.S. Department of Health and Human Services created the Office of Minority Health (OMH) (www.omhrc.gov) and the Center of Cultural and Linguistic Competence in Healthcare (www.omhrc.gov/templates/browse.aspx?lvl=2&lvlid=16). These sites are two examples where a provider can find resources on statistics and education or surveys and assessments. The National Center for Complementary and Alternative Medicine, a division of the National Institute of Health (nccam.nih.gov), has useful information and evidence about many complementary and alternative therapies—some of which are available in other languages—that are used by women especially from certain cultures.**

Additional content available at
www.ashp.org/womenshealth

Race and Ethnic Influences in Women's Health

The race and ethnic diversity of the U.S. will continue to experience much growth over the next 50 years.[1] The U.S. 2000 Census categorized people into either American Indian and Alaska Native, Asian, Black or African Americans, Native Hawaiian and Other Pacific Islander, White, or "some other race" race group and into only one ethnic group—Hispanic or Latino (female form Latina).[31] Other ethnic groups were only captured through the country of origin.

While not every woman will identify with characteristics found among persons of her race or ethnicity, some common features exist within these cultural groups that are relevant to women's health, healthcare decision making, and healthcare delivery. Only a few races and ethnic groups are included in this review. These comments are made as points for initiating discussion and understanding general cultural traits that need to be confirmed or rejected for each patient. Highlights of some race and ethnic differences in communication, family structure, and healthcare decision making are found in Table 2-1. (See Web Resources for Influence of Ethnic Culture on Communications with a Pharmacist Patient Case.)

AMERICAN INDIAN AND ALASKA NATIVE

Demographics/Background

In the 2000 U.S. census, about 0.9% of the population identified themselves as being an American Indian or Alaska Native (more than 560 tribes and 200 languages) with 40% being multiracial.[5,23,42] Racism, discrimination, and mistrust have contributed to low self-esteem and high poverty rates in American Indians and Alaska Natives.[42,43]

Role of Women

Some American Indian and Alaska Native cultures are matriarchal partially related to the great respect of women as the life givers. Women might consult with their husbands about health decisions out of respect for their role in the family.[44] In 33% of American Indian/Alaska Native households, women are the head of household.[42]

Health Beliefs

American Indians and Alaska Natives may believe in "original" medicine.[45] In original medicine, everything in the world has a spirit—from a rock, herb, and animal to a human being—all originating from one creator. Body, mind, and spirit are one. Therefore, American Indians and Alaska Natives may show great respect for life, honor, and integrity. Illness results from an imbalance of life forces, thus spirituality and restoring harmony play important roles in healing.[23,46]

Herbal and alternative therapies such as smudging, dancing, chanting, and drumming may be preferred for treatments.[47] Sweat lodges may be places of prayer and spiritual healing. When using an herb, an offering may also be given. Western medications are usually combined with indigenous therapies and only used after receiving sufficient information about them. Use of a medicine healer and indigenous therapies might not be conveyed to the Western-medicine provider unless specifically asked. Part of this reticence relates to the U.S. declaring herbal therapies illegal in the past, which was corrected with the 1978 passage of the Indian Religious Freedom Act. In this culture, aggressive use of technology and end of life sustaining therapies might not be desired.

Mistrust of the healthcare system may be related to past injustices by the U.S. government such as placement on reservations, disease transmission from settlers, the removal of Indian children from families into government run boarding schools, and reported sterilizations of American Indian and Alaska Native women receiving care through the Indian Health Service in the 1970s.[43,48,49] Because boarding school records were incomplete, not kept or destroyed, many children and adults do not know their heritage or health history.

Disease Prevalence/Incidence

American Indians and Alaska Natives have a high prevalence of certain diseases such as alcoholism, AIDS, cardiovascular diseases, depression, diabetes, obesity, and suicide.[6,42,50,51] Mortality is greater in American Indian and Alaska Native people for conditions such as breast cancer and diabetes. American Indian and Alaska Native women have the highest age-adjusted death rate from diabetes and although they have a low incidence of breast cancer, they experience a poor, 5-year survival rate.[50]

Some American Indians and Alaska Natives have been stereotyped to have problems with alcohol and tobacco use. In general Whites report greater alcohol use than American Indians and Alaska Natives (57% vs. 42%, respectively).[51] However, American Indian and Alaska Native people report binge drinking (33% vs. 23%, respectively) and list heavy alcohol use (11.5% vs. 7.4%, respectively) more frequently than Whites.

Tobacco may be important to American Indians and Alaska Natives and could be required to communicate with the spirit for wisdom and to treat individual patients. Studies show that American Indians and Alaska Natives have the highest prevalence of smoking (42% vs. 31% for Whites).[4] But, these reports do not acknowledge the spiritual use of tobacco at most ceremonies and healing practices.

ARAB AMERICAN

Demographics/Background

Approximately 1.2 million citizens listed Arab ancestry in the 2000 U.S. census (3.5 million with an expanded definition as determined by a private survey).[52,53] Arab Americans come have various religious backgrounds (e.g., about 63% Christian faith) and diverse countries of origin (e.g., the Middle East and North Africa).[54]

Role of Women

The role of women of Arab descent will vary by country of origin, religion, and degree of acculturation to the U.S. Some Arab women will keep their body and face fully covered and stay at home with little decision-making power. Others are college-educated and are equal with their spouse when working and socializing outside of the home. These roles vary and are not based solely on the woman's desire to wear the *hijab* (head scarf). Some women of Arab descent might come with their husbands to the clinic or pharmacy for healthcare and healthcare decision making.[55] Daughters may be expected to assist their non-English speaking, Arab-American mothers when accessing healthcare services.

Health Beliefs

Health beliefs may be based predominantly on religious beliefs (e.g., Muslim, Christian). Because a Western-style approach to healthcare exists in many Arab countries, use of the U.S. healthcare system exists with beliefs consistent with the biomedical model for treatment.[56] Frequently women will prefer female healthcare providers, but because health and wellness are highly revered, opposite gender providers can be used.[55] Special considerations for some women might exist for physical examination, especially for the area between the breasts and knees. Herbal therapies are frequently used along with prayer. Cures are often expected and can result in doctor shopping if not achieved.

Disease Prevalence/Incidence

Information about health issues for this group is just emerging, partly related to this cultural group not being included in past epidemiologic surveys and not being considered a major ethnic group in the U.S. census tabulation reports. Arab Americans have the highest prevalence of diabetes among U.S. cultural groups, with obesity being a concern as well.[57]

Smoking is a highly prevalent social habit and includes the use of a *narghileh* (water pipe). Thus, asking only about cigarette use may underestimate tobacco use. Some Arab Americans can have some degree of post-traumatic stress disorder from personal or family atrocities resulting in physical and mental illness.[58] Frequently, mental health issues will not be discussed because they may be considered to be taboo, nonexistence problems or family embarrassments.[55]

ASIAN AMERICAN

Demographics/Background

Asian Americans are a rapidly growing segment of the U.S. (currently 3.6% increasing to 8% in 2050[32,59]) population with cultural ties to over 20 Asian countries and more than 100 different languages.[42,60] Over two thirds of Asian Americans are foreign born.[42]

Role of Women

The role of the woman in the family will vary among Asian cultures. However, the family is often involved in family decision making.[42] Many Asian cultures also demonstrate respect for authority and desire to preserve harmony among groups.

Health Beliefs

Some Asian cultures identify more with health and illness related to an imbalance of cold (yin) and hot (yang) or results from angering the spirits than with the biomedical model.[4] Asian cultures may include acupuncture, moxibustion (based on heat as a therapeutic agent), and sacrifice to spirits as forms of healing. Hmong women might not access early prenatal care because they may not view pregnancy as an illness.[42] Herbal remedies are commonly used in many Asian cultures and can be a part of the Asian woman's personal treatment considerations.

Disease Prevalence/Incidence

Women of Asian heritage enjoy the highest life expectancy of all groups of women. However, some health issues affect women of Asian descent in disparate numbers.[6,50] For example, cancers are the leading cause of mortality among Asian women.[9] Upon immigration to the U.S., Asian women's breast cancer risks increase up to 80%. Cervical cancer affects Vietnamese women at rates nearly 5 times higher than among White women. Among new immigrant Asian women, hepatitis B and tuberculosis are more prevalent.[50] Women immigrants of Asian descent have an increased risk of developing diabetes compared to White women. Almost three quarters of Asian women who are postmenopausal do not take adequate intakes of calcium.

BLACK AND AFRICAN AMERICAN

Demographics/Background

Currently Blacks from all countries of origin represent 12.3% of the U.S. with 8% foreign born.[31,32,42] By 2050, they will represent 14.6% of the U.S. population.[5] Some black African Americans and African Caribbeans have a lineage connected to slavery. Three variables are thought to contribute the most to the health of this population—genetics, health-related behaviors, and environmental and sociopolitical conditions (such as racism).[42] Disparities in access and usage and disease prevalence among Blacks are largely due to a history of racial discrimination and racism and poverty.[42] Poverty affects nearly 25% of all Black Americans and influences health by leading to inadequate housing, increased exposure to environmental toxins and communicable diseases, violence, and decreased access to proper nutrition and healthcare.[42]

Role of Women

Women have a major role in the family, with many women having strong and resilient roles in the family. Intergenerational living arrangements are common with many grandmothers and or other relatives providing the care for children. Family can be biological or fictive (nonbiological). Single-parent, female-headed homes comprise 44% of all Black family households.[42]

Health Beliefs

Blacks sometimes have significant mistrust of the U.S. health system stemming from past violations.[61,62] For example, Blacks may be familiar with the Tuskegee studies when the U.S. government withheld syphilis therapy from Black men resulting in disease spread and shortened lifespans.[42]

Health beliefs of African Americans can be related to religion (often Christian or Muslim) or tribal heritage.[4,62,63] The health beliefs of other Blacks will be dependent on many things such as their country of origin. Illness can result from fate or punishment for sins. Blacks with strong religious beliefs might put their health into God's hands and thereby can feel less empowered to cure or control disease through diet, exercise, and medications. However, overall the more religious the person, the better the physical and mental health.[61] For some Blacks, healthcare preferences might include denial, prayer, and alternative therapies with Western medicine least preferred.[51,62] Sometimes healthcare information and advice is obtained from family and friends before healthcare providers.[62] The use of herbal therapy and alternative medicine such as folk medicine or voodoo in some Black populations stems from heritage, lack of U.S. healthcare access, or conscious choice.[4] At the end of life, African Americans might choose aggressive therapies and not withhold life-sustaining treatments.[36,51]

Disease Prevalence/Incidence

Some health conditions are more unique to Black women such as sickle cell disease whereas other conditions such as cardiovascular and cerebrovascular disease, metabolic syndrome, and some sexually transmitted diseases have a higher prevalence and more negative outcomes.[6,50] Blacks with health insurance are still offered less preventive healthcare and procedures for diagnosis and treatment.[42] Infant mortality is 2 times higher and maternal mortality 4 times higher for Black women vs. White women.[65] Of great concern is the infant mortality rate for Black women with a college education, which is 2.7 times that of White college-educated women and worse than White women without a high school education.[66] Black women present with later stages and more aggressive forms of breast cancer, which is partially attributed to mistrust and hope for divine intervention.[62,67]

HISPANIC/LATINA

Demographics/Background

The Hispanic population makes up the largest ethnic group within the U.S. (12.5%); represented by Mexican Americans (66%), Central and South Americans (13%), Puerto Ricans (9.4%), Cubans (4%), and other Hispanic groups.[32,68] Each subculture has its own unique traits. The Hispanic population is the fastest growing group estimated to represent 24% of the U.S. by 2050.[59] In general, U.S. Hispanics are younger (median age 27.4 years vs. non-Hispanics 40.5 years), experience a large educational gap (high school education 58.4% vs. non-Hispanic Whites 90%), and self-identify as Christians.[68] The Hispanic population has a high percentage of families living in poverty (21.8% vs. non-Hispanics 8.3%).[42,68] Lack of U.S. citizenship can also add stress to the family.[42]

Role of Women

The role of the Hispanic/Latina woman is very important. She is responsible for the nuclear and extended family's health, frequently putting her health needs last or ignoring them. In caring for the health of the younger Hispanic woman, the importance of family (including extended family), family planning needs, food preparation, and prenatal care should be recognized. It is not uncommon for Hispanic households to be headed by a woman as found in nearly 40% of Puerto Rican, 24% of Central and South American, 20% of Mexican American, and 17% of Cuban households.[42]

Health Beliefs

Health beliefs might be related to the balance and harmony of the body, mind, and spirit.[4,68] In seeking healthcare, Hispanics may expect healthcare providers to be respectful (*respeto*) and personable (*personalismo*) in order to gain their trust (*confianza*).[68]

As with many other race and ethnic groups, Hispanics may seek complementary and alternative medicine along with Western medical treatment.[68] People from the culture might be accustomed to praying and/or consulting with an older woman in the neighborhood who is knowledgeable of folk illnesses and their treatments.[4,68] These women can be family members or good friends who are trusted by the community and might be a community healer (e.g., curandera or santera). Herbal products and teas may be used and seen as natural or safe. This belief can be dangerous as too much chamomile tea (*té de manzanilla*) during pregnancy can increase uterine contractions.[68]

In many Latin American countries, medications can be purchased without a prescription. Therefore, it is possible that pharmacists might be viewed as a reliable source for not only medication information but medications.

Disease Prevalence/Incidence

Several unique health disparities and issues are prevalent among Hispanic women.[6,42] Obesity and low physical activity are more prevalent among Mexican Americans.[42] Hispanic women experience the highest rates of death from liver cirrhosis. They have the second highest rates of cervical cancer among women groups. Women of Hispanic origin have at least a 6 times greater case rate of AIDS than white non-Hispanic women. Over half (53%) of Hispanic women have reported symptoms of depression.[68] Among Mexican-American women, the prevalence of diabetes is 50% higher than among white women.[42]

NON-HISPANIC WHITE

Demographics/Background

The White culture is currently the predominant U.S. culture (81% of the population, decreasing to 72% by 2050).[59] All White people are descendents of immigrants to the U.S., an important fact frequently overlooked. Many White marriages have occurred between ethnic cultures creating culturally diverse women (e.g., a White woman with Irish, German, and Italian backgrounds).

Role of Women

Over the last half century, the White woman's role has expanded from a more traditional wife, mother, and home keeper to include college-educated and outside of home employment. With these changes has come increased use of childcare and residence geographically separated from relatives.

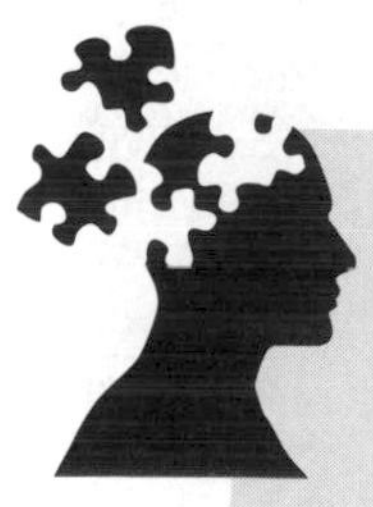

Therapeutic Challenge:

How does the training of a Native American healer and Curandera compare to traditional U.S. healthcare training?

Health Beliefs

The White culture is quite diverse and factors such as socioeconomic status (e.g., issues associated with class, education, and income) and religious beliefs can change preferences for healing options. The health belief of many White women would include the biomedical model with some influences from her religious beliefs. Illness generally results from disease but could be influenced by other cultural or social influences.[23] Thus, White patients often seek Western college- and professionally-trained healthcare providers first for diagnosis and treatment. Many Whites rely heavily on medications sometimes over or in addition to lifestyle changes, prayer, or herbal products. Health information may come primarily from reading literature vs. conversations with family or friends. In the past, many Whites have had total belief in the physician's opinion. However, with access to information, feminist influences, and patient-centered care, many White women actively question and challenge medical advice. High use and reliance on technology, plastic surgery, and dermatology exist.[23,69]

Disease Prevalence/Incidence

White women might have less disease and better survival than women of other race and ethnic backgrounds because on average this culture has more education, higher incomes, more health insurance, and greater access and use of the health system. White women have the highest use of infertility therapies, potentially related to the above reasons.[51] Privileges, such as access to healthcare, might also lead to negative consequences. For example, White women might complain more about menopausal symptoms, perhaps because they have read more about the condition or have more opportunities to discuss symptoms with care providers, and thus have a greater likelihood of receiving treatment for such symptoms.[70] For some health statistics, White women do worse, such as smoking more during pregnancy than the other race and ethnic groups evaluated in the study.[51]

NEW IMMIGRANT POPULATIONS

Demographics/Background

Approximately 34.5 million (12%) U.S. residents are foreign born of which most (74%) are naturalized citizens, legal permanent residents, refugees, or legal nonimmigrants.[71] Most immigrant families have children who are U.S. citizens. About half of the new immigrant population is female.[72] Immigrants represent all levels of education and socioeconomic status upon arrival in the U.S. Immigrants participate

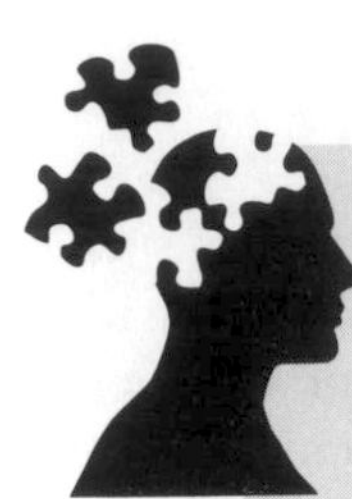

Therapeutic Challenge:

Describe how your health beliefs and practices are influenced by your race and ethnic cultures.

actively in the economy of the U.S. with 81% of immigrant families having at least one full-time worker in the family.[71] However, over half of immigrant families are considered to be low income.

Health Issues

Immigrants face unique healthcare problems primarily related to poor access to healthcare services. Further, many encounter linguistic and cultural barriers when entering the healthcare system.[71] Women without U.S. citizenship status compared to U.S. born citizens or naturalized citizens were 2–3 times more likely to have no usual source of healthcare, 3–4 times more likely to have no health insurance, and about 2–3 times more likely to not have visited with a healthcare professional in the past year.[72]

Racial and Ethnic Influences on Healthcare

In summary, given the diversity in races and ethnicity in the U.S., it is important for healthcare providers to acknowledge how these cultural differences may affect women's health and determine how they influence healthcare decisions and outcomes. Differences in disease prevalence, gender roles, health beliefs, and other factors can influence how women approach and utilize healthcare.

Religious Influences in Women's Health

Religion or spirituality is a part of many women's culture mix and can play a major role in shaping her and her family's health beliefs, decisions, and practices. The majority of U.S. residents have a religious belief (Table 2-2).[73] Some women have spiritual beliefs, believing in a superior being or force, but lack a formalized religion orientation whereas others have no religious or spiritual beliefs.

Health beliefs and behaviors surrounding antenatal care, contraception, fertility, and menopause can be influenced by religion. For example, religion may influence a women's preference to have a female obstetrician/gynecologist (OB/GYN).[74] In one study, 61% of the women preferred a female provider, with specific preferences dependent on religious background (mean percentage preferring a female provider—Muslim: 89%, Hindu: 74%, Jewish: 58%, Catholic: 58%, and Protestant: 56%).

Table 2-2. Religions Practiced in the United States in 2007[73]

Religion	% U.S. Adult Population
Christianity	78.4%
Judaism	1.7%
Buddhism	0.7%
Muslim/Islam	0.6%
Hinduism	0.4%
Other faiths	6.2%
Unaffiliated	16.1%
Don't know/refused	0.8%

The goal of this section is not to provide all the information a provider needs to care for women from various religious or spiritual beliefs. Rather, it is to give insight into the variability of beliefs influenced by religion and depict the importance of understanding a woman's religious beliefs when providing healthcare. An overview of three diverse religions (i.e., Catholicism, Islam, and Hinduism) is presented in this chapter with some information on Buddhism and Judaism in Table 2-3.[26,56,75-78] The specific religion sections were coauthored with practitioners of each faith. This information represents general beliefs from doctrines of the religion. Each woman chooses the degree to which she practices her beliefs, which can change over time and vary per condition (e.g., child vs. adult health issue, acute vs. chronic condition). Furthermore, certain groups within these religions (e.g., orthodox/conservative vs. liberal, different Christian religions vs. Catholicism) may also have different beliefs. Assuming a woman has a certain belief based on her stated religion would be a stereotype; however, conducting a conversation to determine her specific beliefs is a way to use a generalization to improve care. This information serves as a starting point for learning about the influences of religion in women's health and healthcare. (See Web Resources for more information on Religious Influences on Select Women's Health Issues.)

Additional content available at
www.ashp.org/womenshealth

Table 2-3. Religious Influences on Select Women's Health Issues[26,56,75-80]

	Buddhism[a,b]	Hinduism[a]	Islam[a]	Judaism[a,c]	Roman Catholic[a]
Abortion	Patient's condition determines; pray to Buddha afterwards	No policy; however, soul is born at conception	Ensoulment begins at 120 days; not accepted except for special circumstances such as rape and maternal health	Generally forbidden except to save life of the mother	Prohibited; if life of mother is in danger save child first
Birth control	Acceptable; true Buddhists do not engage, in sexual activity,[b] no restriction for "followers"	Acceptable	Acceptable but cannot be irreversible	Generally forbidden but can be permissible after couple already has children or for certain health reasons	Natural means only
Fertility therapy	Acceptable	Acceptable	Acceptable for legally married couples	Some forms encouraged, but under rabbinic review	Drugs allowed to encourage ovulation or resolve sexual dysfunction; sperm migration assistance allowed; prohibited techniques include in vitro fertilization, sperm banks, freezing of embryos, and artificial insemination

Note: See Web Resources for more information on Religious Influences on Select Women's Health Issues.

[a]Based on doctrine with information provided by scholars within each religion. An individual might interpret and/or follow the teachings differently.

[b]"True Buddhists" or Buddhist monks follow all the guiding principles such as no love (family), no greed (monetary possessions), no lies, no killing, no hatred, no fear, love for all living beings, self-sacrificing, etc. Most Buddhist people are "followers" who follow the general teachings, do the readings, and believe in afterlife, but they follow these rules to a less strict extent. For example, followers can get married and have children.

[c]Traditional Jews may submit questions regarding all but the most routine healthcare choices to a competent rabbinic authority, because slightly changed circumstances might result in dramatic variations in permissibility under Jewish law and medical ethics. An attending chaplain, if Orthodox, should know whom to contact for authoritative opinions on a given subject.

CATHOLICISM

Brief Background

Catholicism is the first Christian religion after which many other Christian religions were developed with varying dogma and healthcare beliefs. People are created in the image and likeness of God with freedom (free will), intelligence (rational being), and the capacity for relationship.[79,80] They are created woman and man, each possessing a unity of soul (spiritual) and body (physical). The spiritual is perceived through the body.

Health, Illness, Healthcare Usage, and Complementary and Alternative Medicine

Catholics are instructed to ask for God's help through prayer and reception of the sacraments of the faith to aid in the healing process. Individuals are encouraged to take an active role in their health in a manner consistent with their faith and that treats the whole person.

The Catholic Church supports the use of both healthcare providers and religious healers. Catholics are instructed to only choose treatments consistent with the doctrines of the Catholic Church; however, variability in compliance with Catholic instruction exists.[79] Treatment options include most traditional practices such as surgery (except abortion) blood transfusions, and prescription medications (except contraceptives). Treatments may also include alternative medical practices such as herbal products, acupuncture, and mind body interventions except hypnosis.

In the case of terminal illness, advanced directives (e.g., decisions about aggressive use of technology, pain medications, nutrition) are recommended, medications for pain and comfort are permitted, and hospice assistance is encouraged. Only basic treatments such as nutrition and hydration are required until natural death, while extraordinary treatments such as intubation might be declined. Any treatment that hastens death (e.g., assisted suicide) is viewed as contradictory to the faith and is never allowed.[79]

Family Decisions, Concepts of Life, and Reproductive Health

Women throughout their lives can make their own healthcare decisions but frequently do so in consult with husband and family and sometimes seek religious opinion. Per doctrine, sexual intercourse occurs only within marriage.

All human life is sacred and needs to be cared for from the moment of conception until natural death. In the Catholic faith, life begins in the womb at the moment of conception when the sperm unites with the egg. According to Catholic teachings, contraceptives (barrier, chemical or surgical) to prevent or space births are prohibited; however, practice varies among Catholic women. Spacing of children is allowed with natural family planning, which monitors basal temperature, vaginal mucus consistency, and cervix changes to determine the wife's fertility (see Chapter 18: Family Planning and Nonhormonal Contraception).[79] The deliberate taking of a human life, which the Church considers abortion and assisted suicide, is condemned.

Other beliefs in the Catholic Church also influence women's health and decision making. Medications are allowed to encourage ovulation or treat sexual dysfunction. Techniques such as in vitro fertilization, sperm banks, the freezing of human embryos, artificial insemination, and surrogate parenting are prohibited. These techniques are viewed by the Catholic Church to separate the sexual act from procreation.[79] As a woman ages, hormonal supplements are allowed to treat menopausal symptoms. Given these various examples of Catholic beliefs influencing health, a healthcare provider should first determine a Catholic woman's specific beliefs rather than assume she abides by all Catholic doctrine to help tailor medication education and solve medication-related problems.

ISLAM

Brief Background

Islam is one of the fastest growing religions in the U.S. and is a faith prevalent among most races.[81-83] "Islam is a mosaic and is not a monolith."[84] The Shiites and Sunnis, the two major branches of the Islamic faith, have some different religious practices among themselves. Both groups have the same Quran, but their corpus of Hadith (sayings of Muhammad) differs. Other differences can be related to political and economic issues.

Health, Illness, Healthcare Usage, and Complementary and Alternative Medicine

In accordance with Islamic teachings, God gave human beings the gift of healing.[56] Some illnesses are believed to be tests not punishments from Allah, but most illnesses have an explainable physical cause. Every illness has (or will have) a cure. Only death has no cure. Muslims generally believe in the power of divine intervention (theurgic power) of the Quran. Many Muslims appreciate the presence of an *imam* (male spiritual leader) or Quran memorizer (hafiz) to pray for their health. They find the reading of verses to have a healing effect. Muslims are comfortable with modern medicine and might embrace any system that has evidence of healing or promises cure. Many Muslims prefer alternative medicine especially as practiced in their prior countries or use alternative medicine except superstition and witchcraft to complement conventional medicine.

Many Arab and some non-Arab Muslims emphasize gender separation. This separation can be important in selecting healthcare providers. Devout women after puberty might prefer female physicians and healthcare personnel, especially if the care involves touching, cleansing or treatment between the breasts and the knee.[55,74,85] The rule of necessity allows women to expose parts of their body to strangers from the opposite gender only to the degree necessary. Because seeking the best healthcare is the goal, some U.S. Muslim women might accept male providers for basic healthcare needs, but they would be more comfortable with a female provider.[85]

Depending on the country or region that a Muslim woman is from, she might use a head covering such as a scarf (*hijab*) or a veil (*niqab*), decide not to follow the requirement of head covering, or begin to do so later in life.[55] Muslim women might prefer for healthcare personnel especially male providers to not see them with their hair uncovered and might wish to sleep with a head scarf in the hospital. Some Muslim women have reported to be more comfortable in situations with male providers who avoid hand shaking and eye contact.

Healthcare providers' understanding of Muslim food restrictions is important for selecting and adjusting medications as well as educating and counseling patients about their diet and medications related to health conditions such as diabetes, cholesterol, and hypertension. Most Muslims do not eat pork, meat, or derivative products that do not pass Muslim slaughtering standards (*halal*) except when they face starvation. Although many Muslims do not consume alcohol or other intoxicants except when necessary for therapeutic purposes, not all Muslims follow the ideals of "no alcohol" and other restrictions. Some Muslims prefer to not use medications with alcohol or pork gelatin (e.g., capsules) unless no alternative can be found. Some schools of faith also disallow crayfish and shrimp or scavengers of the sea.

During Ramadan, the holiest of the Muslim lunar months, Muslims fast (unless exempted) from dawn, which is 90 minutes before sunrise, to dusk, which is immediately after sunset for Sunni Muslims and 15–20 minutes after sunset for Shia Muslims. Their observance of this special holiday can influence medication management. For example, diabetes medication doses might need to be changed during the fasting period and potentially greater insulin doses are needed when the fast is broken at sunset and larger than usual evening meal quantities are sometimes ingested.[86] Injections are not considered to break the fast.

Allah desires ease, not difficulty, for the believers, and so Muslims are concerned with taking care of chronic diseases and suffering. Women who experience menopause are allowed to use medication to alleviate symptoms such as mood changes and hot flushes. Managing pain should be encouraged. However, when medications cloud a person's judgment, patients may need counseling about their daily prayers and frequently require chaplains or imams to guide them through this period.

Family Decisions, Concepts of Life, and Reproductive Health

Learning about the Muslim family structure can help the healthcare provider understand communication dynamics when providing health and medication information. Some Muslim families are very democratic whereas others leave the decision to male elders or an imam to decide. Many families depend on an imam for a religious perspective. They regard the opinion of some imams as binding. Usually Muslim women will not make decisions without consulting husbands and husbands generally do not make decisions without conferring with their wives and her family. Given dynamics within the family, female patients may prefer for medication information to be passed through their husband or even an older son, particularly if the pharmacist is male.[85] Some Muslims use nonverbal expressions to show approval or disapproval. Adult children generally make decisions for parents, especially when frail.

Procreation and establishing a lineage are strongly favored in the Islamic faith and influence beliefs regarding reproductive health. Life starts 120 days after conception when ensoulment of the fetus occurs. The heartbeat after 4 weeks is not proof of personhood. A human must look human.

Most married couples feel contraception or birth control methods (e.g., oral contraceptives) are allowed, especially if they are not irreversible or injurious to their health.[55,87] The use of contraception should be consensual. Irreversible methods are allowed only when necessity dictates. Contraception and family planning should prevent unwanted pregnancies. Abortion is not allowed unless the life of the mother is at risk or in some cases if the fetus is severely deformed.[56] Many scholars allow abortion before the 120-day period in the case of forced rape or rape during war. Other scholars encourage giving the child up for adoption.

Medications that aid fertility are welcomed if no harmful side effects exist.[55,56] In vitro fertilization and artificial insemination of the ova and sperm cells of legally married couples are allowed. Sunni scholars unanimously agree that surrogate parenting or "all cases introducing third parties into a marriage, whether a womb, an egg, a sperm, or a cloning cell, is not permissible."[88] Some Shia scholars have allowed surrogacy arguing that surrogacy would prevent the discontinuation of progeny.

As a person nears the end of life or is terminally ill, the family should conduct themselves with dignity in the presence of the patient. The patient can be indulged (e.g., giving a person with diabetes a sweet dish). Some families do not discuss the seriousness of the disease in the presence of the patient as an act of mercy and thus are the decision makers for that person. Although initially this might be viewed by some providers as against a patient's autonomy, the provider needs to understand the cultural issues and consequences.[89] Going against family and cultural wishes is seen as eliminating hope and the drive to live from the patient.

In general, the healthcare provider who recognizes the religious influences on the Muslim women's health and who acts with sensitivity should be able to gain trust with the patient over time. The pharmacist and healthcare provider might not know all of the answers, but should be equipped to understand the patient's situation, seek additional information and resources, and find culturally appropriate alternatives.

HINDUISM

Brief Background

The Hindu religion is possibly the oldest spiritual tradition.[90] The most renowned scripture is the Bhagavad Gita or Song of God.[91] In Hinduism, the soul evolves through different species of life including germs, vegetation, insects, birds, and animals to the human body.[92-94] Consciousness is the energy of the soul. Reincarnation continues as long as the soul has material aspirations and worldly attachments that separate it from love of God.[95]

Health, Illness, Healthcare Usage, and Complementary and Alternative Medicine

The Vedic sages encourage Hindus to live in harmony with self, one's family, community, mother earth, and God to maintain a healthy life balance.[90] The Vedic literature stresses spiritual realization to aid physical and mental health.[92] Illness might occur due to past negative actions in the previous life, by an irregular lifestyle, intoxication and illicit drugs, negative or polluted environments, and poor nutrition. Medicine and the healing herbs are regarded as an aspect of the divine.[96] Healthcare practitioners are highly honored in Hindu society.

The typical Hindu woman of Indian origin honors the principles of chastity to her husband. She is, therefore, more inclined and responsive to a medical examination by a female healthcare provider.[74] She tends to be shy and conservative about bodily exposure but is articulate, congenial, and very polite in her interactions with others.

The Vedic literature describes dietary and social habits that are acceptable.[90,97,98] Because all life is sacred (i.e., everything is the energy of God), Vedic sages recommend followers to be nonviolent. For this reason, a great majority of Hindus are strict vegetarians avoiding all types of meat, fish, and eggs in their diet. The Vedic literature also highly recommends a vegetarian diet as an aid to spiritual, emotional, and physical health. One is permitted by scripture to eat nonvegetarian foods excluding the consumption of cows if there are no vegetarian foods available in one's country. Thus, fish oils would not be a good recommendation for lipid control because other medications are available.

The Vedic literature also advises serious spiritual followers to avoid all forms of intoxication and recreational drugs.[92] These activities root the soul in a bodily attachment and can also reduce mental and physical strength. Abstention helps increase spiritual, emotional, and physical well being.

Hindus have no problem using modern medicines or technologies. Modern medicine shares an equal footing with the natural tradition known as Ayurvedic (meaning "knowledge of life") medicine. The Ayurvedic process is based on creating a perfect harmonious balance of mind, body, and soul.[99] Ayurvedic diagnosis is conducted through pulse analysis and observing external symptoms such as the conditions of the tongue, eyes, stool, and urine. Ayurvedic medicine has many remedies for chronic illnesses and uses massage, meditation, and Hatha Yoga—a system of breathing techniques and physical postures to create good health and well being. Homeopathy is also frequently used by Hindus.

Although the Vedic attitude is that one should always consider the time and circumstance in making decisions, there are preferences in healthcare. If someone is suffering from a chronic condition and requires a blood transfusion to be saved, blood from a vegetarian donor would be preferred. In administering prescription drugs to a Hindu, vegetarian-based medications would also be desirable, especially avoiding gelatin capsules or any products that contain animal or fish extracts.

Family Decisions, Concepts of Life, and Reproductive Health

Some Hindus consider their culture matriarchal. The Hindu wife is supposed to see her spouse as a part and parcel of the divine, and the husband should view his partner likewise. Many women now share equally with their spouses domestically, professionally, and spiritually.

The principle of divinity is also followed in sexual union. The Vedic literature advises serious spiritual followers to avoid sexual activity outside of marriage.[100] Orthodox Hindu couples will even prepare themselves spiritually on the day of conception by first meditating on God. The consciousness of the parents at the time of conception will attract a particular soul into their lives. Life begins at conception due to the presence of the soul (consciousness).

Many secular healthcare professionals in India are now promoting family planning and contraception due to overpopulation. Some Hindu couples may prefer natural family planning and condoms vs. contraception medications. The Vedic literature does not condone abortion due to the belief that the soul is present in the body from the time of conception and teaches that aborting the fetus can create negative karma for the couple in a future life.[101]

In vitro fertilization or surrogate parenting is left to the discretion of individuals but is likely not implemented by a Hindu couple. Hindus often view infertility or impotency as a spiritual karmic condition. Childless couples will often approach an enlightened mystic or priest for his blessings. The mystic will then give spiritual remedies to counteract the karma of their childless condition.

As a woman becomes older, the Vedas recommend a woman experiencing menopause or the later years of life to increase spiritual activity by absorbing her mind in love of God and guiding the younger family members.[100] Ayurvedic remedies are available to relieve hormonal changes.[99]

The end of life for many Hindus is considered to be a most important time because the quality of actions throughout life and consciousness at life's end help to determine the Hindu believer's next existence.[89] Hindus may pray for a healthy state of mind at that crucial juncture when all the bodily organs and functions are shutting down. Hindus might deny pain treatment that clouds judgment because scriptures suggest that pain should be endured.[93] They generally do not favor the modern idea of prolonging life at all costs in a dysfunctional physical condition.

Caring for the dying might be seen as a family responsibility as opposed to a healthcare provider's responsibility.[90,93] At the end of life, several rituals may be important to the patient and family members including chants and recitations from the Bhagavad Gita.[93] Many Hindus will return to India to specific holy places to pass their last days.

Healthcare providers working with the female Hindu patient can work toward creating a more positive patient encounter by taking into consideration the woman's views on what constitutes life, beliefs of reincarnation, and preferences for nonanimal or fish-based medications. During end-of-life care and pain management, healthcare providers will need to be sensitive to the use of pain medication and the desire for some families wanting greater involvement in caring for their loved one.

RELIGIOUS INFLUENCES ON HEALTHCARE

Healthcare providers should recognize that religious beliefs can affect women's health. Religion influences the role a woman has within the culture, views regarding life, contraception, and fertility treatments and decision making. Women's beliefs can also affect their receptiveness to medication therapies and their desire to have a religious or spiritual leader involved in their treatment and care.

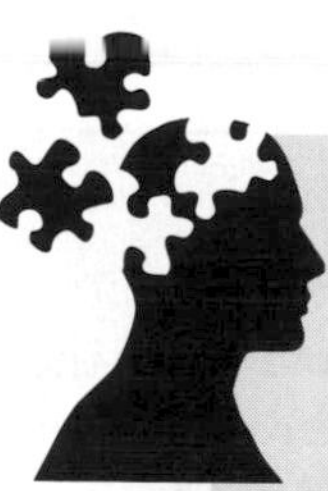

Therapeutic Challenge:

Which of your health beliefs are influenced by religious or spiritual beliefs? If you follow a religion, how do your healthcare beliefs compare to your religion's dogma? Pick either Catholicism, Islam, or Hinduism and contrast that religion's healthcare beliefs with your own beliefs. When you are providing care for a person with different religion influenced healthcare beliefs from your own, how would the difference influence your care and/or decisions?

CASE PRESENTATION

Patient Case: Part 2

Various factors could have influenced J.B.'s reaction. She might have been embarrassed due to her family raising her to be modest about her sexuality, because she is relatively young, or simply because she did not want to attend the session. She could be sexually active without her parents knowing and is concerned about confidentiality. Perhaps her religious or race/ethnic beliefs are against premarital sex and/or the use of oral contraceptives. She could feel that the way the policies were implemented in the school violated her religious and or race/ethnic beliefs and is embarrassed by the situation.

Changes in the approach to care by the clinic providers should occur. The school district's policies might not have been implemented in a way that respected the privacy and individual needs of the students and their families. An interactive session might have been more acceptable vs. a one-sided counseling session. The school clinic protocol might need to be adapted to allow for students to not attend the sex education or allow a parent to attend. There could be false beliefs in the community about the necessity of the HPV and hepatitis B vaccines. The pharmacist might need to adapt the style of patient assessment and education regarding use of birth control to reflect student and family religious and race/ethnic beliefs and cultural influences in making healthcare decisions.

Summary

As the U.S. demographics continue to change, all healthcare providers should recognize and value the increased beauty and benefits of a diverse nation. This growing diversity presents challenges for the healthcare providers to individualize and maximize medication use and treatment outcomes. Respecting and understanding cultural diversity has become a necessity in healthcare including pharmacy and medical practice. To begin working with women from diverse cultures, healthcare providers should start by understanding their own cultures and beliefs and learning about a variety of issues related to women in their communities from different races, ethnicities, and religions. Providers can then adapt their approach to care using culturally-specific communication styles and resources to identify and minimize health disparities. While healthcare providers cannot know everything about all cultures, they should be able to practice with the perspective that women from diverse backgrounds have unique health and medication needs. Healthcare providers should be able to appreciate and identify when cultural issues are affecting the care of their patients and have tools to address and resolve care and medication use problems that arise.

References

Additional content available at
www.ashp.org/womenshealth

3 Socioeconomics

Margaret B. Artz, Ph.D., R.Ph.; Mary E. S. Indritz, Ph.D., R.Ph., FASHP; Kathryn E. Peek, MS, MA, Ph.D.; Joslyn W. Fisher, MD, MPH, FACP; Barbara W. K. Yee, Ph.D.

Learning Objectives

1. Describe the various demographic, economic, and social factors influencing a woman's health.
2. Explain marital, education, and workforce changes influencing a woman's life, health, and healthcare.
3. Compare the similarities and differences of healthcare including access in urban and rural areas.
4. Assist a woman with obtaining medical and prescription drug coverage plans according to age.
5. Identify areas of insurance disparities.
6. Explain the impact of public policy on healthcare for women.
7. Examine the importance self-management plays in a woman's health.

This chapter examines how various demographic, economic, and social forces affect the health of women over their lifecycle. The phrase **socioeconomic status** (SES) is often used to encompass these elements. SES is defined as "a broad concept referring to the placement of persons, families, households and census (land) tracts or other aggregates with respect to the capacity to create or consume goods valued in our society."[1] Simply stated, SES encompasses the characteristics of the individual and of the individual's environment such as age, gender, race, ethnicity, marital status, income level, education, **insurance** coverage, access-to-care, occupation, place of residence, and number of children. While a few SES elements are stable (e.g., age, ethnicity), most elements are dynamic. This makes the influence of SES interesting, challenging, and vital to not only understanding the health of women but providing healthcare.

Other elements influencing a woman's health include her roles, **self-management,** family support systems, public health initiatives, public policy, and **disparities.** Women have multiple roles—each one important—and on which our society depends greatly. As a wife, mother, caregiver, wage earner or homemaker, how a woman manages her roles in tandem with taking care of herself depends on many of the SES elements described above, as well as the social support of her family, community and employer. While these roles shift over a woman's lifetime, one aspect remains constant: women need to take care of themselves (their health) in order to fulfill these roles or acquire new ones.

To assist women in their healthcare needs, pharmacists and other healthcare professionals are valuable resources. Pharmacists with an understanding of SES influences on health status can broaden their pharmaceutical care counseling options to include behavior modifications and self-management options, which are realistically applicable to the current health and SES of the patient.

Demographics

GENDER, AGE, AND HEALTHCARE UTILIZATION

Several positive attributes contribute to women's greater use of healthcare resources than men. Women have babies, live longer, and are more likely to seek medical care compared to men.[2] Besides reproduction and menopause, women have a larger burden of chronic disease leading to a greater use of hormones, analgesics, and psychotropic medications.[3] Consequently, women account for 60% of prescription drug expenditures overall and, in the 65 years and older population, account for up to 70% of

CASE PRESENTATION

Patient Case: Part 1

M.S. and her husband are third generation dairy farmers living on the family farm with their children, ages 12, 10, and 7 years. The nearest town with a clinic is 30 miles away; the nearest hospital 60 miles away. M.S. works as a high school administrative assistant in the next county. M.S.'s job provides medical insurance for the family but has no prescription benefits. M.S.'s elderly parents live nearby. She visits them weekly to make sure they have groceries, clean clothes, a clean house, and their medications. Her husband recently injured his back, which required hiring a neighbor to help work the farm. Their 7-year-old son has asthma that has progressively worsened. At her son's last medical exam, the family doctor told M.S. that switching her son to a nebulizer medication and two inhalers was necessary to get his asthma under control. He wrote the prescriptions, but M.S. has not filled them because money is tight. Their 12-year-old daughter has started middle school and the same doctor is strongly suggesting she receive the HPV vaccine. The vaccine is not only an expense they would have to cover but heightens their awareness of their daughter's possibility of a sex life at this young age.

M.S.'s sister lives in the "big city" and her problems weigh on M.S.'s mind as well. Her sister has just finished her postmastectomy radiation therapy, learned she has lost her accountant job due to downsizing, and must pay high COBRA payments to continue health insurance coverage. M.S. feels isolated and stressed with caring for her family, struggling to make the farm payments, and not missing work when her son gets sick. The stress is starting to take its toll on M.S.'s physical health. She has trouble sleeping and menstruates every 2 weeks, sometimes bleeding heavily for 5 days at a time, leaving her even more exhausted. M.S. wonders how much more she can ask of her husband, older children, employer, and herself in keeping everything together.

prescription drug use ($6.93 billion); spending over a billion dollars more annually for prescription medications than men ($5.77 billion).[3,4] As women and men age, differences in health expenditures become similar.

ETHNICITY

Of the more than 143 million women in the U.S., 29% belong to race and ethnic minority groups.[5] *Race* is the group assignment based on genetics/biology. *Ethnicity* is a group of people that has a unique set of shared characteristics based on culture or national origin. Race groups are categorized by the U.S. Census Bureau and listed in descending order of the size of their populations from the 2000 census: White, Black or African American, Asian, American Indian or Alaska Native, Native Hawaiian or Other Pacific Islander.[5] In the 2000 Census, citizens could select one or more races for the first time. Ethnicity is currently categorized as Hispanic/Latino or Not Hispanic/Latino; with members from various races. Additionally, each minority group is diverse, with different cultures and languages, SES, health insurance eligibility, immigration status, and acculturation. For example, a Black woman could have roots going back to Africa and also to Brazil, and, therefore, considers herself a member of the Black or African American race and of Hispanic ethnicity.

Though many women experience health problems, compared to White women minority women are in poorer health, use fewer health services, and encounter more barriers to healthcare.[5] Some minority women perceive the healthcare system as being hostile and insensitive. Education, income and acculturation appear to have positive influences: the longer a minority woman lives in the U.S., the more her access to healthcare improves. In all race groups, women who are married and with at least a high school education have high preventative screening rates (e.g., Pap tests, mammograms, blood pressure, immunizations).

From 1997 to 2008, the percent of persons of all ages with a usual place to go for medical care has remained steady at approximately 86%. Of three ethnic/race groups (Not Hispanic White, Not Hispanic Black, Hispanic), Hispanic persons are least likely to have a place of usual care (77%).[6] In most surveys asking this question, "usual place" does not include a hospital emergency room. Minority women face additional obstacles when seeking clinic-based healthcare: finding a physician who speaks/understands their language or one who has been trained in cultural competency and provides adequate preventive care counseling. Conversely, women in some cultures are more apt to seek traditional, folk medicine or spiritual healing first.

MARITAL STATUS

According to 2000 U.S. Census, of all women aged 15 years and older almost 50% are married; White women are nearly twice as likely as Black women to be married.[7,8] Marital status (e.g., divorce, separation) influences the use and cost of healthcare utilization.[9,10] While there is evidence to the contrary, generally, being married for women as well as for men is associated with being healthier (lower morbidity and mortality) than being single, in all age groups and controlling for other SES elements (race, ethnicity, education, income, etc.).[8,11,12] Marital status influences on health include household composition, better economic well-being, spousal encouragement of healthy eating and physical activity, and emotional and social fulfillment.[13-21]

CHILDREN

Many industrialized nations have problems with low birthrates and aging populations. When birth rates are low, there are fewer people in the future ready to fill jobs, pay taxes and support the previous generation. Since the 1970s, this trend has also been seen in the U.S. However, in 2000, the total fertility rate (TFR) moved above "replacement" (the rate at which a given generation can exactly replace itself) for the first time in almost 30 years.[22] Each race and Hispanic origin group also had increases in TFRs; as a group, Hispanic women had a higher TFR (3.1). However within this ethnic group, TFR varied between Mexican women (3.3), Puerto Rican women (2.6), and Cuban women (1.9).[22]

Being an unwed teenage mother carries a risk of worsening health: single women under 20 years at the time of their first baby's birth report higher rates of heart disease, lung disease and cancer in midlife.[23] Poorer health could stem from the lowered chance of future marriage and lower economic status carrying into midlife. Of note, births to teenage White, Black, Hispanic, Asian, and Pacific Islanders declined in 2000.[22]

EDUCATION

Education and employment are important factors with respect to earning potential and SES. A woman needs at least a high school education and training to adequately provide for herself, her health, and her future. Of women ages 25 years and older with no high school diploma, only one third are employed; with a high school diploma, 54% are employed. As education increases so does employment rates: some college but no degree, 64% are employed; an associate's degree, 71% are employed; a bachelor's or higher degree, 73% are employed.[24]

Since 1976, female undergraduate and graduate college enrollments have surpassed male enrollments.[25] A major milestone was reached in 2004 when White, Black, and Hispanic women attained higher enrollment rates in college than their male counterparts.[25] In the health professions, gender has shifted to include more women over the past several decades. Women account for 49% of medical students with similar percents for osteopathic medicine and dentistry. Thirty years ago, only 47% of pharmacy students were women; in 2005, 64% were women.[26] Male nurses now make up 10% of the nursing **workforce.**[26]

PLACE OF RESIDENCE

Historically, with the titles "housewife" and "homemaker" to represent the nurturing spirit of the woman who resides there with her family, a woman has been connected to "home." The community surrounding where a woman lives supplies both the support system as well as the healthcare services offered. This section examines the influences of urban and rural residence and what the healthcare professional, clinic, and hospital options have on a woman's health status.

Urban and Rural Areas

In addition to city, state, and zip code, place of residence is also described in terms of how many people reside in a county. The Urban Influence Code of the United States Department of Agriculture's Economic Research Service classifies a metropolitan (urban) county as inhabiting 1 million or more people. A small metropolitan county inhabits less than 1 million people. All other counties are considered nonmetropolitan (rural), with distinctions whether or not the county has a city with a population of 10,000 residents or more.[27]

Population and gender differences exist with residency. Approximately 35% of the U.S. population lives in the South, 23% each in the West and Midwest, and 19% in the Northeast.[27] (See Web Resources for United States Counties by Region and Urbanization Level, 1990.)

Additional content available at
www.ashp.org/womenshealth

While most counties in the U.S. are considered nonmetropolitan (rural), 80% of the population lives in large and small metropolitan areas. Women outnumber men in most states (Figure 3-1).[28] Except for upstate New York and the Florida panhandle, counties with low male-to-female ratios concentrate in the Northeast and South regions, while the West has high male-to-female ratios.

Figure 3-1. U.S. population male to female ratios (adapted).[28]

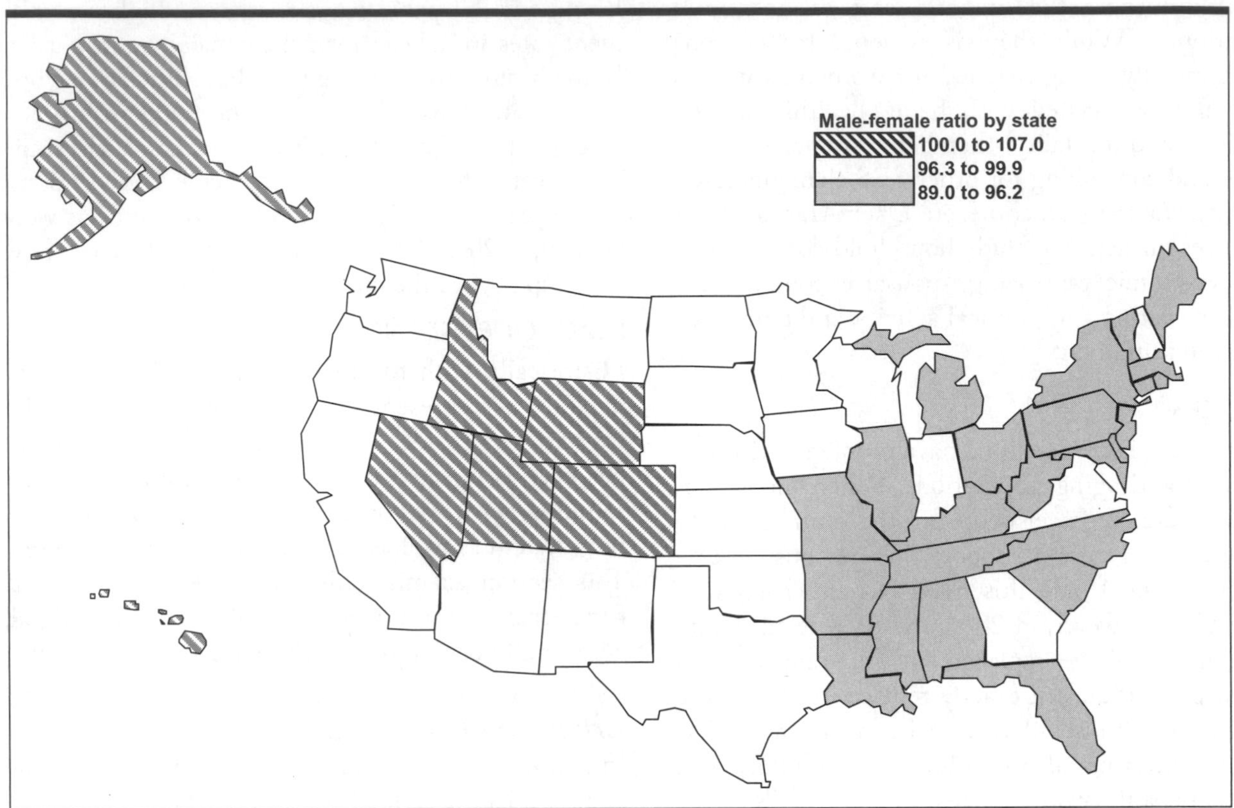

Minorities comprise 44% of the West, 37% of the South, 28% of the Northeast, and 20% of the Midwest. Not Hispanic Blacks are most likely to live in the South, while Asians, Hispanics, and American Indians are most likely to live in the West.[25] Regarding urbanization, Blacks, Asians, and Hispanics more often live in central metropolitan areas than Not Hispanic Whites or American Indians. A large percentage of Not Hispanic Whites and Asians live in suburbs. In contrast, 39% of the American Indian population lives in rural areas.[29] The profiles for women of color are similar to the minority population as a whole. The large majority of Asian and Pacific Islander women are urban residents. Alaska Native, American Indian, African American/Black, and Hispanic/Latina women are found in both rural and urban areas.[30]

Commonalities exist between persons living in remote rural and urban inner-city areas: poverty, high death rates, and high rates of chronic disease.[27] In either region, families headed by women have the highest rates of poverty (40% in rural, 34% in urban areas).[31,32] In general, when compared to metropolitan residents, rural residents tend to be older, poorer, and less educated.[33-39] Possible reasons for these socioeconomic differences include dependence on agriculture, economic downturn due to decreasing business opportunities and business decline, and departure of younger generations to urban areas.

Economics

The money a woman has, whether earned by her or available to her, influences her decisions for preventative, acute, and chronic care services for herself and her family, as well as her healthy lifestyle options. This section provides background into the various areas of economics that impact healthcare for women: career and job options, position levels, and related benefits.

WORKFORCE, EMPLOYMENT OPTIONS, AND SALARY

The female workforce is 67 million, representing 46% of the total U.S. workforce. Of working women, 75% work full-time.[40] According to the 2006 Current Population Survey, compared to men, women generally earn 37% less in sales occupations, 25% less in professional and technical occupations, 20% less in service jobs, and 12% less in office and administrative support positions. (See Web Resources for Median Income Estimates by Occupation).[24,41]

Additional content available at
www.ashp.org/womenshealth

Furthermore, employment opportunities and incomes have steadily increased among African Americans; still, in 2006, the South had a slightly higher poverty rate (14%) than the Northeast, Midwest, and West (each region with approximately 12%).[36]

In the last 40 years, more women increasingly have entered scientific, professional, and healthcare fields. Women provide a majority of the professional-level jobs as well as occupying office and administrative support jobs (75%) and service work (58%).[40] The office support and service fields may or may not require post–high school education, have fewer opportunities for advancement, and have low salaries. Until 2014, jobs related to the service industry and those considered professional-level are projected to increase. Within the professional-level group, careers will be in education, training, library, healthcare practitioners and technicians, and mathematical and computer occupations.[24] The nursing profession will have the largest growth while manufacturing jobs will decrease.[24,40,42]

Currently, the top 10 occupations with the highest median weekly earnings among women working full-time, in order of highest to lower earnings, are pharmacists, chief executives, lawyers, physicians, computer/information systems managers, computer software engineers, psychologists, physical therapists, management analysts, computer programmers, and human resource managers.[24] In the next decade, a college degree will be required for the fastest-growing occupations (e.g., nursing, computer software engineering, teaching).[24,43]

Women have increased their visibility in upper management; however, the percentage increase is small (5.1% of senior executive positions in the 500 largest U.S. companies in 1999 compared to 2.6% in 1996). To gain in leadership positions, women need more role models, more business schools actively pursuing women students, and corporate cultures more involved in advancing women. While upper management positions may be prized for their higher income and prestige, the opposite can occur: some upper management women leave their jobs to focus on children and family life. Some women see management positions as too intense, stressful, competitive, and/or not as rewarding as motherhood.[44,45]

EMPLOYMENT BENEFITS

Important benefits accompany employment that directly affect women: paid sick days, maternity/family leave, and health insurance. Paid sick days and maternity/family leave offer women a safety net in balancing work and family. Currently, 22 million working women do not receive sick day benefits as paid sick days; this is especially true in part-time or low-paying jobs. Paid sick days are benefits more likely offered by large firms and in professional and management-related occupations. In the retail trade (sales) and accommodations/food service industries, areas that employ the most women, almost 9 million women, lack paid sick days.[46] Women whose employer offers paid family leave are more likely to work full-time, be in professional or management occupations, and/or work for large firms.

Employers who offer paid sick days find their employees are more likely to stay home if sick, thereby reducing the spread of illness in the workforce and improving productivity. Healthcare expenditures are reduced because sick children recover more quickly when a parent stays home to care for them.[47] Forty-nine percent of working mothers miss work when a child is sick with a minor illness (e.g., cold, car infection) compared with 30% of working fathers.[46] According to the U.S. Department of Labor, only 8% of all U.S. workers in the private sector receive paid family leave to care for a newborn or other family member.[48] Many companies offer unpaid family leave. Although no federal laws require employers to give paid maternity leave, there are laws that give women rights based on a temporary disability perspective.[48]

Thus, a working woman who is also poor has hard choices when she has no paid sick day benefit. When she or her child is sick, either she loses pay by staying home, leaves a sick child home alone and or goes to work sick.[46] While women at all income levels face this situation, more than one fourth of low income women delay getting healthcare because they are unable to take time off from work.[46] To manage family and work responsibilities, employed women with children often work nonstandard periods (i.e., weekends, afternoons, and evenings). This is especially true for single mothers, especially if the children are under the age of 5.

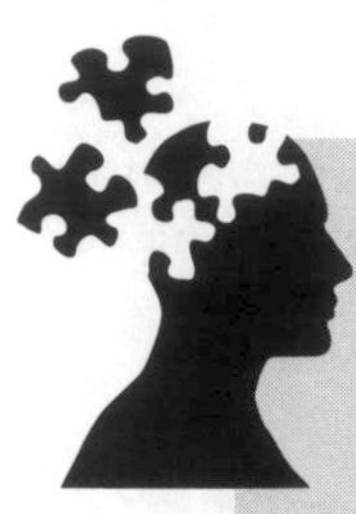

Therapeutic Challenge:

What is the maternity leave policy at your worksite? Does it vary if you are a healthcare provider, technician or administrator? What are the maternity leave policies of other countries such as Canada? Sweden? During a maternity leave, is the woman's medication insurance still viable? Does she need to go on disability insurance during this time?

Health and Prescription Drug Insurance Coverage

Most but not all women have insurance coverage. Women ages 15–44 years received healthcare services through private insurance (65%), Medicaid (12%) or were uninsured (20%) (Figure 3-2).[49] Women who have health insurance are more apt to receive primary, specialty, and preventive care services.[50] For example, in 2003 the annual median healthcare spending for insured women ages 18–64 years was $1,844 compared to $847 spent for men.[51] The insurance options differ in a variety of ways—in the level of coverage and in who provides the coverage.

INSURANCE

Insurance is a contract designed to compensate some or all future services in exchange for a periodic payment (a premium). The term health insurance usually means basic coverage of hospital (inpatient) and medical (outpatient) services, excluding prescription and durable medical products. Health insurance can be categorized by payor type: public (government-sponsored) or private (nongovernment) coverage (Table 3-1).[36,45-46,50,52-54] Public health insurance includes plans funded by any form of government (federal, state, local, military, Indian Health Service). Private health insurance is coverage provided as a benefit through employment or through direct purchase from a private company. Insurance can also be defined by how it is financed or what it covers: fee-for-service vs. managed-care, catastrophic coverage vs. full or partial coverage (Table 3-1).[36,45,46,50,52-54]

Figure 3-2. Health insurance coverage of all women (N = 62 million) of reproductive age (15–44 years), 2006.[48]

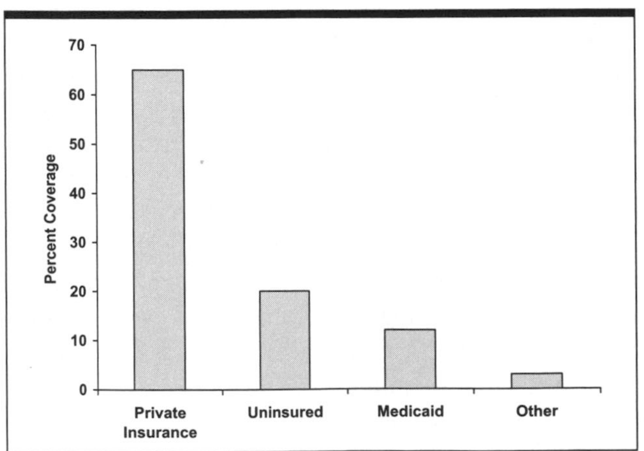

Public Insurance

The most well-known U.S. public insurances are Medicare and Medicaid established with the 1965 Social Security Act Amendments (SSAA) (Table 3-1).[36,45,46,50,52-54] The federally administered Medicare program covers most, but not all, hospital, medical and prescription services for persons age 65 years or older, persons younger than 65 years with certain disabilities, and persons of any age with end-stage renal disease. The U.S. Medicaid system is managed by the Centers for Medicare and Medicaid Services (CMS) and is a state-administered program covering healthcare services to eligible low-income individuals and families. Each state sets Medicaid eligibility guidelines. Medicaid enrollment in particular, plays an important role in rural America as 16% of rural residents have Medicaid coverage compared to 10% of urban residents.[55] Other government sponsored health insurance programs cover military personnel and Native Americans (Table 3-1).

More women than men are covered by public insurance (Medicare and Medicaid). Women are more likely to qualify for Medicaid because they are poorer and more likely to meet eligibility criteria (low-income, have children, pregnant or disabled).[50] Medicaid plays a critical role for the 62 million U.S. women of reproductive age. In 2006, about 70% of Medicaid beneficiaries above the age of 14 years were girls and women. Further, while Medicaid provides more than half of the public dollars allocated for family planning, these services constitute less than 1% of total Medicaid expenditures.[49]

The state legislatures determine annually or biannually what to cover and who is eligible for Medicaid services. Thus income criteria for Medicaid eligibility and specific services offered varies from state to state. This control over Medicaid disproportionately affects

Table 3-1. Types and Characteristics of Health Insurance[a]

Type of Insurance	Financing	Coverage	Components	Other Information
Public—Medicare (established with the Social Security Act Amendments in 1965) (Part D: established in 2003)	Sponsored by federal government, administered by Centers for Medicaid and Medicare Services (CMS) through private insurance providers	In 2006, 14% of U.S. population covered by Medicare[51] Most healthcare services for persons age 65 years and older Persons under age 65 years with certain disabilities Patients with end stage renal disease	Part A (all over 65 years are eligible): hospital care, hospice, skilled nursing facilities, home healthcare Part B: supplementary insurance, insured must pay premiums for physician and outpatient services including physical and occupational therapy, supplies Part D (optional): provides prescription drug coverage, most participants have to pay premium and deductibles	http://www.medicare.gov
Public—Medicaid (established with the Social Securrity Act Amendments in 1965)	Sponsored by federal government, administered by individual states (each state determines eligibility and covered services)	Eligible low-income individuals and families In 2006, approximately 13% of the U.S. population was covered by Medicaid[36] 75% of Medicaid recipients are women[44] 10% of all U.S. women under age 65 years covered by Medicaid[44]	May cover hospital costs, outpatient costs, prenatal care, family planning, prescription drugs, home health services	Medicaid is not the same as "welfare" Medicaid coverage varies by state Medicaid finances 41% of all births in U.S.[11] http://www.cms.hhs.gov/medicaid
Public—Civilian Health and Medical Program of the Uniformed Services (TRICARE/CHAMPUS/VA)	Funded and administered by Department of Veterans Affairs (VA)	3.6% of U.S. covered[52] 1.7 million women veterans (6% to 7% of all veterans)[52] Eligible veterans, their dependents, survivors	Depending on eligibility and enrolled plan type, covered services include inpatient and outpatient services, prescription drugs, dental, vision, and mental health	Center for Women Veterans http://www1.va.gov/womenvet/
Public—Indian Health Service (IHS)	Funded through the federal Department of Health and Human Services (DHHS)	557 tribes in 35 states eligible American Indians and Alaska Natives[45]	Non-Indian women who are pregnant with an eligible Indian's child also can receive healthcare services from the IHS	Pharmacists may have access to the patient's entire health record including labs, immunizations, and medical problems, which can facilitate assessment, management, and counseling on medication therapy Training and student loan (reimbursement) opportunities for pharmacy students exist with IHS http://www.pharmacy.ihs.gov/

(*Continued on next page*)

Type of Insurance	Financing	Coverage	Components	Other Information
Public—State Children's Health Insurance Program (SCHIP) (established by Title XXI of Social Security Act in 1997)	Financed by federal and state government, administered by states (each state determines eligibility, payment to providers, and covered services)	Healthcare to poor children whose parents do not qualify for Medicaid	In most states, SCHIP covers doctor visits, immunizations, hospitalization and emergency room visits and to a variable degree prescription medications for eligible children	http://www.insurekidsnow.gov
Private Insurance	Fee for service Managed care: Health maintenance organizations (HMO), preferred provider organizations (PPO), or point of service (POS) Association-based (through a trade or professional group) High-risk pools			
Group-Based, Employment-Based	Employer-based, discounted because of group pricing—may be paid by employer fully, partially or by employee via payroll deduction	60% U.S. covered by employment-based health insurance[49,53]	Variable services covered—hospital, outpatient, prescriptions May or may not be offered to part-time employees or dependents	Women are more frequently dependents covered by their spouse's employer-based insurance. Infrequently, men or families are covered under the wife's plan
Direct Purchase, Private	Private insurance companies	9% U.S. population covered by direct-purchase health insurance (only 6% of women)[49,53]		Women may directly purchase insurance because they might be self-employed, ran out of insurance extension benefits, or may not have employer-offered insurance
Workers' Compensation Insurance	Employer financed, state administered		Covers medical care incurred in work-related injury or compensation for temporary or permanent disabilities due to work-related injury	
COBRA	Consolidated Omnibus Budget Reconciliation Act (COBRA) of 1986 Individual may need to pay entire premium		Coverage when employee loses/leaves job or changes to part-time; employers of certain size business must offer eligible employees the opportunity to continue with employer's or former employer's group health coverage for limited time	
Prescription Drug Assistance	Some states, charities, and pharmaceutical companies have special programs for eligible people		For those who have no access to private or public assistance	http://www.disabilityresources.org/RX.html

(*Continued on next page*)

Type of Insurance	Financing	Coverage	Components	Other Information
College/Student Health Insurance	Covered by college/ institution, organizational (i.e., American College Student Association), parents			
FMLA (Family Medical Leave Act of 1993)	Employer-based health coverage		Eligible employees may receive health insurance coverage for 12-wk leave during any 1-yr period for newborn, adopted child, or sick family member	
Disability Insurance	May be personal/ individual purchase or employer or union-based insurance	Rarely covers 100% salary 19% of women have some disability (2000 U.S. Census Bureau) Women are much more likely than similarly aged men to become disabled for 90 days or more	May be short (temporary) or long-term disability	Some states have laws that require companies to cover temporary disability benefits during family medical leave (FMLA) http://hrc.nwlc.org/Policy-Indicators/Womens-Access-to-Health-Care-Services/Temporary-Disability-Insurance.aspx Disabled women are less likely to be employed and if employed, earn less on average than disabled men (Center for Research on Women with Disabilities [CROWD]) http://www.bcm.edu/crowd/?PMID=1330 http://www.census.gov/hhes/www/disability/data_title.html#2000
Social Security Disability Insurance (SSDI) or Supplemental Security Income (SSI)	U.S. Social Security Administration	SSDI: Eligible only if unable to be employed in any type of work and if disability expected to last ≥12 mo SSI: Based on disability and financial status	If qualified and approved, SSDI will be paid after 6th mo of disability	http://www.ssa.gov/
Medical Coverage Through Automobile Insurance	May be individual purchase; may be employer-purchased when work is driving or many hours in vehicle	Medical payments (MedPay) Pays for medical expenses for insured and passengers after an accident Personal injury protection (PIP): Covers medical, hospital, and funeral expenses, lost wages of insured, insured's passengers, and pedestrians if struck by insured	MedPay and PIP are similar as they both pay medical bills for injuries due to a vehicle accident, regardless of fault PIP coverage and limits vary by state; some states even allow insurances to offer a variety of PIPs UM is required in many states UIM is only required in a few states.	State laws on MedPay, PIP, UM, and UIM coverages vary; not all states require automobile medical liability coverage; check state's insurance commissioner's office http://www.naic.org/state_web_map.htm

(*Continued on next page*)

Type of Insurance	Financing	Coverage	Components	Other Information
		Uninsured coverage (UM): Pays medical bills for accidents caused by an uninsured driver or for victims of a hit-and-run		
		Underinsured coverage (UIM): Applies when a person who causes an accident does not have adequate insurance		

[a]All information on table obtained and summarized from websites listed under other information.

women and the percent that have insurance coverage. For example, Medicaid covers prenatal, delivery, and postpartum care for up to 60 days for all women with incomes up to 133% of the federal poverty level. In order to meet budget shortfalls, state legislatures may change income requirements for pregnancy-related services making eligibility more difficult for some pregnant women.

Between 3–4 million U.S. women obtain family planning services provided through Medicaid each year. Federal guidelines for Medicaid family planning benefits stipulate counseling and patient education; examination and treatment by medical professionals; laboratory exams and tests; medically-approved methods, procedures, pharmaceutical supplies, and devices to prevent conception; and infertility services including sterilization reversals. Under CMS policy, abortion can not be claimed as a Medicaid service except in cases of rape or incest or if the woman's life is endangered if the pregnancy were carried to term.

Medicaid Family Planning Expansions

Building on the expansion of Medicaid eligibility for pregnancy-related services, more than half of the states have applied for and received permission from CMS to extend family planning eligibility to women with incomes ranging from 133% to 200% of the federal poverty level.[49] To receive the eligibility waiver, states are required to add primary care services for newly eligible women and demonstrate to CMS that family planning services, as well as primary care for thousands of additional women, does not result in increased federal expenditures. In fact, evidence demonstrates that providing family planning plus primary care services costs less than providing pregnancy-related services to beneficiaries who otherwise become pregnant and eligible for Medicaid-funded prenatal, delivery, and postnatal care.[56]

Private Insurance: Employer-Covered

Employers provide health insurance to 62% of women, either through a woman's job or as dependent coverage. Characteristics of women under 65 years who are insured through employer-based insurance: White, age 25 years and older, high school education or greater, a full-time job, and good-to-excellent health status.[54] Women participate less in employer-covered health plans (80%) than their male counterparts (89%) because women are more likely to work part-time (and not be eligible), have lower incomes (and not have enough money for premiums), or are covered by a spouse or partner.[50] When women rely on spouses or partners for coverage, they are susceptible to losing coverage. This coverage loss happens when spouses or partners lose their job or die, the employer ceases family coverage, the premium becomes a financial burden, or in divorce/separation.

In an employer-covered plan, the premium for the health insurance is discounted because the risk is spread among all employees. Some employers offer healthcare coverage to part-time employees but often the coverage is less generous than that offered to full-time employees and might have higher premiums.[36]

Direct-Purchase Insurance Programs

Women (or men) can purchase private, direct-purchase health insurance for various reasons: self-employed, work for a company not offering health insurance, or has left employer and run out of insurance extension benefits. In 2006, only 9% of the

U.S. population was covered by direct-purchase health insurance; only 6% of women chose direct-purchase insurance.[36,50] Compared to employer-based health insurance, private insurance has higher premiums and limited coverage. Persons aged 50 years or older might find it harder to buy private health insurance or need to pay higher than normal premiums, especially if the insurer requires a medical exam or if the applicant has a serious or chronic medical problem.

Various options exist for direct-purchase health insurance (Table 3-1). One option is for the insured to pay a portion of the cost for each service. Another option is for the insured to enroll in a plan where there are restrictions on whom to see and where services are rendered. A third option is where the insured buys insurance at a better rate through a trade or professional association. A last option is a high-risk health insurance plan insuring individuals who have previously been refused insurance and carries extremely high premiums with limited coverage.

There remains a gender difference in health management and outcomes despite similar insurance benefits and access to services. For example, among managed care patients, women received beta-blockers significantly less often than men after a myocardial infarction.[57] While reporting better asthma care measures, women within a managed care organization reported worse health status and more use of asthma-relieving medications.[58] Compared to men, women in managed care plans were more likely to report problems with their healthcare, particularly regarding access to specialists such as obstetrician-gynecologists.[59]

Disability

Disability is defined in many ways and does not always mean the person is unhealthy or unable to live or enjoy a full healthy life. As the definition of disability evolves over time, it is important when reviewing disability statistics to know how the data source defines and measures disability. In the past, disability was seen more as a debilitating physical or mental condition and programs were designed to provide financial support. Presently, physical and mental problems, as well as barriers in the environment that prevent social functioning, are factors in determining one's disability with more programs being designed to support independence and improve social involvement.[60]

From 1997 to 2008, the prevalence of disability in the U.S. population has remained consistent at approximately 18%.[61] Depending on the disability definition, between 20 to 28 million U.S. women have a disability with the most common conditions related to back disorders, arthritis, heart disease, respiratory problems, and high blood pressures.[62]

Disability insurance is not a medical health insurance. It is a benefit that provides income during times when a person is unable to work due to a disability-defined health problem or an accident. There are two types of disability policies one may purchase: short-term and long-term. Definitions of disability, amount of financial benefit, and length of coverage vary depending on the policy. Generally, short-term coverage lasts for several months to 2 years and long-term ranges from several years to remaining lifetime. Disability insurances may be provided as a benefit (free or discounted) by an employer, can be purchased as an individual, or are available through federal programs.

In the U.S., two prominent federal disability programs administered by the Social Security Administration are the Social Security Disability (SSD) program and the Supplemental Security Income (SSI) program. The SSD is funded by Social Security taxes and is a monthly cash benefit applying to persons (and certain family members) who meet explicit criteria: have worked long enough, have paid Social Security taxes, have a medical condition that meets SSD's disability definition, and are unable to work for a certain length of time.[63] The SSI is funded by general/personal income/corporation/other tax revenues and not by Social Security taxes, and its benefits are not based on prior work history. SSI pays monthly benefits to disabled or blind persons based on financial need.[64]

Medical Coverage Through Automobile Insurance

Some states require automobile insurance to include medical coverage related to injuries to the driver or occupants resulting from an accident. This type of medical insurance may also provide coverage if one is injured by a vehicle or riding in another person's vehicle. Depending on an individual state law, medical coverage may be available as medical payments coverage (MEDPAY) or personal injury protection (PIP). The MEDPAY and PIP coverages are similar, but PIP also reimburses for lost wages and child care. Because medical and disability costs are often covered in other policies, buying medical coverage through an automobile insurance is often redundant and an added expense considering its limited scope.

PIP may be beneficial for persons who do not have regular health insurance that adequately covers expenses of a car-related injury, persons who regularly carpool, or often drive with passengers.

UNINSURED

Even with all the types of healthcare insurance available, in 2006 and in 2007, 42 million (16%) of the U.S. population under the age of 65 years were not covered by health insurance.[36,65] Of the uninsured in 2006, 10% were White, 16% were Asian, 21% were Black, and 34% were Hispanic/Latino.[36] Using averages for years 2004 to 2006, more than 30% of American Indians or Alaska Natives had no health insurance; more than 21% of Native Hawaiians or Other Pacific Islanders were without health coverage.[66]

Characteristics related to high percentages of uninsured persons are Hispanic, living in the South and West regions of the U.S., ages of 18–24 years, no high school diploma, and single.[65] A large majority of the uninsured are employed or have working family members; yet, they are unable to obtain insurance due to cost (i.e., high employer-sponsored insurance premiums or no employer-sponsored insurance available or not eligible for employer-sponsored insurance, working part-time or newly-employed).[67]

Characteristics of women who are uninsured (17 million) mirror those of the total uninsured population: young (19–24 years), near poor, ethnic (Latina, Native American or Eskimo, immigrant), and no high school diploma. Uninsured women often delay medical and pharmaceutical care, as well as delay or ignore female preventative care (mammograms, Papanicolaou (PAP) tests, immunizations, etc.).[49,68] This lack of preventative care contributes to the delayed diagnosis and worse prognosis for uninsured women with breast and cervical cancer.[69] Women, particularly uninsured women, receive worse care for chronic diseases including controlling elevated lipid and blood sugar concentrations.[70] In addition to the physical health consequences of increased morbidity and mortality due to being uninsured, the lack of insurance contributes to psychological sequelae including anxiety, depression and familial stress.

Other significant costs are associated with being uninsured. One in three uninsured Americans was unable to fill a prescription due to cost. One study found that 42% of uninsured women did not fill a prescription due to cost, at some time, compared to 18% of insured women. Moreover, almost 20% of the uninsured use the emergency room as their usual source of care, compared to 3% of persons with health insurance.[67] Relying on an emergency department for regular medical care is not only more costly than care through a clinic practice, but overuse in this manner delays critical care to those who are in need. In the U.S., almost $100 billion dollars is spent each year to provide uninsured persons with healthcare—for conditions that often could have been prevented or treated more efficiently with an earlier diagnosis.[71] Uninsured people are more likely to be hospitalized for an avoidable condition, with hospitals uncompensated for about $34 billion worth of this care.[71]

One in five uninsured persons live in rural areas as employers in rural areas are more likely to be in small businesses and less likely to offer health benefits.[72] Rural residents who do have insurance are more likely to be covered by a public insurance such as Medicaid or Medicare.[34] Compared to rural men, rural women are less likely to have health insurance due to lack of employment and poverty.[73] Because coverage through public insurance can have time limitations, women are especially vulnerable (e.g., have children, no spouse or partner) and unable to prepare for its discontinuance.

Furthermore, communities suffer high costs from supporting residents who have no health insurance. For example, employers face lost productivity and early worker disability due to adverse outcomes in the uninsured population. In areas where there are high levels of uninsured persons, delivery capacity could diminish as providers and hospitals cut back, shut down, or move.[74]

OTHER HEALTHCARE MODELS

Many experts propose various models for **universal healthcare.** Universal healthcare can be defined as a basic guarantee of healthcare to all (i.e., in the context of a nation's citizens). The U.S. is the only industrialized country lacking some form of universal healthcare; a number of models for delivering healthcare in a more universal manner have been proposed. A single-payer healthcare system implies financing by one source—usually the federal government. A multipayer system involves a "single-payer" option along with allowing other options such as private insurance. The tax-credit plans provide a credit for health insurance expenditures in the amount that an individual would have to pay for their federal taxes. This system would likely benefit employed workers without employer-based health insurance; however, would not cover those with lower incomes, non–tax payers, and hence not be "universal."

BREAST AND CERVICAL CANCER SCREENING

The U.S. Centers for Disease Control and Prevention (CDC) provides access to breast and cervical cancer screening for low-income, uninsured, and underinsured women through the National Breast and Cervical Cancer Early Detection Program (NBCCEDP) created in 1990 by a Congressional act. This specific public policy program is one of the largest efforts in chronic disease prevention and control ever undertaken by a federal agency. Women at or below 250% of the federal poverty level are eligible; ages 18–64 years for cervical cancer screening and ages 40–64 years for breast cancer screening. Services include clinical breast exams, mammograms, PAP tests, further diagnostic testing for abnormal screenings, surgical consultations, and referrals. Since 2000, states have been able to offer access to treatment for women in the NBCCEDP through Medicaid.[65] An estimated 8% to 11% of U.S. women are eligible to receive NBCCEDP services. Through 2006, the program has served more than 3 million women and provided more than 7.2 million screening exams.[75]

Medical Savings Accounts are tax-free savings accounts created through employers (or potentially the government) to use for the purchase of an insurance plan and/or medical costs. This type of system might be particularly problematic for women because it does not eliminate the issue of paying high out-of-pocket costs for medical care and prescriptions and also might be a disincentive to primary preventive care.

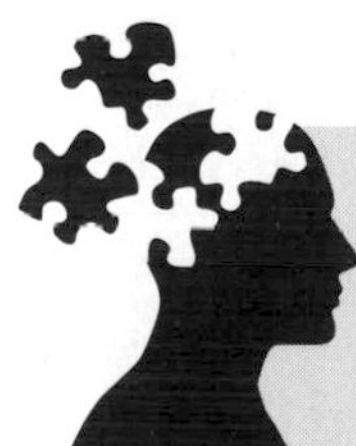

Therapeutic Challenge:

A mother comes into the pharmacy asking which of her family's medications are essential. Her husband lost his job and they no longer have health and medication insurance and quite possibly will lose their home. She needs to conserve money wherever she can. What can you do to help this woman and her family?

There are advantages and disadvantages to each proposal. Further research is needed to elucidate the factors such as insurance status and healthcare delivery systems influencing health disparities and impacting women's health.

Access-to-Care

To visit a doctor, pharmacy, dentist, or other healthcare provider, a person must usually be able to get to the clinic or hospital. Thus, transportation can be a major barrier to obtaining healthcare services in both urban and rural areas. Although most families have one or more cars, large cities can have inadequate mass transit options and low-income, inner-city residents without personal transportation have difficulty getting to physicians although clinics may be near.[76] Rural residents travel longer distances to receive basic healthcare and are thus less likely to receive regular medical checkups and preventive screening.[33,34] Coupled with inclement weather, travel time, inadequate road maintenance, the burden of travel and distance is often one of the main reasons rural residents delay or not seek care at all.

Disparities in health outcomes and healthcare access or treatment have been attributed to discrimination, differential care, and/or lower quality of treatment due to race/ethnicity, gender, age, type or absence of insurance, and poverty.[77] Immigrant populations can further experience language and cultural barriers to healthcare, and have difficulty navigating our complex health service system.[78] Despite the rapidly growing diversity of America, the limited number of ethnic and minority healthcare professionals makes it more difficult for a woman of color to find a practitioner of her same ethnicity. Care is also hindered by linguistic access (limited English speaking skills and health literacy), failure to provide greater patient choice, and less satisfaction with healthcare.[79]

Access-to-care is also influenced by the number and types of healthcare professionals available in a region. Urban counties have a greater supply of healthcare providers compared to rural counties even though 20% of Americans live in rural areas.[80,81] For example, the ratio of physicians to population in urban counties is 136% higher than that in rural counties, the ratio of dentists is 150%, and the ratio of hospital-based registered nurses is 130% of the rural ratio.[82] In a 1999 study, the ratio of pharmacists to population is lower in rural areas, with only 66 pharmacists per 100,000 people, compared to 78 pharmacists per 100,000 nationwide.[83] However, the pharmacist ratio is worse in some states more than others. For example, in Texas, the pharmacist supply ratio in 2005, per 100,000 population was 53 compared to 77 in urban areas.[84] The reasons for the greater numbers of medical professionals and healthcare facilities in urban areas are varied. Medical specialties and expensive technology require a substantial population to support them.[85] Most medical, dental, nursing, and pharmacy schools are located in urban areas. Technology, family and employment opportunities are better in urban areas.

This shortage of healthcare professionals and facilities in rural areas places stresses on both the healthcare providers and their patients. For example, in 2007, of the 2,000 rural communities where there was only one pharmacy and it was independently-owned, there was no other pharmacy available to patients within 10 miles. Pharmacy owners face shrinking reimbursements intended to reduce costs for commercial insurance, Medicaid, and Medicare as well as competition with mail order pharmacy.[86] When the pharmacy is located in a remote location, it is difficult to stay in business if insurance coverage severely limits prescription payment.[87] Yet as the U.S. population ages, the utilization of medical services and prescription drugs creates more of a demand for healthcare professionals. These multiple challenges have led to providing nontraditional methods of medical and pharmaceutical care delivery: higher rates of immunizations by pharmacists, the use of telemedicine, and more recently, telepharmacy.

Psychiatrists and midlevel mental health professionals are mainly located in urban areas. Shortages of these professionals in rural areas leave women needing mental health or emotional support with options of ministers, self-help groups, family or friends.[73] Farm women have high risks of depression as they juggle hard physical labor, financial concerns, and family obligations with little time to attend to emotional needs. Even when family practitioners are available, they fail to detect depression in one out of two of their depressed patients compared to urban family physicians.[73] Further, if a rural woman does have health insurance, the likelihood it covers psychotherapy is small.[88]

Thus, rural medical and pharmacy practitioners enjoy a broad scope of practice and greater autonomy than urban practitioners. Unfortunately, long shifts with fewer support personnel and inadequate relief help puts stress on remote rural practitioners. These stresses account for only 26% of rural family physicians being women.[89] To attract practitioners, many medical and pharmacy schools have integrated rural programs into their training or rotations in order to provide future practitioners the experience of rural healthcare opportunities.

Because of sustained shortages, rural communities have readily accepted less expensive, midlevel providers as alternatives to physicians in supplying primary care services. And while most nurse practitioners and physician assistants are women, only 20% of them work in rural communities leaving rural women also less access to female midlevel providers.[90-94] Opportunities exist for rural pharmacists to broaden their practices to include specialty areas such as chronic disease management, anticoagulation monitoring, nutritional counseling, and hospice medication coordination, as well as to expand their collaborative agreements with physicians to improve healthcare for all citizens including women.

Self-Management in the Context of Family

SES elements influence a woman's health via physical and emotional reactions to life's circumstances (e.g., multiple stressors of income, discrimination, and occupational stagnation). Multiple roles, job pressure, and emotional isolation are identified as major factors in the rates of disease.[95] While some stress is natural and keeps a woman alert and productive, prolonged distress can be detrimental, causing unhealthy changes in the body and lowering resistance to illness. In one model, internal harmony and a proper psychosocial atmosphere maintained health through internal balance—especially when tailored to a woman's particular background, bodily reactions, habits, and personal situation.[95] For example, in many Native American tribes, health means "balance" of body and spirit.

Self-management is defined as a rational, cognitive-behavioral approach to change where the person uses behaviors and tools to improve balance in one's life.[96] Tools for self-management include coping, lifestyle choices, support systems, and regular medical visits. Practically-speaking, self-management enables a woman to deal with trouble using her accumulated resources of experience, natural abilities, learned skills, and personal strengths and assets to emphasize and enhance her wellness. Wisely saying "no" is a very liberating step in gaining peace of mind and a sense of security rather than being overwhelmed or overcommitted. Rewards (e.g., putting something fun on the "to do" list or scheduling personal time) are necessary for acknowledging accomplishments and bringing balance to life.

Coping behaviors are mechanisms for addressing an immediate problem; they are well-reasoned or intuitive, slow to form or fast reactions, or healthy or detrimental in nature. Examples of these behaviors range from exercise to relieve frustration, working more hours to pay for babysitters or housecleaning, bringing a home health nurse to help with care giving, using alcohol in excess, or ignoring a situation altogether. Some coping behaviors become counterproductive and impractical; opposing goals become incompatible when attempted at the same time.

Lifestyle choices of self-management include conscious decisions about what a woman wants her life to be now and in the future. Most often these choices center on family and career and can include marriage, decisions to have children, whether to work and if so, full-time vs. part-time employment. Career aspirations and the sacrifices involved to meet or defer them are choices affecting a woman's lifestyle.

Use of support systems is self-management behavior ensuing after some thought. A woman may be in, or on the verge of, a crisis situation and actively seeks help from outside the family. Examples of this include finding child or adult daycare, contacting local disease-specific associations (e.g., Alzheimer's Association, Cancer Society, hospice, social services, local church or school, food shelf, etc.). Self-management behaviors addressing health needs include regular health screening and monitoring of chronic conditions (i.e., high blood pressure, diabetes). Taking these steps may be hard for a woman who is dealing with many responsibilities. A pharmacist or healthcare provider having knowledge about available assistance programs (free mammograms/blood pressure/diabetic screenings, early childhood screenings, available adult daycares) can easily insert this information into a counseling moment or discussion in a nonjudgmental manner.

SELF-MANAGEMENT IN VIEW OF MARRIAGE AND WITH CHILDREN

Most women make a conscious choice to have a child. Some women find motherhood brings contentment while others feel out of place and conflicted. When babies are born, some women have a period when they find it difficult to adapt to the changes in the relationships and environment. Despite a plethora of childrearing books available, most women do not receive formal training in parenting.[97] In extreme cases after childbirth, some women have difficult times leading to low self-esteem, loss of interest in activities and people, and postpartum depression. Most women find informal support through family members and close friends.

While men are equal partners in parenting, women do relatively more childcare; some women experience a decline in marital satisfaction when their expectations about sharing childcare responsibilities are not met.[97] Examples of self-management involve arranging for adequate childcare, which may involve family or neighbors or daycare environments, so a woman can have a relaxing time out with friends or partner. These respites are positive experiences with most women seeing them as necessary replenishments helping them be good mothers.[98] Self-management is putting self first in order to be the best self to others.

SELF-MANAGEMENT IN VIEW OF CARING FOR AILING FAMILY MEMBERS

More women (12%) manage the care of their children and spouses while being a caregiver of an aging parent or relative as compared to men (8%).[54] Often, women struggle alone to care for elderly family members before seeking help; sometimes disagreements among family members add to the pressures. Caring for elderly parents places stress on a woman: shifts of parent and child relationships, along with additional responsibilities, can leave a woman feeling overwhelmed, discouraged, isolated, angry or depressed.[99] Women may be forced to quit their jobs, use their own vacation or sick leave or take leave without pay to care for elderly relatives. This leaves women with fewer resources and the family burden may negatively impact income, job advancement, and pension for retirement. While leaving a job to provide care so a parent can live outside a facility may sound ideal, often a woman becomes more stressed and more depressed after giving up her job.[99]

Caregiving brings joy and fulfillment to many, but for others, it can be physically and emotionally draining. Furthermore, caregiving may affect health: one half of female caregivers have a chronic health condition and 25% report fair to poor health.[50]

Many activities performed by caregivers are time-consuming: 80% to 90% do housework, shopping, transportation, and run errands.[54] Making meals, insurance paperwork, and choosing a physician are performed by 65% of caregivers; almost 60% administer medication; and more than 40% help with bathing, dressing, and feeding. Twenty-nine percent of women spend more than 40 hours per week and 27% of women spend 11–14 hours per week caring for a sick family member.

Self-management behaviors are critical when taking care of an elderly parent. These behaviors include getting enough rest, short periods of time away from the person with illness, and a support system of friends and professionals. Professional resources, such as an adult daycare center, scheduled home care, support groups, nursing home care or counseling, help the caregiver shoulder the burden. Caregivers also need to identify the emotions being experienced, accept them as part of being human, and find a friend, relative or professional who will listen and help caregivers not dwell on the negativity.[100]

SELF-MANAGEMENT IN VIEW OF RACE/ ETHNICITY, MINORITY STATUS, AND CULTURE

In many cultures, women's natural abilities of loving and nurturing place them as primary caregivers.[54] The expectations of family and intergenerational care giving are greater among minority and immigrant families, but resources and ability to provide such care are diminishing.[16] In a 2001 American Association of Retired Persons (AARP) survey, Asians, Blacks, and Hispanics were more likely to have three generations living under one roof. Further, Asians (42%) were more likely to care for an older relative than Hispanics (34%), Blacks (28%), and Whites (19%).[101]

Lifelong experiences with racism, ageism, minority status, and stigma of different cultural health beliefs influence what self-management behaviors are practiced, or what support systems are used, by minority women. For instance, women of color might feel little personal power because they experience an erosion of self-efficacy or perceptions of control. Some minority women (Hispanic, Asian, Native American, and African American) might choose to react to life or health stresses through religious support, guidance of friends or elders.[102] Some cultures expect women to care for a parent in the home. For women of color who also are poor, using money for

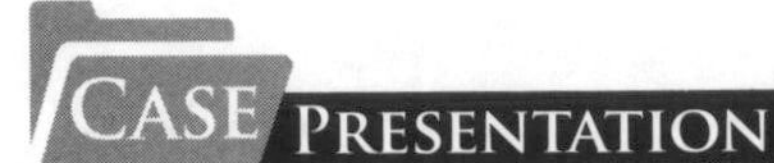

Patient Case: Part 2

With a check from the grain mill, M.S. is able to pay the neighbor but there is not enough money to get her son's new prescriptions filled. M.S. has her son's prescriptions on her mind as she picks up medicine for her parents from the pharmacy close to their home. The pharmacist is a childhood friend of hers and M.S. is happy to find him behind the counter. As M.S. pays for her parents' prescriptions, she comments it would be nice to have an option like Medicaid for children. The pharmacist asks her why and M.S. shyly brings out her son's new prescriptions and says that although she knows this new regimen will help, she cannot afford to fill them at this time.

The pharmacist tells M.S. she has several options to consider: have the doctor change the regimen to something affordable, have the pharmacist contact the drug manufacturers to see if they have a patient assistance program, or apply for the SCHIP program to cover M.S.'s children. The pharmacist gives this information to M.S. in an informational and natural way and says that if she wants more information about the assistance programs, s/he would be glad to download the information from the internet websites and mail it to her.

M.S. thanks the pharmacist and thinks about the conversation on her way to her parents' home. Later that night, after getting her parents' house cleaned and the laundry done, M.S. drives home to talk to her husband. Despite his pride, her husband does feel M.S. ought to follow-up on these options. They both decide to try the first option—calling the doctor to see if there are less expensive drugs available.

The next day after work, M.S. stops at her pharmacy and talks to the new pharmacist. The new pharmacist seems approachable and M.S. feels safe talking to her. M.S. quietly tells the new pharmacist of her son's new prescriptions and the options her pharmacist friend mentioned. The new pharmacist listens, pulls up her son's care plan and reviews his current medications. The new pharmacist agrees with her pharmacist friend's suggestions and asks M.S. if any of the other children have medical concerns. M.S. then mentions her daughter's need for an HPV vaccine and asks the new pharmacist if that is truly necessary at that age. The new pharmacist discusses the importance of preventive care and the benefits related to the vaccine. The new pharmacist looking at M.S.'s tired face, asks if there is any other way she can help. At this kindness, M.S. shares her problems with her menstrual cycle, her immediate family's struggles, and taking care of her parents. For a stoic woman like M.S., this comes out slowly, softly, and with great difficulty.

The new pharmacist connects the preventive care conversation for M.S.'s daughter to the need for preventive care for M.S. and suggests M.S. contact her doctor for a complete physical and reminds her exams are covered by her employer's insurance program. The new pharmacist asks that M.S. write a list of concerns to take in when she has the physical to make sure her irregular menstrual cycle and sleeplessness are not due to something more than stress. The new pharmacist also points out M.S. can care for her family better if she herself is in good health. Also, by taking care of herself, M.S. is teaching her children the importance of self-management.

Asking for help and taking care of her own needs require effort on M.S.'s part. Just discussing her concerns with the new pharmacist gave M.S. hope about her son's medicines and lightened the burden she had been carrying. The next day, the new pharmacist placed a call to the son's physician to find out if he had either drug samples or could switch to lower cost alternative medications. Once she hears from the physician, the new pharmacist will know if she needs to pursue the next options. Her goal is to get the son his asthma medications by the end of this week. In M.S.'s care plan, the new pharmacist notes some additional services (e.g., companion service for parents, physical therapy for her husband, lifestyle changes, and social support network) to improve M.S.'s quality of life and decrease her stress level.

professional help does not make sense; money must be used on basics like food and clothing or transportation.[103] A pharmacist or healthcare provider who understands what women of color experience emotionally and the constant reshuffling of priorities as crises arise, can provide better support, recommendations, and services to each woman's unique situation.

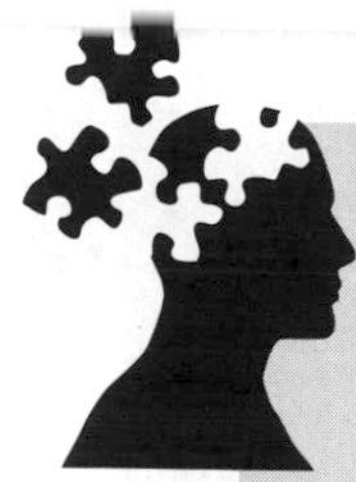

Therapeutic Challenge:

What can be done to help caregivers cope with family health needs, including both nonpharmacologic and pharmacologic therapies/options? What are the expectations within your family and extended family for caregiving? Are there differences based on sex? How do your family's views differ from family views from a different culture?

Summary

Pharmacists and healthcare providers can be an integral figure in the promotion and achievement of a woman's good health. Being healthy is important for women throughout their life—along with balancing family, work, and activities. This chapter provides socioeconomic status-related concepts to help deliver pharmaceutical and healthcare from a broader perspective than strictly biomedical. With better understanding about how the various influences of socioeconomic status, education, family, job, insurance, and public policy play in women's health status, healthcare providers are equipped to identify and suggest more applicable solutions to health problems patients present. Furthermore, the introduction of self-management techniques provides another perspective of behaviors that can promote and keep women healthy. Together the patient and her healthcare team can build a personal strategy that works within the woman's current environment and resources she can implement toward being healthy.

References

Additional content available at
www.ashp.org/womenshealth

4 Psychosocial Factors

Heather E. Dillaway, Ph.D.; Catherine L. Lysack, Ph.D., OT(C)

Learning Objectives

1. Differentiate between biological and psychosocial perspectives and their impacts on women's health.
2. Define gender, gender norms, and a gendered society and explain how each makes a difference in women's health.
3. Explain how women's health can be shaped by gendered roles, gendered communication differences, women's reproductive experiences, body image, and women's experiences of sexuality and intimate relationships.
4. Discuss why women with disabilities, minority status, or low income might face unique experiences of health and illness.
5. Incorporate the unique health concerns of women across their lifespan into therapeutic care plans.

This chapter concentrates on psychosocial issues in women's health. First, this chapter defines a **psychosocial perspective** on women's health and introduces information about how women's health is influenced by the roles women fill, the ways in which women and men understand femininity and masculinity and learn to interact with each other, and the unique reproductive potential of women. Second, this chapter focuses on the major health concerns of women across four major developmental transitions: childhood and adolescence, young adulthood, midlife, and late life. Topics discussed are wide ranging and include beauty norms and body image, women as nurturers and caregivers, unique characteristics of women in paid work and healthcare settings, and physical frailty and economic vulnerability. The chapter includes a table with suggestions for how women, pharmacists, and other healthcare providers can work to improve and advocate for women's health, well-being, and healing.

The Role of Gender and the Social Environment in Shaping Women's Health

Gender forms the backdrop for all of the psychosocial issues discussed in this chapter. *Gender* refers to the social and psychological traits and behaviors that are expected of women and men because of the ideas that are attached to their biological sex.[1] Often the terms *sex* and *gender* are used interchangeably, but *gender* refers to social ideas and expectations about individuals' characteristics (femininity or masculinity), not individuals' biological differences (female or male). Gender is the result of social forces and expectations, and does not flow inherently from being born with a particular set of chromosomes. For instance, there is nothing in the human genetic code that should predispose women to wearing makeup and a dress while men wear a suit and tie. Similarly, why should women be expected to choose teaching and nursing as professions instead of engineering, economics, or physics?[2,3]

Like most countries, the U.S. is a **gendered society.** This means that girls are, from the minute they are born, taught to think and act in particular ways, and grow up having very different experiences than boys because of the ways in which they are socialized.[1] Parents will dress their girls in pink and give them dolls to play with while the boys are dressed in blue and given toy trucks. These differences persist beyond infancy and childhood. Girls and women are treated differently than boys and men by parents, teachers, coworkers, bosses, and healthcare providers, and they are exposed to very different messages. For example, why do so many people still think that mothers are the most appropriate parent to stay home and care for young children, even when the father has the option of paid parental leave?[4-7]

CASE PRESENTATION

Patient Case: Part 1

C.V. (Hispanic professional woman, age 54 years) is juggling significant work and family responsibilities. A single mother of two after her husband died in the Desert Storm war, she is also the primary caregiver for her elderly father. Caring for her family is a high priority for C.V. At work, she is a successful manager at an insurance company, but she would like to further her education and find a more rewarding job that pays more and offers more flexibility. C.V.'s boss is a career woman with no children, and C.V. feels her boss doesn't understand her need to put her family first. She also wonders if her boss views choices about work and family balance differently because of ethnicity differences. Although C.V. would love to explore other career options, she feels insecure and trapped by time. She takes shortcuts with her eating habits and ignores her exercise routine to devote what little time she has to her son's basketball games and her daughter's dance recitals. She recently moved her 72-year-old father into a nursing facility and visits him several times a week to help him adjust; this too cuts into C.V.'s time for herself. In the past few months, she has had trouble sleeping, a problem she attributes to the stresses related to juggling her work and family roles. In the past year, she realizes that she may be starting menopause; her insomnia is sometimes caused by night sweats. She also recognizes she may have early signs of osteoporosis, like her late mother. She is working hard to alter her diet and adhere to her physician's recommendations about more exercise, calcium, and vitamin D, knowing her family needs her and feeling she needs to be healthy for them. Prioritizing her own health needs is hard.

Is it because society believes women make better caregivers than men?[8-10] Do we have scientific evidence of this, or is it simply a gender misperception?

The idea of gender is important to discussions of health because gender is directly related to one's rights and privileges relative to others. The reality of gender is that in many situations, men enjoy more power and opportunity than women, just like straight men and women have more power and opportunity than persons who are gay, lesbian, and transgendered.[1,8,11] And because science now shows that one's opportunities and privileges can have a cumulative effect on one's health and illness across the lifespan, it is critical to appreciate how this occurs.[12-14]

The effects of gender and living in a gendered society have both direct and indirect effects on women's and men's health. For example, women are socialized to put others' needs before their own.[6,7,15] Girls and women are also socialized to take fewer risks than boys and men socially, physically, and economically.[14,16] Women might eventually put their mental and physical health at risk if they feel powerless to change their jobs or other aspects of their lives that are dissatisfying to them. Over the long term, these stressors will exert a negative effect and limit women's ability to be healthy and be a role model for their families. If women and men realize how they are influenced by the social world, they can begin to understand the psychosocial processes by which gender, **gender norms,** and gender experiences affect health, well-being, and healing.

GENDER ROLES

As noted and discussed in the preceding chapters, women are assigned particular roles in society. First and foremost, women are defined as nurturers and caregivers and are given primary responsibility for raising children, tending to partners' emotional needs, and caring for elderly parents.[17,18] Adult women can be caring for as many as three different generations at the same time: their own minor children, their husbands, and their ailing parents and husband's parents. Daughters outnumber sons three to one as the main caregivers of elderly parents. Some researchers refer to these women as the **sandwich generation.**[17,18] The responsibility of caregiving is generally placed on women because both men and women believe women are good nurturers, yet the constant nature of caregiving work and the multiple caregiving activities that women hold can mean that women are attentive to others' health needs to the detriment of their own. Mothers, for instance, schedule regular doctor's appointments for children and aging parents yet ignore their own health needs.[17,19] Caregiving activities can be physically harmful too.[19] For instance, women can acquire physical injuries from lifting and providing care to aging parents.[20] Prioritizing others' needs over their own also leaves women isolated from social support networks (i.e., friends, exercise groups, meetings with coworkers after work hours), an important means by which stress is diminished.[7,21]

In addition to caregiving responsibilities, the majority of women and mothers are in the labor force at least part-time.[22] Women also tend to be employed in service sector jobs (e.g., telecommunications, health services, food services, banking, reception and clerical work, and retail and sales). The concept of gender reasserts itself here because many of these jobs are considered more suitable for women because society defines women as naturally more sensitive, more helpful, and better listeners than men.[1,23] Unfortunately, these jobs tend to hold less prestige and power, and thus have fewer economic benefits (e.g., lower salary, fewer vacation days and paid leave, poorer health insurance).[8] Second, regardless of what job a woman has, female employees more often than male employees are expected to engage in **emotional work** to make other coworkers and clients/customers feel more comfortable (that is, continually displaying positive affect and responding to customer/client emotions but suppressing one's own).[8,15]

Paid workplaces reflect the fact that the majority of workers are men, rendering women's unique needs (e.g., during pregnancy or breast-feeding, for example) problematic.[24,25] This challenge exists in the boardrooms of big city law firms and corporations just as it does in the kitchens of rural truck stops; many women feel they are relegated to second-class status after men. Women's over-representation in low-quality jobs and the expectation that they put the needs of others above their own negatively affects their health and well-being.[26] Women in minimum-wage service jobs are also at a significant disadvantage when it comes to purchasing the most nutritious food, finding a job at which their employer provides a healthy workplace, and living in a safe and secure (more expensive) neighborhood. Years of research shows that chronic exposure to these types of environmental challenges with an inherently social dimension has significant negative and lasting consequences for the health of individuals and society as a whole.[12,13,27,28] New clinical research is even beginning to show how gender-related social disadvantage is passed on from generation to generation through low-birth-weight babies, who are in turn disadvantaged vis-à-vis a range of important health outcomes.[29] In this way, gender is not just important for social reasons; these social reasons are changing people's basic physiology and their ability to secure optimal health.

Gender and the social determinants of health are not only an issue for women with low socioeconomic status. Challenges to good health and well-being are present, although different, for women of higher socioeconomic status. For instance, the pressures of climbing the corporate ladder and achieving a certain lifestyle can take a toll on health. Lack of balance is a common complaint of many women today as they work to juggle work and other life priorities.[30] Having to be in a work environment in which there are few women (e.g., an executive boardroom) also means that a woman is in the spotlight and under pressure more often. Skyrocketing rates of stress-related illnesses like anxiety and depression—but also cardiovascular disease and high blood pressure in both men and women—are evidence of these pressures. Excess production of the hormone cortisol is thought to be the mechanism for these negative conditions.[12] Further, although financial resources can pay for many things that help to offset the stressors women confront, money cannot erase all work-related or family-related stressors. Stress is at the root of many physical and mental health conditions, and stress can require medical and pharmaceutical interventions.[31]

THE WORLD HEALTH ORGANIZATION'S COMMISSION ON SOCIAL DETERMINANTS OF HEALTH

The World Health Organization (WHO)'s Commission on Social Determinants of Health suggests that "being a man or a woman has a significant impact on health, as a result of both biological and gender-related differences."[13] Some psychosocial factors that inhibit women's health, according to WHO, include "unequal power relationships between men and women; social norms that decrease education and paid employment opportunities; an exclusive focus on women's reproductive roles; and potential or actual experience of physical, sexual and emotional violence."[13] WHO suggests that women's health can be improved by ensuring things like fair and decent employment for both women and men.[13] WHO works with organizations around the world to improve gender-related health. For instance, since 1995, WHO has teamed with numerous civil rights, governmental, and consumer organizations and workers' unions to help stop the spread of sweatshop industries across the world, thus helping many low-paid workers (quite often women and children) escape terrible working conditions.[13]

GENDERED COMMUNICATION

Women and men learn to communicate differently from birth, and some scholars go so far as to say that women and men have been misunderstanding each

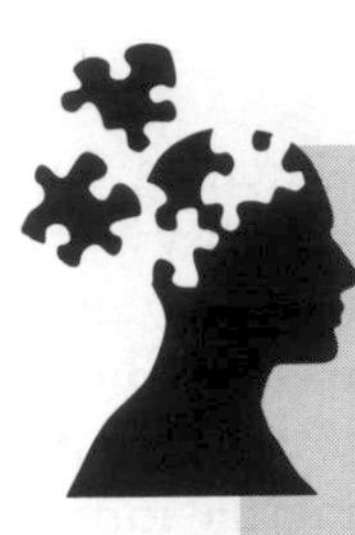

Therapeutic Challenge:

How does gendered communication influence patients' discussions with healthcare providers about their medications (e.g., understanding of patient education, asking of questions)?

other and talking at cross-purposes for generations.[23] Research shows that men talk to report or give information.[23] Men talk about things—business, food, sports—rather than people. Men convey facts and focus on solving problems. Women, on the other hand, talk to get information and gain rapport.[23] Women convey feelings and details that men do not learn to share. Women are quicker to ask for and accept help, and they attempt to cooperate in conversation. These differences can lead to misunderstanding and conflict between the genders within social or intimate relationships and in professional and medical settings. Women talk more within intimate relationships than men, for instance, and desire to share feelings and life's details more than men do. Yet, in public or professional settings, men tend to talk more, as well as interrupt and gain back the floor more than women. Women are sometimes hesitant in public and professional situations to go against someone else's ideas or arguments. Frequently, women take a less active role in group meetings at work and remain more submissive than men in one-on-one meetings with bosses, doctors, and others in powerful positions.[32]

More women are now in business and professions like medicine, engineering, and pharmacy than ever before. The presence of women has transformed the contemporary workplace as employers and employees alike realize how the style of communication used by many women can be advantageous to the bottom line of the organization.[33] Communication in the healthcare environment is also becoming more attuned to gender differences, although difficulties are still present.[8,32] For example, communication difficulties between women and their doctors affect women's access to healthcare treatment as well as their satisfaction with care received. Women are not always willing to interrupt their doctor, especially a male doctor, to assert their own opinion about a health concern or to extend a doctor's visit in order to ask another question about their health and disclose another symptom.[8,32] When women disclose symptoms or other information about their health conditions, they often describe them in different and more negative terms than men, including more feelings and details in the conversation than doctors expect to hear.[34] In these situations, doctors sometimes assume women are just complaining and do not have real symptoms.[8] This can result in misdiagnosis or a protracted period before diagnosis, as some male doctors might dismiss or trivialize women's concerns. Misinterpretations sometimes lead to missed opportunities to respond to female patients' fears and concerns. Doctors and other healthcare providers are even less likely to understand women's portrayal of symptoms when talking to women of different race, ethnic, social-class, and age groups, as each group might have a different way of phrasing their descriptions of symptoms or relating to people in positions of power. Within hospital settings, this often means that female patients often gain greater rapport with nurses than doctors.[9] These communication difficulties have driven many women to find a doctor and other healthcare providers who are also women. As more women enter the health professions, this is becoming easier to do.

When women are misunderstood by intimate partners, coworkers, bosses, and healthcare providers, their physical and mental health suffers. Still, the fact that women are good listeners and are more willing to ask for and accept help means that they may be easier to educate and help than male patients. As is shown in Table 4-1, there are many ways in which pharmacists and other healthcare professionals can remind women to take care of themselves and start solving their own health problems or conditions.[17,35-42] Further, because women are apt to value intimate relationships, they are receptive to developing longer-term relationships with all their healthcare providers. These relationships begin through conversations that bring knowledge and attention to specific women's health issues. The following examples show how healthcare providers, including pharmacists, might begin to develop relationships with their female patients and help individual women with gendered health issues:

- Sponsor "Back to School" events at community pharmacies near high schools and colleges that include in-store education materials focused on sexually transmitted diseases and birth control.
- Partner with a hospital or local doctor's office to hold free seminars on emotional well-being.

Table 4-1. Key Psychosocial Health Issues and Solutions Across Women's Life Stages[a]

Life Stage	Significant Psychosocial Health Issues	Activities and Web Resources for Healthier Living
Childhood and Adolescence		
Body Image, Healthy Weight	53% of American girls are "unhappy with their bodies"; this grows to 78% by the time girls reach age 17.[35] **http://www.mediafamily.org/facts/facts_mediaeffect.shtml** The average adult dress size in the U.S. is now a size 12, but 98% of fashion models are thinner than this.[36] **http://www.empoweredparents.com/mini/t4.htm**	Utilize programs like the Dove Campaign for Real Beauty, which is one example of the cosmetic's industry effort to challenge consumers to think about the unrealistic images of female beauty and pressures to be something different than "real." **http://www.campaignforrealbeauty.com/home.asp** Encourage women to feel positively about their bodies. **http://www.womenshealth.gov/bodyimage/** Emphasize healthy eating guides **http://www.health.gov/dietaryguidelines/**
Young Womanhood		
Exercise	Women's top reason for not exercising is that they are too busy taking care of others to take care of themselves.[37] **http://www.scienceblog.com/community/older/2003/G/20035504.html**	Use national holidays and health awareness days (e.g., Mother's Day, Osteoporosis Prevention Day) to strengthen public education efforts by linking with local fitness and healthy living events going on in the community (e.g., walking or running to prevent breast cancer, dragon boat races, etc.). Use every opportunity to communicate healthy lifestyle behaviors (e.g., proper nutrition, exercise, smoking cessation, and alcohol use limits). **http://www.commonwealthfund.org/publications/publications_show.htm?doc_id=221554**
Violence	Two thirds of all rape and sexual assaults are committed by men whom the female victims know.[38] **http://mchb.hrsa.gov/whusa_06/**	Ask for and use walk-to-car programs on campus and elsewhere. Enroll in a self-defense course. Partner with women's and citizens' group to improve public education and change workplace policies and society's laws. Screen for intimate partner violence in healthcare settings. **http://www.cdc.gov/NCIPC/pub-res/ipv_and_sv_screening.htm**
Mental Health	Depression affects twice as many women as men, yet only half of all women who report serious psychological distress receive any type of treatment or counseling.[38] **http://mchb.hrsa.gov/whusa_06/**	Educate women on how normal it can be to have a range of emotions and moods, especially when going through major life transitions (e.g., geographical moves, school changes, job changes, entry into motherhood, marriage, divorce, children's exit from the homes, or death of a loved one). Also, give women information about when to seek help for these feelings. Partner with pharmacies, pharmaceutical companies, local doctor's offices, and hospitals to offer free seminars on emotional well-being and strategies for maintaining a healthy personal outlook. **http://www.womenshealth.gov/pub/** **http://www.nlm.nih.gov/medlineplus/mentalhealth.html** **http://mentalhealth.about.com/**

(*Continued on next page*)

Life Stage	Significant Psychosocial Health Issues	Activities and Web Resources for Healthier Living
Midlife/Middle Age		
Divorce	In 2000, for example, more than 3 million women ages 45 to 54 years and another 1.8 million women ages 55 to 64 years were divorced.[17,39] **http://www.census.gov/prod/2004pubs/p20-553.pdf**	Educate women through pamphlets and posters about their rights in a divorce, and the common issues that arise in a divorce (e.g., alimony and child support, custody and visitation, property division). **http://www.divorcenet.com/** **http://www.womansdivorce.com/** Encourage women to be concerned about their economic futures, especially when going through major life changes such as divorce. **http://www.wiserwomen.org/portal/**
Income	Women earn only 75% of what men earn.[40] **http://www.womensmedia.com/new/Lips-Hilary-gender-wage-gap.shtml**	Educate and advocate within one's profession regarding gender wage gaps and leadership positions in higher education and professional associations. **http://www.theannals.com/cgi/content/full/40/5/952** Remind women that they can advocate for themselves, in that they can ask for raises and promotions and negotiate higher salaries for themselves at the time of hire.
Older Women		
Poverty	Retired women are twice as likely to be poor as retired men.[41,42] **http://escholarship.bc.edu/retirement_papers/13**	Encourage women to learn more about the financial impact of retirement, their Medicare coverage, etc. **http://www.wiserwomen.org/pdf_files/ebook/completeebook.pdf** Assist women to find resources such as free legal aid, a local cash assistance office, food banks, soup kitchens, thrift shops and secondhand stores, and housing shelters. Put together a list of resources for impoverished women, and post these lists in plain sight. Volunteer a few hours of your time at a local food bank, soup kitchen, thrift store, shelter, or indigent care clinic or pharmacy.
Community Involvement	Women of all ages can volunteer their time to social causes. There are also plenty of organizations that work to solve many of the psychosocial problems highlighted in this chapter, and individuals can participate in any of these efforts to help women. **www.DoSomething.org/volunteer** **www.volunteermatch.org**	Volunteer, either locally or globally, and receive a tremendous boost to physical and mental health, improve self-esteem, and receive greater social support. **http://senior-leisure-activities.suite101.com/article.cfm/opportunities_for_active_seniors**

[a]Websites accessed March 8, 2009.

- Distribute pamphlets during National Osteoporosis Prevention Week that include information about fitness and healthy eating, in addition to advertisements about calcium and vitamin D supplements.
- Cooperate with a local seniors' health advocacy organization to cosponsor distribution of coupons for bone density screenings for low-income women.

A Broad Understanding of Women's Health and Reproduction

Women's health is sometimes considered equivalent to **reproductive health** because women's biological capacities to reproduce (e.g., the ability to conceive, carry a baby to term, and birth a baby) still tend to be used to define who women are.[16] As this book shows, women's health includes much more, including but not limited to cardiovascular health, bone and joint health, physical and cognitive function, and emotional well-being. Reproductive health is also more complex than just the experience of conception, pregnancy, and childbirth. The other reasons why women might go to a women's health clinic, for example, must be considered. Women's reproductive health comprises an entire range of experiences and issues, including concerns about sexually transmitted diseases and infections, fear of pregnancy after a missed dose of an oral contraceptive, postpartum depression, mood swings and abdominal cramps related to menstrual cycles, worries about being able to conceive a child and how in vitro fertilization might work, concerns about a family history of breast cancer, discomfort with male physicians who perform Papanicolaou (Pap) and other gynecologic tests, menstrual irregularity on the early stages of menopause, and vaginal discomfort at any age. Although continued advancements in the medical sciences can improve the treatment of women's major health concerns, both emotional and physical health concerns and consequences will arise with every one of the experiences and decisions above.

PSYCHOSOCIAL DIMENSIONS OF WOMEN'S REPRODUCTIVE HEALTH

While most reproductive processes or experiences involve physical health considerations, they also include some impact on emotional health. The impact on women's emotional health is often a result of psychosocial issues. The extreme emotional toll that infertility problems and treatments have on women, for instance, is partially created by societal norms that suggest to women that motherhood is mandatory.[6,43,44] In recent times, changing social norms are allowing women the choice to be childless without stigma and, similarly, to feel that being an adoptive mother is just as legitimate and personally fulfilling as having one's own biological child. Women's perceptions and social experiences of reproductive events and processes can be as diverse as the women themselves. Even though reproductive processes (e.g., menstrual periods, sexual episodes) are part of everyday life, women sometimes do experience additional emotional pressures because of the very existence of their reproductive capacities and/or because of social definitions of these capacities. For instance, gender norms suggest to women and men that women should have the primary responsibility to use contraception, not men.[45] Women are also expected to hide the evidence of normal reproductive processes like menstruation, breast-feeding, and menopause.[46,47] Social science research has been important here, documenting how some men do not understand women's menstrual cycles or their menstrual and premenstrual symptoms. Research has even shown how uncomfortable men are viewing feminine hygiene products in stores and in advertising.[47] Because of men's expectations and attitudes, women learn to control their reproductive bodies so they appear "normal" to men at all times, and men as well as other women do not see what they don't want to. Pressures to engage in these normalizing behaviors take a toll on emotional and physical well-being. For example, women of varying ages can become involved in excessive hygiene routines to mask menstruation (e.g., shaving or waxing, douching, increased showering or washing, wearing more perfume or body spray) or menopause (e.g., dressing in layers or changing clothes to hide the evidence of sweating, applying deodorant multiple times a day). New mothers may engage in extremely strict dieting behaviors as they fight to lose their baby weight, minimizing nutrients in the breast milk, both of which can affect their health in negative ways. Reproductive health is often assumed to be just a private concern of women, but it is a public concern that needs greater attention from healthcare providers.[48] Pharmacists and other healthcare providers could step into the above scenarios fairly easily to make sure women understand the side effects of certain routines, dieting aids, or hygiene products and to ensure that women know a bit more about what is normal during these reproductive **life stages**.

WOMEN'S SEXUALITY AND INTIMATE RELATIONSHIPS

Throughout history, social norms have shaped how women should think and behave sexually and in intimate relationships.[49] Until very recently, women have been seen as procreative beings and were not supposed to be desirous of sex for themselves, or even have their own sexual identities. Women have also been held responsible over time for keeping men happy within heterosexual relationships, with diminished attention paid to their own sexual desires, behaviors, or identities. Today, women still face considerable pressure as they negotiate gendered ideas about how they should act and think about sexual desire, behavior, relationships, and themselves as sexual beings. For instance, social norms suggest to women that they should be sexy in their physical appearance, sexually available but not too available, and desirous but not too desirous.[50,51] Some women also feel pressure to be in committed relationships because being single is not acceptable for women, especially as they age.[52] Premenopausal women must always deal with the threat of pregnancy when they do engage in sexual activity. Yet, norms are changing, opening up spaces for women to define their own sexual identities and be much more assertive and independent in their sexual encounters. Television shows like *Friends* and *Sex in the City,* for example, have challenged the way society views women and their sexuality. Female characters on these programs are strong, successful, independent, smart, and sexy, and they encourage contemporary changes in social mores. These women are not supposed to be victims of men; rather, they are self-reliant and express their sexual desires openly and unapologetically.

Times are changing, and women are claiming their place beside men as just as deserving of a sexual identity and sexual pleasure.[47] Nowhere is this more evident than in advertising that targets older couples. Perhaps the aging of the baby boomers can be credited with this effect. Advertisements for Viagra®, Cialis®, and K-Y® Yours + Mine® for example, are breaking down long-held societal views that older adults are not sexually active. In some commercials, women are asking their men to seek erectile dysfunction medications. Data show that postmenopausal women, far from being postsex, are actually more sexually active and obtaining more enjoyment from sex because the fear of pregnancy is gone.[53]

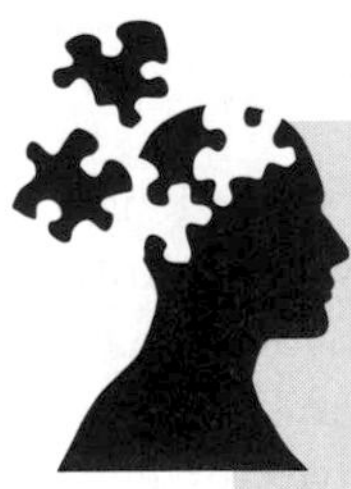

Therapeutic Challenge:

How can healthcare professionals, including pharmacists, help individual women think about their reproductive and sexual health in positive ways?

ADDITIONAL ISSUES

Race and ethnic differences are important in determining how psychosocial stressors affect women's reproductive health and sexuality, even though these differences are minimally discussed in this chapter. For instance, because of access issues, communication problems, and distrust of medical institutions, women of color are more likely to receive late diagnosis for reproductive diseases for which white women might normally receive early treatment.[8,54,55] Because of a legacy of discrimination in the U.S. within the healthcare system (e.g., the Tuskegee Syphilis Study involving black men and rampant sterilization of minority women in the early to mid 1900s), black women in particular still distrust reproductive healthcare providers.[8,11] More generally, women of color also often lack access to educational materials about normal reproduction as well as a wide range of different reproductive healthcare options because of a lack of good health insurance and quality healthcare providers in their area.[8,11,53] Finally, immigrant women of color who speak English as a second language can confront even greater communication problems and access issues, and may therefore be at even greater biopsychosocial health risks as a result.[8,56] To read more on the issues of ethnicity and healthcare, please refer to Chapter 2: Race, Ethnic, and Religious Issues.

Lesbian and bisexual women also face unique reproductive concerns as they attempt to access technologies that give them the potential for biological motherhood.[8,57-59] It is important to keep in mind the variety of reproductive and sexuality experiences created as a result of the identity differences among women and, therefore, the different health needs that individual groups of women might have. Chapter 5: Issues in Lesbian, Bisexual, and Transgender Healthcare illustrates some of these points further.

Women have unique experiences in this gendered world that can eventually affect their emotional and physical health. The above examples of women's gendered roles, communication differences between women and men, influence of cultural characteristics, and how women's health goes beyond a narrow definition of reproductive health experiences underscore the importance of attending to the social expectations and desires of woman at all ages. A sense of control, self-efficacy, and empowerment are as positively linked to health-promoting behaviors as stress and powerlessness are linked to unhealthy activities and routines.

Common Psychosocial Issues at Different Life-Course Stages

The first section of the chapter identified and described specific stressors on women that are caused by the fact that women live in a gendered society. This second section turns to key health concerns that women experience at different ages and life stages and highlights the psychosocial dimensions of these concerns that deserve increased attention by healthcare professionals.

FEMALE CHILDHOOD AND ADOLESCENCE

Childhood and adolescence—that is, youth—is generally considered a time of health, innocence, and freedom. Although this is true to a certain extent, this life stage is also fraught with unique challenges related to human development (physiological and psychological) and, therefore, health risks. Especially in adolescence (typically defined as a period of life ranging from age 12 to 19 years old), a multitude of emotional and physical well-being issues arise.[17] For instance, as adolescent girls gain independence from the home and from parents, they are at greater risk of substance abuse (especially smoking), motor vehicle injuries, sports injuries, emotional bullying (a growing problem among girls as well as boys), and physical fights or other violence in school settings.

Human personality is largely shaped during childhood and adolescence.[8,17,47] Self-confidence, self-esteem, and social assertiveness, for example, are critical components of development. Because of the uncertainty of life at this stage, adolescents may experience emotional health problems and identity issues, which can lead to low self-esteem, depression, and, in extreme cases, suicide. By age 13 years, more than twice as many girls as boys are depressed, a proportion that persists into adulthood.[60] Research has also shown that girls have a tendency to form cliques, which can be a major source of peer pressure on girls. Some experts believe the pressure to conform to standards of dress and behavior has grown over the last few decades and that girls' cliques can be as great a force for negative self-image as boys' bullying is for boys. These pressures take a significant toll. Suicide is the third leading cause of adolescent death, behind only accidents and homicides.[17] Although boys are more likely than girls to succeed in suicide attempts (perhaps because they tend to use more lethal methods), girls think about and attempt suicide about twice as often as boys.[61] On this issue alone there are incredible opportunities to educate and talk to girls about emotional well-being and self-esteem, and all healthcare providers, including pharmacists, are well suited to join in these conversations.

Contributing to these differences in self-image and self-worth is the fact that girls must come to terms with a changing and maturing body as puberty occurs. Menarche represents an important transition for girls, but it changes their physical appearance and bodily awareness, which can be quite life altering. Research shows that around puberty, girls realize that they are sexual beings and that others are now gazing on their physical bodies.[62] The risk for sexual assault and harassment increases at this time, and girls must quickly learn how to deal with boys and men and their interactions regarding their bodies.

Additionally, learning about sexual intercourse, sexual intimacy, contraception, and the threat of pregnancy can put significant pressures on girls. The combination of biological readiness, increased sex drive, and willingness to take risks can put adolescents in risky sexual situations, leading to teenage pregnancy and sexually transmitted diseases.[17] On the flip side, girls can be educated quite quickly on how to have positive experiences about their growing sexuality. Issues of privacy, appropriate sex education, and the maturity of adolescents to make informed decisions about their health come to the fore. In addition, some sexually active adolescent girls want to use birth control and do so without their parent's knowledge. How should the healthcare professional respond when an adolescent girl requests contraceptives? Who should have the authority to make such health-related decisions for adolescents, and based on what criteria? These are important questions for all healthcare providers, including pharmacists.

A related psychosocial issue is the role that beauty norms and a culture of thinness play in young women's attitudes and decision making in the context of their health. Much research suggests that women are defined—and their attitudes are shaped by—their physical appearance. In the U.S., researchers have argued that the contemporary standard for female beauty dictates slenderness/thinness, youth, whiteness, upper-class status, and "no noticeable physical imperfections or disabilities."[50] Among these dictates, a youthful thin appearance is probably the most important. Surprising to some is the fact that research shows that young girls are keenly aware of these pressures and find ways to curb weight gain early on, such as beginning to smoke around age 12 or 13 years, binging and purging, dieting, and using laxatives.[17,47] Girls learn at a young age that their identity is closely linked to their physical appearance. There is evidence, for example, that middle school and high school girls often discuss their appearances first when asked what they like or dislike most about themselves, whereas their male counterparts cite their talents or abilities.[63]

In response to this societal problem, healthcare professionals have an important opportunity to become engaged in education and awareness campaigns. Ways to engage in safe dieting and healthy exercise need to be encouraged, and young women need to be reminded not to abuse over-the-counter health and beauty aids, laxatives, or weight loss or dieting aids in order to lose weight. Adolescents may be more likely to listen to a healthcare provider, such as pharmacist, than their parents, teachers, or counselors about this important issue. Thus, in-store posters, pamphlets, and friendly reminders to eat, exercise, and use over-the-counter drugs in healthy ways could go a long way to promote female adolescent health.

YOUNG WOMANHOOD

The pressure to conform to society's ideals of feminine beauty is just as strong in young adulthood. Young women are at their reproductive peak in their 20s and early 30s.[64] Men, too, are at their physical and sexual prime, and a great deal of men's attention to women reflects this. The psychosocial dimensions of what it means to be beautiful and attractive to the opposite sex are in full display, and therefore much of what was discussed in the previous section still holds true here. The cosmetics industry and media images once again come to the fore. Women's magazines tend to showcase clothing that is a size 0 or size 2 when the average female body is a size 12 or even size 14.[8,36,46,50] Women's magazines also tend to define female beauty in specific ways: for example, flawless white skin, a perfect white smile, and large round breasts. The image does not meet reality, and women who fall short of this artificial image feel it necessary to spend exorbitant amounts of money, time, and emotional energy on their physical bodies.[46,47,50,65,66]

Excessive dieting, cosmetic surgery, and expensive fitness regimens are all examples of women's efforts to recreate their bodies to fit gendered beauty standards. A recent press release from the American Academy of Cosmetic Surgery reports that even with a small increase in the number of male patients, 79% of patients undergoing surgery between 2002 and 2006 were women.[67] These behaviors are often physically and emotionally stressful, not to mention expensive, and they carry serious physical health risks. Inadequate government regulation in the cosmetic surgery industry, for example, is thought to be a factor in unacceptable infection and mortality rates.

Social pressures women feel are also implicated in the rates of eating disorders among women.[8,46,50] Anorexia and bulimia are increasing as women are confronted by strict norms of thinness.[8,50,68] As explained in Chapter 31: Nutrition and Eating Disorders, these disorders stem directly from a general cultural norm of excessive female dieting in the face of these beauty norms. Research has shown that "women's self-esteem and happiness are significantly associated with their physical appearance; no relationship exists for men as a group."[50]

Campaigns by healthcare providers can help raise public awareness of these issues by engaging in education campaigns (as mentioned in the last section) and by working diligently one on one with their patients. In addition, in pharmacy settings, a pharmacist must be alert to unusual numbers of diet products being purchased by girls or young women, because

THE DOVE® CAMPAIGN FOR REAL WOMEN

In 2004, Dove® launched its Campaign for Real Beauty and Self-Esteem Fund, a global effort by this hygiene product company to "make more women feel beautiful every day by widening stereotypical views of beauty."[69] Part of this long-term campaign includes the use of real women, not professional models, of all shapes, sizes, races, and ages in advertisements for Dove® products. Most of these advertisements also include excerpts from actual interviews with women about their bodies in an attempt to challenge society's beauty ideals and a narrow one-size-fits-all standard. In 2007, Dove® teamed up with the entertainment industry to provide girls with a reality check and help them realize that the women they see on television and in movies represent an unrealistic standard.[69] Part of this latter campaign is providing self-esteem workshops and online tools for mothers and daughters to help girls build self-esteem. Regardless of the critiques of the Dove® campaign, any general attempt to help girls think more positively about their bodies is laudable.

this may signal an eating disorder. Likewise, unusual numbers of prescriptions for pain medication and sleep aids may signal a major undiagnosed life stressor in need of professional medical attention.

Psychosocial dimensions of women's health are also evident in situations in which young adult and midlife women undertake well-advised medical treatments and interventions. Consider the situation of mastectomy after breast cancer. Women who lose a breast often report feeling like they are "less of a woman" with the loss of their breast. The experience of losing a breast appears to strike at the heart of what it means to be a woman. Even when breast prostheses are adopted and people do not know of the loss of this part of the woman's body, some women report a profound feeling that they are "damaged goods" and less acceptable to their significant other than before, when they were "whole."[70] Research documents high depression rates among women with concerns about their physical appearance meeting societal and gender norms.[47,50]

Other health risks related to personal security (considered by many to be a fundamental human right) usually start in young adulthood and have psychosocial dimensions as well as physical trauma and sequelae. Statistics show that nearly one third of American women report being physically or sexually abused by a boyfriend or husband at some point in their lives.[71] Abuse can include threats, the destruction of property, rape, murder, emotional cruelty, fondling/grabbing, restriction of behavior, obscene phone calls, and stalking/harassing behavior.[8] In 2001, women accounted for 85% of victims of intimate partner violence.[71] Feminist scholars suggest that the prevalence of **violence against women** is directly related to the fact that our society condones men's power and control over women.[8]

Unfortunately, abuse and violence are topics that are neither frequently discussed nor dealt with. There is a stigma attached to abuse, just as there is a stigma attached to mental illness. Many women think abuse "only happens to someone else . . . it won't happen to me." Yet the facts suggest that violence and abuse can affect all women at all ages and levels of socioeconomic status. According to a research report by the American Association of University Women Educational Foundation, nearly two thirds (62%) of the 2000 college students they surveyed in 2005 said they had been subjected to **sexual harassment** while at college.[72] Most of the students experienced noncontact forms of harassment, such as crude jokes, remarks, and gestures, but nearly one third said the harassment involved physical contact. Although a growing number of women also harass their peers, two thirds of harassers are men.[73]

The greatest barrier to confronting violence and abuse is a general societal complacency about stopping this violence. The number-one reason that sexual harassment and abuse are not reported to the authorities is that women feel afraid that they will not be believed, and the threat of repeated violence keeps them silent.[73] Many women will try to cope with their psychological pain in private by using alcohol and drugs and misusing over-the-counter and prescription medications.

Solutions exist to address many of these problems. Because women frequently are embarrassed or afraid to report violence against them, healthcare and other professionals, such as teachers and workplace supervisors, have become proactive to ask about personal safety. They need to not only be far more alert to this issue but prepared to act. Grade school teachers are now better trained to identify and report suspected child abuse. College health centers have counseling and educational awareness campaigns related to date rape and other sexual abuses. More women's shelters and other protective services provide support groups, legal services, and housing opportunities for women who have been abused than in the past. Still, pharmacists, like all other healthcare professionals, must be aware that feelings of shame and social exclusion after abuse and violence can be profound, and women will not find disclosure of abuse easy. At the patient-pharmacist level, this means being vigilant to signs of violence, abuse, depression, and substance abuse and learning to develop sufficient rapport and communication skills to be effective healthcare providers.

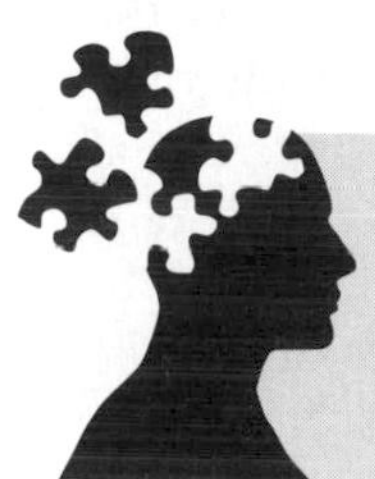

Therapeutic Challenge:

What local and state services can you suggest to a patient who has experienced date rape or other forms of sexual harassment?

MIDLIFE HEALTH AND IDENTITY

Midlife has been described recently as the "last uncharted territory" of the life course.[74] Researchers have concentrated on understanding childhood, adolescence, and, more recently, old age, but the middle years have been virtually ignored, even though they compose the longest part of the lifespan.[74] Perhaps this is because, in a gendered society, women are simply seen to be continuing what they were doing in younger womanhood and nothing more. Yet, by midlife (roughly 40 through 65 years of age), some women will be advancing in their jobs, accepting job promotions that take them and their families across the country or the world. Other women may be finished raising their children and looking forward to a new phase of life with greater personal autonomy. Some women may go through divorce and find themselves single and dating again in their 50s. Others may find intimate partners for the first time at midlife; some may just be beginning their families after successful careers. Some even find themselves actively raising and supporting grandchildren. These role changes, dependent on women's ability to fulfill them, can have either a significant positive or negative impact on their health and well-being. Important physical changes also occur at midlife that have psychosocial dimensions.

As Chapter 32: Overweight and Obesity explains, obesity not only increases for women in adulthood and middle age as the physiology of women's bodies change, but also as they prioritize others' needs over their own and forgo their own nutrition and exercise.[15,17-19,74-76] Some suggest that the speeding up of work and family life coupled with tendency toward sedentary pastimes (e.g., watching TV) is the cause of obesity. Midlife is also the time when both men and women begin to experience some physical wear and tear related to age. Chronic physical health conditions can emerge at this life stage. Women tend to have a higher likelihood of multiple chronic conditions than men.[8,16] Cardiovascular disease, arthritis, diabetes, some bowel diseases, and depression all tend to emerge or become more serious in middle age.[8,73,77-79]

At midlife, women will also experience the onset of reproductive aging or menopause (see Chapter 17: Menopause). Historically, women viewed menopause negatively, as a time of loss of their reproductive capacity. Coinciding as it often did with the departure of children, some women would experience the empty-nest syndrome, a loss of their mothering role as children grew up and left home. Menopause can pose some troublesome symptoms for some women, but there are remedies for these symptoms that include hormone therapy and other pharmacologic treatments, as well as more natural alternatives like herbal teas and a variety of natural supplements and alternative medicines (see Chapter 17: Menopause). Additionally, not all women view menopause as negative. On the contrary, recent social science literature reports that women now define reproductive aging as a time of sexual liberation and freedom from menstrual hygiene routines and fears of pregnancy.[53] In the same way, watching grown children establish themselves in their careers and form their own families can cause celebration, pride, and increased freedom for midlife women. Many women in their 40s, 50s, and 60s may contemplate returning to a career they put on hold, undertake a new business venture that they never had time for before, or expand their volunteer activities.

Separate emotional concerns arise at midlife too, as women deal with transitions into and out of other important social roles and relationships.[17,18] As stated at the outset of this chapter, midlife may bring new caregiving responsibilities, including care for ailing parents.[17] Midlife also commonly includes changing intimate relationships, caused by things such as divorce, remarriage, and death.[74] For instance, some women may finally realize the true nature of their existing intimate relationships at midlife and be more willing in this life stage to exit bad relationships. Because of their longer life expectancy, women also become widowed more often than men do in midlife.[74] In 2000, for example, more than 3 million women ages 45 to 54 years and another 1.8 million women ages 55 to 64 years were divorced; another 725,000 women ages 45 to 54 years and 1.4 million women ages 55 to 64 years were widowed.[17] Thus, many women experience being single again in midlife and must either start dating or become accustomed to a new single life.[53,74]

Changing relationships, particularly divorce and widowhood, can be economically devastating for women. A middle-aged woman who becomes divorced will face significant challenges in finding employment at a rate of pay that replaces her prior income and lifestyle.[80] Although the situation is changing slowly as women participate in the paid workforce for longer periods (and thereby qualify for company pensions and social security), women in all age groups still earn less than men, and they have significantly less wealth accumulated than men of equivalent ages as they approach old age.[40] This affects their ability to have adequate health insurance and prescription coverage.

For both women and men, midlife includes a rethinking of life goals as individuals "look back on what they have accomplished, evaluate their

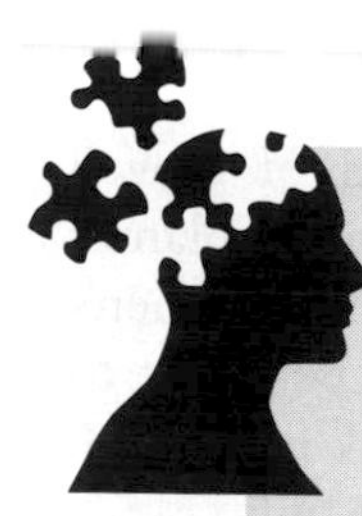

Therapeutic Challenge:

What unique things do women at midlife need to know about prescription medications and healthy living that younger women do not? How can healthcare providers adjust their interactions with patients to account for the age and life stage of women they are treating?

happiness, and make significant adjustments based on what they want for the next phase of their life."[17] Some women may decide to keep working because they are at the peaks of their careers at midlife or need the economic security. Alternatively, middle-aged women may want to think about their own retirement, but their changing roles, responsibilities, and relationships may prevent them from actually doing so as economic stability remains forefront in their minds. In these times, individual women need to be reminded to prioritize physical and emotional health and well-being. This is a time when healthcare providers could step in to help women remember their bodily and emotional needs. Women who are going through life changes may forget to engage in healthy eating habits, attend regular doctors' visits for preventive care, and find ways to lower stress and maintain good levels of self esteem. At these times, too, pharmacists might also see women use more prescription drugs and over-the-counter aids to deal with chronic health conditions, stress-induced sleep changes, or weight gain. Just as in the case of young women and adolescents, then, midlife women could benefit from in-store awareness campaigns that remind them of tips for healthy living and healthy use of over-the-counter products and prescription drugs.

LATE-LIFE TRANSITIONS

Other challenges to health and well-being emerge as women advance in years and encounter major transitions, such as retirement, the death of a spouse, increased frailty or **disability,** or changes in living situation. For instance, a prevalent myth in society is that retirement is a special time of enjoyment with close family and grandchildren, and an opportunity to pursue long desired interests. For some, with good health and adequate economic resources, this can be their reality. A quick glance at the travel section of the newspaper will confirm a myriad of travel options geared toward older adults and increasingly toward older and single women. More opportunities for unpaid contributions of older adults exist with volunteer organizations. However, not all older persons have the ability to pursue their desired activities in retirement. Given the employment mobility of today's society, children and grandchildren can be geographically distant from grandparents, making regular interactions less likely.

Financial limitations can also be present. A report from the Women's Institute for a Secure Retirement stated that in 2004, the median income for retired women was $12,080, compared with men's income of $21,102.[41] The report describes how several factors conspire to reduce the retirement income of older women, which, in turn, puts them at a health disadvantage. First, as mentioned earlier, women earn less than men throughout life: three out of five working women in America today earn less than $30,000 per year.[41] These women are not able to save for retirement. Second, half of all women work in traditionally female, relatively low-paid jobs without pensions. Thus, these women will need to rely solely on social security and family support. Third, women still exit the paid workforce for longer than men (10 years for women [e.g., childcare, parent caregiver] vs. 1 year for men [e.g., health reasons]).[41] In addition, women who come to rely exclusively on survivor benefits after their husband's death are surprised to learn they will only receive about 50% of their husband's full pension. This means that if the husband dies first (as they ordinarily do), the surviving wife could find it difficult to manage. Out-of-pocket medical expenses including prescription drugs alone can whittle away a woman's pension.[41,81,82] Chapter 3: Socioeconomics offers additional information about women's economic situations.

Women born in the U.S. today can expect to live up to 10 years longer than men, on average.[39] Among other things, this means they must learn to cope with becoming widows. Widowhood is stressful. Research shows that women who are recent widows (widowed in the past year) have substantially higher rates of depressed mood, decreased social functioning, poorer mental health, and limited physical functioning for up to 3 years after the husband's death when compared with women of the same age who are not recently widowed.[83] Because women at all ages are already at a twofold risk of depression as compared with men, healthcare professionals need to be especially alert to the signs of depression after bereavement.

Additional challenges facing women are chronic health conditions and disabilities, which increase with age.[77,78] Two common, age-related health conditions that affect older women in unique ways are cardiovascular disease and depression. Older women's increased risk of cardiovascular disease and stroke presents an interesting example for those interested in sex-based and gender-based health differences (see Chapter 30: Cardiovascular Disease and Chapter 41: Neurological Disorders).

Cardiovascular Disease and Neurologic Disorders

Research now shows, for example, that because of sex-based differences in physiology, the signs and symptoms of some diseases are different for women as compared with men. A heart attack, for example, can feel like acid reflux or dizziness much more often in women and not the classic "clutch the heart" experience characteristic in the male paradigm.[84] In the case of stroke, women are more likely than men to experience an altered mental state (e.g., confusion) instead of the classic symptoms of stroke (blurred vision and incoherent speech). The consequence is under-recognition of heart attacks and strokes when they occur and thus delayed treatment. Because women who have a stroke or a heart attack are often older and living alone, the absence of a family member in the home when the crisis occurs further lengthens the time between the acute event and reaching the emergency department for care.

The case of depression is also important (see Chapter 34: Mental Health). Sex-based differences in the rates of depression between men and women at all ages are well documented and are likely due to differences in women's hormones in combination with differences in metabolism.[78] But gender-based dimensions of depression also exist and include the social expectations about who should ask for help and when and how. For example, women are more willing than men to seek treatment for health conditions such as depression. This is positive because depression is a treatable mental illness, and prognosis is better with early intervention.

Despite positive health-seeking behaviors in general, newly widowed women are at increased risk for depression and may not be willing or cognizant enough to ask for help for depression at its onset. Perhaps the newly widowed woman does not want to acknowledge publicly how much her husband's death has affected her (and thus may forgo or postpone treatment).[85] Alternatively, a new widow might not realize that depression after the death of a loved one can be a medical emergency and, instead, blames herself for not being able to handle it. Thus, women's families and healthcare providers must be ready to recognize the early signs of depression. Chapter 34: Mental Health discusses these issues more fully.

Fortunately, both men's and women's awareness of these sex- and gender-based differences (see Chapter 7: Sex and Gender Differences) are increasing, with greater women's health emphasis paying dividends in individual health. For example, women's rates of participation in recommended preventive health screenings like mammography are increased when gender is directly considered in the planning and delivery of services.[78]

Heightened attention to women's health issues and their appropriate treatment is timely given that women live longer than men and have fewer resources in old age to deal with age-related declines. Older widowed women, for example, will be on their own to negotiate declining vision and hearing, as well as physical mobility issues, including driving retirement. Nearly one million Americans stop driving every year for health reasons.[86] Many of these Americans are older women, who tend to retire from driving at an earlier age and in better health than men. Coupled with their longevity, estimates suggest that women are likely to need at least 10 years of transportation support after they stop driving a motor vehicle. Although this may be an appropriate course of action from a safety perspective, driving retirement has negative consequences. First, one's activities of daily living are significantly curtailed (e.g., grocery shopping, attending family functions, keeping medical appointments). Second, as research is beginning to show, giving up driving can result in significant social isolation that can lead to loneliness and depression.[86] Although some alternative transportation options do exist, they are often not as senior-friendly (i.e., safe, accessible) as they could be and are frequently unavailable in rural communities.

To some extent, society has responded to the demographic reality of increasing numbers of older adults. We see more public buildings with wheelchair ramps, streets with wider sidewalks and more brightly lit crosswalks, even low-rise city buses that can accommodate persons using mobility devices like walkers and wheelchairs.[87] Legislation and policy have played an important role in reshaping our environment to facilitate the full inclusion and social participation of older adults and persons with disabilities in our communities.

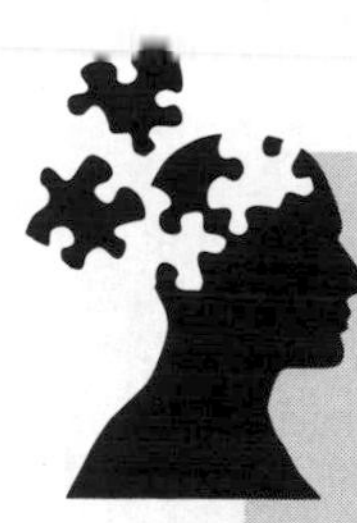

Therapeutic Challenge:

Are there ways to ensure privacy during patient interactions? What type of consultation space would put the patient most at ease? Are there topics that the healthcare provider should raise that an older woman herself might not be comfortable raising?

For older women dealing with age-related health concerns, it is essential that buildings and services be senior friendly. Yet many healthcare settings, including hospitals and pharmacies, pose barriers that reduce the quality and accessibility of healthcare services.[78,82,87] Research has shown, for example, that less than half of women with spinal cord injury receive regular gynecologic care because their physician's office doors are too narrow to get through in a wheelchair or because their physician's examination table did not adjust to accommodate women who were unable to climb on the table themselves.[76] Barriers like this exist for older adults in other contexts. For example, most pharmacy counters are designed for people who stand, thus forcing pharmacists to literally talk down to a patient in a wheelchair. This not only decreases the confidentiality of the conversation but may perpetuate the power imbalance that exists between the "authoritative expert" and the patient. Coming around the counter and crouching down to be eye to eye with the person in the wheelchair is advisable. Pharmacists need to be aware that the manner in which they communicate will shape the message their patients hear. Pharmacists should think about how and where medication counseling sessions are conducted, how various physical and sensory impairments common in advanced age (e.g., decreased hearing, decreased vision) affect understanding, and especially how a trusting and respectful professional relationship will positively influence patients' health behaviors.

An older woman is unlikely to feel comfortable talking about the more private details of her health or health insurance status in the same way that a young woman might not like to be seen purchasing birth control when her friends are in the store. Because many pharmacists sell durable medical equipment, they should also know how to be comfortable discussing personal self-care routines associated with various chronic health conditions and disabilities. Healthcare providers should also speak directly to the older person/customer, not to the younger or able-bodied person accompanying them. Asking respectful questions, listening, and asking permission to touch the person are also good rules of thumb.

Finally, women in older age are likely to undertake at least one major household move. Some will downsize for reasons of physical frailty, others will move to be nearer their family, and still others will be seeking an active retirement community that meets their social and leisure needs. Among the population 75 years and older, 50% of women are living alone, compared with 23% of men.[39] However, it would be a mistake to think that the majority of older women cannot care for themselves and will need formal care. Despite the undisputed graying of the nation, only 7.4% of Americans aged 75 years and older lived in a nursing home in 2006, contrary to popular and social beliefs.[39] Social factors are powerful in shaping perceptions and beliefs about older individuals. The image of older women that many younger people hold reflects biases and assumptions about women who lose their value once they are no longer reproductive or beautiful, or when they are no longer employed and living independently. These views speak to the **ageism** present in society today that is being tested and may be reformed soon. Despite the recent financial crisis, the baby boom generation is the healthiest and wealthiest cohort of older adults ever and includes more professional and educated women than in any previous generation. These women will undoubtedly remake outdated ways of thinking about age and portray more positive images about what it means to have good health and a good life in old age.

This section has described how some common psychosocial issues affect women's health across

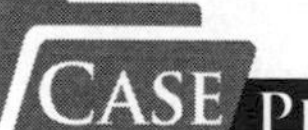

CASE PRESENTATION

Patient Case: Part 2

C.V. is working hard to meet the competing demands of paid work, single parenthood, and elder care. Although she chooses to put her family first, she still feels frustrated by her lack of assertiveness at work and her endless cycle of stress and fatigue. C.V. is exploring some new options, however. She is expanding her social support network and finding more time for herself. She has also accepted her brother's offer to take turns watching the kids. This has been fun for the children and strengthened C.V.'s bonds with her

(Continued on next page)

brother. C.V. has also learned that helping others can be an effective stress reducer. C.V. and her children have participated in two environmental cleanup activities in their town and are thinking about other ways to contribute to their community. At this last outing, C.V. met Andrew, a divorced father of two teenaged boys. They have shared mutual interests and have agreed to get together for coffee soon. Buoyed by these small successes and her growing self-confidence, C.V. has decided to take better advantage of the continuing education opportunities offered by her company. Although she realizes it will take time and there are no guarantees, she is ready to build her skills to give herself the best chance at finding a better job.

Not long ago, C.V. stopped at her neighborhood pharmacy to ask some questions about vitamins, osteoporosis, and her family history of heart disease. She had to make an appointment and return when the pharmacist was available, but she did that, and now feels better informed about the prescriptions she takes and what other natural and over-the-counter product options she has to help promote healthy living. The pictures of full-bodied healthy women in the healthy living posters in the pharmacy helped her accept her physique and motivated her to improve her diet as well. She also realizes that rather than trying to take prescription sleep aids to deal with recent insomnia, it is healthier to try to reduce emotional stresses and find herbal and dietary remedies for the night sweats. C.V. also recently asked her brother to take on more of the caregiving workload, and he agreed. She recognizes that her daughter is entering puberty and will soon begin to menstruate, and that she needs to mirror positive and healthy routines for her daughter's benefit, if not her own. She also knows her son can learn positive things from his mother's health regimens and from simply being aware of women's health issues. Thus, she is changing some of her daily routines to allow both of her children to witness healthy living.

C.V.'s case is also influenced by race and ethnic cultural characteristics. C.V.'s concerns for health and well-being, as well as for her family and paid-work choices, could be analyzed through a lens of race-ethnic or economic inequality. For instance, why does she feel she might be treated differently by her boss because of her race-ethnic background? What is her experience of interactions with doctors and other healthcare providers, and does her race-ethnic background come up in these interactions? Does she have good health insurance? Is she wary of unnecessary medications specifically because of her cultural background?

Even with this case's potential race and ethnic variations, C.V.'s situation is not that different from that of many middle-aged, midcareer women. Her case amplifies the ways in which gender roles, socialization, and powerful images in society shape women's decisions that, in turn, influence their health.

the lifespan and how women at each life stage have unique concerns. While some issues of health and well-being are different depending on a woman's specific life stage, others are common concerns across life stages (e.g., depression, self-esteem, body image).

Summary

This chapter has only touched the surface of the types of psychosocial issues that affect women's health, but it points readers toward the importance of the roles women fill, gendered communication differences, women's varied experiences with reproduction and sexuality, the effects of beauty norms on girls and women, the prevalence of gendered violence, and the relative economic vulnerability of women, which in turn affects health. It should be evident, however, that not all women experience biological issues, psychosocial issues, or health and illness in the same ways. As suggested in this chapter, women who lack economic resources and stability will face more challenges, just as visible minorities and women with disabilities do. A critical issue is health insurance and the diminished quality of care available to women who are poor. For these women, normal preventive healthcare can be nonexistent and good health becomes a luxury.

Although it may be difficult to eradicate gender norms in the U.S. in the near future, healthcare providers and others who serve women must take seriously the types of psychosocial issues highlighted in this chapter. Providing different groups of women with information about their health and well-being should be the goal of all healthcare professionals. Helping individual women navigate various psychosocial contexts and unique life stages should be a challenge that healthcare professionals embrace as well.

References

Additional content available at ***www.ashp.org/womenshealth***

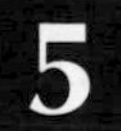

5 Issues in Lesbian, Bisexual, and Transgender Healthcare

Wendy B. Bostwick, Ph.D., MPH; Katherine A. O'Hanlan, MD, FACOG, FACS, SGO; Perry Silverschanz, Ph.D., MSW

Learning Objectives

1. Define and contrast sexual orientation and gender identity.
2. Discuss health disparities among sexual-minority women and transgender women and men.
3. Enumerate reasons for health disparities.
4. Identify pharmacological issues for transgender patients.
5. Improve culturally competency skills to enhance care for persons with varying sexual orientations and gender identities.

In the past 30 years, an upsurge in research devoted to the health and healthcare of **lesbian,** gay, **bisexual,** and **transgender** persons (LGBT) has occurred. Importantly, much of this research has shifted from utilizing a pathological lens, through which nonheterosexuality was viewed as an illness, to employing a more descriptive and theoretical lens, which recognizes a natural spectrum of diversity in human **sexual orientation** and **gender identity.** This new wave of research can provide healthcare professionals with a better understanding of some of the health behaviors and health needs of LGBT populations and ways to eliminate healthcare disparities and improve healthcare delivery and outcomes.

This chapter will focus on some of the better-researched and articulated health needs of lesbian, bisexual, and transgender populations. Lesbian and bisexual women share common concerns with all women about their health across the lifespan. The differences across groups do not lie within a variation in biological processes or any innate physiological dissimilarity. Rather, they are often the manifestation of particular social and cultural processes that lesbian and bisexual women are exposed to and experience. For transgender populations some unique issues exist that will be highlighted. This chapter will also discuss some of the knowledge necessary to provide these groups with a basic level of culturally appropriate and competent care.

Definitions and Population Estimates

Sex is usually used to refer to a person's biological sex, that is, a classification according to anatomy and/or presumed reproductive capability. Terms such as *male* or *female* are usually used in reference to a person's sex. Gender, traditionally a classification as a woman or man, encompasses differential social roles, meanings, and the cultural expectations that societies attach to the sexes (see Table 5-1 for a list of relevant terms).[1,2] Both sex and gender have traditionally been conceptualized as dimorphic (i.e., either male or female, man or woman), thus having only two expressions of structure or function, but more recently "male" and "female" have been represented as the endpoints on a continuum of human expression, rather than the only possibilities.[3]

Sexual orientation is one aspect of a person's sexuality and is generally thought to be comprised of at least three dimensions: sexual identity, **sexual attraction,** and **sexual behavior.**[4] The terms *lesbian* (or gay) and *bisexual* refer to a woman's sexual orientation identification, that is, the **sexual identity** she identifies for herself. Generally, lesbians (or gay women) are those whose primary emotional and sexual attractions

Case Presentation

Patient Case: Part 1

A tall person with long hair approaches the pharmacy counter to fill a prescription. When asked for a name, the person says "Linda Smith" in a deep voice and hands over a prescription benefit card. The name on the card reads "Lawrence Smith." Confused, the pharmacist carefully eyes both Linda and the card multiple times before asking Linda for other identification. Linda produces a driver's license that reads "Linda Smith." Flustered, the pharmacist asks, "Is this prescription for your wife?" "No," says Linda, "it's for me. I changed my name and haven't received my new insurance card yet."

"So you're Lawrence *and* Linda?" the pharmacist asks. Linda, noting that two other customers have arrived, leans in and says softly that she is just Linda, and asks if she could please get her prescription filled. "No problem, sir," replies the pharmacist, hurrying to process the order so that Linda will leave the pharmacy as soon as possible. After Linda departs, the next client steps up and says derisively "What was *that* about?" and the pharmacist replies "We get all kinds in here!"

are toward other women, whereas bisexual women are emotionally and sexually attracted to women and men. Identifying as bisexual does not mean that a woman is involved with multiple partners simultaneously or that her emotions and desires are 50-50, nor does a woman's identity necessarily define her sexual behavior (that is, a self-identified lesbian could be engaged in sexual activity with a man).

How sexual orientation is measured (i.e., how the question is asked) must be evaluated because it will affect estimates of the size of the population of lesbian and bisexual women in the U.S. In national surveys, between 4.4% to 13.4% of women report some same-gender sexual attraction, 4.5% to 11% report having had same-gender sexual behavior since puberty, yet only 0.9% to 1.3% identify as lesbian, and 0.5% to 3% identify as bisexual.[4,5] While 3% of the population may seem small, it translates into nearly 9 million bisexual women in the U.S. and represents only those who felt comfortable enough to reveal their sexual orientation to a stranger (as in a telephone interview or paper-and-pencil survey). In this chapter the term ***sexual minority*** includes all types of nonheterosexual women, whether due to their self-identity, sexual behavior, or patterns of attraction.

While lesbian- and bisexual-identified women share many similar experiences with each other and with other sexual minority women, in that they are all women and all are sexual minorities, distinctions exist between the groups. Therefore providers should not assume that their health issues and healthcare needs are always equivalent. Some women may identify as heterosexual even though they have a history of sexual behavior with other women, and some women change their identity over time or choose no identity label at all, regardless of their sexual behavior.[6] Therefore, if sexual behavior is relevant to a person's healthcare needs, providers need to ask about behavior specifically, in addition to asking about sexual orientation identity. Of note, the terms described here are not used or understood by all lay and healthcare providers, and a variety of social and cultural factors can play a role in how a sexual minority woman ultimately chooses to identify herself.

Gender expression (or **gender presentation**) refers to how a person represents her/his gender, as in her/his dress or mannerisms—for example, women can appear androgynous to hyperfeminine. Gender identity refers to a person's innermost sense of being a man or woman, irrespective of biological sex or genital anatomy. Gender identity is distinct from sexual orientation, and one does not determine the other; thus, the sexual orientation of a transgender individual can be heterosexual, bisexual, lesbian, or gay.

For most people, their gender identity matches their birth sex; those who experience a mismatch between their internal sense of self and their body are often referred to as having gender identity dysphoria. A commonly used term to describe an incongruence between gender identity or expression and birth sex is *transgender.* Transgender people may identify as a transgender, woman, man, with neither gender, or feel as though they embody a mixed-gender self (e.g., "bigender" or "gender-queer"). A transgender man is someone who may have female sex characteristics but self-identifies as a man, whereas a transgender woman may have male sex characteristics but self-identifies as a woman.

A **transsexual** individual is one type of transgender person, one who physically and/or medically transitions to the other sex in order to relieve the debilitating distress resulting from body dysphoria or an overwhelming internal sense of the body being the wrong sex. Transition comprises many life-changing decisions in legal, social, and often medical realms. Medical interventions are often but

Table 5-1. Common Terminology Related to Sexual Minorities[1,2]

Term	Definition
Bisexual	An identity label used by some people whose emotional and sexual attractions are for both women and men.
FTM	Acronym for female-to-male transgender or transsexual person. Also "trans man." Typically referred to with male pronouns (he, him).
Gender	The social and cultural categories of *woman* and *man*.
Gender expression	An individual's presentation of her/his gender through clothing, behavior, mannerisms, etc.
Gender identity	A person's sense of being a woman or man, irrespective of biological sex.
Gender presentation	See gender expression.
Hermaphroditism	An older term for intersex; see intersex definition.
Intersex	Condition in which a person is born with both male and female genitalia or reproductive organs, or with ambiguous genitalia. Previously referred to as hermaphroditism, intersex is now the preferred term.
Lesbian (gay woman)	An identity label used by some women whose primary emotional and sexual attractions are toward other women.
MTF	Acronym for male-to-female transgender or transsexual person. Also "trans woman." Typically referred to with female pronouns (she, her).
Sex	Typically refers to anatomy and biology, traditionally includes only two classifications: female or male.
Sex confirmation surgery	Also known as sex reassignment surgery, procedure(s) in which the body is altered to bring it into alignment with a person's gender identity.
Sexual attraction	Feelings of sexual desire and/or fantasy, which may or may not relate to sexual behavior.
Sexual behavior	Behavioral aspect of sexuality, distinct from sexual identity and attraction. These dimensions are not always congruent (e.g., some women who have sex with women do not label themselves as lesbian or bisexual).
Sexual identity	How people label themselves with regard to their sexuality (e.g., lesbian, heterosexual, asexual, etc.).
Sexual minority	An umbrella term used to describe those whose sexual identity, behavior, or attraction renders them a minority in a predominantly heterosexual population.
Sexual orientation	One aspect of a person's sexuality, involving sexual attraction, sexual identity, and sexual behavior.
Transgender	An umbrella term for persons whose gender identity or gender expression is not congruent with their birth sex, including those who identify with neither (or both) female and male sex.
Transsexual	A transgender person who has transitioned to the other sex, or who wishes to. Not all transsexual people access medical services (such as hormones or surgery).

not always required to align the body with a person's internal experience to achieve congruence, and might include hormone therapy, surgery, or other procedures. Male-to-female **(MTF)** transsexuals might require, for example, female hormones, breast augmentation, electrolysis, facial feminization surgery, or genital surgery. Female-to-male **(FTM)** transsexuals might require male hormones, breast removal and chest reconstruction ("top" surgery), or genital surgery ("bottom" surgery). Transition can also facilitate social acceptance of the person's expressed **gender.** In addition to transsexual people, some transgender persons undergo hormonal and surgical interventions. Some find medical intervention unnecessary for achieving internal congruence; for most, the procedures are not affordable, or, more rarely, could be medically contraindicated. Regardless of their surgical or medical status, all transgender or transsexual persons share a common desire to be seen as who they are and should be referred to by the pronouns of their identified genders. When in doubt, ask the person which pronouns are preferred.

Note that in addition to transgender women, transgender men (FTM) are included in this chapter because many retain some female physiology and biology, which can affect pharmacokinetics and pharmacodynamics. For example, while some transsexual men have undergone total hysterectomy with oophorectomy and therefore have no endogenous estrogens, many other transgender men have had no surgical or hormonal interventions and retain functional female organs. Thus a transgendered man with female anatomy could still experience menopause or develop uterine cancer.

The prevalence of transgender people in the population is unknown. One study estimated the prevalence of transsexuality at 1:11,900 men (i.e., male-to-female; MTFs) and 1:30,400 women (i.e., female-to-male; FTMs), based on the number of people who were diagnosed and treated at a major clinic in the Netherlands between 1987 and 1990.[7] These figures probably greatly underestimate the true prevalence, especially of transsexual men (FTMs), as many do not access formal providers. More recent calculations using U.S. data have suggested that there could be closer to 1 in 500 persons in the population who are transgender or transsexual.[8]

The term ***intersex*** (formerly **hermaphroditism,** a term now considered offensive by many) refers to neither sexual orientation nor gender identity. Intersex individuals are born with anatomic development that renders the infant's genitals indiscernible as either male or female. Some anomalies of chromosomes or the endocrine system result in ambiguous external genitalia at birth, sometimes with internal and/or external sexual characteristics of both sexes.[3,9] Recent literature has grouped these congenital conditions together under the term *disorders of sex development* (DSD).[10] There are a diversity of surgical, medical, and psychosocial issues associated with DSDs. While some may overlap with those of lesbian, bisexual, and transgender people, a full exploration of these issues is beyond the scope of the current chapter.

Because agreement and consistent definitions in these areas do not exist and are evolving, review of the literature should include attention to the definitions used in the study. Thus the impact of different definitions should be considered when comparing results, drawing conclusions, or making policies.

Health Disparities

At the most fundamental level, sexual minority women's general health issues are similar to those of all women. In terms of physiology and pharmacology, no evidence to date suggests that biology differs by sexual orientation such that prescribing guidelines, side effects, contraindications, or metabolic processes (including hormone profiles) would be different for this population of women. That said, evidence suggests certain health behaviors and health conditions might be more prevalent among lesbian and bisexual women. A number of health disparities have been identified among transgender women (MTF) and men (FTM) as well. In reviewing the literature, the emphasis here is on conditions that might be treated pharmacologically or that involve the use of prescription drugs in LBT people.

An important caveat is that there is not an extensive body of rigorous literature devoted to the health issues of lesbian, bisexual, or transgender populations. While this continues to change, particularly as federal funding priorities shift, the LGBT research to date must be considered within the context of some notable methodological limitations. The overall prevalence of these often hidden populations is low, rendering very small samples among studies utilizing random sampling and making recruitment difficult in targeted studies. In addition, studies among transgender persons are universally based on convenience samples, such that findings from most studies cannot be generalized to the entire transgender population. Nevertheless, findings from most studies tend to be in accord with one in another and provide a compelling body of evidence demonstrating stark health disparities between transgender groups and others.

ALCOHOL USE

In the field of LGBT research, one of the more frequently studied areas is substance-use patterns and behaviors, specifically alcohol use.[11] While sexual

FROM "ILLNESS" TO HEALTH

For many the modern LGBT health movement began with the removal of homosexuality from the American Psychological Association's (APA) official list of mental health disorders in 1973. "Homosexuality per se implies no impairment in judgment, stability, reliability, or general social and vocational capabilities. Further, the American Psychological Association urges all mental health professionals to take the lead in removing the stigma of mental illness that has long been associated with homosexual orientations."[12] This groundbreaking action, which suggested that homosexuality was not in and of itself a mental illness, was an important step in depathologizing lesbian, bisexual, and gay people. The door was opened for research that focused on the health needs of these communities, rather than a continual focus on *why* people were lesbian, gay, or bisexual. While much has been accomplished in the past 37 years as a result of the APA's actions, the need for advocacy, education, and policy around LGBT health issues still exists. A number of national organizations focus on these issues and are good sources of information and resources. These organizations include

The National Coalition for LGBT Health
www.lgbthealth.net

The Gay and Lesbian Medical Association
www.glma.org

The Human Rights Campaign
www.hrc.org

The National Lesbian and Gay Task Force
www.thetaskforce.org

minority women may not necessarily drink more in terms of quantity, numerous studies have shown that sexual minority women are less likely to abstain from alcohol use and are more likely to report behaviors related to problem drinking when compared to heterosexual women.[13-18]

In one of the few national studies to date that inquired about sexual identity and utilized diagnostic criteria, researchers found that lesbian and bisexual women had more problems resulting from drinking and were more likely to report past participation in substance-abuse treatment.[19] In terms of *DSM-IV* alcohol dependence, lesbian women were 7 times more likely to meet the criteria, and bisexual women were over 6 times as likely as heterosexual women to meet the criteria for alcohol dependence. A meta-analysis of studies related to mental health and substance-use problems found that sexual minority women were 3.5 times more likely to report any substance-use disorder in their lifetime.[20] Information on resolving substance-use problems is described in Chapter 36: Substance-Use Disorders.

Minimal data have been published on transgender people's use of alcohol. Given that transgender people face as much if not more social stigmatization than lesbians and bisexual women, the risks for alcohol use are likely greater in these populations. Nearly a third of MTFs and FTMs in one study revealed past substance-abuse problems, and almost all characterized that abuse as attempts to cope with distress related to their transgender status.[21]

A recent web survey compared transgender persons, lesbians, bisexual, and heterosexual women in a nationally diverse sample, finding that transgender people, lesbians, and bisexual women all reported significantly more past difficulties with alcohol than heterosexual women, though current alcohol problems were similar among all groups.[22-24] A recent comprehensive survey of transgender people across the state of Virginia found that FTMs were more than twice as likely to report past problems with alcohol (39%) than MTFs (18%).[25] Asked if they needed help getting treatment for alcohol problems, 29% of MTFs and 41% of FTMs surveyed in Philadelphia said yes; thus it is possible that alcohol abuse is a greater risk for FTMs than MTFs.[26]

No reliable estimates describe how often sexual minority women or transgender groups rely on pharmacological interventions (e.g., disulfiram, naltrexone) to reduce their drinking or remain abstinent. However, there are data documenting that more sexual minority women are in recovery than heterosexual women and that they were more likely to have sought treatment related to alcohol problems.[27,28] This might include the use of medical interventions. For transgender persons, because it is difficult to find treatment that is inclusive and accepting of differing gender identities, it is even more difficult to estimate use of pharmacotherapeutic aids for recovery or abstinence.[29]

SMOKING

Recent studies consistently demonstrate higher rates of smoking among sexual minority women as compared to heterosexuals. For example, among Californians, smoking rates of lesbian and bisexual women were over twice that of heterosexual women.[30] In addition, heterosexual women were more likely to report that they had never smoked. These findings are consistent with another California-based study, in which 25% of both lesbians and bisexual women reported current smoking, as compared to 15% of heterosexual women.[31] Lower income and less education were common predictors of smoking among lesbian and bisexual (and gay) populations, similar to predictors for the general population.

Elevated rates of smoking put sexual minority women at higher risk for cancer and cardiovascular disease, and therefore, targeted prevention and cessation efforts are needed. Currently, no reliable estimates determine how often sexual minority women rely on pharmacological interventions to quit smoking (e.g., bupropion, nicotine replacement therapies, varenicline).

Similar to the dearth of information on alcohol use by transgender people, data on smoking are scarcer. In the Virginia study mentioned above, 59% of MTFs and 75% of FTMs reported tobacco use.[25] A San Francisco Bay area sample of MTFs had a similar rate of smoking (57%), a rate higher than nontransgender clients of the same agency.[32]

In addition to the risks usually associated with tobacco, transgender persons who smoke may face additional issues. The combination of tobacco use and hormone therapy can aggravate the possibility of cardiovascular, thromboembolism, and other diseases.[33] Physicians sometimes deny transgender patients hormones if they smoke, citing the potential for increased risks. Surgeons sometimes insist that patients stop smoking before they will agree to perform surgery (to promote better healing); thus, the pharmacist can encounter transgender people who desire to quit and may seem especially concerned about the effectiveness of pharmacological interventions or the speed with which they work.

MENTAL HEALTH

A growing body of evidence has demonstrated that sexual minority women may be at heightened risk for mental health disorders and problems.[15,17,20,34-36] In a study that examined possible sexual identity-related differences in the prevalence of mental disorders using diagnostic criteria, lesbian and bisexual women reported significantly higher rates of generalized anxiety disorder than heterosexual women, but the two groups did not differ in terms of major depression, panic disorder, distress, or self-reports of mental health problems. However, in a study that utilized data from the National Comorbidity Survey, the authors found that women with same-sex sexual partners were significantly more likely than women with other-sex partners to meet *DSM-III-R* criteria for any mood or anxiety disorder.[36] The fact that one study used identity-based criteria to define sexual-minority women and the other used behavioral criteria could explain the conflicting findings but also highlights the importance of attending to how information is gathered, both in research and by healthcare providers.

The issue of measurement is highlighted in a recent study that reports on national prevalence estimates of *DSM-IV* mood and anxiety disorders among sexual minorities in the U.S.[37] This study included the three different dimensions of sexual orientation that were previously noted: sexual behavior, sexual attraction, and sexual identity. It was very clear that compared to women who identified as heterosexual, bisexual- and lesbian-identified women were at higher risk of both mood and anxiety disorders over their lifetime. Bisexual women in particular were twice as likely to report both lifetime and past-year mood and anxiety disorders.

Bisexual behavior was also associated with a two-fold increase in mental health disorders when compared to women who reported lifetime heterosexual behavior. Interestingly, same-sex behavior was not a risk factor among women in this study and, in some instances, was associated with lower levels of mental health disorders. Treatment options for mental health disorders are described in Chapter 34: Mental Health.

Findings across many studies consistently suggest that lesbian and bisexual women are more likely to have sought mental health treatment than heterosexual women.[38-41] Unfortunately, information related to the use of psychiatric medications among sexual minority women is scarce. Lesbians in the Nurses' Health study were twice as likely to have used antidepressants although another study found no differences between lesbians and heterosexual women.[42,43] In a college-aged sample, bisexual women were more likely than heterosexual women to have ever been prescribed antidepressants.[44]

Many studies report high percentages of transgender persons with depression. For example, a study of San Franciscan transgender and transsexual people found that 62% of the MTFs and 55% of the FTMs scored in the clinically depressed range on the Center for Epidemiological Studies Depression Scale (CES-D).[45] Higher CES-D scores were also associated with risky sex behaviors in MTF transgender youth.[46] Approximately 60% of participants (both MTFs and FTMs) across a number of studies reported having contemplated suicide, with a third to a half of those who had considered suicide actually having attempted it.[25,47,48] At odds with findings representing poorer mental health in transgender individuals is a large diverse internet study with 37% of transgender persons reporting having had serious thoughts of suicide, statistically the same rate as lesbians (31%) and psychosocially matched heterosexual women (25%) in the same study.[22] Additionally, a retrospective case file analysis of transsexual patients who were treated at a gender clinic between 1980 and 1995 for gender dysphoria found no evidence of comorbidity with any major psychiatric diagnosis.[21] The difference in mental health reports could stem from the demographic differences across samples, and as with much research, results may only pertain to those who participated—not the broader transgender community.

FERTILITY AND PREGNANCY

Many providers caring for lesbian and bisexual patients may not view them as potentially fertile women who might desire to create a family. However, just like heterosexual women, lesbian and bisexual women bear children and experience similar pharmacologic and pharmacotherapeutic issues related to prenatal and postnatal care. Lesbian women, however, might be more likely to rely on alternative insemination technologies to reproduce, particularly donor insemination.[49,50] Issues relevant to seeking assisted reproductive technologies (see Chapter 22: Infertility) are likely similar for all women, regardless of sexual orientation. However, as noted, several health risks are more prevalent in lesbian and bisexual woman than in the heterosexual women and, if present, pose risks to pregnancy. Alcohol and tobacco use should be firmly discouraged. Achieving a normal body mass index and improving nutritional intake should be addressed preconception. Finally, depression and anxiety should be specifically discussed during both antepartum and postpartum care and aggressively managed.

TRANSGENDER POPULATIONS

Additional issues that are important for transgender populations include gynecological/urological care and HIV/AIDS. Female-to-male transgender persons sometimes retain female body parts and continue to produce female sex hormones that can interfere with exogenous testosterone or other medications. Male-to-female persons who have had **sex confirmation** surgery will still retain the prostate gland, although small and less likely to become cancerous this can be overlooked during physical exams. Female-bodied FTMs often resist gynecological care because of body dysphoria, severe atrophic pain during exams, or the discomfort of being a man and entering a space dedicated to female care. Both FTMs and MTFs sometimes have difficulty finding healthcare providers who are knowledgeable and sensitive to their unique issues and bodies; thus, transgender people may be more likely to have undiagnosed conditions or chronic conditions that are not fully treated. Even when actively seeking treatment, attitudes of providers are crucial for transgender people. The documentary *Southern Comfort* depicts the last year in the life of a transgender man rejected by two dozen doctors who refused to treat his ovarian cancer, of which he subsequently died.[51]

HIV infection has been reported to be higher in MTFs than in men who have sex with men (MSM), though most government reporting agencies have not distinguished between the two populations. A recent systematic review of the literature found 29 studies with HIV positive rates in MTFs ranging from zero to 68% and reported that the rate of new infections was higher for MTFs than other groups (for treatment of HIV/AIDs, see Chapter 38: Sexually Transmitted and Infectious Diseases).[52]

Rates of HIV infection among FTMs were reported as much lower (0% to 3%), but these figures represent only five studies.[53] Other studies have reported that the rate of risky sexual behaviors by FTMs can be as high or higher than those of MTFs and that FTMs are less likely to get tested for the virus.[25,26,54,55]

For those providers, particularly pharmacists, that come into contact with transgender persons, not only is it important to understand their overall health issues and disparities, but it is also important to have special knowledge of pharmacologic interventions and treatments. Table 5-2 provides the reader with the expected change related to use of these medications (see Chapter 17: Menopause for estrogen therapy; Chapter 35: Sexual Disorders for testosterone therapy; and Web Resources for Common Prescription Medications Administered to Transgender People).[56-58] This information should not be considered comprehensive and readers interested in the pharmacology and pharmacotherapeutics of transgender care are strongly

Table 5-2. Common Prescription Medications Administered to Transgender People[56-58,a]

Estrogen (MTF patients)	Spironolactone (MTF patients)	Testosterone (FTM patients)
Clinical Effects Permanent Breast development Reversible Loss of erections Softening of skin Redistribution of body fat Testicular atrophy	*Clinical Effects* Permanent Breast development Testicular atrophy Reversible Loss of erections	*Clinical Effects* Permanent Increased body hair Deeper voice Baldness Clitoral enlargement Reversible Cessation of menses Libido changes Increased muscle mass Acne Increased facial hair

FTM = female to male; MTF = male to female.

[a]Minimal information related to medication use for transgender people; mostly information is extrapolated from use in nontransgendered patients (i.e., testosterone for men, estrogen for women). See Chapter 17: Menopause for full information about hormone therapy; Chapter 35: Sexual Disorders for full information about testosterone therapy; and Web Resources for Common Prescription Medications Administered to Transgender People.

encouraged to seek additional sources. The healthcare provider should also be aware that some of these products are bought via nonlicensed pharmacies (e.g., on the street, via a website, or made from the raw product obtained from chemical manufacturers).[59]

Additional content available at
www.ashp.org/womenshealth

Reasons for Health Disparities

The previous sections have detailed a number of areas in which lesbian, bisexual, and/or transgender people's health fares more poorly than heterosexual and nontransgender women. While it is important to know about these differences, it is equally important to understand why these disparities exist.

As mentioned previously, no evidence suggests that lesbian, bisexual, or other sexual-minority women differ from heterosexual women physically, endocrinologically, or genetically in such a way that their health would differ. Rather, to the extent that they exist, disparities in health outcomes are best understood as a product of the social and cultural environment in which sexual minority women are situated. The same is true for transgender persons, who face an even more disapproving social climate than do sexual-minority women.

Sexual-minority and transgender people are often targets of prejudice, discrimination, and hostility. Negative attitudes and behaviors against lesbian, gay, and bisexual people (sometimes referred to as "homophobia" or "biphobia") or the assumption that everyone is heterosexual (often referred to as "heterosexism") are manifested both at the individual and at the institutional level. For example, sexual-minority

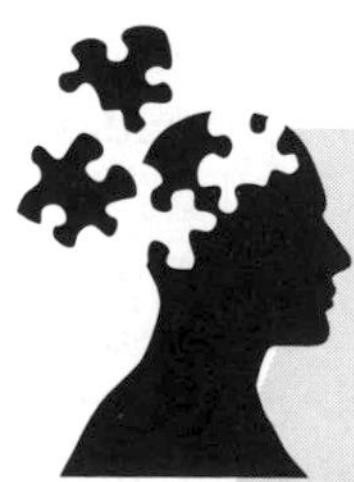

Therapeutic Challenge:

An example of a good website for transgender health is http://www.trans-health.com. What are some other good websites that you would recommend to a layperson about estrogen, spironolactone, and testosterone therapy?

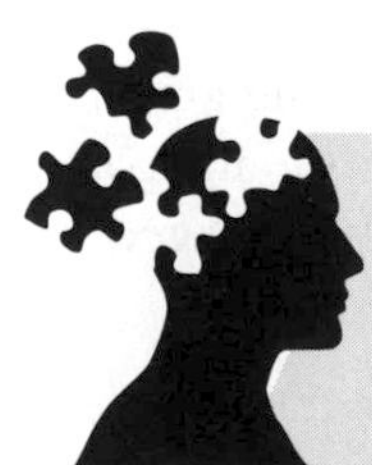

Therapeutic Challenge:

One of your coworkers makes a joke about a lesbian, knowing well that another coworker is a lesbian. How would you rectify this behavior and increase culturally competent behaviors between staff members within your healthcare practice?

and transgender people suffer from discrimination in housing, employment, and basic civil rights, as well as experiencing harassment and even violence at the hands of others.[60,61]

The Kaiser Family Foundation reported that three quarters of lesbians and gay men surveyed had experienced hostile or discriminatory treatment, 74% had experienced verbal abuse, and 32% had experienced physical violence solely due to their sexual orientation. Over 80% thought "a lot" of prejudice existed against them and that the government did too little to protect them; most feeling helpless due to their lack of popular support.[62]

These experiences of discrimination are best understood as stressors in the lives of lesbian, bisexual, and transgender women and men, and can have consequences for health behaviors and health outcomes. Some refer to this as "minority stress" or the additional social stress resulting from being part of a marginalized or stigmatized minority.[20] This is in addition to the sexism that women encounter and the racism and sexism that women of color also face. The connection between excess life stress and poor physical and mental health outcomes has been well documented.[63,64] The negative health consequences of homophobia and sexual minority stress have also been documented by numerous authors.[65-67] In one study, depression and mental distress were more common in lesbians and gay men who reported discrimination due to their orientation.[34] When the data were analyzed adjusting for these experiences, the rates of mental distress were the same as heterosexuals, suggesting that the experience of discrimination might be a potent contributor to mental health disparities.

One of the first studies to explore the connections between heterosexism, healthcare, and health outcomes detailed how poor treatment or insensitivity by medical professionals specifically can start a chain of events that ultimately results in negative health consequences.[68] When patients experience disdain from healthcare providers, it can alienate them from the entire medical system, reducing their utilization of screening modalities, potentially leading to higher morbidity and mortality from infections, cancers, and heart disease.[69] Deferring healthcare until symptoms become severe is a frequent response to disdainful treatment. Quite simply, based on previous bad experiences in healthcare settings, some lesbian women have reported delaying routine care, such as mammography or other screening, or avoid seeking

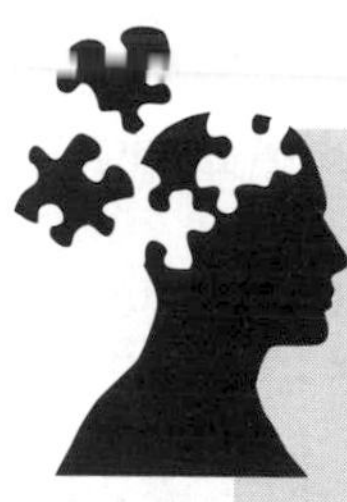

Therapeutic Challenge:

What local, state, and national resources are available about LGBT issues and LGBT friendly providers and pharmacies?

healthcare altogether.[70,71] In one study of lesbians' health-related experiences, 44% of participants had basically stopped seeking healthcare based on negative experiences, such as being shamed about their sexuality, having their partners ignored or dismissed when discussing medical treatment options, and being subjected to the heterosexist assumptions of providers.[72] Noted one woman "There was just no way to escape their oppressive heterosexual assumptions and it never seemed safe enough for me to speak up, so I decided to stop seeing doctors. I haven't had any healthcare in seven years."[72]

Institutional barriers to quality healthcare for sexual minority women and transgender men also exist. Many women cannot access their partner's employee benefits, including health insurance, if they are not legally married to their partners. As of this writing, at least 40 states prohibit same-sex marriage, and the federal Defense of Marriage Act precludes any federal marriage benefits, such as social security, from being conferred to same sex couples. While a growing number of employers offer same-sex partner benefits, even then, in some states it is against the law to provide unmarried couples with benefits (e.g., Michigan). Because the legality of marriage for transsexual people varies from state to state, in a couple where one person is transgender or transsexual, the ability of either partner to cover the other on their health insurance policy remains unclear. Even employers who offer same-sex partner benefits may not be willing to cover an employee's transgender partner, depending on how they view the transgender person's sex (i.e., are they a same-sex couple because he was female at birth? Or are they an other-sex couple because that's how they appear?).

One of the only studies to specifically explore the issue of health insurance coverage among sex-same couples found that sexual minority women, but not sexual minority men, were significantly less likely to have health insurance, to have seen a doctor in the past year, and to have a usual source of care than were women in other-sex couples.[73] Furthermore, they were more likely to report having unmet medical needs due to the cost of care.

In addition to lack of access to health insurance, nonheterosexual and transgender people must often contend with a wide variety of health professionals who at best are uneducated about their health concerns, and who at worst are openly hostile and discriminatory. Studies show that lesbians have experienced ostracism, rough treatment, and derogatory comments from their medical caregivers.[70,71] These experiences, and/or a perception of negative attitudes on the part of providers, can cause patients to withhold medically relevant information or to hesitate in returning for or obtaining routine health maintenance visits. Surveys of physicians and nursing professionals confirm that about 30% of caregivers experience discomfort providing care to lesbian patients and received little training about issues of sexual orientation.[74-77] A more recent survey found that though lessened, negative attitudes toward sexual minority persons persist among physicians.[78]

One of the few studies that touched on interactions with pharmacists' reported stories of six female-to-male transsexuals' experience of barriers at every level of care.[79] One participant detailed his experience of attempting to get his testosterone prescription filled, and noted that while doing so the pharmacists "were smirking at each other and laughing and elbowing each other because they knew what we were there for, and they thought it was hilarious..."[78]

In addition to uneducated and sometimes hostile providers, the lack of rigorous scientific research devoted to the health issues of sexual-minority women and transgender people makes it difficult to ascertain whether or not these populations are receiving appropriate healthcare.

The release of the Institute of Medicine's 1999 report *Lesbian Health* began a change in the federal healthcare research treatment of lesbians.[80] A panel of experts was convened to determine whether lesbians in the U.S. comprised a special population that deserved research focus and funding from the National Institutes of Health. Among other things, the Committee recommended that government funding be set aside for

- population-based studies to determine incidence of cancer, heart disease, infectious diseases, mental illness, and their attendant risk factors in the lesbian population
- investigation of effective health promotion methods to encourage breast and cervical cancer screening, utilization of mental and medical healthcare facilities, and smoking cessation programs
- studies of the impact of prejudice and discrimination and the necessary coping and resiliency patterns

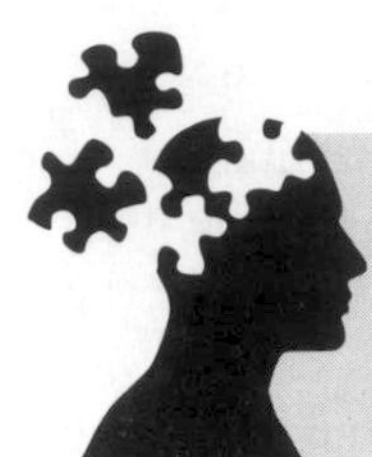

Therapeutic Challenge:

How would you plan a study to determine if prejudice and discrimination were felt by your LGBT patients?

Recommendations also included that ongoing public health surveys include questions asking about sexual orientation, and that medical-specialty associations and training programs disseminate information on lesbian health to healthcare providers, researchers, and to the public. In addition, surveys should include questions about birth sex and current gender identity, and training programs should educate providers about all sexual minority and transgender issues. To date, some progress has been made to implement IOM recommendations on the governmental realm, including federal funding to support more research into the health status and health needs of LGBT groups.

Culturally Competent Care with LGBT Clients

Healthcare professionals will come in contact with a wide range of people in their careers. Providing the best possible care is not solely about possessing empirical knowledge related to standard protocols or dispensing medication. Rather, it also entails the capacity to interact with a diversity of persons and the ability to provide culturally sensitive and appropriate services whenever possible. Cultural competence is predicated on knowledge, beliefs, attitudes, and skills that allow providers to interact effectively with a variety of different populations and cultures (see Chapter 2: Race, Ethnic, and Religious Issues).[81] Cultural competency as it pertains to sexual minority or transgender populations requires awareness of population-specific issues and concerns, corresponding sensitivity to these issues, and ultimately the provision of services that evince such awareness and sensitivity. It is important to note, however, that cultural competency is not a static or linear process. Rather, maintaining a level of competency vis-a-vis diverse populations requires ongoing skill-building, knowledge acquisition, and possibly behavioral change.

At the most basic level, awareness might mean remaining cognizant that not all people are heterosexual and that some women identify as lesbian, bisexual, or transgender, regardless of appearance, age, race, or geographic location. For instance, while large cities might have highly visible lesbian and gay communities, in reality many sexual minority women and transgender persons reside in large and small, urban and rural communities all over the U.S. Data from the 2000 census showed that there are same-sex couples living in 99% of counties in the U.S.[82]

This awareness should in turn foster sensitivity to the needs of sexual minority and transgender patients. This sensitivity pertains not only to specific healthcare needs or issues, but rather, to the larger milieu of provider-patient interaction. For example, terminology and language are important signifiers of a basic level of cultural competence, as well as inclusive care. Language should reflect a nonheterosexist bias: don't assume that a female patient has a husband or a boyfriend, but instead ask about a significant other or partner. For any forms that might be required, options for relationship status should include more than just married, divorced, widowed or single; "living with a partner" or "in a committed relationship" are options that recognize a variety of relationships, without privileging heterosexuality.

Sensitivity to language is perhaps even more of an issue when working with transgender patients. Again, if there are health-focused informational forms that people need to complete, offering more than just a male/female option is an important step toward creating an inclusive environment. In addition to male and female for denoting sex, forms should include FTM and MTF. Including these options on forms signals an aware and approachable provider who can focus on the health issues at hand.

Transgender persons often struggle with others accepting their self-identified gender as legitimate—a struggle that pervades both personal and professional interactions. Therefore, using the preferred pronoun of the person is very important to the provision of culturally competent care to transgender populations. Whenever possible the provider should follow the lead of the patient in this regard. Many transgender persons still have state-issued identification or even health insurance cards that are not consistent with their current name or gender, which can cause confusion. When in doubt, ask the patient the name and pronoun by which she or he prefers to be addressed, and use that pronoun in the chart that other providers can reference.

Healthcare providers should keep records secure from those who do not need personal information and respect the needs of patients for privacy and confidentiality. Of course this is important for all patients, but in many cases, transgender people sometimes face serious consequences if their information is carelessly shared.

While a good rule of thumb is to not assume that all people are heterosexual, by the same token, providers should not assume a patient's sexual orientation based on stereotypes. The most important thing in developing and practicing cultural competency is to retain an open mind, while providing all patients with respectful and thoughtful care.

Cultural competence also entails being familiar with population-specific resources. This could mean that the provider educates her or himself about sexual minority and/or transgender resources in the community. Such resources include general information resources, such as national gay and lesbian information hotlines, as well as contact information for the local LGBT community center. Especially useful information might include a compilation of LGBT-friendly providers in the area, as LGBT persons often encounter hostility from healthcare professionals. A sensitive and aware healthcare provider can gain the trust of a patient and learn of difficulties with particular providers; being able to suggest other more LGBT-friendly providers would be a great service.

While knowledge is a necessary component of cultural awareness, cultural sensitivity, cultural competence, and taking action to reduce disparities or to address health inequalities are also a significant part of the equation as well. This may mean advocating for inclusive policies, working to change policies and procedures that are discriminatory, creating guidelines for the provision of culturally competent care, and/or educating staff and coworkers. Additionally, participating in ongoing training related to cultural competence, as well as trainings on the medical and pharmacological needs of special populations, is also a way to demonstrate a commitment to providing the best possible care to patients.

BENEFITS OF CULTURALLY COMPETENT CARE

There are numerous benefits resulting from the provision of culturally competent care in all health sectors including pharmacy practice. At the most basic level, culturally competent care fulfills the

CASE PRESENTATION

Patient Case: Part 2

In this case, Linda was a transsexual woman, transitioning from male to female. Not all of her identity documents had yet been corrected since her name change. The pharmacist was unprepared for a transgender patient, and loudly reiterated the confusion by addressing Linda as "sir." This signaled to the other patients that the pharmacist was uncomfortable with a gender variant patient, which offered an opening for one of them to make a hostile remark. The pharmacist's reply further reinforced the impression that the exchange with Linda was strange and abnormal and did nothing to convey acceptance, tolerance, or culturally competency. The pharmacist's flustered state prevented her/him from counseling Linda on how to take the medication or to ask whether she was taking any other medications or supplements, which might interfere with its efficacy. This could result in an attenuated therapeutic response or perhaps dangerous side effects if Linda were taking two interactive medications—a possibility the pharmacist neglected to determine.

A more culturally appropriate interaction might have looked like this: A tall person with long hair approaches the counter, gives the name "Linda Smith" and hands over a prescription benefit card that reads "Lawrence Smith." The pharmacist politely asks "Is this your card?" and Linda says "Yes, I changed my name and haven't received my new insurance card yet." The pharmacist then asks which name Linda prefers and enters it into the pharmacy profile. After filling the prescription, she has Linda move to a private consultation area, asks Linda if she's ever taken the medication before, whether she is taking other medications, and instructs her on its use. The pharmacist also double-checks with Linda whether the gender marker listed in the pharmacy's records should be *M* or *F*. After remarking to Linda that the pharmacy is glad to have her as a customer and hopes she returns, the pharmacist returns to help the next patient in line. If a pharmacist is culturally competent, inappropriate comments by staff and patients should be addressed. In response to the other patient's comment, the pharmacist should mention that all patient pharmacist interactions are confidential and all patients are valued at that pharmacy.

healthcare provider's professional obligation, particularly for those working at community-based pharmacies with the greatest contact with patients. Perhaps more importantly, the provision of services that respect the unique needs of sexual minority and transgender patients will contribute to better rapport and more trusting relationships, which in turn can increase patient satisfaction and overall health outcomes. In addition, according to the National Center for Cultural Competence, providing healthcare services that are sensitive to cultural differences can help to reduce health disparities, improve the overall quality of services and care, and meet numerous guidelines and regulatory and accreditation mandates.[83]

Cultural competence in healthcare settings is about providing the best care possible to patients irrespective of sexual orientation, gender identity, sex, race, age, and a host of other characteristics. Competency in one area doesn't assure competency in another, and thus achieving cultural competency is a lifelong learning process that requires providers to be open to learning and have an ongoing commitment to providing quality care.

Summary

This chapter has provided a brief overview of some of the health needs and concerns of lesbian and bisexual women and transgender women and men. Although this chapter focused on LBT issues, many of the issues are similar to the gay male population and also warrant attention to better care and elimination of health disparities. With this basic foundational overview of some of the health concerns and health disparities among sexual minority women and transgender persons, as well as information on some key aspects of providing culturally appropriate and competent care, the healthcare provider should be able to improve the health and healthcare outcomes of people with varying sexual orientations and gender expressions.

References

Additional content available at ***www.ashp.org/womenshealth***

SECTION TWO

Female Biology, Physiology, and Wellness

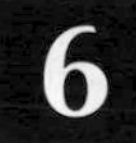

6 Anatomy and Physiology

Alicia B. Forinash, Pharm.D., BCPS, CCD; Evelyn S. Becker, Pharm.D., MA; Norma J. Owens, Pharm.D., BCPS, FCCP

Learning Objectives

1. Describe conception and pre-embryonic development.
2. Delineate changes that occur in girls during embryonic and fetal development, infancy, childhood, adolescence, puberty, and menarche.
3. Explain hormonal control of the menstrual cycle and changes during menopause.
4. Educate a woman about the hormonal and physiologic changes and placental development associated with pregnancy.
5. Relate age-induced changes that occur in major organ systems to the efficacy and safety of medications during the senior years.

This chapter will provide an overview of the female life cycle from conception to old age. The series of biological events that occur during a lifetime can be divided into groups of developmental changes. Prenatal development begins with the union of sperm and egg. This chapter shall begin with a brief overview of **gametogenesis,** factors that affect and result in fertilization, and follow the journey of the fertilized egg through implantation and embryonic development. Fetal development begins during the ninth week and continues until birth. The postnatal developmental stages of infancy, childhood, and adolescence ultimately result in structural and functional changes that mark the beginning of reproductive maturity: **menarche.** The menstrual cycle persists throughout the reproductive life of a woman, which is more extensively covered in Section 3. The maternal experience of pregnancy will be only briefly discussed in this overview as it is examined in greater detail in Section 5. **Perimenopause** and **menopause** are indicative of the end of reproductive capacity, briefly presented here and in detail in Chapter 17: Menopause. Aging is a continuous process that results in decreased functioning later in life. Additional sex-specific aspects of physiology and pathophysiology are explored in greater detail in the clinical chapters in Sections 3–7. Thus, this chapter will provide the framework on which to build in subsequent chapters.

Reproductive-Tract Anatomy of Women

The major anatomic structures that compose the female reproductive tract are the ovaries, fallopian tubes, uterus, and vagina (Figure 6-1). Eggs mature in the ovaries and are released into the fallopian tube on a cyclic basis. Fertilization occurs in the fallopian tubes, and implantation takes place in the uterus, which has been hormonally prepared for its arrival. In the absence of fertilization, this lining is shed in the monthly menstrual flow. Further discussion of these various areas and roles within menstruation and pregnancy are described below.

OOGENESIS, CONCEPTION, AND PRE-EMBRYONIC DEVELOPMENT

Preparation of the Gametes

Production of **gametes** involves two types of cell division. Mitosis, which involves one nuclear and one cytoplasmic division, produces cells identical to the parent cell. Mitosis occurs during the preparation of the gametes, spermatogonia, and oogonia for the next type of division, **meiosis.** Meiosis involves two divisions of nuclear and cytoplasmic material, resulting in the production of four cells, each with half the chromosome number of the adult (haploid number). **Spermatogenesis** normally produces four viable spermatozoa,

Case Presentation

Patient Case: Part 1

"I just found out I'm pregnant!"

HPI: B.F., a 28-year-old woman who is currently at 6 weeks of gestation, is at the pharmacy with some questions about pregnancy. She states she is having trouble tolerating her prenatal vitamin because of nausea and wonders if she really needs to take it. She describes the nausea as a little bothersome but she denies vomiting. She says she is concerned because her friend just had a baby with spina bifida. She asks if discontinuing the vitamin will put the baby at risk for spina bifida. She is also concerned about fetal risk because she had two glasses of wine at a company party 1 month ago before she knew she was pregnant.

PMH: Healthy.

Family history: Mother—hypertension, hypothyroidism; father—osteoarthritis.

Social history: Social alcohol intake before pregnancy, denies tobacco and illegal substance use.

Medications: Prenatal vitamin one tablet by mouth once daily (started 3 months ago).

Allergies: None.

Vitals: BP 118/68 mm Hg, HR 68 bpm, RR 16/min, weight 140 lb.

Laboratory values: Significant findings include (+) hCG, TSH 2.5 milli-International Units/L, HIV nonreactive; complete blood count, chemistry panel, and urinalysis were within normal limits.

whereas **oogenesis,** when completed, produces only one viable egg. In humans, oogenesis begins during early fetal development. By the 12th week of development, the oogonia have undergone several mitotic divisions and enter the first meiotic prophase. These primary **oocytes** are enclosed by support cells to form a capsule called a primordial follicle; however, most of these primordial follicles will degenerate by birth. In response to hormonal stimulation at puberty, the primordial follicles mature into primary follicles. The oocyte and the follicle cells secrete a glycoprotein layer, the **zona pellucida,** which separates the oocyte from the follicular cells.

Only one follicle attains primacy per month to become the graafian follicle.[1] The ovulatory surge stimulates the graafian follicle to resume meiosis and form the secondary oocyte, which is released at ovulation. Because oogenesis involves unequal cytoplasmic division, each meiotic stage produces only one viable oocyte and one polar body. Immediately beneath the egg membrane are cortical granules. These will be important in preventing **polyspermy.**[2] Menopause is the cessation of oocyte maturation. In contrast, spermatogenesis does not begin until the onset of puberty but continues until death.

Sex is determined by the specific combination of female and male gametes. All (normal) ova contain an X chromosome. Theoretically, in men, half the gametes contain an X chromosome and half contain a Y chromosome. Thus, it is the man who determines the sex of the resultant offspring (i.e., girl = XX and boy = XY).

Sperm Migration and Capacitation

Few of the 175,000 to 300 million sperm in the ejaculate ever reach an egg.[3,4] Fertilization must occur in the distal portion of the fallopian tubes, and many sperm do not make it that far. Some migrate up the wrong tube, whereas others are destroyed by acid in the female tract. Sperm propel forward in the female tract through the movement of the flagella. Although female orgasm is not required for fertilization, muscular contractions of the uterus may aid in the movement of sperm. Before fertilization can occur, a series of functional changes, known as capacitation, must occur to allow the sperm to penetrate the zona pellucida of the egg. The toughened sperm must be altered so that the head becomes more permeable to calcium ions.[5]

The egg is released into the fallopian tube before the second meiotic division is completed. When a spermatozoan reaches an oocyte, it binds to the membrane, inducing the **acrosome reaction,** during which hyaluronidase and proteinases (acrosins) are released by the sperm. These enzymes clear a path through the zona pellucida. When the spermatozoan reaches the oocyte, the membranes of the two cells fuse. **Polyploidy** (greater than a diploid chromosome number) is prevented by two separate reactions. One occurs quickly when, upon binding of a sperm, sodium channels open, depolarizing the egg membrane, and preventing entrance of other sperm. Penetration of the egg also stimulates the release of cortical granules from just beneath the zona pellucida. These granules produce secretions that swell and form a fertilization membrane that prevents further penetration.[5] After penetration, the egg completes the second meiotic division. The male and female pronuclei will then fuse, producing a diploid **zygote** that contains one **allele** for each gene from each parent.

The resultant zygote then undergoes several mitotic divisions. This process, cleavage, produces a ball

Figure 6-1. Relationships between sex hormones and anatomy.

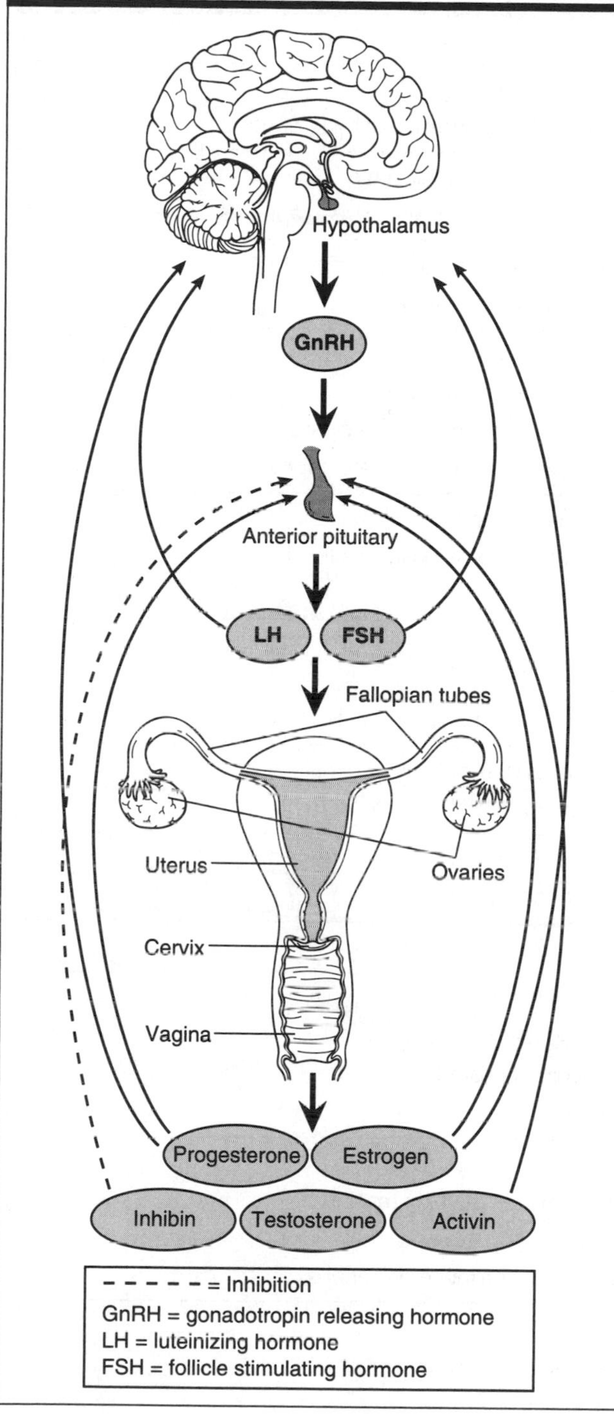

of cells called **blastomeres** that are genetically identical and **pluripotent.** Because they are, as yet, undifferentiated, these cells could theoretically be coaxed into differentiating into specific cell types. There is a great deal of interest and controversy in the use of these embryonic stem cells or blastomeres because of their potential as a source of specialized human tissue for transplantation and treatment of disease.[6,7]

Approximately 72 hours after ovulation, the **conceptus** has traveled down the fallopian tube, reached the 16-cell stage called the **morula,** and entered the uterine cavity, where additional divisions occur. In approximately 4–5 days, the morula will consist of almost 100 cells. The zona pellucida disintegrates, and the morula is now referred to as the **blastocyst,** which is a hollow ball of cells. The outer layer is the **trophoblast,** which will form the fetal contribution to the placenta. The inner cell mass, **embryoblast,** will give rise to the embryo proper.

In the U.S., 12 in 100 births are twins.[8] Monozygotic twinning may occur when the inner cell mass splits. The two resulting embryos have the same chromosomes and are genetically identical. Dizygotic twins are no more closely related than siblings and occur when two ova are released simultaneously and both are fertilized. Monozygotic twins account for 4 in 1,000 births, and dizygotic twins account for 8 in 1,000 births.[8] The rate of dizygotic twinning increases with maternal age from 0.3% at age 20 to 1.4% at ages 35–40.[9] The rate of dizygotic twins is highest among black women (10–40 per 1,000 births) and lowest for Asian women (2 per 1,000 births).[10]

Implantation and Hormonal Changes

About 6 days after ovulation (Table 6-1), the blastocyst usually attaches to the endometrial lining of the uterus; however, implantation can occur wherever the blastocyst finds a vascularized area. Implantation in the fallopian tube or even outside the female reproductive area results in an ectopic pregnancy, which can be life threatening for the pregnant woman. Ectopic pregnancies typically occur when there is an obstruction in the fallopian tube.[11]

During the process of implantation in the uterus, the blastocyst essentially buries itself in the endometrium; a part of the trophoblast extends root-like structures that digest the endometrial cells. The endometrial tissue then grows over the invading cells. This process forms the basis for subsequent early nutrition for the embryo. Implantation requires about 1 week.

The trophoblast also secretes human chorionic hormone (hCG). The hCG stimulates the corpus luteum of the ovary to continue its production of estrogen and progesterone, thereby maintaining the endometrial lining. Estrogen and progesterone also inhibit the pituitary gland. By the end of the second month, the trophoblast has become the **chorion,** the outermost of the fetal extraembryonic membranes,

Table 6-1. Embryonic and Fetal Development by Weeks of Pregnancy

Week	Gestational Changes
Embryonic Phase	
Week 1 (day 1–7 postfertilization)	Fertilization; cleavage Blastocyst implants in endometrial lining of uterus
Week 2	Trophoblast grows to form placenta Embryonic disc flattens; primitive streak appears
Week 3 (First missed menstrual period)	Notochord appears; gastrulation begins Neural grove and somites appear
Week 4	Embryo measures 4 mm Heart bulges and begins to beat Branchial arches form; neural tube closes Ear buds (otic pits) and hepatic plate appear
Week 5	Embryo measures 8 mm Optic cups and lens form, nasal pits form Limb buds form
Week 6	Embryo measures13 mm Lungs begin to form Arms and legs lengthen, digits (webbed) appear
Week 7	Embryo measures18 mm All essential organs have begun to form
Week 8	Embryo measures30 mm Facial features continue to develop
Fetal stage	
Weeks 9–12	Fetus measures 8 cm Head makes up half of fetal body Genitals well differentiated Face well formed
Weeks 13–16	Fetus measures about15 cm Fetus actively moves; sucking motions Lanugo covers transparent skin Liver and pancreas produce secretions
Week 19	Fetus reaches 20 cm Eyebrows, lashes, fingernails appear "Quickening" occurs Fetal heartbeat can be heard with stethoscope
Week 23	Fetus reaches 28 cm and weighs about 725 g Alveoli form; startle reflex present
Week 27	Fetus is 38 cm, weighs about 1.2 kg Nervous system controls some body functions Baby may survive if born

(*Continued on next page*)

Week	Gestational Changes
Week 31	Fetus is 38–43 cm and weighs about 2 kg Body fat increases Bones fully developed but soft
Week 35	Fetus is 40–48 cm and weighs 2.5–3 kg Baby born at 36 weeks has good chance of surviving
Weeks 36–39	Fetus is 48–53 cm; lanugo mostly gone Fetus is considered full term at week 37

and will begin secretion of progesterone, which makes the corpus luteum unnecessary. During the remainder of the pregnancy, the ovary remains dormant.

Prenatal Nutrition and Placenta

During the early stages of fetal development, the embryo is nourished by the trophoblast that secretes enzymes to digest the energy-rich decidual cells of the endometrium. This source of nutrition persists for the first 8 weeks of development. The placenta begins to develop at 11 days after conception and takes over the nutrition function by 9 weeks. Formation of the placenta involves extension of the chorionic villi into the endometrium. Pools of free blood develop around the villi that merge to form the placental sinus. Rapid growth of the villi produces mesenchymal cells that develop into blood vessels. As the pregnancy proceeds, the chorionic villi branch out extensively and are surrounded by maternal blood in the placental sinus. This is the site of gas exchange, where oxygen passes by simple diffusion into the fetal circulation and carbon dioxide is removed. Electrolytes and lipophilic substances also move across the placental membranes via simple diffusion. Glucose moves by facilitated diffusion; amino acids move by active transport. As the placental membranes grow, they become stretched thinner, thereby increasing permeability.

The placenta is about 20 cm in diameter and 3 cm in thickness. The surface facing the fetus gives rise to the umbilical cord, which contains three vessels. The two umbilical arteries carry deoxygenated, waste-laden blood to the maternal circulation for elimination. The umbilical arteries flank the umbilical vein, which carries oxygen and nutrient-rich blood from the maternal circulation directly to the fetal liver. Some of this blood is filtered by the fetal liver, but much of it passes into the ductus venosus, which leads directly to the inferior vena cava and then to the heart.

The placenta fulfills a number of functions in addition to the nutritional, respiratory, and excretory roles described above. The placenta promotes blood flow at the implantation site by secretion of angiogenic factors and promotion of vasodilation.[12] It stores carbohydrates, iron, and calcium, which can be released when fetal demands exceed maternal supply. The placenta also transports some maternal antibodies (e.g., immunoglobulin G) into the fetal circulation to confer passive immunity. Estrogen, progesterone, lactogen, growth hormone, leptin, ghrelin, and relaxin are secreted by the placenta.[13] Placental development appears to be both highly adaptable and highly regulated.[5,14]

The placenta is also permeable to nicotine, alcohol, many drugs, and chemicals, as well as some bacteria and viruses. The negative effects of nicotine and alcohol on fetal development have been well documented and are discussed in Chapter 36: Substance-Use Disorders. The adjective *teratogenic* is used to describe organic molecules known to cause fetal abnormalities. These include a number of over-the-counter and prescription medications and substances of abuse, which are described generally in Chapter 23: Drug Principles in Pregnancy and Lactation and specifically in some clinical chapters. Some viruses and bacteria are known to cross the placenta, and some can lead to serious fetal deformities and possibly death. These include, but are not limited to, human immunodeficiency virus (HIV), cytomegalovirus, rubella, and bacteria that are responsible for causing gonorrhea and syphilis (Chapter 38: Sexually Transmitted and Infectious Diseases). A protozoan, *Toxoplasma*, which is relatively harmless in adults, can have devastating effects on fetal development.[5] Thus, women who are pregnant are not to empty cat litter boxes, a common site for *Toxoplasma*.

The placenta has both maternal (endometrial) and fetal (chorionic) components. The chorion is entirely fetal in origin. Cells from the chorion can be removed by chorionic villus biopsy and examined for genetic abnormalities (Chapter 27: Prenatal Diagnosis). The fetus also produces three additional membranes; the **amnion,** yolk sac, and allantois. The formation of the fetal embryonic membranes reflects the phylogenetic history of all vertebrates. All vertebrate embryos develop in a watery environment. In terrestrial vertebrates (amniotes), the embryo floats in a fluid-filled sac, the amnion. The amnion persists in mammals, completely surrounding the embryo and becoming filled with amniotic fluid filtered from the maternal circulation, which protects the fetus during gestation. During the gestational period, fetal cells routinely slough off into the amniotic fluid, which can be accessed through amniocentesis and analyzed for birth defects and genetic abnormalities. Egg-laying vertebrates have a yolk sac to gather nutrition from the yolk, a function rendered useless in placental mammals. The yolk sac serves a hematopoietic function in early development and contributes to the formation of the digestive tract in humans. The allantois, which arises as an outpocketing from the yolk sac, forms the proximal portion of the umbilical cord in humans but performs respiratory and excretory functions in egg-laying amniotes.[15]

Embryonic Development

GASTRULATION

Weeks 2–8 of pregnancy constitute the embryonic phase (Table 6-1). The onset of this phase is marked by a process called **gastrulation.** The amniotic cavity forms during the second week as fluid begins to accumulate between the cells that make up the embryonic disk and the overlying trophoblast. Another space separates the embryo with its attached amnion from the outer wall of the blastocyst, now called the chorion. All cells in the inner cell mass of the blastocyst are identical as no differentiation has occurred. Gastrulation requires cells to change position relative to one another. Cells move inward along a narrow line called the primitive streak. The cells that move inward become the embryonic endoderm, whereas those on the outer surface become the ectoderm. Finally, a third layer forms between the ectoderm and endoderm called the mesoderm. Each of these germ layers will form a specific part of the developing embryo (Table 6-2). Once gastrulation is complete, the fate of the cells has been determined.

ORGANOGENESIS

The nervous system is among the first organ systems to develop. The movement of cells internally, which marks the onset of gastrulation, stimulates the overlying ectoderm to form neural tissue.[16] The neural ridges and folds are visible on the dorsal surface. The edges of the neural folds will fuse to form the neural tube by the third week of development. The anterior (superior) portion of the neural tube will differentiate into the five parts of the embryonic brain: telencephalon, diencephalon, mesencephalon, metencephalon, and myelencephalon. The optic vesicles protrude from the diencephalon. They will form the optic nerve, retina, and iris. The posterior (inferior) portion of the neural tube forms the spinal cord. The hollow center of the neural tube remains as the ventricles of the brain. The ectoderm will also form the epidermis, lens, and cornea of the eye and contribute to several glands. Many congenital malformations result from incomplete closure of the neural tube, including **spina bifida** and **meningoceles.** A number of neural tube defects can be diagnosed by detection of alpha-fetoprotein in the amniotic fluid (Chapter 27: Prenatal Diagnosis). The rate of neural tube defects appears to be correlated with low folic acid concentrations in the mother, although the role played by folic acid in normal neural tube development remains unknown.[17,18]

Immediately below the developing neural tube lies the notochord; this mesodermally derived embryonic structure will form the vertebrae. The mesoderm forms or contributes to almost every organ system

Table 6-2. Results of Gastrulation

Germ Layer	Tissues Formed
Ectoderm	Nervous system and sense organs
Mesoderm	Skeleton (bone, cartilage)
	Muscles
	Circulatory system
	Excretory system
	Reproductive system
	Dermis
	Muscle layers surround digestive tract
	Peritoneal membranes
Endoderm	Lining of digestive tract
	Organs that develop as outgrowths of digestive tract (liver, pancreas, lungs)

except the nervous system. Bands of tissue called somites appear on either side of the developing neural tube. These will form muscles. The pharyngeal arches that form the future face, neck, mouth, and nose begin to form by day 21.

The circulatory system begins to form early in development. The heart begins as a hollow tube, developing from the confluence of early blood vessels (sinus venosus). The posterior portion will become the atria; the anterior part, the ventricles. The heart begins to beat at about 22 days. Septa form, creating a right and left atrium and ventricle. The opening between the atria persists throughout fetal development as the foramen ovale. This structure, along with the ductus arteriosus, a connection between the pulmonary trunk and aorta, diverts blood flow from the fetal lungs to the placenta. Endoderm will form the mucosal lining of the digestive system.[19]

During the third week, primordial germ cells, which arise from mesodermal cells surrounding the yolk sac, begin to migrate to the genital ridges. Gonads in both sexes develop from embryonic mesoderm by the sixth week of development, but they are generic. Sexual differentiation of genetic boy begins at the end of the sixth week, when a specific gene on the Y chromosome, the SRY gene, is expressed. This gene codes for a protein that regulates formation of male genitalia. In the absence of the SRY gene product, an ovary containing ovarian follicles will develop. Mutations in this gene may produce genetic boys with female external genitalia and rudimentary testes.[20] The SRY gene also makes a protein that affects dopamine concentrations in the brain. Men are more prone to development of dopamine-related diseases, such as Parkinson disease and schizophrenia.[21]

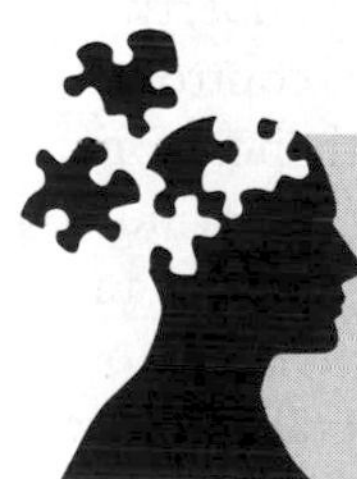

Therapeutic Challenge:

Some antiseizure medications can increase the risk of neural tube defects. Furthermore, discontinuation of antiseizure medications during a pregnancy can pose a risk to both the fetus and the pregnant woman. Healthcare providers have duties to avoid harm. How should parents be educated about these harms? How does one balance the risks to both the fetus and pregnant woman?

Lateral to the presumptive gonads are two tubes: the müllerian (paramesonephric) duct and the mesonephric duct. In male fetuses, müllerian-inhibiting substance causes degeneration of the müllerian duct, and the mesonephric duct differentiates into the paired ductus deferens. In female fetuses, the müllerian duct will develop into the fallopian tube, and the mesonephric duct degenerates. The ducts from both sides of the body fuse in the inferior portion of the pelvic cavity to become the uterus. By 8 weeks of development, the ovaries (or testes) are clearly differentiated, although external genitalia are not yet distinguishable.[22] The external genitalia develop from a genital tubercle that in female fetuses gives rise to the clitoris and in male fetuses becomes the penis. Urethral folds extending from the tubercle will become the labia.

Some babies are born with "ambiguous genitalia." For example, some newborns can genetically be male with testes present in the groin area but have female external genitalia. Parents may be asked to choose a sex assignment for their child. Male sex assignment would involve surgeries along with testosterone treatment. Female sex assignment would require hormone therapy but less invasive surgery. The dilemma for parents is to choose a sex for a newborn without knowing anything about the child. The chapters on the effect of development and sex differences on diseases and drugs and the lesbian, bisexual, and transgender healthcare issues provide some additional information, but a complete discussion of ambiguous and multiple sex genitalia and the issues of the child's and adult's sex throughout life is beyond the scope of this book.

By the end of the first 8 weeks of the prenatal period, all organ systems have begun to form. This period is most critical for the developing embryo. The embryo is also particularly susceptible to the effects of alcohol, medications, radiation, and nutritional deficiencies during this time.[5] Spontaneous abortions (miscarriages) that occur during the first trimester are usually caused by major genetic defects or congenital abnormalities in the embryo.

Fetal Development

The ninth week through birth makes up the fetal period. The transition from embryo to fetus is marked by the onset of ossification in the cartilaginous skeleton. At 9 weeks, the fetus weighs about 5 g and is about 3 cm long. The head makes up nearly half of

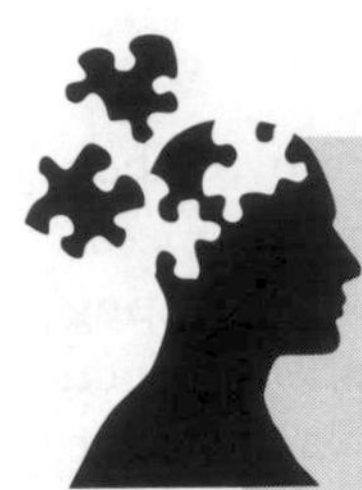

Therapeutic Challenge:

How can you determine if a girl is growing similar to average growth rates?

body. Limbs are now distinct, and digits are formed. Major blood vessels form.[23]

By the third month, the kidneys have begun to function. Urine is formed and excreted into the amniotic fluid, and hematopoiesis begins in the fetal bone marrow. During the first trimester, the head and brain grow rapidly. Now, body growth accelerates. Although cardiac activity is visible by a vaginal probe on a real-time ultrasound around 6 weeks, a heartbeat can be heard by Doppler by the end of the third month.[24] Although fetal movement is occurring, it cannot, as yet, be detected by the pregnant woman. Brain waves are measurable by electroencephalogram by the end of 12 weeks. By the onset of the second trimester, the placenta takes over as the producer of the hormones necessary to maintain the pregnancy.

During the fourth month, ossification continues. The demand for calcium to support bone growth is very high now. The lungs are formed but collapsed and nonfunctional. Rapid development of body systems progresses.

At 5 months, the fetus weighs about 200 g and is more than 20 cm long. Muscle movements become more pronounced and can be felt by the pregnant woman **(quickening).** The skin is fully formed but cannot yet perform all of its adult functions. The eyes are sensitive to light. Fine hair **(lanugo)** covers the body.

During the sixth month, substantial weight gain occurs. By the end of the sixth month, the completion of the second trimester, the fetus weighs 550–800 g and is 27–35 cm long. The skin is wrinkled. Alveolar cells in the lungs begin to produce surfactant.

By the end of the seventh month, the head is more proportionate to the rest of the body. A fetus at this stage can survive independently outside the womb. The fetus assumes an upside-down position.

During the eighth month, growth continues as subcutaneous fat is deposited and the skin becomes less wrinkled. By the end of the eighth month, the fetus weighs 2,000–2,300 g and is 41–45 cm long.

Growth continues during the ninth month. The fetus fills the uterine cavity, making movement difficult. Nails grow, and the lanugo is shed. Average birth weight is 3,200–3,400 g (7–7.5 lb), but birth weights vary as a result of maternal, fetal, and placental factors.[25] Low birth weight increases the risk for perinatal mortality. The birthing process is covered in Chapter 28: Labor and Delivery.

Postnatal Development

INFANCY, CHILDHOOD, AND ADOLESCENCE

Human growth from birth to adulthood can be divided into stages: infancy includes the first 2 years of life, childhood extends from years 2–10, and adolescence begins with puberty and continues until approximately 18 years of age. Infancy, early childhood, and adolescence are characterized by growth and development. Growth occurs when cells divide or when existing cells increase in size. Development refers to the emergence of new structures or functions. Both of these processes continue throughout these periods, at varying rates. Pharmacokinetics of medications can also change as growth and development occur and are discussed in Chapter 7: Sex and Gender Differences. Furthermore, growth and development can result in the appearance of new behaviors. For example, the ability of an infant to see and grasp a toy requires the growth and development of motor neurons, skeletal muscles, the visual cortex, and retinal cells.

Different tissues grow and develop at different rates. The growth of the nervous system is disproportionately rapid during prenatal and early postnatal periods. At birth, the brain has already attained 25% of its adult size, and by age 5, it is almost 90% complete. Neurons do not generally divide once formed, but they do enlarge and establish new connections, dramatically increasing the number of synapses. Other tissues develop more slowly. In general, overall body growth is rapid during the first 4 years, tapers off somewhat, and then accelerates during puberty.

Growth and metabolic patterns are controlled, in part, by changes in hormones: growth hormone, thyroxine, and the sex hormones. Growth hormone stimulates protein synthesis in most tissues and causes growth of the long bones by stimulating osteogenic activity. Thyroxine regulates metabolic rate and remains high throughout infancy and early childhood. The sex hormones bring about sex-specific changes before and during puberty. Girls experience an increase in the secretion of adrenal androgens (adrenarche) around age 7 or 8 years.

An accelerated growth spurt that accompanies puberty produces a rapid increase in height: 2.5–4 inches in girls.[25] Girls begin their adolescent growth spurt and attain peak growth rates earlier than boys. The average onset of the adolescent growth spurt in girls is at 11–14 years; in boys, it is at 12–16 years.

The sex hormones produce differences in skeletal growth. Testosterone causes the bones of the chest and shoulders to grow rapidly; estrogen causes growth of the pelvic bones. These hormones also influence muscle and fat composition of the body, with estrogen stimulating fat deposition and testosterone affecting muscle mass. The sex hormones, of course, influence the appearance of secondary sex characteristics. Stimulation by estrogen, progesterone, and growth hormone brings about the appearance of breast buds (thelarche) between the ages of 8 and 13 years. Estrogen, along with adrenal androgens, stimulates the development of pubic hair (typically ages 8–14 years) followed by axillary hair (pubarche).[25]

Both estrogen and progesterone contribute to the onset of the first menstrual flow (typically ages 10–16 years).[26,27] The last century has witnessed a decline in the average age for the onset of menarche. The average age for a girl born in 1900 to begin menstruation was 14 years; in contrast, a girl born today will probably begin to menstruate by age 12–13 years. Earlier maturation is described by some as a secular trend and is often attributed to improved nutrition and environmental conditions. However, the decline in the age at onset of puberty during the last century has been observed among all socioeconomic classes. Increases in migration and consequent variations in genetic makeup might also have contributed to early maturation.

MENARCHE AND THE MENSTRUAL CYCLE

Menarche is defined as the onset of menstrual bleeding, which defines the beginning of reproductive life. It is preceded by thelarche and pubarche. Rising concentrations of gonadotropin-releasing hormone (GnRH) released by the hypothalamus stimulate the anterior pituitary gland to release follicle-stimulating hormone (FSH) and luteinizing hormone (LH) (Figure 6-1). The FSH targets the ovary, stimulating the release of estrogen, inhibin, and some androgens. Concentrations of FSH and LH rise sharply during the early teens. Estrogens (estradiol and estrone) stimulate breast development and fat deposition, increase growth hormone and height, and widen the pelvis. The ovary also produces a small amount of androgens (0.5 mg/day) that contribute to hair growth and libido.

During the menstrual cycle, hormone concentrations fluctuate, whereas in men, sex-hormone concentrations remain fairly constant. The menstrual cycle is ultimately controlled by the hypothalamus, the secretions of which stimulate the anterior pituitary gland to produce hormones that target the ovaries (Figure 6-1 and Table 6-3). The ovaries, in turn, produce hormones that target the uterus but also inhibit the hypothalamus. This cycling of hormones is controlled by feedback inhibition such that high concentrations of ovarian hormone, inhibin, decrease the secretion of hormones, particularly FSH, from the anterior pituitary. This feedback loop constitutes the hypothalamic–pituitary–ovarian (H-P-O) axis.

The menstrual cycle is divided into the follicular and luteal phases (Figure 6-2). The menstrual cycle begins at day 1 with menstrual bleeding and lasts an average of 28 days. The actual cycle length can vary from woman to woman as well as each cycle of the same woman. The normal cycle length is 23–35 days. Cycle length is particularly variable the first few years after menarche as well as during perimenopause (the few years leading up to menopause). The remainder of this chapter will refer to a cycle length of 28 days. Each half of the cycle lasts approximately 14 days, although this can vary as well. Additional information about the normal cycle and menstrual abnormalities can be found in Section 3. Variations in the length of time of each phase of the cycle may contribute to infertility in some women (Chapter 22: Infertility).[28,29]

The first half of the cycle, which occurs from the first day of menstrual bleeding until ovulation, is defined as the follicular phase, because during this time the follicle is developing inside of the ovary. The FSH produced by the anterior pituitary controls this part of the cycle and stimulates maturation of the primary follicle in preparation for ovulation. The mature oocyte typically is 21–23 mm.[29] Estrogen is synthesized by the follicular cells in response to FSH stimulation. The estrogen secreted by each follicle increases the number of FSH receptors on that follicle, thereby making its own cells more sensitive to FSH. Thus, the most mature follicle gets stimulated at the expense of the others. That follicle will then release its mature oocyte while the other, less sensitive follicles degenerate and form scar tissue, referred to as *atresia*. Estrogen and FSH also stimulate the mature follicle to produce LH receptors.

Estrogen concentrations begin to increase around day 8 and peak around day 12. The estrogen peak stimulates the pulsatile secretion of GnRH by the hypothalamus, which, in turn, produces a surge in

Figure 6-2. Menstrual cycle.

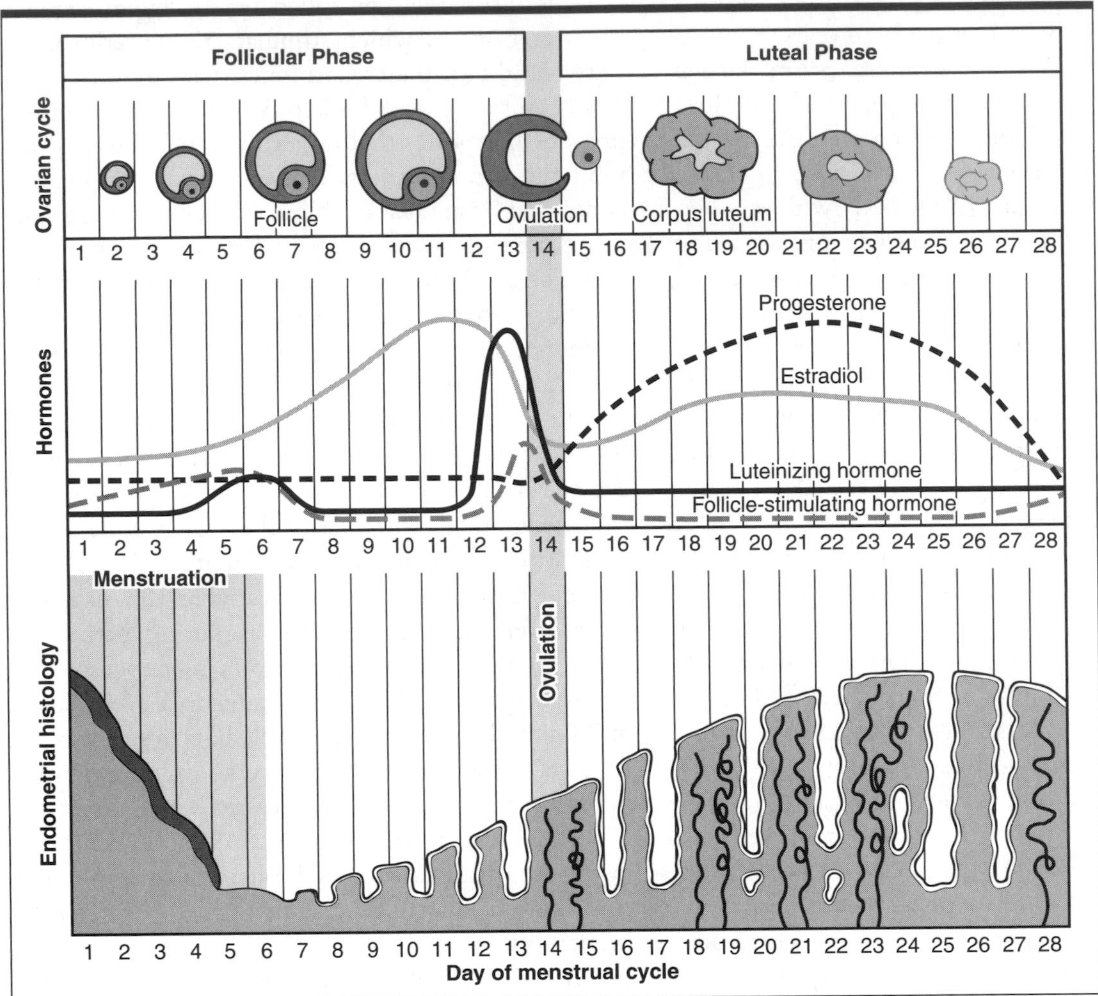

FSH and LH concentrations, with LH concentrations rising more sharply but in a pulsatile release. Luteinizing hormone has several roles within the cycle. To begin, LH inhibits oocyte maturation–inhibiting substance; this allows the follicle to continue maturation through meiosis in preparation for potential fertilization.[30] The LH increases blood flow in the follicle and stimulates production of enzymes that weaken the ovary wall to facilitate release of the egg from the mature follicle. A structure called a stigma appears on the surface of the follicle. Follicular fluid escapes, carrying the oocyte with it. The oocyte will be picked up by the fimbriae, fingerlike projections of the fallopian tubes. Ovulation typically occurs on day 14 of a 28-day cycle. After ovulation, the egg remains viable for fertilization for 24 hours. Immature or smaller-sized ovulated oocytes can be a potential cause for infertility.[28] For the first 2 years following menarche, many of the cycles are anovulatory because LH is not produced.[30,31]

Luteinizing hormone is the hormone responsible for the second half—or luteal phase—of the menstrual cycle. After ovulation, the corpus luteum, which is what remains of the now-empty follicle, produces estrogen, progesterone, and testosterone as a result of stimulation by LH. Lutein cells in the corpus luteum also produce inhibin, a hormone that inhibits FSH production by the pituitary gland. In the luteal phase, estrogen concentrations decline but begin to increase again around cycle day 20 and peak around cycle day 25. In the uterus, estrogen is responsible for increasing the number of endometrial cells, production of progesterone receptors, and blood flow. Progesterone concentrations begin to rise and peak around cycle day 22. The role of progesterone during the cycle is also to build up the uterine lining. The uterine blood flow increases and the lining thickens to allow for implantation to occur. If fertilization does not occur within 10–12 days after ovulation, the corpus luteum begins to degrade, which results in decreased estrogen and progesterone produc-

Table 6-3. Hormones in Women During Menstruation

Hormone	Produced By	Target	Role
Gonadotropin-releasing hormone (GnRH)	Hypothalamus	Anterior pituitary	Stimulates the anterior pituitary to produce FSH and LH
Follicle-stimulating hormone (FSH)	Anterior pituitary	Ovary	Oocyte maturation
Inhibin	Dominant follicle	Anterior pituitary	The dominant follicle produces inhibin to decrease FSH production from the anterior pituitary
Luteinizing hormone (LH)	Anterior pituitary	Ovary	Matures oocyte to stimulate ovulation
Estrogen (primarily estradiol)	Ovary	Various tissues	At menarche, encourages breast, hair, bone, and muscle growth Throughout reproductive years: maintains female sexual physical characteristics, related behaviors, and reproductive organs; stimulates cyclic uterine lining growth and repair
Progesterone	Ovary and corpus luteum	Uterus	Thickens uterine lining to prepare for potential implantation
Testosterone	Ovary and adrenal gland	Ovary	Precursor to estrogen production (primarily estradiol)

tion. Without high progesterone concentrations, the thickened uterine lining cannot be maintained and is thus shed, resulting in menstrual bleeding. The corpus luteum atrophies (producing the corpus albicans), and negative inhibition of the H-P-O axis ceases. The first day of discharge marks day 1 of a new cycle. The vaginal discharge consists of blood, serous fluid, and endometrial tissue. The presence of fibrinolysins prevents clotting of the menstrual fluid.[5]

If implantation does occur, the implanted embryo begins producing hCG, which maintains the uterine lining and corpus luteum. The corpus luteum begins producing hormone concentrations to help support the pregnancy until the placenta is capable of hormone production. Stimulated by LH, the corpus luteum secretes progesterone, which continues the preparation of the endometrium for pregnancy, inhibits the contraction of the uterus, and inhibits the development of a new follicle.

Pregnancy

Preparation for pregnancy begins early in the life cycle of an adolescent and continues through the reproductive ages. All of the eggs have begun development by birth, awaiting only the hormonal stimulus that signals the onset of sexual maturity.

Many changes occur in a pregnant woman during the 9-month gestation period. The female body adapts to the needs of the growing embryo and then fetus through changes in weight and physiology. Metabolic demands throughout pregnancy increase approximately 300 kcal/day above the woman's prepregnancy need. Overall, in the course of pregnancy, women of normal body mass index (BMI)should gain 25–35 lb, whereas underweight women should gain 27.5–40 lb and overweight women should gain 15–25 lb.[32-36] Women who deviate markedly from recommended weight during pregnancy are at higher risk for maternal and neonatal complications. These include abnormal fetal size for gestational age, cesarean deliveries, **pre-eclampsia** (Chapter 26: High-Risk Pregnancies), and postpartum obesity. A significant portion of peripartum weight gain occurs during the third trimester, when women will gain approximately 1 lb/week while the developing fetus gains approximately 0.5 lb/week. For a woman who has gained 30 lb during pregnancy, her increased weight can be estimated as 7.5 lb for the baby, 1.5 lb for the placenta, 2 lb for amniotic fluid, 2 lb for the enlarged uterus, 2 lb for enlarged breasts, 8 lb for increased bodily fluid, and 7 lb for maternal storage.[37] The remaining weight after delivery is stored in the maternal body and should slowly be lost within 1 year of delivery. Women who have returned to prepregnancy weight within 6–12 months postpartum are more likely to maintain normal BMI long term.[36,38,39]

Likewise in pregnancy, many physiological changes occur. The total amount of fluid in the body increases 40% to 50%, approximately 8 additional liters, by the end of the pregnancy.[40] To maintain adequate perfusion with the increased blood volume, cardiac output increases at around 10–20 weeks of gestation; however, as early as 5 weeks of gestation, cardiac output begins to increase in response to a decrease in systemic resistance and an acceleration of 10 beats/minute in heart rate. Glomerular filtration rates increase by an average of 30 mL/min in patients with normal prepregnancy kidney function because of cardiac output and contribution of fetal waste. Many of these changes results in changes in the pharmacokinetic handling of medications (Chapter 7: Sex and Gender Differences and Chapter 23: Drug Principles in Pregnancy and Lactation). In the skin, increased estrogen and progesterone concentrations can stimulate melanocyte-stimulating hormone to produce several pigment changes. In fact, many pregnant women will develop linea nigra, a dark line in the midline of the abdomen; chloasma, darkened skin underneath the eyes; darkened areola (breast nipples); or darkened genital skin. After pregnancy, the pigment changes in the skin usually returns to prepregnancy pigmentation.[37]

As expected, the uterus itself increases drastically during pregnancy. A nonpregnant uterine cavity can hold up to 10 mL but increases to 5–20 L at pregnancy term. The uterine walls increase in thickness during early pregnancy because of high estrogen and progesterone concentrations but thin to ≤1.5 cm in late pregnancy, which allows for fetal movements to be easily detected. The shape of the uterus changes from a pear shape in a nonpregnant woman to an ovoid shape that protrudes from the pelvic and abdominal cavity during pregnancy. The length of the fundus of the uterus, the fundal height, is measured from the top of the uterus to the pubic bone during pregnancy to monitor fetal growth.[37] Because the enlarged uterus is capable of compressing the vena cava, women after 20 weeks of gestation should no longer sleep on their backs.

As the uterus enlarges, organs within the abdominal cavity have less space. In the pulmonary system, the diaphragm is shifted upward by 4 cm; however, the ribs increase in circumference by 5 cm to maintain lung volume.[41] In fact, tidal volume, ventilation, inspiratory capacity, and pulmonary blood flow increase as a result of decreased airway resistance, progesterone, and fetal contribution. On the other hand, vital capacity and inspiratory reserve volume remain unchanged, but total lung capacity, residual volume, functional residual capacity, and expiratory reserve volume decrease during pregnancy. Maternal blood has a higher oxygenation level because of the increased amount of inspired oxygen, increased hemoglobin, and increased cardiac output. However, third-trimester serum oxygen concentrations are significantly lowered compared with postpartum women because of declining hemoglobin concentrations in the third trimester. Because of ventilation changes, carbon dioxide concentrations are increased, creating a respiratory alkalosis, which is thought to cause increased maternal dyspnea. In response, the kidneys increase bicarbonate excretion to maintain the acid-base balance.[37,41] The expanding uterus may impinge on the stomach, producing an increased incidence of reflux. The decreased abdominal space and increased hormone concentrations can contribute to constipation. Peripheral edema is common during pregnancy as a result of decreased plasma osmolality, increased vasopressin, and decreased blood circulation in the lower vena cava from the enlarged uterus.[37]

Placental hormones produced during pregnancy are responsible for many of the physiologic changes during pregnancy. Elevated estrogen concentrations are responsible for increasing the uterine lining and strength of the uterine tissue throughout the pregnancy. The increased estrogen concentrations can lead to other changes during pregnancy, including nausea/vomiting (Chapter 24: Conditions Associated with Pregnancy) for more details). Progesterone helps prevent premature uterine contractions, forms a cervical mucous plug that decreases the risk for infection during pregnancy, and develops the milk glands in the breast. For women with a history of preterm deliveries, injectable progesterone, 17-alpha hydroxyprogesterone caproate, can be administered to prevent uterine contractions (Chapter 28: Labor and Delivery).[42,43] High concentrations of estrogen, progesterone, and testosterone have a negative feedback effect on the hypothalamus and pituitary gland, resulting in low FSH and LH concentrations throughout pregnancy. Breast tissue increases in response to estrogen simulation to facilitate subsequent milk production. Also, placental lactogen, progesterone, and prolactin are responsible for developing and preparing mammary glands for milk production. However, milk ejection is not stimulated until postpartum secretion of oxytocin by the posterior pituitary gland. Placental relaxin prepares the cervix for dilation by softening it and relaxes pelvic connective tissue to allow for the pelvis to widen in preparation for labor.

Menopause

Perhaps the most dramatic sex differences in age-related function are found in the reproductive system. Decline of reproductive capacity occurs earlier in women than in men. In men, reproductive decline is gradual, and they are able to father children well into old age. For women, starting at menarche, the number of primary ovarian follicles declines, with marked reduction after age 40 years.

As women approach their late 40s and early 50s, all of the primary follicles have been ovulated or undergone atresia, which prevents future menstrual cycles. Absent follicles in the ovaries removes the source of premenopausal estradiol, progesterone, and inhibin. With absence of inhibin, the H-P-O axis increases production of GnRH, which increases FSH and LH production. Because the ovaries cannot respond to the FSH and LH production, those concentrations remain elevated in postmenopausal women. Postmenopausal estrogen is predominately estrone, which is derived from adipose tissue. Therefore, obese postmenopausal women will have higher estrone levels and less risk for osteoporosis. Refer to Chapter 17: Menopause for more discussion.

Menopause is a developmental process that occurs as ovarian function drops.[44] The World Health Organization defines menopause as the permanent cessation of menstruation resulting from the loss of follicular activity. As a woman's cycle length increases and the time between periods increases, she may experience symptoms related to fluctuating estrogen and progesterone concentrations, such as hot flushes, mood changes, insomnia, vaginal dryness, and **dyspareunia.** Perimenopause is the time frame from cycle length varying by more than 7 days until 1 year after the final menstrual cycle.[45] Postmenopause is the time after the last menstrual cycle; this includes

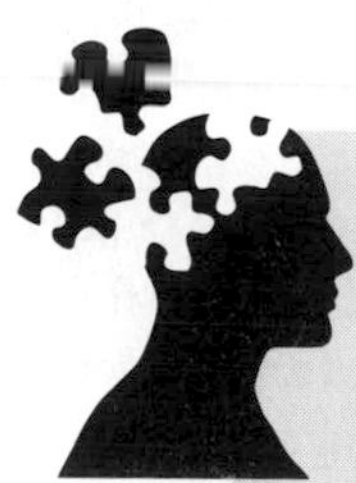

Therapeutic Challenge:

What is the usefulness and accuracy of FSH, LH, and inhibin concentration monitoring during perimenopause?

1 year of perimenopause. Figure 17-1, in Chapter 17: Menopause, explains this further. Follicular production of estrogen declines rapidly and is associated with postmenopausal symptoms of hot flushes and vaginal dryness.

The Older Woman

Women live longer than men and thus generally find themselves single in their later years. For individuals born in 2005, men can expect to live 75.2 years vs. 80.4 years for women.[45,46] In general, the characteristics of individuals who live to very old age include a family history of very old age, avoidance of obesity, adherence to a healthy diet, participation in exercise, and avoidance of cigarette smoking.[47]

More than two thirds of centenarians in the U.S. are women. Longitudinal studies of this group reveal that male centenarians are more often than female centenarians to be independent and cognitively intact. The "compression of morbidity hypothesis" postulates that individuals living to very old age delay morbidity from disease until the end of their lives.[48] However, recent evaluation of the New England Centenarian Study suggests that one third of centenarians had a chronic disease, such as heart disease, diagnosed in their mid-80s.[49] Centenarians living into very old age with morbidity ("survivors") vs. those living into very old age without morbidity ("delayers") are still more likely to be women than men. A key distinction in this research is the difference between disability and morbidity. A significant number of centenarians are able to adapt to disability for more than 15 years. This work suggests that some individuals compress disability (retain function) while others compress morbidity (avoid disease) and that both concepts are important to successful aging. In both situations, men are more likely than women to have higher physical and mental function at very old age. This sex difference could be due to an adaptive ability of women to live with disability from chronic illness.[49] The socioeconomics and psychosocial aspects of aging can be found in the respective chapters in Section 1.

AGING THEORIES

Aging is a biological process of slow, progressive, and accumulated decline throughout cells and tissues that results in a loss of function, disease, and death. There are three principal theories to explain aging: "wear and tear," genetics, and hormonal and nutrient deficiency. The wear-and-tear theory posits that aging of the cells is due to a lack of repair from the accumulating damage of free radicals or repetitive use.[50] Most free radicals are the end result of adenosine triphosphate synthesis in cells. As people age, more free radicals are formed and are more likely to leak out of the mitochondria and damage deoxyribonucleic acid (DNA). Free radical damage is interrelated with the pattern of gene expression that changes between an old vs. a young cell. As cells divide, the long piece of DNA on the end of the chromosome called the telomere shortens, leading to slight changes in gene expression on the chromosome.

In addition to changes in gene expression, another theory postulates that aging is genetically programmed so that a genome will activate at a certain point, leading to self-destructive cellular actions. This could be because some genes are essential for early development but may be detrimental to the life cycle over a long period. Current research about the genetic control of aging is partly derived from calorie restriction research in yeast, fruit flies, and earthworms with families of genes that are preserved in the evolutionary tree of mammals and humans. Calorie restriction increases the expression of the SIR2 family of mammalian genes, which repress apoptosis, increase cellular stress resistance, and decrease some endocrine actions related to insulin and fat storage. There is overlap between different families of genes that are linked to aging and might reflect a cascade of actions.[51]

A number of hormones and nutrients decline with aging coincident with the onset of degenerative changes, chronic diseases, and functional loss. In women, loss of estrogen and progesterone during menopause is an important example of age-associated hormone loss. Growth hormone and dehydroepiandrosterone, the largest component of adrenal gland secretions, are also dramatically lower in older women and men. Concentrations of 25-hydroxyvitamin D are frequently below normal values in older people, which probably play an etiologic role in the frailty syndrome leading to functional loss.

Most likely, no one theory will fully explain all of the components of aging. A combination of genetic deficiency conditions and molecular damage may overlap and contribute to a complex process.[47]

AGE-RELATED PHYSIOLOGIC CHANGES

Aging involves changes at the molecular level that affect a number of organ systems. Certain body cells, notably nerve and muscle cells, lose their ability to divide once differentiated. In tissues that contain these cell types, cell numbers and tissue mass decline over the years. Aging also results in a decreased capacity to respond to environmental changes, producing more organ dysfunction. Significant changes also occur in collagen and elastin fibers found in connective tissue. These tissues tend to lose their ability to retain water and tend to become calcified.

Most organ systems are affected in some way by aging. The skin becomes thinner because cell division is declining in the epidermis. In the hypodermis, fat accumulation declines as a result of low estrogen concentrations. The distribution of melanocytes changes, which can produce pigmented areas known as aging spots. A decrease in the numbers of collagen and elastin fibers in the dermis makes the skin less resilient and thus prone to wrinkles and sagging. In the musculoskeletal system, cell loss reduces muscle mass and, consequently, muscle strength. There is a progressive loss of cardiac muscle and decline in stroke volume as women age. Calcium loss in bone is far more significant in aging women, particularly after menopause, than aging men. As a result, osteoporosis (discussed in Chapter 40: Bone and Joint Disorders) is far more prevalent in women (65%) than in men (21%) older than age 65 years.[25] As the alveoli become less resilient, ventilation declines. Neuronal transmission in the nervous system declines with age as the myelin sheath thins and neurotransmitter concentrations decline. Portions of the brain, notably the cerebellum, lose mass with advanced age. Decreases in peristalsis and enzyme secretion cause age-related declines in the ability to absorb nutrients. Basal metabolism rates fall, as does the production of insulin, although this change may be associated with aging rather than caused by aging. Other examples can be found in Table 6-4.[52]

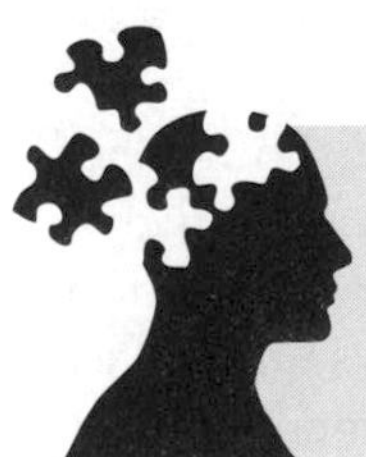

Therapeutic Challenge:

What role do antioxidants have in terms of delaying or slowing aging?

Table 6-4. Age-Induced Changes in Anatomy and Physiology

Organ System	Manifestation
Body composition	↓ Total body water ↓ Lean body mass ↑ Body fat ↔ or ↓ Serum albumin ↑ α_1-Acid glycoprotein (↔ or ↑ by several disease states)
Cardiovascular	↓ Myocardial sensitivity to β-adrenergic stimulation ↓ Baroreceptor activity ↓ Cardiac output ↑ Total peripheral resistance
Central nervous system	↓ Weight and volume of the brain Alterations in several aspects of cognition
Endocrine	Thyroid gland atrophies with age Increased incidence of diabetes mellitus, thyroid disease Menopause
Gastrointestinal	↑ Gastric pH ↓ Gastrointestinal blood flow Delayed gastric emptying Slowed intestinal transit
Genitourinary	Atrophy of the vagina due to decreased estrogen Age-related changes may predispose to incontinence
Immune	↓ Cell-mediated immunity
Liver	↓ Hepatic size ↓ Hepatic blood flow
Oral	Altered dentition ↓ Ability to taste sweetness, sourness, bitterness
Pulmonary	↓ Respiratory muscle strength ↓ Chest wall compliance ↓ Total alveolar surface ↓ Vital capacity ↓ Maximal breathing capacity
Renal	↓ Glomerular filtration rate ↓ Renal blood flow ↑ Filtration fraction ↓ Tubular secretory function ↓ Renal mass
Sensory	↓ Accommodation of the lens of the eye, causing farsightedness Presbycusis (loss of auditory acuity) ↓ Conduction velocity
Skeletal	Loss of skeletal bone mass (osteopenia)
Skin/hair	Skin dryness, wrinkling, changes in pigmentation, epithelial thinning, loss of dermal thickness ↓ Number of hair follicles ↓ Number of melanocytes in hair bulbs

Source: Adapted from reference 52.

CASE PRESENTATION

Patient Case: Part 2

Pregnancy Health Maintenance

Assessment: B.F.'s nutrient needs will increase during pregnancy to allow for proper fetal development with minimal loss from the mother. The patient consumed two alcoholic beverages around the time of conception (2 weeks of gestation). The amount of alcohol ingested by B.F. early in the pregnancy is unlikely to be a concern because major malformations that occur during gastrulation will most likely result in miscarriage.

Recommendation: Continue the prenatal vitamin daily. Administering the vitamin with a meal or small snack can improve tolerability of the vitamin. B.F. should be advised to avoid alcohol during the rest of her pregnancy.

Rationale: Most prenatal vitamins will produce appropriate vitamin and mineral concentrations during pregnancy.

Monitoring: Patient weight at each visit; specific nutrient concentrations will be drawn per clinic protocol and as symptoms dictate.

Patient education: Information on the risks of fetal alcohol exposure can be given to the patient as well as a list of foods with high calcium, iron, and other nutrient requirements.

Risk of Neural Tube Defects

Assessment: The patient has a low risk of neural tube defects like spina bifida because she has been taking folic acid for at least 1 month before conception.

Recommendation: The patient can have testing for neural tube defects with an alpha-fetoprotein level in a quad screen at 15–16 weeks of gestation.

Rationale: The neural tube has already closed at this point in pregnancy.

Monitoring: Antenatal testing per B.F.'s clinic protocol.

Patient education: Explain the early development of the neural tube and compliment on starting folic acid before conception.

Nausea

Assessment: The nausea is likely from the high estrogen concentrations during pregnancy. She has not vomited.

Recommendation: She can administer her vitamin as above and add some nonpharmacologic treatments to reduce nausea. She can avoid any triggers that make the nausea worse and try eating smaller low-fat meals and drink cold fluids. Herbals and prescription therapy also exist if nonpharmacologic therapy is insufficient.[53]

Rationale: Nonpharmacologic therapy poses no risks, but if not controlled, poor nutrition would have greater negative consequences than potential side effects from herbal and prescription medications that have documented efficacy for this condition.

Monitoring: Symptoms and patient weight at each visit.

Patient education: Reassure the mother that this symptom is very common during pregnancy and generally resolves in the first trimester or early part of the second trimester.

Summary

The continuum of development experienced by a woman throughout her life cycle affect her physical and mental well-being. Genetic, environmental, and hormonal differences affect fetal development, postnatal development, reproductive life, and aging. The unique aspects of female anatomy and physiology can be applied to an understanding of the therapeutic needs during each stage of the woman's life cycle.

References

Additional content available at
www.ashp.org/womenshealth

7 Sex and Gender Differences

Norma J. Owens, Pharm.D., BCPS, FCCP; Alicia B. Forinash, Pharm.D., BCPS, CCD; Kelly L. Matson, BSN, Pharm.D.

Learning Objectives

1. Distinguish between the terms sex and gender to foster their correct usage.
2. Describe sex/gender differences in disease presentation, morbidity, and mortality.
3. Analyze the differences in disease epidemiology and presentation in women for common conditions.
4. Apply the changes in drug pharmacokinetics and pharmacodynamics across a woman's lifespan to individualize medication therapy.
5. Evaluate the potential reasons for the differences in adverse drug effects between women and men.

To achieve optimal pharmacotherapy in women, healthcare providers must understand the effect of **sex** and **gender** on diseases and medications. Presently, the scientific evidence has documented many sex/gender differences that are clinically important to healthcare providers. This chapter is an overview of sex/gender differences with an emphasis on pharmacokinetics and pharmacodynamics. Some of the more important differences in biology that are due to sex will be highlighted, as well as some differences in epidemiology of common diseases in women vs. men. Within the other clinical chapters, further exploration and details are provided for sex/gender differences. Recommendations for individualizing pharmacotherapy to account for sex/gender differences are also provided in those chapters.

Terminology

The sex and gender of a person, whether woman or man, profoundly affects her/his biology, behavior, perceptions (e.g., self, life), and health. *Sex* is a biologic classification determined by reproductive organs and is usually the result of having two X chromosomes for women, or one X and one Y chromosome for men. Sexual differences between women and men manifest not only at a reproductive level in the person, but are also expressed at basic cellular and molecular levels. *Gender,* on the other hand, is a person's outward expression (i.e., clothing, behavior, etc.) of being a woman or man and is influenced by society, the environment, and personal cultural beliefs and experiences.[1] Confusion about the correct use of these terms—sex vs. gender—occurs in both the scientific and lay press. When the two terms are used interchangeably or incorrectly, barriers are created as a result of misunderstandings that require clarification and result in slowed progress for research in this area.

The Institute of Medicine Report on Sex as a Contributor to Human Health

In 2001, the Institute of Medicine released a publication that explored the sexual differences in many diseases from genetic, physiologic, and environmental perspectives.[1] Many examples were reviewed that show how sex affects the physiology and epidemiology of diseases and how sex influences the drugs used to treat diseases in women and men. Three consistent topics were woven throughout this publication, including the importance of sex as a biologic characteristic, the improvement in research knowledge on the biology of sex differences, and an acknowledgment of barriers that exist for those who conduct research in this area.[1]

CASE PRESENTATION

Patient Case: Part 1

M.A. is a pleasant, sleepy, 87-year-old Lebanese woman who lives at home with her daughter, son-in-law, and two grandchildren. M.A. has been a U.S. citizen for the last 30 years and fully understands the English language. She presents for follow-up care at your geriatric care clinic with no specific symptoms. The daughter accompanies M.A. to the appointment and reports that her mother is less steady on her feet and seems more confused in the morning. The daughter further describes that her mother is often groggy and asks the clinic pharmacist to evaluate her medication regimen. Three months ago, M.A. was started on ziprasidone for afternoon and evening agitation that was believed to be due to her Alzheimer's disease.

HPI: M.A. has a history of multiple medical conditions that include diabetes mellitus type 2, osteoarthritis of knees and left hip, hypertension, atrial fibrillation, and probable Alzheimer's disease.

PMH: M.A. has a pacemaker for a history of a cardiac arrhythmia.

Family and social history: M.A. was married at 21 years of age and remained married until her husband's death 3 years ago. M.A. became confused and disoriented after the death of her husband and subsequently moved to her daughter's house, where she presently resides.

Medications: Aspirin 81 mg daily, Coumadin 4 mg daily, calcium with vitamin D supplements 2 times daily with food, glyburide 5 mg daily, lisinopril 5 mg daily, acetaminophen 1,000 mg 3 times daily, donepezil 10 mg at bedtime, ziprasidone 40 mg at bedtime, and docusate 200 mg at bedtime.

Allergies: No known drug allergies.

Vital signs: Blood pressure 128/74 mm Hg (without postural changes), heart rate 76 beats/minute, afebrile, and respirations 16/minute. M.A. weighs 48 kg and is 5 feet tall.

Physical exam: M.A.'s physical exam is unchanged from her last visit 3 months ago. Her cardiac, pulmonary, and gastrointestinal exams are normal. M.A. continues to have a small amount of swelling and hypertrophy of both knees with good strength in all extremities. M.A. is not able to cooperate with the Mini Mental State Exam (MMSE) because of sedation. Her MMSE from 3 months ago was 25/30.

All labs are normal with the following significant findings: sodium 139 mEq/L, potassium 4.3 mEq/L, blood urea nitrogen 28 mg/dL, creatinine 1.2 mg/dL, glucose 102 mg/dL, A1C 5.4%, and the international normalized ratio (INR) 2.7.

At a cellular level, differences in basic biochemical processes exist that are the result of X or Y chromosome characteristics, which might be independent of hormonal differences between women and men. For instance, testosterone is presumed to be the reason men have a larger skeletal and muscle mass than women even though the effect of testosterone on genes has not been determined.[2] Recently, gene expression in human skeletal muscle was explored by examining common skeletal and muscle genes in healthy women and men.[2] The women and men in this study were from two age groups: a younger group between 20 and 29 years and an older group between 65 and 75 years of age. Both the younger and older women had a twofold higher expression of two important genes than men: one that encodes growth factor proteins and another that regulates myostatin activity. The growth factor receptor bound 10 gene (GRB10) inhibits insulin-like growth factor signals, whereas the activin A receptor IIB gene (ACVR2B) increases the effect of myostatin, which significantly influences muscle size.[2] Even though the women were from both pre- and postmenopausal age groups, their high expression of GRB10 and ACVR2B was consistent. This research is generating hypotheses that can be tested to further understand the sexual differences in the biology of women and men. In addition, research at the molecular and cellular level helps us to understand one of the premises of the Institute of Medicine report: that "every cell has a sex."[1] This is an important fact to both understand and control for in all aspects of research that will be applied to healthcare in people.

Language may serve as an example of a sex difference that extends from cellular biology and human function through recovery from disease. Women are believed to use both cerebral hemispheres for language, whereas men have a localized organization in the left hemisphere.[3] Echoplanar functional magnetic resonance imaging was used to study the language differences between 19 healthy women and 19 men.[3] Tests of **orthographic, phonologic,** and **semantic language** skills were done equally well between the women and men. The women used both the right and left inferior frontal gyrus to complete these tasks, whereas the imaging scans showed that the men had markedly localized activity in the left inferior frontal gyrus.[3] This difference in language organization in the brain may explain why women are more likely to recover speech than men after a left-sided stroke.[1] However, even though there may be evidence for improved speech recovery in one specific type of stroke, overall, women have poorer recovery from stroke than men. For instance, in a prospective cohort of 373 patients with stroke in Michigan, at 3 months after hospital discharge, women were less likely to achieve independence in activities of daily living, to improve stroke quality of life measures, and to improve scores of thinking, language, and energy.[4] To provide better healthcare for women and men, healthcare providers need to understand the sex differences in biology and disease epidemiology, as well as the social factors that influence the spectrum of illness and recovery. Although sex might explain most of these differences, gender is also important when weighing the role of social influences on disease presentation, treatment, and recovery.

Sex/Gender Differences in Mortality

Men have higher age-adjusted death rates for all causes combined, as well as for almost every specific cause, than women.[5] Cardiac disease has been the number-one cause of death for both women and men since the 1950s (Table 7-1).[5-7] However, for both women and men, the death rate for cardiac disease has declined 64% from 1950.[5] Men continue to have significantly higher death rates for cardiac disease than women (260.9 vs. 172.3 per 100,000 people, respectively in 2005).[5]

Both women and men have sex-specific cancers as the leading cancer diagnosis; however, both sexes are more likely to die as a result of lung cancer (Table 7-1). The overall age-adjusted death rate for cancer declined by 15% for both women and men from 1990 to 2005.[5] This improvement is predominately due to gains in successful treatment of cancer in younger women and men.

In the U.S., disparities in mortality statistics exist by race and sex (Figure 7-1 and Figure 7-2).[5] For men, the disparities in mortality values by race are mainly due to injuries and violence.

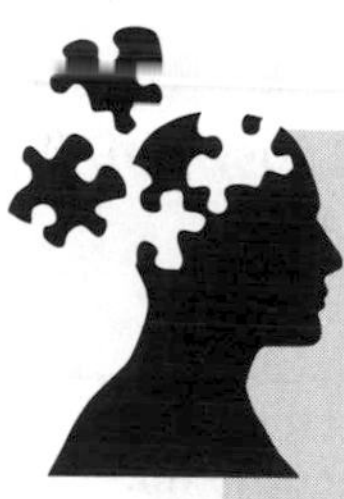

Therapeutic Challenge:

Many women are more fearful of dying from breast cancer than cardiovascular disease. Why is this? How can women be educated and motivated to follow heart-healthy lifestyles to prevent cardiovascular disease and death?

Sex/Gender Differences in Disease Morbidity

Although many similarities are found with causes of death, many diseases affect women and men differently. The incidence of cardiovascular disease is similar between women and men, but women with cardiovascular disease tend to be 10–15 years older than men upon diagnosis and are more likely to die from myocardial infarctions (see Chapter 30: Cardiovascular Disease).[6,7] Women also present with different symptoms of angina. Instead of having the classic angina symptoms of left-sided chest pain or pressure, women more commonly report nausea, indigestion, chest discomfort, upper back and jaw pain, and profound exhaustion. Because of these differences in presentation, standard treatments for acute myocardial infarctions like aspirin, beta-blockers, thrombolytics, and percutaneous transluminal coronary angioplasty are not provided as often to women. More recently, differences in standard treatments between women and men with cardiovascular disease have diminished significantly.[6,7] Women also have a higher mortality rate with coronary artery bypass grafts, higher bleeding rates with thrombolytic therapy, and lower success rates with initial angiography.[7]

The rate of cigarette smoking has declined in men but increased in women even though evidence suggests that women may be more susceptible to lung damage from cigarette smoking. Women who smoke have a significantly higher diagnosis rate for lung cancer despite differences in smoking history and body size (see Chapter 36: Substance-Use Disorders).[1,6,8,9] Another disease strongly linked to cigarette smoking, chronic obstructive lung disease, is the leading cause of death worldwide, and the actual number of deaths in women are greater than in men.[10] The rate of cigarette smoking by women in developing countries continues to rise. Women are

Table 7-1. Differences in Leading Causes of Death, Cancer Diagnosis, and Cancer Death in the U.S. Between Women And Men[a,5-7]

Women		Men	
Leading Causes of Death	**Deaths (per/100,000 U.S. Residents)**	**Leading Causes of Death**	**Deaths (per/100,000 U.S. Residents)**
1. Heart disease	172.3	1. Heart disease	260.9
2. Cancer	155.6	2. Cancer	225.1
3. Stroke	45.6	3. Unintentional injuries	54.2
4. Chronic lower respiratory diseases	38.1	4. Stroke	46.9
5. Alzheimer's disease	36.1	5. Chronic lower respiratory diseases	51.2
6. Unintentional injuries	25.0	6. Diabetes	28.4
7. Diabetes	21.6	7. Influenza and pneumonia	23.9
8. Influenza and pneumonia	17.9	8. Suicide	18.0
9. Kidney disease	14.6	9. Kidney disease	13.8
10. Septicemia	12.3	10. Alzheimer's disease	13.1
Leading Cancer Diagnosis	**New Cases (per/100,000 U.S. Residents)**	**Leading Cancer Diagnosis**	**New Cases (per/100,000 U.S. Residents)**
1. Breast	121.0	1. Prostate	159.3
2. Lung	47.2	2. Lung	69.3
3. Colorectal	40.7	3. Colorectal	54.8
Leading Causes of Cancer Death	**Cancer Deaths (per/100,000 U.S. Residents)**	**Leading Causes of Cancer Death**	**Cancer Deaths (per/100,000 U.S. Residents)**
1. Lung	40.5	1. Lung	69.0
2. Breast	24.1	2. Prostate	24.5
3. Colorectal	14.8	3. Colorectal	20.9

[a]Age-adjusted death and incidence rates per 100,000 U.S. resident population in 2005.

more susceptible to lung damage from some of the other causes for chronic obstructive lung disease, such as pollution and occupational exposure.[11] Women are not diagnosed as early with chronic obstructive lung disease, nor do they receive treatment that successfully controls their pulmonary symptoms as often as men.[11]

Common bone and joint diseases, such as osteoporosis and osteoarthritis, primarily affect women (see Chapter 40: Bone and Joint Disorders). Of the 10 million patients diagnosed with osteoporosis, 80% are women.[12] Osteoporosis also has appreciable morbidity differences between the sexes. In patients older than 50 years, 50% of women will suffer an osteoporosis-related fracture as compared with 25% of men. These fractures tend to be devastating, because 20% of patients with a hip fracture die within 1 year.[12] Osteoarthritis affects more than 16 million people in the U.S. and is the leading cause of disability in older women.[13] Some evidence suggests that women do not receive surgical joint replacement as often as men, even though women have greater disease severity. In a population-based study in Canada, 48,218 residents with hip or knee pain were

Figure 7-1. Life expectancy by sex and race.[5]

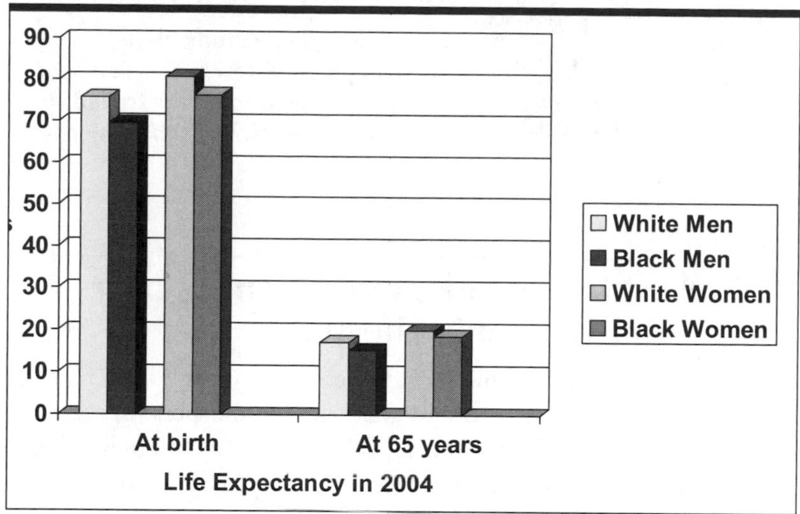

evaluated for the use of total joint arthroplasty.[14] After adjustments for disease prevalence and willingness to undergo surgery, women were 3 times more likely as men to have a medical need for surgery but were less likely to talk with their physicians about surgery (adjusted odds ratio 0.63; $p < 0.01$) or to undergo arthroplasty (adjusted odds ratio 0.78; $p < 0.001$).[14] In Canada, where access to healthcare is more equal than in the U.S., it is hard to explain the large disparity in arthroplasty rates for women with osteoarthritis. Some gender-based reasons could exist, such as a fear in women to experience any amount of disability from surgery, given that they tend to either live alone or to be caretakers of family. Women and men might perceive surgical risk and pain differently. The results could also suggest a possibility of unconscious selection bias by the healthcare providers.[14] Education directed at all individuals about osteoarthritis and osteoporosis and their treatments is needed to ensure optimal patient outcomes.

Many immunological diseases occur more often in women than men (see Chapter 37: Immunity and Autoimmune Diseases and Chapter 41: Neurological Disorders). Women are afflicted with rheumatoid

Figure 7-2. Age-adjusted death rates by sex and race in 2005.[5]

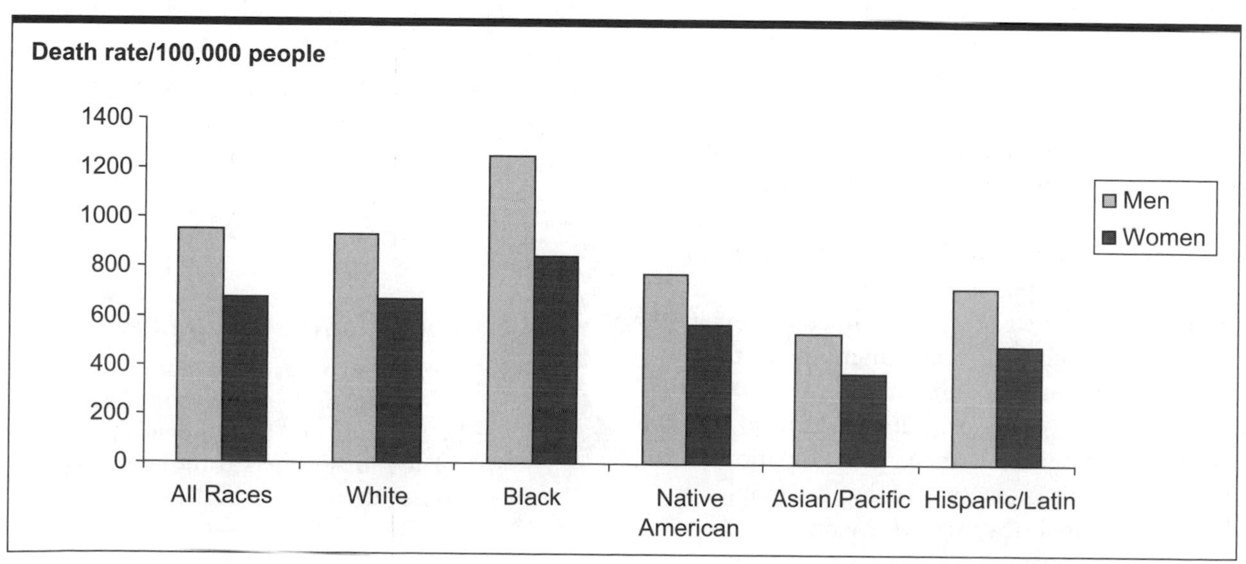

arthritis, scleroderma, myasthenia gravis, and multiple sclerosis at a rate that is 2–3 times greater than that for men.[1] There are even larger differences in the rates of occurrence for systemic lupus erythematosus, Hashimoto thyroiditis, Graves' disease, autoimmune hepatitis, and primary biliary cirrhosis, with women experiencing these diseases up to 10 times more often than men.[1,15] The reason for the marked differences in occurrence in autoimmune diseases between women and men is controversial and confounded by sex, biology, and rate of exposure of agents in the environment that might induce disease. Because women and men have a similar immune response after immunization and to treatment of infection, sex-based causes are under investigation.[15]

Some immune-based diseases fluctuate in severity during times of hormonal change in women, leading to theories that circulating estrogen plays a role in the severity of disease. Case reports support the notion that during states of hormone castration or supplementation, disease remission or exacerbation may occur. For instance, patients with rheumatoid arthritis and multiple sclerosis may enter disease remission during pregnancy.[16] One theory to explain the hormonal effect suggests that estrogen is permissive to growth of autoimmune clones of cells, placing girls and women at risk during a time of environmental exposure.[17] The X chromosome in women might also be a possible reason for the differences in disease by inactivation, modulation, or imprinting of genetic information. Lupus remains an active model of research to explain sex differences because of the marked male-to-female ratio of disease occurrence, long latency period for disease expression, and genetic risk factors. One proposed theory suggests three sequential steps that begin at conception and culminate during menarche. First, a girl may be at risk because of genetics or through in utero factors, and she is subsequently exposed to an etiologic agent, such as a virus, during childhood. The final step would occur during puberty, when estrogen may permit autoimmunity (or a lack of testosterone to restrain autoimmunity), leading to the development of clinical symptoms of lupus in young women.[18]

Even though investigating the effect of sex in health-related research is a recent phenomena, there are presently many known differences in disease incidence, presentation, diagnosis, and treatment outcome between women and men. Consideration of the influence of this powerful biologic variable is needed for the optimal healthcare for women.

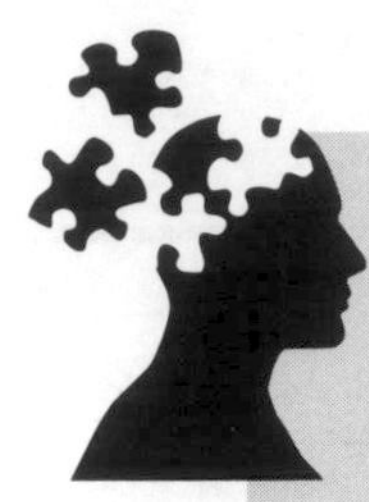

Therapeutic Challenge:

When evaluating a study about sex (biological) differences, what confounders need to be controlled to eliminate gender (social) differences?

Pharmacokinetic Changes over a Women's Lifespan

Pharmacokinetic parameters vary for many reasons related to age and maturity of the person, sex, and genetic background (Table 7-2).[1,19-54] Sex-related differences in pharmacokinetics will include both chromosomal and hormonal differences. The following section will summarize pharmacokinetics in infants, girls, menstruating women, pregnancy and childbirth, and elderly women. Oftentimes, sex-related effects on pharmacokinetics are not well investigated, requiring the healthcare provider to make dosing decisions based on data published exclusively in men or data that are combined for both women and men.

INFANTS AND CHILDREN COMPARED WITH ADULTS

The basic pharmacokinetic properties of absorption, distribution, metabolism, and elimination are strongly influenced by pediatric growth and development, which affects medication dosing for girls. There are no known sex differences in pharmacokinetics at this age. At birth, the pH of the stomach is neutral; however, acid production begins within minutes of delivery in full-term infants. By 48 hours following birth, the gastric pH decreases to 3. Then, over the next 24 hours, the pH returns to neutral and remains neutral for the following 10 days.[19] Thereafter, gastric pH steadily decreases through the first 2 years of life until it reaches adult values. Preterm infants' initial

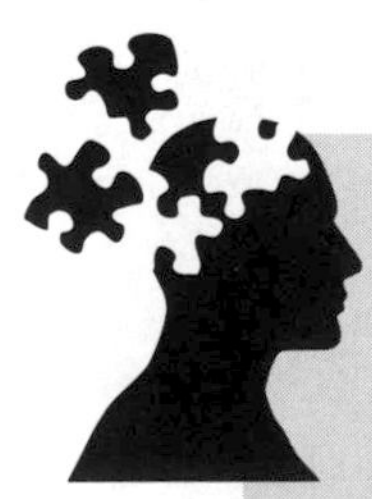

Therapeutic Challenge:

What type of research, data collection, and analyses are required by the Food and Drug Administration related to age and sex for new drug approvals?

Table 7-2. Pharmacokinetic and Physiologic Changes Associated with Age, Menstrual Cycle, Pregnancy, and Sex Differences

	Changes in Pediatrics	Changes During Menstrual Cycle	Changes During Pregnancy	Changes in Elderly Women	Changes Due to Sex[a]
Absorption	↓ Gastric pH[19] Gastric emptying time reaches adult times by 6–8 mo[20,21] ↑ Skin absorption in infants[19,21,22] ↑ Rectal pH[23]	No change[23,26,27]	↓ Motility and intestinal blood flow[31] ↑ Gastric pH[31]	↑ Gastric pH ↓ Gastric emptying time ↓ Gastrointestinal blood flow ↓ or unknown percutaneous absorption[36,37]	↓ Gastric emptying time[38-40]
Distribution	↑ Volume of distribution for hydrophilic medications[20] ↓ Protein binding[21]	No change[28-30]	↑ Blood volume ↓ Serum albumin levels Thinning of fetal-maternal barrier[32,33]	↓ Volume of distribution for hydrophilic medications ↑ Volume distribution for lipophilic medications ↓ Protein binding[36,37]	↑ Volume of distribution for lipophilic medications[1,41] ↓ Volume of distribution for hydrophilic medications[1,41]
Metabolism	Phase I[b] and II[c] metabolism immature until 1 year of age[24]	Variable effects[30]	Phase I: ↑ Hydrolysis (phenytoin) ↓ Oxidation (theophylline) ↓ CYP1A2 ↑ CYP2A6 ↑ CYP2C9 ↓ CYP2C19 ↑ CYP2D6 (third trimester) ↑ CYP3A4[34] Phase II: No change	Phase I: Variable influence on CYP activity[36,37] Phase II: No change	Phase I: ↑ Oxidation (benzodiazepines)[41-48] No change oxidation[41-48] No difference CYP3A4 isoenzyme[43,44,49,50] ↑ CYP1A2[44,50] ↑ CYP2D6[44,50-52] No change in other CYP isoenzymes[33] Phase II: ↓ Conjugation (benzodiazepines)[41-53]
Renal Elimination	GFR matures by 2 years of age[22,25]	↓ GFR in early follicular phase ↑ GFR in luteal phase[23,26,27]	↑ Renal blood flow and GFR[31-35]	↓ Creatinine clearance[36]	↓ Creatinine clearance[54]

GFR = glomerular filtration rate; CYP = liver isoenzymes.
[a]Women compared with men.
[b]Phase I metabolism includes oxidation, hydrolysis, and reduction.
[c]Phase II metabolism includes conjugation, glucuronidation, sulfation, and acetylation.

acid production and following changes are delayed up to 2 weeks. Gastric emptying is delayed for the first few days after birth in all newborns because of a lack of peristalsis and reduced gastric motility.[20,21] However, in infants 6–8 months of age, gastric motility has reached adult values.[21] Other factors to consider in intestinal drug absorption are immaturity of gut mucosa leading to increased permeability, immature biliary function, reduced first-pass metabolism, and variable microbial colonization.[22] Intramuscular administration is unreliable in neonates because of decreased peripheral perfusion and muscular contraction.[21] Additionally, neonates have less muscle mass, which is associated with severe pain at the injection site. Absorption through the skin in neonates, especially premature infants, is faster and higher because of an undeveloped epidermal barrier, increased skin hydration, and increased surface area relative to weight.[19,21,22]

Rectal absorption has limited changes that are due to maturation. Rectal pH in children is alkaline but is close to neutral in adults.[21] However, bioavailability may be affected by the first-pass effect. The degree of first-pass metabolism of a rectal-administered drug is determined by local venous drainage and the site of drug delivery. Drugs administered high in the rectum are directly metabolized by the liver, whereas administration in the lower rectum results in local absorption of the drug, which is then delivered systemically before passing through the liver.[25]

In comparison with children and adults, total body water in infants is high (80% to 90% of body weight), whereas adipose content is low (10% to 15% of body weight). The amount of total body water decreases to 55% to 60% by adulthood.[20] Extracellular water content is also different; 45% of body weight in neonates is extracellular compared with 20% in adults, which correlates with larger volume of distribution for hydrophilic drugs. Age-related distribution changes are also observed in protein binding, which is reduced in neonates and infants. Binding proteins in this population are low in concentration and have a lower capacity to bind.[21]

Birth results in dramatic changes in the hepatic circulation and oxygen tension, which may affect hepatic function within the neonatal period.[24] Biliary excretion and hepatocellular uptake are inefficient, and phase I (oxidation) and phase II (conjugation) metabolic enzymes are immature.[24] However, in vitro data showed that by 2 months of age, significant amounts and activity of metabolic enzymes were present, and by 1 year of life, they were fully matured.[21,22,24]

Unlike metabolism, maturation of renal function begins during fetal development. Nephrogenesis begins at 9 weeks of gestation, is completed by 34 weeks of gestation, and is followed by postnatal renal blood flow changes. As renal blood flow increases, glomerular filtration rate (GFR) increases during the first few weeks of life from 2–4 mL/min/1.73 m^2 at birth to 70 mL/min/1.73 m^2 in full-term infants and only 20 mL/min/1.73 m^2 in preterm infants.[22] Premature infants have reduced renal function at birth, and nephrogenesis will continue after delivery. Glomerular filtration rate may exceed adult values on a kilogram basis around 3 months of age, and it has been shown that glomerular filtration takes approximately 2 years to mature. After 2 years, GFR capacity is similar in children and adults.[25] Tubular secretion is decreased at birth but reaches adult values in about 1 year.

MENSTRUAL CYCLE-RELATED CHANGES

Limited information has been published in the literature to document the effects of a woman's menstrual cycle on drug pharmacokinetics. Some of these changes are summarized in Table 7-2 and also discussed in Chapter 10: Menstrual Cycle. During menstruation, varying effects on gastric emptying time have been reported, but these changes do not appear to significantly affect drug absorption.[23,26] Protein binding or volume of distribution changes during the menstrual cycle do not affect drug concentrations for ranitidine, theophylline, phenytoin, or nitrazepam.[27-29] With respect to metabolism, several small studies demonstrated that fluctuating hormone concentration during the menstrual cycle produced variable affects on cytochrome P450 enzyme metabolism.[27] Creatinine clearance decreased by 4% to 20% during the first week of the menstrual cycle compared with the luteal phase, although no clinically significant changes occurred for amikacin, theophylline, or tobramycin concentrations.[28-30,32,33] Despite these potential pharmacokinetic changes, none have resulted in any clinically significant effects on medications (i.e., no dosage adjustments).[27]

PREGNANCY-RELATED CHANGES

Several changes occur during pregnancy that affect pharmacokinetics (see Chapter 23: Drug Principles in Pregnancy and Lactation) that may result in increased or decreased drug concentrations (Table 7-2). Elevated serum estrogen concentrations decrease gastrointestinal motility and increase intestinal blood flow, which increases drug absorption. Drug distribution may increase during pregnancy because of a 40% to 50% increase in blood volume and increased distribution to the fetal circulation from thinning of the placental barrier. Hepatic metabolism can increase and decrease during pregnancy. Progesterone elevations can stimulate increased metabolism of drugs such as phenytoin, resulting in lower concentrations. On the other hand, medications like theophylline can compete with high estrogen and progesterone concentrations for metabolism, resulting in higher drug concentrations. Renal function increases by 25% to 50% during pregnancy from increased cardiac output, which results in an elevated creatinine clearance.[31-35] These changes can affect drug concentrations of renally eliminated medications, with dosage adjustments required as function continues to change throughout the pregnancy. Many medications, particularly drugs with a narrow therapeutic index, require more frequent monitoring during pregnancy.

ELDERLY WOMEN

Aging produces significant changes in drug pharmacokinetics that are correlated to changes in physiology. Pharmacokinetic changes that may be related to sex can not usually be separated from pharmacokinetic changes that are due to age, even though the sex differences persist as women get older.

Older people have an increase in gastric pH, a delay in gastric emptying time, and reduced gastrointestinal blood flow.[37] However, because most drugs are absorbed through passive diffusion, these age-related physiologic changes in the gastrointestinal track do not lead to significant changes in the bioavailability of most drugs. Older women continue to have a higher bioavailability for drugs that undergo CYP3A4 metabolism and p-glycoprotein transport, such as midazolam and verapamil.[36] Percutaneous absorption may be less in older people using transdermal drug delivery systems because of atrophy of the epidermis, thinning of the dermis, and a decrease in skin lipid content. Sex-related differences in percutaneous absorption have not been investigated between older women and men, but caution should be exercised for older women who lack a sufficient fat layer (because of physical size or weight) to appropriately absorb medications from transdermal drug-delivery systems.

Drug distribution can be altered in seniors because of changes in body composition that include a decrease in body water content, an increase in body fat, and a decrease in serum albumin. These age-related changes occur in both women and men.[36,37] In addition, older women and men weigh less than younger adults, and white and Asian elderly women tend to weigh the least in comparison with other groups. This has an impact on initial loading doses for older women who are physically small and who are receiving drugs with a narrow therapeutic window like digoxin, antiarrhythmics, and certain antibiotics. Because of a smaller volume of distribution, loading doses in older women should be individualized based on weight. For drugs that are particularly fat soluble, such as the benzodiazepines, the increase in total body fat leads to a larger volume of distribution and longer elimination half-life. Drug distribution may also be altered because of changes in serum albumin and α_1-acid glycoprotein concentrations leading to a higher proportion of the free fraction of bound drugs.[37] These changes do not generally affect maintenance dosing of the high-protein-bound and low-extraction-ratio drug phenytoin, but they do create a need to interpret the serum concentrations differently.[36]

Elimination of drugs is less in older people, as well as being generally lower in women. A reduction in liver blood flow will lead to a decrease in metabolism for drugs that are dependent on hepatic blood flow, such as morphine, propranolol, and some hydroxymethylglutaryl coenzyme A reductase inhibitors (e.g., simvastatin).[37] Changes related to aging and sex in metabolism through phase I cytochrome P450 pathways are more complex and are not well studied in older women.[36] Drug elimination by phase II pathways is probably not significantly different between older vs. younger people or by sex. Recent work suggests that reductions in metabolism of drugs through CYP450 enzymes is more related to alcohol intake, smoking cigarettes, genetic differences, and underlying liver disease than to age or sex.

Renal function does decline progressively with age and continues to be further decreased in elderly women vs. elderly men, resulting in the need to lower dosages of renally eliminated drugs. Renal function should be estimated with an acceptable equation—such as the Cockcroft-Gault formula, which adjusts for renal function changes related to both age and sex—to determine the extent of dosing adjustment needed. An ideal formula is not available to estimate creatinine clearance, particularly in older women who may be physically small or have a low serum creatinine. Adjustment of the Cockcroft-Gault formula for body surface area can minimize some of the estimation error.[36] Generally, the formulas are used to estimate renal function to place an older woman into mild, moderate, or severe categories so that proper dosing of medications can occur.

Pharmacokinetic Differences That Are Due to Sex

Several differences exist between women and men in pharmacokinetic properties (Table 7-2). Differences in bioavailability, distribution, metabolism, and renal elimination related to sex differences are often

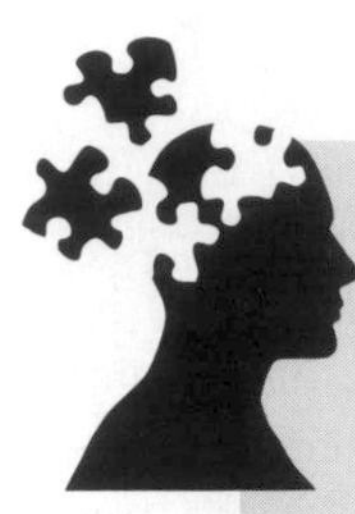

Therapeutic Challenge:

What impact do the age-related changes have on dosing, efficacy, and safety of opioids in seniors, especially agents such as propoxyphene and meperidine? How do age-related pharmacokinetic changes influence medications placed on the Beer's list of inappropriate medications that should not be used in seniors?[55]

ascribed to variation in body weight, plasma volume, plasma protein levels, cytochrome P450 activity, α_1-acid glycoprotein activity, and renal clearance.

Drug absorption factors, such as gastric emptying, transporters, and enzymes, have both similarities and differences between the sexes; however, clinical significance of this data has not been determined. To begin, gastric emptying time of both liquids and solids is slower in women, but no difference exists in small intestine emptying time; however, the clinical significance for medications absorbed in the stomach is unknown.[36,38-40] Absorption for most medications is not significantly changed, because most drug absorption occurs in the small intestine.[1,38] Changes in gastric enzymes responsible for drug metabolism are best demonstrated in women, in whom alcohol dehydrogenase activity is lower, leading to higher concentrations of serum alcohol compared with men even after controlling for differences in body size.[56,57]

Differences between women and men in the expression of transporter proteins that influence drug absorption are conflicting. Early literature had disagreement with respect to P-glycoprotein concentration expression between women and men; however, recent work failed to find sex differences when using fexofenadine as a probe for P-glycoprotein.[56] Another recent study analyzing overall sex differences using Western blot technology confirmed that no difference exists between the sexes with P-glycoprotein expression.[43]

The volume of distribution of medications can vary depending on the lipid solubility of the drug and its protein-binding characteristics. Women have a higher percentage of body fat and, as a result, lipophilic medications have a larger volume of distribution.[1,41] Some drugs that are more water soluble, like levofloxacin, fleroxacin, ofloxacin, and fluconazole, have been noted to have higher serum concentrations, even with adjustments for body mass. This difference may account for an increased incidence of adverse effects of fluoroquinolones in women.[44-47] Serum albumin does not seem to vary by sex; however, α_1-acid glycoprotein may change in relation to estrogen. Examples of how this may affect drug dosing are not clear.

Several differences exist between the sexes with respect to drug metabolism. Women tend to oxidize faster and conjugate slower but reduce similarly; however, nonbenzodiazepine medications metabolized via oxidation did not demonstrate a difference between women and men.[41,42,48] With cytochrome P450 enzyme metabolism, no overall difference exists between the sexes for activity for the enzyme family 3A.[43,44,49,50] However, when additional medications are administered that can induce CYP3A activity, women may have greater induction of intestinal activity than men, but the clinical significance of this is unknown.[49] Additionally, St. John's wort seems to induce CYP3A4 in women by about 90% vs. 50% in men.[53] Less information is available about the cytochrome P450 isoenzyme 1A2, but clearance might be higher in men than women with respect to clozapine and caffeine.[45,50] Sex differences do not appear in the 2C9 family of enzymes.[44,45-51] Women tended to have higher activity for 2D6 when the probe drug metoprolol was used. Similarly, in patients with high expression for 2D6, women have higher activity, but the clinical significance of these findings is unknown.[44,50-52]

Finally, variations with renal drug excretion have been noted between women and men, which may result in clinically significant differences and risks for adverse events. Women have lower serum creatinine concentrations and creatinine clearance compared with men.[54] Although some equations for calculating creatinine clearance, like the Cockcroft-Gault, adjust for differences in women, many medications do not have separate dosing recommendations for the sexes. The differences in renal function are clinically important because they may increase the risk of adverse events, as with bleeding risk from glycoprotein IIb/IIIa inhibitors in women.[58]

Pharmacodynamic Differences That Are Due to Sex

Sex-related differences in pharmacodynamics are less documented than sex-induced changes in pharmacokinetics. Often, pharmacodynamic differences are considered only when a higher rate of adverse drug reactions in women is noticed. Even when a pharmacodynamic difference in women may be a likely cause for a different pharmacologic response, the pharmacokinetic and pharmacogenetic influences are difficult to separate from the pharmacodynamic. Overall differences in the use of a medication between women and men add further bias and confusion when interpreting adverse drug reaction data. The U.S. General Accounting Office published a report on drugs withdrawn from the market for safety reasons from 1997 to 2001. Of the 10 withdrawn medications, eight had higher reported adverse reactions in women than men, and of those eight drugs, four medications likely had a pharmacologic reason for the difference in adverse event (terfenadine, astemizole, mibefradil, and cisapride).[59] QTc-prolongation and torsades de pointes are frequently reported adverse drug reactions for a number of drugs that may not share any chemical similarity. Women have a baseline-corrected QT interval (QTc) that is longer than men, which may add an additional risk factor.[60,61] There are drugs known to have significant differences in adverse reaction profiles between women and men (see Web Resources for Examples of Adverse Drug Reactions Reported to Occur at a Higher Rate in Women).[58,61-70]

Additional content available at
www.ashp.org/womenshealth

Some data suggest that women suffer a higher rate of death when treated with digoxin for chronic heart failure.[71] In a post hoc analysis of the Digitalis Investigation Group Trial, women who were treated with digoxin suffered a rate of death that was higher than men; an adjusted odds ratio of 1.23 (95% confidence interval 1.02–1.47). Men received an average digoxin dose of 0.25 mg and women received 0.22 mg. After adjustment for body mass index, the dose of digoxin was slightly higher for the men than women (0.0093 vs. 0.0084 mg per unit of body mass index, respectively), but digoxin serum concentrations were slightly higher for women than men at 1 month (0.9 ng/mL vs. 0.8 ng/mL, respectively).[71] The serum concentrations of digoxin were the same in women and men at 1 year (0.6 ng/mL), and there were no differences in digoxin toxicity between women and men. The increase in death in women treated with digoxin could be related to pharmacokinetics, pharmacodynamics, or a combination of the two.

Women may respond differently than men when aspirin is used for primary prevention of heart disease and stroke. In a large primary prevention trial, 100 mg of aspirin every other day for 10 years reduced the risk of stroke but not the risk for myocardial infarction or death from cardiovascular disease.[72] Aspirin used in a similar fashion in men is effective in reducing the risk for myocardial infarction and death from cardiovascular disease but not stroke.[73] This opposite finding for women vs. men may be due to sex-based pharmacodynamics. Aspirin reduces platelet aggregation more in men than women in in vitro studies.[74] This effect may be related to the presence of testosterone.

Finally, particular caution must be employed when using drug treatments that place older women at risk for bleeding. Older women who need anticoagulation with warfarin have a higher rate of hemorrhage, even after adjustment for INR, which is likely due to age, genetics, and sex-related changes in pharmacokinetics, pharmacodynamics, and pharmacogenetics.[63] These differences are adjusted in present algorithms that individualize warfarin dosing by reducing the warfarin dosage for all three of these variables. Older women have also experienced higher rates of hemorrhage from thrombolytics, low-molecular-weight heparin, and glycoprotein IIb/IIIa inhibitors.[58,75] The precise cause of the high rate of drug-induced bleeding in older women is not known, but for glycoprotein IIb/IIIa inhibitors, it is likely due to a failure to appropriately adjust the drug dosage based on renal function.[58]

Summary

Many differences exist between disease incidence, presentation, diagnosis, and outcome to treatment between women and men. Many of these differences are due to the biological consequences of sex, although gender can contribute to and influence diagnosis and treatment differences. Women also have differences in drug pharmacokinetics that occur as they mature and enter adolescence, and that continue

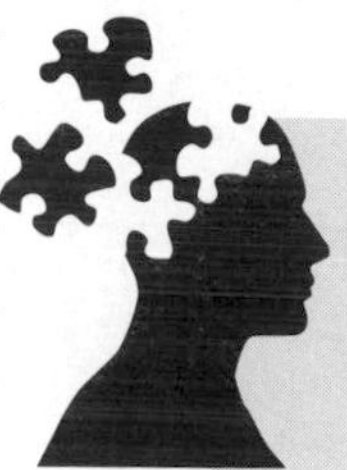

Therapeutic Challenge:

What other medications have pharmacodynamic differences between the sexes?

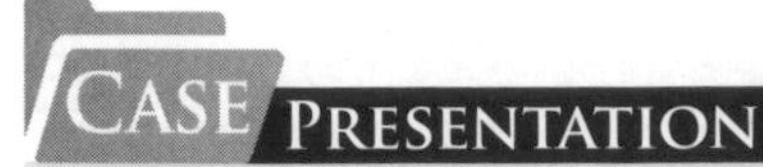

Case Presentation

Patient Case: Part 2

Diabetes

Assessment: Presently, M.A.'s diabetes is under control; she has a normal blood sugar and meets treatment guidelines for an A1C <7%. Her creatinine clearance is estimated to be 25 mL/min with the Cockcroft-Gault equation.

Recommendation: Decrease the dosage of glyburide to 2.5 mg daily.

Rationale: Glyburide is metabolized to a renally excreted active metabolite. It is not known if M.A. has impairment in liver function related to sex or age. Although creatinine clearances are not precise in seniors, because of the estimated value, her age, and small size, she most likely has compromised renal function. Hypoglycemia related to accumulated concentrations of glyburide could contribute to this patient's symptoms of unsteadiness and confusion.

Monitoring: Home blood glucose checked and recorded daily at varying times and A1C. Review patient's home glucose values and an A1C in 3 months.

Patient education: Both patient and family need to be able to recognize and respond to low blood-glucose concentrations.

Cardiovascular Diseases

Assessment: M.A.'s blood pressure is at goal values of <130/80 mm Hg, and she does not experience postural effects upon standing. M.A.'s heart rate is controlled. Her INR is within normal range, but she is receiving duplicative anticoagulation therapy.

Recommendation: Continue treatment of her hypertension with lisinopril. Refer her to a cardiologist for discontinuation of Coumadin or aspirin.

Rationale: The use of both aspirin and Coumadin is not recommended because the combination in an older woman will increase the likelihood of bleeding.

Monitoring: Blood pressure and bleeding. Because M.A.'s blood pressure is controlled, every 6–12-month checks should be adequate. The patient should check for signs of bleeding on a daily basis.

Patient education: Both patient and family need to be able to recognize and respond to signs of minor and major bleeding.

Osteoarthritis and Osteoporosis

Assessment: M.A. is receiving a total daily dosage of 3 g of acetaminophen for osteoarthritis management and calcium with vitamin D supplements for osteoporosis prevention. M.A. does not report pain, although her mobility is reported to be limited.

Recommendation: Refer M.A. to a physical therapist for assessment and possible implementation of a therapeutic walking regimen. In this older woman, a trial of a lower dosage of acetaminophen (650 mg 3 times daily) is recommended. Continue the calcium with vitamin D supplementation. Ask family if they would like to have a DXA (dual energy absorptiometry) test done to assess her bone mineral density and need for additional medication.

Rationale: It is not known if either age- or sex-related changes in metabolism affect the use of acetaminophen in this case; some limited evidence suggests that acetaminophen is metabolized less in older individuals and less in women than men. M.A. has normal liver function tests.

Monitoring: Pain and mobility limitations; liver function tests. Follow-up at routine scheduled clinic visits for osteoarthritis pain assessment and liver function tests as needed while she receives acetaminophen on a regular basis.

Patient education: Advise the patient and family to avoid taking more than 3 g of acetaminophen from all sources daily; encourage walking to maintain mobility.

Alzheimer's Disease

Assessment: M.A. has increased confusion, which could be related to disease, medications, and or environment.

Recommendation: No change in Alzheimer's medication. Decrease the dosage of ziprasidone, using a tapering process until the drug can be discontinued.

Rationale: M.A.'s MMSE score was within normal limits 3 months ago. Alzheimer's disease is a slowly progressing disease; the confusion is most likely not related to disease deterioration and does not warrant additional Alzheimer's medications at this time. The use of atypical antipsychotics for agitation in a patient with dementia is controversial and may lead to an increase in mortality. Ziprasidone is also metabolized by the cytochrome P450 2D6 family of isoenzymes. There are no reports of decreased metabolism of ziprasidone related to age or sex, although this drug has QT prolongation as a side effect. In addition, ziprasidone is a likely cause of increased sedation and confusion in this setting. Nonpharmacologic therapies, such as creating a serene environment and using a consistent daily structure, should be tried first for behavior management, which were not done in this case (beyond scope of this chapter).

Monitoring: Night-time agitation, daytime sedation and confusion. Weekly contact with the family to assess for changes in mental state and mood.

Patient education: Affirm with the family that Alzheimer's disease is a slowly progressive condition and that any abrupt changes in M.A.'s status should be reported to their healthcare provider.

through their older years, from both sex, hormonal, and maturation influences. Some pharmacokinetic differences are significant and place women at an increased risk for adverse drug reactions. Pharmacodynamic changes are also important, although less well studied, and explain some of the differences in treatment outcome and adverse effects seen in women. Healthcare providers must carefully weigh the influence of sex on drug and disease parameters to create optimal pharmacotherapy regimens in women.

References

Additional content available at
www.ashp.org/womenshealth

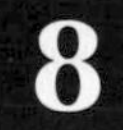

8 Health and Wellness

Kelly L. Matson, BSN, Pharm.D.; Alicia B. Forinash, Pharm.D., BCPS, CCD;
Norma J. Owens, Pharm.D., BCPS, FCCP

Learning Objectives

1. Describe the role and outcomes of health organizations and governmental agencies in setting public health policy and implementing health and wellness initiatives that affect children and women.
2. Advise children and women about health screenings and exams, vaccinations, and other preventive health recommendations.
3. Educate children and women about appropriate dietary and exercise recommendations.
4. Utilize innovative stress management methods to improve wellness.

The profile of diseases contributing profoundly to illness, disability, and death among Americans has changed dramatically during the last 100 years.[1] Chronic diseases such as cardiovascular disease, cancer, and diabetes are among the most prevalent, costly, and preventable of all **health** problems currently within the U.S. Seven out of every 10 Americans who die each year, more than 1.7 million people, will die of a chronic disease. As healthcare costs continually rise due to the problem of the growing number of Americans with chronic diseases, healthcare must shift from disease-centered management to prevention of chronic diseases through the promotion of health and **wellness.** Prevention has already demonstrated cost effectiveness in healthcare. Furthermore, national awareness of chronic diseases can also stimulate the promotion of health and wellness by starting the dialogue of prevention.[2] National health observances are organized both locally and nationally into devoted days (e.g., National Smoke Out Day), weeks (e.g., National Poison Prevention Week), and months (e.g., Breast Cancer Month) to provide information regarding health concerns. These examples of successful prevention approaches should be looked on as ways to promote a healthier nation and to direct additional strategies that address other public health concerns in the U.S.

The goal of this chapter is to provide an overview of health and wellness issues that closely affect children and women of all ages and the role of healthcare providers in educating and supporting women's health concerns. Preventive health, nutrition, physical activity, and stress management will be discussed as well as the public policies that guide their management. Other children's and women's health and wellness topics, such as mental health, substance abuse, and environmental protection will not be covered; however, many of the clinical chapters discuss prevention of these and many other conditions.

Preventive Health and Wellness

The World Health Organization (WHO) defines health as the complete physical, mental and social well-being of a person, not just the absence of disease.[3] Chronic disease burdens many Americans within the U.S. as 44% of persons have one chronic medical condition and 13% have three or more.[4] The Centers for Disease Control and Prevention (CDC) have established the National Center for Chronic Disease Prevention and Health Promotion (NCCDPHP), an agency that monitors the health of U.S. citizens, supports programs to promote healthy behaviors, and conducts chronic disease research for better understanding of their prevention.[1] With NCCDPHP and its partnership with individual state health and education agencies and other voluntary, private and federal organizations, the U.S. is moving

Case Presentation

Patient Case: Part 1

B.C. is a 48-year-old, African-American, single mother who lives with her 13-year-old daughter, K.C. B.C. has a very busy schedule, as she works as an assistant manager of a clothing retail store and also attends community college in the evenings two nights a week. She is working on getting her master's in business administration as she would like to advance her career. However, she feels overwhelmed with both her work and school commitments and caring for her daughter. Recently, K.C.'s school work has started to decline since starting middle school and B.C. has been worried about her academic success. In the past, K.C has excelled at school and her other activities: girl scouts, tap dance and flute lessons. B.C. tries to make time for K.C.'s studies and activities. However, she feels she cannot give K.C. enough time that she needs and is thinking about enrolling her into an after-school study program.

In addition, B.C.'s health is also weighing on her mind, as she is scheduled for her annual check-up. She knows she has gained weight, 15 lb, over the last year. She has tried to diet and exercise; however, with both K.C.'s and her schedules, they usually do not have time for grocery shopping, let alone well-balanced meals and routine exercise. She has noticed that their eating habits have contributed to K.C.'s additional weight gain and is also worried about her health. Recently at K.C.'s last check-up, the pediatrician discussed K.C.'s risk for obesity and the possibility of future diabetes and cardiovascular disease. B.C. is aware of her family history of diabetes and heart disease as she and her own mother both have Type 2 diabetes and high cholesterol. The pediatrician also recommended K.C. receive the Tdap and HPV vaccines, which raises additional vaccine concerns for B.C regarding her daughter's sexual activity. B.C. knows she needs to make her and K.C.'s health a priority, but she just doesn't have the time.

B.C. did visit her physician and stops by the pharmacy to drop off her prescriptions. She is beside herself as she has learned at the physician's office that her diabetes has not been well-controlled over the past year and she is going to need additional medication to manage her blood sugars. Her physician recommended diet and exercise again, which B.C. recognizes. She just doesn't know where she can find the time to meal plan, to shop, to cook, to walk and lift weights, all the while being a coworker, a student, and a mom.

As she makes her way to the pharmacy counter, B.C. sees her community pharmacist. They share a hello, but the pharmacist can see B.C. is anxious. He asks what is troubling her and B.C. explains about her high stress level, her health concerns for both K.C. and her, and now the new prescription for her diabetes. The pharmacist asks if B.C. has time to talk as he would like to sit down and discuss some ways to help. B.C. is late for class, but says she come by tomorrow after work.

in the direction of preventing chronic disease as the first step of chronic disease management. This paradigm shift can improve children's and women's health and wellness, and extend their life expectancies by advances in preventative health. Areas of awareness include the most prevalent chronic diseases currently in the U.S. (i.e., diabetes, cancer, heart disease and stroke, as well as arthritis, obesity, and tobacco use). Additionally, health promotion in specific age and gender groups (i.e., youth, women and the aging) are also being pursued. These recommendations encompass nutrition, exercise, stress management, health screenings, vaccinations and dental measures that begin at birth and continue throughout life (Table 8-1).[5-30]

Prevention has already demonstrated cost effectiveness in healthcare. For every $1 spent on preconception care programs for women with diabetes, health costs can be reduced by up to $5.19 by preventing costly complications in both mothers and babies.[1] A mammogram every 2 years for women aged 50–69 years old costs only about $9,000 per year of life saved, which compares favorably with other widely used clinical preventive services.[1] Other preventable health screenings also have documentation of positive outcomes beyond the cost of the health screening program in women. Cervical screenings or pap (Papanicolaou) smears (Table 8-1) have been one of the most successful screening programs.[19] Cervical cancer was the leading cause of cancer death in American women in the 1930s. However, widespread cervical cytology screening has decreased the incidence and mortality dramatically, and the annual incidence rate is still eight cases per 100,000 women.[31] Screening for cholesterol, blood pressure, and blood glucose are also essential for disease detection, awareness, prevention, and management in women, especially for heart health.[32-35] According

Table 8-1. Preventative Health Recommendations for Women from Birth to Death

	Age in Years								Comments[a]
	Birth–9	10–19	20–29	30–39	40–49	50–59	60–69	≥70	
Vaccinations[b]									
Haemophilus influenzae type b[5]	✓								Series of four injections unless PRP-OMP is administered at ages 2 and 4 mo, then the 6 mo dose is not needed
Hepatitis A[5]	✓								Series of two injections
Hepatitis B[5]	✓								Series of three injections
Human papillomavirus[5,6]		✓	✓						Series of three injections; should be completed between 11–26 yr
Influenza[5,6]	✓	✓	✓	✓	✓	✓	✓	✓	Recommended yearly
Measles, mumps, rubella[5]	✓								Primary series of two injections
Meningococcal[5]		✓							One injection for primary series
Pneumococcal conjugate (PCV)[5]	✓								Series of four injections
Pneumococcal polysaccharide (PPV)[65]							✓		One injection after 65 yr old; some patients recommended to receive prior to age 65 yr
Inactive polio[5]	✓								Series of four injections
Rotavirus[5]	✓								Series of three oral doses unless Rotarix is used at 2 and 4 mo, then 6 mo dose is not needed
Tetanus, diptheria, pertussis (DTaP)[5]	✓								Primary series of five injections
Tetanus and diptheria (Td)[5,6] Tetanus, diptheria, pertussis (Tdap)[5,6]		✓	✓	✓	✓	✓	✓	✓	One injection per booster every 10 yr; substitute Tdap for one Td up to age 64 yr
Varicella[5]	✓								Series of two injections
Zoster[6]							✓		One injection
Screening									
Colon screening[7]						✓	✓	✓	
Cholesterol (fasting lab)[8,9]	✓	✓	✓	✓	✓	✓	✓	✓	Children at higher risk (i.e., positive family history of dyslipidemia or premature CVD) or have CVD risk factors should start at 2 yr of age but no later than age 10 yr; start routine screening at age 20 yr

(*Continued on next page*)

	Birth–9	10–19	20–29	30–39	40–49	50–59	60–69	≥70	Comments[a]
				Age in Years					
Blood pressure[10-13]	✓	✓	✓	✓	✓	✓	✓	✓	Annual screening starting at age 3 yr or earlier if risk factors (i.e., CHD, prematurity, etc.)
Blood glucose[14]					✓	✓	✓	✓	Start at age 45 yr old, then every 3 yr
Thyroid (TSH)[15]				✓	✓	✓	✓	✓	Start at age 35 yr old, then every 5 yr
DXA[16]							✓		Indicated earlier for women at high risk or if fracture after age 50 yr
Clinical breast exam[17]			✓	✓	✓	✓	✓	✓	Optional
Self breast exam[17]			✓	✓	✓	✓	✓	✓	Optional
Mammogram[17,18]					✓	✓	✓	✓	Every 1–2 yr[c]
PAP smear and pelvic exam[19]			✓	✓	✓	✓	✓	✓	Every 1–3 yr if sexually active or older than 21 yr; starting at age 65 yr discuss with healthcare professional
Eye exam[20,21]	✓		✓	✓	✓	✓	✓	✓	Vision should be checked once between 0–5 yr, then at least once between ages 20–29 yr and at least twice between ages 30–39 yr; every 2 yr after age 40 yr
Hearing exam[22,23]	✓	✓	✓	✓	✓	✓	✓	✓	Screen once during newborn period and again before entering school; every 10 yr starting at age 18 yr old until age 49 yr old, then every 3 yr (≥50 yr old)
Mole exam[24]			✓	✓	✓	✓	✓	✓	Every 3 yr starting at age 20 yr, then every yr starting age 40 yr
Yearly well patient check-up	✓	✓	✓	✓	✓	✓	✓	✓	Well child check-ups needed more often when child is <2 yr old

(*Continued on next page*)

	Age in Years								Comments[a]
	Birth–9	10–19	20–29	30–39	40–49	50–59	60–69	≥70	
Dental									
Dental visits every 6 mo[25,26]	✓	✓	✓	✓	✓	✓	✓	✓	Infants at higher risk of early dental caries should be referred to a dentist as early as 6 mo of age and no later than 6 mo after the first tooth erupts or 12 mo of age (whichever comes first); certain diseases[d] and/or medications[e] require more frequent monitoring or precautions prior to visits
Brushing teeth at least twice daily[25]	✓	✓	✓	✓	✓	✓	✓	✓	
Flossing teeth daily[25]	✓	✓	✓	✓	✓	✓	✓	✓	

DXA = dual energy absorptiometry (bone mineral density measurement); Pap = Papanicolaou, TSH = thyroid stimulating hormone.

[a]For specific recommendations refer to the various recommendations and guidelines referenced within Table 8-2. If vaccinations are not given as scheduled or the series is not completed, or the patient is immunocompromised or has certain chronic diseases see the specific recommendations for problem solving.
[b]Vaccination schedules are updated annually. For current recommendations refer to the CDC website (www.cdc.gov/vaccines). For current schedules and for catch-up immunizations and high risk group recommendations and or other risk factor information.
[c]American Geriatrics Society recommends every 1–2 years up through age 85 years for women "with average or better and life expectancy of at least 5 years" and continued screening for those women over age of 85 years "in excellent health and functional status."
[d]Prosthetic cardiac valve, previous infective endocarditis, congenital heart disease (CHD), unrepaired cyanotic CHD (including palliative shunts and conduits), completely repaired congenital heart defect with prosthetic material or device, whether placed by surgery or by catheter intervention, during the first 6 months after the procedure, repaired CHD with residual defects at the site or adjacent to the site of a prosthetic patch or prosthetic device (which inhibit endothelialization), cardiac transplantation recipients who develop cardiac valvulopathy, joint replacement patients in the first 2 years after replacement or immunocompromised/immunosuppressed.[27-28]
[e]Bisphosphonates, anticoagulants, seizure medications.[29-30]

to the Department of Health and Human Services (DHHS), one in three women die from heart disease, and in 2003 almost twice the number of women died of cardiovascular disease (i.e., heart disease and stroke) than of all cancers combined.[36] Healthcare providers thus need to actively include prevention in their treatment plans and patient discussions.

Nutrition

BREASTFEEDING, INFANT FORMULAS, AND SUPPLEMENTS

Human or breast milk for years has been recognized as a vital source of nutrition and enhanced immunity for infants. With technological advances, commercially available infant formulas became popular within developed societies. Not until recently has human milk made a comeback as the "ideal method of feeding and nurturing infants" as described by the U.S. Surgeon General and the American Academy of Pediatrics (AAP).[37,38] Commercial infant formulas do not provide the health, nutritional, immunologic, psychological, social, economic, and environmental benefits of breast milk. Scientific research from around the world has provided evidence that human milk decreased the incidence and severity of bacteremia, bacterial meningitis, respiratory tract infections, otitis media, and gastrointestinal illness such as diarrhea and necrotizing enterocolitis in the infant.[38] Other health benefits documented include decreased rates of sudden infant death syndrome within the first year of life, and reduction in the incidence of diabetes Type 1 and 2, overweight and obesity, hyperlipidemia, lymphoma, leukemia, and asthma in older children and adults that were previously breastfed. Human milk has also been associated with increased cognitive development and analgesia. Specifically for mothers, decreased postpartum recovery time (i.e., shortening of bleeding time, prompt reduction of the uterus to normal nonpregnant size and state after delivery, and earlier return to prepregnancy weight) and facilitation of a close bond with their child are direct benefits of breastfeeding. Mothers who breastfed also have benefits throughout their lives with decreased risk of breast and ovarian cancer and possibly decreased risk of hip fractures and osteoporosis after menopause.

Within society, using human milk plays an important economic and environmental role. Breastfeeding allows for a potential reduction in the annual U.S. healthcare costs of $3.6 billion; decreased costs in public health programs such as Special Supplemental Nutrition Program for Women, Infants, and Children (WIC); decreased parental employee absenteeism and associated lost of family's income; decreased environmental burden for disposal of formula containers; and decreased energy demands for production and transportation of commercially available infant formulas.[38]

Mothers who are unable to breastfeed their infants can still rely on formula as a good alternative to achieve infant nutritional goals. Many varieties of formulas exist on the market; however, the most common are milk-based and soy-based products.[39,40] Milk-based formulas are prepared from nonfat cow's milk and vegetable oils with added carbohydrates to resemble human milk components. Soy-based formulas are made from soy-protein isolate and are considered cow milk and lactose free.[40] Soy formulas are recommended for children of vegetarian families, management of lactose intolerance and potentially for infants with IgE-mediated allergies. However, milk and/or soy formulas have no proven benefit for the prevention of colic or atopic disease and should not be considered for very low birth weight premature infants or infants with documented protein-induced enterocolitis. In addition, both types of formulas are supplemented with docosahexaenoic acid (DHA) and arachidonic acid (ARA).[39,40] Docosahexaenoic acid and ARA are long-chain polyunsaturated fatty acids, which studies suggest help to support brain and eye development in infants, especially premature infants.[41] Though these long-chain polyunsaturated fatty acids are abundant in human milk, maternal diet can affect their concentrations in infants both in utero and during lactation.[39] Recently marketed supplements for pregnant and lactating mothers contain 200 mg DHA to increase maternal and subsequently infant dietary intake; however, more information is needed before DHA is routinely recommended. Most infant formulas are also fortified with taurine and L-carnitine, as these amino acids are considered conditionally essential amino acids during infancy.[39,40] The infant is unable to make taurine or L-carnitine from ingested proteins due to immature biochemical pathways in the liver. Taurine supplementation may help fat absorption and brain and eye development in preterm infants, while L-carnitine may decrease the incidence of muscle weakness and cardiomyopathy, both seen in carnitine deficiency.[39,42]

Most importantly, infants less than 6 months old should be exclusively fed with human milk or formula for optimal growth and development.[14] Furthermore, exclusive breastfeeding for the first 6 months of life provides continuing protection against diarrhea and respiratory tract infections, including otitis media and pneumonia.[38,43] Water and juice regardless of climate should not be given until 6 months old. Foods rich in iron may also be introduced around 6 months of age; the most common initial supplement is iron-enriched rice cereal. Iron-rich cereal should be offered only once daily in 1–2 teaspoonfuls and continued daily until infant becomes accustomed to it.[38,44] Although breastfeeding past 1 year is not the norm in the U.S., some mothers continue to breastfeed past infancy, which provides continued immune protection and better social adjustment for children.[43] Studies have shown no evidence of psychological or developmental harm from breastfeeding into the third year of life or longer.[38]

Vitamin supplementation is also important within the first year of life. Vitamin D oral supplementation is usually started within the first few days of life in breastfed or partially breastfed infants and continued through childhood.[45] Iron oral supplements are started by 6 weeks of age in the breastfed infant and continued until fortified cow's milk is introduced usually at 1 year of age.[38] However, infants fed commercially available infant formulas do not require supplements since they have already been added to the products. Fluoride supplementation is also recommended for infants 6 months to 3 years of age whose drinking water concentration is less than 0.3 ppm.[38] Fluoride dosing based on its concentration in drinking water can be found at the AAP website (www.aap.org).[46]

CHILDHOOD RECOMMENDATIONS

After breastfeeding, families need to begin good nutrition and healthy eating habits. The American Heart Association's Dietary Recommendation for Children and Adolescents recommend a diet for those aged 2 years and older that incorporates fruits and vegetables, whole grains, low-fat and nonfat dairy products, beans, fish, and lean meat.[47] This recommendation is championed by the revision of the food guide pyramid, MyPyramid, which includes physical activity, moderation, proportionality, variety, personalization, and a need for more individualized approach to improving diet and lifestyle.[48] MyPyramid offers guidance by providing recommended food amounts in cups or ounces and other hints to limit intake of high-fat, high-calorie foods, as well as, providing interactive web tools to help enhance education.

To prevent overweight and obesity, *Healthy People 2010* recommends establishing good eating habits with education beginning in school.[49] Curricula within schools encourage specific healthy eating behavior and provide students skills to adopt and maintain those dietary behaviors. The curriculum should include discussions regarding meals and snacks, food labels, exercise, diet, food safety, body size acceptance, and the food guide pyramid. Additionally, middle and high school students should review dietary guidelines, information about eating disorders, healthy weight maintenance, and influences on food choices. Additionally, the United States Department of Agriculture (USDA) has established standards requiring schools to plan menus that meet the dietary guidelines, but those standards do not apply to a la carte foods, school stores, vending machines, or foods brought from home. Advocacy is needed to enlist policy makers and local school officials to support healthy lifestyle for all children and ways to decrease the availability of foods and beverages with little nutritional value within the community.[50] Though many of the current recommendations are governmental and school-based, families also have the added responsibility to be aware of the vast nutritional information, make wise food choices for their children, and help support community decisions to help slow childhood obesity rates.

WOMEN RECOMMENDATIONS

For women, the USDA in 2005 created new adult dietary guidelines that recommend habits of eating a diet high in fruits, vegetables, whole grains, and low-fat sources of dairy foods. The recommendations also include balancing food with one's activity level to maintain a healthy weight and limiting the intake of salt, saturated fat, trans saturated fat, cholesterol, and sugar.[51] This approach represents a shift of dietary recommendations from primarily preventing nutrient deficiencies to the current efforts to promote health and prevent disease. These recommendations are based largely on the scientific evidence that has shown a relationship between poor diet and sedentary lifestyle to cardiovascular disease, diabetes, hypertension, cerebrovascular disease, osteoarthritis, osteoporosis, and some forms of cancer. Utilizing the interactive website, MyPyramid, can also create personalized and gender-based dietary guidelines for women in order that they can achieve and maintain health within a normal weight based on their food intake and activity level.[48] Furthermore, certain vitamins and minerals play an essential role in women's health issues such as the prevention of osteoporosis and neural tube defects during the early stages of pregnancy. Vitamin D, calcium, folate, and iron recommendations (Table 8-2) vary based on a women's age and whether she is pregnant or lactating.[39,45,52-54]

To determine a normal weight, women can use a few different sources. In 1943, the Metropolitan Life Insurance Company published widely used height and weight tables for women and men aged 25–59 years stratified by frame size.[55,56] These tables were revised in 1983 with the listed weights described as "desirable" although many have used these weight values as ideal weights.[57] The weight values were determined from mortality data with the desirable weights correlated with lowest mortality. Most medical literature today utilizes the body mass index (BMI) to categorize weight.[58] Women above a BMI of 25 kg/m^2 are considered overweight and are at greater risk for diabetes, hypertension, and cardiovascular disease. However, BMI is a unisex value and might not accurately reflect weight categories at the low ends. For instance, women and men with a BMI less than 19 are considered underweight, which might be a reasonable cutoff number for most women but is considered an unreasonably low cutoff value for men.[59]

As women age, energy needs start to decline as their metabolism slows and they get less physical exercise.[60] Nutrition in the elderly population becomes more difficult as they must eat more nutrient dense food to achieve dietary requirements, while eating less to maintain their weight. Again as with younger women, calcium, vitamin D, and folate supplementation are

Table 8-2. Vitamin D, Calcium, Folate, and Iron Daily Recommendations for Children and Women[39,45,52-54]

	AGE							
	0–6 mo	**7–12 mo**	**1–3 yr**	**4–8 yr**	**9–13 yr**	**14–18 yr**	**19–50 yr**	**>50 yr**
Vitamin D	400 units	400 units	400 units	400 units	400 units	400 units	200 units	800–1,000 units
Pregnancy/ Lactation						400 units	400 units	
Calcium	210 mg	270 mg	500 mg	800 mg	1,300 mg	1,300 mg	1,000 mg	1,200 mg
Pregnancy/ Lactation						1,300 mg	1,000 mg	
Folate	65 mcg	80 mcg	150 mcg	200 mcg	300 mcg	400 mcg	400 mcg	400 mcg
Pregnancy						600 mcg	600 mcg	
Lactation						500 mcg	500 mcg	
Iron	0.27 mg	11 mg	7 mg	10 mg	8 mg	15 mg	18 mg	8 mg
Pregnancy						27 mg	27 mg	
Lactation						10 mg	9 mg	

equally important in elderly women (Table 8-2).[16,52,53] In addition, women's desire to eat may also decline as they age. Appetite loss can be from many different causes such as dental problems, including poorly fitting dentures and gum disease, decrease senses of taste and smell, difficultly swallowing and chewing as well as low income, illness, medication interference, depression, and lack of socialization. Many seniors live alone and may not bother with preparing well-balanced and nutritious meals. Thus, nutritional assistance (e.g., Meals on Wheels) becomes essential for both socialization and proper nutrition. The Meals on Wheels program is federally funded and provides meals to seniors aged 60 years and older that reside in the community, cannot prepare their own meals at home, live alone, and qualify for a waiver program such as Medicaid.[61,62]

Physical Activity

Since health can be improved with exercise, most wellness, prevention and treatment care plans include recommendations for increased physical activity.[63] Sometimes the quantity and type of exercise required to maintain health is difficult to determine. When reviewing literature in this area, care must be taken to evaluate the goals and specific exercise program, as well as health outcomes.

CHILDREN AND ADOLESCENTS

As children and adolescents spend more time in sedentary activities such as television viewing and internet activities, greater focus is being placed on efforts to increase exercise in this age group.[50] For children and adolescents, weight bearing exercise is needed as it promotes normal skeletal development. In addition, *Healthy People 2010* states that moderate physical activity for at least 30 minutes on five or more of the previous 7 days is recommended for adolescent girls and boys.[64] However, in 1999 only 27% of 9th–12th graders met the weekly recommendation (*Healthy People 2010* target goal is 35% by 2010, which is actually a low benchmark). Physical education is the primary source of exercise and fitness instruction. However, public and private schools have decreased requirements for daily physical education recently (individual states determine physical education requirements for students). *Healthy People 2010* recommends increasing the proportion of adolescents who participate in school-driven physical education to 50% and increasing the proportion of private and public schools that require daily physical education for all students to 25% for grades 7–8 and 5% for grades 9–12. Families need to be aware and monitor their children's physical activity. They should encourage and establish a priority of exercise in daily activities whether unstructured play at home, in school, in child care settings, with their parents, or throughout the community.[50] Lastly, adults should limit total media time to recommended amounts, which are less than 2 hours per day for children and adolescents, and no media time for children younger than 2 years to help promote healthier behaviors.[65]

ADULTS

The American College of Sports Medicine in conjunction with the American Heart Association recommend that to maintain health and reduce the risk of chronic diseases like coronary artery disease, both women and men should perform at least 30 minutes of moderate intensity physical activity on 5 days each week.[66] Moderate intensity physical activity is aerobic in nature and is roughly equated to a brisk walk that accelerates the heart rate. The current guidelines also recommend that muscle strengthening activity helps maintain physical independence and should be performed at least twice a week and consist of 8–10 exercises with weights that work major muscle groups. However, to lower weight or prevent weight gain, no clear consensus for physical activity recommendations exists. When coupled with a healthy diet, the USDA guidelines recommend women should perform 60 minutes of moderate to vigorous activity most days of the week to prevent weight gain associated with aging and to sustain weight loss, they should perform 60–90 minutes of moderate to vigorous activity most days of the week.[51]

Exercise to improve balance is particularly important for older women at risk for injury related to falls. Older women who experience falls often lose independence and can suffer an early death.[67] Evidence suggests that perhaps both muscle strengthening exercise, as well as balance training may help prevent falls. A recent meta-analysis evaluated randomized controlled trials testing exercise to improve balance and found statistically significant benefits for exercises that involved gait, balance and balance coordination, and muscle strengthening. The majority of participants in this research were women over the age of 75 years. In addition to walking and muscle strengthening through weight training, exercise programs involving Tai-Chi and yoga are other exercises that can be used to improve balance. Physical activity, as well as, novel mental activity has been reported to also help maintain and improve cognitive health (i.e., learning, memory, decision-making and planning) in older women.[68] Aging women may experience a slower pace of learning and need for new information repeated, which are normal changes in cognitive function. However, women who experience a decline in cognition health might have a higher risk of dementia and Alzheimer's disease later in life.[68]

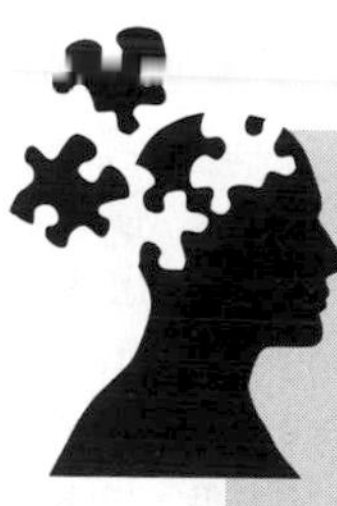

Therapeutic Challenge:

Are you achieving the daily recommended exercise standards? What materials and resources can you use to educate and motivate yourself and your patients to implement and sustain good exercise practices?

Vaccinations

CHILDREN AND ADOLESCENTS

Immunization schedules are constantly changing to reflect new discoveries such human papillomavirus (HPV) vaccine and additional vaccine data (Table 8-1). Human papillomavirus vaccine, which was approved in 2006, protects against four different types of HPV that are responsible for 70% of cervical cancer and 90% of genital warts (Chapter 46: Cervical Cancer).[69] Tetanus toxoid, reduced diphtheria toxoid, and acellular pertussis (Tdap) vaccine was also added in 2006 to the adolescent and adult schedules.[5,6] The Tdap vaccine helps to reduce pertussis morbidity in the above populations and also to reduce transmission of pertussis to infants.[70,71] Currently, every adolescent girl and adult of a child who is vulnerable to other vaccine-preventable diseases should be informed and educated regarding the most current immunizations and any specific state policies directed to this public health initiative. To determine the latest in immunizations, the CDC website (www.cdc.gov/vaccines) should be consulted.[5,6]

ADULTS

Many vaccinations need to be continued throughout life (Table 8-1) or started if not received in childhood. For example, the use of Tdap in adults offers an opportunity to reduce the burden of pertussis in the U.S. By replacing an adult dose of Td (i.e., tetanus booster) with Tdap, the vaccinated adult is protected against pertussis, as well as decreasing exposure of infants to the disease.[71] Additionally, a single dose of the 23-valent pneumococcal vaccine is routinely recommended for elderly patients over the age of 65 years to reduce invasive disease (i.e., bacteremia, meningitis, pneumonia) in this population.[72,73]

Stress Management

Stress and its negative impact on health and wellbeing are growing problems in the U.S. for both women and men of all ages.[74,75] Stress can come about by sexual orientation and sexuality pressures, a traumatic accident, death or emergency situation, but it is also associated with daily life including school, work, and family issues. Additional information and resources to overcome some areas of stress are in Chapter 4: Psychosocial Factors.

CHILDREN AND ADOLESCENTS

Children are under more stress than ever before due to their family's hurried lifestyle as well as increased focus on academic preparation.[76] Increased pressures during childhood and adolescence may even contribute to depression and decrease coping skills in the future. For children, child-driven, unscheduled play is essential to their development, by giving them time to be creative and independent and to decompress and reflect. For older children and adolescents, limiting the need for perfectionism and supporting a balance of organized activities and academics with free time can help reduce their stress and anxiety.

WOMEN

As women, their roles as wife, mother, caregiver, friend, and or worker may put them at risk for stress-related health issues. Employment and family responsibilities are two stressors that have been highly associated with women.[74,75,77] In a national survey, women have reported higher levels of occupational stress and stress-related illness than employed men and in another survey, 60% of women stated job stress was their number-one problem.[75] Job stressors commonly include work overload, poor interpersonal relations, and/or underutilization of skills. However, working women may also be subject to sex-specific occupational stressors such as sex discrimination and the difficulty of combining work and family. Sex discrimination is defined as inequitable treatment based on gender and includes discriminatory hiring and promotion practices, salary differentials, and sexual harassment. Women who are affected by discrimination in regards to financial and career advancement have reported more frequent physical and psychological symptoms, more physician visits, and more thoughts of leaving or changing jobs.[75] Harassment of women at work also has been associated with psychological (e.g., depression, anxiety, feelings of guilt and shame) and physical (e.g., headaches, gastrointestinal and sleep disorders) symptoms, as well as, a negative job attitude, absenteeism, and even voluntary withdrawal from employment.

In addition, family responsibilities combined with the responsibilities of work life likely add to women's stress level. Though women over 20 years of age make up 58% of the employed U.S. population, they still remain the primary caregivers at home.[75,78] Women are more likely to address children's needs or have elder care responsibilities, all the while still tending to household chores, making their stress levels likely greater than that of men.[75] Recent research indicates professional women with higher job and family workloads have increased burden of psychological stress.

Women are not always mindful of stress and the effects on their health, thus stress management can be underutilized and or challenging.[77] Various ways exist to help alleviate and handle stressful situations. Overall wellness such as eating right, exercising, and getting enough sleep (i.e., 7–9 hours per night) can decrease stress levels and lower the risk of stress-related illness.[77,79] In addition, organizing time and establishing limits, whether keeping a "to-do" list or journal or setting aside at least 15 minutes each day for one's self, can also manage stress.[77] Women tend to react to stress by finding support in other female friends and if needed, professional help for psychological and physical symptoms. They also tend to care for their children in times of stress, which consequently may increase levels of oxytocin. Estrogen may boost the effects of oxytocin, which may further enhance its calming effect. Additionally, more women are turning to complementary and alternative medicine (CAM) (Chapter 9: Medication Use and Complimentary and Alternative Therapy) for stress management. Acupuncture and acupressure, massage therapy, exercise (e.g., yoga, tai chi), reflexology, herbal or natural products, and spiritual healing methods are all increasing in popularity for various women's health issues.[77,80,81] Additionally, some CAM therapies have shown some benefit to treat pregnancy associated conditions, decrease labor pain, and improve symptom management for menopause and breast cancer.[80-83] For occupational stress, workplace changes such as enforced sex discrimination policies and family support programs, including flexible work schedules and child care assistance can improve job commitment and reduce stress in women.[75]

Violence and Abuse

CHILDREN AND ADOLESCENTS

Violence and abuse can affect anyone (Chapter 4: Psychosocial Factors). In 2006, 3.6 million children were maltreated in the U.S., including all types of abuse and neglect.[84] Children under 4 years of age are at the greatest risk for severe injury and death from maltreatment. Stressful factors such as family history of violence, alcohol and drug abuse, chronic health problems, poverty, and violence in the community can increase the risk of childhood abuse and neglect. A Department of Social Services referral to evaluate the safety of children is essential if maltreatment is suspected. Women between the ages of 15 and 54 years are at the highest risk of violence and abuse.[85]

WOMEN

Violence against women includes intimate partner violence, sexual violence, and other forms of violence committed against women by acquaintances or strangers. Statistics according to the National Violence Against Women survey state 1.5 million women are raped and or physically assaulted by an intimate partner each year and nearly two thirds of women have been raped, physically assaulted, or stalked since age 18 years by a current or former husband, cohabiting partner, boyfriend, or date.[86] To prevent violence against women requires support and contribution from several organizations, from federal agencies and local and state health departments to nonprofits and academic institutions. Organizations may collect data, educate regarding risk factors, develop prevention strategies, and ensure resources reach those women in need. Many resources can be found locally, as well as the CDC and National Online Resource Center on Violence Against Women websites. Visits to healthcare providers usually include an assessment related to women's personal safety, in addition to acute, preventive, and chronic care.

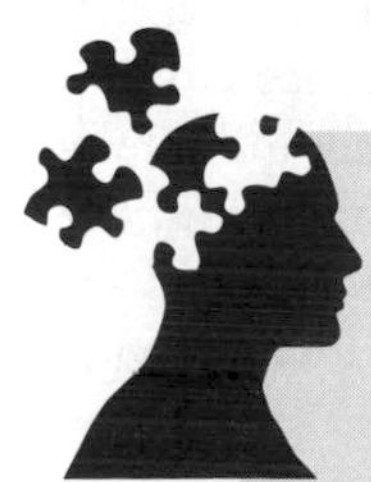

Therapeutic Challenge:

What resources exist on college campuses for students experiencing violence and sexual abuse?

Other Preventive Health Measures

CHILDREN AND ADOLESCENTS

For children, well-patient visits are included in the preventive health recommendations and begin typically 2 weeks after birth, then every 2–3 months during the first 2 years, and finally yearly throughout life to monitor physical, social, and psychological development, as well as to administer vaccines and screen and educate for injury and abuse. For families of young children, educating them regarding sleep position of infants is essential for the prevention of sudden infant death syndrome (SIDS). Infants should always be placed on their back for sleep and their sleep surface should be firm and free of soft bedding (i.e., pillows, quilts, comforters) and stuffed toys.[87] Additionally, the CDC website provides families information on childhood injuries and has safety recommendations on sports and play activities, water activities, and unintentional poisonings.[84] Most importantly regarding children's recreational sports is bicycle and all-terrain vehicle (ATV) safety. Among children's sport activities, bicycle injuries are the leading cause of emergency room visits and two thirds of related bicycle injuries are traumatic brain injuries.[88] Properly-fitted bicycle helmets are effective devices to prevent serious brain injuries and also a *Healthy People 2010* objective. In addition, ATVs can be dangerous, with injuries ranging from thermal burns to shoulder, knee, leg, and head injuries.[89] To prevent severe injuries and death from ATV accidents, motorcycle helmets, eye protection, and protective reflective clothing should be worn during their use. Additionally, parents should not allow street use or nighttime riding of vehicles. The CDC also provides substantial information on other topics such as teenage suicide.[84] Automobile safety is a major concern for children. Child passenger seats are mandatory for all children. Rear-facing seats are recommended for children until 1 year of age and 20 lb in weight.[90] When children reach 1 year and 20 lb, they may move to a forward-facing safety seat. Once they have outgrown the forward-facing seat (i.e., approximately 40 lb), booster seats are then recommended for children until reaching 4'9". Lastly, children should remain in the back seat with lap and shoulder belt until the age of 13 years.

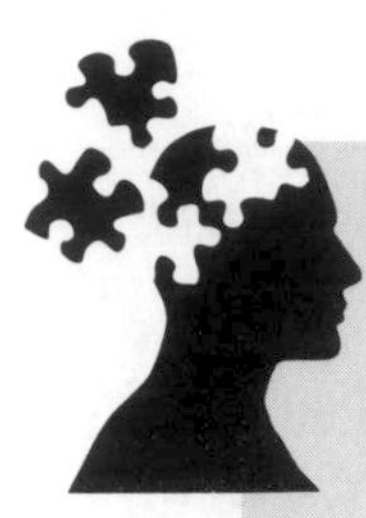

Therapeutic Challenge:

What is the telephone number of your local poison information center? What patient education materials do they have for poisoning prevention?

ADULTS

Many preventive health practices carryover into adulthood. Automobile safety for women also involves safety belt use, as well as evaluation of driving habits and number of accidents. Women drivers have a higher seat belt use rate and lower rates of speeding and crash involvement than men overall, but more older drivers are women.[91] For older women concerned with their ability to continue driving an automobile safely, the American Association of Automobiles offers an interactive self assessment program called Roadwise Review™ that can be administered in the privacy of one's home.[84] This program is a validated assessment of skills and attributes needed to safely drive including leg strength, head and neck flexibility, visual acuity, working memory, and visualization parameters.

Preventable health screenings such as cervical screenings and pap (Papanicolaou) smears (Table 8-1) have been documented to improve health outcomes in women. Cervical screenings and pap smears have been one of the most successful screening programs.[19,31] Screening for cholesterol, blood pressure, and blood glucose are essential for health prevention in women, especially heart health.[32-36] In addition, women should maintain healthy weight, limit stress and alcohol consumption, and eliminate tobacco from their daily lives. Preventing and eliminating substance abuse is very important to wellness and is covered in detail in Chapter 36: Substance-Use Disorders. Daily low dose aspirin is also recommended for women at high risk (i.e., with acute coronary syndrome and/or coronary artery disease), or with diabetes or a past myocardial infarction (MI).[92,93] However, a recent study suggested that primary prevention with daily aspirin for cardiovascular events in women may only decrease ischemic stroke risk but not MI (Chapter 30: Cardiovascular Disease).[92] The CDC also provides substantial information on how to protect women in other ways such as suicide and fall prevention in older women.[84]

Public Policy Related to Children's and Women's Wellness and Preventive Health Services

As healthcare shifts from treatment of diseases and illnesses to prevention of chronic diseases, the U.S.'s public policy for wellness and preventive services must continue to expand. Currently, the U.S. Preventive Services Task Force (USPSTF) is a leading independent panel of experts in prevention within the U.S. private sector that focuses on healthcare screening, counseling, and preventive medications for all citizens. They first convened in 1984 by the U.S. Public Health Service and since 1998 are sponsored by the Agency for Healthcare Research and Quality under DHHS. The USPSTF represents the gold standard for clinical preventive services for the U.S. based on age, gender, and risk factors for disease. Their mission is to make recommendations for routine preventive care in clinical practice and to identify research needs in preventive health.[94] Though the USPSTF is a principal organization with the U.S., other agencies and organizations also provide guidance to preventive healthcare policies for both women and children.

For almost 80 years, the American Academy of Pediatrics has established itself as an organization dedicated "to attain optimal physical, mental and social health and well-being for all infants, children, adolescents and young adults."[95] As an organization of pediatricians, they have been the leader in developing policy statements and clinical practice guidelines and reports addressing children's special developmental and health needs. In addition, several governmental agencies also have guided policy and health services of children, including the DHHS, the National Institutes of Health (NIH), the Food and Drug Administration (FDA), and the CDC. Based on the above agencies' efforts, routine childhood immunizations have achieved significant success. More than 95% protection against vaccine-preventable diseases, such as diphtheria, tetanus, pertussis, measles, mumps, rubella, and poliomyelitis, has been documented to date.[96] Vaccination of children and adults alike provides the goal of disease prevention and the decrease in its related morbidity and mortality. Vaccination also aids in the ultimate goal of world-wide eradication of disease.

Moreover for women, the last 20 years has brought a significant body of literature that has described important differences in healthcare related to sex, gender, and gender-bias (Chapter 7: Sex and Gender Differences). In an effort to rectify the lack of knowledge in health issues related to women, the U.S. Surgeon General's Office has made the elimination of health disparities a public health priority for the U.S.[97] In 1991, the FDA Office on Women's Health (OWH) was created within the DHHS with a mission to "provide leadership to promote health equity for women and girls through sex/gender-specific approaches."[94] One major role for both the OWH and the NIH Office of Research on Women's Health (ORWH) is to coordinate programs and plans on women's health across federal agencies and departments.[94,98] One important outcome to this work has been the funding of National Centers of Excellence in Women's Health (CoEs) located in more than 20 academic centers across the country as well as in the community. The purpose of the CoEs is to connect research, medical training, prevention and public health initiatives, and community outreach in women's health.

To help guide overall health and wellness across the lifespan, an U.S. initiative began in 1979 with the report, *Healthy People: The Surgeon General's Report on Health Promotion and Disease Prevention.*[99] The first report outlined five national goals to decrease premature deaths and increase the quality of life for older Americans. Now the overall goal is to increase the quality and years of healthy life for all ages and to eliminate all health disparities. The initiatives result in policy formation and mandates to achieve goals to improve public health. Healthy People, as the initiative is now referred to, is a broad-based collaborative effort between government, private, public, and nonprofit institutions and is currently working to achieve the objectives for 2010 and develop updated and new goals for 2020. The national disease prevention and health promotion goals are set with measurable outcomes to be achieved within 10 years. The 10 leading health categories in the 2010 policy were physical activity; overweight and obesity; tobacco use; substance abuse; responsible sexual behavior; mental health; injury and violence; environmental quality; immunization; and access to healthcare.

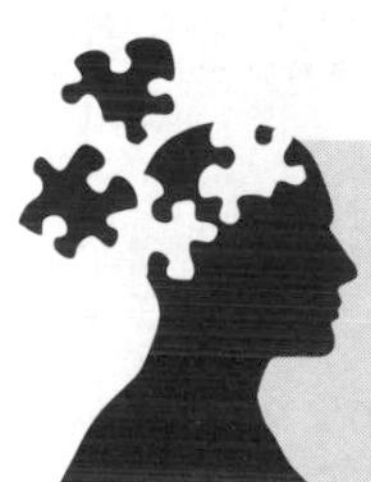

Therapeutic Challenge:

Which *Healthy People 2010* goals have been achieved? For the goals that have not been achieved what can you do to help the U.S. achieve each of these targets?

Healthcare Provider Roles in Children's and Women's Health

Further resources from local and national organizations have been established to promote wellness and safety throughout life, which are informative programs for patients but also helpful for healthcare providers.[48,99,100-109](See Web Resources for Examples of Wellness Resources.)

Additional content available at
www.ashp.org/womenshealth

All healthcare providers have a responsibility to educate and support women and children throughout their life in regards to their health and wellness. They can aid in diet, exercise, and stress-management recommendations. They can counsel patients on routine preventive checkups, but in addition, pharmacists can perform certain laboratory screenings such as cholesterol and blood glucose monitoring to assist disease-state management in the local community pharmacies. Healthcare providers can participate in camps for children with specific diseases or special needs or educate parents on safe and effective medication use in children. A successful pharmacist-based program is tobacco cessation, where pharmacists have reported increased rates of patients who have quit smoking.[110,111] As an immunization advocate, healthcare providers, especially pharmacists in the community can inform and motivate patients to understand disease risk and receive vaccines.[112] Additionally, they can also facilitate immunizations by hosting other healthcare professionals who vaccinate within their community pharmacies or they can become a certified immunizer to improve vaccination rates if consistent with state law.[112-114] Moreover, healthcare providers can also aid in patients' health and understanding of medications by volunteering at community events and health fairs, as well as participating in medication brown bags. In addition, healthcare providers can advocate for patients by participating in legislative issues to best serve their community and also participate in national health professional organizations or sponsor their own patient education programs and other various health- and wellness-related initiatives.

An Example of a Major Public Health Initiative

Current increases in childhood obesity have stimulated aggressive public health campaigns to achieve consensus childhood weight goals. Ideal weight and percentile ranges for weight disorders for children and adolescents are determined using CDC growth charts for BMI based on their sex and age (Table 8-3).[115,116] Based on National Health and Nutrition Examination Survey (NHANES) data from 2003–2004, 13.9% of children aged 2–5 years, 18.8% of children aged 6–11 years, and 17.4% of adolescents aged 12–19 years in the U.S. are overweight.[49,50,117] Race and ethnicity influence obesity prevalences, as Hispanic children have the highest obesity rates (31%), followed by African-American children (20%), Caucasian children (15%), and Asian children (11%).[118] In the U.S., obesity prevalence among children and adolescents has doubled in the past two decades, and more recent data indicate obesity prevalence rates increased to 20% to 30%, respectively for children and adolescents aged 6–11 years and 12–19 years old, when including children at risk for obesity (BMI >85th percentile).[119] The *Healthy People 2010* target goal is to reduce the percentage of overweight children and adolescents to 5% since obesity is associated with significant childhood health problems including dyslipidemia, hypertension, type 2 diabetes, and psychological stress.[49,50] For instance, one study reported children with a BMI <85th percentile had a 2.6% prevalence of hypertension, while obese children (BMI ≥95th percentile) had a 10.7% prevalence of hypertension.[118] Obesity is also an early risk factor for morbidity and mortality in adulthood.[50] Additional programs, such as the USDA's Eat Smart, Play Hard campaign, for reducing obesity are to improve accessibility of nutritional information, nutrition education, nutrition counseling and related services, and provide healthier foods in a variety of settings (Chapter 31: Nutrition and Eating Disorders and Chapter 32: Overweight and Obesity).[49,120]

Table 8-3. Body Mass Index Ranges[115,116]

Weight Classification	Children (2–20 yr)	Adults (>20 yr)
Underweight	<5th percentile	Below 18.5
Healthy weight	5th to <85th percentile	18.5–24.9
Overweight	85th to <95th percentile	25–29.9
Obese	≥95th percentile	30 and above

BMI formula: weight (kg)/[height (m)]^2.

Case Presentation

Patient Case: Part 2

Assessment: B.C. has hypercholesterolemia and Type 2 diabetes mellitus. After a primary care visit, she has documented weight gain of 15 lb and uncontrolled blood glucose concentrations. Additionally, she is experiencing increased stress in her busy life and is having trouble coping with her daily activities and her healthcare needs.

Plan: Establish nutrition and physical activity plan through the MyPyramid website for weight loss. Develop better organizational skills and establish limits to daily activities to include at least 15–30 minutes of free time.

Rationale: By using MyPyramid for a nutrition and exercise plan, it allows her an interactive and personal tool to help B.C. promote her health and wellness through weight and disease-state management of her diabetes and high cholesterol. Better organization will help manage daily tasks such as meal planning, shopping, and cooking as well as schedule time for physical activity. By establishing some free time in her schedule, it should also help manage her stress and free her daily schedule for exercise or another leisure activity with her daughter.

Monitoring: B.C. should continue to monitor her daily blood glucose levels. She should schedule an appointment with her primary care physician or pharmacist for follow-up blood glucose and A1C levels and monitoring of side effects and or other concerns of her new diabetic medication. Weight loss and maintenance plans should also be determined and discussed at follow-up visits for continued success or additional changes to regimen if needed. Stress management should further be evaluated at follow-up and if needed additional help from healthcare professionals should be encouraged.

Patient education: Healthcare provider should identify with B.C.'s weight management struggles and her daily stresses. It should be explained to B.C. that health and wellness are related to nutrition, physical activity, stress management, and small changes to daily activities.

Assessment: K.C. is a 13-year-old female teenager who is at risk for obesity from growth chart documentation at her last pediatrician's check-up. She also is in need of recommended routine Tdap and HPV immunizations based on her age. Additionally, her academic studies have declined since starting middle school.

Plan: Recommend Tdap and HPV vaccinations at this time, either at pediatrician's office or a pharmacy. Develop better organizational skills and establish limits to daily activities to include at least 15–30 minutes of free time. Establish nutrition and physical activity plan with mother through the MyPyramid website for weight management.

Rationale: Immunization with Tdap instead of previously routine Td booster is essential to help decrease her risk of pertussis. Her immunity has waned since childhood vaccinations and pertussis rates in adolescents are on the rise. Immunization with HPV vaccine has benefits against virus strains that causes most cervical cancers and genital warts and should be given prior to sexual activity for the best efficacy. By developing organizational skills, K.C. may have more time for academic studies, which may be needed given starting a new school and the challenges she may have with additional coursework. However, also establishing some free time to her schedule should help manage her potential stress and free her daily schedule for exercise or time with mother for support.

Monitoring: Follow-up visit to a healthcare professional for weight maintenance with a recommended weight-for-age growth chart should be scheduled in 6 months. Stress management should further be evaluated at follow-up and if needed additional help from healthcare professional or school educator should be encouraged. Lastly, providers and family should maintain up-to-date records of immunizations.

Patient education: Healthcare provider can identify with weight and school stress concerns. Again an explanation to K.C. about her health and wellness and its relationship to nutrition, physical activity and stress management, and small changes to her daily activities will help manage her overall health currently and for the future should be included.

Summary

Children and women require unique care throughout their lives, whether diet and exercise, stress management, or other health preventive measures. In turn, governmental agencies and their health policies have been established to eliminate disparities within children's and women's health and wellness. Overall, all healthcare providers should play a role within these special populations. However, pharmacists, given their accessibility to their community, can promote health education and disease prevention and management readily, helping to support and encourage health and wellness in beginning in childhood and carried throughout life.

References

Additional content available at
www.ashp.org/womenshealth

9 Medication Use and Complementary and Alternative Therapy

Mary L. Chavez, B.S.Pharm., Pharm.D., FAACP; Leslie A. Shimp, Pharm.D., MS; Philip J. Gregory, Pharm.D.

Learning Objectives

1. Compare the use of conventional medications with the use complementary and alternative therapies in women and men.
2. Know the herbals/dietary supplements commonly used by women.
3. Apply a simple method that can be used to assess the risk vs. benefit of using complementary and alternative therapies.
4. Recommend selected resources for information on complementary and alternative therapies to laypeople and healthcare providers.

The hardest years in life are those between ten and seventy.

~Helen Hayes (two-time, Academy Award–winning American actress at age 73 years)

Human longevity in the U.S. has dramatically increased over the past century due, in part, to the tremendous advances in medicine, public health, science, and technology.[1] Although life expectancy has increased for both sexes, women experience greater longevity (i.e., women currently live 5.8 years longer than men) but with more morbidity than men over their lifetime.[2] In other words, the longer life a woman experiences can be of poorer quality due to worsening health.[1]

Studies have shown that women use medical services (including medications) and **complementary and alternative medicine (CAM)** more often than men and girls and women ages 12 years and older take more prescription and nonprescription medications than men of the same age.[3,4] According to surveys, CAM use rates are also higher for women than men.[5]

The National Center for Complementary and Alternative Medicine (NCCAM) of the National Institutes of Health (NIH) classifies CAM into several broad categories. These include whole medical systems (e.g., traditional Chinese medicine and ayurveda) or specific practices such as mind-body medicine (e.g., meditation, yoga, tai chi), biologically-based practices (e.g., **herbs**, vitamins, foods used for medicinal purposes), manipulative and body-based practices (e.g., massage, chiropractic, and osteopathic manipulation), and energy medicine (e.g., Reiki, magnetic fields).[6] Women's health needs and values concerning self care and CAM should be integrated into all medical and pharmacy care plans. An understanding of medication use and CAM is needed in order to appropriately provide good care and counseling to women and to individuals under their care. (See Web Resources for Major Types of Complementary and Alternative Therapies.)

Additional content available at ***www.ashp.org/womenshealth***

This chapter examines how various demographic, cultural, social, and economic factors and health concerns influence the use of prescription medicine, CAM, and self care by women. To assist laypeople and healthcare providers to make appropriate decisions about CAM, the available guidelines for this area will be examined. Resources to obtain accurate

Case Presentation

Patient Case: Part 1

L.F. is a 27-year-old Native American physical therapist who is in the pharmacy asking to speak with the pharmacist about some symptoms she is experiencing. The symptoms she describes are irritability and being easily angered, sometimes about events that typically do not result in the same intensity of feelings that she currently has been experiencing. She feels much more stressed and has a tendency to cry easily when feeling stressed. These symptoms occur especially during the week prior to her menstrual period. In addition she notes abdominal bloating and a craving for carbohydrate foods like potato chips. The symptoms that especially bother her are the emotional symptoms. She describes them as bothersome but not severe. Based on what she has read, she thinks she might have premenstrual syndrome (PMS). She would like to know what she might do to relieve these symptoms and has heard from her mother and aunts that there are some herbs that are good for PMS. The pharmacist asked more questions and discovered the following:

Medical history: Hypertension
Allergies in fall
Migraines (which occur about once every 2 months or so)

Social history: About 3 cups of coffee and two 16-ounce cola beverages daily
1–2 glasses of wine once or twice a week and beer occasionally on the weekend
½ pack of cigarettes daily (knows she should quit)

Medications: Hydrochlorothiazide 25 mg daily
Triamcinolone two sprays each nostril daily beginning in early fall
Multivitamin daily
Excedrin (acetaminophen, aspirin, and caffeine)

Allergies: NKDA

Vitals: BP 120/80 mmHg, HR 70 bpm, height: 5′4″, weight: 145 lb

information on the efficacy and safety of CAM will also be discussed. Specific use of prescription and CAM for women's health is described in the clinically oriented chapters in Sections 3 to 7.

The Impact of Women on the Healthcare System

Across the lifespan, girls and women have many questions starting at puberty about menstruation, PMS, and eating disorders. Later questions change to concerns about loss of sexual desire, cardiovascular disease, osteoporosis, breast, cervical, ovarian, or endometrial cancer, menopause, and Alzheimer's disease. Although breast cancer is often a major concern of women, heart disease and lung cancer are the main killers of both women and men age 65 years and over.[7] Further discussion of how sex and gender influence health is discussed in Chapter 7: Sex and Gender Differences.

Women have a dominant impact on the healthcare system for a variety of reasons. Besides taking care of themselves, women are often the chief executive of the household. This role includes managing the family's health, including scheduling medical appointments, filling prescriptions, and administering medications. In fact, women make more physician visits, more healthcare decisions, undergo more hospital procedures, and spend two of every three healthcare dollars in the U.S.[8] The impact of women on the healthcare system cannot be overstated.

Despite women having a more active role in healthcare, 50% of women are dissatisfied with the healthcare they receive.[9] Many women feel that they do not receive adequate educational support or have enough social support to implement adequate lifestyle changes to improve their health. Women have expressed that they want their healthcare provider to demonstrate respect and they want to be in partnership with their healthcare provider. Focus groups have found that women feel their healthcare is often limited or haphazard. Some women feel there is often a lack of privacy and respect.[9,10] As an example, women expressed that they are uncomfortable having to provide personal information in public areas, which could theoretically extend to the pharmacy counter.[9,10]

Compared to men, women prefer to take a more active role in healthcare.[7] Women are more likely to prefer a patient-centered approach to gather health-related information that provides various options for treatment. In a study involving patient preference for participation in medical decision making, it was determined that women are more likely to prefer an active role in health-related, decision-making processes compared to men who more often prefer physician-directed care.[7]

Surveys assessing reasons why individuals use CAM find higher usage is associated with persons who want to have a proactive role in their healthcare and possess a holistic health perspective rather than being dissatisfied with conventional medicine. Rather than expecting CAM to be more efficacious than conventional care, research suggests that users of CAM want a medical system that goes beyond simply managing symptoms.[12]

Self-Care

Self-care for health problems is common. It is estimated that 57% of all health problems are treated with nonprescription therapies.[13] An increase in the number of nonprescription products on the market as well as an increased use of herbs, other **dietary supplements,** and CAM over the last two decades have supported and encouraged self-care of health symptoms and conditions.

Prescription and Complementary Medicine Studies

For many of the next sections, data from studies on prescription and CAM use will be described. Although these studies are helpful to understand use and problems, each study has limitations that the healthcare provider should understand when extrapolating this data to practice. Even with limitations, medication use data help understand and resolve medication use issues and develop policy.

For all studies, design issues and confounders can influence the results. The exact prevalence and reason for medication and CAM use are difficult to assess. Large chain pharmacy databases provide valuable information but medication procurement from competitor local and mail order pharmacies and important medications such as over-the-counter, herbs, and supplement products would not be included. Discrepancy between the prescribing of medications and CAM and actual consumption/use by patients is another potential confounder. When consumption is evaluated, various definitions for adherence and persistence of use are employed. Furthermore, most medication use databases are not linked to medication indications. Most research studies on medication and CAM use also do not capture indications.

The results of surveys of medication and CAM use sometimes are questioned due to possible methodological flaws such as data collection methods, use of combination products, lack of power, and other confounders. One objection is that the classification of CAM is too broad and that some therapies should be considered conventional medicine. For example, use of multiple vitamins or prayer was considered CAM by some surveys. Many practitioners do not consider these to be CAM. Also, some CAM therapies cannot be well defined and may have different meanings to different people, such as spiritual healing.[14] Some studies rely on current and past medication and CAM use recall. The sensitivity and specificity of this means of data collection are unknown. The ability of Danish nurses to self-report hormone therapy use in two time frames was 78.4% (95% CI 75.4–81.4) for past use (1993) and 98.4% (95% CI 97.8–98.9) for current use (1999) when compared to actual prescription reimbursement data.[15] Because this sample represented healthcare professionals, the ability to extrapolate these findings to other groups might be limited and higher than nonmedical laypeople's medication recall. The use of telephone surveys by individuals who only speak English can limit findings. Recently, a survey of five types of CAM usage during the menopause transition across cohorts of White, Japanese, Chinese, Hispanic, and African-American women was conducted.[16] Participants were questioned in their own language. The researchers found that White and Japanese women had the highest rates of CAM use (60%), followed by Chinese (46%), African American (40%), and Hispanic (20%) women. Women who used postmenopausal hormone therapy (HT) used more CAM compared to women who did not use HT, regardless of ethnicity and symptoms.

Prescription Medication Use

USE BY AGE AND GENDER IN CHILDREN

Medication use does not generally vary by age in childhood but begins to vary in adulthood. For children under the age of 18 years, the number of medications dispensed is overall equivalent (OR = 0.95 – 1.05) between sexes.[17] Stimulant medications are more commonly dispensed to young boys (<18 years) compared to young girls, which is consistent with the higher prevalence of attention deficit hyperactivity disorder (ADHD) in male children. [18]

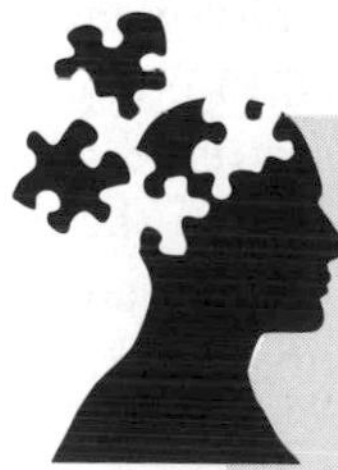

Therapeutic Challenge:

You wish to determine the most commonly used herbal medications in your practice to make sure all healthcare providers are well versed in the efficacy and safety of these herbs. How would you design the study?

USE BY AGE AND GENDER IN ADULTS

As women age, their medication use becomes higher than in men creating some sex/gender differences. Analysis of a large national pharmacy chain database revealed more medications were dispensed to women compared to men, especially during the reproductive years.[11] Twelve groups of medications had higher female/male ratios (defined as greater than one standard deviation difference). In all adult age groups, women received more antibiotics, antihistamines, sympathomimetics, benzodiazepines, antidepressants, phenothiazines, diuretics, thyroid drugs, propoxyphene, and acetaminophen compared to men. Medications almost exclusively used by the female gender were oral contraceptives, estrogens, progestogens, tamoxifen, and estrogen agonists/antagonists. The study did not compare use of medication between genders in patients ≥75 years of age because the majority of subjects in this age group were women. Men were dispensed more antianginals, anticoagulants, antihypertensives, and cardiac glycosides compared to women. Medications dispensed almost solely to men included sildenafil, terazosin, and allopurinol. Other research based on epidemiological data suggested the increased use of antianxiety and antidepressants in women 18 years and older could be due to women having more acute and chronic conditions such as major depression, anxiety, and painful condition.[19] Another factor, could be the propensity of men to shun healthcare. [20]

USE BY AGE AND GENDER IN SENIORS

In a study of gender differences in use and expenditures of prescription drugs in both Medicare- and privately-insured older adults aged 65 years and older, senior women spent approximately $1,178 for medications, which is about 17% more than expenditures by senior men. [21] Senior women constituted 50.7% of the U.S. population in 2005 and had average annual aggregate expenditures for prescribed medicines of $6.93 billion compared to $5.77 billion for senior men.

A random telephone survey of community-living adults (n = 2590, 22.8% adults ≥65 years) throughout the U.S. was performed during February 1998 to December 1999 to determine medication use (i.e., prescription, nonprescription, vitamin/mineral and dietary supplements) during the preceding week.[22] Use of some medication was age- and gender-related. Greater use in women than men was reported in every age group, except for persons 65 years of age who took 10 medications, where the prevalence of use was the same for men and women. Aspirin was used less often for cardiovascular prophylaxis in older women (51%) compared to older men (58%). Senior women more frequently used levothyroxine, amlodipine, hydrochlorothiazide, triamterene, and diltiazem compared to senior men. Atorvastatin, furosemide, warfarin and digoxin were more commonly used by senior men as compared to senior women. Diuretics and antihypertensives were more commonly used in both senior men and women compared to the younger groups. Ibuprofen and caffeine (not including caffeine in beverages or food) were more frequently used by young people.

USE DURING PREGNANCY AND LACTATION

Every year, approximately 6 million women become pregnant in the U.S., resulting in more than 4 million births.[23] The limited information on the safety of medication use during pregnancy is a critical issue for women's healthcare (see Chapter 23: Drug Principles in Pregnancy and Lactation).[24] Several studies show that pregnant women are prescribed one or more drugs during the course of pregnancy.[25,26] Using retrospective data of automated databases of eight health maintenance organizations in the U.S., researchers estimated that 64% of pregnant women (totaling >152,000 deliveries) were prescribed at least one medication. Of these, 3.4% received a category D drug (i.e., positive evidence exists for fetal risk, but potential benefit may warrant use) and 1.1% received a category X drug (i.e., positive evidence exists for fetal risk, and the risk clearly outweighs any benefit), as classified by the U.S. Food and Drug Administration (FDA) risk classification system.[26] Of note, this classification scheme is being revised. The results of this study are confirmed by other large studies in which the majority of pregnant women were prescribed a prescription drug (up to 68%), with up to 4% of women being prescribed a category D or X drug.[25-30] This risk appears to also occur in other countries as a retrospective, register-based cohort study of three nationwide-linked registers in Finland found that 20.4% of women received at least one drug classified as potentially harmful during pregnancy, and up to 3% received at least one drug classified as clearly harmful.[31] The results of these studies underscore the importance and need to understand the effects of these medications on the developing fetus and on the pregnant woman and for women to consult with educated healthcare providers about safe medication use during these times.

The frequency of medication use in breastfeeding women is not well documented. In a survey of 549 mothers at well-baby clinics in the Netherlands, 82.1% of mothers breastfed and 65.9% had concurrently used prescription drugs while breastfeeding.[32] Compared to women who did not breastfeed, the pattern of drug use differed: oral contraceptives, iron preparations, drugs for peptic ulcer, and several psychotropic drugs were more frequently used by nonbreastfeeding women. Vitamins and homeopathic remedies were more frequently used by breastfeeding women. Breastfeeding women tended to avoid drug use or discontinued breastfeeding when they received a prescription medication. These data underscore the fact that all breastfeeding women should receive advice on the appropriateness of using medications while breastfeeding.

Complementary and Alternative Medicine (CAM) Therapies

The National Center for Complementary and Alternative Medicine (NCCAM) created definitions for the various types of therapies and also greatly increased the number and quality of research in this area.[33,34] They defined an **alternative provider** or practitioner as someone who is knowledgeable about a specific alternative health therapy, provides care or gives advice about its use, and usually receives payment for her or his services. For some therapies, the provider might have received formal training and might be certified by a licensing board or related professional association. For example, a practitioner of biofeedback, biofeedback therapist, has usually received training in psychology and physiology and can be certified by the Biofeedback Certification Institute of America. To also help with research efforts, CAM has been divided into the following categories: whole medical systems, mind-body medicine, biologically-based practices, manipulative and body-based practices, and energy medicine. Teaching of the concepts and sometimes the actual CAM practices are beginning to appear within health-care professional curricula and training.

WHOLE MEDICAL SYSTEMS

Whole medical systems include practices such as ayurveda, traditional Chinese medicine, homeopathy, folk medicine, and naturopathy. Ayurveda is a comprehensive system of medicine, developed in India over 5,000 years ago and places equal emphasis on body, mind, and spirit. The goal is to restore the natural harmony of the individual. An ayurvedic doctor identifies an individual's "constitution" or overall health profile by ascertaining the patient's metabolic body type (Vata, Pitta, or Kapha) through a series of personal history questions. Then the patient's "constitution" becomes the foundation for a specific treatment plan designed to guide the individual back into harmony with his or her environment. This plan may include dietary changes, exercise, yoga, meditation, massage, herbal tonics, and other remedies.

Traditional Chinese medicine includes acupuncture, moxibustion, herbs, natural products, massage, and manipulation. Acupuncture is based on the theory that health is determined by a balanced flow of energy (*chi* or *qi*), which is thought to be present in all living organisms. This life energy circulates throughout the body along a series of energy pathways (meridians). Each of these meridians is linked to specific internal organs and organ systems. Within this system of energy pathways, there are over 1,000 acupoints that can be stimulated through the insertion of needles. This practice is thought to help correct and rebalance the flow of life energy and restore health. Acupuncture has been used to treat health problems and conditions ranging from the common cold to addiction and chronic fatigue syndrome. Moxibustion is the use of heat at the acupuncture points created by burning the herb moxa.

Homeopathic treatment is based on the theory that any substance that can produce symptoms of disease or illness in a healthy person can cure those symptoms in a sick person. For example, someone suffering from insomnia may be given a homeopathic dose of coffee. Administered in diluted form, homeopathic remedies are derived from many natural sources including plants, metals, and minerals. Numbering in the thousands, these remedies have been used to treat a wide variety of ailments including seasonal allergies, asthma, influenza, headaches, and indigestion.

Folk medicine systems of healing such as *Curanderismo* and Native American healing have persisted since the beginning of culture and flourished long before the development of conventional medicine. Folk healers usually participate in a training regimen of observation and imitation, with healing often considered a gift passed down through several generations of a family. Folk healers may employ a range of remedies including prayer, healing touch, or laying on of hands, charms, herbal teas or tinctures, magic rituals, and others. Folk healers are found in all cultures and operate under a variety of names and labels.

Naturopathy is a broad system of medicine based on the theory that the body is a self-regulating mechanism with the natural ability to maintain a state of health and wellness. Naturopathic doctors, who generally reject invasive techniques and the use of synthetic drugs, try to cure illness and disease by harnessing the body's natural healing powers. This is done with the use of various alternative and traditional techniques, including herbal medicine, homeopathic treatment, massage, dietary supplements, and other physical therapies.

MIND-BODY MEDICINE

Mind-body medicine such as biofeedback, deep breathing, guided imagery, and yoga focuses on the interactions between the brain, mind, body, and behavior. Biofeedback teaches clients, through the use of simple electronic devices, how to consciously regulate normally unconscious bodily functions (e.g., breathing, heart rate, blood pressure) to improve overall health. Biofeedback has been used to reduce stress, eliminate headaches, recondition injured muscles, control asthmatic attacks, and relieve pain. Deep breathing involves slow, deep inhalation through the nose, usually for a count of 10, followed by slow and complete exhalation for a similar count. To help quiet the mind, one generally concentrates fully on breathing and counting through each cycle. The process may be repeated 5–10 times, several times a day.

Guided imagery involves a series of relaxation techniques followed by the visualization of detailed images, usually calm and peaceful in nature. If used for treatment, the client may visualize her/his body as healthy, strong, and free of the specific problem or condition. Sessions conducted in groups or one-on-one are typically 20–30 minutes, and may be practiced several times a week. Guided imagery has been advocated for a number of chronic conditions including headaches, stress, high blood pressure, and anxiety.

Hypnosis involves an altered state of consciousness and is characterized by increased responsiveness to suggestion. The hypnotic state is attained by first relaxing the body and then shifting the client's attention toward a narrow range of objects or ideas as suggested by the hypnotist or hypnotherapist. The procedure is used to access various levels of the mind to effect positive changes in a person's behavior and to treat numerous health conditions. For example, hypnosis has been used to lose weight, improve sleep, stop smoking, and reduce pain and stress.

Yoga combines breathing exercises, physical postures, and meditation to calm the nervous system and balance body, mind, and spirit. Yoga has been practiced for over 5,000 years. It is thought to prevent specific diseases and maladies by keeping the energy meridians (see acupuncture) open and life energy (qi) flowing. Usually performed in classes, sessions are conducted at least once a week and for approximately 45 minutes. Yoga has been used to lower blood pressure, reduce stress, and improve coordination, flexibility, concentration, sleep, and digestion. It has also been used as supplementary therapy for such diverse conditions as cancer, diabetes, asthma, and AIDS.

BIOLOGICALLY-BASED PRACTICES

Biologically-based practices include dietary supplements, functional foods, and special diets. **Dietary supplements** are natural products including vitamins, minerals, and other natural products that are taken by mouth and contain a dietary ingredient intended to supplement the diet. They include herbs or herbal medicine as single herbs or mixtures, other botanical products such as soy or flax products, and dietary substances such as enzymes and **glandulars.** Among the most popular are echinacea, ginkgo, ginseng, feverfew, garlic, kava kava, and saw palmetto. Garlic, for example, has been used to treat fevers, sore throats, digestive ailments, hardening of the arteries, and other health problems and conditions.

In contrast to dietary supplements, **nutraceuticals** or functional foods are components of the usual diet that may have biologically active components (e.g., polyphenols, phytoestrogens, fish oils, carotenoids) that may provide health benefits beyond basic nutrition. Examples of some functional foods include soy, nuts, chocolate, and cranberries.

Some examples of CAM diets include the Ornish diet, which is a high-fiber, low-fat, vegetarian diet that promotes weight loss and health by controlling what one eats, not by restricting the intake of calories. Fruits, beans, grains, and vegetables can be eaten at all meals, while nonfat dairy products such as skim milk, nonfat cheeses, and egg whites are to be consumed in moderation. Products such as oils, avocados, nuts and seeds, and meats of all kinds are avoided. The Pritikin diet or Pritikin Principle is another diet that is a low-fat diet emphasizing the consumption of foods with a large volume of fiber and water including many vegetables, fruits, beans, and natural, unprocessed grains.

MANIPULATIVE AND BODY-BASED PRACTICES

Manipulative and body-based practices include such practices as chiropractic care, massage therapy, meditation, progressive relaxation, and tai chi. Chiropractic care involves the adjustment of the spine and joints to influence the body's nervous system and natural defense mechanisms to alleviate pain and improve general health. It is primarily used to treat back problems, headaches, nerve inflammation, muscle spasms, and other injuries and traumas.

Massage therapy involves pressing, rubbing, and otherwise manipulating muscles and other soft tissues of the body causing them to relax and lengthen and allowing pain-relieving oxygen and blood to flow to the affected area. Using their hands and sometimes feet, elbows, and forearms, massage therapists use over 75 different methods, such as Swedish massage, deep-tissue massage, neuromuscular massage, and manual lymph drainage. Massage is considered effective for relieving any type of pain in the body's soft tissue, including back, neck, and shoulder pain, headaches, bursitis, and tendonitis.

Meditation is use of mental calmness and physical relaxation and is achieved by suspending the stream of thoughts that normally occupy the mind. Generally performed once or twice a day for approximately 20 minutes at a time, meditation is used to reduce stress, alter hormone levels, and elevate one's mood. In addition, a person experienced in meditation can achieve a reduction in blood pressure, adrenaline levels, heart rate, and skin temperature.

Progressive relaxation therapy involves the successive tensing and relaxing of each of the 15 major muscle groups. Performed lying down, one generally begins with the head and progresses downward, tensing each muscle as tightly as possible for a count of 5 to 10 and then releasing it completely. Often combined with deep breathing, progressive relaxation is particularly useful for reducing stress, relieving tension, and inducing sleep.

Tai chi is a Chinese self-defense discipline and low-intensity, low-impact exercise regimen used for health, relaxation, and self-exploration. Usually performed daily, tai chi exercises include a set of forms, with each form comprising a series of body positions connected into one continuous movement. A single form may include up to 100 positions and may take as long as 20 minutes to complete. Some of the proposed benefits of tai chi include improved concentration, circulation, balance, and posture, reduction of stress, and prevention of osteoporosis.

ENERGY MEDICINE

Energy medicine is a form of CAM that deals with two types of energy fields: veritable, which can be measured, and putative, which is not measurable. Veritable energies use mechanical vibrations such as sound and electromagnetic forces, such as visible light, magnetism, monochromatic radiation such as laser beams, and rays from other parts of the electromagnetic spectrum. Putative energy fields are based on the concept that human beings are infused with a subtle form of energy. Examples are Reiki and qi gong.

Reiki helps the body's ability to heal itself through the flow and focusing of healing energy. During treatment, this healing energy is channeled through the hands of a practitioner into the client's body to restore a normal energy balance and health. Energy healing therapy has been used to treat a wide variety of ailments and health problems and is often used in conjunction with other alternative and conventional medical treatments.

Qi gong is an ancient Chinese discipline that combines the use of gentle physical movements, mental focus, and deep breathing designed to integrate the mind, body, and spirit, and to stimulate the flow of vital life energy (qi). Directed toward specific parts of the body, qi gong exercises are normally performed two or more times a week for 30 minutes at a time and have been used to treat a variety of ailments including asthma, arthritis, stress, lower back pain, allergies, diabetes, headaches, heart disease, hypertension, and chronic pain.

Complementary and Alternative Therapy Use

OVERALL USE

Use of CAM has risen dramatically in the U.S. in recent years. Increased coverage by the media and in the lay press might have fueled some of this interest.[34-36] A 1990 national survey of prevalence, cost, and patterns of use of CAM found that 34% of U.S. adults use some form of CAM.[35] In 1997, use had risen to approximately 42%.[36] Results of a 2002 cross-sectional health status survey of >30,000 adults living throughout the U.S. conducted by NCCAM and the National Center for Health Statistics (part of the Centers for Disease Control and Prevention) found that 36% of adults used at least one of 19 different CAM therapies in the prior 12 months.[6] The most commonly used CAM therapies were prayer for one's own health (43%), prayer for another person's health (24%), natural products (19%), deep breathing exercises (10%), chiropractic care (8%), yoga (5%), massage (5%), and diet-based therapies (4%). These studies support previous data suggesting that women tend to take a proactive role in managing their health and pursuing self-care treatments. Women can have an important impact on whether other family members use CAM. Not surprisingly, children with a medical condition such as cancer are significantly more likely to receive CAM therapies if such therapies are used by the parent.[37,38] A mother's attitude toward these therapies and resultant use of them might substantially impact the use of these therapies by other family members.

When use of CAM in 2002 was compared to use in 2007, the National Center for Health Statistics survey found that overall use among adults remained relatively steady with 36% of adults in the U.S. using CAM in 2002 and 38% in 2007.[34] Nonvitamin, nonmineral dietary supplements were the most commonly used CAM therapy among adults. In 2007, the CAM therapies most commonly used by U.S. adults were nonvitamin, nonmineral, natural products (17.7%), deep breathing exercises (12.7%), meditation (9.4%), chiropractic or osteopathic manipulation (8.6%), massage (8.3%), and yoga (6.1%). In 2007 CAM use was more prevalent among women, adults aged 30–69 years old, adults with higher levels of education, adults who were not poor, adults living in the West, former smokers, and adults who were hospitalized in the last year, which is consistent with results from the 2002 National Health Interview Survey (NHIS).

USE IN CHILDREN BY AGE, GENDER AND RACE/ETHNICITY

Older surveys on use of CAM among U.S. children under 18 years of age found use was less prevalent compared to adult use rates; with estimated usage from 1.6% to 15%.[37] In December 2008, the NCCAM and the National Center for Health Statistics released new findings on Americans' use of CAM. The NHIS asked selected adult respondents about CAM use by children in their households.[34] Overall, approximately 12% of children used at least one of 10 forms of CAM. Use was greater in children whose parents used CAM (23.9%), in adolescents aged 12–17 years of age (16.4%) compared to younger children, in white children (12.8%) compared to Hispanic children (7.9%) and black children (5.9%), in children whose parents had higher education levels defined as more than high school (14.7%), in children with six or more health conditions (23.8%), and children whose families delayed conventional care because of cost (16.9%).

USE BY WOMEN

CAM therapies are commonly used for specific female conditions such as PMS and menopause. A survey of 1,826 women in Wellington, New Zealand found 85% of menstruating women reported PMS and 81% of these women used some type of self-help defined as treatment not prescribed or recommended by a physician.[38] In a similar survey of women living in Great Britain, up to 75% of women contacted alternative medicine agencies for management of their PMS symptoms.[39] In a survey of 4,402 women who were recruited in the Menopause Epidemiology Study during April 2005, 60% sought healthcare for menopausal symptoms.[40] The most frequently reported menopause symptoms were vasomotor symptoms across all races/ethnicities. Over 61% of women reported using some type of menopausal therapy in their lifetime, with 33.7% using hormone therapy (oral, patch, or cream), 12.2% using CAM, and 15.5% using both types of therapies.

Women are the most frequent users of CAM based on total group and also across all race/ethnic groups. A survey of Asian Americans found that a total of 47% of women used CAM compared to 38% of Asian American men.[41] In another study 89% of Hispanic women used CAM compared to 38% of Hispanic men.[42] A telephone survey conducted in 2001 of 808 U.S. women 18 years and older assessed the use of 11 CAM categories during the year prior to the survey.[3] Women were asked about use of CAM for 16 health-related conditions over the life cycle. Over half (53%) of the respondents used CAM. The most common health condition for which CAM was used was painful conditions (i.e., back pain, joint pain, or headaches). Other conditions for which CAM was commonly used were pregnancy-related conditions, menstrual symptoms, and menopausal symptoms. CAM was less commonly used for cancer, heart disease, osteoporosis, and uterine fibroids. The most commonly used CAMs were vitamins, nutritional supplements, and herbals. The majority of women disclosed use of CAM to their doctor but approximately 23% of women used CAM for pregnancy-related conditions without informing their healthcare provider. Nutritional supplements and herbals were often used along with prescription and over-the-counter medications.

Herb and Dietary Supplements

USE IN CHILDREN

A few studies have specifically looked at children and use of herbs and supplements. Analysis of nationally representative data from the 1999–2002 National Health and Nutrition Examination Survey (NHANES) found that between 1999–2002, 31.8% of children used dietary supplements with the lowest rates in infants younger than 1 year (11.9%).[43] The highest rate of use was in children ages 4 to 8 years (48.5%). The most commonly used dietary supplements were vitamins and minerals. The highest use was in non-Hispanic white children (38.1%) and Mexican-American children (22.4%), and the lowest use in non-Hispanic black children (18.8%).

USE IN ADULTS

Over the last two decades, the use of herbals and other dietary supplements has gained in popularity.

It was estimated that Americans spent $5.1 billion on herbal remedies in 1997. From 1990 to 1997, use of these therapies grew by 380%.[36] However, statistics and demographic characteristics of herbal/dietary supplement use vary. Results of the 2002 National Interview Survey found that 18.9% of those surveyed used at least one herbal supplement in the previous year.[44] The most commonly used herbal supplements were echinacea (40%), ginseng (24%), ginkgo (21%), and garlic (20%). In 2007, the most commonly used nonvitamin, nonmineral, natural products used by adults for health reasons in the past 30 days were fish oil, omega 3 or docosahexaenoic acid (DHA) (37.4%), glucosamine (19.9%), echinacea (19.8%), flaxseed oil (15.9%), and ginseng (14.1%).[34]

All types of consumers are often using natural products unsupervised without sufficient information on indication, dosage, adverse effects, and drug interactions, and often in combination with prescription medications.[36] Of concern, 51% of users do not discuss use with a medical professional.[44] Disclosure rates to physicians were significantly lower in men, younger adults, and in race and ethnic minorities.[44] From 1994 to 1998, the FDA received more than 800 adverse events reports attributed to the use of the dietary supplement ephedra or *ma huang*. In 2004, the NIH reported more than 16,000 adverse events associated with ephedra, and the FDA banned dietary supplements containing this plant-based supplement.[45] Adverse events associated with *Ephedra sinica* included heart palpitation, myocardial infarctions, and stroke. Drug interactions involving a number of herbals and dietary supplements such as St. John's wort are also becoming increasingly well documented.[46] It is, therefore, imperative that all healthcare providers become informed about the current scientific evidence regarding these CAM therapies.

USE BY WOMEN

Many women use herbals and other dietary supplements throughout their life cycle. Herbals and other dietary supplements have a long history of use for gynecological and other female functional disorders. Historically, herbals have been used for a wide range of female medical conditions including breast pain, dysmenorrhea, PMS, menstrual irregularities, infertility, nausea, and vomiting in pregnancy, postpartum hemorrhage, decreased libido, and menopausal symptoms.[47]

Many women turn to herbs and dietary supplements for PMS and menopausal symptoms for a variety of reasons. One of the primary reasons is that many women are concerned about adverse effects and drug interactions with conventional drug therapy. The most common dietary supplements and herbals used for treatment of PMS include calcium, chasteberry, evening primrose oil, vitamin E, magnesium, vitamin B_6, ginkgo, black cohosh, and dong quai.[39] The exact number of women who use herbals and dietary supplements for perimenopausal and menopausal symptoms remains to be determined. Herbal and dietary supplements used for treatment of menopausal symptoms include soy and soy protein, red clover, black cohosh, wild yam cream, dehydroepiandrosterone (DHEA), vitamin E, kava, St. John's wort, evening primrose oil, melatonin, vitamin E, and S-adenosyl-L-methionine (SAMe).[48] Individual studies suggest a limited benefit of some therapies although in most cases more research is needed.

Bioidentical hormone therapy (BHT) is a commonly used form of CAM for treatment of menopausal symptoms.[49] The BHT uses bioidentical hormones or chemically modified plant extracts that are structurally similar to human endogenous hormones. The BHTs are commercially available or can be compounded into various dosages forms. Compounded BHT products may contain estriol, estrone, estradiol, testosterone, micronized progesterone, and DHEA. Compounded BHTs are promoted as a natural, safer, and sometimes more efficacious than conventional HT. However, there is lack of evidence to support such claims. Furthermore, some of these compounding facilities have been closed by the FDA for poor manufacturing practices. Compounded BHTs lack quality controlled studies that examine the pharmacokinetics, safety, and efficacy of these products. Many promoters of compounded BHTs tailor BHT products based on saliva tests or blood sera concentrations to pre- or perimenopausal concentrations, the accuracy of all these labs have not been fully established. This is contrary to evidence-based guidelines, which support prescribing the lowest dose for the shortest duration of HT individually according to the women's symptoms (see Chapter 17: Menopause).[50] Until data are available, most experts recommend considering the safety and efficacy of these products similar to prescription products, many of which are natural products.

USE DURING PREGNANCY

Minimal data exist for the safety and efficacy of herbs and supplements to fetus and mother. One study conducted in 1999–2000 found that 13% of pregnant women use herbal or dietary supplements to maintain a healthy pregnancy or treat common conditions such as gastrointestinal discomfort or respiratory symptoms.[51] A survey of 578 pregnant women in rural West Virginia reported that 45% of respondents had used herbs and other dietary supplements during pregnancy.[52] The risks of herbals/dietary supplements during pregnancy remains to be determined.[53] Therefore, the use of herbals/dietary supplements during pregnancy should generally be discouraged.

Reasons for Complementary Medicine Use

Many laypeople are already using CAM. The issue is not whether people should use CAM, rather what is the efficacy and safety of CAM and how to integrate with traditional care. A number of factors are thought to influence the use of CAM.[54] First, CAM is seen as a "natural approach" in contrast to the "chemical" approach of medications. Most individuals use CAM not because of dissatisfaction with conventional therapy, but because the CAM therapies are more congruent with their values and beliefs toward health and life and might be an integral component of their cultural beliefs. Many individuals use herbal products and dietary supplements concurrently with prescription medications.[36] The majority of CAM users (79%) perceive the combination of CAM and conventional therapy to be superior to either alone.[36] Sometimes use of herbs and dietary supplements as well as other CAM modalities represents a different philosophical approach with their use as preventive or wellness care and therapy, which addresses more than just the physical aspects of health.[6] Many consumers appreciate the "holistic" side of CAM therapy as they believe it treats the mind, body, spirit, and emotion. Some patients feel that conventional medicine is too impersonal or limited to only the physical aspect of health.[55] Many patients do not disclose use of CAM therapies, including use of herbal products and dietary supplements, to healthcare providers.[36] There are three common reasons that patients do not inform their healthcare provider about use of CAM: 1) fear of disapproval or a negative response such as the suggestion that use be stopped; 2) patients do not feel that conventional practitioners are knowledgeable about CAM therapies; and 3) the provider never asked about the use of CAM.[22] Many healthcare providers do not routinely ask patients about use of these agents or discuss nonconventional options for the management of symptoms and health conditions.[56]

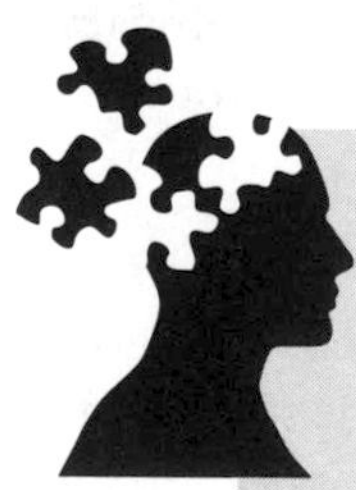

Therapeutic Challenge:

When taking a medication or medical history, how can you increase the patient's comfort and trust to describe all CAM use?

Some people believe that CAM therapies, such as herbs and dietary supplements, are safer. While herbs and dietary supplements are not without side effects and other potential safety issues such as contamination and drug–drug interactions, prescription medications also come with risks. The high profile removal of prescription medications and compounds considered tampered or falsely labeled on the market only increases consumer concern about the safety of prescription medications. A CAM approach is often used if conventional therapy is unsuccessful or associated with perceived unacceptable risks or adverse effects.[6,54] Another factor is direct access to CAM, especially herbs and dietary supplements, which provides consumers the ability to control their own healthcare.[22]

Finally, advertising and access play a role.[57,58] Herbal products are widely advertised on the internet and approximately half of individuals using the internet to obtain health information search for information on CAM therapies.[58] Many CAM providers use direct to consumer advertising. Patients frequently have total control over selection of specific CAM providers vs. having insurance companies dictate who, when, and for how long they can use a provider. However times are changing. Many medical plans pay for some CAM such as massages by physical therapy and services by a chiropractor. Some health plans now also have integrated clinics that provide traditional and nontraditional services.

Guidelines and Recommendations to Healthcare Providers About CAM Use

NEED FOR EDUCATION ON COMPLEMENTARY MEDICINE

Several major organizations have recently issued reports that address the need for improvements in patient–healthcare provider communications, respect for patient autonomy and preferences, and knowledge of CAM to assist patients in evaluating and monitoring these health modalities. The White House

Table 9-1. Guiding Principles to Improve Delivery of Healthcare (White House Commission on Complementary and Alternative Medicine Policy)[59]

- A whole-person orientation in the delivery of healthcare—health involves all aspects of life—mind, body, and spirit
- A commitment to promoting the use of science to help identify safe and effective CAM products
- Respect for individuality and the notion that every person is unique and has the right to healthcare, which is appropriately responsive to him or her and respects his/her preferences
- Recognition of the right to choose treatment—every person has the right to choose freely among safe and effective care or approaches
- Partnerships between patients and healthcare providers are essential for good healthcare

Commission on Complementary and Alternative Medicine Policy convened in 2000 addressed several aspects of complementary and alternative medicine including the education of healthcare professionals about CAM.[59] This commission stated the education and training of healthcare professionals should include information on CAM so providers can discuss and provide guidance to their patients. The commission felt educating healthcare providers about CAM and encouraging the discussion of nonconventional or combined conventional and CAM approaches to healthcare with patients are ways to increase public safety and improve health. The commission had several guiding principles for providers that are advocated as ways to improve the delivery of healthcare (Table 9-1). In a 2003 study, 73% (46 out of 64 respondents) of pharmacy schools/colleges offered instruction in CAM.[60] The most frequently taught content area was herb and other dietary supplements (45 schools).

These guiding principles of the commission on CAM are consistent with thoughts expressed in the Institute of Medicine reports, *Crossing the Quality Chasm: A New Health System for the 21st Century* and *Preventing Medication Errors, 2006*.[61,62] These reports emphasize the importance of better communication between patients and providers, expansion of evidence-based care, improved safety, and dissemination of healthcare information to consumers.[61,62] In addition, the report, *Preventing Medication Errors,* recommends that healthcare providers conduct a systematic review of medication therapy, which includes CAM, for each patient at each patient-provider encounter or at frequent intervals.[62] Table 9-2 provides information on how to advise patients who use CAM therapies.[63]

Table 9-2. How to Advise Patients on the Use of Complementary and Alternative Medicine (CAM) Therapies[63]

Step 1. At initial patient encounter obtain reason for use
Step 2. Advise patient to maintain a diary on effectiveness and side effects
Step 3. Discuss patient's preferences and expectations
Step 4. Review safety and efficacy of the CAM
Step 5. Follow-up with patient

ACCURATE AND COMPLETE MEDICATION HISTORY—KNOWLEDGE OF ALL MEDICINAL PRODUCTS

Given the prevalence of herb and dietary supplement use, healthcare providers must be knowledgeable about these agents and incorporate knowledge of these agents into their patient care activities. Information about all conventional and unconventional therapies a patient is using is required in order to perform an accurate assessment and make appropriate judgments regarding healthcare. Incomplete knowledge of medicinal agents used by a patient can result in flawed decision making. CAM use solely or in conjunction with use of prescription medications can result in adverse effects, drug-herb interactions or additive effects between conventional and CAM products. Use of herbs and dietary supplements may result in symptoms. It is important to determine if use is the cause of a symptom prior to attributing the symptom to another cause. For example, a woman may use chasteberry *(Vitex agnus-castus)* to manage symptoms of PMS. If she were to develop acne it would be important to know that this dermatologic side effect is possible with chasteberry so that it could be determined if use of the herbal product were the cause.[64] Similarly, the possibility of an adverse reaction to the herb should be evaluated in a woman taking black cohosh to treat menopause-related hot flashes who experiences GI upset.[65] In addition, many people use herbs and dietary supplements concurrently with prescription medications so drug-herb/dietary supplement interactions are possible. St. John's wort is one of the most commonly used herbs and it is the herb with the most documented interactions with medications.[66] St. John's wort can cause serotonin syndrome when used in combination with the SSRI antidepressants, can increase the metabolism of various drugs such calcium channel blockers, chemotherapeutic agents and antifungals by inducing the cytochrome P-450 3A4 enzymes, and can reduce the effectiveness of the oral contraceptive. Ginkgo and garlic are also among the most commonly used herbs and each of these herbs has a drug interaction with warfarin and aspirin due to additive antiplatelet effects that can increase the risk for bleeding.[66] Use of herbs and dietary supplements in addition to prescribed therapy for a condition may also indicate a lack of or suboptimal efficacy of the prescription therapy. In a similar way, use of an herb or dietary supplement may indicate poor adherence or misuse resulting in lack of effect from prescribed therapy.

APPLICATION TO PHARMACEUTICAL AND MEDICAL CARE

The provision of pharmaceutical care encompasses several principles that echo the recommendations of these reports.[67] First, the pharmaceutical care model states "The pharmacist has an obligation to ensure effective and safe medication use."[67] When patients use herbs and dietary supplements this principle should also apply to those agents. Healthcare providers should consider all medicinal products (prescription, nonprescription, herbs, and dietary supplements) when advising a patient or conducting a medication therapy assessment. Secondly, an expectation of this model of care is "all medical indications for (drug) therapy are assessed, cared for and evaluated."[67] In other words, the healthcare provider cares for the whole person. This principle implies that the healthcare provider considers all aspects of health—physical, mental, emotional, and spiritual. This thought is expanded in the patient care process of pharmaceutical care that recognizes the individuality of each patient. "Pharmacists recognize that each patient is a complete and complex human being. Pharmacists assess the drug-related needs of each patient from the perspective of that person's unique medication experience."[67] For example, all pharmacists and healthcare providers should inquire about a patient's ability to afford medications and concerns about medications, such as potential adverse effects. In addition, the healthcare provider needs to understand the patient's preferences about medications and the desired approach to healthcare.[68] Effective patient care involves consideration of factors beyond knowledge of the medical condition and the therapeutics of drug therapy. Use of medications occurs in a context and "the pharmacist must understand the patient's medication experience better than all other healthcare providers because it is their primary responsibility to optimize it."[67]

INCREASED KNOWLEDGE OF HERBS AND DIETARY SUPPLEMENTS

Healthcare providers should be knowledgeable about herbs and dietary supplements for several reasons. There is evidence supporting the use of some CAM therapies as useful and effective ways to manage some common medical conditions. For example, the American Heart Association advocates fish oil for the management of hypertriglyceridemia and the American College of Obstetricians and Gynecologists supports the use of ginger for the management of nausea associated with pregnancy.[69,70]

Knowledge of these agents is also useful to formulate recommendations for the management of symptoms for a patient whose preference is to use nondrug therapies and to be able to suggest options for a patient who is already taking multiple medications or for whom conventional therapy has failed or been intolerable.

In addition, healthcare providers should also be able to serve as a source of information about herbs and dietary supplements and to recommend resources and references containing accurate and well-founded/substantiated information on herbs and dietary supplements to patients. Pharmacists should also be able to advise patients on purchasing high-quality products and the certification of herbal products and dietary supplements. In one survey pharmacists were cited as a source of information on herbal products by 23% of consumers.[71] In two other surveys approximately 60% of pharmacists reported that they were often asked about herbal products.[72] However, pharmacists often do not feel that they have sufficient knowledge to advise patients about herbs and dietary supplements or to recognize interactions between herbs and prescription medications.[73,74] Of the pharmacists who reported being asked about herbal products only 2% felt they were always prepared to answer the questions posed by consumers.[72] With CAM therapies part of healthcare professional education, more providers will be competent with these therapies and their integration into care plans.

DOCUMENTATION

Herbs, dietary supplements, and other CAM therapies are not typically recorded in the medical record or pharmacy profile whereas prescription medications are almost always documented. In one study, herbal therapies were documented in the medical record by

Figure 9-1. Evaluation of the Balance Between Effectiveness and Safety[54,a]

		Effectiveness	
		+	--
Risk	+	Weigh possible risk vs. possible benefit; determine if better alternative exists; monitor, especially safety	Avoid or discourage use; monitor, especially safety
	--	Recommend use; monitor	Consider likelihood of benefit; determine if better alternative exists; use may be acceptable but need to monitor for desired effect; monitor, especially effectiveness

Source: Adapted from Figure 7-3, Clinical Risk and Therapeutic Posture. In: Institute of Medicine. *Complementary and Alternative Medicine in the United States*. Washington DC: National Academies Press; 2005.

[a]Discuss strengths and weaknesses of literature including amount available.

fewer than half of prescribers.[75] All providers should make sure medical record charts are comprehensive for CAM therapies and pharmacists should make sure herbs and dietary supplements are entered into pharmacy profiles. Information on use of CAM therapy needs to be available to all healthcare providers.

Implications for Specific Patient Care

ASSESSING RISK VS. BENEFIT

Assistance is needed from healthcare providers to help consumers make informed choices, especially given the limited scientific information available about herbal and supplement therapies. Figure 9-1 depicts a simple but useful tool to help a patient understand the balance between evidence for effectiveness and safety.[54] By comparing the evidence or current knowledge about the safety and effectiveness of an agent it can be placed into one of four categories that are easy to understand by lay persons. A more detailed version of this figure is a component of the Natural Medicines Comprehensive Database.

REPORTING ADVERSE EVENTS RELATED TO CAM THERAPIES

As with conventional drugs, adverse events related to CAM therapies are dramatically underreported. Many barriers exist to adequate reporting of adverse events such as lack of knowledge in how and where to report adverse events, fear of legal ramifications, uncertainty about causality, lack of time or incentive for reporting, and complacency. However, healthcare providers should make every effort to report adverse events related to CAM therapies. Adverse reactions to CAM products can be reported, just like those for conventional medicines, through the FDA MedWatch system at www.accessdata.fda.gov/scripts/medwatch/medwatch-online.htm.

COMMUNICATION

Knowledge of an individual patient is key to providing patient-specific care. A healthcare provider must be able to communicate with her/his patients so as to have a sense for the patient as a person. The healthcare provider should understand the patient's circumstances (e.g., health, health literacy, economic status, living arrangement, cultural and health beliefs). The patient's drug therapy concerns need to be discussed and, if possible, alleviated. Patient preferences with regard to drug therapy are important to designing a care plan. A patient may prefer to use a nondrug therapy or CAM for some symptoms or cost of therapy may be a compelling issue. Knowledge of medication-related behaviors, including adherence and utilization of herbal products and dietary supplements form the foundation for the assessment and recommendations that will be part of the care plan. The patients should be comfortable discussing medication-related behaviors, concerns, preferences, and health beliefs with their healthcare provider.

INVOLVEMENT OF THE PATIENT IN HEALTHCARE

Chronic illness imposes demands on individuals. In addition to taking care of all of the demands of everyday life a person must also accomplish the tasks necessary to the management of her/his illness. In addition, they must deal with the altered image of life imposed by their illness and the associated feelings such as anger, frustration, and depression.[68] *Empowerment* is a term describing helping people to discover their ability to manage illness and improve their health.[76] Healthcare providers can empower their patients by providing them with the knowledge to make rational decisions and involving them in the decisions that affect their health and healthcare, thus giving patients a sense of control. Adherence with drug therapy is improved when patients are involved in determining a care plan and their healthcare goals and health-related beliefs are acknowledged and respected by the healthcare provider.[76]

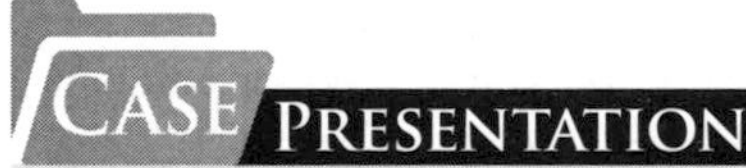

PRESENTATION

Patient Case: Part 2

L.F.'s symptoms are consistent with mild/moderate PMS and self-care is appropriate (see Chapter 13: Premenstrual Syndrome and Premenstrual Dysphoric Disorder). Her hypertension is controlled.

Recommendations

Several self-care options exist for mild/moderate PMS management. Prescription medication is not warranted at this time. She should try one therapy first to see if effective vs. trying many therapies right away. Although her blood pressure is controlled, with her preference for nonprescription products, she could try dietary changes, weight loss, and exercise.

PMS self-care options:

1) Dietary changes—Decrease caffeine intake, decrease salt and sugar intake, moderate/reduced intake of alcohol-containing beverages, increase consumption of complex carbohydrates such as whole-grain foods
2) Social habits—Discontinue, ideally, or reduce tobacco smoking
3) Vitamins and or minerals[82]
   a. Calcium 1,000–1,500 mg daily in divided doses with each dose no more than 500 mg (this agent has the strongest CAM evidence of efficacy for PMS)
   b. Vitamin D 800–1,000 units daily
   c. Vitamin B-6 (pyridoxine) 50–100 mg daily
4) Herbal therapies[82]
   a. Chasteberry *(Vitex agnus)*—Dosing of chasteberry depends on the product used. One formulation of dried fruit extract studied in clinical trials is agnolyt. A dose of agnolyt 4 mg daily is appropriate for the treatment of PMS.
   b. Ginkgo *(Ginkgo biloba)*—80 mg twice daily, starting on the 16th day of the menstrual cycle until the fifth day of the next cycle.
   c. Using Figure 9-1, these two herbs can be compared with regard to evidence for effectiveness and risk/safety. Both agents have some evidence of benefit in relieving some of the emotional symptoms associated with PMS. In comparing risk chasteberry and ginkgo are both generally well tolerated with few side effects and therefore would be rated as having low risk. However, ginkgo has the potential to cause bleeding and is associated with more risk than chasteberry.
5) Hypertension self-care options
   a. DASH diet will reduce blood pressure and may also help to lower cholesterol.[83]
   b. Exercise

Rationale

She should begin to take calcium and vitamin D for 3 months because this regimen has the most data and can also help prevent bone loss. Although blood pressure is controlled, changing diet, weight, and exercise patterns can help control blood pressure without medication and help with long-term wellness (see Chapter 30: Cardiovascular Disease). However, L.F. might wish to use an herbal product first, especially if recommended by a Native American healer.

Monitoring

All the physical and emotional patient symptoms can be monitored, especially those occurring before her menstrual cycle. She could use a calendar to monitor symptoms (see Chapter 13: Premenstrual Syndrome and Premenstrual Dysphoric Disorder). She could have her blood pressure checked at a pharmacy or by a blood pressure cuff for home monitoring.

Follow-up

PMS therapy effects are generally seen with the next menstrual cycle but might take up to three cycles; thus, follow-up should occur in about 3 months. If calcium and vitamin D were not helpful, another CAM therapy such as chasteberry can be tried and then reevaluated in another 3 months.

Patient education

Provide education about triggers of PMS such as stress and options for stress management.

Herb and Dietary Supplement Resources

Finding reliable information on CAM therapies can be a challenge. In general, a shortage exists for reliable information about many of these therapies. Therefore, making informed decisions for both consumers and professionals is difficult. Although there is a lack of high-quality information, a very large amount of poor-quality, commercial information is available, especially on the internet. Hopefully healthcare providers know how to evaluate the reliability of data and resources, but most laypeople probably do not. In order to evaluate web based information resources, NCCAM suggests use of 10 questions.[77] Generally, reliable resources utilize authoritative authors or editors, are fully referenced, and are free from commercial bias or influence. Several resources meet these criteria for conventional drugs, but relatively few exist for CAM therapies. (See Web Resources for 10 Things to Know About Evaluating Medical Resources on the Web, and Resources About Complementary and Alternative Methods of Healing for Consumers and Healthcare Providers).

Additional content available at ***www.ashp.org/womenshealth***

Several studies have evaluated and compared professional resources that provide information on CAM therapies. In a study conducted by a drug information service, Natural Medicines Comprehensive Database was somewhat or very helpful for 82% of questions on CAM therapies compared to 75% with Micromedex.[78] Another drug information center found that Natural Medicines Comprehensive Database provided a direct answer to 61% of CAM-therapy-related questions, Micromedex provided a direct answer 49% of the time, *The Review of Natural Products* provided a direct answer 24% of the time, and the *PDR for Herbal Medicines* provided an answer 21% of the time.[79] Similar to other studies, Natural Medicines Comprehensive Database more consistently provided answers to questions on adverse events compared to other resources.[80]

The Natural Standard database has evidence-based reviews of CAM information including herbals and other dietary supplements, functional foods, diets, complementary practices (modalities), exercises, and medical conditions.[81] It is not as exhaustive as Natural Medicines Comprehensive Database. The database is well referenced with links to PubMed. This database is only available through annly institutional subscription.

Summary

Studies have shown that women are using medications and various CAM for a variety of reasons. More well-conducted clinical studies are needed for both prescription and CAM therapies for women's health conditions. Most lay literature contains anecdotal evidence or opinion rather than scientific support. Consumers are often using natural products unsupervised without sufficient information regarding efficacy, indication, dosages, adverse effects, and drug herb interactions. Many individuals are using CAM in combination with prescription medications without information of potential interactions with natural products and without informing their healthcare providers. Laypeople and healthcare providers need to know how to make informed decisions about the use of all medications and CAM therapies. The same standards of evidence-based medicine should apply to all treatments, whether they are CAM or conventional therapies.

References

Additional content available at ***www.ashp.org/womenshealth***

SECTION THREE

Menstrual Health

10 Menstrual Cycle

Desireé M. McCarthy-Keith, MD, MPH; Alicia Armstrong, MD, MHSCR

Learning Objectives

1. Describe the hypothalamic and pituitary hormones, which are essential for regulation of the menstrual cycle.
2. Define the follicular phase of the menstrual cycle and describe its associated changes in pituitary and ovarian hormone levels.
3. Define the luteal phase of the menstrual cycle and describe its associated changes in pituitary and ovarian hormone levels.
4. Understand the role of follicle-stimulating hormone (FSH) and luteinizing hormone (LH) in follicle development and ovulation.
5. Be familiar with the structural components of the endometrium, and explain its secretory transformation during the menstrual cycle.
6. Understand the role of estrogen and progesterone in the pathophysiology of chronic medical conditions affecting women.

The menstrual cycle involves a highly coordinated series of events, which results in the maturation and release of a single oocyte for fertilization. If the oocyte remains unfertilized, the endometrium is sloughed in preparation for the subsequent menstrual cycle to begin. This process requires the cyclic release of hypothalamic, pituitary, and ovarian hormones, which exert their effects on the uterus and ovary. The synchronized interaction of these hormones is critical to establishing and maintaining the normal menstrual cycle in women from adolescence through the childbearing years until its cessation at menopause.

The phases of the menstrual cycle are governed by the stimulatory and inhibitory effects of the gonadotropins and sex steroids on the pituitary gland and ovary, and an aberration in these physiologic mechanisms leads to menstrual dysfunction. To effectively diagnose and manage the abnormal menstrual cycle, one must first understand the regulation of the normal menstrual cycle and the influence of the menstrual cycle on other medical conditions.

Clinical Presentation

In women, the onset of puberty is marked by **thelarche** or breast development. The final stage in pubertal development, **menarche** or the initiation of menses, occurs within 2 years of thelarche. From the early 1800s to the mid-1950s, the age of menarche for girls in the U.S. occurred at an increasingly lower age.[1] Over the past 50 years, the age of menarche has remained stable in the U.S. and other developed countries. The U.S. National Health and Nutrition Examination Surveys found that the median age of menarche for all girls is 12.43 years; this number is lower in non-Hispanic black girls (12.06 years).[2] Age at menarche varies internationally, and menarche occurs at older ages in girls from some less developed countries. Studies have also shown that girls with higher body mass index (BMI) have earlier onset of menarche. Environmental, socioeconomic, and dietary factors have been suggested as explanations for variation in timing of menarche across populations.[3]

Menses following menarche are usually anovulatory and can occur irregularly for as long as 12–24 months. The interval between the first and second cycles can be particularly irregular, with the first cycle length ranging between 20 and 60 days. As the hypothalamic–pituitary–ovarian axis matures, the cycles become ovulatory and regular. By the third year after menarche, the majority of menstrual cycles occur between 21 and 34 days. Normal cycle length is established by the sixth year after menarche, and the average menstrual cycle occurs every 28 days, with 3–7 days of bleeding.[4,5] Abnormal menstrual cycles occur when the cycle interval occurs <21 days or >35 days, or

CASE PRESENTATION

Patient Case: Part 1

D.M. is a 19-year-old woman with a 4-year history of seizures. She has been compliant with her phenytoin, but has noticed an increase in frequency of seizures around her menses and in the weeks following the onset of menstruation. She is currently a sophomore in college and has recently become sexually active. She wants to improve the control of her epilepsy and to get a recommendation for contraception.

Past medical history: Epilepsy since age 15.

Past obstetric/gynecologic history: Menarche at age 11. Cycles initially occurred every 28–30 days, lasting 4 days until ages 12–15, then menses became irregular every 30–45 days. Pap test 6 months ago was normal. No history of sexually transmitted infections. Using condoms for contraception.

Family history: Mother—hypothyroid; father—diabetes; sister—healthy.

Social history: College sophomore, sexually active for 3 months. Denies tobacco or alcohol use.

Medications: Phenytoin, extended release, 300 mg orally once a day.

Allergies: No known drug allergies.

Vital signs: Height 5′6″, weight 145 lb, BP 132/78, HR 84, Temp. 99.1°F

Physical exam:

General appearance: Well-developed, well-nourished woman with mild hirsutism.

Head, eyes, ears, nose, and throat: Mild gingival hypertrophy.

Remainder of physical exam was unremarkable.

Laboratory evaluation: Urine hCG negative; cultures for gonorrhea and chlamydia both negative; phenytoin level—10 mcg/mL; WBC—5,400/mL^3; hemoglobin 13g/dL; hematocrit 39%; platelet count 254,000/mm^3.

if bleeding is prolonged or excessively heavy. Menstrual disorders will be discussed in detail in Chapter 11: Menstruation Disorders.

In up to 80% of women, premenstrual symptoms develop in the 14 days before menstruation. These changes include emotional lability, irritability, weight gain, bloating, breast tenderness, and headaches. These symptoms are often mild and usually resolve once menstruation begins. Symptoms that are severe and interfere with normal activities are commonly attributed to the premenstrual syndrome (PMS), which will be discussed in Chapter 13: Premenstrual Syndrome and Premenstrual Dysphoric Disorder.

With the exceptions of pregnancy and lactation, regular menses occur throughout a woman's reproductive years until their cessation with menopause. The years of menstrual function span a large portion of a woman's life, and this process is integral to her reproductive health and general health as well.

Normal Physiology of the Menstrual Cycle

Regulation of the menstrual cycle and timing of ovulation are the result of the precise coordination of events between the hypothalamus, pituitary gland, and ovary, or H-P-O axis. We will describe each component of the H-P-O axis, discuss its regulatory role in the menstrual cycle, and then illustrate the interaction of these components along the reproductive axis. Pharmacologic applications related to each component of the axis are listed in Table 10-1.

THE HYPOTHALAMUS

The hypothalamus is located at the base of the brain above the pituitary gland. It controls pituitary function through the secretion of hormones acting on either the anterior or posterior pituitary. The gonadotropins luteinizing hormone (LH) and follicle-stimulating hormone (FSH) are released from the anterior pituitary under the influence of hypothalamic gonadotropin-releasing hormone (GnRH). A direct neuronal connection between the hypothalamus and anterior pituitary does not exist, and GnRH reaches the pituitary via the capillary system of the hypothalamic–hypophyseal portal circulation. These capillaries drain into the portal vessels, which travel along the pituitary stalk to the anterior pituitary. The hypothalamus influences the pituitary through the release of GnRH into the portal circulation. Retrograde flow of pituitary hormones to the hypothalamus also occurs, which allows pituitary feedback on the hypothalamus.

The hypothalamus secretes many different releasing hormones that influence the release of specific pituitary hormones. For the purpose of this chapter, we will only discuss GnRH. Gonadotropin-releasing hormone is secreted in a pulsatile fashion from a specialized network of neurons in the hypothalamus called the GnRH pulse generator. This pulsatile secretion must occur within a narrow critical range in frequency and amplitude for the pulsatile release of

Table 10-1. Reproductive Physiology and Pharmacologic Applications

H-P-O Axis Level	Function	Pharmacologic Applications
Hypothalamus	Initiates puberty through GnRH pulses; regulates FSH and LH secretion	• GnRH antagonists/agonists for suppression of pituitary gonadotropins and reduction of estrogen levels • Pulsatile GnRH, via pump, for induction of ovulation
Pituitary	Secretes FSH and LH necessary for follicular maturation	• Exogenous FSH and LH for ovulation induction in gonadotropin deficiency or superovulation in infertility
Ovary	Produces estrogen and progesterone; provides hormonal control of endometrium	• Oral contraceptive pills for suppression of ovulation • Hormonal therapy for supplementation of low estradiol levels

FSH = follicle stimulating hormone; GnRH = gonadotropin-releasing hormone; H-P-O = hypothalamus, pituitary gland, and ovary; LH = luteinizing hormone.

gonadotropins to occur. Faster GnRH pulse frequencies stimulate LH secretion, whereas slower pulse frequencies favor FSH secretion.[6,7] Enhanced pulsatile secretion of GnRH begins just before puberty. With the onset of puberty, GnRH secretion occurs nocturnally and then progresses to the adult pattern of pulsatile secretion over time. The adult pattern of pulsatility is signaled by the tightly controlled pulsatile secretion of LH and FSH, resulting in oocyte maturation and ovulation of the normal menstrual cycle.

PITUITARY

The pituitary gland is composed of the neurohypophysis (posterior lobe) and adenohypophysis (anterior lobe). The anterior pituitary is composed of multiple cell types, including somatotrophs (growth hormone), lactotrophs (prolactin), thyrotrophs (thyroid-stimulating hormone), and the gonadotrophs, which secrete FSH and LH. Gonadotrophs constitute approximately 15% of the anterior pituitary cells.

FSH is secreted during the early to mid-**follicular phase** of the menstrual cycle and is responsible for follicular development and induction of LH receptors on granulosa cells of the ovary. The primary function of LH is to bind to the theca cells of the ovary and stimulate the conversion of cholesterol to androgens, which then diffuse into the granulosa cell. The primary role of FSH is to bind to receptors on the granulosa cells of the ovary and stimulate the aromatization of the theca-derived androgens (testosterone and androstenedione) to estradiol.

OVARIES

The primary activities of the ovaries are the periodic release of oocytes and the production of estradiol and progesterone. These roles are integrated into the cyclic processes of follicle maturation, ovulation, corpus luteum formation, and corpus luteum regression. At 16–20 weeks of fetal life, the ovaries contain 6 million to 7 million **oogonia;** by birth, this number has declined to 1 million to 2 million. At the time of puberty, approximately 400,000 oocytes remain, and only a fraction of these undergo maturation and ovulation. Follicle-stimulating hormone stimulates follicular maturation within the ovary and then subsequently stimulates the production and secretion of estradiol from the granulosa cell. It also induces the expression of additional FSH receptors on the granulosa cells.[8]

Estradiol influences proliferation of the uterine endometrium in preparation for implantation of the fertilized oocyte. As endometrial proliferation occurs, the spiral arteries become progressively branched and coiled within the stromal layer. Following ovulation, the ruptured follicle develops into the corpus luteum. In response to low levels of LH, the granulosa cells of the corpus luteum produce both estradiol and progesterone.

Progesterone is secreted predominantly in the **luteal phase** of the menstrual cycle by the corpus luteum. Progesterone acts at the level of the hypothalamus to decrease the frequency of the GnRH pulse generator, which subsequently decreases the pulse frequency of LH. Levels of LH are highest immediately preceding the luteal phase because of less frequent, but higher amplitude, pulses of LH.[9]

In the ovary, the growth factor inhibin is secreted mainly by the granulosa cells. Inhibin functions to selectively inhibit FSH secretion from the anterior pituitary.[10-12] Another growth factor, activin, is also secreted from the granulosa cell. In contrast to inhibin, activin is also present in pituitary gonadotrophs.

The role of activin is less well understood, but it is thought to stimulate the secretion of FSH and also to increase the pituitary response to GnRH. The actions of activin are blocked by inhibin.[13,14]

THE ENDOMETRIUM

The endometrium is composed of glandular, vascular, and stromal components. Throughout the menstrual cycle, the endometrium undergoes a precisely coordinated series of events characterized by proliferation, secretion, degeneration, and regeneration. The upper two thirds of the endometrium, the functionalis layer, is the site of proliferative and secretory change in preparation for implantation. The lower one third of the endometrium, the basalis layer, provides the regenerative endometrium after menstrual shedding of the functionalis layer.[15]

The menstrual endometrium is composed of disordered glands, fragmented vessels, and stroma with evidence of necrosis and white cell infiltration. After the functionalis layer is shed, epithelial repair by underlying fibroblasts begins. By day 5–6 of the menstrual cycle, the entire uterine cavity is re-epithelialized, and stromal proliferation begins. The proliferative phase of the endometrium is stimulated by increased secretion of estradiol by maturing ovarian follicles. This estrogen-dominant phase is marked by extensive glandular and stromal growth within the functionalis layer. During this time, the endometrium grows from approximately 0.5 mm to 3.5–5.0 mm in height.[8]

Following ovulation, the endometrium is responsive to the effects of both estrogen and progesterone. During this secretory phase, endometrial growth continues for a few days after ovulation, and then further growth is inhibited through the activity of progesterone on the endometrium. Endometrial glands and vessels continue to proliferate within the confined functionalis layer, which results in increased tortuosity of glands and intensified coiling of the vessels. Glycoproteins, peptides, and immunoglobulins are secreted into the endometrial cavity in preparation for implantation of the blastocyst. In the absence of fertilization and implantation, the corpus luteum regresses, and estrogen and progesterone levels fall. The withdrawal of estrogen and progesterone stimulates vasospasm of the endometrial vessels, which leads to endometrial ischemia, stasis, and, finally, breakdown. The menstrual endometrium is then shed, and the process of endometrial proliferation starts again.

Phases of the Menstrual Cycle

FOLLICULAR PHASE

The follicular phase occurs during the first half of the menstrual cycle and usually spans 10–14 days. The first day of the follicular phase is marked by the onset of menstruation, and the phase ends with ovulation. During the first part of the follicular phase, the endometrium is sloughed as menstrual blood. Once the sloughing is complete, the process of endometrial proliferation begins. Growth of the endometrium during the follicular phase occurs in response to slowly increasing estradiol secretion from the maturing ovarian follicle.

During the follicular phase, FSH secretion increases, and numerous follicles undergo development, with usually one mature follicle proceeding to ovulation. The dominant follicle secretes estradiol, which stimulates further FSH and LH secretion from the pituitary. The follicular phase of the menstrual cycle is characterized by increased pulse frequency of LH, which leads to more frequent, but lower amplitude, pulses and lower LH levels overall. A surge of LH secretion at the end of the follicular phase provokes rupture of the dominant follicle and formation of the corpus luteum. Estradiol and progesterone levels are relatively low during the early follicular phase, but estradiol rises dramatically prior to ovulation.

LUTEAL PHASE

The luteal phase occurs during the second half of the menstrual cycle. This phase begins following ovulation and ends with menstruation. The corpus luteum develops from the ruptured follicle, and its secretion of progesterone results in the increased levels of progesterone during this phase. The corpus luteum also produces estradiol; however, levels are decreased relative to the follicular phase. The endometrium is described as secretory during this phase of the menstrual cycle because of its active secretion of glycoproteins and peptides into the endometrial cavity. Because of negative feedback mechanisms, FSH levels remain relatively low. In the luteal phase, the LH pulse frequency is of higher amplitude but lower frequency, which results in decreased LH levels overall. Although LH levels fall sharply after ovulation, the low levels are critical in maintaining the life of the newly formed corpus luteum. To persist beyond its 14-day lifespan, the corpus luteum requires a new source of the LH-like hormone human chorionic gonadotropin (HCG), which is produced from a successful implantation. In

Figure 10-1. Phases of the Menstrual Cycle

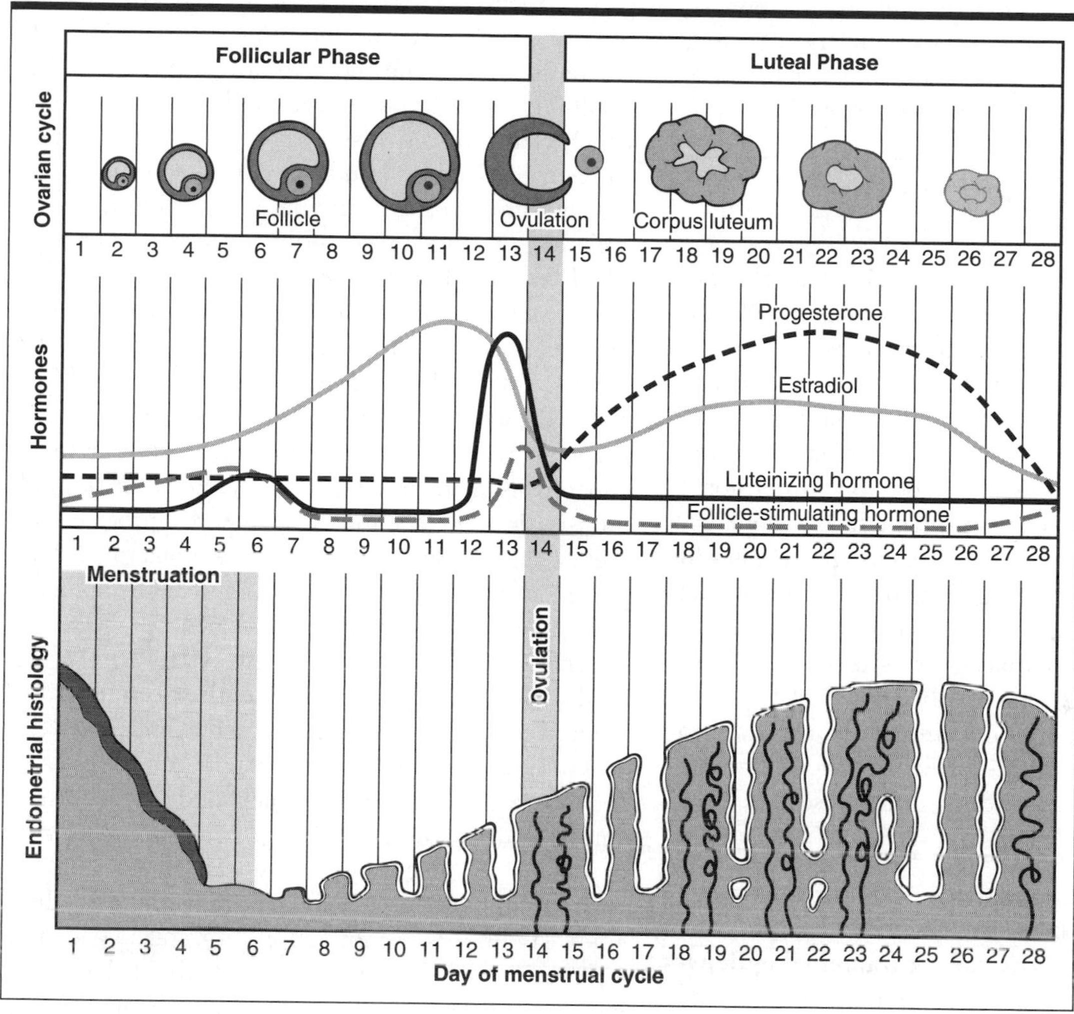

the absence of a continued source of LH, the corpus luteum rapidly regresses (Figure 10-1).[16]

The Menstrual Cycle as a Vital Sign

Throughout their menstrual life, teenage girls and women experience a variety of menstrual-related physical and psychological changes. These symptoms may represent normal ovulatory events or suggest underlying illness that can affect a woman's reproductive and general health. To this end, some propose that the menstrual cycle should be recorded as an additional vital sign in all menstruating female patients undergoing medical evaluation. In the same way that an elevated blood pressure may prompt a risk assessment for cardiovascular disease, an abnormal menstrual cycle should prompt the healthcare provider to evaluate the patient for underlying disease. The American College of Obstetricians and Gynecologists (ACOG) and the American Academy of Pediatrics (AAP) endorse the concept of the menstrual cycle as a vital sign. In 2007, the organizations released a joint committee statement suggesting that including the menstrual cycle as an additional vital sign reinforces its importance in assessing the overall health status of the female patient.[17]

Menarche is an important milestone in a young woman's development. Including the menstrual cycle as a vital sign allows healthcare providers to discuss normal female development and educate adolescent women and their parents about what constitutes a normal menstrual cycle. Menstrual cycles are typically irregular during adolescence, and young girls may be unaware of what represents a normal bleeding pattern. When the concept of the menstrual cycle as a vital sign is established early, young girls are better informed about the irregular menstrual patterns that are common in the first year of menstruation. Educating young girls about the normal menstrual cycle appears to relieve anxiety regarding pubertal development and to reduce negative expectations about this developmental milestone.[18,19]

Medical Conditions and the Menstrual Cycle

Sex-based differences in disease exist, and the exacerbation of certain medical conditions in relation to particular phases of the menstrual cycle is a well-documented phenomenon. Fluctuations in circulating ovarian hormones during ovulation and before menstruation may explain the menstrual-cycle related changes in some disorders. In addition to hormonal variations, theories to explain these effects include cyclic alterations in the immune system and changes in perception of disease brought about by premenstrual mood changes. Menstrual cycle–related changes in epilepsy, migraine, rheumatoid arthritis, diabetes, asthma, and PMS have also been described. As the latter conditions occur commonly in women, it is important to recognize these menstrual-related alterations that significantly affect women's health and disease.

EPILEPSY

Epilepsy can be particularly problematic for women because both the disease and its treatment can alter the menstrual cycle. The term **catamenial epilepsy** refers to seizures that occur more frequently around the time of menses. These seizures can occur just before or in the first few days of the menstrual cycle, and they have been reported in 10% to 72% of women with epilepsy.[20,21] The increased frequency of premenstrual seizures in some women results from the fluctuating levels of the ovarian steroid hormones during the menstrual cycle. In addition to their role in regulation of the menstrual cycle, progesterone and estradiol also demonstrate neuroactive properties. Progesterone is believed to depress seizure-related neurotransmitter activity in the brain. Estradiol increases neuronal metabolism and discharges and promotes the occurrence of seizures.[22,23] In general, catamenial epilepsy appears to result from a relative lack of progesterone, and the frequency of seizures is greatest when the estrogen/progesterone ratio is high. This ratio is highest in the days before ovulation and menstruation and lowest during the luteal phase. The LH pulse frequency has also been demonstrated to be increased or variable in some women with catamenial epilepsy.[22]

Anticonvulsant medications that induce the hepatic cytochrome P450 system increase the metabolism of ovarian steroid hormones and induce the synthesis of sex hormone–binding globulin. This results in lower levels of unbound steroid hormone, which can lead to ovulatory dysfunction and irregular menstrual cycles. Additionally, alterations in the metabolism of anticonvulsants during the menstrual cycle can produce lower serum drug concentrations, which may result in increased seizure frequency.[24,25]

A major factor in the occurrence of catamenial seizures is the relative progesterone deficiency during the luteal phase of the menstrual cycle. Many researchers have demonstrated improved control of perimenstrual epilepsy by adding progesterone to the anticonvulsant regimen during the luteal phase. Administration of intramuscular medroxyprogesterone acetate and vaginal progesterone suppositories have proven to be effective in reducing seizure frequency in some women with established progesterone deficiency.[26-29] Use of the selective estrogen receptor modulator clomiphene citrate has also been described as an effective treatment of catamenial epilepsy.[30]

Optimal treatment of epilepsy requires choosing the most effective anticonvulsant medication for seizure type, increasing the dosage for maximum effect or until side effects become unacceptable, and exhausting monotherapy before adding additional therapies. Traditional monotherapies for epilepsy include phenytoin, carbamazepine, phenobarbital, lamotrigine, and valproic acid. If seizures persist on conventional therapy, then an association with the menstrual cycle should be explored. Catamenial epilepsy can be demonstrated through the association of seizures with the menstrual cycle on a menstrual calendar. A low serum progesterone level in the midluteal phase (days 20–22 of a 28-day cycle) suggests a progesterone deficiency and that progesterone supplementation may be useful. Intramuscular medroxyprogesterone 150 mg every 12 weeks or oral medroxyprogesterone 10 mg daily days 10–26 of the menstrual cycle may be prescribed; however, its tolerability may be limited

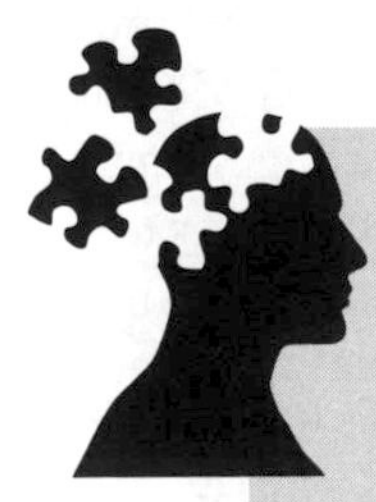

Therapeutic Challenge:

What is the effect of long-term medroxyprogesterone therapy on bone mineral density? Is the effect reversible?

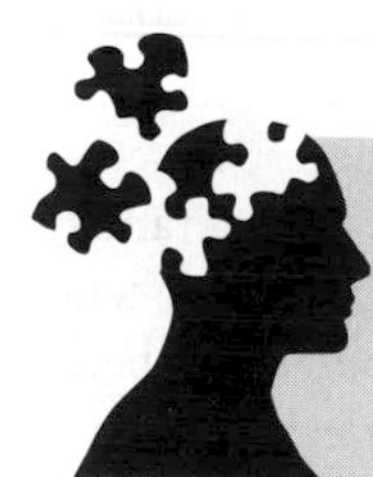

Therapeutic Challenge:

Would a transdermal hormonal contraceptive be a good choice for a woman taking anticonvulsant drugs?

by side effects of hot flashes, irregular bleeding, cessation of menses, and breast tenderness.[24,26] Alternatively, intermittent clobazam or acetazolamide during the perimenstrual period has been suggested.[31,32] The effectiveness of estrogen- and progesterone-containing contraceptives can be affected by anticonvulsant drugs through induction of cytochrome p450 enzyme metabolism. Lower concentrations of estrogens and unbound progesterone are reported in women taking anticonvulsant therapy; therefore, caution should be used in prescribing these medications, and nonhormonal contraceptives should be considered.

MENSTRUAL MIGRAINE

Migraine is a neurologic disorder that affects at least 10% of the general population.[33,34] The frequency of migraine headaches increases after menarche, and they are 2–3 times more common in women than in men. In population-based studies, 50% of women report an association between migraine headaches and the menstrual cycle.[35,36] True menstrual migraines occur in 8% to 14% of women, who experience migraine attacks only at the time of menstruation and are relatively free of migraine at other times during the menstrual cycle.[37-39] The International Headache Society defines menstrual migraine as migraine headache without aura occurring from 2 days before menstruation through the third day of menstrual bleeding in two of three consecutive menstrual cycles. Women must also demonstrate either 1) nausea and/or vomiting or 2) **photophobia** and **phonophobia** at the time of the headache to meet the criteria of menstrual migraine.[40]

The symptoms of migraine occur when a stimulus triggers abnormal neurologic activity in the brainstem. Serotonergic neurons are presumed to be affected in this process, and selective serotonin receptor agonists are effective in prevention and treatment of migraines. Many trigger factors of migraine headache have been described, including stress, sleep disturbance, diet, and hormonal fluctuations.[41] For those women suffering from menstrual migraine, the effect of estrogen withdrawal in the late luteal/early follicular phase of the menstrual cycle plays a significant role in the pathophysiology of this disorder.[42,43] This concept has been supported by delay in migraine attack with premenstrual estrogen supplementation in women with severe menstrual migraine.[40] The role of estrogen withdrawal in migraines has also been demonstrated in women taking oral contraceptive pills (OCPs), as the estrogen withdrawal during the placebo week of OCPs has been associated with increased migraine headaches in some women.[44]

Menstrual migraines typically develop around the onset of menarche, have peak prevalence around age 40, and then decline corresponding to menopause.[45,46] Recent studies support the clinical observation that menstrual migraines are more severe, last longer, and are less responsive to acute and prophylactic treatment than migraines occurring at other times.[39,47] The first step in the treatment of menstrual migraine is to have the woman keep a headache diary for 3 months to establish that there is a correlation between the occurrence of headaches and the menstrual cycle. Once this correlation is determined, nonpharmacologic therapies—such as avoidance of triggers, regular exercise, and biofeedback—are effective treatment options. Regarding pharmacologic options, the triptans have shown clear benefit in the treatment of classic and menstrual migraines and are considered first line for pharmacologic therapy. Initiation of sumatriptan 2 days before menses and continued for 5–6 days is an effective treatment strategy, as are other triptans.[37,40] Estrogen supplementation in the luteal phase has also proven beneficial, but the side effects associated with these medications preclude them from being used more broadly.[49,50] Estrogens are available in oral, injectable, and transdermal preparations. Hormonal prophylaxis with daily oral contraceptive use is an effective therapy in women with no contraindications to estrogen therapy.[37] Investigators have also shown soy-based phytoestrogens to be effective prophylaxis for menstrual migraine attacks.[51,52] Antiemetics and nonsteroidal anti-inflammatory drugs may be added to the treatment regimen for difficult-to-control attacks.

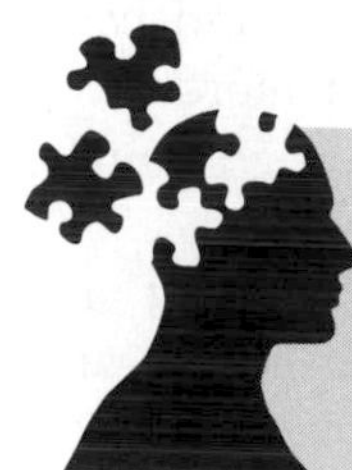

Therapeutic Challenge:

How do soy-based phytoestrogens differ from synthetic estrogens? Is one better than the other?

RHEUMATOID ARTHRITIS

Rheumatoid arthritis (RA) is an autoimmune disorder characterized by chronic inflammation of the joints. Its clinical presentation involves intermittent flares and remissions, often related to morning stiffness and pain. The symptoms of RA are affected by various inflammatory mediators, and the anti-inflammatory actions of both estrogen and progesterone have been linked with the fluctuations in the symptoms of RA.[53,54] In the postovulatory phase of the menstrual cycle, serum concentrations of estrogen and progesterone are increased. Several investigators have described a reduction in symptoms of RA during this phase of the menstrual cycle.[55] This concept is further supported by reports showing a relief of RA symptoms in some women taking progesterone- and estrogen-containing oral contraceptive pills.[56] Some women with RA report an increase in morning stiffness and arthritis pain during the early follicular phase of the menstrual cycle, when estrogen and progesterone levels are relatively low. There have also been reports of a decreased grip strength and increased finger-joint size during the first few days of menstruation, which suggests that low estrogen levels may cause symptom flares in some women with RA.[57] Several investigators have studied estrogen as adjuvant therapy in the treatment of RA; however, their findings have been inconsistent with regard to benefit. In light of conflicting results regarding estrogen and progesterone treatment, only conventional therapies for RA are recommended. For treating practitioners and patients with RA, knowledge of these menstrual-related exacerbations of RA may relieve anxiety regarding the worsening of RA symptoms during menstruation.

DIABETES

A relationship between the menstrual cycle and insulin sensitivity has been described. Some investigators have reported impaired insulin sensitivity in healthy nondiabetic women during the luteal phase of the menstrual cycle.[58] Worsening glycemic control in the luteal phase has been described in women with insulin-dependent diabetes mellitus as well.[59,60] In addition, diabetic ketoacidosis and hypoglycemia have been reported to occur more frequently around the time of menstruation for some women.[61]

The mechanism of the menstrual cycle's effect on glycemic control in women with diabetes is unclear, and findings of poor premenstrual glycemic control in this population are inconsistent.[62] Investigators have attempted to show a correlation between estrogen and progesterone levels and worsening glycemic control; however, this relationship has not been consistently described. Researchers have described worsening glycemic control, paired with elevated estradiol levels, in a small group of women with diabetes, but this finding has not been reproduced.[58] A subgroup of women with insulin-dependent diabetes also report symptoms of PMS, and some investigators have suggested that the food cravings and eating behaviors associated with the PMS may lead to altered diet and hyperglycemia in select patients with diabetes.[62] Although the mechanism of altered glycemic control for some women with diabetes is not well understood, studies of this population suggest that blood glucose management during the luteal phase may warrant closer surveillance than at other times in the menstrual cycle.

Oral hypoglycemic agents and insulin remain the first-line pharmacologic treatments for women with diabetes, but other menstrual-related therapies have also been proposed. Pituitary and ovarian suppression with monthly depot leuprolide acetate 3.75 mg is recommended for women with recurrent life-threatening complications of diabetes, such as cycle-related diabetic ketoacidosis or severe insulin reactions. This treatment should be combined with add-back therapy in the form of conjugated estrogen 0.625 mg/day or oral medroxyprogesterone acetate 2.5 mg/day. Oral contraceptive use in women with diabetes has been associated with impaired glycemic control, and these medications should be used with caution in this population.[63]

ASTHMA

Asthma is a significant chronic respiratory illness in the U.S., which carries considerable morbidity and mortality for affected individuals. In children, the disease is more common in boys, but then becomes more common in girls after puberty. Population-based studies show that rates of hospital admissions for asthma are similar in boys and girls through the teenage years, and then rates become 3 times higher in women than men between ages 20 and 50.[64-66] Premenstrual asthma is estimated to affect up to 40% of women with asthma. After menopause, the incidence of asthma in women falls and matches that of men.[67]

Investigators have hypothesized that fluctuations in sex hormones during the menstrual cycle play a role in the pathophysiology of asthma and lead to periodic worsening of disease severity in women.

This is supported by reports of asthma exacerbations in women in which up to 50% of emergency department visits have occurred during the perimenstrual phase of the menstrual cycle.[68] Further, many women with asthma report worsening asthma symptoms before menstruation, and this premenstrual deterioration in asthma symptoms has been confirmed by decreased peak expiratory flow measurements in women with asthma.[69]

Alhough sex hormones are believed to play a role in premenstrual asthma, the exact mechanism remains unclear. Progesterone levels are relatively high in the luteal phase, and one proposed mechanism is that progesterone reduces the contractility of smooth muscle, producing cyclic changes in airway responsiveness in women with premenstrual asthma. Progesterone-related hyperventilation may contribute to symptomatic deterioration and dyspnea as well. Estradiol is also believed to alter pulmonary function, although its mechanism of action is not well understood.[70] Because of the lack of definitive support for a hormonal cause of premenstrual asthma, some have suggested that premenstrual asthma exacerbations are due to heightened perception of asthma symptoms during the premenstrual period.

Anecdotal treatments of premenstrual asthma with intramuscular progesterone, OCPs, and GnRH analogs have been reported.[71-73] Oral administration of estradiol 2 mg daily during the premenstrual period is an effective treatment for severe premenstrual asthma. Mild, well-controlled premenstrual asthma does not appear to respond to oral estradiol therapy.[74,75] Corticosteroids and beta-adrenergic agonists remain first-line therapy for the treatment of premenstrual asthma.

Guidelines/Position Statement

In the opinion of both ACOG and AAP, the menstrual cycle is an important indicator of wellness, and it should be used as an additional vital sign in reproductive-aged women.[17]

Summary

From menarche to menopause, the menstrual cycle is characterized by diverse physiological, psychological, and physical changes in women. The detailed processes of folliculogenesis, ovulation, and menstruation rely on the coordinated interaction of the sex hormones with the hypothalamus, pituitary, ovary, and uterus. The stimulatory and inhibitory effects

CASE PRESENTATION

Patient Case: Part 2

D.M. is experiencing perimenstrual worsening of her epilepsy. On exam, she has evidence of prolonged phenytoin therapy with hirsutism and gingival hypertrophy. She is on a relatively low dosage, and her phenytoin level is low normal (therapeutic range: 10–20 mcg/mL).

Recommendation:

1) Increase phenytoin to improve control of seizures (recommended dosage 4–7 mg/kg/day). Repeat phenytoin level 4 weeks after dosage increase, and check complete blood count every 4–12 months.
2) Counsel D.M. regarding pregnancy and sexually transmitted disease (STD) prevention. Prescribe depo-medroxyprogesterone 150 mg intramuscularly every 3 months for contraception. Continue condom use for STD prevention.

Rationale: D.M. is on a starting dosage of phenytoin, which has not been adjusted since her seizure disorder was diagnosed. Her seizures may be better controlled with an increased dosage of this medication, and she should be monitored to ensure that her phenytoin levels are within the therapeutic range. Common side effects of phenytoin therapy are hirsutism and gingival hypertrophy. A serious but less common side effect is low blood counts; thus, D.M. should have complete blood count evaluation to screen for this complication of therapy. Alternatively, she could be switched to a newer treatment—such as lamotrigine, oxcarbazepine, or topiramate—that has demonstrated efficacy as monotherapy for patients with persistent seizures or side effects on other anticonvulsant medications.

Regarding contraception, the progestin-only depot medroxyprogesterone is an excellent option for D.M. because of its ease of use and limited interaction with her phenytoin therapy. Estrogens may increase phenytoin levels; therefore estrogen-containing contraceptives (oral or transdermal preparations) may not be a good option for her. Alternatively, phenytoin therapy can decrease the efficacy of estrogen-containing contraceptives.[24] Evaluation of a young, sexually active woman should always include assessment for high-risk sexual behavior, screening for STD, and counseling regarding pregnancy and STD prevention. Anticonvulsant medications can be continued during pregnancy if necessary for the control of persistent seizure activity. Lamotrigine, carbamazepine, phenytoin, and oxcarbazepine are all therapeutic options; however, drug levels should be monitored because of alterations in clearance and concentrations of these medications during pregnancy. Congenital malformations also have been reported in association with some anticonvulsant medications, so an assessment of risks and benefits is in order before a therapy is chosen.

of the pituitary and ovarian hormones are evident at every level of the hypothalamic–pituitary–ovarian axis. The effects of these hormones are also demonstrated in the cyclic worsening of certain medical conditions during the follicular or luteal phases of the menstrual cycle. The menstrual cycle is a critical vital sign for adolescent girls and women, and it plays a central role in women's wellness and disease. Women should be educated early about the importance of the menstrual cycle as an indicator of overall health and about its effect on other diseases. The impact of the menstrual cycle on diseases such as epilepsy, diabetes, migraines, rheumatoid arthritis, and asthma must be considered when managing these conditions in the reproductive-aged woman.

References

Additional content available at
www.ashp.org/womenshealth

11 Menstruation Disorders

Somjate Manipalviratn, MD; Alicia Armstrong, MD, MHSCR

Learning Objectives

1. To understand pathophysiology of menstrual disorders.
2. To understand clinical presentation of common menstrual disorders.
3. To understand basic investigation in women with menstrual disorders.
4. To understand roles of common pharmacologic and nonpharmacologic management of women with menstrual disorders.
5. To understand pharmacodynamics and pharmacokinetics of common drugs used for treatment of menstrual disorders.
6. To understand medical management of women with menstrual disorders.

Menstrual disorders, particularly abnormal uterine bleeding, are extremely common gynecologic disorders. Abnormal uterine bleeding is responsible for 20% of gynecologic visits. It is estimated that 30% of women will report heavy menses or menorrhagia each year.[1,2] Although the prevalence of absence or cessation of menses (amenorrhea) is as high as 14%, after excluding pregnancy, lactation, and menopause, the prevalence of amenorrhea is approximately 3% to 4%.[3,4] In contrast, the prevalence of infrequent menses (oligomenorrhea) is as high as 11% in adolescence.[4] Menstrual disorders such as heavy and irregular menses are clinically important because they are the indication for two thirds of hysterectomies and nearly 25% of gynecologic operations.[1,2]

Menstrual disorders are most prevalent during the early reproductive years (perimenarche) and in women older than age 45 (perimenopause). Problems with the menstrual cycle are the leading reason for doctor visits by teenagers. As many as 75% of perimenarchal adolescents may experience abnormalities in their menstrual cycles, which may include the unexpected cessation of their menses (amenorrhea) or changes in the timing, amount, and duration of their menses.[5] Menstrual irregularities in adolescence are thought to be the result of slow maturation of the hypothalamic–pituitary–ovarian axis and can last 2–5 years after menarche.[6] Menstrual abnormalities are equally common in perimenopause. Nearly 75% of gynecologic consultations that occur in perimenopausal and postmenopausal women are due to abnormal uterine bleeding.[7]

Menstrual disorders are generally viewed as disorders of regularity, duration, frequency, and amount of menstrual blood flow. Abnormal menses are typically described using terminologies in the glossary (Table 11-1). This chapter will focus on the three common menstrual disorders: amenorrhea, oligomenorrhea, and menorrhagia.

Table 11-1. Terminologies of Abnormal Menstrual Blood Flow

Type of Abnormal Menstrual Blood Flow	Definition
Amenorrhea	Absence of menstrual bleeding
Oligomenorrhea	Menstrual cycle interval >35 days
Polymenorrhea	Menstrual cycle interval <24 days
Menorrhagia	Regular menstrual bleeding with blood loss >80 mL per cycle or prolonged menstrual bleeding >7 days
Metrorrhagia	Irregular menstrual bleeding
Menometrorrhagia	Heavy menstrual bleeding occurring at irregular intervals

Case Presentation

Patient Case: Part 1

HPI: A 28-year-old white female patient presents with a chief symptom of heavy menses. Patient reports that for the last 3 months, menses have become heavier, with several episodes of soiling clothing. Previously, she reports a moderate flow, with the heaviest days on day 1 and 2 and a total duration of 5–6 days. She previously used four to five tampons/day. Currently, her menses are consistently lasting 7 days and recurring every 28 days. She reports that days 1–3 are heavy and require seven to eight tampons per day. She reports that in addition to having a "heavy flow," she also passes clots that are comparable in size to a silver dollar. She denies any severe abdominal cramping, change in bowel or bladder habits, or nausea or vomiting associated with menses. She reports increased fatigue and intermittent lightheadedness for the past 2–3 weeks.

Obstetric history: Two pregnancies, one full-term delivery, and one spontaneous miscarriage. She had one full-term delivered naturally at 37 weeks productive of 6-lb, 7-oz boy. Her pregnancy was uncomplicated.

Gynecologic history: She reports menarche at 12 years of age. Last menstrual period (LMP) occurred 1 week before presentation. Menses are regular, lasting 7 days and recurring every 28 days. The patient is sexually active with her husband. Her Pap tests are up to date. She has a history of one abnormal Pap of low-grade squamous intraepithelial lesion (LGSIL), a precancerous lesion, in 2003 that resolved spontaneously. No history of other sexually transmitted diseases. She reports four lifetime partners. She is currently using barrier devices for contraception.

Past medical history: Exercise-induced asthma and seasonal allergies.

Past surgical history: Tonsillectomy at 3 years of age.

Social history: Patient has been an elementary school teacher for past 2 years. Married for 3 years. Reports smoking three to five cigarettes/day. She drinks one glass of wine/month. She denies any illicit drug use.

Family history: No family history of bleeding disorders or irregular menses.

Medications: Allegra, multivitamin, and albuterol as needed.

Allergies: No known drug allergies.

Review of systems: The patient reports fatigue and lightheadedness for 4–5 weeks. She denies any temperature intolerance or recent weight loss or gain. She denies any unusual life stressors.

Physical examination:

Vitals: Temp 98.7°F; RR 12/min; BP (supine128/68 mm Hg, standing 120/62 mm Hg); HR (supine 78 beats/min, standing 83 beats/min).

Body mass index: 30 kg/m^2.

General: Well developed, well nourished, and appears her stated age.

HEENT: Pupils equally round and reactive to light, extraocular movements intact, pale conjunctiva.

Cardiovascular: Regular rate and rhythm with normal S1/S2 heart sounds and no murmurs, rubs, or gallops.

Pulmonary: Clear to auscultation bilaterally, no rhonchi, wheezing, or crackles.

Abdomen: Mildly obese, soft, nontender, nondistended, bowel sounds present.

Extremities: No clubbing, cyanosis, or edema.

Speculum exam: Vaginal vault with minimal physiologic discharge, normal appearance of vaginal wall. Cervix looks normal. Squamocolumnar junction (the region in the uterine cervix in which the squamous lining of the vagina is replaced by the columnar epithelium typical of the body of the uterus and which is a common site of neoplastic change) appears smooth, with no obvious areas of friability.

Bimanual exam: Small, regular, nontender, anteverted uterus with no adnexal fullness or tenderness. No cervical motion tenderness.

Laboratory values:

Wet prep: Negative for infection.

Gonorrhea/chlamydia probe: Negative.

Urine ß-hCG (pregnancy test): Negative.

Complete blood count (CBC): White blood cell (WBC) 8,300/mm^3 (normal 4,500–10,000 cells/mm^3); hemoglobin (Hgb) 9 g/dL (normal 12–15 g/dL); hematocrit (Hct) 28% (normal 36–44%; platelets (Plt) 285,000/mm^3 (normal 100,000≠450,000/mm^3); thyroid-stimulating hormone (TSH) 2.86 milliunits/L (normal 0.25–4.30 milliunits/mL).

Serum iron studies: Serum iron (Fe) 38 mcg/dL (normal 65–150 mcg/dL); ferritin 15 ng/dL (normal 3–300 ng/dL; total iron binding capacity (TIBC) 615 mcg/dL (normal 250–420 mcg/dL).

Pap test: Adequate sample. No abnormal cells detected. No evidence of precancerous or cancerous lesions.

Imaging: Transvaginal ultrasound—the uterus measures 8.2 x 4.1 x 6.1 cm. No focal deformities/irregularities of the uterus are noted. The uterine echo texture is homogenous. Endometrium is triple layer in appearance with a thickness of 6 mm. The left ovary measures 2.1 x 1.4 x 1.9 cm. The right ovary measures 1.8 x 3.0 x 2.1 cm. Several small follicles are seen bilaterally. Both ovaries do not have polycystic appearance. There are no adnexal masses.

Assessment: 28-year-old woman with regular, excessive menstrual bleeding and anemia secondary to iron deficiency.

Pathophysiology

AMENORRHEA

Amenorrhea is the absence or abnormal cessation of menses. Primary amenorrhea is defined as having no menstrual bleeding by the age of 16 in the presence of normal growth and development of secondary sexual characteristics or by the age of 14 in the absence of growth and development of secondary sexual characteristics.[8] Secondary amenorrhea is defined as the absence of periods for a length of time equivalent to a total of at least three of the previous cycle intervals or 6 months of amenorrhea in women who have been menstruating.[8] Nevertheless, the clinical approach of women with either primary or secondary amenorrhea is similar.

Physiology of normal menstruation is described in detail in Chapter 10: Menstrual Cycle. Briefly, the presence of normal menstruation depends on normal hormonal control from the ovary, which is under the control of anterior pituitary, hypothalamus, and central nervous system. An endometrium that is responsive to ovarian hormonal input is necessary for cyclic menses. The outflow tract (uterus and vagina) must be patent to allow menstrual blood flow. Basic physiologic control of normal menstruation is divided into four compartments: 1) uterus and outflow tract, 2) ovary, 3) anterior pituitary gland, and 4) hypothalamus and central nervous system. Disruption in any one of the four compartments can result in amenorrhea (Table 11-2).

Compartment I: Disorders of Uterus and Outflow Tract

The uterus, specifically the endometrium, is the end organ that responds to hormonal changes resulting in cyclic withdrawal bleeding. Any abnormalities of uterus, endometrium, or the outflow tract can cause

Table 11-2. Common Causes of Amenorrhea Classified by Compartments

	Diseases
Compartment I: Disorders of uterus and outflow tract	• Asherman's syndrome • Müllerian anomalies • Müllerian agenesis • Androgen insensitivity syndrome
Compartment II: Disorders of ovary	• Primary ovarian insufficiency (natural vs. iatrogenic) • Resistant ovary syndrome • Turner's syndrome • Gonadal dysgenesis • Gonadal agenesis
Compartment III: Disorders of anterior pituitary gland	• Hyperprolactinemia • Pituitary adenoma (functioning vs. nonfunctioning) • Empty sella syndrome • Sheehan's syndrome
Compartment IV: Disorders of hypothalamus and central nervous system	• Dysfunctional hypothalamic amenorrhea (stress, exercise induced, nutritional related, psuedocyesis) • Kallmann syndrome • Idiopathic hypogonadotropic hypogonadism

amenorrhea. Müllerian agenesis, the absence of internal genital organs that are derived from the müllerian duct in embryo, is a relatively common cause of primary amenorrhea. Women with this disorder usually have an absence of the uterus, fallopian tubes, and upper vagina. However, they have normal functional ovaries and have a normal 46,XX karyotype. The exact cause of müllerian agenesis is unknown; however, the likely causes are mutations of the gene for antimüllerian hormone or the gene for antimüllerian hormone receptor.[8] Müllerian agenesis is frequently associated with urologic and skeletal abnormalities.

Like müllerian agenesis, androgen insensitivity syndrome causes amenorrhea in women because of the absence of internal genital organs. Women with androgen insensitivity have a normal male karyotype, 46,XY. They are phenotypically female but have male gonads that produce testosterone and antimüllerian hormone. The development of müllerian ducts in the embryo is inhibited by antimüllerian hormone, resulting in the absence of female internal genital organs. Because they do not respond to androgens, they have female external genitalia and a normal female phenotype.

There are various abnormalities of müllerian duct development that can cause an obstruction of the outflow tract which results in amenorrhea, although regular cyclic shedding of the endometrium occurs. Such anomalies include imperforate hymen, transverse vaginal septum, cervical agenesis, and vaginal agenesis. By having cyclic endometrial shedding and blood accumulated above the site of obstruction, these women usually have cyclic abdominal pain. Other causes of obstruction of the outflow tract include trauma to the genital organs, such as cervical stenosis.

Lack of a functional endometrium will result in amenorrhea. Congenital absence or hypoplasia of the endometrium is rare. Destruction of functional endometrium that is due to aggressive uterine curettage is more common. Intrauterine adhesions, or **Asherman's syndrome,** can partially or completely obliterate the endometrial cavity, resulting in decreased menstrual blood flow or amenorrhea. In addition to curettage, any surgery involving the uterine cavity can cause Asherman's syndrome. Although rare, infection of the endometrium can impair endometrial function, resulting in amenorrhea.

Compartment II: Disorders of Ovary

The ovary is the source of estrogen and progesterone that controls the cyclic changes of the endometrium. Absence of ovarian function can result in either primary or secondary amenorrhea. Amenorrhea from the absence of ovarian function is often classified as hypergonadotropic hypogonadism: high follicle-stimulating hormone (FSH), and luteinizing hormone (LH), but low estradiol levels. Primary ovarian insufficiency—loss of ovarian function before the age of 40—is a common disorder of the ovary leading to amenorrhea. There is an early depletion of ovarian follicles in women with primary ovarian insufficiency.[9] Besides iatrogenic causes such as radiation and chemotherapy, the etiology of most cases of primary ovarian insufficiency is unknown. Some chromosomal abnormalities can cause primary ovarian insufficiency, most commonly 45 XO, 47 XXY, and **mosaicism.** Two functioning X chromosomes appear to be necessary for normal ovarian function.[10] Autoimmune inflammation and infections such as mumps oophoritis can also cause primary ovarian insufficiency.

Gonadal dysgenesis is a condition of abnormal development of the gonad presenting as streaks of connective tissue without germ cells. This can occur with normal XX and XY karyotypes (pure gonadal dysgenesis) and a variety of abnormal karyotypes, most commonly **Turner's syndrome** and mosaicism. The cause is unclear; either germ cells do not form, do not interact normally with the gonadal ridge, or undergo accelerated atresia. Gonadal agenesis is even more uncommon. The cause of gonadal agenesis is not known but could be the result of a viral or metabolic alteration in early gestation that resulted in agenesis of the gonads. The resistant ovary syndrome is a rare condition in which patients present like ovarian failure, having hypergonadotropic amenorrhea, but ovarian follicles are present without autoimmune inflammation. This could be viewed as a category of primary ovarian insufficiency.

Compartment III: Disorders of Anterior Pituitary Gland

The anterior pituitary gland is the source of trophic hormones that stimulate other endocrine glands. Gonadotropin (FSH and LH) and prolactin are major hormones from the anterior pituitary gland that play roles in menstrual control. FSH and LH control ovarian follicular growth and ovulation, respectively. Without follicular growth and ovulation, menstruation does not occur. Disorders that impair the function of gonadotropes (cells in the anterior pituitary gland that produce and secrete FSH and LH) can cause amenorrhea. Adenomas of the pituitary gland, lymphocytic hypophysitis, **Sheehan's syndrome,** and surgery or radiation of pituitary gland can destroy gonadotropes, leading to amenorrhea.

Increased levels of prolactin or hyperprolactinemia cause menstrual abnormalities by inhibiting pulsatile gonadotropin-releasing hormone (GnRH) secretion from the hypothalamus. Hyperprolactinemia can be caused by a prolactin-producing pituitary adenoma or hyperplasia of the lactotrophs. As prolactin is under the negative control of dopamine from hypothalamus, any tumor that compresses the pituitary stalk will remove this negative control of prolactin, resulting in a rise in prolactin level. In addition to disorders of the pituitary gland, hypothyroidism can also cause amenorrhea by stimulating prolactin production as a result of thyrotropin-releasing hormone stimulation of the lactotrophs. The degree of menstrual pattern alteration correlates with prolactin level. Prolactin levels are highest in women with amenorrhea compared to those with oligomenorrhea and normal menstrual cycles.[11,12]

Compartment IV: Disorders of Hypothalamus and Central Nervous System

Gonadotropin-releasing hormone is synthesized and released from the hypothalamus in a pulsatile fashion to control the release of FSH and LH in the pituitary gland. A deficiency in GnRH pulsatile secretion causes a hypogonadotropic hypogonadal state (low FSH and LH and low estrogen), resulting in anovulation. The degree of alteration in hypothalamic function determines the degree of menstrual patterns abnormalities, from no change of menstrual cycle to oligomenorrhea and amenorrhea in women with profound suppression of hypothalamic function. As the hypothalamus is a part of central nervous system, inputs from the brain have an influence on its function. Psychological stress, weight changes, poor nutritional status, and excessive exercise can cause functional suppression of the hypothalamus. The pathophysiologic mechanism of functional hypothalamic suppression is unclear. It is postulated that alteration in corticotropin-releasing hormone, endogenous opioid, and dopamine released in response to stress results in the pathophysiology of hypothalamic amenorrhea.[8] Neuropeptide Y, which is secreted from the arcuate nucleus in the hypothalamus, may be the link between the nutritional status and gonadal function.[13] Neuropeptide Y stimulates eating behavior and inhibits gonadotropin secretion, presumably by suppression of GnRH pulses. In a starvation state, neuropeptide Y level increases dramatically, which in turn could suppress GnRH secretion.[13] Neuropeptide Y level has been shown to be elevated in the cerebrospinal fluid of anorexic women.[14]

Kallmann syndrome is a congenital hypothalamic hypogonadotropic hypogonadism that is usually associated with a diminished sense of smell or inability to smell, anosmia, or hyposmia. In the embryo, GnRH neurons and olfactory neurons develop from the same area: the olfactory placode. The failure of these cells to penetrate the forebrain prevents successful migration of GnRH neurons to hypothalamus. This syndrome is caused by an X-linked mutation or deletion of KAL gene on the short arm of the X chromosome that encodes a protein responsible for neuronal migration.[8] These women present with primary amenorrhea, lack of secondary sexual characteristics, and anosmia.

OLIGOMENORRHEA

Oligomenorrhea is infrequent menstruation characterized by having a menstrual cycle interval longer than 35 days. Oligomenorrhea is caused by dysfunction of hypothalamic–pituitary–ovarian axis. Oligomenorrhea and amenorrhea can be viewed as a spectrum of clinical presentations resulting from anovulation. All the disturbances to hypothalamic–pituitary–ovarian axis described in the amenorrhea section; if they are not critical enough to cause amenorrhea, they can result in oligomenorrhea. Generally, in women with oligomenorrhea, periods are mostly light but of variable duration. However, these infrequent periods can be occasionally heavy. The most common cause of prolonged menstrual interval is anovulation. In normal ovulatory women, after ovulation, the dominant ovarian follicle becomes a corpus luteum, which predominantly produces progesterone lasting for 14 days. Regression of the corpus luteum is the key for cyclic endometrial withdrawal bleeding. Progesterone acts on the endometrium to oppose the stimulatory effect of estrogen and stabilize the endometrium. In anovulatory women, there is no progesterone to oppose the stimulatory effect of estrogen, creating an unstable endometrial lining that eventually breaks down and sloughs at an unpredictable time, not in a cyclic fashion. Prolonged unopposed estrogen stimulation of endometrium can cause endometrial hyperplasia or cancer. In anovulatory cycles, estrogen levels can be either high or low. With chronic high levels, there is infrequent heavy bleeding, whereas chronically low levels may result in prolonged light bleeding. Anovulation can be physiologic during the early reproductive years (perimenarche) and the late reproductive years (perimenopause).

Oligomenorrhea is the most common menstrual abnormality in women with hyperthyroidism. Almost 60% of women with hyperthyroidism reported oligomenorrhea or amenorrhea.[15] Menstrual abnormalities may precede thyroid dysfunction. Thyrotoxic women frequently present with increased LH, FSH, and estrogen levels and have an increased gonadotropin response to GnRH.[16] However, the midcycle LH peak is reduced or absent, resulting in anovulation.[16]

Polycystic ovary syndrome is the most common cause of oligomenorrhea. More than 75% of oligomenorrheic women are diagnosed with polycystic ovary syndrome. Women with polycystic ovary syndrome can present with any type of menstrual patterns: normal menstruation, oligomenorrhea, amenorrhea, metrorrhagia, menorrhagia, or menometrorrhagia. The pathophysiology of polycystic ovary syndrome is complex, involving many endocrine systems. (See Chapter 16: Polycystic Ovary Syndrome.)

MENORRHAGIA

Menorrhagia is the term used to describe menstrual disorders characterized by regular bleeding with blood loss >80 mL per cycle or prolonged menstrual bleeding >7 days. Many conditions can be associated with menorrhagia: pelvic pathology (uterine myoma, adenomyosis [endometrial glands located in the muscle of the uterus that cause pain and abnormal bleeding], endometrial polyps, endometrial carcinoma); foreign bodies, such as intrauterine device (IUD); systemic diseases (coagulopathy, hypothyroidism); and dysfunctional uterine bleeding (DUB). This chapter will focus on DUB: excessive bleeding of uterine origin that is not due to pelvic pathology, systemic diseases, or complications of pregnancy. Dysfunctional uterine bleeding is a diagnosis of exclusion. The underlying mechanism of menorrhagia is complex, involving dysregulation of expression and signaling process of various local mediators within the endometrium. As 75% of menstrual blood loss is arteriolar, it is assumed that vascular constriction is responsible for controlling menstrual blood loss. Hemostasis and endometrial regeneration are important to limit the volume of blood loss during menstruation. Vasodilators, vasoconstrictors, and vasculogenic factors (such as **prostaglandins**, matrix metalloproteinases [MMPs] and **vascular endothelial growth factor [VEGF]**) are implicated in the pathogenesis of menorrhagia.

Thromboxane A_2 (TXA_2) and prostacycline (PGI_2) are prostaglandins synthesized by metabolism of arachidonic acid through the cyclo-oxygenase pathway. The balance between these two prostaglandins is critical for maintaining homeostasis.[17] TXA_2 is primarily synthesized in platelets and promotes platelet aggregation and vasoconstriction while PGI_2 is mainly produced in vascular endothelial cells causing vasodilation and inhibition of platelet aggregation.[17] The imbalance between TXA_2 and PGI_2 causes menorrhagia. Endometrial prostaglandin release is greatly influenced by circulating steroid levels. The endometrium from women with menorrhagia has an enhanced synthesis of PGI_2 from arachidonic acid compared with endometrium from normally menstruating women.[18] Ratio of TXA_2:PGI_2 metabolites in endometrium is reduced in patients with menorrhagia.[19] Moreover, there is an increase in prostaglandin E_2 (PGE_2)and PGI_2 receptors, predisposing to vasodilatation in women with menorrhagia.[20]

Matrix metalloproteinases, protease enzymes capable of degrading many kinds of extracellular matrix proteins, play a major role in cell proliferation, migration, differentiation, and angiogenesis during tissue breakdown and remodeling process. Matrix metalloproteinase-2 and MMP-9 are expressed in endometrial blood vessels. Levels of activated MMP-2 and MMP-9 are significantly lower in women with menorrhagia compared with those with normal menstruation.[21] Defective MMP-2 activation has an impact on local VEGF-A levels and thus impaired vessel growth or function, causing menorrhagia. The proliferation and differentiation pattern of the vascular smooth muscle cells around spiral arterioles of the endometrium in women with menorrhagia is reduced. Inhibition of MMP-2 and MMP-9 has been shown to decrease migration of smooth muscle cells to the intimal layer of vessel wall.[22] Besides the effects on angiogenesis, MMP-2 also functions as a vasoconstrictor and a promoter of platelet aggregation.

A study of endometrial gene expression has shown that endometrial bleeding associated factor (ebaf) gene, located on chromosome 1, usually expresses before and during menstrual bleeding. Ebaf gene is strongly expressed in the endometrium of women with menorrhagia and menometrorrhagia.[23] It is hypothesized that the ebaf gene could be implicated in local regulation of the process of endometrial bleeding and menorrhagia.

Diagnostic Evaluation

AMENORRHEA

A careful history and physical examination of amenorrheic patients should help identify the cause of amenorrhea and thereby limit the number of unnecessary investigations. History and physical examination should include the list in Table 11-3. Amenorrhea in the perimenarchal and perimenopausal years is likely the result of anovulation. A history of secondary amenorrhea provides proof of the presence of internal genital organs and rules out congenital outflow tract obstruction. History of extreme stress, excessive exercise, and eating disorders are all suggestive of hypothalamic amenorrhea. A family history of late menarche and early menopause is suggestive of constitutional delay of menarche and primary ovarian insufficiency, respectively. Women with a history or pelvic radiation or chemotherapy are at risk of ovarian failure, whereas women with history of intracranial radiation are at risk of pituitary failure. Many medications, including contraception, can cause amenorrhea, which is reversible on discontinuation of the drug. The presence of breast development demonstrates estrogen action, whereas excessive testosterone secretion is suspected in women with hirsutism or other signs of virilization. Nutritional status can be assessed from physical examination. A thorough examination of external and internal genitalia will detect the abnormalities of uterus and outflow tract.

In this chapter, a single algorithm (Figure 11-1) is used to approach all women with either primary or secondary amenorrhea after pregnancy is excluded. With complete history, physical examination, FSH, TSH, and prolactin and progesterone withdrawal test, common causes of amenorrhea can usually be identified.

Abnormal thyroid function—both hypo- and hyperthyroidism, even with subclinical disease—can cause amenorrhea. This can be diagnosed by measuring TSH levels. Women with hypothyroidism have elevated TSH levels, whereas those with hyperthyroidism have depressed TSH levels. In women with elevated prolactin, if they also have elevated TSH, hyperprolactinemia could result from hypothyroidism and should be managed accordingly. However, prolactin levels associated with primary hypothyroidism are usually <100 ng/mL.[8] A list of drugs that potentially cause hyperprolactinemia is listed in Table 11-4. In women with prolactin levels >100 ng/mL or prolactin levels <100 ng/mL with visual problems or headache, magnetic resonance imagine (MRI) of the pituitary is indicated to rule out tumor of the pituitary gland. However, the utility of an MRI study in women with an elevated prolactin level <100 ng/mL is controversial.[24]

Table 11-3. List of History and Physical Examination for the Evaluation of Amenorrhea

History	Physical Examination
• Menstrual history (primary vs. secondary amenorrhea, age at menarche, menstrual cycle pattern)	• General physical examination
• History of growth and development	• Weight/height
• Sexual history	• Secondary sexual characteristics
• Pregnancy and gynecologic history	• Sign of hyperandrogenism (enlarged clitoris, hirsutism)
• History of galactorrhea	• Presence of galactorrhea
• Contraceptive history	• Dysmorphic features (e.g., Turner's stigmata)
• Underlying medical history	• External genital organ examination
• Surgical history	• Pelvic examination
• History of radiation exposure	
• History of chemotherapy	
• Current and past medications	
• Family history, including mother's age at menarche and menopause, genetic anomalies	
• Amount, type, and intensity of exercise, emotional or psychological stress	
• Weight gain/loss, eating habits, nutritional status	
• Symptoms of thyroid or adrenal diseases	

Figure 11-1. Algorithm for the evaluation of women with amenorrhea.[8]

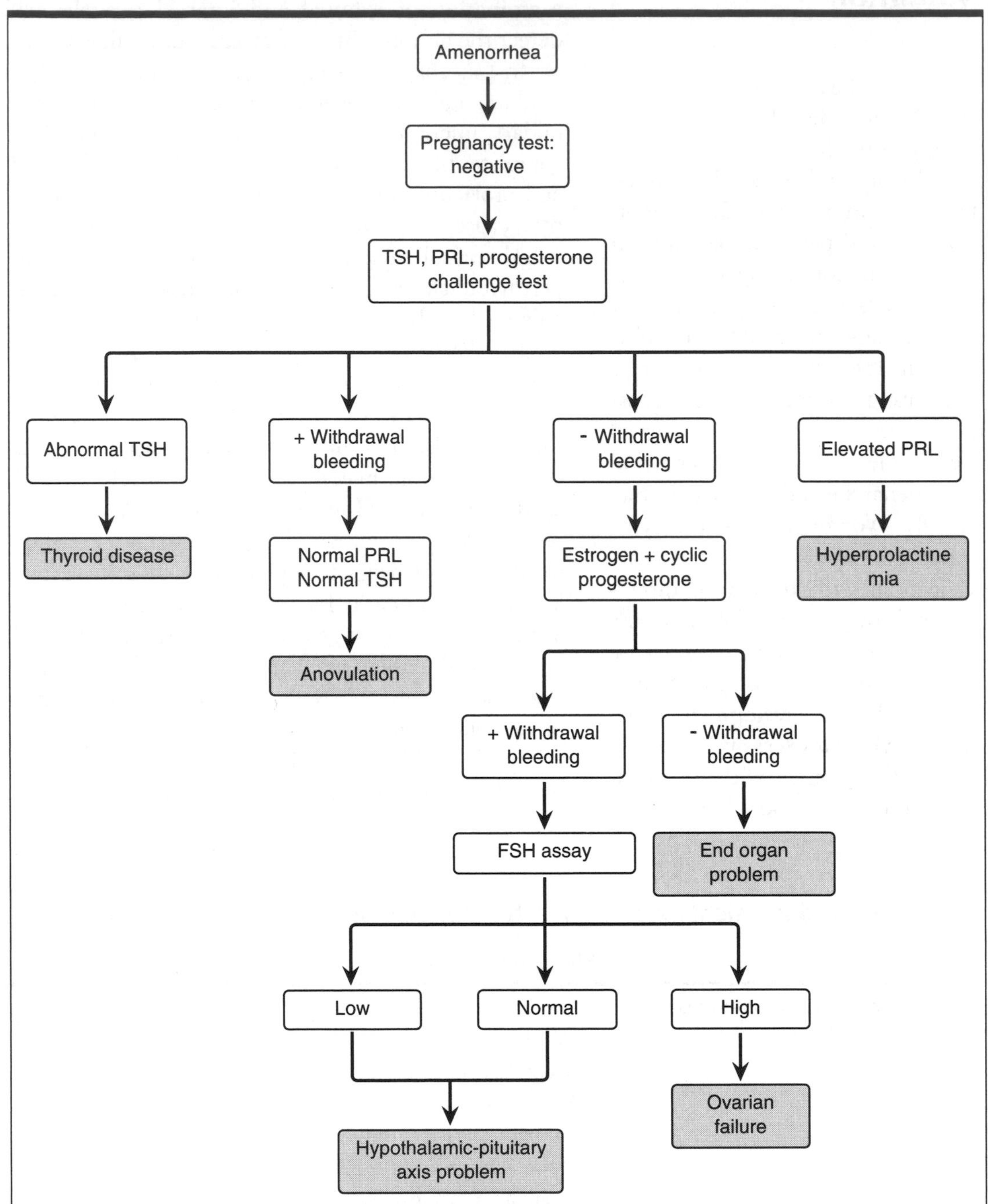

Endogenous estrogen levels, endometrial function, and competence of the outflow tract can be assessed with a progesterone challenge test. A 5-day course of oral progestational agents—300 mg micronized progesterone or 10 mg medroxyprogesterone acetate daily—is given to patients. In the presence of endogenous estrogen, functional endometrium, and a patent outflow tract, patients will have withdrawal bleeding within 2–7 days after the completion of a 5-day course of progestational medications. If TSH and prolactin levels are normal, no further investigation is required, and the diagnosis of anovulation can reliably be made.

In women with negative progesterone challenge test, the next step is to separate those with low endogenous estrogen from those with impairment of the endometrium or the outflow tract. Oral estrogen is given to induce proliferation of endometrium

Table 11-4. List of Medications That Potentially Cause Hyperprolactinemia[24]

Mediations	Mechanism
• Antipsychotics (phenothiazines, butyrophenones, risperidone) • Antidepressant (fluoxetine, tricyclic antidepressants, monoamine oxidase inhibitors) • Antiemetics (domperidone, metoclorpramide) • Antihypertensive (methyldopa, calcium channel blockers, reserpine)	Inhibition of dopamine release
• Opiates	Stimulation of hypothalamic opioid receptors
• Estrogens	Stimulation of lactotrophs
• Verapamil • Protease inhibitors	Unknown

during the initial phase, then it is followed by oral progestational agents to induce secretory change of endometrium, which will slough after the cessation of both hormones. Generally 1.25 mg conjugated estrogens or 2 mg estradiol is given daily for 21 days. Oral progestational agents—either 300 mg micronized progesterone or 10 mg medroxyprogesterone acetate—are given in addition to daily estrogen during the last 5 days. In women with no withdrawal bleeding after a complete course of estrogen and progestogen administration, a problem in the compartment I (uterus, endometrium, and outflow tract) can be diagnosed with confidence. For those with withdrawal bleeding, the uterus, endometrium, and outflow tract are proven intact and functional. The cause of amenorrhea then is due to low estrogen production.

Problems with low endogenous estrogen production can be further categorized into ovarian problems or hypothalamic pituitary problems by measuring FSH level. Those with high FSH level (>20 International Units/L) have ovarian failure, as ovarian follicular growth does not respond to gonadotropin stimulation from the intact pituitary gland. The cause of ovarian failure should be further investigated. Karyotyping should be done in women younger than 30 years who have primary ovarian insufficiency. In women with normal or low FSH level, the problem is in the higher center: either pituitary gland or hypothalamus. Gonadotropin secretion could be impaired because of diseases of gonadotroph itself or the lack of GnRH from the hypothalamus.

OLIGOMENORRHEA

As oligomenorrhea is commonly caused by anovulation, clinical evaluation of women with oligomenorrhea is very similar to those of secondary amenorrhea, which is also a manifestation of anovulation. Pregnancy should be ruled out before further investigating for the cause of oligomenorrhea. Simple blood evaluation of FSH, LH, prolactin, and TSH should be performed as in women with amenorrhea. Both hypothyroidism and hyperthyroidism can cause anovulation and oligomenorrhea. In women with signs and symptoms of hyperandrogenism (acne, hirsutism, and alopecia), serum-free testosterone level should also be measured because the majority of oligomenorrheic women are diagnosed with polycystic ovary syndrome. Ratio of LH:FSH of greater than 2:1 or 3:1 is also suggestive of polycystic ovary syndrome. In patients with anovulation, a detailed pelvic ultrasound should be performed to evaluate the morphology of ovaries and endometrium, as the ovaries commonly have a polycystic appearance and have increased risk of endometrial hyperplasia because of unopposed estrogen stimulation on the endometrium.

MENORRHAGIA

In women with menorrhagia, assessment of the severity of bleeding is one of the top priorities. If the patient is hemodynamically unstable, resuscitation should be initiated before investigating the cause of menorrhagia. Complete history, vital signs, physical examination, and complete blood counts with platelets will help physicians assessing bleeding severity (Table 11-5). Pregnancy must be excluded.

Table 11-5. Clinical Evaluation of Women with Menorrhagia

History	Physical Examination	Investigation
• Onset of bleeding	• Vital signs	• Complete blood count with platelets
• Duration of bleeding	• General physical examination	• Coagulation screening test
• Number of pads/tampons used per day or per cycle	• Pelvic examination	• Serum luteal progesterone
• Presence or absence of blood clots		• Thyroid-stimulating hormone
• Menstrual regularity		• Serum ferritin
• Social/occupational disturbance		• Pregnancy test
• Anemic symptoms (fatigue, fainting, syncope)		• Pelvic ultrasonography
• Underlying medical diseases and bleeding disorders		• Dilatation and curettage (if indicated)
• Contraceptive history		
• Pregnancy history		
• Past and current medication		
• History of systemic bleeding		

Serum ferritin maybe useful if the cause of anemia is questionable. In women with an equivocal amount of menstrual bleeding, a pictorial blood loss assessment chart (Figure 11-2) may be useful to confirm the diagnosis of menorrhagia and monitor response to treatment.[25] A pictorial chart score of 100 or more has a sensitivity and specificity of >85% in diagnosing menorrhagia.[25]

In the evaluation of menstrual disorders, it is important to differentiate ovulatory and anovulatory cycles. Women with regular menstrual cycles every 21–35 days are likely to have ovulatory cycles.

Figure 11-2. Pictorial blood loss assessment chart.[25]

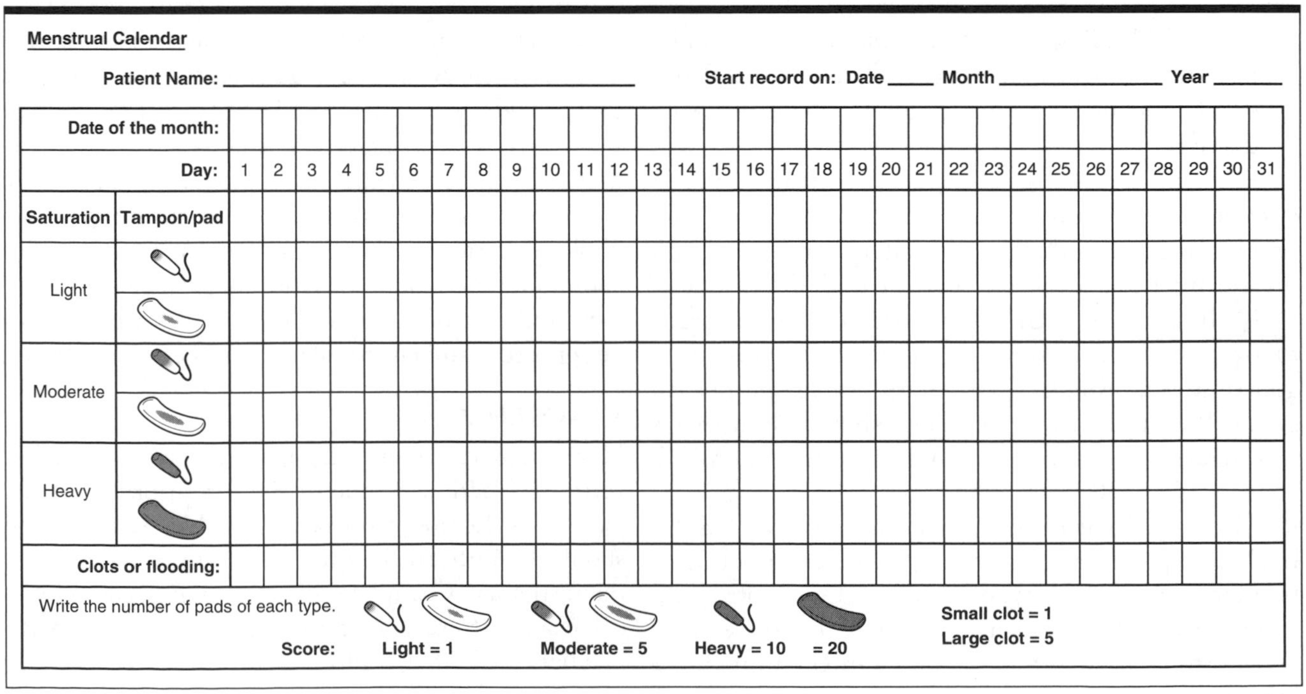

Menstrual Calendar

Patient Name: ____________ Start record on: Date ____ Month ____________ Year ______

Date of the month:																																
	Day:	1	2	3	4	5	6	7	8	9	10	11	12	13	14	15	16	17	18	19	20	21	22	23	24	25	26	27	28	29	30	31
Saturation	Tampon/pad																															
Light																																
Moderate																																
Heavy																																
Clots or flooding:																																

Write the number of pads of each type.

Score: Light = 1 Moderate = 5 Heavy = 10 = 20

Small clot = 1
Large clot = 5

Figure 11-3. Algorithm for the evaluation of women with menorrhagia.

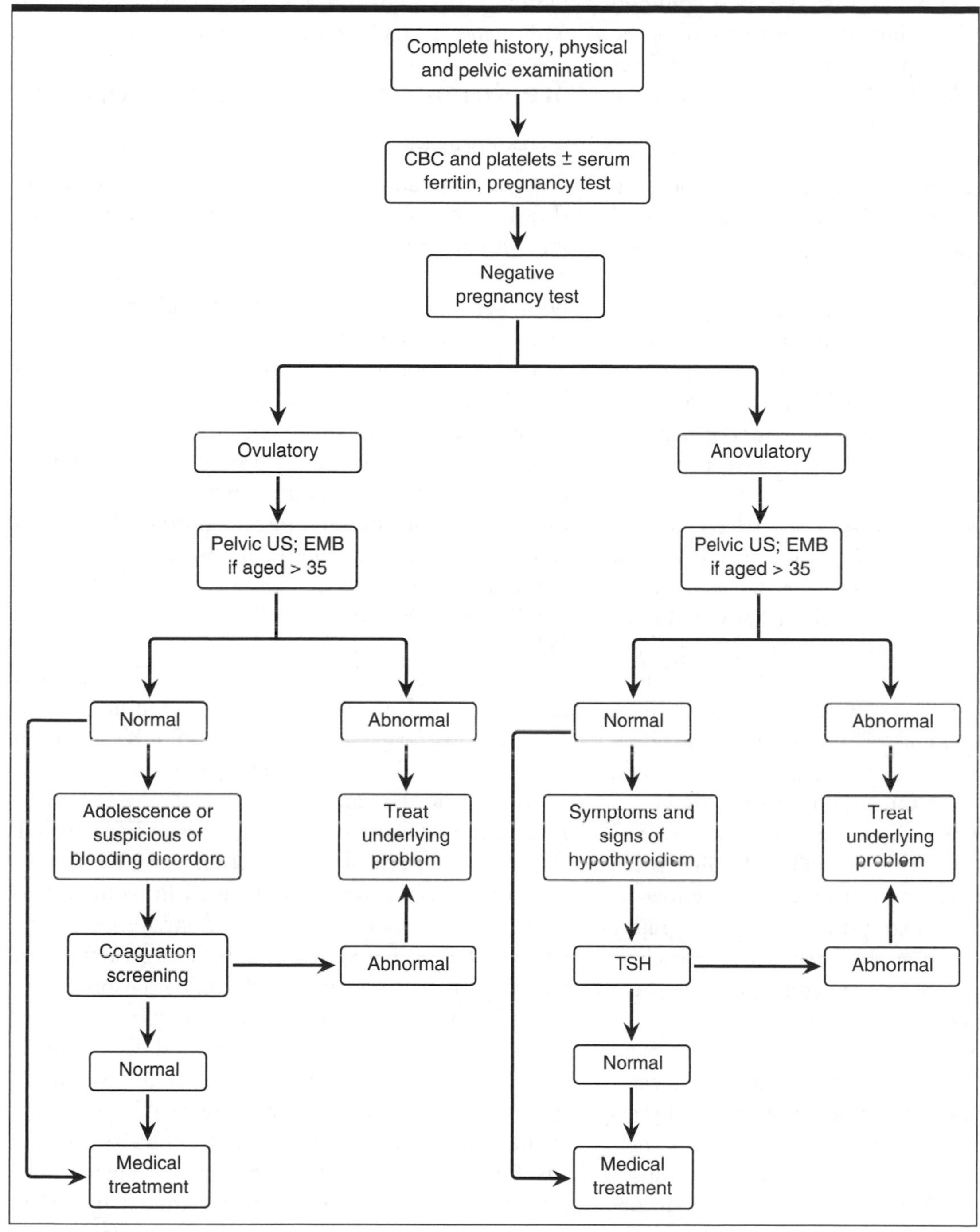

If anovulation is suspected, serum progesterone measurement during the midluteal phase (day 21 of the menstrual cycle) may be useful. A progesterone level >3 ng/mL is reliable evidence of ovulation.[26] Women in the perimenarchal and perimenopausal years and obese women are more likely to have anovulatory bleeding. Menorrhagia may also be seen in women who are anovulatory as a result of severe hypothyroidism.[15] Thyroid-stimulating hormone is a sensitive assay that should detect most cases of thyroid dysfunction. However, as menorrhagia from thyroid disorders is uncommon, screening of thyroid function tests is only indicated in women with symptoms and signs suggestive of hypothyroidism.

Women with coagulation disorders can present with heavy menstrual blood loss. The most common coagulation disorders include thrombocytopenia, idiopathic thrombocytopenic purpura, chronic liver diseases, and von Willebrand's disease. Iatrogenic causes of coagulopathy are also common, such as anticoagulant use and chemotherapy-induced thrombocytopenia. Coagulation screening includes bleeding time, prothrombin time (PT), and activated partial thrombin time (aPTT). Coagulation screening should be performed only if patients have a personal or family history suggesting coagulation problems. Nevertheless, coagulation screening may be appropriate in teenagers presenting with menorrhagia, as the incidence of coagulopathy is as high as 12% to 33%.[6] Moreover, in those presenting with menorrhagia at their first menses, 50% were found to have a coagulation disorder.[27]

Pelvic pathology that causes menorrhagia should be investigated. Bleeding that results from cervical and vaginal pathology can often be detected by direct visualization during a speculum examination or more commonly by cervical or vaginal cytology. Suspected uterine abnormalities should be assessed by ultrasonography to rule out structural abnormalities. Endometrial thickness of >5 mm in postmenopausal women and 12 mm in premenopausal women should alert physician to rule out endometrial pathology.[28] Detailed study of the endometrial cavity can be done by sonohysterography, in which normal saline is infused through the cervix to distend the endometrial cavity during ultrasonography. Sonohysterography better detects lesions in endometrial cavity—such as endometrial polyps and submucous fibroids—than regular ultrasonography.

The American College of Obstetricians and Gynecologists recommends an endometrial assessment to exclude cancer in women older than 35 years who have anovulatory uterine bleeding, as the incidence of endometrial carcinoma increases with age.[29] However, women younger than 35 years who do not respond to medical treatment or have risk factors for endometrial carcinoma (chronic anovulation, diabetes, hypertension, obesity) should be evaluated by endometrial biopsy. Methods of endometrial sampling include dilatation and curettage and endometrial biopsy (with or without hysteroscopy). Hysteroscopically directed endometrial sampling detects a higher percentage of abnormalities compared with traditional dilatation and curettage.[30] Dilatation and curettage may be preferable in the case of active hemorrhage, as it provides both diagnosis and will acutely treat the bleeding. The algorithm for the evaluation of women with menorrhagia is shown in Figure 11-3.

Treatment for Menstrual Disorders

AMENORRHEA AND OLIGOMENORRHEA

The goal of treatment of amenorrhea and oligomenorrhea is to establish regular monthly menstrual bleeding with the resumption of ovulation or to establish a regular uterine withdrawal bleeding by exogenous hormone administration. Besides the disorders of the uterus and outflow tract, the etiologies of amenorrhea and oligomenorrhea are similar—anovulation from hypothalamic–pituitary–ovarian axis dysfunction—so we will discuss the treatment for amenorrhea and oligomenorrhea together. Primary ovarian insufficiency and polycystic ovary syndrome are common causes of amenorrhea and oligomenorrhea. In women who have anovulation and desire for pregnancy, ovulation induction is the treatment of choice. (See Chapter 15: Primary Ovarian Insufficiency and Chapter 16: Polycystic Ovary Syndrome.)

Explanation and reassurance is the initial step of treatment. Behavioral and diet modification to treat the underlying problem should be done in conjunction with medical management. Recovery of hypothalamic dysfunction can be achieved if stress factors and energy imbalance are properly corrected. An increase in caloric consumption and reduction in physical activities are recommended in women who have negative energy balance and strenuous physical activities. This topic is discussed in greater detail in Chapter 31: Nutrition and Eating Disorders. A critical proportion of fat tissue is required to start menarche (27% of body weight) and to maintain regular ovarian cyclicity (22% of body weight).[31] Menstrual irregularities appear reversible once patients return to a normal weight and nutritional status. A study demonstrated a menstrual cycle recovery rate of 70.7% in women with functional hypothalamic amenorrhea.[32] Among those with resumption of menstrual cycle, their body mass index was shown to increase.[32] Moreover, the cyclic menstrual recovery rate of untreated women with functional hypothalamic amenorrhea is as high as 80%.[32]

Estrogen and Progesterone

With an intact uterus, endometrium, and outflow tract, monthly uterine withdrawal bleeding can be induced by cyclic administration of estrogen and progesterone regardless of the cause of amenorrhea. In addition to induction of monthly uterine withdrawal bleeding, administration of estrogen theoretically should prevent bone loss in women with hypothalamic amenorrhea. However, the beneficial effect of estrogen/progesterone on bone mineral density and fracture prevention in women with hypothalamic amenorrhea is inconclusive, unlike the benefit shown in women with primary ovarian insufficiency.[33] In general, estrogen (estradiol valerate 1–2 mg/day or conjugated estrogen 0.625–1.25 mg/day) is given for 21–25 days with progestins (medroxyprogesterone acetate 5 mg/day or norethindrone 0.5 mg/day) during the last 10–14 days of estrogen treatment. The estrogen dosage may have to be increased to stimulate endometrial growth to achieve withdrawal bleeding in some patients. If progestational agents cause side effects, micronized progesterone can be used instead. For easy drug administration, there are various preparations of combined estrogen and progesterone, either for contraception or hormone therapy. In women with anovulation, combined contraceptive regimen is recommended, as these women may have unpredictable ovulation and contraceptive hormones will prevent an unplanned pregnancy. All preparations of combined oral contraceptive pills or contraceptive patches have ethinyl estradiol as estrogen but differ in types of progestins. The cyclic administration of combined oral contraceptive pills or contraceptive patches to manage amenorrhea and oligomonorrhea is the same as for contraception. After pregnancy is ruled out, contraceptive pills or patches can be started immediately and continued for 21–24 days followed by a hormone-free period of 4–7 days, depending on regimens. Patients can expect monthly withdrawal bleeding during the hormone-free period. Detailed discussion of combined oral contraceptive pills, contraceptive patches, and hormone therapy is provided in Chapter 19: Hormonal Contraception.

In women with anovulation, the endometrium is chronically stimulated by endogenous estrogen. Cyclic progestin administration can induce withdrawal bleeding. Progestins act on the endometrium, converting proliferative endometrium to secretory endometrium, which will slough on the cessation of progestin administration. In addition to inducing withdrawal bleeding, progestins, as antiestrogens, also prevent endometrial hyperplasia and carcinoma resulting from chronic unopposed estrogen stimulation in anovulatory women. Progestins have been shown to suppress estrogen-mediated oncogenes transcription.[34] A 5- to 10-day course of either medroxyprogesterone acetate 10 mg/day, dydrogesterone 20 mg/day, or micronized progesterone 300 mg/day can induce withdrawal bleeding of >90% in anovulatory women.[35,36] To induce monthly withdrawal bleeding and prevent endometrial hyperplasia, any orally active progestin should be given 10–14 days each month. Progestins can be started on either the first day of each calendar month or on day 15 after the onset of last withdrawal bleeding. Cyclic progestin is not a contraceptive. Patients should be counseled for proper contraception if pregnancy is not desired.

Dopamine Agonists

A dopamine agonist is the first-line treatment for amenorrhea and oligomenorrhea secondary to hyperprolactinemia with or without a prolactin-producing adenoma. Treatment with a dopamine agonist will induce a resumption of cyclic ovulation and regular menstrual bleeding. Commonly used dopamine agonists for treatment of hyperprolactinemia include bromocriptine, cabergoline, and quinagolide. Bromocriptine and cabergoline are ergot-derived dopamine agonists.[24] Quinagolide is nonergot-derived dopamine agonist having chemical structure similar to apomorphine.[24] Prolactin release and synthesis are generally under tonic negative control of dopamine from hypothalamus. Dopamine agonists act on cell surface dopamine receptor D_1 and D_2. Dopamine receptor D_2 is predominant on lactotroph cells.[37] As other cells in central nervous system and peripheral tissue also have either dopamine receptor D_1, D_2, or both, dopamine agonists that act selectively on the dopamine D_2 receptor will cause fewer side effects compared with nonselective dopamine agonists. Within seconds of exposure, dopamine induces membrane hyperpolarization, resulting in inhibition of prolactin release from secretory granules. Within minutes to hours, dopamine suppresses prolactin gene expression and causes changes in cell morphology.[37] Within days, dopamine inhibits lactotroph proliferation and decreases the size of hypertrophied lactotrophs.[37]

Bromocriptine acts on both dopamine receptors D_1 and D_2, having an agonist effect on the D_2 receptor and both an agonist and antagonist effect on the D_1 receptor.[24] Bromocriptine has the longest history of use for treatment of hyperprolactinemia, with a well-established safety profile and effectiveness. Bromocriptine has a short half-life of 3.3 hours, requiring multiple daily dosing. However, bromocriptine is also available in long-acting formulation—either monthly intramuscular injection or once-daily slow-released oral form.[8] In 22 clinical trials using bromocriptine to treat amenorrhea/galactorrhea associated with hyperprolactinemia without demonstrable pituitary tumor, successful menstrual cycle resumption occurred in 80% of treated women with the average time to initiation of menses of 5.7 weeks.[38] Maximum reduction of serum prolactin level was achieved within the first 4 weeks of treatment.[38] The typical dosage of bromocriptine is 5 mg/day in divided doses and can be titrated up to the maximum of 15–20 mg/day unless limited by its side effects. Treatment should be started with an initial dose of 1.25–2.5 mg at bedtime to minimize side effects. The second dose of 2.5 mg in the morning can generally be started in the second week. More than half of women receiving bromocriptine experience adverse reactions, which are generally mild and transient.[38] These reactions include nausea, dizziness, headache, orthostatic hypotension, fatigue, nasal congestion, abdominal cramps, and, rarely, hallucinations. Approximately 10% of patients cannot tolerate the side effects of bromocriptine, leading to discontinuation of treatment. Vaginal administration of bromocriptine is an alternative route to avoid side effects. Vaginal administration of bromocriptine has been shown to lower serum prolactin level and restore menstrual cycle in women intolerant to oral bromocriptine.[39] Complete drug absorption from the vagina and avoidance of first-pass hepatic metabolism allow the use of lower dose of bromocriptine to achieve therapeutic effects.[8] A 2.5-mg tablet inserted high into vagina at bedtime provides excellent therapeutic effects with few side effects.[8]

Cabergoline also acts on dopamine receptors D_1 and D_2, having a high affinity to the D_2 receptor and a low affinity to the D_1 receptor. Cabergoline has a very long half-life of 65 hours, which provides the advantage of weekly or twice-weekly dosing. Dosage of cabergoline is usually started at 0.25–0.5 mg twice a week. The dosage can be titrated by 0.25 mg twice a week up to 1 mg twice a week every 2–4 months, according to serum prolactin levels. In a study of 221 women with hyperprolactinemic amenorrhea treated with cabergoline, after excluding for pregnancy, 93% of treated women resumed menstruation, with 82% having regular menstrual periods.[40] Menses resumption occurred during the first 8 weeks of therapy.[40] Only 3% of women discontinued cabergoline because of drug intolerance.[40] The common side effects include nausea, headache, dizziness, abdominal pain, vertigo, fatigue, and constipation. This study also showed that cabergoline has a higher response rate and less reported side effects than bromocriptine in treating women with hyperprolactinemic amenorrhea. Like bromocriptine, cabergoline can be administered vaginally in patients who cannot tolerate oral administration.[41] Cabergoline can be used successfully to treat women who are resistant or intolerant to bromocriptine and quinagolide.[42]

Quinagolide is a specific dopamine receptor D_2 agonist that is not an ergot derivative. Quinagolide has a half-life of 22 hours, allowing once-daily administration. The adverse side effects of quinagolide—including nausea, headache, orthostatic hypotension, and fatigue—are milder and more transient than those of bromocriptine. Generally, quinagolide is started at 25 mcg/day at bedtime and is gradually increased to 75 mcg/day over 1 week. The daily dosage can be titrated in steps of 75–150 mcg/day every 4 weeks until achieving therapeutic effects with the maximum dosages of 300 mcg/day. Restoration of menstrual function can be achieved in more than 80% of women with hyperprolactinemic amenorrhea and in more than 50% of those who failed bromocriptine.[43,44] Quinagolide is not currently available in the U.S.

Side effects, intolerance, and treatment failure with one dopamine agonist can usually be solved by switching to another dopamine agoinst.[8]

MENORRHAGIA

The goals of treatment are to reduce monthly menstrual blood loss, correct iron-deficiency anemia, and improve quality of life by either inducing amenorrhea or regular cyclic menstruation with reduced blood loss. Medical therapy is the first-line treatment for those without demonstrable uterine pathology who wish to retain fertility. Surgery is usually reserved for those who failed medical treatment. If specific medical problems, such as bleeding disorders and thyroid dysfunction, are identified, they must be treated along with the treatment of menorrhagia. Iron-rich food and iron supplements should be taken to replenish the depleted iron storage that results from menorrhagia. A daily dose of 60–180 mg of elemental iron is recommended.[45] In the setting of acute severe menorrhagia, high-dose intravenous estrogen, such as conjugated equine estrogen, is highly effective in rapidly controlling uterine bleeding by stabilizing capillary fragility.[46,47] Twenty-five mg of intravenous conjugated equine estrogen given every 3 hours stopped bleeding in 72% of patients within 5 hours of treatment initiation.[46] However, high-dose intravenous conjugated equine estrogen cannot be used long term for this purpose, as heavy bleeding will ensue. Other long-term medical treatment is generally initiated once the acute bleeding episode is under control. Long-term medical treatments are divided into two classes: hormonal and nonhormonal treatment. Common nonhormonal treatment includes nonsteroidal anti-inflammatory drugs (NSAIDs) and antifibrinolytics. Common hormonal treatment includes oral contraceptive pills, progestins, progestin-containing intrauterine system, danazol, and GnRH agonist. The choices of treatment for each particular patient depend on individual preferences and circumstances, such as contraceptive need and associated menstrual symptoms (dysmenorrhea, menstrual migraine, premenstrual symptoms).

Combined Oral Contraceptive Pills

Combined oral contraceptive pills are commonly prescribed for women with menorrhagia who also require cycle control and contraception. The aim of treatment can be either having monthly withdrawal bleeding with reduced blood loss, having fewer withdrawal bleeding episodes, or having amenorrhea, depending on whether the pills are taken in cyclic, extended-cyclic, or continuous fashion, respectively. The combined oral contraceptive pills suppress endometrial growth, thus minimizing menstrual blood loss.[48] Moreover, these drugs cause a reduction in prostacyclin (PGI_2) production favoring platelet aggregation and vasoconstriction.[49] These drugs reduce menstrual blood loss by 40% to 50% and are effective for both ovulatory and anovulatory menorrhagia.[50] In those with anovulation, the combined oral contraceptive pills also improve cycle control. The dosage of oral contraceptive pills for the management of menorrhagia is the same as those aimed for contraception. Traditionally, the active pills are taken continuously for 21 days, followed by a 7-day, hormone-free period. A new combined oral contraceptive regimen offers an extended 91-day cycle by taking the active pills continuously for 84 days, followed by 7 days of inactive pills.[51] To avoid cyclic withdrawal bleeding, the combined oral contraceptive pills can be taken continuously for up to 1 year.[52] However, in the extended cycle regimen, women generally experience unscheduled bleeding or spotting during the first 3 months, which gradually decreases over time.[51,52] There are currently many regimens of extended cycle to reduce the number of bleeding days. For women with active heavy menstrual bleeding, low-dose combined oral contraceptive pills can be started at one tablet 2–4 times a day until bleeding stops, then stepped down to regular dosage of one tablet a day.[53] Antiemetic drugs may be needed during the high dosage of combined oral contraceptive pills. There is anecdotal evidence that monophasic pills are more effective than triphasic pills, the higher-dose preparations are better than the lower-dose ones, and the preparations using mildly androgenic progestins such as levonorgestrel are more effective than those with nonandrogenic progestins.[52] The combined oral contraceptive pills also provide contraception, improve dysmenorrhea, and possibly reduce premenstrual symptoms. Side effects and contraindications are the same as for contraception.

Progestins

Progestins are common medications prescribed for the treatment of menorrhagia. There are two regimens commonly used for the management of menorrhagia: cyclic oral progestin and long-acting intramuscular progestin. Cyclic oral progestin acts in anovulatory women by supplementing endogenous progesterone during the luteal phase, resulting in secretory transformation of the endometrium and leading to synchronized withdrawal bleeding. However, the mechanism of action for those with ovulatory menorrhagia is not clear. For long-acting intramuscular progestin, the goal is to induce endometrial atrophy resulting in amenorrhea. Moreover, long-acting intramuscular progestin also suppresses ovarian steroidogenesis and thus minimizes estrogen stimulation of the endometrium.

The usual cyclic oral regimens are norethindrone 5 mg 3 times a day or medroxyprogesterone acetate 10 mg 3 times a day for 14–21 days for women with anovulatory menorrhagia.[50] These regimens should reduce blood loss by 50% after two cycles of therapy in women with anovulation. However, in women with ovulatory menorrhagia, two thirds of these women do not respond to these regimens after two cycles of treatment.[54] Progestin therapy using norethindrone 5 mg 3 times a day for 21 days each cycle (days 5–26) has shown to be highly effective in reducing menstrual blood loss by 87% compared with pretreatment blood loss in women with regular heavy bleeding.[55] Nevertheless, this regimen is not well tolerated because of its side effects. Only 22% of participants wished to continue this treatment.[55] A Cochrane meta-analysis has shown that cyclic progestin was less effective in reducing menstrual blood loss than tranexamic acid, danazol, and progestin-releasing intrauterine devices.[56] Common side effects of progestins include weight gain, mood change, headaches, and bloating.

Depot medroxyprogesterone acetate (DMPA), a long-acting intramuscular progestin known to cause amenorrhea in women with long-term use for contraception, has been used widely to treat menorrhagia. However, there are no studies of DMPA for the treatment of menorrhagia. The dosage for contraception is 150 mg intramuscularly every 3 months. At contraceptive dosage, DMPA was shown to be useful in preventing moderate to severe menorrhagia in up to 80% of women with iatrogenic thrombocytopenia.[57] However, only 25% to 43% of women using DMPA for contraception achieve amenorrhea at 6 months, and the irregular bleeding at 6 months is high at 76%.[58,59] A small study in thrombocytopenic patients showed that DMPA at a dosage of 100 mg every week for 2 weeks, then every 2 weeks for 4 months, then 200 mg every 4 weeks effectively prevents menorrhagia during episodes of thrombocytopenia in 62% of treated patients.[60] Side effects and contraindications are the same as for contraception.

Nonsteroidal Anti-inflammatory Drugs

An increase in endometrial prostaglandin levels and an alteration in the balance of several prostaglandins toward vasodilatation and antiplatelet aggregation are associated with menorrhagia, as discussed earlier. Nonsteroidal anti-inflammatory drugs inhibit cyclo-oxygenase enzyme, which converts arachidonic acid to prostaglandins, reducing prostaglandin levels overall. Mefenamic acid is the most extensively studied NSAID for the treatment of menorrhagia. Unlike other NSAIDs, mefenamic acid blocks prostaglandin E_2 receptors and inhibits prostaglandin synthesis. Mefenamic acid has been shown to reduce menstrual blood loss by 22% to 46%.[54,61] A Cochrane review has shown that NSAIDs as a group are as effective as luteal phase progestins and oral contraceptive pills but less effective than tranexamic acid and danazol in reducing menstrual blood loss in women with menorrhagia.[62] The other NSAIDs used for the treatment of menorrhagia include naproxen, ibuprofen, flurbiprofen, meclofenamic acid, diclofenac, indomethacin, and acetylsalicylic acid. With limited information, there is no significant difference in terms of efficacy between each individual NSAID.[62] Generally, the optimal dosage of mefenamic acid is 500 mg 3–4 times a day; naproxen is 500 mg for the first dose, then 250 mg 3 times a day; and ibuprofen is 600–1,200 mg/day. The reduction in blood loss is dose related.[50] Treatment is initiated on the first day of menstruation and lasts for the entire menstrual period. As the treatment is required only during the menstrual period, this treatment is suitable for women who desire conception. Nonsteroidal anti-inflammatory drugs are also useful for dysmenorrhea and menstrual migraine. Side effects are generally mild, and the most common are nausea, dyspepsia, diarrhea, headaches, rashes, and dizziness. The gastrointestinal side effects can be minimized by taking drugs with meals. Nonsteroidal anti-inflammatory drugs are contraindicated for women with peptic ulcers. The side effects are not usually a major problem as these medications are taken for only a short time.

Levonorgestrel-Releasing Intrauterine System

Levonorgestrel-releasing intrauterine system (LNG-IUS) initially releases approximately 20 mcg of levonorgestrel daily and gradually falls to 11 mcg/day at the end of 5 years.[63] The intraendometrial concentration of levonorgestrel with the LNG-IUS is 100 and 1,000 times higher than with oral and subdermal implant levonorgestrel, respectively.[63,64] The mechanism of action of LNG-IUS for the treatment of menorrhagia is profound local suppression of endometrial growth causing atrophy. Moreover, a recent study has shown that LNG-IUS demonstrated a local antifibrinolytic activity in the endometrium without affecting systemic hemostasis.[65] The LNG-IUS reduces menstrual blood loss up to 95% at 12 months of treatment.[66,67] Up to 35% of women became amenorrheic at 24 months after the insertion of LNG-IUS.[68] During the first 4 months after LNG-IUS insertion, patients should be counseled for unscheduled spotting and bleeding, which generally decreases dramatically after 4 months. The LNG-IUS also improves dysmenorrhea and provides contraception. The LNG-IUS appears to be the most effective long-term medical treatment compared with other medical therapies used for menorrhagia. It was shown to be more effective than tranexamic acid, flurbiprofen, mefenamic acid, and cyclic 21-day norethindrone in the reduction of menstrual blood loss.[67,69,70] Randomized studies comparing LNG-IUS to hysterectomy and surgical endometrial destruction have shown no difference in the quality-of-life score improvement or patient satisfaction between LNG-IUS and surgical treatments at 1 year.[69] The use of

LNG-IUS is restricted to women whose uterine cavities measure 6–9 cm and are not distorted. The use of LNG-IUS in immunocompromised women is not recommended. The LNG-IUS has a lifespan of 5 years. However, current literature has shown the efficacy of LNG-IUS for up to 7 years.[71] Common side effects of LNG-IUS include intermenstrual bleeding, ovarian cysts, and breast tenderness. Progestogenic side effects are uncommon owing to minimal systemic absorption of hormone.

Gonadotropin-Releasing Hormone Agonists

Gonadotropin-releasing hormone agonists are synthetic analogs of endogenous GnRH. They are modified from the endogenous GnRH decapeptide by changing the amino acids in position 6 and 10, resulting in a longer half-life. During the initial phase, they stimulate the GnRH receptor, causing a rise in FSH and LH secretion. However, as GnRH agonists have a long half-life, GnRH receptor downregulation usually occurs approximately 10–14 days after administration, causing profound suppression of FSH and LH secretion and resulting in a profound hypogonadal stage and amenorrhea. Currently available GnRH agonists are leuprolide, buserelin, nafarelin, histrelin, goserelin, deslorelin, and triptorelin. Each GnRH agonist has many forms of administration. This form of monthly or quarterly injection or implant is suitable for the treatment of menorrhagia. Gonadotropin-releasing hormone agonists are highly effective medical therapy for menorrhagia by inducing amenorrhea in 90% of women.[72] Leuprolide has shown to effectively prevent menstruation during the period of myelosuppression in 73% to 96% of patients who undergo bone marrow transplant.[73,74] Even though menstruation is not 100% suppressed, moderate or severe menorrhagia is completely prevented with the use of a GnRH agonist during the period of myelosuppression.[57] To be more effective in suppressing menstruation, GnRH agonists should be started during the luteal phase. Limitation to the long-term use of GnRH agonists are the hypoestrogenic side effects causing hot flashes, vaginal dryness, insomnia, and, after 6 months of treatment, osteoporosis.[75] If GnRH agonists are given for longer than 6 months, estrogen-progesterone add-back is needed to prevent osteoporosis. Preoperative administration of GnRH agonist before endometrial ablative surgery, hysterectomy, and myomectomy have shown to facilitate surgery and improve the outcomes.[76,77] Gonadotropin-releasing hormone agonists are suitable for short-term management of menorrhagia during the period of temporary myelosuppression or as a preoperative measure.

Danazol

Danazol, a synthetic steroid with antiestrogenic, antiprogestogenic, and mild androgenic properties suppresses the hypothalamic–pituitary–ovarian axis and has a profound direct effect on endometrial tissue. Danazol suppresses endometrial estrogen and progesterone receptors, and leads to endometrial atrophy, reduced menstrual blood loss, and, in some women, amenorrhea. Danazol can reduce menstrual blood loss by as much as 80% in a dose-dependent manner.[2] Danazol also provides a relief of dysmenorrhea and endometriosis. The usual dosage is 100–200 mg twice daily for a maximum of 6 months. At the dosage higher than 400 mg/day, amenorrhea is common.[2] A Cochrane meta-analysis has demonstrated that danazol was more effective than placebo, progestins, NSAIDs, and oral contraceptive pills in reducing menstrual blood loss.[78] Unfortunately, as many as 75% of patients treated with danazol reported unpleasant side effects, such as breast atrophy, acne, weight gain, voice change, irritability/aggression, headache, nausea, vomiting, and musculoskeletal pain; these side effects led to treatment discontinuation.[79] Given this and the fact that danazol is teratogenic and not contraceptive, treatment should be initiated after pregnancy is ruled out, and a nonhormonal method of contraception should be used during treatment.

Antifibrinolytics

Antifibrinolytics are promoted for the treatment of menorrhagia because hemostasis plays an important role in limiting the amount of menstrual blood loss. The balance between fibrin formation and fibrinolysis determines hemostatic status. Women with menorrhagia have an increased level of plasminogen activators (a group of enzymes responsible for fibrinolysis) and increased local fibrinolytic activity.[80] Tranexamic acid is a synthetic derivative of lysine that inhibits fibrin degradation by reversibly binding to lysine binding sites on plasminogen. A Cochrane meta-analysis concluded that treatment with tranexamic acid resulted in a greater reduction in objective menstrual blood loss than NSAIDs, luteal phase progestins, and ethamsylate.[81] Tranexamic acid reduces menstrual blood loss by up to 50%.[61,82] Tranexamic acid is also effective in treating menorrhagia associated with intrauterine contraceptive devices. The commonly prescribed dosage of tranexamic acid is 1.0–1.5 g orally 3 times a day starting on the first day of bleeding for the duration of menstruation. To limit the side effects of tranexamic acid, it should be given only during the first 3 days of the cycle, during which menstrual flow is heavy. Common side effects are gastrointestinal symptoms. Although tranexamic acid minimizes the amount of menstrual blood loss, it has no effect on menstrual duration.[82] Like NSAIDs, tranexamic acid is advisable for treatment of menorrhagia in women who wish to conceive, as it is taken only during the menstrual period, thus avoiding teratogenic concern, and does not disrupt ovulatory cycles. Because tranexamic acid modifies hemostatic balance toward a prothrombotic state, there is a theoretic concern of the risk of venous thromboembolism. Nevertheless, a long-term study in Sweden has shown that the incidence of thrombosis in women treated with tranexamic acid is comparable with the spontaneous frequency of thrombosis in women.[83]

Surgical Treatment

Surgery is indicated for women who have pelvic pathology that causes menorrhagia, such as endometrial polyps, uterine fibroids, and endometrial malignancy. However, in women with dysfunctional uterine bleeding, surgery is indicated for those who fail medical treatment, have contraindication for medical treatment, or have intolerable side effects from medical treatment. Data from a Cochrane analysis showed that 58% of women randomized to medical treatment eventually have surgical treatment by 2 years.[84] Hysterectomy is the surgical treatment for menorrhagia, with a 100% cure rate and a very high level of patient satisfaction. Nevertheless, it is a major operation with significant morbidity and cost.

Endometrial ablation is a surgical procedure that selectively destroys the endometrium, often leading to oligomenorrhea or amenorrhea. Endometrial ablation is a minimally invasive method that is an alternative to hysterectomy in women with menorrhagia. As endometrium can regenerate from the basal layer, the aim of endometrial ablation is to destroy the entire endometrium and up to 3 mm of myometrium.[2] The first generation of endometrial ablation was performed with the use of hysteroscopy to directly visualize the endometrial cavity during the operation, and the endometrium was destroyed with the use of either laser, radiofrequency, or electric or thermal energy source. The second generation of endometrial ablation is a blind technique performed without the use of hysteroscopy. The second generation ablation

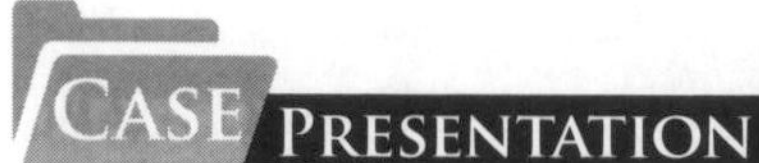

PRESENTATION

Patient Case: Part 2

Diagnosis: Menorrhagia; iron deficiency anemia.

Treatment: The treatment of menorrhagia can be categorized into two main pharmacologic therapies: hormonal vs. nonhormonal. The goal of the patient's therapy is directed toward decreasing the amount of blood loss with each menstrual period. The nonhormonal options include episodic therapy with antifibrinolytics and NSAIDs. The use of these medications would be restricted to the menstrual cycle and discontinued for the remainder of the month. Antifibrinolytics and NSAIDs offer no contraception and do not affect the hormonal regulation of the menstrual cycle.

There are several options for hormonal management of menorrhagia. These options include combined oral contraceptives, DMPA, and LNG-IUS. Although each hormonal method provides contraception, each therapy varies in its mechanism, duration of use, and side effects. Important aspects to consider are effects on monthly menses and the patient's future childbearing plans.

The patient expressed her desire to initiate a therapy that offered contraception, allowed her to continue to have regular menses, and did not delay conception once discontinued. When considering the patient's personal requests and therapeutic options, the most appropriate therapy was combined oral contraceptives pills (OCPs). OCPs will allow the patient to continue to have regular menses with a decrease in the duration and amount of bleeding. In addition, OCPs will allow her to quickly resume childbearing, without a prolonged interval of anovulatory cycles.

In addition to hormonal therapy for the patient's menorrhagia, treatment of her iron deficiency anemia was also needed. The hormonal therapy would successfully decrease the amount of blood loss monthly; however, additional measures would help replete iron stores and accelerate hematopoiesis. Therefore, the patient was also advised to increase dietary consumption of iron-rich foods as well as to supplement her diet with ferrous sulfate 325 mg twice a day.

Follow-up: The patient was advised to follow up in 1 month to assess the response to treatment. During this interval, she will be instructed to maintain a menstrual calendar to document her bleeding history and associated symptoms. The calendar should also document compliance with OCPs and side effects (including nausea, vomiting, and weight gain). The follow-up visit will also provide an opportunity to assess improvement in anemia with a physical exam and report laboratory studies.

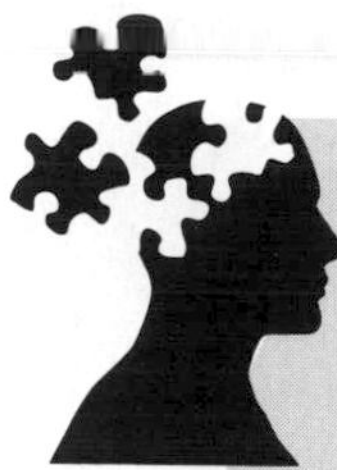

Therapeutic Challenge:

The challenge is to identify medical management that has a favorable risk-benefit ratio, particularly in women who have contraindications to hormonal therapy. Another challenge is to identify treatments of abnormal uterine bleeding that also offer contraception in women who desire a birth control method.

What are the options for menses regulation in a woman with a medical contraindication to estrogen? What are the options for a patient with irregular menses who also needs contraception?

devices require less skill and have a lower risk compared with the first generation. Overall, 25% to 30% of patients have amenorrhea and 45% to 60% have a significant reduction in menstrual flow, giving a satisfaction rate of 75% to 80%.[72] Preoperative endometrial thinning with GnRH agonists or danazol has shown to facilitate surgical procedures and result in higher rates of postoperative amenorrhea.[76] Endometrial ablation is not indicated for those who need future fertility.

Summary

Menstrual disorders are major problems in women of reproductive age from perimenarche to menopause. Nearly all women experience some form of menstrual abnormality at least once in their lifetime. The causes of menstrual disorders can be either from the uterus and outflow tract or hypothalamic–pituitary–ovarian axis. Moreover, menstrual abnormalities could be a clinical manifestation of many systemic disorders that affect other organ systems on a long-term basis. Pregnancy and malignancy must be excluded, as these issues need special attention. The primary systemic disorders causing menstrual abnormalities should be treated properly to resume normal menstrual cycle and to minimize long-term consequences in other organ systems. Treatment of menstrual disorders may be long term, so patients are encouraged to understand the pathophysiology of the problems and the aim of treatment. Most menstrual disorders can be treated successfully with either hormonal or nonhormonal medications. In addition to medical treatment, diet and lifestyle modification are important in some types of menstrual disorders. Surgical treatment is usually reserved for those with anatomic defects, those having pelvic pathology, or those who failed medical treatment.

References

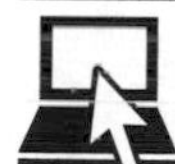

Additional content available at
www.ashp.org/womenshealth

Acknowledgment

We would like to thank Dr. Candice Jones for providing the patient case.

12

Dysmenorrhea

Devra K. Dang, Pharm.D., BCPS, CDE; Fei Wang, M.Sc., Pharm.D., BCPS, FASHP; Karim Anton Calis, Pharm.D., MPH, FASHP, FCCP

Learning Objectives

1. Define primary and secondary dysmenorrhea, and describe the clinical presentation and diagnosis of both conditions.
2. Explain the pathophysiologic mechanisms of primary and secondary dysmenorrhea.
3. Describe nonpharmacologic and pharmacologic treatment options for primary dysmenorrhea and their places in therapy.
4. Review nonpharmacologic and pharmacologic treatment options for secondary dysmenorrhea.
5. Devise a treatment plan for patients with dysmenorrhea, including evaluation, treatment, and monitoring for those with primary dysmenorrhea and appropriate referrals for those with secondary dysmenorrhea.

Dysmenorrhea is defined as painful menstruation of uterine origin and is commonly divided into two categories based on the pathophysiology. Primary dysmenorrhea is painful menstruation that typically begins during adolescence with ovulatory cycles and is not due to any pelvic disease. It is distinguished from secondary dysmenorrhea, which is uncommon during adolescence and results from pelvic organ pathology. Common causes of secondary dysmenorrhea include endometriosis, **uterine fibroids,** adenomyosis, obstructive vaginal or uterine congenital anomalies, and use of intrauterine contraceptive devices.[1,2]

Epidemiology

Primary dysmenorrhea is by far the most common gynecologic symptom among menstruating women. The prevalence of dysmenorrhea is difficult to determine because of different definitions of the condition and different groups of patients studied. However, estimates vary from 60% to 90%.[3-6,7]

About 14% to 15% of adolescent girls report severe pain that interfered with daily functions.[3,4] Dysmenorrhea is the leading cause of recurrent short-term absenteeism from school among adolescent girls in the U.S.[3,5] In several longitudinal studies in women younger than age 30 years, the rates of absenteeism ranged from 34% to 50%.[4,6] In contrast, absence from work occurred in <5% of women older than age 30.[8] The prevalence of primary dysmenorrhea decreases with increasing age, with prevalence being highest in the 20- to 24-year-old age group and decreasing progressively thereafter.[9]

Epidemiologic data suggest that there is a significant correlation of certain risk factors to more severe episodes of primary dysmenorrhea. These risk factors include earlier age at menarche (<12 years), longer cycles or duration of bleeding, heavy menstrual flow, **nulliparity,** and a positive family history. Certain behavioral risk factors have also been associated with dysmenorrhea. Some studies found an association between smoking and dysmenorrhea.[3,4,10,11] Physical activity and alcohol consumption have not been consistently associated with dysmenorrhea.[4,10,11] A recent systematic review found that the risk of dysmenorrhea increased with the number of cigarettes smoked and decreased with use of oral contraceptives, fish intake, physical exercise, being married or in a stable relationship, and higher parity.[12] In a national survey, socioeconomic status was positively associated with dysmenorrhea and race was not. However, even when socioeconomic status was held constant, black students (24%) missed more school because of dysmenorrhea than white students (12%), suggesting that other biological variables, particularly increasing gynecologic

CASE PRESENTATION

Patient Case: Part 1

T. F. is a 19-year-old college sophomore who presents to the university student health clinic for an evaluation of painful menstrual "cramps." She reports that she has been experiencing lower abdominal cramps since last night, when her menstrual cycle started; rates the pain as 8 out of 10 on the pain scale; and has had to miss her morning classes. She also reports lower back pain but denies any other associated symptoms.

HPI: T.F. gives a history of suprapubic and back pain associated with menstrual cycles since **menarche** at age 12. The pain appears during the first day of each menstrual cycle and typically lasts for the next 2 days. The pain is most intense on the first day and has caused her to miss school. She reports that the menstrual pain subsided during high school—when she was on the field hockey team and experienced very light menstrual periods—but has since returned as she is less active in college and her menstrual periods are heavier.

PMH: Occasional mild headaches associated with menses; not sexually active.

Family history: No history of gynecologic conditions in female first-degree relatives.

Social history: Smokes ½ pack of cigarettes per day; denies alcohol or illicit drug use.

Medications: None.

Allergies: None known.

Vital signs: Weight 130 lb; height 5′5″; blood pressure 118/74; pulse 82; temperature 98.6° F; respiration rate 12.

Physical exam: Pelvic exam within normal limits.

Laboratory values: None obtained today; last Pap test 6 months ago within normal limits.

age (i.e., increase of dysmenorrhea with chronological age from 39% of 12-year-old girls to 72% of 17-year-old girls), play a substantial role in the pathogenesis of dysmenorrhea.[3] Despite the high prevalence of dysmenorrhea in adolescents and young adults, many do not seek help from healthcare providers.

Clinical Presentation

Primary dysmenorrhea typically presents in the adolescent years, about 6–12 months after menarche, or when regular ovulatory cycles are established. It is characterized by fluctuating and spasmodic crampy lower abdominal pain (located in the suprapubic area), sometimes referred to as "laborlike" pain, which begins a few hours before or with the onset of menstrual flow. The pains are most intense within the first 24–48 hours of the onset of menstruation, and symptoms may last up to 72 hours. The cramps are frequently accompanied by backache, thigh pain, nausea, vomiting, headache, fatigue, lightheadedness, and increased frequency of defecation in a high percentage of cases.[1,3,9] There is no specific laboratory test required for the diagnosis of primary dysmenorrhea. A typical history of onset of dysmenorrhea with menarche, onset of symptoms with the onset of menstrual flow, duration of menstrual cramping, and absence of any positive findings in the physical examination are the only key diagnostic features.

Secondary dysmenorrhea can occur at any time after menarche but is usually more likely to occur in women after the age of 25. Only about 10% of adolescents and young adults who present with dysmenorrhea have pelvic abnormalities.[13] Secondary dysmenorrhea should be suspected when it arises as a new symptom in a woman in her 30s or 40s. The pain associated with secondary dysmenorrhea usually begins several days or 1–2 weeks before the onset of bleeding and may persist through the end of the menstrual flow.[2] Secondary dysmenorrhea may also be accompanied by other gynecologic symptoms,

Table 12-1. Common Causes of Secondary Dysmenorrhea

• Endometriosis
• Adenomyosis
• Pelvic inflammation
• Uterine fibroids—endometrial polyps
• Ovarian cysts and tumors
• Intrauterine contraceptive devices
• Stenosis of the cervical channel
• Intrauterine adhesions
• Congenital malformations
• Pelvic varicocele
• Allen-Masters syndrome
• Uterine retroversion in fixed position

such as **dyspareunia, menorrhagia,** intermenstrual bleeding, infertility, and postcoital bleeding, depending on the underlying condition.[1] The diagnosis of secondary dysmenorrhea can be ruled in with a history of late onset of dysmenorrhea after no prior history of pain with menstruation; first occurrence after the age of 25; pelvic abnormality on physical examination; heavy menstrual flow or irregular cycles; and little or no response to treatment with nonsteroidal anti-inflammatory drugs (NSAIDs), oral contraceptives, or both.[1] The single most useful diagnostic procedure is laparoscopy. Table 12-1 shows the most important causes of secondary dysmenorrhea.

Pathophysiology

PRIMARY DYSMENORRHEA

Menstrual pain in primary dysmenorrhea is primarily due to factors that affect uterine hypercontractility, reduced uterine blood flow, or increased peripheral nerve hypersensitivity. Prostanoids and possibly eicosanoid and vasopressin secretions during menstruation have been involved in myometrial hypersensitivity, reduced uterine blood flow, and pain associated with primary dysmenorrhea.[14]

Prostaglandins and Leukotrienes

Primary dysmenorrhea, associated with a normal ovulatory cycle and with no pelvic pathology, has a clear physiologic etiology. After ovulation, in response to the production of progesterone, there is a buildup of fatty acids in the phospholipids of the cell membranes. After the onset of progesterone withdrawal before menstruation, these fatty acids, particularly arachidonic acid, are released and initiate a cascade of prostaglandins and leukotrienes in the uterus.[13] These, in turn, induce an inflammatory response that results in abnormal uterine contractions, which reduces uterine blood flow and leads to uterine tissue ischemia and pain.[9] The inflammatory response mediated by prostaglandins can also produce systemic symptoms such as nausea, vomiting, bloating, and headaches.

Current evidence suggests that in most women with primary dysmenorrhea, there is an abnormally high release of prostaglandin $F_{2\alpha}$($PGF_{2\alpha}$) found in menstrual fluid and endometrial tissues. $PGF_{2\alpha}$ causes a potent vasoconstriction and myometrial contraction. The intensity of the menstrual cramps and associated symptoms are directly proportional to the amount of $PGF_{2\alpha}$ released. An abnormal $PGF_{2\alpha}$:PGE_2 ratio has also been associated with primary dysmenorrhea.[9,14]

Despite advances implicating the role of prostaglandins in the etiology of primary dysmenorrhea, there are a number of women with evidence of primary dysmenorrhea who don't have an elevated level of menstrual $PGF_{2\alpha}$. Increased production of menstrual leukotrienes through the 5-lipo-oxygenase enzyme pathway rather than the cyclooxygenase (COX) pathway may account for some forms of dysmenorrhea that are not responsive to NSAID therapy.[9] Leukotrienes have been postulated to cause a hypersensitization of pain fibers in the uterus.[14] High concentrations of leukotrienes have been found in adult women who have dysmenorrhea.[2] These substances are potent vasoconstrictors and inflammatory mediators, although their exact role and mechanism in causing dysmenorrhea is not well established. Figure 12-1 summarizes the biochemical pathways that lead to pain in primary dysmenorrhea.

Vasopressin

The role of vasopressin, a hormone released by the posterior pituitary glands, remains unclear, as studies have shown inconsistent results.[15-17] It is postulated that increased levels of vasopressin during menstruation cause a dysrhythmic uterine contraction that reduces uterine blood flow, leading to uterine hypoxia and myometrial hypersensitivity.[9,17]

SECONDARY DYSMENORRHEA

Secondary dysmenorrhea refers to painful menstruation associated with pelvic abnormalities. A number of common pathologies responsible for secondary dysmenorrhea are presented in 12-1. Secondary dysmenorrhea is more likely to be associated with chronic pelvic pain, midcycle pain (pain maybe continuous or intermittent), dyspareunia, **metrorrhagia,** or menorrhagia. The pathologic mechanism of pain associated with secondary dysmenorrhea is specific to the etiology of the pathologic condition (Table 12-1).

Endometriosis, the most common cause of secondary dysmenorrhea, is the ectopic presence and growth of uterine endometrial tissue outside the uterine cavity. The majority of endometriosis implants are located in the pelvis, with the ovaries being the most common site.[13] The principal manifestations of endometriosis are pelvic pain and infertility. The extent of the pain is influenced primarily by the locations and depth of the implant.[18] Endometriosis is an estrogen-dependent disorder, and an increase in estrogen is likely responsible for increased COX activity and subsequent increased production of prostaglandins. The accumulation of estrogen and

Figure 12-1. Pathophysiology of dysmenorrhea. The inflammatory response is mediated by the following PG and LT shown above. PG = prostaglandin; LT = leukotriene. Reprinted with permission from reference 13.

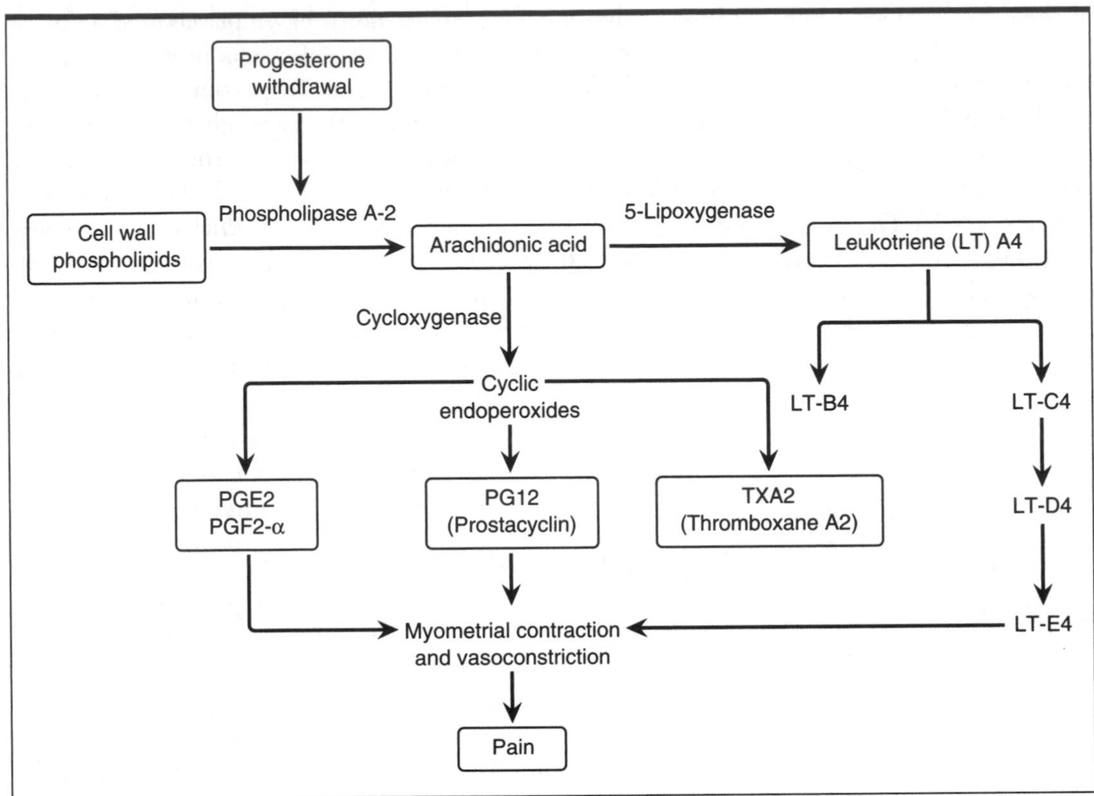

prostaglandin results in a potent inflammatory process and pelvic pain. **Adenomyosis** (endometriosis interna) is another common benign condition of the uterus in which the endometrium (the mucous membrane lining the inside of the uterus) grows into the myometrium (the uterine musculature located just outside the endometrium), causing dysmenorrhea and menorrhagia. Other secondary causes (listed in Table 12-1) that result in any distortion or displacement of normal uterine pathology are commonly associated with chronic pelvic pain, dyspareunia, and disturbances in menstruation.

Diagnosis

The first step in the diagnosis of dysmenorrhea is to obtain a thorough history. The characteristic (location, duration, and severity) of the pain and any associated symptoms (such as bloating and headache), as well as response to any previous pharmacologic or nonpharmacologic treatments, should be assessed. Characteristics of the menstrual cycle (duration, frequency, and menstrual flow) should also be determined. The relationship of the pelvic pain and any accompanying symptom to the menstrual cycle, the timing of the initial onset of symptoms in relation to menarche, as well as family history are important pieces of information that will also assist in the differential between primary and secondary dysmenorrhea. In addition, a thorough gynecologic medical history, taking into account sexual history, pregnancy history, previous pelvic infections, and pelvic abnormalities, should also be evaluated.[14] The presence of pelvic abnormalities suggests secondary dysmenorrhea. In adolescents who do not have a history of sexual activity and who have a clinical presentation clearly consistent with primary dysmenorrhea, a pelvic examination is not necessary.[13] Primary dysmenorrhea is diagnosed based only on a thorough history and not on any laboratory or other diagnostic criteria. By contrast, the diagnosis of the underlying etiology of secondary dysmenorrhea may require imaging studies (such as pelvic ultrasound or laparoscopy), biopsy, or laboratory studies to evaluate for the presence of infections (e.g., sexually transmitted disease), ectopic pregnancy, or other causes.[14]

Guidelines and/or Position Statements

As of this writing, there are no national clinical practice guidelines for the management of primary dysmenorrhea from U.S.-based organizations or professional groups. The Society of Obstetricians and Gynaecologists of Canada (SOGC) has published a consensus guideline on primary dysmenorrhea (available at http://sogc.medical.org/guidelines/index_e.asp#Gynaecology).[19] For the management of secondary dysmenorrhea, guidelines are available for the specific underlying pathology. For example, the American College of Obstetricians and Gynecologists (ACOG) has published guidelines on the medical management of endometriosis.[20] Guidelines for the management of chronic pelvic pain are available from both SOGC and ACOG.[21,22]

Treatment

The therapeutic goals of treating primary dysmenorrhea are to provide symptomatic relief from the pelvic pain and associated symptoms, reduce lost school and work productivity, return the patient to normal activity, and improve her quality of life. The therapeutic goals for treating secondary dysmenorrhea are the same except that the primary treatment goal is to correct the underlying pathophysiology. An algorithm for the general management of dysmenorrhea is provided in Figure 12-2.

NONPHARMACOLOGIC THERAPY

Nonpharmacologic treatment modalities studied for the pain management of primary or secondary dysmenorrhea include continuous, low-level topical heat, transcutaneous electrical nerve stimulation (TENS), and behavioral intervention. The most effective method of these three appears to be topical heat therapy (heating pad, heating patch, or hot water bottle) applied to the painful suprapubic areas. Anecdotally, this is a popular method with patients because of its ease of use and availability. Two randomized, placebo-controlled trials have been conducted using abdominal heat patch or wrap (heated to approximately 40° C [104° F] and worn for either 8 or 12 hours daily from the start of menses) in women with primary dysmenorrhea.[23,24] In the first trial, topical heat therapy (worn as a patch for 12 hours a day) was found to be more effective for pain relief than placebo and as effective as ibuprofen. However, using a heated patch plus ibuprofen did not lead to greater pain relief compared with using ibuprofen alone, although the time to pain relief was approximately 1.3 hours shorter ($p = 0.01$) with the combination compared with ibuprofen alone.[23] In the second study, conducted by the same group of researchers, a heated wrap worn for 8 hours a day provided better pain relief than acetaminophen.[24] Adverse events with heat therapy included mild skin redness that resolved upon removing the heat patch or wrap. TENS is a treatment method that involves applying electrical current at different frequencies to the skin to provide pain relief. It has been studied in a number of acute and chronic painful conditions, including postoperative pain, osteoarthritis, and labor pain. In the management of dysmenorrhea, TENS is thought to provide pain relief by increasing the threshold by which pain signals from the uterus is perceived and by stimulating endorphin release.[9] A Cochrane systematic review found that high-frequency, but not low-frequency, TENS was more effective at pain relief in primary dysmenorrhea than placebo TENS.[25] Adverse effects of high-frequency TENS included muscle tightness and vibration, headaches, and slight redness or burning of the skin. The review concluded that "TENS represents a suitable alternative for women who prefer not to use medication, or wish to minimize their NSAID consumption."[25] A recent Cochrane review of behavioral interventions (using relaxation training, relaxation and biofeedback training, biofeedback with electromyography training, or pain management training) concluded that although there are some data to demonstrate pain reduction with these methods, the evidence is not conclusive given the lower methodological quality of the trials.[26]

PHARMACOLOGIC THERAPY

Pharmacologic therapy is the mainstay for the management of primary dysmenorrhea. NSAIDs are considered by many to be the first-line treatment. NSAIDs are commonly prescribed for primary dysmenorrhea because of their demonstrated efficacy and ability to provide rapid pain relief on a short-term basis. Oral contraceptives also have established efficacy for primary dysmenorrhea and can be another option in patients who are not actively trying

Figure 12-2. Management of dysmenorrhea. Adapted and reprinted with permission from reference 9.

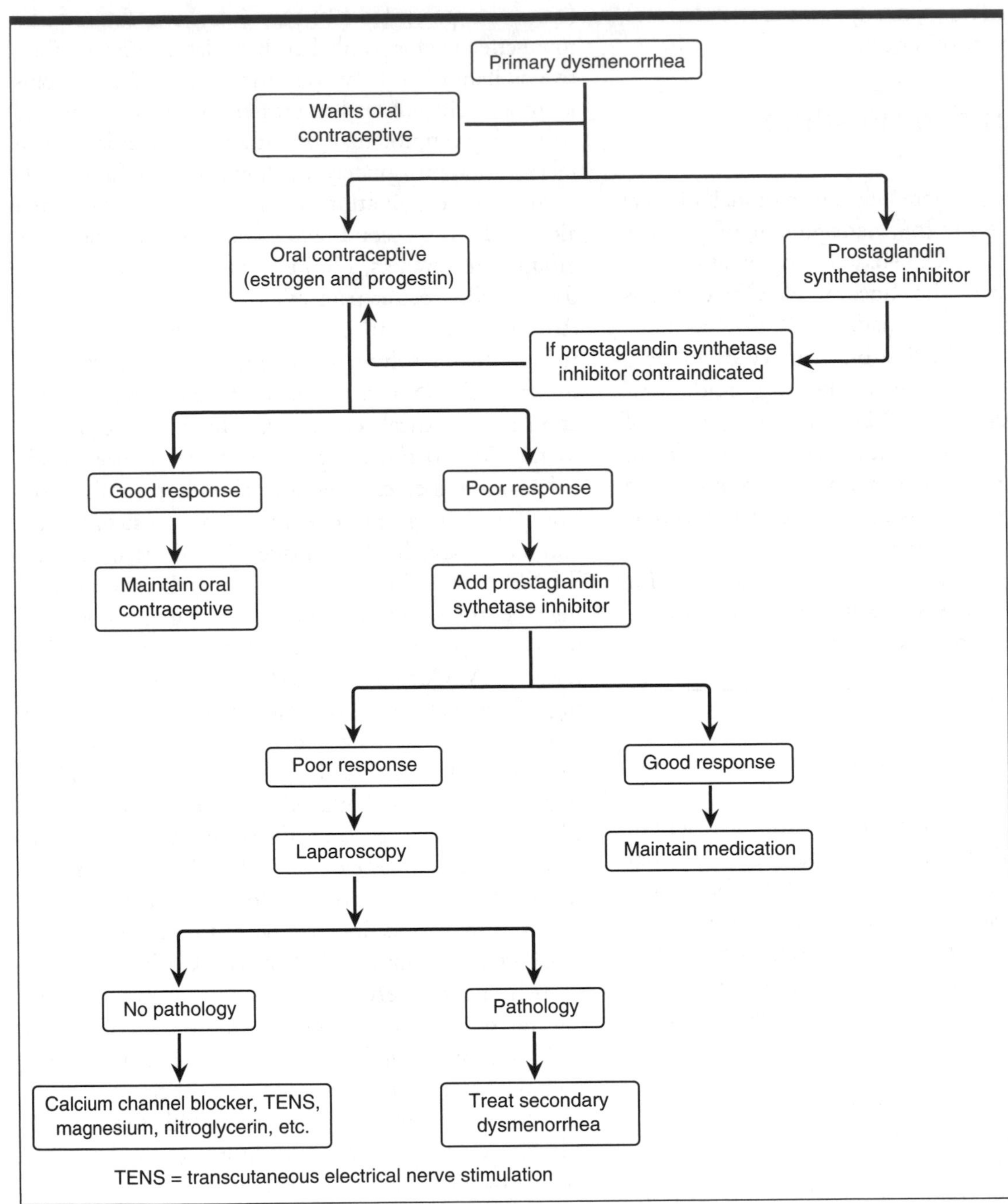

to conceive. To date, studies comparing NSAIDs to oral contraceptives have not been reported.

Nonsteroidal Anti-Inflammatory Drugs

Nonselective NSAIDs inhibit both COX-1 and -2, the enzymes responsible for prostaglandins production, and therefore reduce prostaglandins concentrations throughout the body. NSAIDs have been shown to decrease concentrations of $PGF_{2\alpha}$ in menstrual fluids.[14] Thus, this drug class treats the principal pathophysiology of primary dysmenorrhea. There is extensive evidence for the efficacy of NSAIDs in alleviating the pain of primary dysmenorrhea, starting with clinical trials in the late 1970s. A Cochrane meta-analysis found 63 randomized, placebo-controlled trials and concluded that NSAIDs are significantly more effective than placebo in providing moderate to excellent pain relief.[27] There are no definitive data to show superiority of one nonselective NSAID over another, and, given the mechanism of action, the efficacy is likely a class effect.[27] NSAIDs that are selective COX-2 inhibitors have also been shown to be more effective than placebo—and equally effective as nonselective NSAIDs—in providing pain relief, but because of cardiovascular side effects, only celecoxib is still available on the U.S. market.[28-31] Although a number of significant adverse drug reactions can result from NSAID therapy, the incidence is expected to be low when used only for brief periods in a relatively young and healthy population, such as those with primary dysmenorrhea. The choice of which NSAID to use may be based on the prescriber's experience, the patient's previous experience (efficacy or lack of efficacy) with a particular NSAID, the onset of therapeutic effect, dosing frequency, possibility for adverse reactions, cost, and availability in nonprescription preparations. For optimal efficacy, the NSAID should be taken at the beginning of each cycle and continued on an around-the-clock basis during the first 2–3 days of menses. Table 12-2 lists the characteristics for the most commonly used NSAIDs.

Hormonal Contraceptives

Four types of hormonal contraceptives are available to treat dysmenorrhea: combined (estrogen plus progestin or estrogen plus drospirenone) oral contraceptive, extended-cycle oral contraceptive, depot medroxyprogesterone acetate (DMPA), and the levonorgestrel intrauterine device (LNG-IUD). Regardless of type, all hormonal contraceptives provide pain relief in dysmenorrhea by inhibiting ovulation and decreasing the thickness of the endometrium, thus reducing the endometrial production of prostaglandins as well as menstrual fluid volume. Oral contraceptives have been shown to decrease concentrations of prostaglandins and leukotrienes in menstrual fluid as well as uterine contractility.[32-34] A 2001 Cochrane systematic review concluded that although oral contraceptives with medium-dose estrogen (>35 mcg) were more effective than placebo in providing pain relief in primary dysmenorrhea in several studies, the quality of evidence is weak.[35] However, since then, several randomized, clinical trials have been published that demonstrate pain relief with low-dose (<35 mcg of estrogen) combined oral contraceptives.[36-38] As with NSAID therapy, the side-effect profile of estrogen and progestin combination therapy (Table 12-2) should be carefully considered when selecting appropriate candidates for this therapeutic strategy. Extended-cycle oral contraceptives have not been specifically studied for the management of primary dysmenorrhea, but an observational study reported that significantly more women who used a combined oral contraceptive continuously for 42 to 126 days experienced a reduction in dysmenorrhea compared with women who used the same oral contraceptive on a 21-day cycle. The oral contraceptive used consisted of 30 mcg ethinyl estradiol and 3 mg drospirenone.[39] One study with extended-cycle oral contraceptive in secondary dysmenorrhea has been published. In this study, women with dysmenorrhea from endometriosis experienced significant pain relief with continuous use of a low-dose, monophasic oral contraceptive during the 2 years of therapy.[40]

The majority of efficacy evidence with hormonal contraceptives is with daily oral contraceptives, but several other forms have also been studied. These include the LNG-IUD (Mirena®) and the injectable long-acting DMPA (Depo-Provera®). The mechanism of pain relief with both of these contraceptive methods is thought to be due to **amenorrhea**, a common side effect of therapy. An observational study in women who used the LNG-IUD reported that the percentage of women who experienced menstrual pain decreased from 60% before use to 29% after 36 months of use, and amenorrhea was experienced in 47% of women.[41] In a small trial, women who had the LNG-IUD inserted after laparoscopic treatment of endometriosis lesions experienced a lower rate of moderate or severe dysmenorrhea compared with those who received the surgical treatment only.[42] Use of DMPA has been reported to decrease primary and secondary (endometriosis-related) dysmenorrhea.[43,44] However, no randomized, placebo-controlled clinical trials have been published. The use of DMPA in adolescent and young adult women is also complicated by the fact that the drug decreases bone mineral density, and use for more than 2 years is generally not recommended.[45] Research is needed regarding the efficacy of both of these forms of hormonal contraceptives, extended-cycle oral contraceptives, and non-oral forms of contraceptives (such as the transdermal patch, intravaginal ring, and intradermal implants) in both primary and secondary dysmenorrhea.

Table 12-2. Pharmacologic Treatments of Primary Dysmenorrhea

Drug or Drug Class	Mechanism of Action in Dysmenorrhea	Usual Dosage	Contraindications[a]	Common and/or Major Adverse Reactions
First-line				
Nonsteroidal anti-inflammatory drugs (NSAIDs)	Inhibit cyclooxygenase thereby decreasing prostaglandin concentrations	Best efficacy if taken around-the-clock for the first 48 hr of each menstrual cycle and with an initial loading dose	Patients who have experienced asthma, urticaria, or allergic-type reactions after taking aspirin or other NSAIDs Treatment of peri-operative pain in the setting of coronary artery bypass graft surgery	Gastrointestinal (black box warning): Dyspepsia, ulcer, perforation, and bleeding Cardiovascular (black box warning): Increased blood pressure, thrombotic events, myocardial infarction, stroke Renal: Sodium and water retention, renal failure Hepatic: Transaminase elevations, liver failure (rare) Rare serious skin side effects including rash, exfoliative dermatitis, Stevens-Johnson syndrome, and toxic epidermal necrolysis Pregnancy category D in third trimester (premature closure of ductus arteriosus)
• Ibuprofen[b]		400–800 mg PO 3–4 times daily, max 3,200 mg/day		
• Ketoprofen		25–50 mg PO 3–4 times daily, max 300 mg/day		
• Meclofenamate sodium		100 mg 3 times daily, max 300 mg/day		
• Mefenamic acid		500 mg PO initially then 250–500 mg 4 times daily, max 1,000 mg/day		
• Naproxen[b]		500 mg PO initially then 250–500 mg twice daily, max 1,250 mg/day		
• Diclofenac		100 mg PO initially then 50 mg 3 times daily, max 150 mg/day		
• Celecoxib	Selectively inhibits cyclooxygenase-2 thereby decreasing prostaglandin concentrations	400 mg PO initially, followed by an additional 200 mg dose if needed on the first day; then 200 mg twice daily	Hypersensitivity to sulfonamides Patients who have experienced asthma, urticaria, or allergic-type reactions after taking aspirin or other NSAIDs Treatment of peri-operative pain in the setting of coronary artery bypass graft surgery	Gastrointestinal (black box warning): Dyspepsia, ulcer, perforation, and bleeding Cardiovascular (black box warning): Increased blood pressure, thrombotic events, myocardial infarction, stroke Renal: Sodium and water retention, renal failure Hepatic: Transaminase elevations, liver failure (rare) Rare serious skin side effects including rash, exfoliative dermatitis, Stevens-Johnson syndrome, and toxic epidermal necrolysis Pregnancy category D in third trimester (premature closure of ductus arteriosus)

(*Continued on next page*)

Drug or Drug Class	Mechanism of Action in Dysmenorrhea	Usual Dosage	Contraindications[a]	Common and/or Major Adverse Reactions
Oral combined contraceptive (estrogen + progestin or estrogen + drospirenone)	Inhibits secretions of gonadotropins thereby inhibiting ovulation and decreasing thickness of endometrium	One tablet PO once daily with 0–7 days off per month depending on formulation (doses of estrogen content vary from 20–50 mcg of ethinyl estradiol or 50 mcg of mestranol; doses of progestin component vary depending on the specific progestin used in each product; doses of drospirenone vary depending on the product)	Undiagnosed vaginal bleeding Active thrombophlebitis, or current or past history of thromboembolic disorders, or cerebral vascular disease Major surgery with prolonged immobilization Carcinoma of the endometrium or other known or suspected estrogen-dependent neoplasia Known or suspected breast malignancy Cerebrovascular or coronary artery disease Cholestatic jaundice of pregnancy or jaundice with prior hormonal contraceptive use Hepatic adenomas or carcinomas or active liver disease Diabetes with vascular involvement Headaches with focal neurological symptoms Uncontrolled hypertension Thrombogenic rhythm disorders or valvulopathies Smokers >35 yo Pregnancy Any conditions that predispose to hyperkalemia such as renal dysfunction or adrenal insufficiency (for drospirenone-containing formulations)	Increased blood pressure Nausea Headache Increased blood pressure Weight gain Fluid retention Thromboembolic event Hyperkalemia (with drospirenone-containing contraceptives)
Second-line				
Depot medroxyprogesterone acetate (DMPA)	Inhibits secretions of gonadotropins thereby inhibiting ovulation and decreasing thickness of endometrium	One injection (150 mg intramuscularly or 104 mg subcutaneously) every 13 wk	Pregnancy Undiagnosed vaginal bleeding Known or suspected malignancy of breast Active thrombophlebitis, or current or past history of thromboembolic disorders, or cerebral vascular disease Significant liver disease	Menstrual irregularities (primarily amenorrhea) Decreased bone mineral density (black box warning) that is greater with longer duration of use and may not be reversible, use for >2 yr only if other methods are not adequate Weight gain Fluid retention

(*Continued on next page*)

Drug or Drug Class	Mechanism of Action in Dysmenorrhea	Usual Dosage	Contraindications[a]	Common and/or Major Adverse Reactions
Levonorgestrel-releasing intrauterine device (Mirena)	Inhibits secretions of gonadotropins thereby inhibiting ovulation and decreasing thickness of endometrium	52 mg levonorgestrel, inserted intrauterine; removed after 5 yr	Pregnancy Known or suspected carcinoma of the breast History of ectopic pregnancy or condition that would predispose to ectopic pregnancy Congenital or acquired uterine anomaly including fibroids if they distort the uterine cavity Acute pelvic inflammatory disease (PID) or a history of PID unless there has been a subsequent intrauterine pregnancy Postpartum endometritis or infected abortion in the past 3 mo Known or suspected uterine or cervical neoplasia or unresolved, abnormal Pap smear Genital bleeding of unknown etiology Untreated acute cervicitis or vaginitis, including bacterial vaginosis or other lower genital tract infections until infection is controlled Acute liver disease or liver tumor (benign or malignant) Woman or her partner has multiple sexual partners Conditions associated with increased susceptibility to infections with microorganisms (e.g., leukemia, acquired immune deficiency syndrome [AIDS], and intravenous drug abuse) Genital actinomycosis	Cramps, dizziness, or faintness during insertion Menstrual irregularities (primarily amenorrhea, also spotting and bleeding in between menstrual periods or heavier menstrual flow) Pelvic inflammatory disease Life-threatening infection within the first few days after insertion (rare) Perforation of uterus Expulsion Ovarian cyst

[a]In addition to hypersensitivity to the drug or any of its ingredients.
[b]Also available without a prescription.

Other Pharmacologic Agents

Several other medications have been investigated for the treatment of primary dysmenorrhea. Both aspirin and acetaminophen have been reported to decrease blood concentration of $PGF_{2\alpha}$.[46,47] Both have been demonstrated to be more effective than placebo in providing pain relief but less effective than NSAIDs.[46,48,49] Montelukast, a leukotriene receptor antagonist, taken immediately before the beginning of the menstrual cycle at the Food and Drug Administration–approved dose for asthma, was found to be no more effective than placebo for primary dysmenorrhea symptoms.[50] Two drugs that can relax uterine contractions have been studied for the management of primary dysmenorrhea. The calcium channel blocker nifedipine, given in small doses orally, has been found to produce pain relief in three small older studies but also led to transient facial flushing, increased heart rate, and headache.[51-53] Transdermal nitroglycerin patches (0.1 mg/hr) provided superior pain relief compared with placebo in one trial, but were less effective than diclofenac in another. [54,55] In both studies, the incidence of headache was significantly higher with the nitroglycerin-treated patients.[54,55] The side effects of both nifedipine and nitroglycerine limit their use to patients who have failed first- and second-line treatment options. Treatment options under investigation for primary dysmenorrhea include vitamin K acupuncture point injection, sildenafil, and various oral contraceptive formulations.[56]

DIETARY SUPPLEMENTS AND COMPLEMENTARY AND ALTERNATIVE MEDICINE

Many complementary and alternative medicinal treatment strategies and preparations have been promoted and studied for the treatment of the pain of dysmenorrhea but most lack concrete clinical evidence in the form of randomized clinical trials. A 2001 Cochrane systematic review of herbal and dietary therapies for primary and secondary dysmenorrhea concluded that vitamin B_1 (thiamine) and magnesium, based on a small number of clinical trials, appeared to be effective in reducing pain for patients with primary dysmenorrhea.[57] These findings were based on a short-term, large randomized clinical trial conducted in India with adolescent girls for vitamin B_1, and three small double-blinded clinical trials for magnesium; the authors recommended that more research is needed.[57,58] The dosage of vitamin B_1 used was 100 mg per day for 90 days, but the magnesium dosage and duration varied among the studies. For vitamin B_6, vitamin E, omega-3 fatty acids, or a Japanese herbal preparation called Tokishakuyaku-san, the Cochrane review found only one small randomized clinical trial, for each agent, that investigated their efficacy. Although each study reported that the respective agent was more effective than placebo for pain relief, the sum of evidence is insufficient to recommend any of these treatment strategies.[57] Since this review, two additional clinical trials, both conducted in adolescent girls with primary dysmenorrhea in Iran by the same lead researcher, have been published that reported a significant reduction in pain severity with vitamin E.[59,60] The dosages used were 400 and 500 units of vitamin E per day, starting two days before the start of menses and continuing through the first 3 days of the cycle.[59,60] However, it should be noted that two major meta-analyses of clinical trials with vitamin E conducted in a variety of patient populations concluded that vitamin E supplementation is associated with an increased risk of all-cause mortality.[61,62] Most of the studies included in these meta-analyses were conducted in patients with chronic illnesses, and the findings may not apply to healthy, young women. Nonetheless, increased cardiovascular risk is a concern and should be considered before prescribing vitamin E. A number of case reports published in a journal on traditional Chinese medicine and four small placebo-controlled trials have reported that acupuncture is effective in the treatment of primary or secondary dysmenorrhea.[63-71] One of the placebo-controlled trials, a well-designed study conducted in the U.S., reported a significant reduction in pain in the acupuncture treatment group compared with the sham acupuncture or control groups.[69] Likewise, acupressure has been reported—in four clinical trials conducted in Asia and Iran—to be effective at reducing the pain of primary dysmenorrhea.[72-75] A variety of acupressure methods were used. Manipulation of the lower spine (spinal manipulation) using chiropractic or osteopathic techniques has not been found to be effective for either primary or secondary dysmenorrhea.[76] Overall, there are very limited data to recommend any complementary and alternative medicine pain treatment strategy for either primary or secondary dysmenorrhea, but the data do show promise for the use of vitamin B1, magnesium, acupuncture, and acupressure for pain relief in primary dysmenorrhea. More research is needed regarding exact therapeutic dosing and efficacy, any potential harm of therapy, and in a wider range of patient populations.

SURGERY

The use of NSAIDs and oral contraceptives for the management of primary dysmenorrhea has been reported to be associated with a 20% to 25% failure

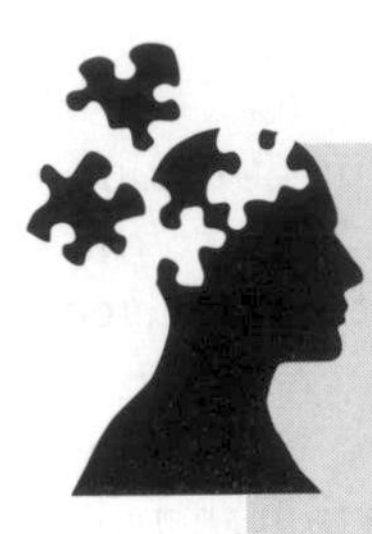

Therapeutic Challenge:

What are the treatment options for patients with primary dysmenorrhea who are not ideal candidates for either NSAIDs or hormonal contraceptives?

rate.[77] In patients who experience treatment-resistant dysmenorrhea, there are two methods of surgical interventions available: laparoscopic uterosacral nerve ablation (LUNA) and presacral neurectomy (PSN). These methods consist of the division (LUNA) or removal (PSN) of nerve fibers near the cervix to reduce uterine pain.[77] A systematic review has been conducted to evaluate the efficacy of both types of surgery.[77] In the treatment of primary dysmenorrhea, LUNA was found to be more effective at providing pain relief than control or no treatment, but PSN was more effective than LUNA. In the treatment of endometriosis, PSN combined with surgery was determined to be more effective than endometriosis surgery alone, whereas LUNA combined with endometriosis surgery did not yield additional pain relief than endometriosis surgical treatment alone. The trials that were evaluated in the systematic review were small and of varying quality. Adverse events reported with LUNA include a decrease in efficacy over time that may be due to regrowth of nerve fibers or rerouting of pain signals, risk of uterine prolapse or bladder dysfunction, and painless pregnancy labor that is due to nerve disruption. Adverse events associated with PSN include constipation, bladder dysfunction, and painless labor. Therefore, the authors of the review recommended that these surgical procedures should only be considered as last-resort treatment options.[78]

SECONDARY DYSMENORRHEA

Most of the above discussion of treatment modalities focused on primary dysmenorrhea. The treatment of secondary dysmenorrhea is more complex, as the treatment options depend on the underlying pathology. Although hormonal contraceptives can lead to pain relief in some patients with secondary dysmenorrhea, the underlying conditions that lead to it, such as endometriosis, should be carefully evaluated and treated by the appropriate gynecologic specialists. See other chapters in this textbook for detailed discussions regarding treatments for endometriosis (Chapter 14: Endometriosis, Chapter 44: Endometrial Cancer, Chapter 45: Ovarian Cancer, and Chapter 46: Cervical Cancer.)

Monitoring and Follow-up

Women treated for primary dysmenorrhea should be monitored for the efficacy of the treatment method to achieve resolution of symptoms and return of daily functioning. Treatment with either NSAIDs or oral contraceptive therapy is recommended for at least three menstrual cycles before changing therapy to another treatment modality if no or inadequate efficacy is experienced.[13] Use of combination therapy has not been studied but may be a reasonable option, especially with the use of adjunctive nonpharmacologic methods, such as topical heat. Monitoring for adverse events must also be performed. Patients who do not respond to NSAIDs or hormonal contraceptive therapy should be evaluated for secondary dysmenorrhea or an organic cause of pelvic pain.

Patient Education

Patients should be counseled on the best way to take pharmacologic therapy to achieve the best therapeutic effect and minimize potential side effects. When treating primary dysmenorrhea, the following patient counseling points should be kept in mind:

- Patients taking NSAIDs should be advised to start therapy at the first day of menses and continue therapy on a scheduled—instead of as-needed—basis for the first 48–72 hours of menstruation, until symptoms subside.
- Patients taking NSAIDs should be advised to take the medication with food to minimize gastrointestinal upset.
- Patients should be aware of the use of adjunctive nonpharmacologic treatments, such as continuous, low-level topical heat therapy and TENS. These treatment strategies may enable reduced use of pharmacologic agents or can be used as alternatives if the pharmacologic agents are contraindicated or not tolerated.
- All patients using pharmacologic therapy should be educated on possible adverse drug reactions and how to monitor for these reactions.

CASE PRESENTATION

Patient Case: Part 2

T.F.'s clinical presentation (symptoms, history of pain onset with the start of menarche, and absence of pelvic pathology on physical exam) is consistent with primary dysmenorrhea. She is prescribed naproxen, to take 500 mg orally starting on the first day of menses each month, then 250–500 mg twice daily (up to a maximum of 1,250 mg per day) on an around-the-clock basis for the duration of the cramping, which she reported as typically lasting for the first 48 hours after onset of menstruation. An NSAID is an appropriate first-line treatment, and this patient does not have any contraindication to its use. Naproxen, available in nonprescription form, was selected because of its rapid onset and long duration of action, enabling twice daily dosing. She was counseled to take naproxen with food to minimize gastrointestinal upset and will be monitored for possible adverse effects (see Table 12-2). T.F. is also advised to use topical heat (a heating pad or heating patches) in combination with the naproxen if needed. She was counseled on the possible benefits of smoking cessation as an additional mean of achieving pain relief. T.F. was scheduled for a follow-up in the student health clinic in 6 weeks, after which she will have experienced another menstrual period and can report on the efficacy of the prescribed treatments. Dosing and frequency of the naproxen can be adjusted, and another NSAID may be tried if T.F. does not respond to naproxen. A low-dose combined oral contraceptive is another option if T.F. does not respond to NSAID therapy.

Summary

Dysmenorrhea is a common gynecologic symptom in women that may lead to significant morbidity yet is under-reported and underdiagnosed. Evaluation of patients presenting with dysmenorrhea should aim to differentiate between primary and secondary dysmenorrhea in order to determine the most optimal management strategy. Treatment options for primary dysmenorrhea include NSAIDs and oral contraceptives. Other forms of hormonal contraceptives and dietary supplements, such as vitamin B1, may be considered, although there is limited evidence regarding their efficacy. Nonpharmacologic treatments, including topical heat therapy and TENS, may be useful as adjunctive therapy in selected patients. The management of secondary dysmenorrhea depends on the underlying pathology and should be determined in consultation with gynecology specialists.

References

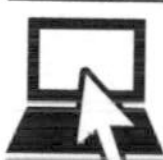

Additional content available at
www.ashp.org/womenshealth

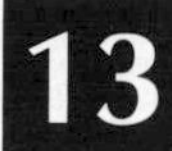

13 Premenstrual Syndrome and Premenstrual Dysphoric Disorder

Teresa M. Bailey, Pharm.D., BCPS, FCCP; Nicole S. Culhane, Pharm.D., BCPS, FCCP

Learning Objectives

1. Identify the signs and symptoms associated with PMS and PMDD.
2. Explain the pathophysiologic theories associated with PMS and PMDD.
3. List criteria used for the diagnosis of PMS and PMDD.
4. Recommend nonpharmacologic and pharmacologic therapy for PMS and PMDD.
5. Monitor treatment of PMS and PMDD for efficacy and toxicity.

In 1931, Robert Frank introduced the term *premenstrual tension* to describe 15 women with a menstrual cyclic occurrence of negative symptoms that disappeared shortly after the onset of menstruation. *Premenstrual tension* was used until the 1950s, when Greene and Dalton broadened the definition to *premenstrual syndrome* (PMS).[1,2] In 1994, the *Diagnostic and Statistical Manual of Mental Disorders, 4th Edition (DSM-IV)* included the term *premenstrual dysphoric disorder* (PMDD).[2]

Although there are no universally accepted definitions for PMS or PMDD, various organizations, such as the World Health Organization (WHO), the American College of Obstetricians and Gynecologists (ACOG), and the American Psychiatric Association (APA), have published definitions. The WHO International Classification of Diseases (ICD) uses ICD-9 code 625.4 for premenstrual tension or premenstrual syndrome and lists PMS and PMDD under this heading. The WHO definition of premenstrual tension syndrome is an unspecified severity of tension, any headache, and/or **molimen** that occurs premenstrually and remits following menses. The WHO definition has no separate diagnostic code for PMS or PMDD. ACOG defines PMS as having at least one related symptom associated with an identifiable dysfunction in social or economic performance that occurs 5 days before menses and remits within 4 days of the onset of menses. The *DSM-IV* defines PMDD as having at least five symptoms, with at least one being depression, anxiety, tension, anger or irritability, or mood swings occurring during the last week before menses and remitting within the few days after the onset of menses. *DSM-IV* criteria states that PMDD is associated with marked interference with work, social activities, or relationships during the past year as compared with PMS.

In general, PMS is the condition that occurs regularly during the luteal phase of the menstrual cycle and disappears during the follicular phase. Symptoms usually start 5–7 days before the onset of menses but may start as early as 12–14 days before menses. Symptoms usually disappear shortly after the onset of menses. The symptoms may be physical, cognitive, emotional, behavioral, or a combination of these.[2] Symptoms may begin any time after menarche and typically increase with age, with women older than age of 30 seeking treatment. The symptoms generally remit after menopause, during pregnancy, or with any other discontinuation of the ovulatory cycle.[2] PMS may be classified as mild, moderate, or severe, and the term *PMDD* generally refers to severe PMS with functional or psychological impairment.[3] PMDD

CASE PRESENTATION

Patient Case: Part 1

Z.Z. is a 32-year-old woman who presents to clinic reporting irritability, crying, mood swings, and fatigue for the past 6 months. She is under more stress since she started a new job 8 months ago. On questioning, Z.Z. states her symptoms seem to "wax and wane" but do not correlate with her menses. She also has breast tenderness approximately 1 week before the start of menses that resolves within 2 days after the start of menses. She has tried a variety of OTC products—such as ibuprofen, black cohosh, and chasteberry—with some relief but still continues to miss work 2–3 days/mo.

PMH: Occasional headaches.

Family history: Mother—migraines; father—hypertension.

Social history: No tobacco, occasional alcohol, walks 30 minutes 3 times/week.

Medications: Ibuprofen one to two tablets as needed for headaches, spermicide with condom for contraception, multivitamin daily, black cohosh and chasteberry daily, calcium with vitamin D daily.

Allergies: NKDA.

Vitals: 5′3″, 124 lb (BMI 22 kg/m^2), BP 124/81, HR 74, Temp 98.6 F, RR 18.

Physical exam: Normal.

Laboratory values: Significant findings include TSH 3.0, WBC 8.0, Hgb 12.0, Hct 36, Plt 350.

Mammogram: Normal.

Pap and pelvic exam: Normal.

relates to severe negative physiological and emotional changes that cause functional impairment during the late luteal phase of the menstrual cycle (approximately days 21–28). When a women suffers not only from somatic symptoms but also mental symptoms severe enough to significantly interfere with social functioning, the diagnosis of PMDD vs. PMS is made.[4]

Both PMS and PMDD are under-recognized and underdiagnosed disorders. It is estimated that 70% to 90% of menstruating women experience some PMS symptoms, whereas the adolescent prevalence of PMS symptoms is estimated to be 51% to 86%.[5,6] According to *DSM-IV*, 3% to 8% of all reproductive age women meet the criteria for PMDD.[5-7] In women 14–24 years old, 5.8% have met the *DSM-IV* criteria for PMDD, and in 36- to 44-year-old women, 6.4% have met the criteria.[5-8] The prevalence of PMS and PMDD is consistent in European countries, the U.S., India, Israel, and China.[7]

Premenstrual impairment may be more severe at home compared with out-of-home occupational and social activities.[7] However, 8% to 16% of women missed work because of PMS in the past year, and of those, 5% to 8% missed more than 14 work days.[9]

PMDD is viewed as a psychiatric and medical syndrome rather than an exacerbation of an underlying psychiatric disorder. It should be noted that depression, bipolar disorder, panic disorder, generalized anxiety disorder, and attention deficit disorder may be exacerbated during the late luteal phase of some women's menstrual cycles.[5] However, the main difference is that women with PMDD will usually be symptom-free except in the luteal phase.

Some suggested risk factors for PMS and PMDD include advancing age, psychosocial factors, and genetic factors. Advancing age (beyond 30 years) has been a suggested risk factor. Older women are more likely and more comfortable reporting and seeking treatment for these symptoms; however, studies have not consistently supported age as a risk factor. There are conflicting data associated with menstrual cycle length and symptom severity.[10] Low parity or women with fewer pregnancies may have a higher incidence of PMDD.[10] Genetic factors may influence the incidence of PMS and PMDD. Studies infer that women whose mothers report PMS (70%) are more likely to develop PMS compared with daughters of unaffected mothers (37%). Studies suggest an inheritable component with an incidence of monozygotic twins (93%) compared with dizygotic twins (44%) and nontwin sisters (31%).[11] However, no actual gene abnormalities have been demonstrated. No difference in personality profile or level of stress has been correlated to the incidence of PMS and PMDD. However, traumatic or major life events and stressors may increase the odds of developing PMDD.[5,10] Seventy percent of women with PMDD also have a history of mood disorders, anxiety disorders, personality disorders, or substance abuse.[10]

Clinical Presentation

At least 200 different premenstrual symptoms have been reported by PMS patients. However, only some of the symptoms are routinely assessed and identified. PMS shares many similar features with other conditions, except PMS is cyclic. As stated previously, symptoms usually start 5–7 days before the onset of menses and usually disappear after the onset of menses. Most common symptoms include tension, depression, bloating, **mastalgia,** headache, and irritability.[7] Symptoms may be further divided into physical (somatic) and psychological (affective). Physical symptoms may include weight gain, breast tenderness, menstrual irregularities, appetite changes, and fatigue. Psychological symptoms may include anxiety, depression, and irritability, with irritability being the most prominent. A more complete list of symptoms appears in Table 13-1.

Pathophysiology

Although the etiology of PMS and PMDD is still unknown, several biological theories exist, such as the involvement of serotonin, reproductive hormones, endogenous opiates, and the role of genetics. The most probable theory is the correlation between sex steroids and central neurotransmitters, primarily the involvement of serotonin.

It is widely accepted that ovarian function is normal among women with PMS and PMDD; however, hormonal fluctuations or exposure may trigger biochemical events to result in PMS and PMDD.[11] Premenstrual symptoms have been absent during menstrual cycles that are spontaneously anovulatory. Furthermore, suppression of ovulation and elimination of gonadal hormone fluctuation with gonadotropin-releasing hormone (GnRH) has relieved PMS symptoms. In addition, PMS and PMDD do not start before menarche or continue beyond menopause.[12] Estrogen, progesterone, and testosterone have also been found to increase serotonergic activity by increasing the number of serotonergic receptors, transport, and uptake. It is suggested that women with PMS and PMDD may be predisposed to an abnormal response of central neurotransmitters to normal ovarian function.[10,13] Therefore, normal declining levels of ovarian steroid hormones in the late luteal phase of the menstrual cycle may affect the brain and peripheral responses to central neurotransmitters, specifically serotonin, because a low central serotonin level is associated with impulsivity, irritability, dysphoria, and increased carbohydrate craving.[10]

Some data suggest that PMDD is related to a hormonal ratio imbalance instead of hormone fluctuation or exposure.[2] For example, when estrogen levels are high in relation to progesterone, PMDD may occur. Other studies have suggested that women with

Table 13-1. American College of Obstetricians and Gynecologists Diagnostic Criteria[18]

Patient reports one or more of the following affective or somatic symptoms during 5 days before menses in each of three prior menstrual cycles:

Affective

- Depression
- Angry outbursts
- Anxiety
- Irritability
- Confusion
- Social withdrawal

Somatic

- Breast tenderness
- Abdominal bloating
- Headache
- Swelling of extremities
- Symptoms relieved within 4 days of menses onset without recurrence until at least cycle day 13
- Symptoms present in absence of any pharmacologic therapy, hormone ingestion, drug or alcohol abuse, or other medical/psychiatric disorders
- Symptoms occur reproducibly during at least two cycles of prospective recording
- Patient experiences identifiable dysfunction in social or economic sphere

PMDD have normal levels of estrogen and progesterone but have an abnormal secretion pattern. Despite these theories, studies have confirmed normal blood levels of ovarian hormones in women regardless of the diagnosis of PMDD.[2] Therefore, the premenstrual symptoms may be independent of the amount of estrogen and progesterone produced by the ovaries, but dependent on how behaviorally or biochemically sensitive the brain is to these hormones.[4]

Decreases in gamma-aminobutyric acid (GABA) activity have been associated with anxiety and depression. Studies have reported low GABA levels and low GABA receptor sensitivity during the late luteal phase in women with PMS and PMDD.[2,10] Therefore, anxiolytics, specifically alprazolam, have been studied and may be beneficial.

Prolactin, growth hormone, thyroid hormone, luteinizing hormone, follicle-stimulating hormone, antidiuretic hormone, insulin, aldosterone, renin-angiotensin, or cortisol have not been associated with PMS and PMDD symptoms. In addition, PMS and PMDD do not appear to be related to vitamin or mineral deficiencies, specifically vitamin A, vitamin E, thiamine, magnesium, pyridoxine or zinc.[5,10]

Diagnosis

Universally accepted diagnostic criteria do not exist for PMS, and there are no definitive diagnostic tests or specific physical findings for either PMS or PMDD. Therefore, the diagnosis of PMS and PMDD is one of exclusion. Initially, a complete medical and psychological history should be performed to rule out underlying disorders such as personal or family psychological and medical disorders. A physical exam should be performed to rule out possible thyroid disease, breast disease, anemia, and pelvic abnormalities. Based on the physical exam and hematologic, hormonal, and chemistry levels, mammography or radiologic imaging may be indicated. Obtaining levels of any reproductive hormones, such as estradiol, progesterone, follicle-stimulating hormone, luteinizing hormone, or testosterone, may be useful to rule out other gynecologic disorders such as endometriosis, but not to diagnose PMS and PMDD.[3] Prospectively charting symptoms on a calendar or diary for three menstrual cycles may be useful to determine if the symptoms occur after ovulation and is recommended to confirm the diagnosis of PMS and PMDD.[14,15]

Validated questionnaires, such as the Premenstrual Experience Assessment (PEA) or the Premenstrual Assessment Form (PAF), may be beneficial to evaluate the severity at one or more points in time. Unfortunately, there is no consensus on the best assessment instrument. Many questionnaires exist, such as the Menstrual Distress Questionnaire (MDQ), the Rating Scale for Premenstrual Tension Syndrome (PMTS), the Calendar of Premenstrual Experiences (COPE), the Daily Record of Severity of Problems (DRSP), and the Premenstrual Symptoms Screening Tool (PSST). All questionnaires have patients rate their PMS symptom severity by either a Likert scale or a visual analog scale. Some questionnaires document prospectively (COPE, DRPS), whereas others document retrospectively (PSST). Some questionnaires assess PMS symptoms at one point in time (PMTS), whereas others assess symptoms daily (COPE, DSRP).[16] An example of a patient diary to prospectively record the frequency and severity of PMS symptoms is in Figure 13-1.

Differential diagnosis is necessary to rule out PMS symptoms that may be attributed to another cause, such as premenstrual exacerbation of a medical condition or psychiatric disorder. Other causes of symptoms similar to PMS may be psychiatric, medical, gynecologic, or psychosocial in nature. Table 13-2 includes a list of conditions that may be included in a differential diagnosis.[16]

AMERICAN COLLEGE OF OBSTETRICIANS AND GYNECOLOGISTS CRITERIA

According to ACOG, PMS is diagnosed if at least one of the affective or somatic symptoms is reported 5 days before the onset of menses in two prospective menstrual cycles. The symptoms must resolve within 4 days of onset of menses and not recur until after day 12 of the cycle. Affective symptoms include depression, angry outbursts, irritability, anxiety, confusion, and social withdrawal. Somatic symptoms consist of breast tenderness, abdominal bloating, headache, and swelling of extremities (Table 13-2).[17,18]

DIAGNOSTIC AND STATISTICAL MANUAL OF MENTAL HEALTH DISORDERS, 4TH EDITION CRITERIA

According to *DSM-IV-TR (text revision)*, PMDD is diagnosed when symptoms occur during the last week of the luteal phase of most menstrual cycles during the previous 12 months and remit within a few days after the onset of menstruation. The symptoms are always absent in the week following menses. A prospective confirmation is necessary for at least two consecutive months. Five of the 11 symptoms must be present, and one of the symptoms must be a primary symptom. There must be impairment of daily functioning in

Figure 13-1. Premenstrual daily symptom diary.

Name: ______________________________ Month: ______________

Write the date in the first row, starting with today. Circle the days of your menstrual period.

Each day, rate the severity of your symptoms: 1 = no symptoms; 2 = mild symptoms; 3 = moderate symptoms; 4 = severe symptoms.

Date																															
Day of the month	1	2	3	4	5	6	7	8	9	10	11	12	13	14	15	16	17	18	19	20	21	22	23	24	25	26	27	28	29	30	31
Irritability or tension																															
Anger or short temper																															
Anxiety or nervousness																															
Depression or sadness																															
Crying or tearfulness																															
Relationship problems																															
Tiredness or lack of energy																															
Insomnia																															
Changes in sexual interest																															
Food cravings or overeating																															
Difficulty concentrating																															
Feeling overwhelmed																															
Headaches																															
Breast tenderness or swelling																															
Back pain																															
Abdominal pain																															
Muscle and joint pain																															
Weight gain																															
Nausea																															
Other (please specify)																															
Other (please specify)																															

Source: Adapted and reprinted with permission from reference 22.

work, school, usual activities, or relationships with others during the luteal phase for the majority of the cycles in the previous year. The symptoms can not represent an exacerbation of another existing disorder.[5,15] (See Web Resources for Research Criteria for Premenstrual Dysphoric Disorder.)

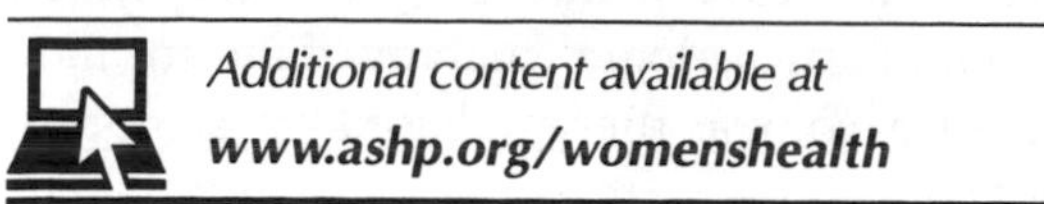

Additional content available at ***www.ashp.org/womenshealth***

Guidelines and Position Statements

The ACOG developed a practice guideline bulletin for the diagnosis, evaluation, and management and treatment of PMS in April 2000.[17] The guideline was the product of a systematic review intended to examine the evidence for treatments of PMS and to guide family practitioners, obstetricians, and gynecologists in making decisions regarding the management of women with PMS. The major outcome considered for

Table 13-2. Differential Diagnosis of Premenstrual Syndrome[5,22,61]

Allergies	Endometriosis
Anemia	Generalized anxiety disorder
Anorexia	Hypothyroidism
Autoimmune disorders	Oral contraceptives
Bipolar	Panic disorder
Bulimia	Perimenopause
Chronic fatigue syndrome	Personality disorder
Depression	Polycystic ovary syndrome
Diabetes	Seizure disorder
Dysmenorrhea	Somatoform disorder
Dysthymia	Substance abuse

the recommended treatments was an improvement in the symptoms of PMS. The ACOG supports a clinical diagnosis, including a complete medical and psychological history and physical examination, with prospective symptom charting to document the timing of symptoms, and recommends a stepwise approach to the management of PMS.

1. *Step 1:* Nonpharmacologic therapy, including behavioral therapy and aerobic exercise, should be used first line for premenstrual symptoms because of convenience and safety. These therapies are rated as Level C recommendations (recommendations based primarily on consensus and expert opinion). The use of dietary supplements, including calcium, magnesium, vitamin E, and vitamin B_6, are rated as Level B recommendations (recommendations based on limited or inconsistent scientific evidence), with the strongest evidence in support of the use of calcium supplements.
2. *Step 2:* Selective serotonin reuptake inhibitors (SSRIs)—including fluoxetine, sertraline, paroxetine, and fluvoxamine—and those medications with some norepinephrine reuptake inhibition, such as clomipramine, should be recommended as first-line pharmacologic therapy for the behavioral symptoms of PMS. These medications are rated as Level A recommendations (recommendations based on good and consistent scientific evidence). Anxiolytics such as alprazolam may be used for women who do not respond to SSRIs (Level B recommendation).
3. *Step 3:* Other Level B recommendations include hormonal ovulation suppression with the use of oral contraceptives, GnRH agonists, and surgical oophorectomy.

A limitation of this bulletin is that it refers to PMS and does not specifically address PMDD. In addition, although the guideline was developed 9 years ago, a review of the literature for this guideline is performed every 18–24 months and was still considered to be up to date as of December 2005. Although more recent evidence is available for some of the level B and C recommendations, the nonpharmacologic therapies and pharmacologic therapies that manage the behavioral as well as the physical symptoms remain first-line therapy for PMS and PMDD.[17]

Treatment

The primary goal for the treatment of PMS and PMDD is the resolution of or significant improvement in symptoms. Significant improvement is generally defined as at least a 50% improvement in symptoms.[19,20] According to studies, improvement in symptoms is generally seen within two to three menstrual cycles.[3,11,13,21] It is important to make certain that patients understand PMS and that they are educated regarding this time frame for symptom improvement and expectations of treatment. If pharmacologic therapy is necessary, the lowest possible dosage is recommended to minimize side effects, eliminate or reduce symptoms, and limit the impact on activities, daily functioning, and relationships.[19,22,23] Discussing these goals with patients is necessary to ensure therapeutic safety and efficacy of the management options.[23]

NONPHARMACOLOGIC THERAPY

Nonpharmacologic therapy for PMS has not been well studied in large, randomized trials, and there is limited evidence to support these recommendations. However, because of minimal side effects, patients should try lifestyle and behavioral modifications before and as an adjunct to pharmacologic therapy. Because it is recommended that patients chart their symptoms for at least two menstrual cycles, it is prudent to initiate these nonpharmacologic recommendations during this time. If PMS symptoms do not resolve or decrease within two to three cycles, continue nonpharmacologic therapy, but strongly consider pharmacologic therapy based on symptom severity.[20,24]

The most common nonpharmacologic interventions for PMS include dietary modifications and exercise. Dietary changes during the luteal phase include limiting the amount of sodium to minimize bloating and fluid retention, and limiting caffeine and alcohol to reduce irritability and insomnia.[20,24,25] Diets rich in complex carbohydrates, such as fruits, vegetables, grains, and cereals, have also demonstrated, in small studies, an improvement in mood symptoms such as depression, tension, anger, and confusion, possibly by increasing tryptophan levels, a precursor to serotonin.[10,19,24,25] Exercise, particularly aerobic, has demonstrated improvement in symptoms, possibly because of the release of endorphins, which are reduced in the late luteal phase of the menstrual cycle.[26] Other interventions that may improve symptoms simply by enhancing overall well-being include relaxation techniques, such as yoga and stress management. Patients are encouraged to schedule more stressful activities during the follicular phase of the menstrual cycle to decrease stress and minimize the effect that PMS symptoms have on daily functioning during symptomatic days of the luteal phase.[10,19] Regularly engaging in relaxation and coping skills, a structured sleep schedule, dietary restrictions, and exercise may prove to be quite beneficial for a patient with PMS.

Dietary Supplements

Dietary supplements, including calcium, magnesium, and vitamins (A, E, B_6), have been studied for the relief of the physical symptoms of PMS. For most dietary supplements, with the exception of calcium, data are limited, and studies have been conducted in relatively small numbers of patients.

Calcium at a dosage of 1,200 mg/day (600 mg twice daily) demonstrated in a well-designed clinical trial to significantly decrease emotional, behavioral, and physical symptoms of PMS in 48% of women over a 3-month period, compared with 30% of women taking placebo, and was well tolerated. More than 50% of women taking calcium had a >50% improvement, and 29% of women had a >75% improvement in symptoms. Calcium should be recommended to women because of the overall safety profile and added benefit for the prevention of osteoporosis.[17,27]

Reduced magnesium levels have been reported in women with PMS.[28] Magnesium in dosages of 200–400 mg daily has been shown to reduce symptoms of bloating and fluid retention over a 2-month period.[29] One small study demonstrated that 360 mg daily, administered during the luteal phase, decreased affective symptoms over a 2-month period.[28] However, a recent double-blind placebo-controlled study of magnesium infusion failed to demonstrate a statistically significant improvement in mood symptoms compared with placebo.[30] Magnesium is well tolerated, with diarrhea being the most common side effect. Because most women do not consume the recommended daily allowance of magnesium (280–300 mg) and because many multivitamins only contain 100 mg of magnesium or less, obtaining a magnesium level may identify whether a woman is magnesium deficient. At a minimum, recommending a daily multivitamin may be prudent for overall health maintenance and may help to alleviate PMS symptoms.[17]

There is limited evidence demonstrating benefit from vitamins for the treatment of PMS. Vitamin B_6 in dosages of 50–100 mg daily has been shown to moderately improve PMS symptoms and depression. Dosages should not exceed 100 mg daily because of the potential risk of peripheral neuropathy at higher dosages.[31] Vitamin E has been shown to improve affective and somatic symptoms, particularly anxiety and irritability, in a randomized, controlled trial of 400 International Units daily administered during the luteal phase.[17] However, vitamin A is not recommended because of the potential for toxicity and limited benefit.[22] The ACOG supports the use of vitamin E because of the potential benefit and minimal risk of harm.[17]

PHARMACOLOGIC THERAPY

Nonhormonal Therapies

Analgesics and Diuretics

Nonsteroidal anti-inflammatory drugs (NSAIDs), such as naproxen and mefanamic acid, and analgesics, such as acetaminophen, are generally used first line to relieve cramping associated with PMS. These medications are most commonly administered during the luteal phase and stopped 1–2 days after menses begins. They are available **over the counter (OTC)** and are well tolerated when taken within dosage recommendations. Educate patients to take NSAIDs with food to minimize risk of stomach upset. Spironolactone, an aldosterone antagonist, dosed 100 mg daily on days 15–28 is the only diuretic that has been shown to have some improvement on somatic and affective symptoms, such as bloating, fluid retention, and breast tenderness.[5,17] In a placebo-controlled study of luteal phase dosing, spironolactone significantly decreased somatic and negative symptoms and improved irritability, depressed mood,

Table 13-3. Medications Used in the Treatment of Premenstrual Syndrome/Premenstrual Dysphoric Disorder

Drug Class	Dosage	Select Side Effects	Role in Therapy
Treatment of PMS			
Calcium	600 mg BID	Constipation; generally well tolerated	Effective for physical and behavioral PMS symptoms and should be tried first line following nonpharmacologic therapy for mild symptoms
Magnesium	200–400 mg daily or 360 mg daily given 14 days before menses	Diarrhea; generally well tolerated	May be effective for PMS symptoms such as bloating and fluid retention and may be tried following nonpharmacologic therapy
Vitamin B_6	50–100 mg daily	Peripheral neuropathy at dosages >100 mg daily	
Vitamin E	400 International Units daily	Generally well tolerated	
NSAIDs		GI upset, nausea, renal dysfunction	Effective at relieving PMS symptoms, such as cramping, headache; should use before initiating prescription medications for mild symptoms
Diuretics Spironolactone	100 mg daily days 15–28	Hyperkalemia; monitor periodically	Effective at reducing PMS symptoms of bloating and breast tenderness; may be used before antidepressants for mild symptoms
Treatment of PMDD			
Antidepressants[a]			
Fluoxetine[b]	10–20 mg	Sexual dysfunction, sleep disturbances (insomnia or drowsiness), nervousness, GI upset, headache	Used first line for PMDD
Sertraline[b]	50–150 mg		
Paroxetine	10–30 mg; 12.5–25 mg CR[b]		
Citalopram	20–40 mg		
Escitalopram	10–20 mg		
Venlafaxine	75–112 mg dosed during the luteal phase or 50–200 mg daily	Headache, potential increase in BP	Second line for PMDD in patients who fail, cannot tolerate, or have contraindications to treatment with SSRIs; recommend before trying other second-line therapies. such as clomipramine or alprazolam, because of more tolerable side-effect profile
Clomipramine	25–75 mg	Blurred vision, dry mouth, constipation, fatigue, headache	Second line for PMDD in patients who fail, cannot tolerate, or have contraindications to treatment with SSRIs because of bothersome side effects

(*Continued on next page*)

Drug Class	Dosage	Select Side Effects	Role in Therapy
Anxiolytics Alprazolam	0.25–1.0 mg TID–QID 6 to 14 days before menses	Sedation, drowsiness	Second line for PMDD in patients who fail, cannot tolerate, or have contraindications to treatment with SSRIs and clomipramine because of potential for addiction
Oral Contraceptives[b] (Ethinyl estradiol 20 mcg/ drospirenone 3 mg)	One tablet daily for 24 days	Nausea, breakthrough bleeding, breast tenderness, mild bloating but generally less than other combinations OCs, potential hyperkalemia (drospirenone 3 mg has similar side effects as 25 mg of spironolactone)	May be used second line for PMDD in patients requesting or requiring contraception and/or before initiating other second-line therapies (clomipramine/ alprazolam)
GnRH agonists Danazol	100–200 mg twice daily	Weight gain, deepening voice, hot flashes, night sweats, atrophic vaginitis, osteoporosis	Third-line therapy for PMDD; reserved for patients with severe PMDD or refractory to other therapies because of cost and side effects
Leuprolide	3.75–7.5 mg IM monthly		

Source: Adapted from references 17, 22, 23, and 46.

BID = twice daily; BP = blood pressure; CR = controlled release; GI = gastrointestinal; GnRH = gonadotropin-releasing hormone; IM = intramuscularly; NSAIDs = nonsteroidal anti-inflammatory drugs; OCs = oral contraceptives; PMDD = premenstrual dysphoric disorder; PMS = premenstrual syndrome; QID = 4 times daily; SSRIs = selective serotonin reuptake inhibitors; TID = 3 times daily.

[a]May be dosed daily or during luteal phase only.
[b]FDA approved.

swelling, breast tenderness, and food cravings.[32] This medication is generally well tolerated and safe at recommended dosages, but potassium levels should be monitored periodically during treatment because of the potential for hyperkalemia (Table 13-3).

Antidepressants

SSRIs are the most common and widely used medications for the treatment of PMDD. Several randomized, controlled trials have demonstrated significant improvements in both physical symptoms and mood with daily dosing as well as luteal phase dosing.[33-41] To date, only three SSRIs—fluoxetine, sertraline, and paroxetine CR—are U.S. Food and Drug Administration (FDA) approved for the treatment of PMDD, with fluoxetine and sertraline having the most supporting data. Fluvoxamine has been studied the least of all of the SSRIs and is generally not recommended. Venlafaxine, a serotonin and norepinephrine reuptake inhibitor, and clomipramine, a norepinephrine reuptake inhibitor, have also demonstrated in small studies to be effective at improving physical and behavioral symptoms.[42-44] All of the antidepressants may be dosed daily or intermittently during the luteal phase. Luteal phase dosing may be more convenient for patients, will minimize side effects, and may increase adherence. Higher dosages have not been shown to be significantly more effective than lower dosages. Thus, the lowest dosage should be administered during days 14–28 of the menstrual cycle. Symptoms generally start to improve within 24–48 hours but may take up to three menstrual cycles to see significant improvements.[5,24] Patients who fail one SSRI may try another SSRI before switching to a second-line therapy.[45,46] One of the most common side effects of SSRIs is sexual dysfunction. Patients must be educated regarding this side effect to prevent premature discontinuation of treatment. However, despite this bothersome side effect and the potential for sleep disturbances and gastrointestinal upset, SSRIs significantly improve physical and behavioral symptoms as well as quality of life in patients with PMDD. Therefore, SSRIs are recommended as first-line agents for the treatment of PMDD.[45]

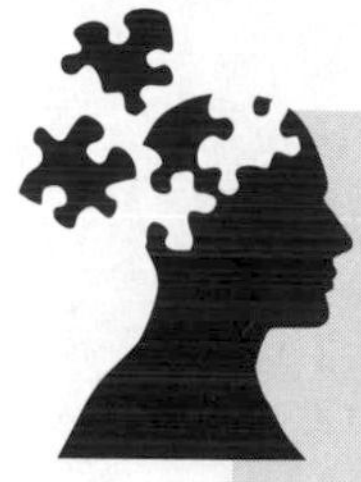

Therapeutic Challenge:

What factors should be considered when choosing luteal phase dosing vs. continuous dosing of SSRIs for PMDD?

Anxiolytics

Benzodiazepines, most commonly alprazolam, have been studied in double-blind placebo-controlled trials for PMS and PMDD and have been shown to be effective for the improvement of PMS symptoms such as tension, irritability, and anxiety. However, alprazolam should be reserved for patients who fail, cannot tolerate, or have contraindications to treatment with SSRIs because of the potential for addiction with extended treatment.[17,46-48]

Hormonal Therapies

Combination Oral Contraceptives

Oral contraceptives pills (OCPs) have been studied for PMS and PMDD with mixed results. Studies with positive results generally demonstrated improvement in physical symptoms and not mood symptoms.[49] It is theorized that the lack of efficacy on mood symptoms of combined OCPs with progestins derived from 19-nortestosterone may be due to side effects from the progestin rather than untreated PMS symptoms.[50] Studies using combined OCPs with a progestin derived from 17α-spironolactone, drospirenone, were conducted. Drospirenone has antiandrogenic and antimineralocorticoid effects and when combined with ethinyl estradiol demonstrated improvement in both physical and mood symptoms. Although the majority of the older studies were open label, two randomized, placebo-controlled trials studying drospirenone 3 mg plus ethinyl estradiol 20 mcg for 24 out of 28 days of the menstrual cycle demonstrated improvements in physical symptoms as shown by changes in the DRSP scale and also in mood symptoms, primarily depression. Improvements in daily functioning and social relationships were also seen.[17,46,50-53] Therefore, OCPs containing drospirenone and low-dose ethinyl estradiol may be used second line for PMDD in patients requesting or requiring contraception or before initiating other second-line therapies, such as clomipramine or alprazolam.

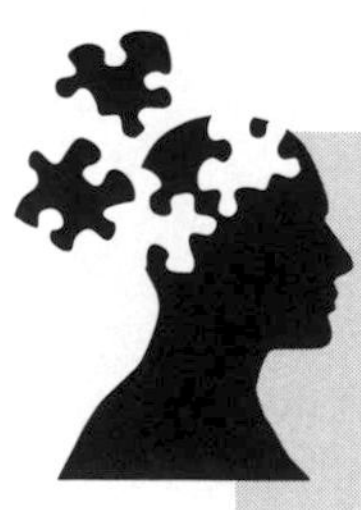

Therapeutic Challenge:

What patient factors and drug factors should be considered when determining whether an OCP is indicated for treating PMDD?

Gonadotropin-Releasing Hormone Agonists

Gonadotropin-releasing hormone agonists are commonly used to suppress ovulation and induce a "medical oophorectomy." Leuprolide and danazol are the GnRH agonists used in the treatment of PMDD. Intramuscular leuprolide (3.75–7.5 mg/mo) has been shown to improve physical symptoms; however, danazol 100–200 mg daily, when dosed in the luteal phase, has only been shown to improve mastalgia and not the general symptoms of PMS. Because these agents have androgenic effects (danazol), inhibit pituitary gonadotropin release, and cause a hypoestrogenic state, menopausal symptoms such as hot flashes, atrophic vaginitis, and osteoporosis are common and concerning side effects. Therefore, these agents should be reserved for last-line therapy in women refractory to other treatments or severe PMDD because of cost and the severity of side effects.[10,17,54-56]

Progesterone

Luteal phase dosing of progesterone either orally or by vaginal suppository has been studied for the treatment of PMS symptoms. Depo-Provera (medroxyprogesterone acetate) has also been used as an alternative to combination oral contraceptives to suppress ovulation. A systematic review failed to demonstrate any benefit of progesterone and other progestins, administered orally or by suppository, over placebo.[57] Therefore, progesterone should not be recommended as a treatment option for PMS and PMDD.

COMPLEMENTARY THERAPY

Several herbal products have been evaluated for the treatment of PMS, including black cohosh, evening primrose oil, chasteberry, soy, ginkgo, and St. John's wort. Black cohosh and evening primrose oil have not been shown to reduce PMS symptoms and should not be recommended. Although chasteberry has been shown to improve physical symptoms, studies were performed using multiple different formulations, making it difficult to recommend a consistent effective dosage. Soy isoflavones have been shown to improve physical symptoms and cramping at a dosage of 68 mg daily.[58] Ginkgo improved breast tenderness and fluid retention, and St. John's wort may be beneficial in treating depressive symptoms. However, ginkgo and St. John's wort have several potential drug interactions. Specifically, St. John's wort interacts with SSRIs and alprazolam, and the combination should be avoided because of the risk of serotonin syndrome. Although some of these products appear efficacious and may be purchased without a prescription, they should not be routinely recommended, and patients need to be counseled regarding the risk of side effects, potential drug interactions, and lack of standardization and regulation of these products.[59]

Other alternative therapies, such as acupuncture and homeopathy, lack evidence of benefit and are not considered treatment options. One small placebo-controlled crossover trial evaluating the effects of chiropractic therapy demonstrated a reduction in PMS symptoms.[60] Although evidence is lacking from treatments such as massage therapy, reflexology, and relaxation, these treatments are safe, help to alleviate stress, and are important components to a healthy lifestyle.[56]

MONITORING AND FOLLOW-UP

Evaluating the outcomes of therapy for PMS and PMDD symptoms primarily focuses on the patient's report of symptom resolution. Ask patients to report the resolution or reduction in symptoms and improvement in daily functioning. Patients can self-evaluate and subjectively monitor the effectiveness of nonpharmacologic and pharmacologic therapy by assessing changes in symptom charting and may use either the PEA or the PAF. Healthcare providers may use the Clinical Global Impressions Scale (CGIS) to objectively monitor for improvement in symptoms and symptom severity with treatment.[19,61] Patients should be evaluated every 2 weeks within 1 month of starting therapy. Improvement in therapy is generally seen within two to three menstrual cycles, and therapy should be discontinued if there is no significant improvement in symptoms despite appropriate dosage titrations. Either luteal symptoms should decrease by 50% or the difference between follicular and luteal phase symptoms should be <30%.[23] Appropriate follow-up for patients with PMS and PMDD should include routine monitoring of subjective parameters, such as side effects and adherence to the therapy regimen. Frequent follow-up, proper monitoring, and education will help to ensure that patients achieve optimal results from any therapy chosen to treat PMS and PMDD symptoms.

PATIENT EDUCATION

Patient education is extremely important when treating a patient for PMS and PMDD. Patients should be educated to continue to chart their symptoms during therapy to self-monitor the improvement or worsening of symptoms in response to therapy or dosage adjustment, to monitor for side effects, and to provide documentation for the healthcare provider.[23] Patients need to be educated on the proper use, potential side effects, and expected therapeutic response with every therapy that is initiated. Several therapies may be necessary, including a combination of nonpharmacologic and pharmacologic, but only one therapy should be added or discontinued at a time to evaluate the response to the change.[19] Evidence suggests that symptoms may gradually worsen over time and that symptoms return when therapy is discontinued. Therefore, patients should be counseled regarding the importance of adherence to therapy and that therapy may last until at least the perimenopausal period.[23]

CASE PRESENTATION

Patient Case: Part 2

Assessment: Z.Z. has PMS, as evidenced by irritability, crying, mood swings, fatigue, breast tenderness approximately 1 week before the start of menses that resolves within 3 days after the start of menses for the last 6 months. Z.Z. has not indicated the severity of social impairment but misses work 2–3 days/mo. Z.Z.'s findings do not suggest thyroid disease, breast disease, anemia, or any pelvic abnormality.

Plan: Goal for the treatment of PMS and PMDD is the resolution of or significant improvement in symptoms.

Recommendation:

1. Continue aerobic exercise.
2. Modify diet if necessary. Dietary changes include limiting the amount of sodium to minimize bloating and fluid retention, and limiting caffeine and alcohol to reduce irritability and insomnia. Diets rich in complex carbohydrates may improve mood symptoms.
3. Continue daily multivitamin to increase the amount of magnesium and vitamin E.
4. Ensure calcium dosage is 600 mg twice daily.
5. Discontinue black cohosh and chasteberry.
6. Initiate sertraline 50 mg daily during days 14–28 of the menstrual cycle.

Rationale: Black cohosh has not been shown to reduce PMS symptoms and should not be recommended. Although chasteberry has been shown to

(Continued on next page)

improve physical symptoms, studies used multiple different formulations, making it difficult to recommend a consistent effective dosage. In addition, the use of herbal products may be cost prohibitive, especially if patients have prescription drug coverage. SSRIs are the most common and widely used medications for the treatment of PMDD. To date, only three SSRIs—fluoxetine, sertraline, and paroxetine CR—are FDA approved for the treatment of PMDD, with fluoxetine and sertraline having the most supporting data. Any of the SSRIs may be initiated in this patient. The choice may be based on patient preference or prescription drug coverage. Luteal phase dosing may be more convenient for patients, will minimize side effects, and may increase adherence. Higher dosages have not been shown to be significantly more effective than lower dosages. Thus, the lowest dosage should be administered during days 14–28 of the menstrual cycle.

Monitoring: PMS symptoms and medication side effects, including sexual dysfunction, sleep disturbances, and gastrointestinal upset. Monitor patients every 2 weeks within 1 month of starting therapy in person or over the phone. Return to primary care provider in 3 months to evaluate efficacy of therapy and assess whether therapy should be continued.

Patient education: Chart PMS symptoms during therapy to self-monitor the improvement or worsening of symptoms in response to therapy or dosage adjustment. Monitor for side effects, especially sexual dysfunction, to prevent premature discontinuation. It is important to stress the importance of adherence to therapy and that therapy may last until perimenopause or menopause.

Summary

The majority of menstruating women experience some PMS symptoms, whereas a small percentage of women meet the *DSM-IV* criteria for PMDD. Although there are no universally accepted definitions for PMS and PMDD, the ACOG has established diagnostic criteria for PMS and the American Psychiatric Association has established diagnostic criteria for PMDD. Furthermore, there is no definitive diagnostic test or specific physical findings for PMS and PMDD. Therefore, the diagnostic process is one of exclusion. A medical and psychological history; symptom charting; physical exam; hematologic, hormonal, and chemistry levels; and mammography or radiologic imaging may be necessary to rule out PMS symptoms that may be attributed to another cause. Once the diagnosis for PMS or PMDD is made, nonpharmacologic therapy, such as behavioral therapy and aerobic exercise, should be encouraged. NSAIDs such as naproxen and mefanamic acid, and analgesics, such as acetaminophen, are generally used first line to relieve cramping associated with PMS. Spironolactone, an aldosterone antagonist, is the only diuretic that has been shown to have some improvement on somatic and affective symptoms. SSRIs significantly improve physical and behavioral symptoms as well as quality of life in patients with PMDD and therefore are first-line agents for the treatment of PMDD. Second-line agents for PMDD include other antidepressants, anxiolytics, combination oral contraceptives that include drospirenone, and, lastly, GnRH agonists. Dietary supplements, such as black cohosh, ginkgo, evening primrose oil, chasteberry, soy, and St. John's wort, are not generally recommended. Several therapies may be necessary, including a combination of nonpharmacologic and pharmacologic therapies, but only one therapy should be added or discontinued at a time to evaluate the response to the change. Significant improvement is generally defined as at least a 50% improvement in symptoms and should be seen within two to three menstrual cycles. Frequent follow-up, proper monitoring, and education will help to ensure that patients achieve optimal results from any therapy chosen to treat PMS and PMDD symptoms.

References

Additional content available at
www.ashp.org/womenshealth

14 Endometriosis

Andrea L. Coffee, Pharm.D., BCPS, MBA; Lazaros G. Lavasidis, MD; Sophia N. Kalantaridou, MD, Ph.D.

Learning Objectives

1. Identify the symptoms/signs that may lead to the diagnosis of endometriosis.
2. Explain the pharmacologic basis for hormonal therapies for endometriosis.
3. Compare and contrast available agents used to treat endometriosis.
4. Formulate a comprehensive clinical plan for a patient with symptomatic endometriosis and not desiring conception.
5. List common patient education points.

Endometriosis, the ectopic displacement of endometrium, is a common disorder of reproductive-age women thought to affect up to 10% of women in this age group.[1] The incidence is even higher in women with pelvic pain, infertility, or both. No one etiology has been proven, and the cause is likely multifactorial. The common symptoms that cause women to seek therapy are **dysmenorrhea,** chronic pelvic pain, **dyspareunia,** and, for some women, infertility.

Etiological Theories

The etiology of endometriosis is unclear. The most widely accepted hypothesis was introduced by Sampson, in 1927; he assumed that retrograde menstruation through the fallopian tubes into the peritoneal cavity is responsible for the appearance of the disease in the pelvis.[2] Subsequently, Meyer, in an effort to explain ovarian endometriosis, proposed that the germinal ovarian epithelium is capable of transformation into endometriotic tissue.[3] To explain peritoneal endometriosis, he suggested that mesothelial stem cells with metaplastic properties are transformed into endometriotic cells.[4] Another theory suggested that endometrial cells use metastatic pathways (both vascular and lymphatic) to implant themselves outside the pelvic area.[5] Also, it has been suggested that peritoneal endometriosis, ovarian endometriosis, and adenomyotic nodules of the rectovaginal septum are three different entities and that deep infiltrating, rectovaginal endometriotic tissue originates from the remnants of the müllerian tissue that is present in the rectovaginal septum.[6]

Recent etiologic approaches correlate the presence of endometriosis with defective cellular immunity procedures.[7,8] It has been suggested that environmental factors may trigger or enhance abnormal immune response and endometriosis development. Finally, it should be mentioned that endometriosis has been reported to occur in various sites of the abdomen after iatrogenic spread of endometrial cells (i.e., during a gynecologic surgery).

Whichever mechanism is responsible, there are likely to be additional factors that determine whether a woman develops endometriosis, including genetic predisposition. Thus, endometriosis is a multifactorial genetic disorder, inherited as a complex genetic trait in which multiple genes conferring disease predisposition interact with one another and the environment to facilitate development of the disease.

Clinical Presentation

Pelvic pain is the most common symptom of endometriosis, occurring in approximately 70% of the cases of referrals to endometriosis centers in the United Kingdom and the US.[9] Usually, it presents with a cyclic character.[10]

CASE PRESENTATION

Patient Case: Part 1

K.G. is a 32-year-old married woman who presents to the outpatient ob-gyn clinic today because of mild left quadrant abdominal pain, which appeared 12 hours before during physical training. Her menarche was at 14, and she initially had regular periods without any dysmenorrhea. She developed moderate-to-severe dysmenorrhea at age 21, and she was placed on oral contraceptives (OCs) for 10 years. She denied any pelvic pain or dysmenorrhea while she was on OCs. She and her husband have unsuccessfully attempted pregnancy for 2 years.

PMH: Hashimoto thyroiditis.

Family history: Father—non-Hodgkin lymphoma; mother—no history of endometriosis.

Social history: No tobacco; drinks one glass of red wine per day.

Medications: Levothyroxine 0.1 mg daily; multivitamin daily.

Vitals: BMI 23 kg/m^2, BP 125/70 mm Hg, HR 68, Temp. 98.4°, RR 17.

Physical examination: Unremarkable; breast examination was normal. On pelvic examination, the uterus was palpable on a retroverted position; a left adnexal mass was suspected.

Transvaginal ultrasound examination revealed a left ovarian mass consistent with **endometrioma,** 4.5 x 5 cm; a small quantity of free fluid in the **Douglas pouch** was also detected. The characteristics of the mass were verified by MRI examination. Because the patient desired conception, she had a hysterosalpingogram, which demonstrated normal uterus, left patent fallopian tube, and obstructed right fallopian tube. CA-125 levels were 75 units/mL (normal range 5–35 units/mL, as was determined by the laboratory). The optimal treatment in this case is surgical removal of the ovarian mass.

Dysmenorrhea occurs in 71% to 76% of cases.[9] It often begins a few hours or a couple of days before menses and continues throughout menses. It may persist for several days afterward. The location is the low abdomen and pelvis, but it can radiate to the thighs and back. It is bilateral and aching; it can also present along with nausea, vomiting, or diarrhea.

Dyspareunia occurs in 44% of cases and may be associated with specific positioning during intercourse, with more intensity during deep penetration and before menstruation.[9] It is may be associated with deep infiltrating nodules at the pouch of Douglas and at the rectovaginal septum. The frequency and severity of pain seems to be related to the depth and volume of infiltration.[11-13]

Infertility is reported in 15% to 20% of cases of endometriosis.[9] In minimal and mild endometriosis (American Society for Reproductive Medicine [ASRM] stages I and II, respectively), other factors are presumed to relate to poor fertility response: e.g., failure in implantation, oocyte abnormalities, or defective embryos. In moderate and severe cases of the disease (ASRM stages III and IV, respectively), infertility may be attributed to the pelvic distortion caused by adhesions and endometriomas.

In adolescents, endometriosis most commonly presents with dysmenorrhea (64% to 94%).[14,15] Other symptoms include intermenstrual pain (36% to 91%), dyspareunia (14% to 25%), and gastrointestinal disturbance (2% to 46%).[15]

Endometriosis is associated more frequently with early menarche (≤11–13 years) and with short menstrual cycle (≤28 days), longer menstruation (≥6 days), heavier bleeding, and spotting before the onset of menses.[16-19] Parity is another characteristic that correlates with endometriosis risk; multiparous women (≥2 births) have a 0.4 odds ratio for developing endometriosis when compared with nulliparous women, but this protective mechanism/effect of pregnancy gradually decreases as the number of years after the last birth increases.[20] A strong relation between first-degree relatives is observed, with a reported sevenfold increased risk for the disease.

The optimal timing for performing the clinical examination seems to be a little before or during menstruation, although this may not be well tolerated by the patient.[21] Although determining the origin of pain would be the ideal goal of clinical examination, this can not be achieved; nevertheless, examining the patient when she is experiencing pain might be helpful in localizing the pain in an effort to aid in the differential diagnosis and treatment. An ovarian tumor or a congenital anomaly of the reproductive tract should also be excluded. A retroverted position of the uterus is a common finding in most cases of endometriosis, although it does not characterize endometriosis by itself. If the retroverted position is due to adhesion formation, the bimanual examination could show that the uterus has reduced or absent mobility. Also, bimanual examination could detect endometriotic nodules, both at the posterior fornix and uterosacral ligaments; endometriomas, in the form of tender or nontender masses in the adnexae; and "fixed" **parametria** to the pelvic sidewall. A vaginorectal examination should be performed to detect nodularity or tenderness at the rectovaginal septum and rectum.

When the endometriotic lesion is located in the gastrointestinal tract (incidence: 3.8% to 37%), symptoms include **dyschezia,** diarrhea, constipation, abnormal bloating, and, rarely, menstrual **catamenial** rectal bleeding.[22,23] The sigmoid is the most frequent area of bowel involvement, followed by the rectum, the ileum, the appendix, and the cecum.[24] Apart from the bowel, endometriotic lesions can be found in the urinary tract, leading to urgency and frequent urination, and hematuria can occur if the lesion is found in the bladder.[25] Rarely, endometriosis is located inside the ureteral wall. If the lesion is transmural, it causes flank pain and obstruction. After some pelvic surgery, some women develop endometriosis in their surgical scar. In these cases, endometriosis presents with intermenstrual or catamenial pain. If the foci lie subdiaphragmatically, it may result in chest pain. In the rare case of pulmonary endometriosis, chest pain, pneumothorax/hemothorax, pleural effusions, or cyclic hemoptysis may occur.[26] Lesions in the brain have caused catamenial headaches, seizures, or subarachnoid hemorrhages.[27,28]

Pathophysiology

ENDOCRINOLOGY OF ENDOMETRIOSIS

Estrogen is a key factor for the development of endometriosis. On the contrary, progesterone seems to inhibit the mitogenic role of estrogens, because it contributes in the reduction of their concentration, both in the eutopic endometrium and the endometriotic implants. Aromatase, a key enzyme in estradiol production, is overexpressed in endometriotic lesions, possibly because of heterozygous mutations on aromatase-gene (CYP19) or initiation of transcriptional overactivity of aromatase promoters.

Progesterone is normally secreted in the eutopic endometrium and acts as antiestrogen by stimulating the expression of 17-β hydroxysteroid dehydrogenase type 2 (17βHSD-2) enzyme in endometrial glandular cells during the luteal phase. This enzyme converts the biologically active estrogen estradiol to the less estrogenic steroid estrone.[29-31] Estradiol is then lowered during the luteal phase, thus contributing in the normal apoptosis of the endometrium. In cases of endometriosis, there is an impaired progesterone effect on 17βHSD-2. This results in a deficient expression of 17βHSD-2 in eutopic endometrium and its marked absence in endometriotic lesions; as a result, there is reduced conversion of estradiol to estrone.[32] On the other hand, 17-βHSD type 1, which converts estrone to estradiol, is present in endometriotic tissues.

Progesterone-mediated development of endometriosis is based on the reduced progesterone responsiveness of the endometrium during the menstrual cycle. This leads to the disruption of the production of local differentiating factors, coded by progesterone-responsive genes (e.g., TGF-β2, TIMP-1, TIMP-3) and significant reduction of endometrial progesterone receptors.[33,34] In fact, in the endometrium of women suffering from endometriosis, there is lack of progesterone receptor B (PR-B) and a significant reduction of progesterone receptor A (PR-A).[35,36] The consequence of this impaired progesterone activity is the deficient apoptosis of the endometriotic tissue and the promotion of matrix metalloproteinase (MMP)-mediated invasion of endometriotic lesions in various peritoneal sites.

Furthermore, on in vitro studies of uterine endothelial cells, estrogen seems to up-regulate prostaglandin E_2 (PGE_2) production through the enhanced expression of the cyclo-oxygenase enzyme type 2 (COX-2). Consequently, a positive feedback loop for nonstop local production of estrogen and PGE_2 is established. All these contributing factors support the proliferative and inflammatory characteristics of endometriosis.

Indeed, peritoneal fluid in women with endometriosis is marked by increased inflammation; there is aberrant expression of a series of cytokines by activated macrophages, such as interleukin (IL)-1, IL-6, IL-8, and tumor necrosis factor (TNF)-α, which contribute to the creation of a microenvironment that is favorable to the establishment and development of peritoneal endometriotic lesions.[37] Macrophages are activated by other peritoneal immune factors, like RANTES (regulated on activation, normal T-cell expressed and secreted).[38] The continuous interaction between the aforementioned immune factors results in a dynamic cross talk that is still being investigated; therefore, whether endometriosis per se leads to inflammation or the opposite is still under discussion. Interestingly, experimental data support either side.[39,40]

ANGIOGENESIS AND ENDOMETRIOSIS

Adequate blood supply is crucial for the survival, implantation, and development of endometriotic lesions. It is difficult to extract sufficient information from in vivo models on vascular infrastructure during endometriosis because of the delayed diagnosis of the disease, but studies have shown that the process is initiated by an "angiogenic switch" based on inflammation.[41] The analogy of the establishment of an endometriotic and metastasizing malignant cell is evident; nevertheless, it seems that malignant tissues do not migrate in large amounts, but in single-cell or small-clamp patterns. On the other hand, endometriotic lesions should maintain their original architecture (stroma, glands), to have the opportunity to implant.

ENDOMETRIOSIS AND CANCER

The relationship between endometriosis and certain types of malignancy is not yet fully understood. Although some characteristics of endometriosis are indicative of malignant procedures, such as the development of both local and distant lesions, as well as the attachment and invasion of other tissues and damage of the target organs, the parameters converting a benign into a malignant entity are largely speculative.[42] Endometriosis-associated ovarian cancer occurs 1.7-fold more frequently (95% confidence interval [CI], 1.2–2.4).[43] Especially if there is a long-standing (≥10 years) history of endometriosis, the incidence of ovarian cancer is reported to be more frequent, by 4.2-fold (95% CI, 2.0–7.7);[44] 60% to 80% of cases of endometriosis-associated ovarian cancer occur in the presence of atypical ovarian endometriosis.[45-47] Of these cases, 25% have a direct continuity of the atypical ovarian endometriosis with ovarian cancer, indicating the presence of a variety of agents contributing to the transformation from a benign to a malignant status.[44]

The presence of endometriosis has been linked with an increased incidence of hematopoietic malignancies as well.[44] (standardized incidence ratio [SIR]: 1.4; 95% CI, 1.0–1.8).[44] This increase has been reported as largely due to the increased incidence of non-Hodgkin lymphoma (SIR: 1.8; 95% CI, 1.2–1.6).

ENVIRONMENTAL EFFECTS

The most common environmental agents associated with endometriosis are dioxins and dioxin-like agents. The most common source for the introduction of these agents to the human body is by ingestion of contaminated food; also, industrial wastes contain a variety of these agents, and potential exposure to them may occur during wartime.

The presence of dioxins and dioxin-like components may affect the establishment and development of endometriosis through the following pathophysiologic pathways: 1) activation of procarcinogens via activation of P-450 isoenzymes, 2) promoted production of proinflammatory growth factors or cytokines, 3) enhancement of estrogenic synthesis, and 4) misexpression of progesterone-dependent remodeling enzymes of the endometrium.[48]

Studies on the effect of environmental agents on endometriosis have been conducted both in human and nonhuman populations. Human population-based studies are not conclusive because they are small numbered and the control groups have not been surgically diagnosed for the presence or absence of the disease.[48] Also, there is not a sufficient estimation of the concentration of the environmental contaminants in peripheral blood.[48] In a study by World Health Organization (WHO), high prevalence of endometriosis was reported in infertile Belgian women, along with high concentrations of dioxins in breast milk.[49] Eighteen percent of infertile women with endometriosis were reported to have a detectable serum TCDD (2,3,7,8-tetrachlorodibenzo-p-dioxin), whereas serum levels of TCDD could be detected only in 3% of infertile women without endometriosis.[50] Animal studies with rhesus monkeys and immune-deficient mice have demonstrated that endometriosis is a disease that may be enhanced by the activity of these environmental compounds.[51-53]

Long-term Complications

Women with long-standing endometriosis often have chronic pain problems. Medical therapy may have to be changed because of adverse effects that are intolerable for the long term. Gonadotropin-releasing hormone (GnRH) agonists with **add-back therapy** have been evaluated for 2 years of use.[54] Because of the risk of adhesions, the ASRM guideline recommends avoiding multiple surgical procedures whenever possible. Clinical situations may require surgical or medical (with GnRH agonists and add-back therapy) retreatment. Women who are seeking pregnancy may spend significant time unable to use any hormonal treatments, as hormonal agents do not improve fertility and women may be following infertility protocols. For those women, the focus is conception instead of pain control. Additionally, these women may seek specialized infertility treatment, which can be expensive and often not covered by health insurance policies. Endometriosis, especially when diagnosed in the early reproductive years, should be treated with a long-term strategy.

Diagnosis

Diagnosis may be considered based on history and pelvic examination findings. Because endometriosis may have a wide range of clinical symptomatology, its differential diagnosis includes a variety of clinical conditions (Table 14-1). Therefore, to be more certain of the diagnosis, other techniques must be employed. Women should be investigated as early as possible if conventional pain medication does not ameliorate their pelvic pain. If not, women will continue to suffer for long periods, and this can significantly impair their quality of life. Although the mean delay between the onset and the diagnosis of endometriosis is 8–12 years, it is not inappropriate to use an empirical, second-line treatment (i.e., GnRH analogs, danazol, progestins) without a definitive diagnosis of the disease.[55,56] On the contrary, it is considered a current therapeutic standard.

SURGICAL

The gold standard for diagnosis is laparoscopic identification of disease.[57] However, diagnostic laparoscopy as the "golden" diagnostic criterion for the detection of endometriotic lesions is not always accurate; a negative diagnostic laparoscopy seems to be highly accurate for excluding endometriosis (overall weighted sensitivity 94% CI, 80% to 98%). A positive laparoscopy is less informative and of limited value when used in isolation (overall weighted specificity 79% CI, 76% to 87%), with a raising predictive ability as the severity of endometriosis increases (0.85 vs. 0.94). This means that a positive laparoscopy for visual detection of endometriosis could be wrong in approximately 50% of cases, resulting in unnecessary treatment and augmentation of expenses. Therefore, additional testing, especially biopsy of the suspected peritoneal lesions, will be required to verify the potential diagnosis of endometriosis.[58]

The American Society for Reproductive Medicine scoring system categorizes the disease as minimal (1–5), mild (6–15), moderate (16–40), or severe (>40).[57] Lesions are assessed as deep or superficial

Table 14-1. Differential Diagnosis of Endometriosis

Symptoms and Finding	Differential Diagnosis
Repeated painful menses (dysmenorrhea)	1) Adenomyosis
	2) Myoma
Painful penetration (dyspareunia)	1) Vaginal atrophy
	2) Reduced lubrication
	3) Sexual abuse/violence
	4) Psychosexual abnormalities
Painful micturition	1) Interstitial cystitis
	2) Urethritis/urethral syndrome
	3) Bladder dyssynergia
Painful defecation (dyschezia)	1) Anal fissure
	2) Irritable bowel syndrome
Generalized pelvic pain	1) Endometritis
	2) Pelvic adhesions
	3) Neoplasms (benign/malignant)
	4) Pelvic inflammatory disease

(*Continued on next page*)

Symptoms and Finding	Differential Diagnosis
	5) Fibromyalgia 6) Fasciitis 7) Herniation
Left-sided pelvic pain	1) Diverticulum 2) Diverticulitis
Right-sided pelvic pain	1) Chronic appendicitis 2) Meckel's diverticulum
Back pain	1) Scoliosis 2) Musculoskeletal tenderness 3) Spondylolisthesis 4) Osteitis pubis
Adnexal mass	1) Hydrosalpinx/pyosalpinx 2) Tubo-ovarian abscess 3) Functional cyst (corpus luteum/hemorrhagic follicular cyst) 4) Ovarian malignancy 5) Ovarian fibroma
Nodularity in the rectum/uterosacral ligaments/vagina	1) Fibroma/extended fibrosis 2) Abscess
Infertility	1) Tubal infection 2) Hydrosalpinx/pyosalpinx 3) Male factor infertility 4) Cervical factor infertility (stenosis, antibodies, sperm, mucus)

in the peritoneum and ovaries. **Posterior cul-de-sac obliteration,** if found, is noted as partial or complete. Adhesions are scored for the ovaries and tubes. The latest version of the ASRM scoring system contains more detail on assessing ovarian endometriotic cysts and cul-de-sac obliteration.

IMAGING TECHNIQUES

For superficial endometriosis, radiologic evaluation of simple endometriotic implants in the surface of the peritoneum or viscera with the use of transvaginal ultrasound is of limited value, and some authors support that it is not detectable.[59,60] Magnetic resonance imaging (MRI) provides a more successful detection of superficial lesions; with the use of thinner sections (5–6 mm instead of 10 mm) and fat saturation techniques, small implants can be more easily detected.[61,62] No diagnostic strategy for detecting and evaluating peritoneal endometriosis is supported by evidence of effectiveness. Therefore, in cases of suspected peritoneal disease, the only effective diagnostic approach is laparoscopic evaluation and, optimally, histologic sampling.

Transrectal ultrasound gives some clues for the existence of deep infiltrating lesions because it can detect thicker uterosacral ligaments and more nodular and irregular appearance of uterosacral ligaments.[63] If MRI is performed, the sensitivity for endometriotic implants ranges from 13% (conventional imaging) to 61% (fat suppression techniques).[61,64] MRI false-positive diagnosis for deep endometriotic implants occurs when anatomic features are misinterpreted, artifacts in MRI are spotted, and previous pelvic surgery has been performed.[65]

To diagnose endometriomas, transvaginal ultrasound detects cysts with low-level internal echoes and echogenic wall foci.[66,67] The differential diagnosis of an endometrioma should include dermoid cyst, teratoma, corpus luteum/lutein cyst, cystic neoplasms (i.e., cystadenoma, carcinoma), tubo-ovarian abscess, and ovarian fibroid. MRI can detect ovarian endometriomas, especially if their size is larger than 2 cm, as well as differentiate if the endometrioma is recent or chronic.[61]

LABORATORY TESTING

There are no reliable serum, peritoneal, or endometrial markers for the diagnosis, prognosis, and follow-up of endometriosis. CA-125 seems to be the most helpful marker for detecting the disease, although its sensitivity (13% to 87%) and specificity (86% to 100%) vary significantly. CA-125 elevations seem to be more reliable when combined with clinical evidence, and they are more useful in detecting moderate to severe endometriosis than minimal to mild, but there is still some debate about which is the optimal period during the menstrual cycle for the measurement of its level. Despite its poor sensitivity, a serum CA-125 level can be predictive of response to medical and surgical treatment; if it remains elevated after treatment, it is associated with lower fertility rates, and the prognosis is poor.[68-70] Also, in cases of ovarian cysts, measuring CA-125 in the cyst's content can be useful for differentiating ovarian endometriomas (>10,000 units/mL) from nonendometriotic benign cysts, like corpus luteum or dermoid cyst.[71] Serum and peritoneal fluid levels of some growth factors, hormones, proteolytic enzymes and their inhibitors, cytokines, and soluble adhesion molecules may be found altered in women with endometriosis, reflecting the impact of the disease on vascular and peritoneal environment, but are not clinically useful currently.

Guidelines and Position Statements

The American Society for Reproductive Medicine released practice recommendations for the treatment of pelvic pain associated with endometriosis in 2006.[72] The recommendations summarize the knowledge regarding different surgical procedures and the hormonal medical therapies. Blinded trials comparing different agents are difficult because of common adverse effects, such as amenorrhea and hot flushes. The practice recommendations state that both medical and surgical treatments are effective, medical therapy following surgical therapy offers longer symptom relief than surgery alone, and endometriosis should be viewed as a chronic disease that requires lifelong management, maximizing medical treatment over repeated surgical procedures.

The European Society for Human Reproduction Special Interest for Endometriosis and Endometrium Guideline Development Group published a guideline on the diagnosis and treatment of endometriosis in 2005.[73] Updated guidelines will be available at http://www.endometriosis.org/guidelines.html. Strength of evidence in the literature is graded A, B, C, D, or good clinical point (per the views of the Guideline Development Group). Diagnosis, surgical and medical therapy, and treatment of infertility are covered in this document. Although definitive diagnosis requires visual inspection of the pelvis at laparoscopy, empiric therapy with hormonal therapy suppressing menstruation for presumptive endometriosis is acceptable. Treatment with ovarian suppression for 6 months reduces endometriosis-associated pain and is a grade A recommendation, with all hormonal agents considered equally effective. Laparoscopic uterine nerve ablation (LUNA) does not give additional benefit to ablation of lesions (grade A). In minimal-mild disease, suppression of ovarian function does not improve fertility, but ablation of endometriotic lesions plus adhesiolysis is effective compared with diagnostic laparoscopy alone (grade A). This guideline is concisely written and easy to use.

The American College of Obstetricians and Gynecologists (ACOG) Practice Bulletin for the medical management of endometriosis is the oldest guideline of these three.[74] Background information on incidence, etiology, clinical manifestations, diagnosis, and the ASRM classification system are reviewed. The summary of data covered is in response to clinical situations. Level A recommendations include that pain relief with a GnRH-agonist for at least 3 months or with danazol for at least 6 months appears to be equally effective in most women. A second recommendation is the importance of add-back therapy (such as progestins alone, progestins and bisphosphonates, estrogens, or nasal calcitonin) to reduce or eliminate GnRH-induced bone mineral loss if GnRH-agonist treatment is effective and thus continued. Level B recommendations include the empiric use of GnRH-agonists for chronic pelvic pain in presumed endometriosis. Treatment with OCs and oral or depot medroxyprogesterone are effective compared with placebo and may be equivalent to more costly regimens. Lastly, estrogen replacement therapy is not contraindicated following hysterectomy and bilateral salpingo-oophorectomy for endometriosis. ACOG also published a criteria set for abdominal hysterectomy with or without adnexectomy for endometriosis.[75]

The Practice Committee of the ASRM has developed a document summarizing the data and making general treatment recommendations on endometriosis and infertility.[76] Data on **fecundity** in women with endometriosis is outlined, plus biologic mechanisms that may have a role in infertility in this patient population is reviewed. Medical therapy has not been shown to improve fecundity in stage I/II disease. Surgical treatment and the role or superovulation and assisted reproductive technology is discussed. The specifics will be outlined in the infertility section.

Treatment Goals

The therapeutic strategy for endometriosis must be determined for each patient individually, based on each patient's needs and symptoms.[77,78] The principal goal in treating endometriosis is the relief of symptoms, shortened time to conception (when desired), and the prevention or delay of disease progression, although for the last, there is still no available strategy. On the other hand, endometriosis has a prevalence of 20% to 50% in cases of infertile women.[12,79,80] For women with pain, surgery usually provides temporary relief; symptoms recur in up to 75% of women within 2 years. Medical treatments have focused on the hormonal alteration of the menstrual cycle in an effort to produce iatrogenic menopause, anovulation, or pseudopregnancy. For those women desiring conception, the objective becomes aiding that goal. The treatment may be combined with the use of assisted reproductive methods, which include controlled ovarian hyperstimulation and intrauterine insemination or in vitro fertilization and embryo transfer. Improving the patient's symptomatology (e.g., pelvic pain) is important for her quality of life.[81] In the adolescent population, the goals of therapy are to suppress pain and preserve fertility; thus the recommendation to continue medical therapy until women desire pregnancy.

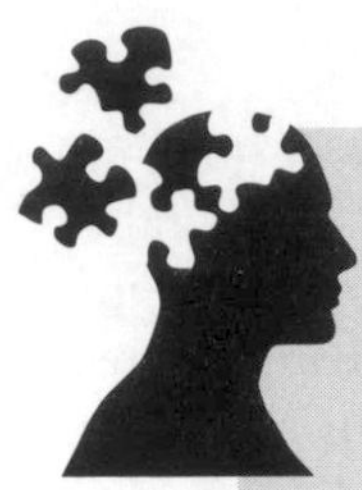

Therapeutic Challenge:

After multiple surgical and medical treatment attempts (OC and progestin therapy), what are the treatment options for young patients with endometriosis and persistent pelvic pain desiring fertility (i.e., when hysterectomy and oophorectomy is not an option)?

Surgical Treatment

INFERTILITY

In infertile women with minimal and mild endometriosis, it has been established that the possibility to achieve spontaneous pregnancy after surgical treatment is increased by 73% in the first 36 weeks after treatment.[82] The increased rate of spontaneous pregnancy occurs regardless of whether access is laparoscopic or open, or of the technique used for the removal of endometriotic lesions (laser/diathermy ablation or excision).[83] Unfortunately, the monthly fecundity rate among women who underwent laparoscopic surgery remains lower than the rate in fertile women (6.1% vs. 20%), supporting the view that the destruction of implants and adhesiolysis does not eliminate all factors by which minimal and mild endometriosis affect the occurrence of spontaneous abortion in infertile women.[82]

In cases of moderate and severe endometriosis, the distortion of pelvic anatomy requires restoration, either by laparoscopic or open surgery, regardless of other infertility factors, but there are no randomized controlled trials (RCTs) to define results of surgical treatment for these stages of endometriosis.[76] It seems, though, that the important factor for determining therapeutic options in cases of endometriosis-related infertility is patient's age. If younger than 35 years, surgical treatment (either excision or ablation of lesions) should be performed, regardless of the ASRM stage of the disease. If older than 35 years, surgical procedure should be selected in cases of no previous fertility surgery (Figure 14-1). Endometrioma-related infertility will be discussed in the section "Endometriomas."

PELVIC PAIN

Pelvic pain associated with endometriosis usually is cyclic; however, the pain may also be continuous. It is common for any type of regional pain syndrome to

Figure 14-1. Surgical treatment of endometriosis-associated infertility.

Surgical Treatment of Endometriosis-associated Infertility

Patient's Age

Age <35 yr
- Minimal/mild endometriosis (ASRM) → Laparoscopic excision/ablation (increased possibility for spontaneous pregnancy)
- Moderate/severe endometriosis (ASRM) → Laparoscopic excision/ablation (probably increased possibility for spontaneous pregnancy-limited data)

Age 35 yr
- No previous fertility surgery → Consider aggressive ART (limited data); Laparoscopic excision/ablation (regardless of ASRM stage)
- Failure(s) in previous fertility surgery → Try aggressive ART (limited data)

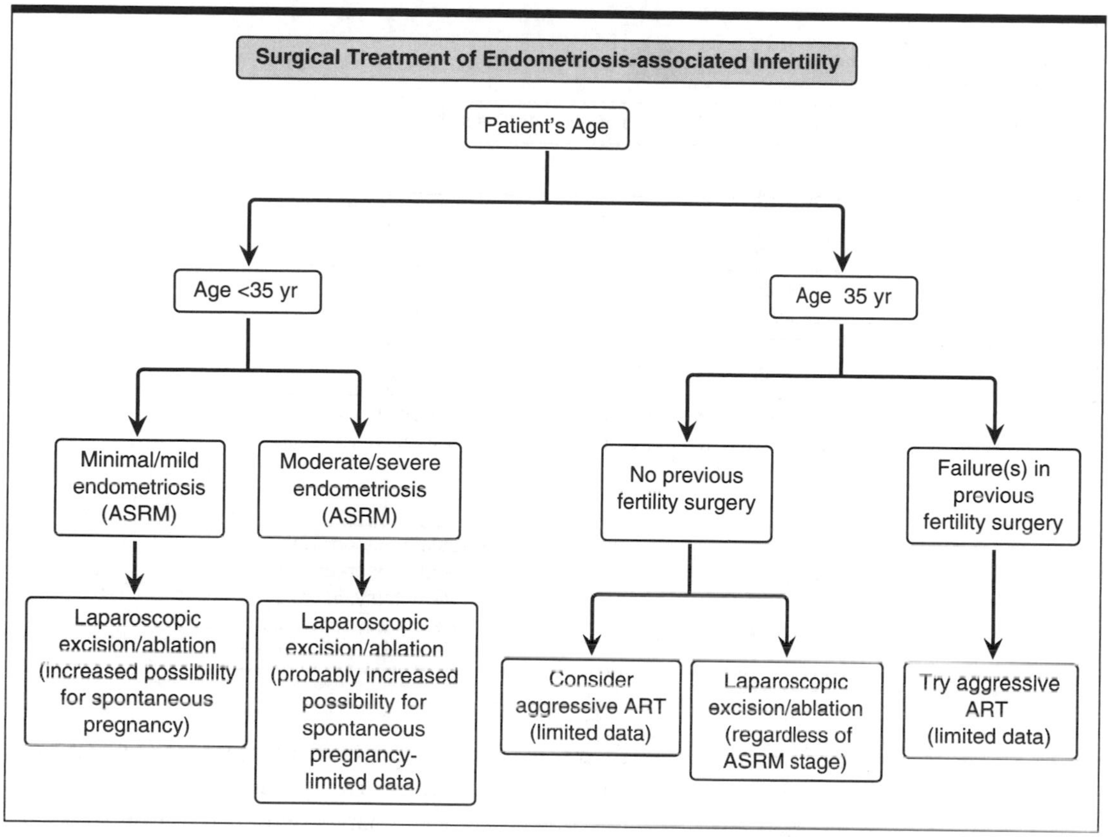

eventually spread to become more systemic and involve the entire body (i.e., transform to **fibromyalgia**).[84] Little is known about the association between the endometriotic lesions and pain. It has been reported that pain is greater in women with deeply infiltrating endometriotic lesions in highly innervated areas than in women with more superficial lesions. It seems that the intensity of pain is determined by the interaction between endometriotic lesions and sensory afferent nerve fibers and not by the type and extension of the implants.[85] The growth of nerve supply into the ectopic endometrial tissue could have a varied and widespread influence on the activity of neurons throughout the central nervous system.[86] The relief of pain after surgical treatment of endometriosis varies from 50% to 95%, but there seems to be greater relief in cases of mild and moderate endometriosis than in cases of minimal endometriosis.[78] Because there is no current globally accepted consensus on the optimal surgical treatment for endometriosis-related pelvic pain, the therapeutic procedures tend to be tailored to the individual needs of each patient.

Laparoscopic access is the best way to treat minimal and mild endometriotic lesions (Figure 14-2), especially in a one-step ("see and treat") procedure. This can be performed by excision, laser ablation, or diathermy ablation of the lesions, but there are not enough data to clarify which technique prevails.[87]

Moderate endometriosis is also treated laparoscopically (Figure 14-2), but data are insufficient to support whether excision, ablation, or adhesiolysis is superior against the others. Severe endometriosis was not included in any trials because withholding treatment from these women was considered unethical.

For women with severe dysmenorrhea, LUNA aims to interrupt nerve fibers in the uterosacral ligaments to diminish pelvic pain derived from the uterus. Seemingly, LUNA by itself has no effect on dysmenorrhea associated with endometriosis; therefore, it offers no benefit in the treatment of endometriosis, beyond those that which can be achieved with conservative surgery alone.[88,89]

Presacral neurectomy aims to interrupt the sympathetic innervation to the uterus at the level of the superior hypogastric plexus. It was shown to reduce midline dysmenorrhea, but the difference was not statistically important; also, it was not reported to improve other forms of chronic pelvic pain.[89]

Figure 14-2. Surgical treatment of endometriosis-associated pain.

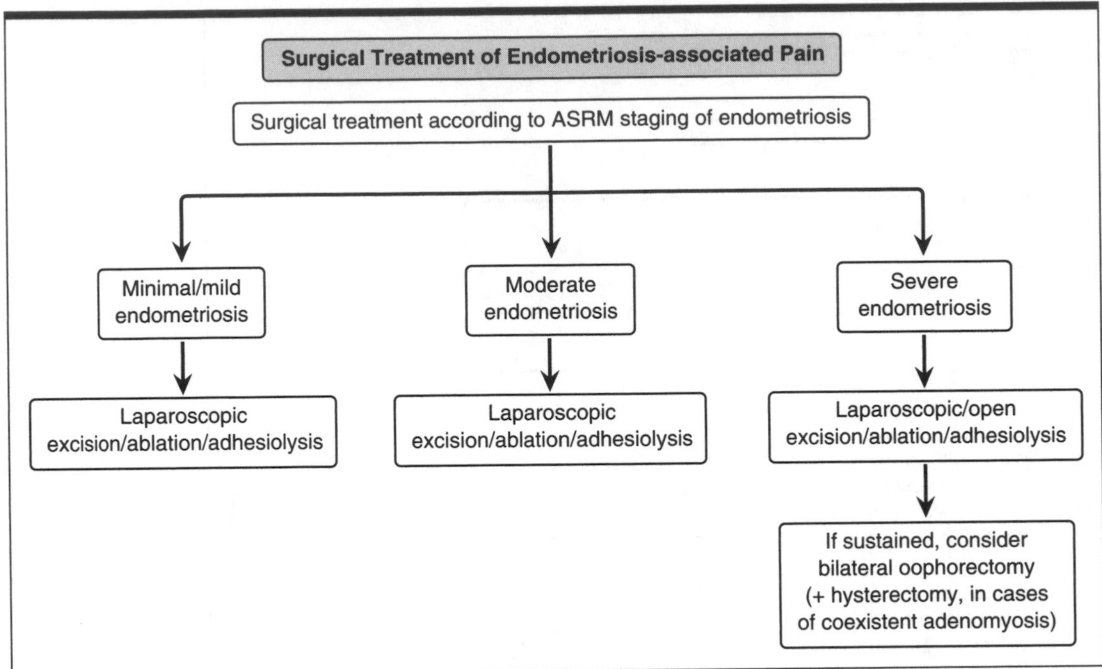

Hysterectomy, with or without bilateral oophorectomy, is usually performed in cases of severe endometriosis when laparoscopy cannot be performed (e.g., because of extended pelvic adhesion formation) and in women with no further wish for childbearing. If performed, all visible endometriotic lesions should be excised simultaneously. If bilateral oophorectomy is performed as well, it may result in as much as 6.1 times less risk of developing recurrent pain and a reduced chance of future surgery.[90,91] Nevertheless, bilateral oophorectomy introduces women to menopause iatrogenically; therefore, this surgical procedure should be regarded as a health consequence and, in cases of endometriosis, should be performed only according to the ACOG criteria set.[75]

In conclusion, a combined approach of laparoscopic laser ablation, adhesiolysis, and uterine nerve ablation seems most advantageous for the treatment of minimal, mild, and moderate endometriosis.[87] The recurrence in a 12-month follow-up reaches 44%. It is very important that the surgeon is adequately trained and experienced, and that there is care both for proper patient selection and use of appropriate equipment.

ENDOMETRIOMAS

The presence of endometriomas is associated with the existence of chronic pelvic pain and infertility; therefore, it is important to treat endometriomas with respect to these two clinical conditions and, if possible, treat them laparoscopically (Figure 14-3). Regardless of their size, endometriomas should be removed, especially if they are involved in cases of chronic pelvic pain. There are various techniques for removing an endometriotic cyst according to their size and the surgeon's technical efficacy (because not all surgeons are capable of performing the same variety of surgical operations with optimal efficacy). It seems, though, that when excision is performed, reoperation rates are lower in comparison with simple **fenestration** and ablation in a 42-month follow-up (23.5% vs. 57.8%, respectively) and also in symptoms like dysmenorrhea, deep dyspareunia, and nonmenstrual pain, compared with fenestration and coagulation.

Laparoscopic excision of the cyst wall is followed by reduced requirement for further surgery and increased rate of spontaneous pregnancy in cases of prior infertility/subfertility, but there is lack of sufficient data as to the effect of any approach on women who subsequently undergo assisted reproduction techniques and on their quality of life.[88,92] In fact, there seems to be no need for surgery before in vitro fertilization–intracytoplasmic sperm injection (IVF-ICSI) cycles, but there are no available RCTs to support this observation.[93] Therefore, treatment should

Figure 14-3. Surgical treatment of endometriomas.

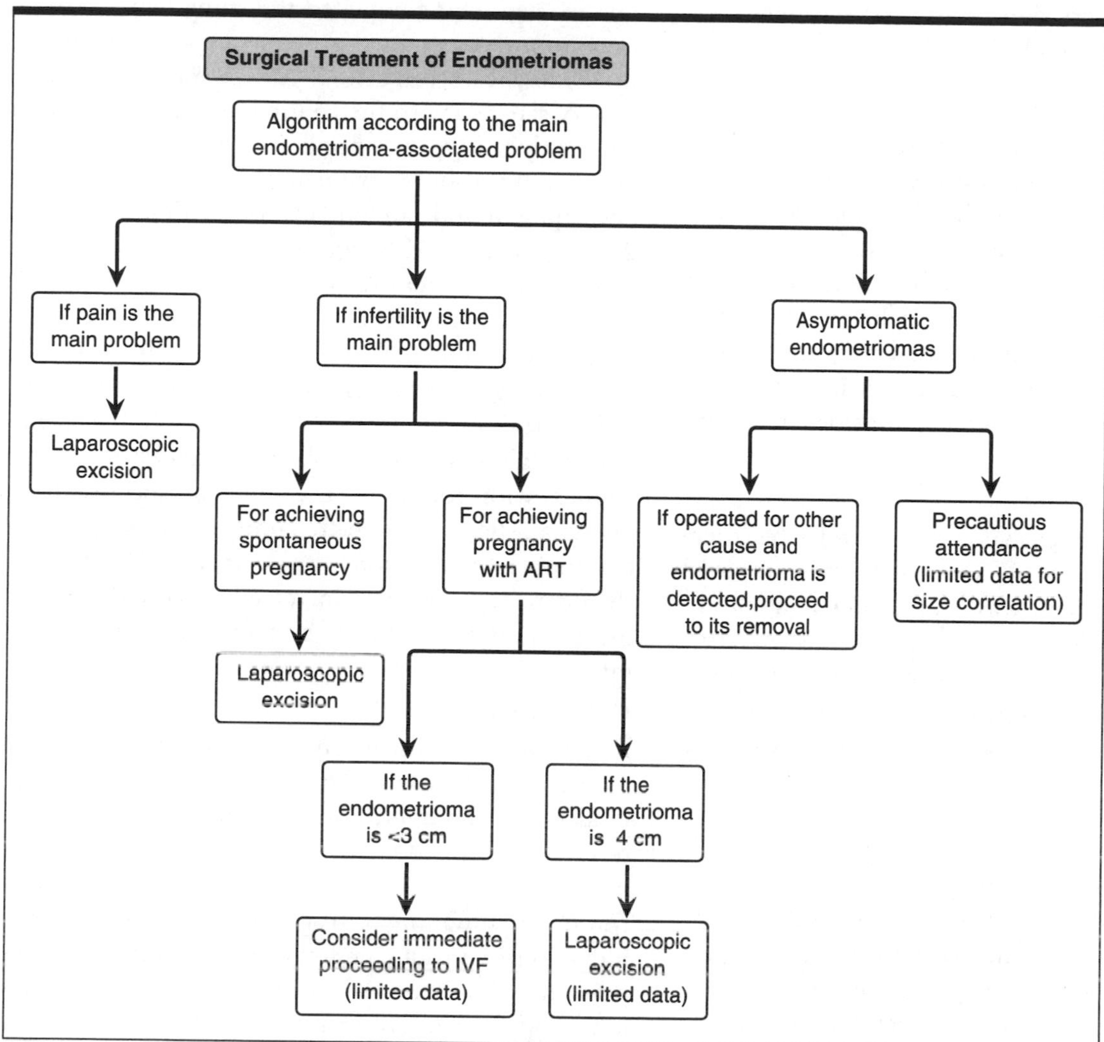

be individualized according to the needs of each patient.

The size of the cyst seems to play an important role in the selection of the appropriate treatment in infertile women with endometriosis who wish to undergo assisted reproduction techniques (Figure 14-3). If the diameter of the cyst is <3 cm, the patient could proceed to IVF immediately, but if it is 4 cm or larger, cystectomy should be performed.[76,88] Nevertheless, cystectomy is related to an increased risk of losing functional ovarian tissue, although current evidence shows that the ovarian tissue next to the cystic wall does not have the follicular pattern observed in normal ovaries.[93-96,97] Therefore, stripping of the cystic wall may not be so harmful or considered to be overtreatment because the tissue adjacent to the cystic wall is probably nonfunctional.

Pharmacologic Treatment

SYMPTOMATIC

One of the initial therapies given for endometriosis is symptomatic therapy with nonsteroidal anti-inflammatory drugs (NSAIDs). Because of the safety and minor adverse effects in healthy reproductive-age women, these agents are used frequently for pelvic pain. Because NSAIDs are the most common treatment for dysmenorrhea, they may be given for the treatment of pelvic pain with or without the diagnosis of endometriosis. Ibuprofen and naproxen sodium are available without a prescription, and women will often try these agents before seeking medical care for the pain or other symptoms of endometriosis. Some suggested NSAIDs are mefenamic acid 500 mg 3 times daily, naproxen 250 mg 2–4 times daily, naproxen sodium 275–550 mg twice daily, ibuprofen 400 mg every 4–6 hours, and diclofenac sodium 50 mg 3 times daily.[98]

HORMONAL

Targeted therapy for endometriosis is currently hormonal manipulation. Because the superiority of one hormonal therapy over another has not been established, therapy is often selected based on cost and side effects.[1,72] Tissue studies have suggested that eutopic and ectopic endometrium has immunologic differences that cause a differential response to hormonal therapy.[99] Blinding in endometriosis studies is difficult because of the differences in side effects and amenorrhea.

Oral Contraceptives

One of the least expensive and most tolerable therapies is combination OCs. Initially, the proposed mechanism of action was initial **decidualization** and growth of endometrial tissue, followed by atrophy of the endometrial tissue, causing a pseudopregnancy state.[100] Several agents studied were at higher dosages than those used today. The commonly used combination OCs today are progestin dominant, and the therapeutic effects are similar to the use of progestins alone. Traditionally, the more androgenic progestins (19-nortestosterone derivatives) have been used, but desogestrel has also been shown effective.[101] A comparative study of the desogestrel OC to cyproterone acetate in women with recurrent moderate to severe pelvic pain after surgical treatment found both agents improved pain scores for dysmenorrhea, deep dyspareunia, and nonmenstrual pelvic pain.

A Cochrane Database Systematic Review of combined OCs for pain associated with endometriosis found only one study that met the criteria.[102] The study compared an OC to a GnRH analogue (or agonist) for 6 months of therapy. The conclusion was that there was no difference in outcomes between the two agents for endometriosis-related pain symptoms. Looking at the specific trial, the findings were that the cyclic OCs were significantly less effective than the GnRH agonist for dysmenorrhea (GnRH agonists usually cause amenorrhea), nearly as effective for dyspareunia, and equally efficacious on nonspecific pelvic pain.[103]

Continuous OC regimens have been used in the treatment of endometriosis, although only one prospective study is available.[56,104] A continuous regimen of desogestrel 0.15 mg and ethinyl estradiol 0.02 mg was used following surgery in 50 women who had recurrent dysmenorrhea with a cyclic regimen. Forty-one women who completed the study had a significant improvement in the frequency and severity of dysmenorrhea. Even after 2 years, 80% were satisfied or very satisfied with the continuous regimen. It does appear that using a continuous OC regimen would be more efficacious as women do have some follicular development and rarely, ovulation, with a traditional 21/7 regimen.[105] Although most of the trials are uncontrolled, treatment recommendations routinely include OCs, both cyclic and continuous, based on a long history of use.

The biggest drawback to any continuous regimen is the breakthrough bleeding that may bother some women, although this problem improves for many women with continued use. In a prospective trial, taking a 3-day hormone-free interval was superior to continuing the hormonal-active tablets.[106] Although the intensity of bleeding increased initially, the bleeding resolved more quickly by taking a hormone-free interval.

Progestins

Progestins are a mainstay of treatment for endometriosis. The proposed mechanism of action is to induce the endometriotic implants into a decidual reaction with endometrial atrophy. Recent studies have shown that progestins act on eutopic endometrium by inhibiting estrogen-induced mitosis and induction of various endometrial enzymes that oppose the stimulatory effect of estrogens, directly inhibit endometrial stromal cell proliferation in vitro, affect the expression of endometrial MMPs, and inhibit angiogenesis by suppressing plasminogen activator activity.[107] Osteen and colleagues reported that endometrial tissue from women with endometriosis showed a partial loss of sensitivity to progesterone compared with tissue from women without endometriosis.[35] Multiple oral progestins have been investigated for the treatment of endometriosis. Unfortunately, most of the trials have a small sample size and are retrospective in nature.

Several observational trials have evaluated oral medroxyprogesterone acetate (MPA) in 3- to 6-month studies. The dosages used were 10, 30, 50, and 100 mg/day. The 100-mg dose was part of a 6-month randomized trial that compared MPA with danazol 800 mg and placebo after surgical excision of endometriosis.[108] There was no difference between the two active agents, but both were significantly better than placebo. The minimal effective dosage of MPA has not been established.

Norethindrone acetate has been analyzed in two observational studies. The dosage in one study was 5–20 mg, increased in 2.5 mg increments. Ninety-four percent of women had overall pain relief, but breakthrough bleeding was high: 57.6% of women.[109] A randomized study compared norethindrone acetate 2.5 mg with a combination OC containing cyproterone acetate in women with recurrent moderate or severe pelvic pain after conservative surgery for symptomatic rectovaginal endometriosis.[110] After 12 months of therapy, dysmenorrhea, deep dyspareunia, nonmenstrual pelvic pain, and dyschezia were reduced without significant between-group differences. Both groups had minor unfavorable lipid changes.

Megestrol acetate was evaluated in a single retrospective study of 29 women. The dose used was 40 mg, and 86% reported improvement, but the duration of therapy was not standardized.[111] There are no published studies of micronized progesterone for the treatment of endometriosis. Dydrogesterone and cyproterone acetate (a derivative of 17α-hydroxyprogesterone with antiandrogenic effects), dienogest, and lynestrenol have shown some benefit but are not available in the U.S.

Because of the higher doses used with oral progestins, side effects such as breakthrough bleeding, weight gain, bloating, edema, and decreased high-density lipoprotein (HDL) cholesterol are not uncommon. Potential benefits to oral progestins include possible long-term use and the low cost.

MPA 150 mg as an intramuscular depot injection given every 3 months has been compared with a control group taking danazol 50 mg daily for 21/28 days plus a monophasic OC.[112] Both groups had a significant decrease in HDL cholesterol. Breakthrough bleeding or spotting was high, with 80% of the depot MPA group compared with 10% of the control group. A lower dose, 104 mg subcutaneous depot MPA, had been compared with leuprolide acetate in two 6-month studies.[113,114] Pain reduction was similar for both groups in each of the studies. Besides the breakthrough bleeding, the MPA groups also had significant bone mineral density loss in the lumbar spine. Bone lost because of depot MPA may be partially reversible. Another injectable progestin, gestrinone, has shown favorable results but is not available in the U.S. Although injectable progestins have shown promise, the decrease in bone mineral density is concerning, and the breakthrough bleeding may be unacceptable to many women.

The levonorgestrel-releasing intrauterine system (LNG-IUS) has also been investigated for the medical treatment of endometriosis, although it is not U.S. Food and Drug Administration (FDA) approved for this indication. A proposed mechanism of action is that LNG concentrations in the peritoneal fluid have a local effect on implants, inducing decidualization.[115] In this study at 6 months, peritoneal fluid concentrations of LNG were approximately two thirds the serum concentrations.[115] The LNG-IUS has been shown to improve rectovaginal endometriosis[116] and significantly decrease visible disease at a second-look laparoscopy after 6 months of treatment.[117] One study compared LNG-IUS with expectant management after laparoscopic surgical management for symptomatic endometriosis and found that 1 year after surgery, the risk of recurrence of moderate or severe dysmenorrhea was significantly lower in the LNG-IUS group.[118]

The LNG-IUS has also been compared with a depot GnRH analogue in women with stages I–IV endometriosis suffering from chronic pelvic pain.[119] The 6-month study found that both treatments were effective, and no differences between the treatments were found. The chronic pelvic pain decreased significantly beginning at the first month of treatment. The LNG-IUS users had a higher bleeding score than the GnRH analogue users. At 6 months, 70% of the LNG-IUS users reported no bleeding compared with 98% of the GnRH analogue users.

The LNG-IUS treatment has some potential therapeutic benefits over treatments in women not desiring conception. Adverse effects are usually mild and do not cause hypoestrogenism and bone loss commonly seen with GnRH agonists. The LNG-IUS does not normally inhibit ovulation. Although there are no long-term studies available, the LNG-IUS is FDA approved for 5 years of contraception and thus may be a very cost-effective therapy in the long term.

Gonadotropin-Releasing Hormone Agonists

GnRH agonists are an effective treatment for endometriosis-related pain, both in placebo-controlled and randomized trials. These agents bind to receptors in the pituitary but have a longer half-life. This results in down-regulation of the pituitary–ovarian axis and hypoestrogenism. The likely beneficial effects are induction of amenorrhea and progressive endometrial atrophy.[120] GnRH agonists are the only agents shown to be effective in women who did not respond to OCs.[121] Women were randomized to leuprolide acetate vs. placebo. The response was superior in those women receiving leuprolide: 80% experienced relief in 3 months.

Available agents in this category are nafarelin acetate nasal spray, a depot formulation of leuprolide acetate injections (1 month and 3 month), and goserelin acetate subcutaneous implant. Common side effects that are due to the hypoestrogenic state are hot flushes, vaginal dryness, decreased libido, mood swings, and a decrease in bone mineral density. Pain relief usually occurs within 1 month of starting therapy.

Women can be treated with add-back therapy of a progestin or an estrogen and progestin to address these adverse effects. The use of add-back therapy is based on the estrogen threshold hypothesis, which states that the amount of estrogen and/or progestogen necessary to prevent hypoestrogenic effects, including hot flushes and bone loss, is less than that which promotes endometriosis.[122] Norethindrone acetate 5 mg/day is the only FDA-approved agent for this use, but estrogen/progestin combinations are also used—conjugated estrogens 0.625 mg plus norethindrone acetate 5 mg or medroxyprogesterone 2.5 mg/day. Additionally, 17-β estradiol has been used as the estrogen in add-back regimens. Oral MPA 100 mg has been used alone. An exception to the estrogen-only recommendation for women after a hysterectomy is to use continuous combined estrogen-progestin therapy for treating menopausal symptoms.[73] Adequate intake of calcium and vitamin D should be emphasized, as well as physical exercise for bone health.

The initial action of GnRH agonists is a flare of follicle-stimulating hormone and luteinizing hormone, which prompts estrogen release and worsening of endometriosis pain. Although initiation of therapy at the onset of menses is common, midluteal administration may produce a more rapid response as high progesterone levels inhibit the release of gonadotropins.[120] The drawback to this method is the possibility of an unidentified pregnancy. Another option is pretreatment with OCs or high-dose progestins for several weeks before the initiation of GnRH agonist therapy.[120] The FDA-approved treatment duration is limited to 6 months, although with the addition of add-back therapy, this is sometimes extended to a year in practice and appears to be safe. Endometriomas cannot be effectively treated with GnRH agonists or other hormonal agents. There are little data on retreatment with this class of drugs.

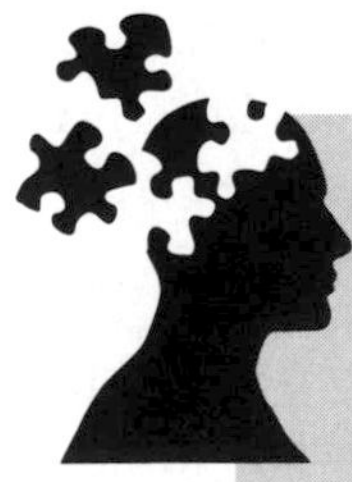

Therapeutic Challenge:

For those women who respond well to GnRH agonist therapy, can therapy be safely administered longer than a year?

Because the utility of GnRH agonists is based on the suppression of pituitary function after initial stimulation, the use of GnRH antagonists seems to be a more direct method. Cetrorelix has been investigated in a short-term study and did achieve pain relief and disease regression in 60% of the cases at follow-up diagnostic laparoscopy.[123]

Danazol

Danazol, a derivative of 17α-ethinyl testosterone, was the first approved treatment for endometriosis in the U.S. The primary mechanism of action is by diminishing the midcycle luteinizing hormone.[99] Serum testosterone is increased, and at the recommended dosage of 600–800 mg/day, there are significant androgenic adverse effects, including hirsutism, mood changes, acne, deepening of the voice, and adverse changes to the lipid profile.[124] Danazol administered vaginally in a dosage of 200 mg daily for 12 months effectively treated dysmenorrhea, dyspareunia, and pelvic pain beginning at 3 months of use in a small study.[125] Alternate routes of administration, including a danazol-impregnated vaginal ring, are under investigation.[100] A summary of commonly used agents is in Table 14-2.

INVESTIGATIONAL AGENTS

The medical treatment of endometriosis continues to be an active area of research. Some of the research continues on drug classes already in clinical use, such as GnRH agonists and progestins. Other agents under investigation include GnRH antagonists, selective estrogen receptor modulators (or estrogen agonist-antagonist), aromatase inhibitors, and selective progesterone receptor modulators. Pentoxifylline (because of immunomodulation properties) was compared with placebo in women following surgery, and no difference in recurrence of pain or pregnancy was found in the two groups.[126] Therapies that target cytokines, angiogenic factors, and MMPs may be possible in the future.

Table 14-2. Therapeutic Agents for Endometriosis

Agent	Category	Dosages	FDA Approved	Comments
Oral contraceptives	Oral contraceptives	One tablet daily; cyclic or extended	No	First-line therapy; inexpensive; no agent proven superior
Medroxyprogesterone acetate (oral)	Progestin	30–100 mg/day	No	Minimal effective dosage unknown
Medroxyprogesterone acetate (SQ)	Progestin	104 mg SQ q 3 mo	Yes	Associated with bone loss with long-term use
Megestrol acetate	Progestin	40 mg/day	No	One small study
Norethindrone acetate	Progestin	2.5–70 mg/day; 15 mg/day approved dosage	Yes	May use for long-term treatment; breakthrough bleeding may require temporary termination
Danazol	Androgen	600–800 mg/day	Yes	Not well tolerated; menopausal and androgenic side effects; barrier contraception needed
Leuprolide acetate	GnRH agonist	3.75 mg IM monthly or 11.25 mg IM q 3 mo	Yes	Recommended duration is 6 mo
Nafarelin acetate	GnRH agonist	400 mcg/day (200 mcg/spray twice daily)	Yes	Recommended duration is 6 mo
Goserelin acetate implant	GnRH agonist	3.6 mg subcutaneous implant every month	Yes	Recommended duration is 6 mo

GnRH = gonadotropin-releasing hormone; IM = intramuscular; SQ = subcutaneous.

MEDICAL TREATMENT FOLLOWING SURGERY

Treatment before surgery with a GnRH agonist has been shown to be of little value, but postoperative treatment with a GnRH agonist for 6 months, but not 3 months, prolonged the pain-free interval.[95,127,128] Women may be started on combination OCs after surgical treatment in hopes of maintaining a response. Extended OCs after surgical therapy was more effective than cyclic OCs.[104]

ADOLESCENTS AND YOUNG WOMEN

Because of the increase in diagnosis of endometriosis in adolescents, ACOG has drafted a document addressing this disease in the adolescent population.[129] Treatment of girls younger than 18 years should be treated empirically with cyclic combination hormone therapy, which the committee defines as OCs, estrogen/progestin patch or vaginal ring, norethindrone acetate, or MPA, and NSAIDs. NSAIDs are important in adolescents, who typically report severe dysmenorrhea. If ineffective, the teen can be offered a diagnostic laparoscopy. In a woman 18 years or older, an ovarian mass or tumor should be ruled out; then she can be offered an empiric trial of GnRH agonist therapy. If the pain subsides with this therapy, a presumptive diagnosis of endometriosis can be made. Once the diagnosis is made in either group—by laparoscopy or in response to GnRH agonist therapy—the use of continuous combination hormone therapy can be used. Surgical treatment of the endometriosis is also performed if a laparoscopy is undertaken. Women older than 16 years and diagnosed by laparoscopy can also be offered GnRH agonist (± add-back) therapy, followed by continuous combined hormone therapy; this can also be offered to young women with continued symptoms on continuous combination hormonal therapy. Continued pain may require laparoscopy with resection of endometriosis or long-term GnRH agonist with add-back therapy.

Because of the adverse effect on bone mineralization, GnRH agonist therapy is not a first-line treatment for adolescents younger than 16 years. Additionally, the use of depot MPA for longer than 2 years has been shown to decrease bone mineral density in adolescents. Also, in a large group of teens, treatment with MPA or depot MPA was the least well tolerated and the least effective on pain symptoms compared with combination OCs, GnRH agonists, and pain medications.[130]

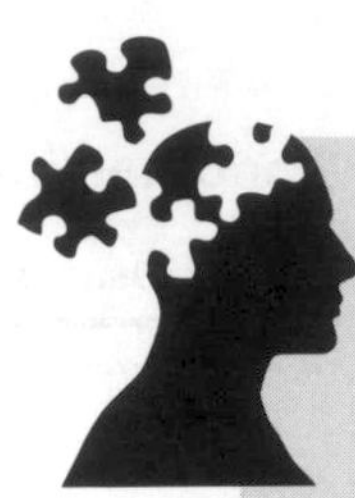

Therapeutic Challenge:

For women with known endometriosis and pelvic pain, is there a treatment regimen that can be used to minimize the time off hormonal therapy before conception? Can factors be identified that increase the odds that assisted-reproduction techniques will be needed for conception (such as IVF-ET)?

Treatment of Infertility

For many women with endometriosis, the goal at some time during their reproductive years will be conception. Decreased fecundity is well documented in women with endometriosis, and many women will seek medical assistance with conception. The treatment of infertility in this patient population is neither straightforward nor fully supported by randomized clinical trials. Although the medical and hormonal therapies for the assisted reproduction techniques can be the same as those used for infertility because of other causes, the use of medical, surgical, or expectant management of the endometriosis must be considered. Unfortunately, the ASRM staging system does not correlate well with the chance of conception after treatment. General recommendations from the Practice Committee of the ASRM are summarized in the following information.[76]

Treatment options are based on a woman's age, duration of infertility, pelvic pain, and stage of endometriosis. If a laparoscopy is undertaken, the surgeon should consider ablating or excising visible lesions. Hormonal therapy of stage I/II disease has not been shown to improve the fecundity of infertile women. Surgical therapy of stage I/II disease found an 8.6% difference in pregnancy rates in favor of treatment.[131] Thus, for every 12 patients with stage I/II disease diagnosed at laparoscopy, there is one additional successful pregnancy after ablation/resection. For those with stage III/IV disease, conservative surgical treatment with laparoscopy and possible laparotomy increase fertility.[132]

Although postoperative hormonal therapy may treat "microscopic disease," it has not been shown to enhance fertility. Fecundity per cycle has been increased in studies using superovulation with gonadotropins and intrauterine insemination. There does appear to be a role for long-term treatment (such as 6 months) with GnRH agonists before initiation of a cycle of in vitro fertilization–embryo transfer (IVF-ET). For women with pain, a laparoscopy may be undertaken more quickly. Because of age-related decrease in fecundity and increase in spontaneous abortion rate after age 35, a more aggressive approach is necessary, such as superovulation with intrauterine insemination or in IVF-EF. A systematic review of the data regarding long-term pituitary downregulation before IVF in women with endometriosis concluded that the administration of GnRH agonists for a period of 3–6 months before IVF or ICSI increases the odds of clinical pregnancy fourfold.[133] Surgical treatment for endometriosis has not been shown to reduce the risk of spontaneous abortions in infertile women.[82]

Monitoring and Follow-up

To assess the effectiveness of therapy, there are three outcomes that can be assessed: the anatomic manifestations of disease, pain symptomatology, and, in some women, fertility outcome.[100] A second-look laparoscopy to assess the anatomic manifestations of disease has been used to evaluate the response to drug therapy in clinical trials but is not used in clinical practice. The value of this has to be tempered with the knowledge that endometriosis may regress on its own and that over time, implant and adhesion regrowth is normal.[100] Last, because of the morbidity associated with a surgical procedure, this is not a common method of assessment. Physical examination findings thought to be due to endometriosis can be repeated on follow-up.

To assess pain—whether dysmenorrhea, deep dyspareunia, nonmenstrual pelvic pain, or dyschezia—a visual analog pain scale is common and easy to use. A large placebo effect—as high as 55% in women with endometriosis—has been noted.[134] A severity score by Biberoglu and Behrman has been used in older studies.[135] The symptoms of dysmenorrhea, nonmenstrual pain, deep dyspareunia, and dyschezia are rated as absent, mild, moderate, or severe based on the impact on a woman's life. Pelvic tenderness and induration on examination are assessed as mild, moderate, or severe. A response to pharmacologic treatment usually takes 1–3 months. Evaluation of response can be tied to prescription refills (for subjective assessments) or office visits, especially for GnRH agonist injections.

Patient Education

Endometriosis can play a significant role in decreasing a woman's quality of life. In the reproductive years, many women are healthy overall, and this may be the only chronic disease of significance that they are treating. These may be the first chronic medications they have to take, and the adverse effects associated with these medications may be difficult to tolerate. Many women suffer from endometriosis pain without treatment other than self-treatment with over-the-counter pain medications. Women often think cyclic pain and symptoms are a normal part of being female. Healthcare providers may need to broach the subject of pelvic pain symptoms before an assessment can be initiated.

Women suffering from endometriosis need to realize that many women are affected by this disease. Women can check the Endometriosis Association website at www.endometriosisassn.org for both support and current information. Women may benefit from local support groups available in larger metropolitan areas; these are listed on the website.

A healthy lifestyle should also be stressed, as exercise may have some benefit on pain symptoms and bone health. Women should also be advised that achieving pregnancy with endometriosis takes longer than women with normal fertility. Therefore, women may want to begin trying for a pregnancy at a younger age and not be hesitant to discuss with their physician when pregnancy is not achieved. Many women want therapy that improves their ability to conceive in the near future and may need referral to their physician or to an infertility treatment program. Women who are not under the care of a physician may benefit from an ovulation predictor kit to better time intercourse.

Patient education points:

- Explain how the diagnosis was made; if a laparoscopy was not involved, this may be necessary in the future.
- Discuss the goals of therapy with the planned treatment: medical or surgical.
- Remind a woman that if she desires conception or wishes to stop trying to conceive, she needs to notify her physician.
- NSAIDs may be used as adjunctive therapy if hormonal therapy is used.
- Explain the estimated duration of treatment (may be indefinite during reproductive years for some therapies).
- Note which therapies are also effective contraceptives or if additional contraception is needed.
- Recommend additional healthy lifestyle behaviors, such as exercise and calcium with vitamin D supplements.
- Notify women of available internet information and support groups.
- Encourage women to use other modalities that may improve pain tolerance, such as massage and yoga.

CASE PRESENTATION

Patient Case: Part 2

Assessment: The optimal treatment in this case is surgical removal of the left cystic ovarian mass. K.G. underwent an operative laparoscopy for the removal of the 4.5 x 5 cm mass. The cystic mass was removed by fenestration and excision of the cystic wall. During the operation, the content of the cystic mass was found to be thick, chocolate fluid; therefore, the mass was suspected to be an endometrioma. Also, severe endometriosis (stage IV) was diagnosed with a score of 42 based on the American Fertility Society Revised Classification of Endometriosis Scoring System. All endometriotic lesions were ablated.

Plan: The patient will be advised to have a levonorgestrel intrauterine system (LNG-IUS) inserted postoperatively. If she does not wish to have an LNG-IUS inserted, she should receive GnRH agonist treatment for 6 months. A transvaginal ultrasound check should

(Continued on next page)

be performed in 12 months postoperatively to exclude recurrence. At 12 months, if the pain persists, a second-look laparoscopy should be performed. Some authors use a CA-125 blood test in 12 months to check the effectiveness of surgical removal of the cyst.

Recommendation:

1. If the patient desires to conceive, she can commence efforts after the end of a 3- to 4-month post-treatment period, during which the menses will probably return to normal.
2. If pregnancy is not achieved within 1 year postoperatively, the patient should have a transvaginal ultrasound to exclude recurrence, and then visit an infertility clinic.

Rationale: Pelvic pain is clearly relieved for many women after surgical treatment of endometriosis, although there are limited data available from randomized controlled trials.[88] When pelvic pain is the main symptom, excision is the optimal treatment for ovarian endometriomas.[92] In cases of coexisting endometriosis, the insertion of LNG-IUS postoperatively has been found to reduce the risk of recurrent moderate-severe dysmenorrheal at 1 year follow-up.[88] If the patient receives GnRH agonist for 6 months, there may be a reduction of pain, but it is not statistically significant for a period of 12 or 24 months postoperatively.[88]

The return to normal menses is usually achieved within the first few months after treatment. If the patient desires to conceive, it is important that she feels ready to commence the effort for conceiving, and normal menses contribute to her reassurance. The effect of endometriomas on fertility is not clearly established. Nevertheless, it should be stressed that the existence of a solitary endometrioma without any surrounding endometriotic lesions is extremely rare. Although data show that pregnancy rates following surgery for endometrioma are 24% to 60% (odds ration [OR] 5.24, CI 1.92–14.27), if pregnancy is not achieved within 1 year, the couple should be considered hypofertile and be referred to an infertility clinic to receive expert assistance.[136] Also, recurrence is possible in 6.4% of cases after surgical removal of the cyst; therefore, a transvaginal ultrasound should be performed 6 and 12 months after surgery to exclude recurrence.[136] If this is not possible, a serum CA-125 measurement could imply the postoperative effectiveness of the procedure, because it is found to be useful in postoperative monitoring.[68-70] As for IVF treatment, it should be stressed that the impact of endometriomata on the outcome of fertility treatment is controversial, as there are studies that failed to support an adverse effect of endometriomata on the IVF techniques.[93]

Monitoring: Lower abdominal pain, change in menses, bloating, or altered bowel habits may imply cyst recurrence or postoperative adhesion formation.

Patient education: Face anxiety derived from a nondefinite diagnosis.

Summary

Endometriosis is a difficult disease with common presentations of dysmenorrhea, noncyclic pelvic pain, dyspareunia, and infertility. Uncommon sites on endometriotic implants can cause pain and cyclic bleeding and are more difficult to diagnose. Pelvic examination findings often suggest endometriosis, but radiologic techniques may also give diagnostic information. Laparoscopic evaluation also allows for the surgical treatment of lesions and adhesions. Current medical therapy is based on hormonal manipulation of a woman's menstrual cycle with OCs, progestins, and GnRH analogues, most commonly. Women unable to conceive in the expected time frame may benefit from assisted-reproduction techniques. Research continues on both factors contributing to endometriotic implants and more medical therapies. Unfortunately, this disease can affect a woman for many years and must be addressed with long-term treatment strategies.

References

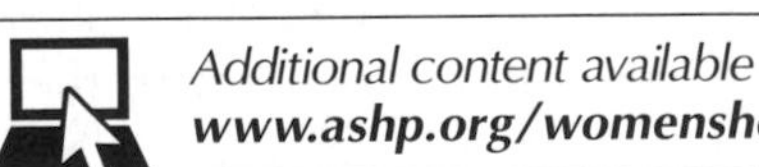

Additional content available at ***www.ashp.org/womenshealth***

15 Primary Ovarian Insufficiency

Sophia N. Kalantaridou, MD, Ph.D.; Lazaros G. Lavasidis, MD; Karim Anton Calis, Pharm.D., MPH, FASHP, FCCP

Learning Objectives

1. Describe criteria used for the diagnosis of primary ovarian insufficiency (POI).
2. Evaluate clinical manifestations and long-term risks associated with POI.
3. Explain the pathophysiologic abnormalities in POI involving sex-steroid deficiency, intermittent ovarian function, and autoimmunity.
4. Describe the clinical pharmacology of agents used in the management of POI, including estrogens, progestogens, androgens, and oral contraceptives (used as hormone replacement).
5. Formulate a comprehensive, long-term treatment and monitoring plan for a patient with POI receiving hormone replacement until the age of natural menopause.

Primary ovarian insufficiency (POI), also referred to as hypergonadotropic hypogonadism or premature ovarian failure, is a condition characterized by sex-steroid deficiency, **amenorrhea, infertility,** and elevated gonadotropins in women younger than 40 years of age.[1] It affects 1% of women by age 40 and 0.1% by age 30.[2] POI occurs in 10% to 28% of women with **primary amenorrhea** and 4% to 18% of women with **secondary amenorrhea.**[2] A cross-sectional survey of 16,065 women aged 40–55 years suggested that the prevalence of POI varies by ethnicity, with women of Asian origin having a lower risk and black Americans a higher risk compared with white Americans.[3] In this study, the prevalence of POI was 1.4% in women of black and Hispanic descent, 1% in white American, 0.5% in Chinese American, and 0.1% in Japanese American women.[3]

At one time, POI was considered irreversible and was described as premature **menopause.** However, menopause is the permanent cessation of menses following the loss of ovarian follicular activity.[4] It is a natural physiologic event in a woman's life that occurs at an average age of 51 years and results from ovarian follicle depletion.[3] In contrast, POI is characterized by intermittent ovarian function, and pregnancy may occur many years after the diagnosis.[1,5]

POI may present as either primary or secondary amenorrhea. When POI presents as primary amenorrhea, approximately 50% of cases will be associated with an abnormal karyotype.[6] Approximately one half of women with POI report a history of oligomenorrhea or dysfunctional uterine bleeding (prodromal POI). POI may also occur acutely, with no warning signs of the approaching disease.

The incidence of familial cases, which suggest a genetic component, varies in several studies from 30% to 12.7%.[7,8] probably because of selection and recall bias. A detailed family history may distinguish between familial and sporadic POI. The risk of developing POI may be higher in female relatives in familial POI as compared with sporadic cases. Early diagnosis of familial predisposition permits prediction of impending POI, and susceptible women are encouraged to consider their reproductive plans and timely scheduling of pregnancy, if appropriate. Fertility is usually normal before the development of POI.

Etiology

POI is a heterogeneous disorder and may occur as a result of decreased initial follicle number, ovarian follicle dysfunction, or ovarian follicle depletion. Indeed, a wide range of defects may lead to POI, including autoimmune, genetic, iatrogenic, and metabolic causes

Table 15-1. Etiology of Primary Ovarian Insufficiency

Idiopathic or karyotypically normal spontaneous premature ovarian failure (the majority of the cases)
Surgically induced premature ovarian failure (following oophorectomy)
Ovarian failure due to chemotherapy of radiation
Autoimmunity a) isolated autoimmune premature ovarian failure or b) as a component of an autoimmune polyglandular syndrome in association with Addison's disease, hypothyroidism, hypoparathyroidism, or mucocutaneous candidiasis (*AIRE* gene mutations; 21q22.3)
X-chromosome defects X-monosomy (Turner's syndrome); X-mosaicism; X chromosome translocations or partial deletions; *FMR1* gene premutations (fragile X premutation, Xq27.3); *FMR2* (Xq28); *BMP15* gene mutation (Xp11.2)
Autosomal chromosome abnormalities *NOG* gene mutations (17q22); *POLG* gene mutations (15q25); Inhibin A variation (2q33-q36)
Gonadotropin and gonadotropin-receptor abnormalities affecting ovarian function FSH-receptor gene mutations (2p21-p16); LH-receptor gene mutations (2p21)
Enzyme deficiencies affecting ovarian function Cholesterol desmolase, 17a-hydroxylase, 17-20 desmolase
Rare syndromes associated with premature ovarian failure Galactosemia (galactose-1-phosphate uridyl transferase, *GALT* gene mutations; 9p13) Blepharophimosis, ptosis, and epicanthus inversus syndrome type 1; autosomal dominant syndrome, in which premature ovarian failure is the predominant syndrome) Perrault's syndrome; familial autosomal recessive premature ovarian failure in association with deafness

(Table 15-1).[9] In most cases (approximately 90%), the etiology of ovarian insufficiency cannot be identified. Rare causes of POI include autoimmune ovarian damage, chromosomal and genetic abnormalities involving the X chromosome or autosomes, and iatrogenic damage following pelvic surgery and cancer therapy (chemotherapy or radiotherapy). A complete discussion regarding the etiology of POF is beyond the scope of this chapter.

A large number of genes have been screened for their potential to cause POI. Genetic abnormalities associated with POI include mutations involving the follicle-stimulated hormone (FSH) receptor (*FSHR*), the galactose-1-phosphate uridyltransferase associated with galactosemia (*GALT*), the forehead transcription factor associated with the blepharophimosis/ptosis/epicanthus inversus syndrome (*FOXL2*), the inhibin A gene (*INHA*), the bone morphogenetic protein 15 (*BMP15*), among others.[9]

It is important to note that POI affects 15% to 22% of women who carry the *FMR1* permutation.[10] An *FMR1* mutation occurs in 0.8% to 7.5% of women with sporadic POI and in approximately 13% of women with a family history of POI (without prior known history of fragile X syndrome).[11] Fragile X syndrome is the most common inherited cause of mental retardation, caused by an expanded CGG trinucleotide repeat in the promoter region of the *FMR1* gene.[12] Normal alleles have approximately 12–44 CGG repeats in this region. Full mutation alleles have more than 200 CGG repeats and are partially or fully hypermethylated, resulting in the inactivation of the *FMR1* gene product, fragile X mental retardation protein. Premutation alleles have 55–200 CGG repeats and do not result in gene inactivation.[12]

Clinical Presentation

In the majority of patients, ovarian insufficiency develops after the establishment of regular menses (secondary amenorrhea). In these cases, symptoms may include hot flushes, night sweats, sleep disturbances, sexual dysfunction and **dyspareunia,** fatigue, problems with concentration and memory, and mood changes. The development of secondary sex charac-

CASE PRESENTATION

Patient Case: Part 1

A.M. is a 22-year-old woman who presents to the reproductive endocrinology clinic with a 5-month history of secondary amenorrhea. During the last month, she had moderate-to-severe hot flushes (five to six episodes per day), which were exacerbated during the night. Her menarche was at age 14. She had regular periods until the last 6 months, when she started having irregular menstrual cycles. Her body mass index is 22.5, and her past medical history is significant for Hashimoto's thyroiditis. Current medications include levothyroxine sodium and a multivitamin. She does not smoke, and she drinks one glass of red wine per day.

Family history: Mother—diabetes; father—hypertension and coronary artery disease.

Physical examination: Unremarkable. Vital signs were stable. Breast and pelvic examinations were normal. Transvaginal ultrasound examination revealed a normal-size uterus with a thin endometrium (2 mm). No follicles were observed in the ovaries.

Laboratory values: Pertinent findings include FSH: 150 milli-International Units/mL; LH: 45 milli-International Units/mL; E_2: 20 pg/mL; TSH: 0.9 milli-International Units/L; FT4: 1.8 ng/dL; anti-TPO: 310 International Units/mL; anti-TG: 80 International Units/mL (normal ranges: FSH:<1–3 prepubertal, 1–11 follicular and luteal phase, 6–26 at ovulation, 30–118 postmenopausal [milli-International Units/mL], LH: <0.15 prepubertal, 0.5–14.5 follicular and luteal phase, 16–84 at ovulation, 17–75 postmenopausal [milli-International Units/mL], E_2: 20–140 early follicular phase –day 5, 100–400 preovulatory peak, 20–160 luteal phase, 35<postmenopausal [pg/mL], TSH: 0.5–4.8 milli-International Units/L, FT4: 0.7–1.85 ng/dL, anti-TPO: <10 International Units/mL, anti-TG: <20 International Units/mL).

teristics is normal in women with secondary amenorrhea. Signs of secondary amenorrhea may include urogenital atrophy.

Primary amenorrhea is not associated with vasomotor symptoms. Signs of primary amenorrhea may include urogenital atrophy and incomplete development of secondary sex characteristics. In patients with primary amenorrhea, stature, signs of Turner's syndrome, and other features of gonadal dysgenesis should be examined.

Pathophysiology

Women with POI sustain estrogen and androgen deficiency for more years than do naturally menopausal women.[13] This deficiency results in a significantly higher risk for osteoporosis and cardiovascular disease.[14-17] In addition, a survey of more than 19,000 women between the ages of 25 and 100 years suggested that ovarian insufficiency occurring before 40 years of age is associated with significantly increased mortality, with the age-adjusted odds ratio for all-cause mortality being 2.14 (95% CI, 1.15–3.99).[18]

A study of 119 women with spontaneous POI showed that 27% (32/119) had hypothyroidism, 2.5% (3/119) had diabetes mellitus, and 2.5% (3/119) had Addison's disease.[19] A 3.2% prevalence of previously undetected adrenal insufficiency has been noted among women with spontaneous POI.[20] Women with spontaneous POI should be tested for these associated endocrine disorders.

Long-term Complications: Osteoporosis and Cardiovascular Disease Risk

OSTEOPOROSIS RISK

Women with normal ovarian function achieve peak femoral neck bone mineral density in their 20s and peak spinal bone mineral density in their 30s.[21] Sex steroids play an important role in maintaining bone mass and cessation of ovarian function results in significant bone loss.[22] Estrogen deficiency is associated with accelerated bone loss that is due to increased bone turnover.

Cross-sectional studies indicate that patients with POI have a more severe bone loss and a significantly greater frequency of vertebral fractures compared with normally menopausal women.[13,23,24] Therefore, a diagnosis of POI in itself is an indication for bone density testing.

The World Health Organization (WHO) defines osteoporosis as a progressive systemic disease characterized by low bone density and microarchitectural deterioration in bone that predisposes to increased bone fragility and fracture.[25] According to

WHO, osteoporosis is defined as a T-score of −2.5 or lower (i.e., bone mineral density that is 2.5 SD or more below the normal mean value for young adults), and osteopenia as a T-score that is greater than −2.5 but less than −1.0.[25] Nevertheless, the WHO criteria for diagnosis of osteoporosis by T-scores apply only to postmenopausal women; these criteria were not intended to be used in young premenopausal women.

We have shown that two thirds of young women with POI have a bone mineral density that has been associated with an increased risk for hip fracture.[15] It is worthwhile noting that 47% of these women had significantly reduced bone mineral density within 1.5 years of their diagnosis despite taking standard hormone therapy.[15] One reason for the loss of bone mass in these young women is that they have menstrual irregularities in the years preceding POI, and menstrual irregularities have been associated with significant bone loss.[26,27] Another reason for the loss of bone mass in these young women with POI on "standard" estrogen therapy is that the standard estrogen dose, which has been designed for normal menopausal women, is generally too low for these young women.[28,29] In addition, androgen deficiency might explain why two thirds of these young women have significantly reduced bone mineral density—associated with a 2.6-fold increased risk for hip fracture—despite taking standard estrogen replacement therapy.[15] Recently, a randomized trial conducted at the National Institutes of Health has shown that a relatively high estrogen dosage (100 mcg/day transdermally) maintains bone mass as well as normal ovarian function in age-matched women with regular menstrual cycles.[30] The addition of physiologic transdermal testosterone replacement to standard estrogen/progestogen therapy does not significantly increase bone mass.[31]

Other bone-protecting agents, such as bisphosphonates and human parathyroid hormone (hPTH), have been evaluated in postmenopausal women with osteoporosis. Safety of these agents for women with POI should be considered. There are no data evaluating the usefulness of bisphosphonates among young women with POI. Bisphosphonates, however, have been evaluated among premenopausal women with primary hyperparathyroidism and in those who receiving glucocorticoid therapy.[32-34]

As previously mentioned, women with POI have a 5% to 10% chance for a spontaneous pregnancy. Bisphosphonates have long-term skeletal retention, and these agents can be released from the skeleton several years later, potentially in a subsequent pregnancy. The effects of bisphosphonates on the developing fetal skeleton are unknown. Bisphosphonates have a category C rating for safety in pregnancy, based on toxic effects at parturition in the rat model.[35] Similarly, a potential safety issue with hPTH is increased risk of osteosarcoma, which was reported in a lifelong carcinogenicity study in a rat model.[36] Therefore, bisphosphonate and hPTH use should be discouraged in young women with POI until appropriately designed studies clarify their safety and efficacy.

CARDIOVASCULAR DISEASE

Women with POI have an increased risk for cardiovascular disease, which may be attributed to the early onset of vascular endothelial dysfunction (a marker of atherosclerosis) associated with sex-steroid deficiency.[16,17,37] Cyclic estrogen/progestogen therapy has been shown to restore endothelial function in these young women.[17]

Previous observational and prospective cohort studies suggested that hormone therapy decreases the risk of cardiovascular disease in early postmenopausal women.[38,39] In contrast, large prospective randomized trials conducted in older postmenopausal women, who were menopausal for more than a decade, showed that hormone therapy increases the risk of cardiovascular disease, mainly during the first year of hormone therapy use.[40-42] These findings have led young women with POI and their physicians to question whether they should initiate or continue hormone therapy. However, there are no prospective data regarding the impact of hormone therapy on cardiovascular disease in women with POI, and a decision regarding hormone therapy in these young women should not be based on studies of hormone therapy in women older than 50 years of age. More importantly, reanalysis of the results from recent randomized trials suggested that a woman's age and the number of years of ovarian dysfunction are potential factors influencing the effects of hormone therapy on cardiovascular disease.[41-44] Indeed, most previous observational and prospective cohort studies of hormone therapy involved the use of estrogen given alone or in cyclic regimens in relatively young postmenopausal women, whereas the more recent randomized studies involved the use of continuous combined hormone therapy in older postmenopausal women. Therefore, it appears that a beneficial effect on cardiovascular disease with hormone therapy can be seen with estrogen alone or cyclic estrogen/progestogen treatment, but not with continuous combined therapy and in young women with POI.[17]

INFERTILITY

Infertility is a major issue for young women with POI. However, women with spontaneous POI produce estrogen intermittently and may ovulate despite the presence of high gonadotropin concentrations.[5] Spontaneous pregnancies have occurred in 5% to 10% of women after the diagnosis of POI.[1] Ovarian function is notably unpredictable, and some residual ovarian activity may be present many years after the initial diagnosis.

Diagnosis of Primary Ovarian Insufficiency

In most cases of amenorrhea, history, physical examination (including a thorough examination of the external and internal genitalia), and measurement of FSH, thyroid-stimulating hormone (TSH), and prolactin will provide the diagnosis.[45] The diagnosis of POI is specifically formed on the presence of amenorrhea for 4 months and the finding of elevated serum FSH levels. In a young girl, evaluation of primary amenorrhea should be initiated when there is a failure to menstruate by age 15 in the presence of normal secondary sexual characteristics, or within 5 years after breast development if that occurs before age 10.[45] Failure to initiate breast development by age 13 also requires evaluation; the presence of breast development provides evidence of prior estrogen action, thus excluding the possibility of an abnormal karyotype that includes the Y chromosome.[45] Gonadal tumors occur in as many as 25% of women with a Y chromosome. As such, the gonads should be removed at the time of diagnosis in order to prevent the development of gonadoblastoma.[46] Secondary amenorrhea lasting 3 months requires evaluation.[45]

LABORATORY TESTING AND DIAGNOSTIC PROCEDURES

The presence of amenorrhea along with elevated serum FSH concentrations in the menopausal range on at least two occasions (drawn at least 1 month apart) are essential elements in the diagnosis of POI. It should be noted that, with the newer assays, 20 milli-International Units/mL is now considered menopausal. The repeated testing is necessary because the natural history of POI can be variable, and ovarian function in affected women can be intermittent and unpredictable. A pregnancy test also is essential in order to exclude the possibility of pregnancy.

A karyotype and *FMR1* testing should be performed in all women experiencing amenorrhea and elevated gonadotropins. Women with POI and alleles in the 45–54 CGG repeat range should be referred for genetic counseling.[12] Indeed, women with a permutation in the *FMR1* gene are at risk of having a child with mental retardation should they conceive spontaneously in the presence of POI.[47] Of note, women with relatives with spontaneous POI should also be referred for genetic counseling.[12] In addition, *FMR1* testing is recommended in some infertile women (especially those with increased FSH levels), egg donors, and patients presenting with a personal or family history of mental retardation, developmental disability, or autism.[12]

Ovarian biopsy and anti-ovarian antibody testing have no proven clinical benefit in POI.[1,48] Baseline bone mineral density testing should be performed in all women with POI, but mammography should be performed annually only after the age of 40 years according to standard guidelines.[4] Additional testing includes thyroid function tests (serum TSH, free T4, and serum thyroid peroxidase autoantibodies) and detection of adrenal antibodies for thyroid and adrenal insufficiency. Testing for adrenal antibodies will identify women with POI who have steroidogenic cell autoimmunity and are at increased risk of adrenal insufficiency, a potentially fatal condition. As noted, approximately 20% of women with spontaneous POI develop autoimmune hypothyroidism, and 4% will test positive for adrenal antibodies. Other tests should be performed as clinically indicated.

Treatment Goals

Treatment goals include cyclic hormone therapy for the prevention of long-term complications of estrogen deficiency and infertility management.

Nonpharmacologic Intervention

Women with POI should follow standard lifestyle interventions measures for osteoporosis prevention, such as adequate weight-bearing exercise (i.e., walking, moderate resistance training), smoking cessation, avoidance of excessive alcohol intake (no more than two drinks/day), and adequate calcium and vitamin D intake.[49] These nonpharmacologic measures should supplement, not replace, hormone therapy.

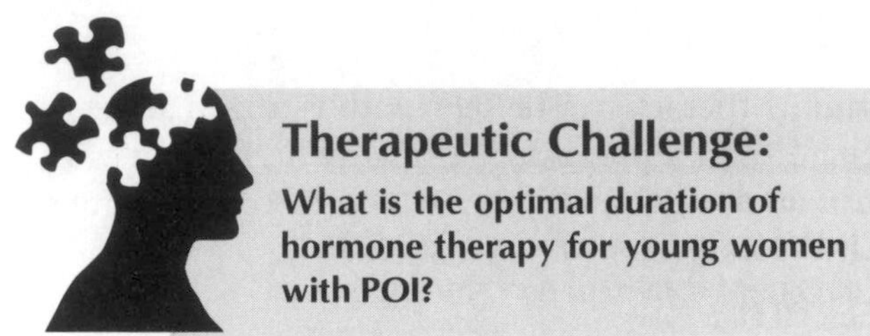

Therapeutic Challenge:
What is the optimal duration of hormone therapy for young women with POI?

Pharmacologic Treatment

CALCIUM AND VITAMIN D

Women with POI should be advised regarding adequate calcium (1,200–1,500 mg/day) and vitamin D (about 800 International Units/day) intake to prevent deficiency. In western society, supplementation is necessary in many cases because of inadequate sun exposure and dietary intake.

HORMONE THERAPY

Women with POI need exogenous sex steroids to compensate for the decreased production by their ovaries. Indeed, for young women with POI, hormone therapy is "true replacement" of ovarian hormones. In these women, physiologic hormone therapy until the age of natural menopause may be necessary for relief of menopausal symptoms (i.e., vasomotor symptoms and urogenital atrophy) and prevention of long-term consequences of sex-steroid deficiency, such as osteoporosis and possibly cardiovascular disease. Practically, there is no alternative to hormone replacement in these young women.[50] Few data are available about possible adverse effects of hormone therapy in young women with POI, but there are no data to suggest an increased risk of breast cancer.[50,51] A study of a French cohort of postmenopausal women suggests that when natural progesterone is used instead of synthetic progestogens in hormone therapy, the risk of breast cancer is not increased.[52] The main concern about hormone therapy in young women with POI appears to be the prothrombotic risk. Recent data indicate that oral but not transdermal estrogen is associated with an increased risk for venous thromboembolism in postmenopausal women.[53] Therefore, until additional data are available, transdermal estrogen and oral natural progesterone can be recommended as a first-line therapy in women with POI.

A wide range of estrogen and progestogen regimens are available for hormone replacement, including oral, transdermal, subcutaneous, and vaginal routes of administration (Tables 15-2 and 15-3). The estrogen/progestogen regimen should be based on individual needs and individual preferences. Estrogens administered in usual replacement doses do not suppress spontaneous follicular activity or ovulation and do not prevent spontaneous conceptions. Most pregnancies have occurred during or following hormone replacement. Optimal hormone therapy should consider whether the patient has primary or secondary amenorrhea.

Primary Amenorrhea—Induction of Puberty

Young girls with primary amenorrhea in whom secondary sex characteristics have failed to develop should initially be exposed to very low doses of estrogen in an attempt to mimic the gradual pubertal maturation process.[54] Treatment should begin around the age of 12 years in order to permit the normal pace of puberty. Estradiol treatment usually begins at 10% to 12% of the adult replacement dose (Table 15-2). To allow for normal breast and uterine development, it is best to delay the addition of progestogens at least 2 years after starting estrogen or until breakthrough bleeding occurs. The oral contraceptive use should be avoided for induction of puberty, because the synthetic estrogen doses are much too high (even in the low-estrogen products).

Secondary Amenorrhea—Cyclic Hormone Therapy

Because women with POI can have spontaneous pregnancies, cyclic regimens of hormone therapy that produce regular, predictable menstrual flow patterns—mimicking the menses of age-matched women with normal ovarian function—should be used, instead of continuous combined hormone therapy that results in the absence of menses.[1] Consequently, if these young patients miss an expected menses, they should be tested for pregnancy and instructed to discontinue the hormone therapy.

Daily serum measurements of estradiol in regularly menstruating women indicate that the mean estradiol level over the menstrual cycle is approximately 100 pg/mL.[55] Indeed, in women with POI (mean age = 32 years), hormone therapy using a transdermal patch of estradiol (100 mcg/day—i.e., a dosage about twice as much as the standard dosage given to older women experiencing natural menopause; Table 15-2) resulted in comparable estradiol levels to those of age-matched women with normal

Table 15-2. Estrogen Replacement for Young Women with Primary Ovarian Insufficiency

Regimen	Suggested Dose for Young Women with Primary Ovarian Insufficiency	"Standard" Dose for Peri- and Early Post-menopausal Women	Suggested Low-Dose for Postmenopausal Women	Comments
Oral estrogens				
Conjugated equine estrogens	1.25 mg	0.625 mg	0.3 or 0.45 mg	Orally administered estrogens (once daily) stimulate the synthesis of hepatic proteins and increase the circulating concentrations of sex-hormone binding globulin, which, in turn, may compromise the bioavailability of androgens and estrogens
Synthetic conjugated estrogens	1.25 mg	0.625 mg	0.3 mg	
-Estropipate (piperazine estrone sulfate)	1.25 mg	0.625 mg	0.3 mg	
Ethinyl estradiol	10 mcg	5 mcg	2.5 mcg	
Micronized 17β-estradiol	2 mg	1 mg	0.25 or 0.5 mg	
Parenteral estrogens				
Transdermal 17β-estradiol (once or twice weekly)	100-mcg patch	50-mcg patch	25-mcg patch	Women with elevated triglyceride concentrations or significant liver function abnormalities may benefit from parenteral therapy Parenteral therapy may be associated with a lower risk for thromboembolic disease than oral treatment
Intranasal 17β-estradiol (once daily)	300 mcg per nostril	150 mcg per nostril		
Implanted 17β-estradiol pellets subcutaneously (every 6 months)	100 mg	50 mg		
Percutaneous 17β-estradiol (emulsion; gel; once daily)	0.08 mg (gel) 0.10 mg (emulsion)	0.04 mg (gel) 0.05 mg (emulsion)		

ovarian function.[13] This dosage should be adjusted to avoid hot flushes (which might require an increase in the estrogen dose) or breast tenderness (which might require a decrease in the estrogen dose).

In women with POI and an intact uterus, a progestogen should be added for endometrial protection, whereas women who have undergone hysterectomy should receive estrogen alone.[4] Therefore, cyclic progestogen should be added, at a dosage equivalent to 10 mg of medroxyprogesterone acetate for the last 12–14 days of each 28-day cycle (Table 15-3). In older postmenopausal women, this regimen has been shown to adequately protect the endometrium in combination with estrogen treatment.[56] Progestogen administration less frequently than each 28-day cycle has been associated with endometrial hyperplasia, and if this is preferred by the patient, she must be informed of the need for appropriate monitoring.[57] Finally, some women may prefer the use of oral contraceptives instead of "postmenopausal regimens." Generally this is not recommended, and it should be noted that some oral contraceptives are not an effective means of birth control in women with POI.[1]

Equivalent oral and parenteral estrogens have comparable effects on hot flushes and bone mineral density.[4] Women with secondary amenorrhea who have estrogen deficiency for 12 months or longer should also initially be given low-dose estrogen therapy to avoid adverse effects such as breast tenderness and nausea. Women with a brief history of secondary amenorrhea are less likely to experience side effects from hormone therapy if they are given a reduced dose for the first month of therapy followed by a full dose from the second month onward.

Table 15-3. Progestogens for Endometrial Protection

Regimens	Suggested Dose for Young Women with Primary Ovarian Insufficiency	"Standard" Dose For Peri- and Early Postmenopausal Women
Oral progestogens (once daily)		
Medroxyprogesterone acetate	10 mg	5–10 mg
Dydrogesterone	20 mg	10–20 mg
Norethindrone	1 mg	0.7–1 mg
Norethisterone acetate	10 mg	5–10 mg
Micronized progesterone	200 mg	200 mg
Norgestrel	0.15 mg	0.15 mg
Levonorgestrel	150 mcg	150 mcg
Parenteral progestogens		
Transdermal norethindrone acetate (twice a week)[b]	250 mcg	250 mcg
Vaginal progesterone 4% (once daily)	45 mg	45 mg

[a]Cyclic administration; 12–14 days per calendar month.
[b]In combination with transdermal estradiol (50 mcg): estradiol alone for days 1–14, followed by estradiol/norethindrone acetate (50 mcg/250 mcg) for days 15–28.

Androgen Therapy

The normal functioning ovary is an important source of estrogen as well as androgen production. Young women with POI have lower testosterone concentrations compared with normal ovulatory women.[13] Nevertheless, physiologic testosterone replacement failed to improve bone mineral density and sexual function in women with POI receiving estrogen/progestogen replacement.[31,58,59]

Infertility Treatment

As previously mentioned, women with POI have a 5% to 10% chance for spontaneous pregnancy. There are no proven therapies to improve ovarian function and increase fertility rates in women with POI.[60] A small placebo-controlled study suggested that pretreatment with ethinyl estradiol may improve the success of rate of ovulation induction with exogenous gonadotropins in women with POI.[61] Larger studies with adequate power are needed to confirm this finding. The use of corticosteroids for ovulation induction has provided conflicting results in women with POI.[62–64]

Presently, assisted conception with donated oocytes is the only well-documented way to achieve pregnancy.[65] An important issue for oocyte donation is the need for *FMR1* testing.[12] This is particularly important in women with POI who are tempted to ask for oocyte donation from a relative who may also carry a fragile X permutation and who might be at risk for donating an oocyte with a full fragile X mutation. Embryo cryopreservation has been used in cases in which ovarian insufficiency is anticipated because of impending cancer treatment. In some cases, chemotherapy or radiotherapy has been delayed until after ovulation induction and in vitro fertilization.[66]

Recently, a successful pregnancy has been reported following ovarian transplantation between monozygotic twins discordant for POI.[67]

With the discovery of markers identifying the development of ovarian insufficiency many years before

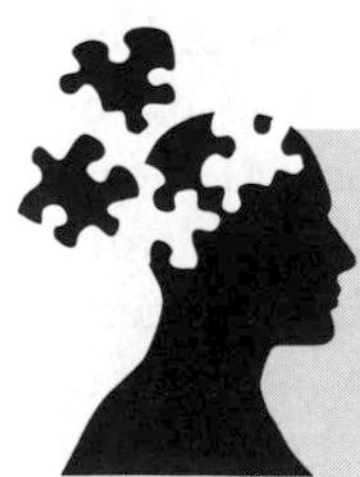

Therapeutic Challenge:

Under what circumstances would an androgen regimen be a good choice for a woman with POI and low androgen levels?

the establishment of the disease, oocyte or ovarian tissue cryopreservation (which are currently experimental procedures) have been proposed as new options in the management of infertility.[68,69]

Monitoring and Follow-up

Women with POI should be monitored annually for their response to treatment, and their compliance with hormone therapy should be regularly assessed. Initially, after the young woman begins hormone therapy, a brief follow-up visit 6 weeks after initiation of hormone therapy may be useful to discuss patient concerns about the treatment and to evaluate the patient for symptom relief, adverse effects, and patterns of withdrawal bleeding. Additional follow-up should be determined based on the patient's initial response to therapy and the need for any modification of the regimen. The persistence of hot flushes may require the increase in the estrogen dose. However, oral estrogens produce a marked dose-dependent increase in sex-hormone binding globulin (SHBG) levels; switching to parenteral therapy may alleviate menopausal symptoms by decreasing SHBG concentrations and, thus, increasing bioavailable estrogen. On the other hand, the presence of breast tenderness or nausea may require the decrease in the estrogen dose. Endometrial biopsy should be considered in women with POI taking cyclic hormone therapy as clinically indicated. Women with POI should also be evaluated continuously for the presence of signs and symptoms of associated autoimmune endocrine disorders, such as hypothyroidism, adrenal insufficiency, and diabetes mellitus. At present there are no guidelines for follow-up bone mineral density testing. However, in women with significant bone loss, repeat testing should be performed as clinically indicated.

Patient Education

Young women find the diagnosis of POI particularly traumatic and frequently need extensive emotional and psychological support. These young women may experience a sense of helplessness, and physicians may play a role in alleviating this. A healthy lifestyle should be stressed, as well as exercise and adequate calcium and vitamin D intake.

Many women with POI benefit from meeting other women with this condition; therefore, referral to an organization such as the Premature Ovarian Failure (POF) Support Group can be helpful (http://pofsupport.org).

CASE PRESENTATION

Patient Case: Part 2

Assessment: A karyotype and *FMR1* testing were performed with normal results (karyotype: 46,XX; *FMR1* testing revealed 34 CGG repeats in this region). Antiadrenal antibody testing by indirect immunofluorescence was negative. Bone mineral density at the lumbar spine was normal (T-score: –0.1).

Plan: A.M. was advised to start taking transdermal estradiol therapy (100 mcg/day) along with oral natural progesterone (200 mg/day) for the last 12 days of each 28-day cycle. She was also advised to get adequate exercise and increase her calcium and vitamin D intake. Because at present the patient wants to avoid pregnancy, the possibility of a spontaneous conception was discussed. A scheduled visit was planned 6 weeks later to discuss hormone therapy–related issues (adherence, response to therapy, and potential adverse effects). Follow-up for osteoporosis prevention and associated endocrine disorders was discussed.

Once endocrine and emotional health issues regarding POI are addressed, women with POI are ready to move forward to make decisions about reproduction. Apart from assisted reproduction, options may include child-free living and adoption.

Summary

POI is not an early natural menopause. Most affected women produce estrogen intermittently and may ovulate despite the presence of high gonadotropin concentrations. However, these women sustain sex-steroid deficiency for more years than do naturally menopausal women, resulting in a significantly higher risk for osteoporosis and cardiovascular disease. Furthermore, women with POI have more severe menopausal symptoms than women with natural menopause. These young women should be treated with hormone therapy to compensate for the decreased ovarian production of sex steroids. Practically, there is no alternative to hormone therapy in young women with POI. At present, there are no guidelines for the management of young women with POI, and data from prospective clinical trials are lacking.

Because women with POI can have spontaneous pregnancies, cyclic regimens of hormone therapy that produce regular, predictable menstrual flow patterns—mimicking the menses of age-matched women with normal ovarian function—should be used. Findings from recent randomized trials in postmenopausal women are not applicable to young women with POI because postmenopausal women who take hormone therapy prolong their exposure to estrogen beyond the average age of completion of their reproductive phase. Women with POI need long-term follow-up for the presence of associated endocrine disorders and for general health maintenance, including osteoporosis prevention.

References

Additional content available at
www.ashp.org/womenshealth

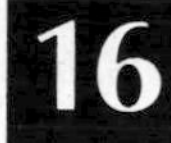

16 Polycystic Ovary Syndrome

Laura Marie Borgelt, Pharm.D., FCCP, BCPS; Kai I. Cheang, Pharm.D., M.Sc., BCPS, FCCP

Learning Objectives

1. Describe criteria used for the diagnosis of polycystic ovary syndrome (PCOS).
2. Evaluate clinical manifestations and long-term risks associated with PCOS.
3. Explain the pathophysiologic abnormalities in PCOS involving gonadotropin secretion, androgen production, and insulin resistance with hyperinsulinemia.
4. Compare and contrast medications used for the treatment of PCOS, including oral contraceptives, insulin sensitizers, antiandrogens, and ovulation-induction agents.
5. Formulate a comprehensive clinical plan including nonpharmacologic and pharmacologic therapy for a patient with PCOS.

Polycystic ovary syndrome (PCOS) affects approximately 6% to 8% (or 1 in 15) women of reproductive age, making it the most common endocrine abnormality and the leading cause of anovulatory **infertility** for this age group.[1] The clinical presentation will vary among individual women and can make management intriguing, complex, and challenging. Women with PCOS may have poor self-image because of hirsutism, acne (which can cause scarring), or obesity despite rigorous diet and exercise plans. The syndrome can also have major impact throughout life on the reproductive, metabolic, and cardiovascular health of affected women. Healthcare providers are well aligned to interact with this patient population by providing assessment and assisting in the decision-making process for appropriate treatment.

This syndrome was first described in 1935 by Stein and Leventhal when they reported infertility and amenorrhea in seven women with enlarged cystic ovaries.[2] Stein later added excessive male-patterned hair growth and obesity to the description.[3] Although it has been called Stein-Leventhal syndrome, polycystic ovary, polycystic ovarian disease, hyperandrogenic chronic anovulatory syndrome, and functional ovarian **hyperandrogenism**, the name *polycystic ovary syndrome* has been widely accepted to describe the heterogeneous nature of this disorder.

Clinical Presentation

Women with PCOS typically have a clinical presentation that involves hyperandrogenism, menstrual disturbances, and possible obesity. Common clinical signs of hyperandrogenism include hirsutism, acne, and alopecia. Hirsutism is the most common of these characteristics and occurs in 60% to 70% of women with PCOS.[4] It is defined as an excess of thickly pigmented body hair in a male distribution and commonly found on the upper lip, around the chin, on lower abdomen, around the nipples, on the inner aspects of the thighs, and on the lower back. Acne affects 15% to 25% of women with PCOS, but this incidence may not be different from the general population. Alopecia presents as scalp hair loss in the crown and vertex areas and occurs in approximately 5% of the PCOS population.[5]

Ovulatory dysfunction in PCOS is typically described as **oligo-ovulation** or **anovulation**, which means the patient has irregular menstrual cycles (eight or fewer per year). Overall, 60% to 85% of patients with PCOS and oligoovulation have menstrual dysfunction, usually oligomenorrhea or amenorrhea.[1] These menstrual disturbances usually begin in the peripubertal years. A laboratory finding that may provide evidence for irregular ovulation and menses is an increased luteinizing hormone (LH) to follicle-stimulating hormone (FSH) ratio greater than 2 or 3; however, LH and FSH levels

CASE PRESENTATION

Patient Case: Part 1

J.C. is a 24-year-old obese woman who presents to clinic today for a co-consult for suspected PCOS with a physician and clinical pharmacist. She has mild hair growth above her upper lip, mild acne, and a history of irregular menstrual periods. Her irregular periods were not bothersome until the last 2 years when she and her husband have tried to get pregnant. She is interested in learning more about why they may be having difficulty and what treatments are available to help her become pregnant. Her husband has been checked, and he has a normal semen analysis.

HPI: Since age 12, J.C. has had six to seven periods per year that occur every 30 to 90 days. When she does have a period, she considers them to be normal, without pain or excessive bleeding. She states that the hair on her upper lip has always been bothersome, but she gets it waxed routinely. She struggles with her obesity because she has been unable to lose weight despite walking vigorously for 20 minutes 5 days/week over the past 6 months.

PMH: Occasional headaches when stressed.

Family history: Mother—diabetes, hypertension; father—diabetes, hypertension, dyslipidemia.

Social history: No tobacco, occasional alcohol, walks 20 min five days/week.

Medications: Benzoyl peroxide 5% topical twice daily; acetaminophen 1,000 mg as needed for headaches; multivitamin daily.

Allergies: No known drug allergies.

Vitals: 5′7″, 195 lb, body mass index (BMI) 30.5, blood pressure 114/80, heart rate 70, temperature 98.6°F, respiration rate 18.

Physical exam: Normal, with the exception of noted excessive facial hair, mild acne, and acanthosis nigricans.

Laboratory values: Pertinent findings include fasting glucose 102 mg/dL, total cholesterol 236, low-density lipoprotein 150 mg/dL, high-density lipoprotein 40 mg/dL, triglyceride 210 mg/dL, serum creatinine 0.9 mg/dL.

fluctuate throughout the menstrual cycle so this measurement may be inaccurate and is not considered diagnostic for PCOS.[4]

Obesity occurs in approximately 30% to 60% of women with PCOS.[1] A pattern of central or abdominal obesity is typically seen, which is a risk factor for many obesity-related health risks (e.g., diabetes, heart disease), worsens other clinical features of PCOS (e.g., anovulation, hyperandrogenism), and suggests that insulin resistance may be present.[6] Therefore, lifestyle modification with appropriate diet and exercise is a foundation of treatment for many patients with PCOS.

Pathophysiology

The pathophysiology of PCOS is complex and important to understand for appropriate treatment decisions. The primary defect in PCOS is unknown, but there appear to be three possible mechanisms acting alone or synergistically to create the presentation seen with PCOS. These mechanisms include inappropriate gonadotropin secretion, insulin resistance with hyperinsulinemia, and excessive androgen production. These mechanisms are closely integrated, as seen in Figure 16-1.

A genetic basis for PCOS has been postulated, but its mode of transmission is unclear.[7] Hypotheses have ranged from an autosomal dominant model to a polygenic model with genetic-environmental interactions. More than 50 candidate genes have been proposed as potential contributors to PCOS.

GONADOTROPIN SECRETION

In normal menstrual cycles, the hypothalamus produces a neurohormone called gonadotropin-releasing hormone (GnRH), which regulates the release of FSH and LH from the anterior pituitary in a pulsatile fashion every 60–90 minutes. FSH stimulates growth of ovarian follicles, and LH is critical for ovulation and sex steroid production. Typically, when FSH concentrations rise, a small group of follicles develop, then a dominant follicle emerges in the follicular phase. Estrogen concentrations also rise during this time and create an LH surge to cause ovulation. In the luteal phase that follows, progesterone is synthesized and secreted, which is necessary for successful implantation of an embryo. If pregnancy does not occur, progesterone concentrations decrease and menstruation occurs.

In PCOS, there is an increased frequency of GnRH stimulation, which results in an increase in LH pulse frequency and amplitude; FSH secretion remains normal. The development of a dominant follicle does not occur because LH secretion occurs before a dominant follicle can emerge. Therefore, a woman is left with several immature follicles and will not

Figure 16-1. Pathophysiology of PCOS.

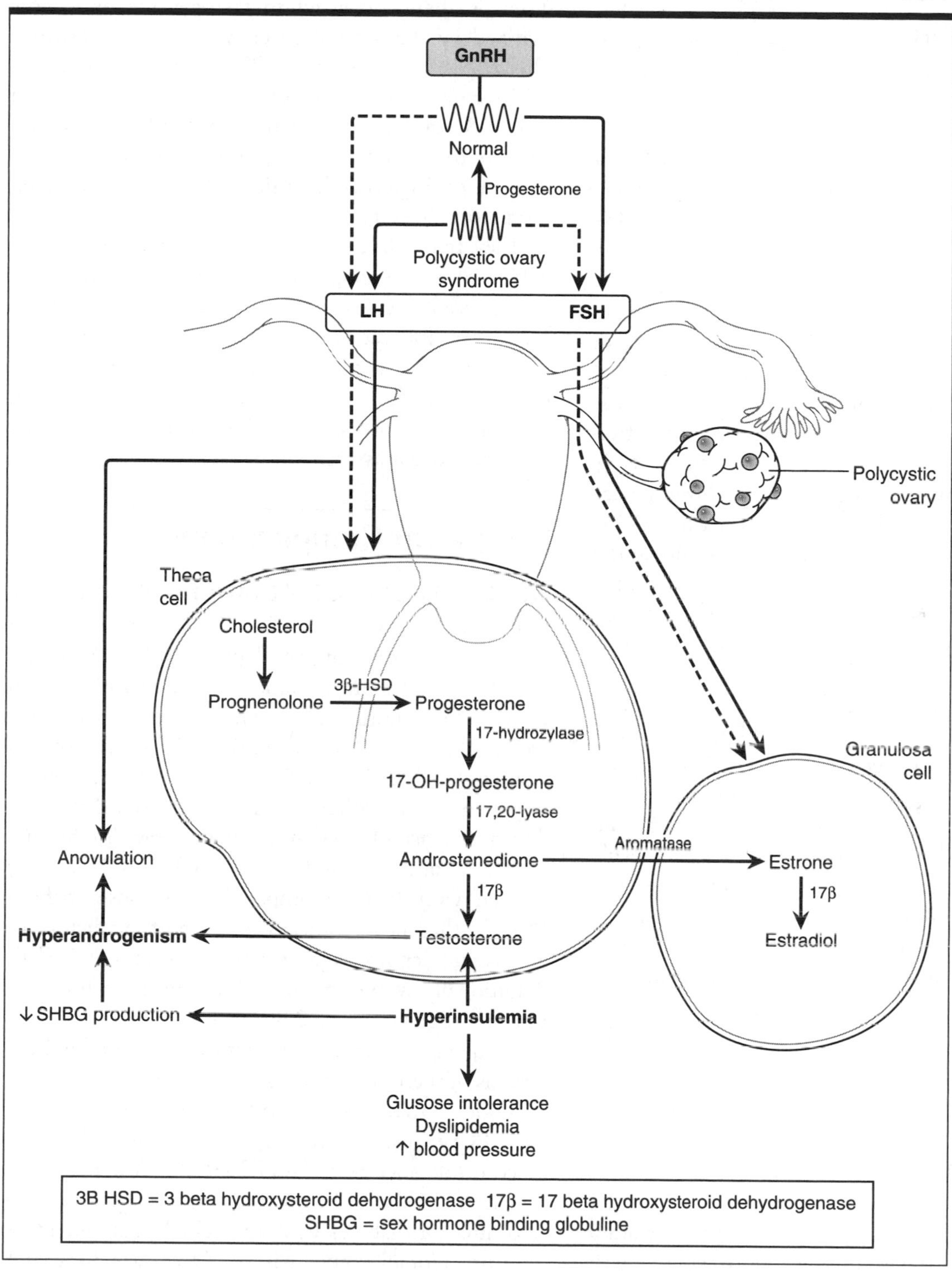

typically ovulate. It is unclear whether the abnormal pulse frequency of GnRH is an intrinsic problem in the GnRH pulse generator or a result of relatively low progesterone concentrations from infrequent ovulation.[8] A woman with this abnormality does not enter the luteal phase of her menstrual cycle, leaving estrogen unopposed. This can create endometrial hyperplasia and increase risk for endometrial cancer. Increased LH stimulation also leads to increased steroidogenesis in the ovary, leading to excess androgen production.

INSULIN RESISTANCE

In addition to gonadotropin secretion, another mechanism for increased androgen production in the ovary is through insulin resistance. Insulin resistance with compensatory hyperinsulinemia occurs in 50% to 70% of women with PCOS.[1] Insulin resistance can occur in both obese and nonobese women and is associated with reproductive and metabolic abnormalities in PCOS. Although the nature of insulin resistance in PCOS is currently unclear, defects that have been implicated include insulin receptor or postreceptor signal transduction, altered adipocyte lipolysis, decreased GLUT-4 glucose transporters in adipocytes, and impaired release of a D-chiro-inositol mediator.[9-18] Regardless of the mechanism, it appears that insulin resistance in PCOS is a selective, tissue-specific process whereby insulin sensitivity is increased in the ovarian androgenic pathway (causing hyperandrogenism). However, in other tissues involved in carbohydrate metabolism, specifically in the fat and muscle, there is tissue resistance to insulin. Hyperinsulinemia results through the compensatory increase in insulin secretion to maintain euglycemia secondary to insulin resistance.

Insulin acts directly and indirectly in PCOS. In the ovary, insulin alone or with LH increases androgen production in theca cells. In the liver, insulin inhibits synthesis of sex-hormone binding globulin (SHBG), which binds to testosterone, causing an increase in the free fraction of androgens available for biologic activity. Therefore, hyperinsulinemia is a major contributor to hyperandrogenism and **hyperandrogenemia** in PCOS. Treatments targeted to improve insulin resistance in women with PCOS have shown improvements in ovulatory function, hirsutism, androgen levels, and metabolic profiles.[19,20] Indirectly, insulin may enhance the amplitude of LH pulses, advancing further the gonadotropin secretion defect in PCOS.[21]

EXCESS ANDROGEN PRODUCTION

Androgen production occurs in the theca cell of the ovary to facilitate follicular growth while estradiol synthesis occurs in the granulosa cell. In women with PCOS, hypersecretion of LH and insulin increase the production of androgens in the theca cell causing abnormal sex steroid synthesis, hyperandrogenism, and hyperandrogenemia. The dysregulation in steroid synthesis and metabolism is believed to primarily result from a dysfunction of the cytochrome P450c17 enzyme in the ovaries, an enzyme with 17-hydroxylase and 17,20-lyase activities that are required to form androstenedione.[8,22] Androstenedione is then converted to testosterone or is aromatized by the aromatase enzyme to form estrone. Theca cells in women with PCOS are more efficient at the conversion to testosterone than normal theca cells.[23] A similar steroid pathway simultaneously occurs in the adrenal cortex, and when hyperandrogenism or hyperinsulinemic states exist, androgen production is exacerbated.

Elevated androgen levels are seen in approximately 60% to 80% of women with PCOS, evidenced mostly as increased free testosterone concentrations.[4] However, assays for testosterone tend to be highly variable and inaccurate, so measurement of androgen concentrations, if used, should be used with other additional criteria for diagnosis. Clinical assessment will be the primary tool for assessment of excess androgen.

Long-term Complications

IMPAIRED GLUCOSE TOLERANCE AND DIABETES

Studies have shown that women with PCOS have a higher prevalence of impaired glucose tolerance (IGT), diabetes, and insulin resistance compared with women without the syndrome.[24] A family history further increases the risk of these conditions. In a study of 254 women with PCOS, 38.6% were found to have either impaired glucose tolerance or undiagnosed diabetes.[25] The prevalence of IGT and diabetes was significantly higher in both obese and nonobese (BMI <27 km/m^2) women with PCOS compared with those without PCOS. The most clinically important predictors of glucose intolerance were waist-to-hip ratio and BMI. Additionally, women with PCOS who have IGT appear to progress to type 2 diabetes at higher rates than the general population.[24] Therefore, screening and diagnosis of these conditions are important.

Glucose tolerance should be assessed in all women with PCOS using a fasting and 2-hour oral (75 g) glucose tolerance test (OGTT).[24] The American Association of Clinical Endocrinologists suggests routine screening for diabetes with an OGTT that should be performed for all women with PCOS by age 30 years.[26] The Androgen Excess and PCOS Society recommends routine screening for IGT with an OGTT in all women with PCOS, and screenings should be repeated at least every 2 years.[27] The American Diabetes Association or World Health Organization criteria should be followed to appropriately diagnose IGT or diabetes. Insulin concentrations are typically not obtained in clinical settings because insulin assays

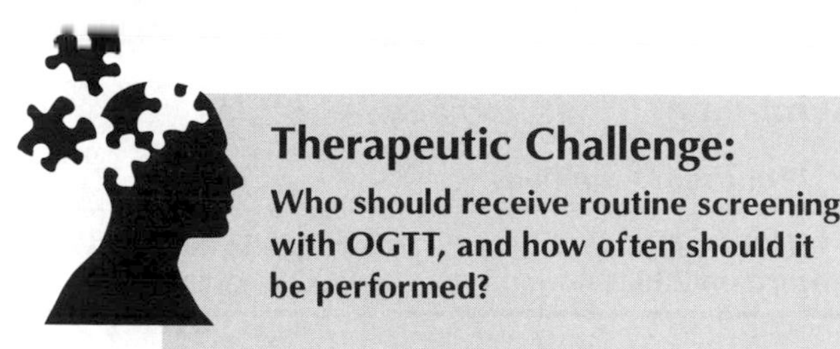

are not standardized and determination of insulin levels is not helpful in the management of PCOS.

Despite endorsement from professional societies for screening with an OGTT in women with PCOS, there is still considerate debate about whether all women with PCOS should be screened or whether the test should be restricted to PCOS women with other metabolic abnormalities, such as obesity. In addition, the optimal frequency of repeat screenings needs to be further evaluated.

METABOLIC SYNDROME AND CARDIOVASCULAR RISK

Approximately 30% to 50% of women with PCOS have the metabolic syndrome using the National Cholesterol Education Panel-Adult Treatment Panel III (NCEP-ATP III) criteria.[28-31] The rates in women with PCOS are significantly higher compared with the general U.S. population (45% vs. 6% ages 20–29 years, 53% vs. 14% ages 30–39 years) and are independent of body weight.[28] It is believed that insulin resistance is the primary contributing factor to metabolic syndrome in women with PCOS.[32] Insulin resistance in the metabolic syndrome has been associated with a twofold increased risk of cardiovascular disease and fivefold increased risk of type 2 diabetes.[33] Characteristics of the metabolic syndrome seen in women with PCOS include low high-density lipoprotein cholesterol (HDL-C) (68%), increased BMI and waist circumference (67%), high blood pressure (45%), hypertriglyceridemia (35%), and elevated fasting glucose (4%).[29] Elevated fasting insulin concentrations, obesity, and a family history of diabetes also appear to confer a higher risk of metabolic syndrome in women with PCOS.[31]

Women with PCOS have a higher prevalence of cardiovascular risk factors, including hypertension, dyslipidemia, and surrogate markers for early atherosclerosis (e.g., increased C-reactive protein concentrations) compared with women without PCOS.[32] Postmenopausal women with PCOS have a twofold increased risk of hypertension compared with age-matched controls.[34] Dyslipidemia in women with PCOS typically presents as decreased HDL-C, elevated triglycerides, elevated low-density lipoprotein cholesterol (LDL-C), and higher LDL-to-HDL ratios.[35] Women with PCOS may have more atherogenic, small, dense LDL-C compared with controls, and this substantially increases cardiovascular risk.[36] Surrogate markers for early atherosclerosis and cardiovascular disease, impaired endothelial dysfunction, and other markers of cardiovascular risk (e.g., coronary artery calcifications, carotid intima-media thickness) are also elevated in women with PCOS.[32] It appears that increased cardiovascular risk exists, with a recent study demonstrating an approximate twofold increase in cardiovascular events in postmenopausal women with a history of PCOS compared with those without PCOS.[37] Cardiovascular studies have not demonstrated an increase in overall mortality, but the methodology of these studies has been debated.

OBSTRUCTIVE SLEEP APNEA

Obstructive sleep apnea is cessation of breathing that occurs during sleep. Patients may not be aware they have symptoms of sleep apnea, such as snoring and a gasping or snorting when breathing resumes. Obstructive sleep apnea causes sleep disruption and daytime fatigue. The prevalence of obstructive sleep apnea in PCOS is higher than expected and cannot be explained by obesity alone.[38-40] The strongest predictor of sleep apnea appears to be insulin resistance, more so than age, BMI, or the circulating testosterone concentration.[38]

ENDOMETRIAL HYPERPLASIA AND CANCER

Anovulation in PCOS causes prolonged exposure of estrogen to the endometrium without the appropriate exposure to progesterone. Therefore, PCOS is recognized as a risk factor for endometrial hyperplasia. It is unknown if this translates into an increased risk for endometrial cancer because it is a rare occurrence in women of this age (4% of all cases of women <40 years).[41] It is considered prudent management to induce artificial withdrawal bleeds at least every 3 months in women with PCOS and amenorrhea or oligomenorrhea to prevent endometrial hyperplasia.[42] If this is not done, ultrasound scans can also be used to measure endometrial thickness and morphology every 6–12 months.

Diagnosis of PCOS

The diagnosis of PCOS can be difficult because presenting signs and symptoms vary among women. Additionally, precise and uniform criteria for diagnosis have not been established. Major diagnostic

Table 16-1. Criteria for Defining Polycystic Ovary Syndrome

Clinical Criteria	Proposed Definitions: NIH 1990[43]	ESHRE/ASRM (Rotterdam 2003)[44]	Androgen Excess and PCOS Society[4]
1. Hyperandrogenism or hyperandrogenemia	X	X	X
2. Oligo-ovulation or anovulation	X	X	X
3. Polycystic ovaries (by ultrasound)		X	
4. Exclusion of related disorders	X	X	X
Diagnostic criteria	**1, 2, and 4**	**2 of first 3 criteria and 4**	**1, 2, and 4**

Source: NIH, National Institutes of Health; ESHRE, European Society for Human Reproduction and Embryology; ASRM, American Society for Reproductive Medicine.

criteria for PCOS have been proposed by three different organizations (Table 16-1).

The initial criteria were developed in 1990 during an expert conference sponsored by the National Institutes of Health (NIH) and National Institute of Child Health and Human Development (NICHD). They concluded that the major criteria for PCOS should include (in order of importance) 1) hyperandrogenism (clinical signs of hyperandrogenism, such as hirsutism) and/or hyperandrogenemia (biochemical signs of hyperandrogenism, such as elevated testosterone levels); 2) oligo-ovulation (infrequent or irregular ovulation with fewer than nine menses per year); and 3) exclusion of other known disorders, such as hyperprolactinemia, thyroid abnormalities, and congenital adrenal hyperplasia.[43] Another set of diagnostic criteria for PCOS was proposed at an expert conference in Rotterdam sponsored by the European Society for Human Reproduction and Embryology (ESHRE) and the American Society for Reproductive Medicine (ASRM) in 2003.[44] They concluded that the presence of two of the following three features after exclusion of related disorders confirmed the diagnosis of PCOS: 1) oligo-ovulation or anovulation, 2) clinical and/or biochemical signs of hyperandrogenism, or 3) polycystic ovaries (as evidenced by 12 or more small follicles in one ovary on ultrasound examination). Great controversy exists about whether women fitting this new Rotterdam definition are metabolically similar to those identified using the 1990 NICHD guidelines. In addition, most U.S. centers lack the radiologic expertise to satisfactorily assess the ovaries on ultrasound in the highly rigorous manner required by the guidelines. The third criteria were defined by a task force of the Androgen Excess and PCOS Society in 2006.[4] They concluded that hyperandrogenism and/or hyperandrogenemia (highest priority) and ovarian dysfunction as evidenced by oligo-ovulation and/or polycystic ovaries must be present after exclusion of other androgen excess or related disorders. There are advantages and disadvantages to each of the criteria proposed, but it is clear that the definition of and diagnostic criteria for PCOS will continue to evolve.

Before a diagnosis of PCOS can be made, a detailed history, physical, and laboratory testing have to be performed to exclude other related disorders. A history suggestive of PCOS includes chronic anovulation with mild to moderate clinical signs of hyperandrogenism (e.g., hirsutism, hair loss, acne), usually with onset at puberty or after weight gain. Hypothalamic anovulation can be ruled out by a detailed history of lifestyle and psychosocial problems, whereas premature ovarian failure can be ruled out by menstrual history and FSH concentrations. In addition, very high testosterone and dehydroepiandrosterone sulfate concentrations, when associated with virilizing clinical signs, may suggest an androgen-secreting neoplasm of ovarian or adrenal origins, respectively. Other laboratory assessments should include prolactin, thyroid-stimulating hormone, and 17-hydroxyprogesterone concentrations to rule out hyperprolactinemia, hypothyroidism, and congenital adrenal hyperplasia, respectively. PCOS is primarily diagnosed by clinical assessment; however, a transvaginal ultrasound can be performed to determine if polycystic ovaries are present, defined as more than eight follicles per ovary that are <10 mm (usually 2–8 mm) in diameter or ovarian volume >10 mL.

Guidelines and Position Statements

Guidelines and position statements exist regarding diagnosis of PCOS (discussed above), but no guideline or position statement sufficiently addresses treatment or other aspects of PCOS.

Treatment Goals

The primary goals for PCOS are to maintain a normal endometrium, block the actions of androgens on target tissues, reduce insulin resistance and hyperinsulinemia, reduce weight, and prevent long-term complications. Other goals of treatment in patients with PCOS may include prevention of pregnancy, correcting anovulation or oligo-ovulation, and/or improving fertility.

Treatment goals should encompass both long- and short-term targets because response to nonpharmacologic and pharmacologic therapy is slow, often requiring 3–9 months. Setting long-term goals can minimize the risk for future complications, and specifying short-term goals can improve motivation and adherence to therapy.

Nonpharmacologic Treatment

WEIGHT LOSS

Weight-reduction programs designed for a modest weight loss (5% to 10%) with the incorporation of fitness are effective in improving ovulation and metabolic disease in women with PCOS. A minimum 5% weight loss has consistently demonstrated restoration of menstrual cyclicity and ovulation in overweight and obese women with PCOS.[8,45,46] Weight loss improves pregnancy rates and reduces miscarriage rates in women with PCOS.[47] When lifestyle modification is implemented, free testosterone concentrations decrease, but the effect on acne and hirsutism are not often reported.[6] Obesity in PCOS is associated with a higher risk of developing endometrial cancer, but there is very limited evidence to determine the impact of weight loss on the incidence of endometrial cancer.[8] Studies of weight loss in women without PCOS indicate a 25% to 50% reduced risk of endometrial cancer, so it is logical that addressing weight reduction in women with PCOS may lower the risk as well.[48,49] Studies specifically evaluating cardiovascular improvements with weight loss in women with PCOS are limited, but improvements in dyslipidemia and insulin sensitivity have been noted.

DIET

Although there is not one specific diet proven to be ideal for women with PCOS, a diet low in saturated fat and high in fiber from mostly low-glycemic-index-carbohydrate foods may be suitable and is recommended.[6,50] Low-glycemic-index foods include bran cereals, mixed grain breads, broccoli, peppers, lentils, and soy. High-glycemic-index foods (i.e., those that should be minimized) include white rice and bread, potatoes, chips, and foods containing simple sugars (e.g., juice). In women with PCOS, oral glucose intake caused larger fluctuations in plasma glucose and increased hyperinsulinemia; protein was found to be a preferred nutrient over glucose.[51] Diet should be individualized in women with PCOS to promote adherence and achieve specific goals.

EXERCISE

Exercise is a key component in the attainment and maintenance of weight loss. Exercise with muscle strengthening improves insulin sensitivity, a benefit for women with PCOS.[6] The American Heart Association recommends 1 hour daily of physical activity for weight reduction and 30 minutes daily for all adults. The American Diabetes Association recommends at least 150 minutes per week of moderate to vigorous activity spread over at least 3 days for individuals with IGT and 1 hour daily of exercise for long-term weight loss.

Diet and exercise are efficient, cost-effective, and safe ways to produce weight loss and improve the endocrine and metabolic parameters of PCOS. Weight reduction should be considered first-line therapy in all overweight or obese women with PCOS. It is important to note that even in controlled settings with motivated participants in clinical trials, attrition rates of lifestyle modification have been high, with 26% to

39% discontinuation in women with PCOS over 1–4 months compared with 8% to 9% discontinuation in patients without PCOS over 4 months.[46,52-54] It should be stressed that frequent, continued follow-up is necessary for sustained weight loss.

Pharmacologic Therapy

Successful treatment of PCOS requires an understanding of presenting symptoms and patient-specific goals. For example, sexually active women who are hirsute and do not desire pregnancy may benefit from hormonal contraception. Women with glucose impairment or diabetes may benefit from insulin sensitizer therapy. Women wanting to improve fertility may need ovulation induction agents. Fortunately, several different pharmacologic options are available for women with PCOS (Table 16-2).

ORAL CONTRACEPTIVES

A combined oral contraceptive (COC) containing an estrogen and progestin is the treatment of choice for women seeking menstrual cyclicity, relief of acne and hirsutism, and pregnancy prevention. The estrogen component of the COC suppresses LH, resulting in a reduction of androgen production as well as increased hepatic production of SHBG, which reduces free testosterone. The progestin components in COCs possess variable androgenic effects, so COC selection is important.

COC therapy in PCOS should be initiated with a formulation that contains a low or very low dose of estrogen (≤35 mcg ethinyl estradiol) and a low androgen or antiandrogen progestin. Most COCs have low or very low estrogen doses. Desogestrel and norgestimate are low androgen progestins, and drospirenone is an antiandrogen. These COCs are

Table 16-2. Selected Treatment Options for Polycystic Ovary Syndrome

Drug Class (Example)	Purpose of Therapy	Mechanism of Action	Effective Dosage	Select Side Effects	Pregnancy Category
Combined oral contraceptive (estrogen and progestin)	Menstrual cyclicity, hirsutism, acne	Suppresses LH (and FSH) and thus ovarian androgen	1 tablet orally daily for 21 (or 24) days, then 7-day (or 4-day) pill-free interval	Breast tenderness, breakthrough bleeding, mood swings, libido changes	X
Progestins (medroxyprogesterone)	Menstrual cyclicity	Creates withdrawal bleeding by transforming proliferative endometrium into secretory endometrium	5–10 mg orally daily for 10–14 days at least every 3 mo	Breakthrough bleeding, spotting, mood swings	X
Biguanide (metformin)	Menstrual cyclicity, ovulation induction, hirsutism, acne, insulin lowering	Decreases hepatic glucose production, secondarily reducing insulin levels; may have direct effects on steroidogenesis	500 mg orally 3 times daily (up to 2,550 mg/day)	Gastrointestinal problems, diarrhea, abdominal pain, weight loss	B
Thiazolidinediones (pioglitazone or rosiglitazone)	Menstrual cyclicity, ovulation induction, hirsutism, acne, insulin lowering	Improve insulin sensitivity at target-tissue level (muscle, adipocyte); may have direct effects on steroidogenesis	Pioglitazone: 45 mg orally daily Rosiglitazone: 4 mg orally twice daily	Edema, headache, fatigue, weight gain	C
Antiandrogen (spironolactone)	Hirsutism, acne	Inhibit androgens from binding to androgen receptor	50–100 mg orally twice daily	Hyperkalemia, polymenorrhea, headache, fatigue	C

(*Continued on next page*)

Drug Class (Example)	Purpose of Therapy	Mechanism of Action	Effective Dosage	Select Side Effects	Pregnancy Category
Antiestrogen (clomiphene citrate)	Ovulation induction	Increases GnRH secretion, which induces rise in FSH and LH	50 mg orally daily for 5 days; may increase up to 150 mg in subsequent cycles; not recommended to exceed six total cycles	Vasomotor symptoms, gastrointestinal problems	X
Antiprotozoal (eflornithine)	Hirsutism	Irreversible inhibitor of ornithine decarboxylase, which catalyzes the conversion of ornithine to polyamines necessary for cell growth and differentiation of the hair follicle	13.9% cream, topical application to facial area twice daily	Mild irritation and folliculitis	C

LH = luteinizing hormone; FSH = follicle-stimulating hormone; GnRH = gonadotropin-releasing hormone.

especially beneficial in women with hirsutism and acne.

A COC can be taken in various ways for menstrual cyclicity. For monthly cycles, a patient can take a 21/7 regimen (21 days active pill, 7 days inactive pill) or a 24/4 regimen (24 days active pill, 4 days inactive pill). Although not specifically evaluated in patients with PCOS, monophasic COCs (those containing the same amounts of estrogen and progestin throughout the cycle) can be used in an extended manner. This means that the active pills are taken daily on a continuous basis with no inactive pills, and women will not have a menstrual cycle. Regardless of the COC selected, a long-term benefit is a 50% reduction in endometrial cancer risk, even up to two decades after discontinuation.[55-57]

The effects of COCs on insulin resistance, glucose tolerance, and lipids should be considered when choosing a progestin.[58,59] COCs should be used with caution in those who have insulin resistance, a high propensity to develop type 2 diabetes, or abnormal lipid profiles. Additionally, hyperkalemia has been noted in patients using COCs containing drospirenone and should be used cautiously in patients susceptible to increased potassium concentrations.

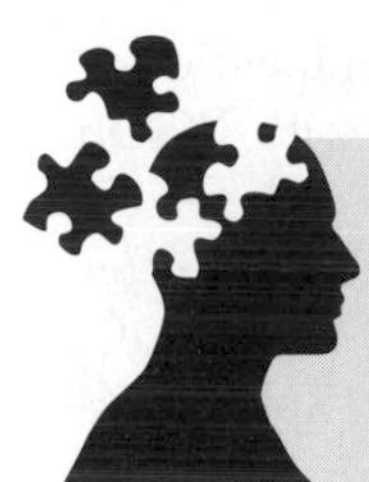

Therapeutic Challenge:

How might COCs interact with the metabolic manifestations in PCOS, and does their benefit outweigh their risk?

INSULIN SENSITIZERS

Insulin sensitizers reduce insulin levels and can ameliorate the consequences of hyperinsulinemia and hyperandrogenemia. Currently available insulin sensitizers include metformin, rosiglitazone, and pioglitazone. More efficacy data are available for metformin than the thiazolidinediones in patients with PCOS. In addition, most pregnancy outcome data in humans are reported for patients taking metformin and suggest that it is not teratogenic. For these reasons, metformin tends to be the preferred insulin sensitizer for women with PCOS.

Metformin

Metformin inhibits hepatic glucose output and reduces insulin concentrations and androgen production in the ovary. Metformin also appears to influence ovarian steroidogenesis directly.[60] Most studies demonstrate that metformin improves menstrual cyclicity, ovulation, and fertility in both obese and lean patients with PCOS.[61] In one study of nonobese women with PCOS, metformin was superior for ovulation induction compared with rosiglitazone.[62] Metformin has been considered in ovulation induction protocols and may be very effective when used alone or with clomiphene citrate for ovulation.[63,64]

Metformin has been shown to improve pregnancy outcomes. In a retrospective study, women with PCOS who achieved pregnancy while receiving metformin and continued taking metformin throughout their pregnancy had lower rates of early pregnancy loss (EPL), as compared with women with PCOS who conceived but were never exposed to metformin.[65] Other evidence suggests that metformin may not need to be administered throughout pregnancy, but only during conception, to confer protection from EPL.[66] However, metformin use for prevention of EPL is controversial, as metformin did not result in lower rates of EPL in the largest prospective study to date.[67]

Current data indicate that metformin use is not teratogenic. Pregnancy and fetal outcomes of women with PCOS who took metformin throughout pregnancy have been described in several historical cohorts.[68-70] Metformin use during pregnancy was not associated with maternal lactic acidosis nor neonatal or maternal hypoglycemia.[69,70] In infants studied up to 18 months of life, metformin did not appear to affect birth weight, length, motor-social development, or growth.[70] In addition, metformin use throughout pregnancy may reduce the incidence of gestational diabetes in the mother.[70,71]

Data also indicate that insulin and free testosterone concentrations may be decreased 20% to 50% with metformin in women with PCOS.[72,73] Metformin may also reduce BMI, especially in obese patients.[61] However, its efficacy in established hirsutism may be limited, and hirsutism should not be the sole indication for using metformin.[61] In women with PCOS whose hirsutism has been improved by antiandrogen treatment, it may be feasible to use metformin for maintenance of clinical improvement.

The minimal effective dosage of metformin in PCOS is 500 mg 3 times daily. It should be titrated slowly to this dosage and then evaluated for efficacy. Dosages up to 2,000 mg daily or 2,550 mg daily may be necessary for individual circumstances. Typical transient, dose-related side effects include diarrhea, nausea, vomiting, and abdominal bloating, but do not require discontinuation of the drug. Serum creatinine should be evaluated at least annually and when clinically prudent (e.g., some cause for change in renal function) in women using metformin; it is contraindicated in women who have a serum creatinine >1.4 mg/dL.[74]

Therapeutic Challenge:

If metformin is used for ovulation induction and pregnancy occurs, should metformin be stopped, continued for the first trimester, or continued for the entire pregnancy?

Thiazolidinediones

Rosiglitazone and pioglitazone have been evaluated in women with PCOS, but relatively few studies have been published. Thiazolidinediones improve insulin action in the liver, skeletal muscle, and adipose tissue and appear to directly affect ovarian steroid synthesis.[75] Rosiglitazone and pioglitazone reduce insulin and androgen concentrations and have modest effects on hirsutism.[8] Rosiglitazone has demonstrated significantly better ovulation rates in women with PCOS compared with placebo, but not better than metformin.[62] Other abstracts have indicated that rosiglitazone may be beneficial for menstrual regularity, hyperandrogenism, and insulin sensitivity. Pioglitazone was as effective as metformin in small studies of women with PCOS and may be especially beneficial when used in combination with metformin for clinical and biochemical improvements.[76,77]

Recommended dosages for rosiglitazone and pioglitazone are up to 4 mg twice daily and up to 45 mg once daily, respectively. Adverse effects include edema, headache, fatigue, potential liver enzyme elevations, and weight gain. Liver enzymes should be measured before initiation of treatment and periodically thereafter. Rosiglitazone also appears to have a negative effect on the lipid profile, an unwanted parameter considering the potential long-term consequences of PCOS. Clinical experiences with the thiazolidinediones during conception and pregnancy have not yet been reported; they are pregnancy category C. Thus, this class of agents should be used with caution in women with PCOS not taking contraception.

AGENTS FOR HIRSUTISM

Antiandrogenic agents are potential therapeutic options for hirsutism and acne in women with PCOS. However, antiandrogens are not approved for female hirsutism or acne in the U.S. They are often used off label alone or in combination with COCs for moderate to severe hirsutism or acne. Spironolactone is an antiandrogen often used for hirsutism, but drospirenone is also an antiandrogen found in COCs, is structurally related to spironolactone, and has been evaluated in the long-term treatment of hirsutism.[78] Spironolactone reduces hair growth in women with PCOS by 40% to 88% and may take 6–9 months for improvement.[79] The usual effective spironolactone dosage is 50–100 mg twice daily for 6–12 months. It is recommended that spironolactone be used with COCs to avoid teratogenicity and polymenorrhea (more frequent menses) and provide additional benefit for the signs and symptoms of PCOS.

Eflornithine hydrochloride cream 13.9% is an agent that has also been used for hirsutism in women with PCOS. It is an irreversible inhibitor of ornithine decarboxylase that helps to slow hair growth. Therefore, it reduces the amount of unwanted facial hair by slowing terminal hair growth, but does not remove the hair. It is applied twice daily to the affected areas of the face.

OVULATION INDUCTION AGENTS

Clomiphene Citrate

Clomiphene citrate is the ovulation induction agent of choice in women with PCOS. Ovulation induction occurs in 50% to 80% and conception occurs in 35% to 40% of women with PCOS using clomiphene citrate. Essentially, clomiphene citrate helps to correct the gonadotropin secretion abnormality in PCOS by providing an antiestrogenic effect on the hypothalamus. GnRH secretion is increased, which leads to increased LH and FSH production. The increased FSH concentrations cause appropriate follicle development and estrogen secretion, which produces a positive feedback on the hypothalamic-pituitary system to create an LH surge for ovulation.

The usual initial dosage of clomiphene citrate is 50 mg orally daily for 5 days, initiated on day 5 after the start of a spontaneous or progestin-induced menses. Ovulation is then confirmed through laboratory testing or ultrasound monitoring. If ovulation does not occur, experts recommend a dosage increase to 100 mg daily, and subsequently to 150 mg daily (for 5 days) in the next cycles. However, dosages >100 mg daily for 5 days are not recommended by the manufacturers.[80] A repeat cycle can occur as early as 30 days after the previous cycle as long as pregnancy has not occurred. If conception does not occur, most patients can attempt three to four cycles before considering another regimen. Long-term cyclic therapy is not recommended beyond a total of six cycles because of potential ovarian cancer risk. Most women respond to clomiphene citrate within three to four ovulatory cycles, but 5% to 10% demonstrate clomiphene resistance and need to consider other options.[47,80]

It had previously been suggested that the combination of clomiphene citrate plus metformin produced higher ovulation rates than either agent alone.[63] However, live-birth rates had not been evaluated until recently. In a randomized controlled study to determine live-birth rates in 626 women with PCOS taking metformin, clomiphene citrate, or both, as initial therapy for ovulation induction and pregnancy, the live-birth rate was 22.5% in the clomiphene citrate group, 7.2% in the metformin group, and 26.8% in the combination group (p <0.001 for metformin vs. clomiphene citrate and combination therapy).[67] The authors concluded that clomiphene citrate was superior to metformin in achieving live birth rates, but it should be noted that multiple births occurred in 6% (3/50) of live births. This study suggests that the combination of metformin and clomiphene citrate is not superior to clomiphene alone as the initial therapy in women with PCOS seeking pregnancy.

Other Agents and Procedures

Other regimens for ovulation induction include metformin (alone or in combination with clomiphene citrate), dexamethasone (in combination with clomiphene citrate), aromatase inhibitors (e.g., letrozole, anastrozole), ovarian drilling, or controlled ovarian stimulation with gonadotropins.[81-84] In clomiphene-resistant patients, combination clomiphene citrate and metformin would be an appropriate next step.[80] If that did not prove successful, then the following alternatives could be tried: dexamethasone 0.25 mg at bedtime can be used in combination with clomiphene citrate, aromatase inhibitors, ovarian drilling, administration of gonadotropins, or in vitro fertilization.[80]

Monitoring and Follow-up

Women with PCOS should be monitored for clinical signs or symptoms at least annually and more frequently when changes in appearance, menstrual cycles, or medication occur. Several laboratory tests are needed initially to rule out other possible disorders, but all of these tests do not require routine monitoring once the diagnosis of PCOS has been made. Routine laboratory tests include an OGTT (at least every 2 years) and fasting lipid panel to detect any endocrine or metabolic abnormalities. Appropriate follow-up for women with PCOS may include quality-of-life measures, laboratory monitoring when necessary (e.g., testosterone), and medication adherence monitoring.

Patient Education

Adherence to therapeutic regimens for PCOS can often be difficult, especially because the drug(s) can take weeks to months for improvements to occur. The emotional and physical factors of PCOS can also affect the ability of women to follow appropriate regimens. Treatment regimens can fail when women are not educated about the rationale for therapy (e.g., using an insulin sensitizer for PCOS) or the importance of adhering to therapy for an extended time. Women need to be counseled on side effects of medications and potential alternatives if they occur. Women should also be referred to appropriate healthcare providers when issues such as infertility arise.

CASE PRESENTATION

Patient Case: Part 2

Assessment: J.C. has PCOS as evidenced by irregular menstrual periods (oligomenorrhea) and clinical signs of hyperandrogenism (acne, facial hair). In addition, J.C. has impaired fasting glucose, and her glucose tolerance status should be further evaluated. J.C. is using benzoyl peroxide for acne, but her desire for fertility is not being addressed with current regimen.

Recommendation:

- Weight loss of at least 5% through diet and exercise.
- Clomiphene citrate 50 mg orally daily for 5 days, started on day 5 after a spontaneous or progestin-induced menses. Dosage may be increased to 100 mg daily if unresponsive.
- Perform OGTT to determine presence of IGT.

Rationale: Weight loss has been shown to have positive impact on ovulation. Both clomiphene citrate and metformin are viable options in this patient, but clomiphene citrate is preferred based on comparative clinical trial for live-birth rates. OGTT will provide information about the presence of IGT and potential risk for diabetes in the future.

Monitoring: Weight loss; ovulation; side effects of clomiphene citrate, including hot flashes, bloating, nausea, vomiting.

Patient education: Eat diet low in saturated fat and high in fiber from mostly low-glycemic-index carbohydrate foods. Perform physical activity 30–60 minutes daily (with physician approval and guidance). Goal weight loss is at least 5% of body weight (10 lb). For clomiphene citrate, multiple gestation is possible, therapy should not extend beyond four to six cycles, and potential side effects should be reviewed. She should return at least monthly for monitoring of her lifestyle compliance.

Summary

Women with PCOS exhibit unique clinical features and have individual concerns that should be addressed when making treatment recommendations. Assessment of women with PCOS should include gathering relevant medical information, such as menstrual history, signs and symptoms of hyperandrogenism, time course of symptoms, weight history, previous agents tried, and family history. If PCOS is suspected, laboratory assessments should be performed to rule out any other related disorders. The criteria for PCOS include hyperandrogenism or hyperandrogenemia, anovulation or oligo-ovulation, and/or polycystic ovaries. Once a diagnosis has been made, recommendations about treatment must consider the patient's desires and motivation to attain individualized goals. Figure 16-2 displays various treatment options and preferences when addressing patient priorities.

In any obese patient, weight loss is a first step to improve many of the clinical and biochemical endocrine and metabolic abnormalities in PCOS. If contraception is desired, COCs will improve menstrual cycles and hyperandrogenism. If contraception is not needed, metformin will address menstrual cyclicity, hyperandrogenism, and insulin resistance. Other agents like thiazolidinediones could be used if contraindications or serious side effects were present with metformin or COCs. Hirsutism can be targeted with COCs or antiandrogens. If pregnancy is desired, clomiphene citrate would be a first-line pharmacologic option for ovulation induction. Other alternatives—including metformin, dexamethasone, aromatase inhibitors, gonadotropins, ovarian drilling, or in vitro fertilization—can be considered if clomiphene citrate alone is not effective.

Appropriate follow-up for women with PCOS may include efficacy of current treatment, quality-of-life measures, and medication adherence monitoring.

Figure 16-2. Treatment Algorithms for PCOS.
(Adapted from *Drugs*. 2006;66:910. Copyright ©Adis Data Informations BV.)

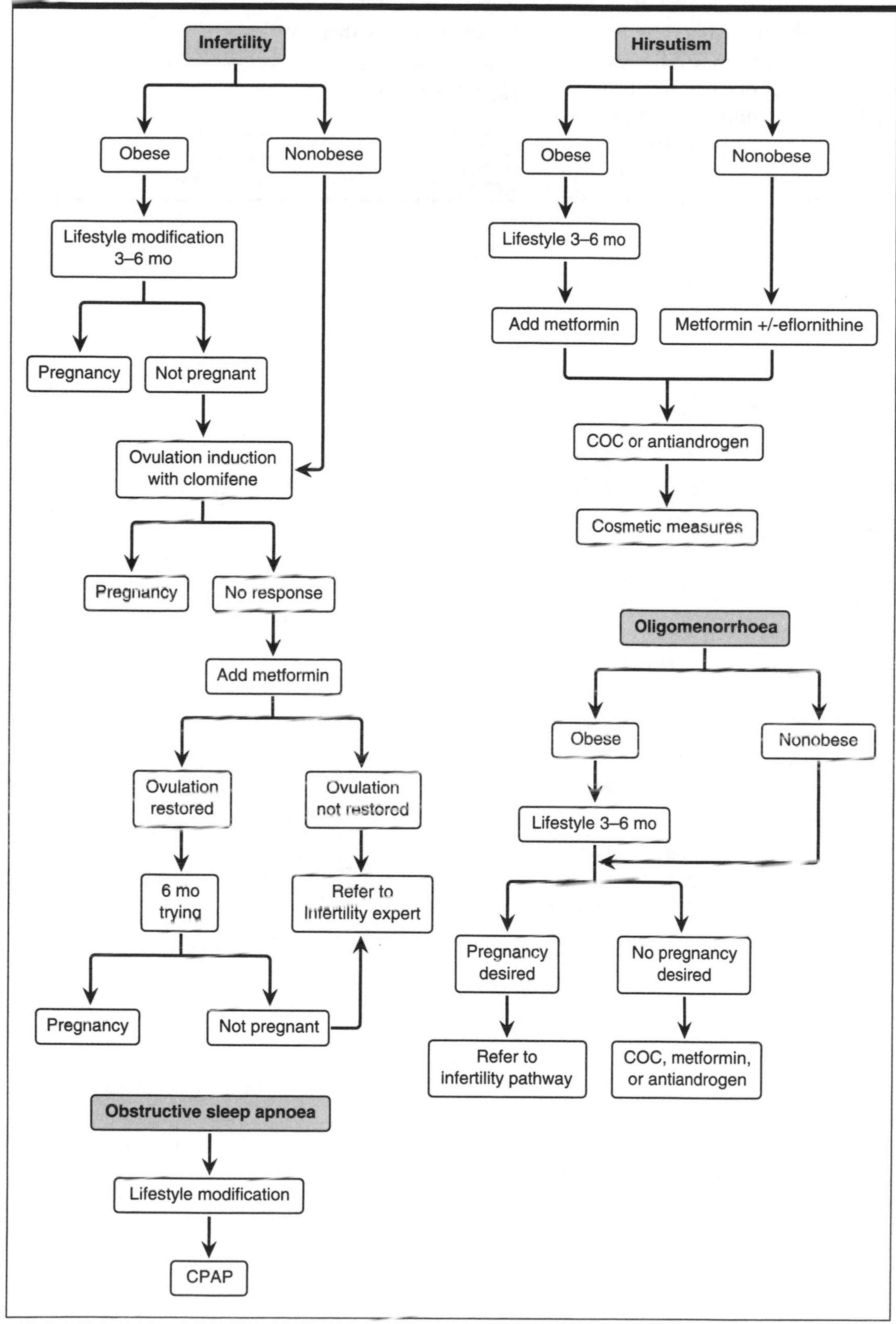

Essential routine laboratory monitoring includes fasting lipid profiles and screening for IGT or frank diabetes. Long-term consequences include IGT, type 2 diabetes, hypertension, dyslipidemia, endometrial hyperplasia, and obstructive sleep apnea; however, an increased mortality risk has not been established.

Women with PCOS have a multifaceted disorder that requires individualized attention. Patient history, laboratory assessment, and appropriate therapy selection should be performed while considering the specific needs of patients. Providers should be educators, facilitators, and empathetic listeners to help women with PCOS become informed and actively engaged in their therapy plan.

References

Additional content available at
www.ashp.org/womenshealth

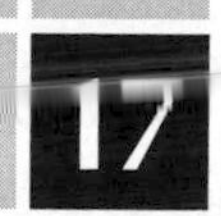

17 Menopause

Fiona Jane, MBBS; Susan R. Davis, MBBS, Ph.D., FRACP

Learning Objectives

1. Describe the hormone changes through the menopause transition.
2. Identify the factors in a woman's history that need to be considered before starting hormone therapy.
3. Explain which nonpharmacologic treatments can be effective in perimenopause and menopause.
4. Compare and contrast the pharmacologic agents used for treating symptoms in perimenopause and menopause.
5. State the major side effects of hormonal and nonhormonal therapies used to treat menopausal symptoms.
6. Evaluate the risks/harm of estrogen and progesterone therapies, alone or in combination.

Understanding menopause is important. With increased longevity has come the challenges that face women growing old. Menopause is not only associated with symptoms that range from bothersome to extremely distressing, but is also accompanied by hormonal changes that adversely affect several nonreproductive systems. Thus, we need to understand the biology of menopause and its short- and long-term sequelae, and consider therapeutic options.

In 1000 B.C., the average life expectancy at birth was merely 18 years, with few women surviving to age 40 and beyond.[1] However, even in ancient times, a handful of women did survive until menopause occurred. Menopause was recognized and documented by Aristotle (384–322 B.C.) who observed that menstruation ceased in a woman at the age of 40.[2] Knowledge of the female gonads in the ancient Mediterranean world has also been reported, with ancient Egyptians performing oophorectomy on human females for the possible purpose of contraception.[3,4] The first clinical experiment reported on the removal of human female ovaries was conducted by Percival Pott in 1775.[5] He observed that bilateral oophorectomy of a young woman was followed by shrinkage of her breasts and cessation of her menses.

Today, **natural menopause** is a recognized consequence of natural ovarian aging and is formally defined as the time of the last menstrual period in a woman who has not had a hysterectomy. Thus, it is usually diagnosed some time after it has actually occurred. The menopausal transition begins with variation in menstrual cycle length and ends after 12 months of **amenorrhea.** The stages of the menopause have been classified according to a woman's reported bleeding pattern, supported by changes in pituitary follicle-stimulating hormone levels (FSH).[6] **Perimenopause,** which means "around menopause," describes the time from which menses become irregular and FSH levels have increased until 12 months after the last menstrual bleed. The term *postmenopause* is applied to women who have not experienced a menstrual bleed for at least 12 months.

Defining menopause in a woman who has had a hysterectomy before the natural cessation of ovarian function requires measurement of the pituitary gonadotropin FSH, which should be elevated with a concurrently low estradiol level. The real clinical challenge is the determination of the menopausal status of a woman using systemic steroid contraception, which not only suppresses menses but also suppresses FSH production and endogenous estradiol. In most instances, however, such classification is academic rather than clinically required. Surgical menopause refers to menopause induced by removal of both ovaries before natural menopause. Menopause is considered to be premature when it occurs in a woman before the age of 40 years. Spontaneous premature ovarian failure affects 1% of women by age 40 and 0.1% by age 30.

CASE PRESENTATION

Patient Case: Part 1

B.B. is a 54-year-old woman who attends the clinic to discuss the issue of osteopenia diagnosed on a routine bone density scan.

HPI: Her menses ceased at the age of 51 years, and she only ever experienced mild flushes and sweats. She has never taken hormone therapy. She does not suffer from migraines or high blood pressure, and she is on treatment for high cholesterol.

It is recommended that bone-sparing agents are not appropriate for osteopenia and that it would be reasonable to repeat her bone density after 24 months of calcium and vitamin D. B.B. then raises the issue of other menopausal symptoms. She reports that she has problems sleeping, is often anxious and irritable, experiences vaginal dryness with intercourse, and has lost interest in sex. She reports that no one has ever offered her hormone therapy and she would like to know if this would alleviate her symptoms and what the inherent risks might be for her as an individual.

Family history: Her mother is alive at 85 years and has never had a fracture. Her father died of a stroke at 70. There is no family history of estrogen-dependent malignancies.

Social history: B.B. is married, has two children aged 31 and 28 years, is a nonsmoker, and drinks little alcohol, and assists her husband in their real estate business. She tries to walk most days.

Medications: She is currently taking vitamin D and calcium, as well as black cohosh and pravastatin.

Bone mineral density: T score lumbar spine L1–L4 = −1.9, neck of femur = −1.7, vitamin D is 75 nmol/L. Her lipid profile is normal on medication.

Physiology of Menopause

The young ovary consists of incompletely developed ova or germ cells surrounded by specialized hormone-producing cells, which form a supportive structure. The follicular cells, which produce estrogen, encase the developing ova in multiple little nests or follicles. Before birth, the ovaries of a healthy 20-week-old fetus contain approximately 7.5 million immature ova. By birth, this number has fallen to 2 million, and by puberty, only about 300,000 remain. Menopause occurs when there is extensive deterioration of the follicular cells and the immature ova within. Thus, the necessary sex hormones can no longer be produced and fertilizable ova can no longer develop. Blood levels of the hormones estrogen and progesterone fall, and women at this time may experience symptoms of estrogen insufficiency.

It is not understood why so many ova are necessary in the first place or what determines their loss. When the number of healthy ova reaches 25,000, at approximately 37 years of age, the rate of loss accelerates, culminating in menopause at the average age of 51.5 years.[7] When the rate at which the ova disappear is accelerated earlier—either spontaneously or by environmental factors, such as cigarette smoking—menopause occurs earlier.

Estradiol, progesterone, and testosterone are the main steroid hormones produced by the ovaries under the direction of the pituitary gland. The pituitary produces FSH, which acts on the ovaries to stimulate the development of a mature egg every 28 days, and luteinizing hormone (LH), which stimulates ovulation. This pituitary function in turn is controlled by the hypothalamus, which acts as the master control box for reproductive function.

When the integrity of the ovarian follicular cells deteriorates, estradiol levels fall, and this change is detected by both the hypothalamus and the pituitary gland. In addition, the production by the ovaries of a protein called inhibin diminishes. The pituitary gland responds by producing greater amounts of both FSH and LH in an attempt to drive ovarian function. Therefore, as menopause approaches, blood levels of inhibin decline, and FSH and LH levels rise. Serum estradiol levels remain relatively unchanged or may increase approaching menopause but are usually well preserved until late perimenopause. This is presumed to be in response to elevated FSH levels.[8] However, the menopause transition is characterized by marked, and often dramatic, variations in FSH and estradiol levels such that measurements of these hormones are unreliable guides to menopausal status.[8]

Estrogen biosynthesis is catalyzed by aromatase cytochrome P450.[9] Following menopause, estradiol is primarily produced in extragonadal sites and acts locally at these sites as a paracrine or even intracrine hormone.[10,11] These sites include the mesenchymal cells of adipose tissue, osteoblasts and chondrocytes of bone, the vascular endothelium and aortic smooth muscle cells, and numerous sites in the brain.[11] Within these sites, aromatase action can generate high levels of estradiol locally without significantly affecting circulating levels. Circulating levels of estrogens in postmenopausal women thus reflect "spillover" of estradiol into the circulation from the peripheral tissues in which estradiol is being produced and where it acts.[11]

In contrast to the fall in estradiol during menopause, total and free testosterone (T) levels, as well as dehydroepiandrosterone sulfate (DHEAS) and androstenedione, decline with age, and an effect of natural menopause on circulating androgen levels is not seen.[12-14] Thus, specific tissue effects of natural menopause cannot be attributed to loss of androgenic hormone production. However, women who have had their ovaries surgically removed, or who have had their ovaries damaged by chemotherapy or radiotherapy, or who have ovarian gonadotropin suppression will have loss of ovarian androgen production as a result.

The fall in estradiol at menopause has effects on nonreproductive tissues. There are two estrogen receptors (ERs), ERα and ERβ, expressed in varying amounts in the brain, vascular tissues, bone, cartilage, urogenital tract, and so forth. The ligand-binding domains of both ERs are capacious and promiscuous and are thus able to accept a variety of ligands, which may act as agonists or antagonists, or elicit mixed agonist/antagonist responses. This has been attributed to the unique three-dimensional conformation induced by the binding of the ligand to the ER, which in turn determines how the ligand-bound receptor will behave.[15] This complex molecular biology explains why plant chemicals (phytoestrogens), environmental chemicals (xenoestrogens), and the new class of therapeutic compounds known as estrogen agonist/antagonists (EAAs) can activate the ERs. Furthermore, we know that growth factors and other such compounds can activate the ERα in the N-terminal region of the receptor (known as the AF1 region) and elicit estrogenlike actions without acting as traditional ligands, therefore not actually being estrogens in the classical sense.

Women experience menopause because there is a decline in fertility with aging in female primates, but menopause—or the total end to reproductive capacity in the middle of life—is virtually unique to human females. Evolutionary biologists believe menopause developed at a very early stage in human evolution, probably as long as 1.5 million years ago. This is most likely as a result of natural selection, such that women survived longer if they became infertile during mid-adulthood. Thus, in early human evolution, women who lost their fertility at an earlier stage were not only protected from the increasing health risks of additional pregnancies, nutritional deficiencies, exhaustion, and risk of maternal death, but were able to fully devote themselves to nurturing and protecting their highly dependent offspring. Menopause is believed to have occurred much earlier in the past than today: probably as early as age 35–40 years. Over thousands of years of evolution, menopause has gradually occurred later in female adult life in the context of increasing human life expectancy.[16]

The greatest predictor of the age at which a woman will experience menopause is the age at which her mother went through menopause. Factors associated with the likelihood of an earlier menopause include smoking cigarettes, hysterectomy, and a family history of early menopause.

Clinical Presentation

Menstrual irregularity is considered to be the earliest indication of the menopause transition (perimenopause).[6] Because of the hormone fluctuations leading up to and around the time of menopause, women may experience intermittent symptoms ranging from hot flushes and night sweats when estradiol levels fall to breast tenderness and swelling and heavy or irregular bleeding when estradiol levels rise in response to FHS drive. Commonly reported symptoms are listed in Table 17-1. Women may experience none of these symptoms, or several. Symptoms of menopausal hormonal changes may start several years before menopause, even whilst regular periods are occurring due to the changing hormone levels. Symptoms may last for few to many years in some women. There is no cutoff age at which menopausal symptoms begin or end.

Hot flashes and night sweats (vasomotor symptoms) are the most common presenting symptoms of women experiencing menopause.[6] Vasomotor symptoms occur in almost 80% of postmenopausal women, and 25% of women report these symptoms as being severe.[17,18] Hispanic and black women are more likely to have vasomotor symptoms than white women, with Asian women being the least likely to report flushes or sweats.[19] Vasomotor symptoms are also more common in smokers, in women with greater body mass, and after surgical menopause.[19] Typically, hot flashes are characterized by increased peripheral blood flow, increased heart rate, skin conductance, and sweating. The precise physiology remains elusive, but clearly the onset of flashes and

Table 17-1. Estimated Prevalence of Menopausal Symptoms[a]

	Premenopause	Perimenopause	Postmenopause
Hot flashes and night sweats	14% to 51%	35% to 50%	30% to 80%
Vaginal dryness	4% to 22%	7% to 39%	17% to 30%
Sleep disturbance	16% to 42%	39% to 47%	35% to 60%
Mood symptoms	8% to 37%	11% to 21%	8% to 38%
Urinary symptoms	10% to 36%	11% to 21%	8% to 38%

Source: Adapted from reference 46.

[a]Annals of Internal Medicine.

sweats are a result of central effects of diminished sex steroid action in the thermoregulatory center of the brain. Higher FSH levels are associated with hot flushes, as are fluctuations of both estradiol and FSH.[20] The fact that vasomotor symptoms are due to estrogen withdrawal and that exogenous estrogen alleviates vasomotor symptoms is not controversial.

Change in sleep quality is a hallmark of menopause. Although more common among women with vasomotor symptoms, disturbed sleep architecture may occur independently of vasomotor symptoms. The three forms of sleep disorders associated with menopause include insomnia/depression, sleep-disordered breathing, and fibromyalgia.[21] The mechanism underlying this change in sleep pattern is not known; however, treatment of insomnia may be an important indication for **hormone therapy** (HT).

There is increasing evidence that depression is a menopausal symptom experienced by some women. Women with a history of depression are more likely to report depressed mood during the menopausal transition and are also likely to experience vasomotor symptoms.[20]

Arthralgia (joint pain and stiffness) is a common menopausal symptom that occurs with increasing frequency as women progress though the menopausal stages, with the occurrence being associated with increasing FSH levels.[20] The strongest evidence that arthralgia is a consequence of estrogen depletion is the high incidence of arthralgia in women treated with aromatase enzyme inhibitors after breast cancer.[22]

At least 50% of postmenopausal women suffer symptoms of urogenital atrophy, including vaginal dryness, dyspareunia, recurrent urinary tract infections, and urge and stress incontinence.[23] Incontinence is not a life-threatening condition, but it can severely impair quality of life and in many instances result in incapacitation.[24] ERs have been demonstrated in the distal urethra, bladder trigone, pelvic muscles, and ligamentum rotundum.[25] In postmenopausal women, unwinding of the urethral submucosal venous plexus and a reduction in vessel number, an increase in connective tissue volume, and a reduction in nerve density have each been reported.[26-28] Oophorectomy results in ultrastructure changes in the detrusor muscle, some of which are reversed with estrogen treatment.[29] Whether the findings from animal models and cross-sectional studies reflect estrogen lack, aging, vascular disease, or other underlying pathophysiology is not known. A systematic meta-analysis reported a beneficial effect of estrogen on incontinence, particularly urge incontinence.[30] In contrast, data from two randomized controlled trials (RCTs) indicate that exogenous estrogen therapy may worsen urinary incontinence.[31,32] This in vitro vs. in vivo discrepancy, and the conflicting findings of different clinical trials, highlights the need for further research to determine the effects of estrogen deprivation on the urogenital tract.

Although bone loss is not a presenting symptom as such, many postmenopausal women will present to their doctor to discuss the findings of a routine bone density study. There is level 1 evidence (evidence from systematic reviews or large, high-quality RCTs) that estrogen insufficiency results in bone loss and increased osteoporotic fracture risk in postmenopausal women, which can be prevented with estrogen therapy.[33-37] Estrogen therapy has been shown to reduce bone turnover, increase bone mineral density (BMD), and decrease vertebral fracture rates by up to 40%.[37-39] Available data indicate the menopause-related BMD decrement is very evident during the first year since menopause (lumbar spine: −8.1%/year; forearm: −3.4%/year), and progressively decreases, according to a logarithmic function usually settling at a rate of −1% to −2% per annum, with considerable interindividual variation.[34,40]

Diagnosis of Menopause

For naturally menopausal women not using exogenous hormones, the primary criteria for defining the stages of the menopause transition are based on menstrual bleeding.[6] The Stages of Reproductive Aging Workshop suggested that the menopausal transition could be characterized by specific stages (the STRAW classification).[6] The transition years are described in two stages by STRAW, with early transition being variable cycle length and increased FSH and late transition being >60 days of amenorrhea and increased FSH. The postmenopausal period is described as early (up to 5 years from the final menstrual period) and late (beyond 5 years). Research supports an interval of amenorrhea of 60 days or more as highly predictive of the onset of the late menopausal transition.[41] Hence, for women with an intact uterus, the menopause transition is diagnosed clinically by change in the bleeding pattern and eventually amenorrhea.

This approach is not useful for women who cannot report their menstrual pattern because of prior hysterectomy or endometrial ablation or use of a **progestogen** intrauterine device, or for women who are using systemic hormonal contraception. Hormone measurement may be useful in the former group, but such measures are uninformative for the latter.[42] For young women with amenorrhea, premature ovarian failure is a diagnosis that requires the measurement of estradiol and gonadotropins. A flow chart developed by Bell et al. provides a pragmatic approach to the menopausal status classification of clinical research study participants that allows for women who have gynecologic circumstances that mask their natural menstrual pattern (Figure 17-1).[43]

The laboratory testing that confirms menopause is an elevated FSH in the setting of a low estradiol level. However, in the early menopause transition, serum FSH and estradiol may be very erratic. Specific cutoff levels vary considerably between laboratories according to the assays used. Biochemical testing is only required for women who cannot describe their underlying cycle or perhaps for younger women with amenorrhea for whom the differential diagnosis may include hyperprolactinemia, exercise- or weight-loss–induced amenorrhea, and so forth. The diagnosis of premature ovarian failure requires at least 4 months of amenorrhea and two to three serum FSH values >40 milli-International Units/mL, obtained at least 1 month apart, in women <40 years of age. The only way to determine if a woman using systemic steroid contraception in her late 40s or early 50s is menopausal is to have her cease the treatment and evaluate her after 6–8 weeks for recurrence of natural menses and symptoms. If menses have not recurred, consider measurement of FSH and estradiol.

Treatment Goals and Guidelines

The primary reason for instituting treatment of a menopausal woman is to alleviate symptoms that impair her quality of life and to optimize health and well-being, both short and long term. The latter includes addressing issues such as prevention of bone loss, cardiovascular disease, and diabetes risk.

Several learned societies have produced menopause treatment guidelines that are clinical consensus statements that do not always reflect the most recent research evidence and cannot always be applied to other populations.[44-46] Hence, these need to be considered in the context of the available knowledge at the time they were produced.

Nonpharmacologic Management Approaches for Menopausal Symptoms

A systematic review of the published quality trials of complementary and alternative medical approaches to the management of menopausal symptoms reported insufficient data to support the consistent effectiveness of such approaches.[47] However, individual trials and clinical guidelines do indicate that some women experiencing mild menopausal symptoms may gain relief by dietary modification and lifestyle changes, such as reduction in smoking, caffeine, and alcohol; stress management; and increased exercise. A recent Cochrane review concluded that evidence to support a benefit of exercise for the treatment of vasomotor symptoms is lacking.[48,49] Acupuncture has not been shown to have a meaningful effect on vasomotor symptoms in quality trials.[47] Strong evidence to support benefits from either relaxation or training in breathing techniques are lacking.[47]

Figure 17-1. Flow chart illustrating a pragmatic approach to the menopausal status classification of clinical research study participants that allows for women who have gynecologic circumstances that mask their natural menstrual pattern.

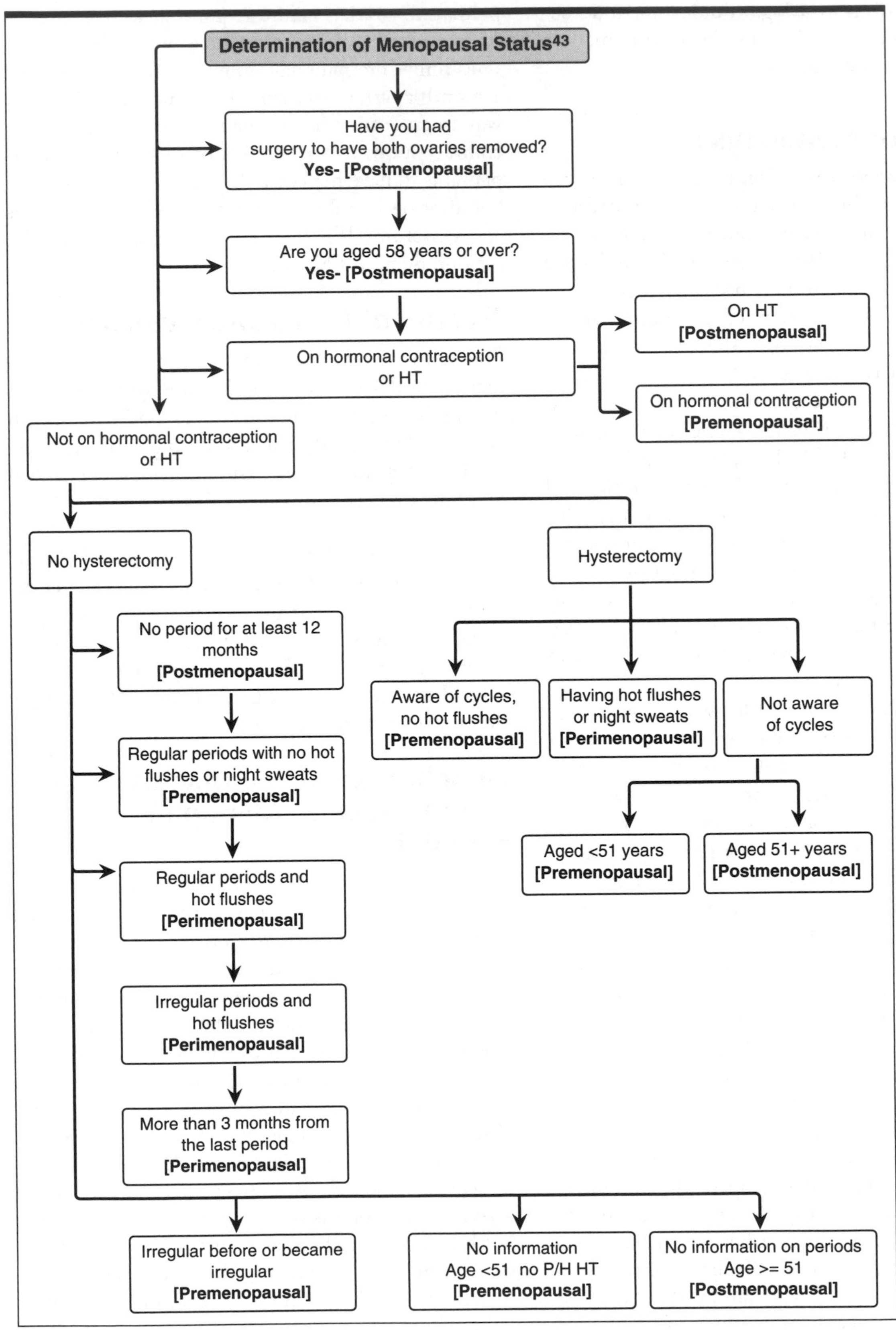

Management of Perimenopause

Treatment for the symptomatic perimenopausal woman who finds her symptoms distressing, is directed at controlling irregular cycling and heavy bleeding, ensuring contraception if required, and providing relief from other symptoms at the lowest effective dosage. Improvement in quality of life is what most of these women are seeking, and advice on dietary and lifestyle modifications as well as pharmacologic and nonpharmacologic treatment is important.

For the perimenopausal woman needing contraception (see also Chapter 19: Hormonal Contraception), the combined oral contraceptive pill provides contraception, regular predictable and lighter withdrawal bleeds, and relief from vasomotor and other symptoms. It also preserves bone density, helps prevent ovarian and endometrial cancer, and treats acne that can occur at this time. Each woman's risks must be assessed to determine the suitability of this approach even though the dosage of hormones is low. This should include smoking status, blood pressure, lipid profile, migraine aura history, deep vein thrombosis and cardiovascular risk, and family history. A low-dose oral contraceptive pill containing 20 mcg of ethinyl estradiol and a progestin such as levonorgestrel 100 mcg or drosperinone 3 mg should be used to minimize cardiovascular risk, will be effective for both contraception and cycle control, and is used as first-line treatment.[50] Vasomotor symptoms should reduce over 2–3 months, and symptoms in the pill-free week can be managed by eliminating the placebo tablets or adding a low dose of supplemental estrogen. In some countries, weekly transdermal, monthly injectable, or monthly intravaginal contraceptive options will provide the same benefits with cyclic bleeding. Women can transition from the contraceptive hormone therapy to HT when contraception is no longer required.

In the menopause transition, the ovaries have variable activity that is due to fluctuating FSH levels, resulting in random hypo- and then hyperestrogenic states. During the late menopause transition phase, the endometrium is stimulated by the increase in estrogen production. The levonorgestrel-releasing intrauterine device (LNG-IUD) provides contraception at this time if required, as well as suppressing the endometrium. Although initially spotting is not uncommon after insertion, about 80% of women will become amenorrheic at 1 year.[51] The direct delivery of low-dose progestogen to the uterus provides contraception, treatment of menorrhagia, and endometrial protection when combined with continuous oral or transdermal estrogen, and the LNG-IUD can be left in situ for 5 years. The low dosage minimizes the side effects.[51]

Low-dose hormone therapy (LD-HT) has been studied in women not needing contraception.[52] It has been shown to control both irregular bleeding and vasomotor symptoms. The lower dosage of HT compared with conventional dosing of HT may be effective because these perimenopausal women maintain some ovarian function and endogenous estrogen production. The low dosing means a lower rate of side effects, as well as preventing reported fluctuations in endogenous estrogen concentrations, which are able to trigger vasomotor symptoms. It is taken cyclically with 17β-estradiol for 14 days, followed by 14 tablets of 17β-estradiol and progestogen (days 15–28 of a 28 day cycle). Ultralow-dose transdermal estrogen at 14 mcg/day has been shown to have a bone-sparing effect, and this is enhanced by adding a progestogen (e.g., MPA or NETA).[53]

Oral progestogen-only regimens (medroxyprogesterone acetate and micronized progesterone) have been shown to provide relief from hot flushes when given in high dosages, as well as to prevent endometrial hyperplasia. However, side effects of the progestogen—such as weight gain, mastalgia, fluid retention, vaginal discharge, and dry mouth—can be a problem at these dosages. Short-term use may be applicable in women who do not want to take estrogen. It can be used cyclically for the first 12–14 days of the cycle and produces predictable bleeding in the majority of women.

Androgen therapy can be considered in women showing signs and symptoms of androgen insufficiency in addition to other hormonal and nonhormonal therapies or as a sole therapeutic agent.

Women unable to use—or who choose not to use—HT in perimenopause may get some relief from other treatments—e.g., selective serotonin or noradrenaline reuptake inhibitors, gabapentin, clonidine, or tibolone—although effects are less than for estrogen.

Estrogen +/− Progestogen Therapy for the Treatment of Menopausal Symptoms

The primary use of HT is to alleviate symptoms of the menopause—namely hot flashes, night sweats, sleep disturbance, arthralgia, and vaginal dryness—and therefore improve the quality of life of women who without HT find these symptoms intolerable. For women with an intact uterus, progestogen therapy is taken with estrogen to protect the lining of the uterus from overstimulation by estrogen. This can be cyclic for 14 days out of a monthly cycle, or as continuous-combined HT when both the estrogen and progestogen are taken every day. Cyclic HT results in scheduled menstrual bleeding, whereas no bleeding occurs with continuous-combined HT in 90% of women after 12 months. If breakthrough bleeding is persistent or prolonged, then investigation of the endometrium is required. For women who have undergone a hysterectomy, the administration of estrogen therapy alone is appropriate.

FORMULATIONS AND ROUTES OF ADMINISTRATION

The most widely used estrogen preparation in North America in postmenopausal women is oral conjugated equine estrogen (CEE). Other oral estrogen preparations include synthetically derived piperazine estrone sulfate, estriol, micronized estradiol, and estradiol valerate. Estradiol may also be given transdermally as a patch or gel, as a slow-release percutaneous implant, and, more recently, as an intranasal spray. Intravaginal estrogens include topical estradiol in the form of a ring or pessary, estriol in pessary or cream form, and dienoestrol and conjugated estrogens in the form of creams. The available therapies and dosage ranges are listed in Table 17-2. Specific dosage recommendations will vary based on patient-specific needs and are beyond the scope of this chapter.

In postmenopausal women, estrone sulfate circulates in concentrations 10–25 times greater than estrone or estradiol.[54] Estrone sulfate has a long plasma half-life and slow clearance rate and thus acts as a reservoir for the formation of estradiol and estrone in target tissues.[55] In their unsulfated forms, estradiol and estrone are partly bound to sex hormone–binding globulin (SHBG), and variations in the plasma level of SHBG significantly affect the amount of free or bioavailable estradiol to a greater extent than estrone, as well as bioavailable testosterone.[56] This has significant therapeutic implications. Oral micronized estradiol and other oral estrogen preparations may result in up to 10-fold higher levels of circulating estrone sulfate than transdermally administered estradiol at comparable or even higher dosages.[55,57] Estrogen-sensitive target tissues, such as breast and endometrium, have high capacity to metabolize estrone sulfate to estradiol. This may be a prime mechanism by which concentrations of estrone and estradiol in breast cancer tissue are severalfold greater than circulating levels.[58] Orally administered estrogen therapy also increases SHBG to a greater extent than nonorally administered estrogens,[59] and this may result in a clinically significant reduction in bioavailable testosterone. Thus, it would seem that the prescription of oral estrogen therapy should be at the lowest available dosage to minimize effects on circulating estrone sulfate and SHBG. Consistent with this, lower-dose combinations of micronized estradiol and norethisterone acetate are associated with equivalent symptom relief as higher-dose combinations but lower rates of mastalgia and vaginal bleeding.[60]

Nonoral estrogen administration results in a more physiologic balance between estradiol and estrone. It can be very useful for women with elevated triglyceride levels or significant liver function abnormalities. Nonoral therapy is also less likely to affect SHBG. Transdermal patches or gels deliver estradiol to the general venous circulation at a continuous rate. Local skin reactions to the patches occur in about 5% of women who use matrix (estrogen in adhesive) patches. The incidence of skin irritation diminishes when women rotate the application site. Percutaneous gel preparations are convenient and have been available in France for more than 20 years. Estradiol pellets (implants) containing pure crystalline 17β-estradiol have been available for more than 50 years. They are inserted subcutaneously into the anterior abdominal wall or buttock. Pellets are difficult to remove and may continue to release estradiol for a long time after insertion. Thus, implantation should not be repeated until the serum estradiol levels have fallen to a value similar to that seen in a premenopausal women during the early to midphase of the menstrual cycle. An intranasal 17β-estradiol spray, which enables pulsatile therapy in a single-daily or twice-daily dosage, has been developed for use in postmenopausal women and is now available in some countries. Vaginal rings are a sustained delivery system composed of a biologically inert liquid polymer matrix with pure crystalline estradiol that maintains adequate estradiol levels. Vaginal estrogens have been used for treatment of vaginal dryness and atrophy. At low dosages, local application can reverse menopausal vaginal changes, and there is little to no significant absorption into the circulation.

PROGESTOGEN THERAPY

The addition of a progestogen to estrogen for a postmenopausal woman with an intact uterus is required to protect against endometrial hyperplasia and endometrial carcinoma. Duration of progestogen use remains under debate; however, this becomes a moot

Table 17-2. Dosage Ranges for Differing Hormone Replacement Therapies

PERIMENOPAUSE TREATMENT OPTIONS				
Estrogens Progestogens				
Low-dose oral contraceptive pill	20 mcg ethinyl estradiol	100 mcg levonorgestrel or 3 mg drosperinone		
Cyclic hormone therapy	1–2 mg estradiol	0.5–1 mg norethisterone acetate		
Vaginal ring	15 mcg ethinyl estradiol	120 mcg etonogestrol		
Levonorgestrel intrauterine device		Mirena 20 mcg/24-hr levonorgestrel initially		
MENOPAUSE TREATMENT OPTIONS				
Estrogens	High	Standard	Low	Ultralow
Conjugated equine estrogens	1.25 mg	0.625 mg	0.3 mg	
Micronized 17β-estradiol	4.0 mg	2.0 mg	1.0 mg	0.5 mg
Estradiol valerate		2.0 mg	1.0 mg	
Piperazine estrone sulfate	1.25 mg	0.625 mg		
Transdermal 17β-estradiol	100 mcg	50 mcg	25 mcg	14 mcg[a]
Subcutaneous implant estradiol	100 mg	50 mg	20 mg	
Local/topical -estriol -estradiol		1 mg/g 25 mcg	0.5 mg	 10 mcg
Gel estradiol		1 mg/1 g		
Nasal spray estradiol hemihydrate		150 mcg/actuation		
Progestogens				
Norethisterone acetate	1 mg	0.5 mg		
Medroxyprogesterone acetate	10 mg	2.5–5 mg	1.5 mg	
Drospirenone		2 mg		
Other				
Tibolone		2.5 mg		
Levonorgestrel intrauterine device		Mirena 20 mcg/24-hr levonorgestrel initially or MLS 10 mcg/24-hr levonorgestrel initially		

[a]14 mcg 17β-estradiol is indicated only for prevention of osteoporosis.

point if women abandon HT use because of progestogen side effects or unwillingness to resume menstrual bleeding. Indeed, epidemiologic data indicate alarmingly high rates of endometrial hyperplasia and cancer among women supposedly on adequate cyclic regimens, indicating that either in reality compliance is poor or that endometrial protection is inadequate, or both.[61]

In addition to the issue of progestogen duration, as in the case of estrogen, the route of administration and dosage remain controversial and in need of clarification. Oral administration of progesterone is convenient; however, the oral micronized form is rapidly metabolized and inactivated in the liver. Therefore, high dosages must be administered to achieve adequate circulating blood levels. Synthetic progestogens are more resistant to hepatic metabolism. Hence, lower dosages can be used to achieve the desired endometrial effect. Yet there is up to a 10-fold variation in the bioavailability of the various progestogens following oral administration.[62] Side effects are reported by a small but significant number of women with both progesterone and synthetic progestin therapy. Natural micronized progesterone taken orally may induce sedation and undesirable hypnotic effects, and synthetic progestins may cause adverse mood effects in some women. Intramuscular progesterone administration results in predictable circulating levels, but the injection is painful and inconvenient. The vaginal route results in therapeutic levels in the endometrium. Vaginal gels and tablets of micronized progesterone are commonly used in in vitro fertilization protocols. Transvaginal progesterone used in an alternate-day regimen for 12 days has been shown to be effective as part of a cyclic HT regimen. But long term, this route of administration is inconvenient and unsatisfactory for most women. A vaginal levonorgestrel-impregnated intrauterine device is available in some countries and in appropriate circumstances is an excellent option for progestogen effects to be achieved in the endometrium with minimization of systemic side effects.

Progestogens can also be administered transdermally as a cream, patch, or gel. Currently in combination with estradiol, norethindrone is available in a patch using either a sequential or cyclic regimen. Nonprescription progesterone creams are widely available and are being used by many women with the belief that this treatment will preserve bone, act as an alternative to HT, may be substituted for synthetic progestogens in HT regimes, and alleviate menstrual and premenstrual symptoms. Some but not all studies indicate that if a sufficient amount of transdermal progesterone can be administered, it may alleviate vasomotor symptoms and afford endometrial protection short term, but long-term benefit and safety need to be established. There is no evidence that transdermal progesterone prevents bone loss.[63-65]

MANAGING CLINICAL SIDE EFFECTS

Common adverse effects of estrogen include nausea, headache, breast tenderness, and, when given with a progestogen, erratic or sometimes heavy bleeding. Cyclic estrogen-progestogen therapy is recommended for women who have not experienced 12 months of amenorrhea. Initiating therapy with the lowest dosage of estrogen often will minimize breast tenderness, unscheduled bleeding, and potentially other adverse effects. Transdermal or transvaginal estrogen is less likely than oral estrogen to cause nausea and headache. Also, transdermal estrogen is associated with a lower incidence of breast tenderness and deep vein thrombosis than oral estrogen. Changing from one estrogen regimen to another in many cases can alleviate certain adverse effects.

EFFECTIVENESS

Estrogen therapy alleviates vasomotor symptoms and the other commonly reported symptoms of menopause in 96% of women.[46] There is still some controversy as to whether systemic estrogen therapy alleviates symptoms of urogenital atrophy. A previous meta-analysis supports the use of systemic estrogen for this purpose; on the other hand, the Nurses' Health Study, an observational study, suggested that HT may worsen urinary incontinence.[30,32] However, most healthcare providers still believe that vaginal administration of estrogen is effective in alleviating vaginal dryness and atrophy, and is safe and acceptable to women.

DURATION OF THERAPY

The Women's Health Initiative (WHI) Study was a major, 15-year, research initiative undertaken in the U.S. funded by the National Institutes of Health to address the most common causes of death, disability, and poor quality of life in postmenopausal women.[37,66] Two arms of this study were dedicated to the evaluation of postmenopausal HT. Commencing in 1997, the HT studies were designed to determine whether the long-term use of oral HT in women aged 50–79 years at baseline would prevent heart disease, osteoporosis, and colon cancer and/or cause breast cancer. They were not designed to address the benefits of HT for the relief of menopausal symptoms. Only 10% of women in these studies were younger than 55 years (i.e., the population of interest in terms of HT benefit and risk), and the study was not powered to evaluate this subgroup. The combined oral CEE plus medroxyprogesterone acetate (MPA) therapy arm of the study was stopped in 2002 after an average of 5.2 years of participation.[37] This was because the slightly greater rate of invasive breast cancer in the combined hormone-treated women reached the safety level determined by the study monitoring committee. The CEE-only arm of the WHI study, intended to run until 2005, was stopped prematurely in 2004, after 7 years, because the rate of

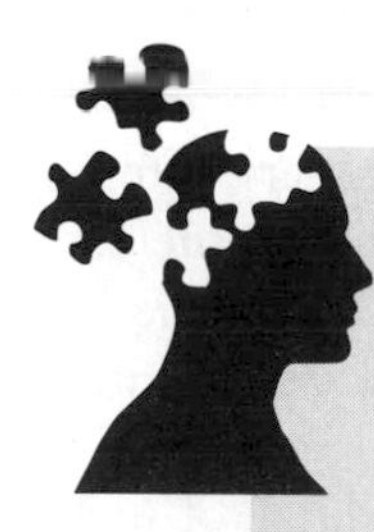

Therapeutic Challenge:

How might a trial be designed to answer questions about HT that were not addressed in the WHI (e.g., younger menopausal population, menopausal symptoms)?

strokes in women randomized to CEE exceeded the rate in women randomized to placebo therapy.[66] After complete data collection and analysis, neither of the stopping points for each of these studies achieved statistical significance.

The Women's Health Initiative has attracted widespread debate as to whether it was a primary intervention study and concern regarding the discrepancy in unblinding between the two groups (approximately 6% in the placebo group and 43% in the HT group).[67] Nonetheless, WHI provides a wealth of valuable information regarding the benefits and risks of continuous combined oral HT and oral estrogen in postmenopausal women aged >50 years. Data from WHI are subject to ongoing analysis.

Following the publication of the initial negative findings of the WHI studies, the general recommendation has been that estrogen +/− progestogen should be used at the lowest dosage for the shortest possible treatment period and ideally in most women for <5 years. The issue of duration of therapy remains controversial. It is the authors' view that the decision to continue therapy is that of the woman being treated, as only she can determine how significant the benefits are to her in terms of quality of life and what risks she is prepared to accept. However, this is in the setting that the user of HT is fully informed of the evidence for risk, and she should discuss this with her health professional every 6–12 months. Thus, some survivors of breast cancer with intolerable vasomotor or mood symptoms may elect to take HT after treatment of their breast cancer and after therapies without hormones have been tried because they have reached a decision that quality of life is more important than length of life.

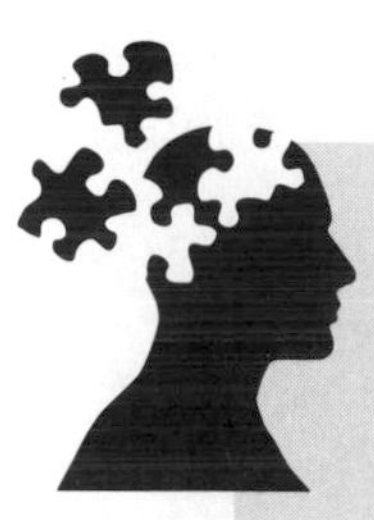

Therapeutic Challenge:

What were the absolute and relative risks of the outcomes in the WHI, and how does that influence how you communicate with women about HT?

BENEFITS VS. RISKS OF ESTROGEN +/− PROGESTOGEN THERAPY

Osteoporosis is a significant cause of morbidity and mortality in postmenopausal women (see also Chapter 40: Bone and Joint Disorders). At age 50, a woman has a 60% lifetime risk of sustaining an osteoporotic fracture and a 16% risk of hip fracture.[68] These risks are partly attributable to the accelerated bone loss, which occurs after menopause as a result of estrogen deficiency. Hormone therapy reduces bone turnover, increases BMD, and decreases vertebral and hip fracture rates by as much as 35%.[39] Importantly, the beneficial skeletal effects of estrogen therapy are not attenuated by increased age.[69] Progestogen therapy does not appear to enhance the effects of estrogen on BMD.

With regard to the effects of estrogen on fracture rates, in the WHI study comparing the effects of CEE 0.625 mg plus MPA 2.5 mg vs. placebo, the absolute risk of all fractures was reduced by 44 per 10,000 HT users per year and that of hip fractures by 5 per 10,000 HT users per year.[37] Despite these findings, this study population was not selected for on the basis of osteoporosis risk. If HT is stopped, bone loss resumes.[38] For the most effective protection against fracture, if HT is used, HT should either be started at menopause and continued long term or started later in life when the risk of fracture is greater.[70] Alternatively, HT may be initiated to manage menopausal symptoms with progression to other agents as women age.

There is strong epidemiologic evidence that HT use is associated with a lower rate of colorectal cancer.[71,72] This has been verified in the combined estrogen progestogen trials, but not with estrogen-only therapy.[37,66]

Accumulation of abdominal fat is associated with an increase in risk for the development of insulin resistance, hyperlipidemia, and hypertension, and therefore cardiovascular disease.[73,74] With respect to body composition, it has been reported that menopause is accompanied by a transition from a gynoid to an android central-type pattern of body fat distribution and an increase in total body fat and hence insulin resistance.[75] Parenteral estrogen therapy is associated with a reduction in central abdominal fat.[76,77] In a large population-based study, current users of postmenopausal hormones had a relative risk of noninsulin-dependent diabetes mellitus (NIDDM) of 0.80 (95% confidence interval [CI], 0.67–0.96) as compared with never users, after adjustment for age and body mass index (BMI).[78] Consistent with this, women treated with HT in WHI had a lower rate of the development of NIDDM.

With respect to HT and the risk of breast cancer, in the combined HT arm of WHI, women treated with CEE-MPA had a 1.26-fold greater risk of invasive breast cancer than women treated with placebo (an absolute risk of eight extra cases/10,000 women/year). However, 12,305 women in the study had not used HT before commencing the study, and for these women, the risk of breast cancer was not increased (relative risk 1.05). Counterintuitively, a family history of breast cancer did not increase the risk of developing breast cancer with HT. Furthermore, mortality resulting from breast cancer was not increased with HT use.[79]

For the CEE-alone vs. placebo arm, the hazard ratio for invasive breast cancer was 0.77 (95% CI, 0.59–1.01) after a mean follow-up of 6.8 years.[66] Consistent with this finding, several studies have indicated that the concurrent use of a progestogen may confer a significantly greater risk of breast cancer than the use of estrogen alone.[80,81] The extrapolation of these findings has been that progestogens increase breast cancer risk when given with estrogen. But of note, 40% of women in the estrogen-only study had undergone bilateral oophorectomy vs. 0.3% of women in the combined HT study. This might in part explain the different breast cancer risks noted in the two groups.

Research into the effects of HT on ovarian cancer has had significant methodological limitations, relying primarily on subject recall of past HT use.[82,83] Overall, the absolute risk of ovarian cancer in HT users remains very small and may be isolated to long-term unopposed estrogen therapy. In addition, many of the women in these observational cohort studies were likely on higher estrogen dosages than what is currently recommended. Additional data are required to clarify the risk of ovarian cancer with short- and long-term combined HT use.

Women who have undergone a premature surgical menopause have double the risk of coronary artery disease compared with those who have undergone natural menopause.[84] (See also Chapter 30: Cardiovascular Disease.) However, the extent to which estrogen insufficiency contributes to this increased risk is uncertain. Estrogen-only therapy is associated with a reduced rate of coronary artery calcification in young postmenopausal women.[85] Consistent with this, for women aged 50–59 years at enrollment into the WHI studies, there was no increase in risk of CHD, stroke, or global mortality.[86] In the Women's Oestrogen and Stroke Trial, of 664 postmenopausal women commenced on 1 mg 17β estradiol or placebo within weeks of a stroke, there was an increase in strokes during the first 6 months, and strokes tended to be more severe in the estradiol group.[87] In the Heart and Estrogen/progestin Replacement Study (HERS), combined continuous HT had no effect on stroke risk in postmenopausal women.[88] Clearly, the risk of stroke is increased in older women, and HT should not be commenced for primary or secondary prevention.

Oral estrogen therapy is consistently associated with a two- to threefold increase in risk of venous thromboembolism (VTE).[66,88] This risk is increased further after major surgery or hospital admission. Increasing age and BMI are additional risk factors. However, for women aged 50–59 years who have a BMI of <25, the rate of VTE in the WHI study was similar to that noted for the control group. Transdermal estrogen does not appear to increase the risk of VTE, although this has not been evaluated in a large RCT.[89]

PRECAUTIONS/CONTRAINDICATIONS

The absolute contraindications to estrogen +/− progestogen therapy include undiagnosed vaginal bleeding and current treatment of a hormone-dependent malignancy. Past estrogen-dependent malignancy is a strong relative contraindication for HT, and some would consider this to be an absolute contraindication to treatment. Other important relative contraindications for the initiation of HT include past VTE disease (oral estrogen in a fully anticoagulated individual may be acceptable as may be transdermal estrogen), frequent migraine with aura (which in itself is a risk factor for stroke),

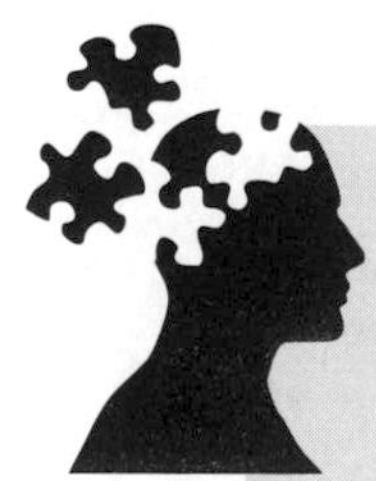

Therapeutic Challenge:

What impact does HT have on dementia? Sleep? Neuropsychiatric disorders (e.g., depression)?

active endometriosis, severe liver disease, unstable major systemic disease, being older than the age of 65 years, or a strong family history of breast cancer.

MONITORING AND FOLLOW-UP

All women using systemic HT should be medically re-evaluated every 6 months, and the need for ongoing HT and the formulation and dosage requirement should be reconsidered. All women should undergo a routine general health and breast check. Review of personal and family history of osteoporosis, breast cancer, migraines, VTE, and cardiovascular risks is important. Investigations should be individually assessed with biannual mammography and breast ultrasound when indicated; vaginal ultrasound or endometrial biopsy if there is any excessive or prolonged bleeding 3–6 months after commencing HT; and bone densitometry measurement (dual-energy x-ray absorptiometry [DEXA]) when indicated.[90]

Testosterone Therapy

Testosterone levels decline in women before menopause and do not appear to change across menopause.[13,14] There has been considerable interest in testosterone supplementation for the treatment of low libido in postmenopausal women. A Cochrane review of studies of the use of testosterone in postmenopausal women for low libido to 2003 concluded that there are benefits in terms of improved sexual function with the addition of testosterone to standard postmenopausal HT.[91] Commonly used formulations include esterified estrogens and methyltestosterone. Large RCTs in both surgically menopausal and naturally menopausal women, for whom the frequency of satisfactory sexual events was the primary endpoint, demonstrate that treatment with the transdermal testosterone patch, which delivers 300 mcg of testosterone per day (but not the patch delivering 450 mcg/day) significantly increased the number of self-reported sexually satisfying events per month when compared with placebo.[92-95] These studies also demonstrated significant improvements in desire, arousal, responsiveness, orgasm, pleasure, and satisfaction.

An analysis of data from a number of these studies combined indicates that women with an SHBG level above 160 nmol/L or taking CEE are unlikely to benefit from testosterone therapy.[96] The former is because testosterone binds to SHBG with high affinity, such that having an elevated SHBG results in a very low free or bioavailable testosterone. The interaction between CEE therapy and exogenous testosterone is unclear, but it may be that a component of CEE interferes with the binding of testosterone to the androgen receptor in addition to increasing SHBG.

The link between postmenopausal estrogen-progestogen use and breast cancer has created a level of concern regarding the use of testosterone in women. Testosterone has been widely used by women as an unapproved therapy for decades. There is no evidence from studies of premenopausal women and postmenopausal women using systemic estrogen treated with testosterone for up to 24 months, or studies of women with chronic androgen excess because of polycystic ovarian syndrome (PCOS), that elevated testosterone levels, even above what is considered physiologically normal, are associated with altered breast cancer risk.[97,98] Primate and human studies suggest that testosterone may in fact protect the breast from estrogen-induced breast cell proliferation.[99-101] However, this is an area of considerable controversy that needs to be addressed in postmarketing surveillance research. There is also no evidence that in women without insulin resistance, testosterone adversely affects cardiovascular disease risk.[102] However, uncertainty as to the consequences of restoring testosterone levels to those of premenopausal women in women who are many years past menopause remains. Now that testosterone patch therapy (Intrinsa®) has been approved for surgically menopausal women with hypoactive sexual desire disorder despite estrogen therapy (other than CEE) in Europe, these data will eventually be forthcoming from postmarketing-surveillance studies of women in the community.

Tibolone

Tibolone is a synthetic steroid possessing a 3 keto-group with a 7α methyl group that is in widespread use in Europe and Asia-Pacific countries as an alternative to conventional estrogen or estrogen/progestogen therapy. It has been described as a prodrug, as following ingestion, it is quickly metabolized in the gastrointestinal tract to two estrogenic metabolites, 3α and β which then circulate predominantly in their sulfated inactive forms.[103] These metabolites only become estrogenically active when desulfated by the sulfatase enzyme in target tissues. Tibolone itself and its 3β metabolite may also be converted to a Δ4-isomer by the enzyme 3β-hydroxysteroid dehydrogenase (HSD)-isomerase.[103] The Δ4-isomer can bind and transactivate the progesterone receptor and the androgen receptor such that in the endometrium tibolone exerts a predominantly progestogenic effect.[103] Tibolone alleviates postmenopausal vasomotor symptoms without stimulating the endometrium.[104,105] Thus, a progestogen is not required, and cyclic bleeding is not induced. In addition to having weak androgenic effects, tibolone significantly lowers SHBG and increases circulating free testosterone, further adding to its androgenicity.[106]

In osteoporotic women older than age 60 years, tibolone significantly reduces the incidence of vertebral and nonvertebral fractures (relative hazard [RH] 0.55, 95% CI, 0.41–0.74; p <0.001 and 0.74, 95% CI 0.58–0.93; p = 0.01, respectively) and is associated with a reduced risk of breast cancer (RH 0.32; 95% CI, 0.13–0.80; p = 0.02) and colon cancer (RH 0.31; 95% CI, 0.10–0.96; p = 0.04) (Level A).[107] The incidence of breast tenderness with tibolone is low, and mammographic density does not generally increase.[108,109,110] Tibolone has been associated with an increased risk of stroke in older women, but this has not been observed in multiple RCTs of younger women.[111,112] Tibolone also does not increase the risk of venous thromboembolic disease or coronary heart disease events (Level A).[107,113] There have been conflicting reports in the literature about the endometrial safety of tibolone. In a large RCT comparing tibolone 1.25 mg and 2.5 mg to CCE/MPA, tibolone did not induce endometrial hyperplasia or carcinoma in postmenopausal women, and it is associated with a better vaginal bleeding profile than CEE/MPA.[111] In addition, rates of breakthrough bleeding after commencement of tibolone are low.[114] Tibolone improves sexual well being in postmenopausal women presenting with low libido, with greater improvements in desire arousal and satisfaction and receptiveness than seen for transdermal estrogen-progestin therapy.[112]

Alternative and Nonhormonal Therapies

ESTROGEN AGONISTS/ANTAGONISTS

Estrogen agonists/antagonists (EAAs) are a class of compounds that exhibit selective estrogenic and antiestrogenic activities in differing tissues as a result of their binding to the ERs. Our understanding of the consequences of the interactions between various ligands (such as EAAs) with ERα and β has been enhanced by the crystal structures of the ERα and β ligand–binding domains (LBD) complexed with several ligands. Although agonists and antagonists bind at the same site within the core of the LBD, each induces specific conformations in the transactivation domain, known as AF-2. The effect of each ligand on the positioning of helix 12 provides a structural mechanism by which a ligand may act as an agonist or antagonist. The binding of estradiol to the LBD places helix 12 in an agonist position such that coactivators can bind the complex and transcription is activated. EAAs such as tamoxifen and raloxifene in vitro distinctly place helix 12 in an antagonist position.[15] Raloxifene exhibits estrogen agonist activity on bone and lipids, and antagonist activity on breast and the endometrium. Raloxifene prevents vertebral fractures in postmenopausal osteoporotic women.[115] Like oral estrogen, raloxifene increases the risk of VTE.[115] However, raloxifene reduces the risk of invasive breast cancer.[116] Unfortunately, both tamoxifen and raloxifene have the tendency to cause rather than alleviate hot flushes and vaginal dryness. There is preliminary evidence that raloxifene can be combined with estrogen therapy, and further studies looking at EAA-estradiol combinations are under way.[117]

DEHYDROEPIANDROSTERONE

Dehydroepiandrosterone (DHEA) and its sulfate ester, DHEAS, are the most abundant circulating sex-steroid hormones in women. The production of DHEA and DHEAS increases at the age of 6–8 years as a consequence of the maturation of the zona reticularis of the adrenal cortex with the resultant initiation of **adrenarche.**[118] Maximal values of circulating DHEAS are achieved between the ages of 20 and 30 years. Thereafter, serum DHEA and DHEAS steadily decline, resulting in widespread speculation that the age-related decline in these C19 steroids results in loss of well-being, deterioration in cognition, and lowered libido.[119-122] It has been proposed that restoration of serum DHEA to the levels found in young people may be beneficial.[122] A number of studies of DHEA therapy have been published, but the results are inconsistent. A review of the literature concluded that evidence to support either benefit or safety of DHEA supplementation for otherwise healthy perimenopausal or postmenopausal women is lacking and that further research into the use of DHEA is warranted.[123] A recent RCT has reported no beneficial effect of DHEA 50 mg per day orally on sexual function, general well being, or menopausal symptoms in postmenopausal women presenting with low libido.[124]

PHYTOESTROGENS

Plant constituents with a phenol structure similar to estrogen are known as phyto (plant) estrogens. These compounds, found in a wide variety of edible plants, may display both estrogenic and antiestrogenic effects. Earlier epidemiologic studies, primarily comparing Asian and Western populations, were interpreted to indicate that consumption of a phytoestrogen-rich diet may ameliorate estrogen deficiency symptoms in postmenopausal women and may protect against breast cancer, bone loss, and cardiovascular disease.[125] Consequently, there was a movement toward increased consumption of phytoestrogen-rich foods, and tablet formulations of concentrated isoflavone extracts were heavily promoted.

Phytoestrogens do not simply mimic the effects of human steroidal estrogen but exhibit both similar and divergent actions. The ultimate actions of these compounds in specific cells is determined by many factors, including the relative levels of the estrogen receptors ERα and β and the diverse mix of coactivators and corepressors present in any given cell type. Effects vary according to the phytoestrogen studied, cell line, tissue, species, and response being evaluated.

Systematic reviews of intervention studies question the validity of the proposed benefits of phytoestrogen supplementation, with little data in postmenopausal women to support a role for phytoestrogens as an alternative for conventional HT.[126,127] Meanwhile, the effects of phytoestrogens on the breast remain unclear.

BLACK COHOSH

Black cohosh *(Cimicifuga racemosa,* also known as *Actaea racemosa*) is North American native plant. It has common usage internationally for the treatment of hot flushes and sweats experienced by postmenopausal women. Overall, results of RCTs do not suggest black cohosh is useful in the treatment of hot flushes.[47] However, results differ between trials.

There have been a number of case reports linking black cohosh to acute hepatitis requiring liver transplant after a few weeks of treatment.[128] Women considering the use of black cohosh should have their liver function checked by blood testing before starting this herb and periodically during treatment.[129] Safety beyond 6 months is unknown, as are the clinical effects of black cohosh on the breast.

CLONIDINE

Women who flush appear to have greater sympathetic nervous system activity, and the drug clonidine, a centrally acting α-adrenergic antihypertensive, may act by elevating the "flush threshold." Clonidine 50–150 mcg twice daily has been used for many years to alleviate hot flushes with limited effectiveness.[47] Some women experience side effects at very low dosages (dry mouth). Generally, most women do not find clonidine useful.

GABAPENTIN

Gabapentin was developed for the treatment of epilepsy. It is also used for neurogenic pain, restless-leg syndrome, essential tremor, bipolar disorder, and migraine prevention. However, dosages of 300–900 mg at night have been shown to be efficacious in reducing the frequency and severity of hot flushes.[130-132] More somatic symptoms were reported with gabapentin than with estrogen or placebo; however, it is still represents a nonhormonal alternative to estrogen for some women.

SEROTONIN REUPTAKE INHIBITORS

Selective serotonin reuptake inhibitors (SSRIs) have been studied as alternatives to estrogen to reduce hot flushes and improve mood disorders in women unable to use HT. Studies of venlafaxine, a serotonergic-noradrenergic reuptake inhibitor, and paroxetine, an SSRI, indicate a moderate reduction in vasomotor symptoms with dosages of 37.5–75 mg and 12.5–25 mg per day, respectively.[133-135] Both therapies may cause nausea and insomnia. In addition, venlafaxine may cause dry mouth, constipation, and decreased appetite, whereas paroxetine may cause headaches. Of note is that paroxetine should not be used in combination with tamoxifen, as it may impair conversion of tamoxifen to its active metabolite, endoxifen, by inhibiting the liver enzyme CYP2D6 (P4502D6).[135]

The vasomotor effect appears to be independent of the effect on mood, with relief from hot flushes occurring in the first week; the antidepressant effect manifests after 6–8 weeks. Lowest effective dosage should be used, and when ceasing the drug, the dosage should be tapered.

BIOIDENTICAL HORMONE THERAPY

Some physicians and compounding pharmacists have been promoting "bioidentical" hormonal preparations, which are said to provide a unique mix of estradiol, estrone, and estriol at dosages specifically designed for each woman. For the estrogen doses commonly given in these preparations, no studies have been conducted to establish the lowest effective dosage to treat symptoms or the required dosage of progestogen (progesterone) to be used for endometrial protection. There is no evidence from any published study that transdermally (skin) or buccally (mouth) absorbed progesterone will protect the lining of the uterus from conditions such as uterine cancer. This has culminated in cases of endometrial cancers being reported among users of such therapy.[136] Compounded estrogen creams, lozenges, or troches are also sometimes combined with testosterone or DHEA, or each of these is sometimes prescribed alone.

Again, there is no evidence that any of the dosages of the mixed preparations are safe or effective, and the use of these preparations may carry the same risk-benefit ratio as commercially available estrogen/progesterone therapies.[48] There are no published data on these products, yet some of the compounding pharmacies have issued documents recommending various dosages and equivalent dosages to U.S. Food and Drug Administration–approved estrogen therapies. Evidence for many of these recommendations is lacking.

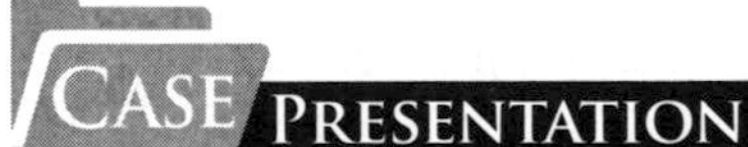

Patient Case: Part 2

B.B. is healthy 54-year-old postmenopausal woman presenting with osteopenia, menopausal symptoms (insomnia and irritable mood), urogenital symptoms (including vaginal atrophy), low libido, and increased risk of cardiovascular disease (history of dyslipidemia [statin medication], and family history risk of stroke).

Plan:

Further assessment at this stage should include a full examination with targeted testing of bloods to include her lipid profile and glucose tolerance. As well, she should have a mammogram and Pap test if she hasn't had one in the last 2 years. B.B. should continue her healthy lifestyle with weight-bearing exercise, a diet rich in calcium, and her calcium/vitamin supplement. Her statin medication should be continued and adjusted if necessary for her dyslipidemia.

She has requested discussion of the use of HT, which should include the advantages and risks for her personally. B.B. would be suitable to try this therapy.

Rationale:

Hormone therapy would alleviate symptoms of insomnia/depression and vaginal dryness, and thus dyspareunia. Increased vaginal lubrication may assist with her sexual desire. HT would help prevent further bone loss and decrease the incidence of vertebral and hip fracture. It may provide a cardioprotective benefit if she commenced HT now, as she is <10 years postmenopausal. This benefit is shown in women younger than age 60.[85,86] The route of administration needs to be considered. A nonoral preparation of estrogen would be preferable to avoid the first-pass hepatic effect of estrogen and thus the undesirable procoagulant effect of oral estrogen.[133]

BB could benefit from a transdermal estrogen patch but would require progestogen supplementation as she has an intact uterus. This will decrease her risk of endometrial hyperplasia and cancer. Progestogen therapy could be delivered orally, in a combined patch, or in the LNG-IUD.

Monitoring and follow-up:

Review in 6 weeks will assess her tolerability of HT, symptom relief, and any side effects. If she has continued symptoms of insomnia and mood changes, consider adding an SSRI. If her libido is still low and causing her distress, this should be further explored.

B.B. will need regular 6-month reviews to assess symptom control, side effects, and risks. Each review is an opportunity to discuss her desire to continue, change, or cease her current therapy.

Summary

Menopause may bring symptoms that are distressing and affect a woman's quality of life. Women may present through the menopause transition and into menopause with symptoms such as menstrual irregularity initially, followed by cessation of menses, hot flushes and night sweats, change in sleep quality, depression, and arthralgias. Fifty percent of women will show symptoms of urogenital atrophy. Some will present with evidence of reduced bone mass. Understanding the pathophysiology helps guide the choice of appropriate management for the individual woman. Mild symptoms can be addressed using nonpharmacologic methods, such as reduction in smoking, coffee, and alcohol; stress management; and increased exercise. Hormonal methods of symptom control may differ between perimenopause and menopause, as contraception is often still a requirement in the former. Therapies that provide contraception and reduce common menopausal symptoms are low-dose oral contraceptives, LNG-IUD, and the vaginal ring. For those needing symptom relief but no contraception, there are low-dose HT and oral progestogen-only regimens.

Once menopause is established, estrogen +/− progestogen therapy can be used to treat women who find their symptoms intolerable. There are a variety of formulations and routes of administration that can influence side effects and risk factors. Changing from one to another may alleviate problem side effects. Although controversial, HT should be used at the lowest possible dose for the shortest amount of time, ideally <5 years. However, some women, fully informed of their risks, may elect to continue HT longer to ensure the quality of life. Informed choices by the patient should be supported. The benefits and risks of estrogen +/− progestogen therapy have been assessed in osteoporosis, NIDDM, breast cancer, ovarian cancer, coronary heart disease, stroke, and VTE. Each woman should be assessed individually for her needs and risk factors. Monitoring should be every 6 months with health checks performed and discussion about the need for ongoing treatment, dosage, and formulation.

Other pharmacologic treatments have been studied for symptoms during menopause, including testosterone, tibolone, SSRIs, serotonin-norepinephrine reuptake inhibitors, phytoestrogens, black cohosh, clonidine, gabapentin, and bioidentical hormones. However, none of these second- or third-line agents are as effective as HT with estrogen +/− progestogen.

Menopause is inevitable, and the management of menopause is individual, based on a woman's symptoms, her general health and risk factors, and her willingness to weigh the benefits and risks of various pharmacologic choices.

References

Additional content available at
www.ashp.org/womenshealth

SECTION FOUR

Contraceptive Methods

18 Family Planning and Nonhormonal Contraception

Jacki S. Witt, JD, MSN, WHNP, CNM; Julie L. Strickland, MD, MPH; Kimberly Thrasher, Pharm.D., BCPS, FCCP, CPP

Learning Objectives

1. Assess the short- and long-term effectiveness and safety for patient-directed and healthcare provider–directed nonhormonal contraception methods, and apply this to an individual's contraceptive planning.
2. Identify individuals who would be ideal candidates for nonhormonal contraceptive methods.
3. Develop counseling information to optimize patient compliance with nonhormonal contraceptive methods.
4. Describe proper instructions for the handling, storage, use, and need to resupply for each type of barrier or spermicidal method.
5. Compare the duration of effect and reversal of fertility for each type of nonhormonal contraceptive method.

Pregnancy prevention by a variety of means has been practiced by almost every culture. Historical evidence of contraceptive use dates back thousands of years and includes behavioral methods (e.g., *coitus interruptus*) as well as mechanical methods (e.g., vaginal sponges and recipes for vaginal inserts that were believed to form an impenetrable barrier to the cervix).

Of significance is the fact that the natural methods involving the recognition of signs and symptoms of fertility are used by women to plan as well as prevent conception. For this reason, knowledge of the "natural" or physiologic signs of female fertility may involve a much broader audience than those interested in contraceptive methods.

The majority of birth control methods in this section are under the control of the woman, which may make them more desirable. With the exception of the nonhormonal intrauterine contraceptive and sterilization by surgery or microinserts, women can decide to stop using any of these methods and can expect an almost immediate return to fertility because there is no disruption of normal hormonal function and no structural or organic change.

With the advent of newer hormonal as well as nonhormonal methods of contraception (see Chapter 19: Hormonal Contraception), many of the reversible nonhormonal options are now practiced infrequently in the U.S. For instance, despite a resurgence of male condom use in the 1980s subsequent to concern with the transmission of sexually transmitted infections (STIs), specifically human immunodeficiency virus (HIV), this method amounts to approximately 18% of total contraception use in the U.S.[1] On the other hand, researchers at *Child Trends* reviewed their data as well as data from the 2002 National Survey of Family Growth and found that use of the male condom by women 15–19 years of age increased from 23% in 1982 to 63% in 1995 at the time of first sex; the use of oral contraceptives remained steady at 8% during the same years of observation.[2] Contraceptive choices differ greatly by patient age, and since the 1980s, the pill and sterilization have become the most frequently used methods of contraception in the U.S., with 50% of women older than 40 years of age choosing sterilization.[1]

Behavioral Methods

Behavioral methods of contraception are patient directed and include options such as abstinence; fertility awareness methods (FAMs) and natural family planning (NFP); coitus interruptus; and the lactation amenorrhea method (LAM).

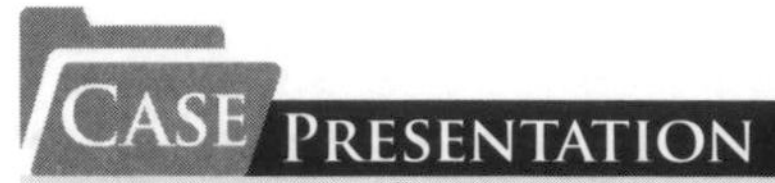

CASE PRESENTATION

Patient Case: Part 1

K.L. is a 34-year-old woman presenting to the clinic for a method of contraception that doesn't involve "using something" at the time of intercourse. She and her partner are currently using condoms, but she says that they are "not very consistent" with their use. She has had four pregnancies: three vaginal births and one spontaneous abortion. She doesn't think she wants any more children but is not interested in anything permanent at this time.

HPI: K.L. wants a method of birth control that is not a "hassle"; she has been on birth control pills in the past but was not successful in taking them daily at the same time. She calls both of her last two pregnancies "pill pregnancies" because she became pregnant while taking oral contraceptives, but she does admit that she had difficulty adhering to the daily schedule. She has also been told that she can't take birth control pills and smoke after she turns 35; she has no plans for smoking cessation at this time. She has used "the shot" (depot medroxyprogesterone acetate) in the past but says that it caused her to gain 30 lb in 1 year.

PMH: Asthma.

PSH: Removal of benign cyst left breast at age 29.

Gynecologic history: No history of STIs or recurrent vaginal infections; normal Pap tests X 3. Menarche was at age 12. First day of last menstrual period was 4 days ago. Menstrual cycles are regular, occur at 30- to 35-day intervals, last about 5 days; denies severe premenstrual symptoms and denies dysmenorrhea, heavy menstrual flow, or clotting with menses.

Family history: Mother (59)—hypertension, arthritis; father (61)—hypertension, diabetes; brother (38)—healthy.

Social history: Smokes ½ ppd; occasional alcohol; works as paralegal in a legal office; swims twice per week for 30 minutes and attends yoga classes twice per week for 1 hour.

Medications: Multivitamin one daily.

Allergies: Penicillin (rash).

Vital signs: 5′3″, 145 lb (BMI 25), BP 138/88, HR 76, RR 16.

Physical exam: Normal, including normal pelvic examination with firm, nontender, uterus.

ABSTINENCE

Description

Sexual abstinence is most often defined as the voluntary avoidance of genital contact. There is some controversy, however, about this definition. For some, abstinence implies having no sexual experiences, including masturbation. For others, it means refraining from penetrative sex (anal, oral or vaginal). *Othercourse* or *outercourse* are terms used to describe a variety of sexual acts not involving intercourse.[3-6] Periodic abstinence is required for the FAMs or NFP to be effective.

Effectiveness

If practiced consistently, abstinence is theoretically 100% effective. There are no data available for typical-use effectiveness.

Advantages

Abstinence that includes othercourse or outercourse involves no devices or drugs and can be practiced spontaneously without risk of pregnancy or STIs, as long as no body fluids are exchanged. Temporarily avoiding intercourse for a variety of sexual problems may take performance pressure off one or both partners, especially those with orgasmic difficulty or rapid ejaculation. Some couples report increased emotional intimacy during times of voluntary abstinence.[3-6]

Disadvantages

Abstinence as a method of birth control requires commitment and self-control. Long-term use of abstinence for contraception may be unsatisfying for one or both partners. There may still be a risk for transmitting infections unless all body fluids are avoided.[6-7]

Ideal Candidates

For individuals or couples who want to temporarily avoid intercourse for pregnancy prevention or health problems, this may be an acceptable strategy.

Patient Education and Follow-up

Individuals or couples should be counseled to decide, with their partners, what they will and will not do. If appropriate, women should be educated about condoms and postcoital contraception in case of need.

FERTILITY AWARENESS AND NATURAL FAMILY PLANNING

Description

FAMs and NFP are behavioral methods of contraception that rely on the couple to predict fertile periods in the woman's menstrual cycle and their commitment to abstain from intercourse during those fertile periods. In all of the FAMs, the woman is instructed about signs and symptoms of fertility, and the couple is counseled about the necessity of periodic abstinence to prevent pregnancy. Alternatively, these methods may be used by couples trying to conceive: By using the identified fertile times of the cycle for sexual intercourse, the couple may increase their chances for conception.[8-10] All of the natural approaches to family planning are based on known physiologic changes during the menstrual cycle. Cycle day 1 is the first day of menstrual bleeding; in each cycle there are about 6 days of fertility, beginning 5 days before ovulation and continuing through the 24-hour ovulatory window. The 2 days preceding ovulation are the most fertile days. The human ovum is viable for 12–24 hours after ovulation, and sperm survive for about 3–5 days in estrogen-stimulated cervical mucus. Alterations in this "typical" pattern can change the fertile period in any cycle, and the pattern may change because of lifestyle factors (e.g., smoking or using medications), environmental factors (e.g., illness or stress), or the age of either partner. Practically speaking, there is some probability of fertility throughout the menstrual cycle.[11-13] Table 18-1 is a brief summary of the NFP and other nonhormonal methods.

Table 18-1. Comparison of Nonhormonal Contraceptive Methods: Efficacy Rates, Appropriate Candidates, Contraindications, Advantages, and Disadvantages

Type of Contraceptive	Efficacy Rate (%) (pregnancy/100 women/year)		Appropriate for	Contraindications (relative = R, absolute = A)	Advantages	Disadvantages
	Perfect Use	Typical Use				
Nonprescription						
NFP		3–22	Any reproductive age Religious or philosophical reasons that may limit options	Women with • irregular menstrual cycle (R) • uncooperative partner (A) • history of substance abuse or partner with same (R) • potential for high-risk pregnancy (R) • history of recurrent genital tract infections (R)	Lack of method-related health risks Lack of systemic side effects Sense of enhanced "partnership" among partners	Timed abstinence required No protection from HIV/STIs Lower efficacy rate
Coitus Interruptus		4–27	Any reproductive age	Potential for high-risk pregnancy (R) History of substance abuse or partner with same (R)	Lack of method-related health risks Lack of systemic side effects	No protection from HIV/STIs Lower efficacy rate
LAM	<2	4–7	Any reproductive age "Fully or nearly fully" breast-feeding first 6 mo postpartum	Regular supplementation Infant use of pacifier	Effective High satisfaction No cost	Ovulation may return before return of menses No protection from HIV/STIs

(*Continued on next page*)

Type of Contraceptive	Efficacy Rate (%) (pregnancy/100 women/year)		Appropriate for	Contraindications (relative = R, absolute = A)	Advantages	Disadvantages
	Perfect Use	Typical Use				
Barriers						
Male Condom	2–3	14% to 15%	Any reproductive age Couples who need • immediate contraception • temporary contraception • backup method • extra protection from HIV/STIs	Allergy to latex	No method-related health risks No systemic side effects Inexpensive Protection from HIV/STIs	User dependent Moderately effective Supply must be readily available Male controlled Frequent slippage or breakage
Female Condom	2–5	20–21	Any reproductive age Women who • prefer not to or cannot use hormonal methods • want protection from STIs with partners unwilling to use condoms • prefer not to use IUCs • need immediate contraception • need backup method	Hypersensitivity	No method-related health risks No systemic side effects Female controlled Can be inserted up to 8 hr before intercourse High satisfaction rate Protection from HIV/STIs	Moderately effective User dependent Supply must be readily available
Vaginal Sponge nulliparous women parous women	 9–10 20	 15–16 32–40	Any reproductive age Women who • need a barrier method • prefer not to or cannot use hormonal methods	Allergy to N-9	Protection up to 24 hr after insertion Greater spontaneity allowed	Lacks protection from HIV User dependent
Spermicide	6–15	10–29	Any reproductive age Women who • prefer not to or cannot use hormonal methods • are breast-feeding • need a backup method	Hypersensitivity	Variety of available products Rapid onset of effectiveness No systemic side effects	Lacks protection from HIV Short duration of effectiveness Immediate need to resupply with repeated intercourse User dependent

(*Continued on next page*)

Type of Contraceptive	Efficacy Rate (%) (pregnancy/100 women/year)		Appropriate for	Contraindications (relative = R, absolute = A)	Advantages	Disadvantages
	Perfect Use	Typical Use				
Prescription						
Diaphragm (with spermicide)	6	20	Any reproductive age Women who • prefer not to or cannot use hormonal methods • are with partners who refuse to use condoms • are breast-feeding	Allergy to N-9 Allergy to latex History of TSS	May be inserted 6–8 hr before intercourse May protect from non-HIV STIs No method-related health risks No systemic side effects	Must be properly fitted Lacks protection from HIV User dependent UTI and TSS risk
Cervical Cap			Same as diaphragm	Same as diaphragm	Provides contraception for up to 48 hr after insertion No method-related health risks No systemic side effects	Must be properly fitted Lacks protection from HIV User dependent UTI and TSS risk
nulliparous women	9	15–20				
parous women	25	40				
IUC Copper	<1	<1	Any reproductive age Women who • are >35 yr old and who smoke • are unable to use hormonal methods • are breast-feeding • are postpartum • are postabortion • desire reliable long-term contraception	Nulliparous (R) History of ectopic pregnancy, severe valvular heart disease, severe dysmenorrhea (A) Current PID Known or suspected pregnancy High-risk STIs Undiagnosed genital bleeding Distorted uterine canal Allergy to copper Immunosuppressed	Intercourse independent Reversible, long term Highly effective	Must be properly inserted and removed by healthcare provider High up-front cost Expulsion (10%) Rarely: perforation, infection at time of insertion May ↑ menstrual pain, bleeding Lacks protection from HIV
Sterilization Female (Essure®)		0.2	Any reproductive age Women who • desire contraceptive permanency • desire not to use hormonal methods	Uncertainty in ending fertility Previous TL Known or suspected pregnancy	Highly effective Outpatient setting Minimal anesthesia	Inserted by healthcare provider Timing of insertion dependent on cycle Surgical removal

(*Continued on next page*)

Type of Contraceptive	Efficacy Rate (%) (pregnancy/100 women/year)		Appropriate for	Contraindications (relative = R, absolute = A)	Advantages	Disadvantages
	Perfect Use	Typical Use				
				Placement of <1 insert <6 wk postpartum or postabortion Recent or acute PID Allergy to contrast media or nickel Immunosuppressed	Intercourse independent	Lacks protection from HIV and STIs Women must use another highly effective contraceptive for 3 mo postinsertion
Female (TL)		0.5–1.8	Any reproductive age Women who • desire contraceptive permanency and have completed childbearing • are postpartum • are postabortion Anytime unrelated to pregnancy	Uncertainty in ending fertility	Permanency Immediate contraception Intercourse independent	Surgical complications Lacks protection from HIV and STIs Lack of easy reversibility
Male		0.7–1.1	Women and their male partners who desire contraceptive permanency	Uncertainty in ending fertility	Permanency Intercourse independent Safer and less costly than TL	Surgical complications Lacks protection from HIV and STIs Men remain fertile for several months postprocedure Lack of easy reversibility

HIV = human immunodeficiency virus; IUC = intrauterine contraceptive; LAM = lactational amenorrhea method; N-9 = nonoxynol-9; NFP = natural family planning; PID = pelvic inflammatory disease; STI = sexually transmitted infection; TL = tubal ligation; TSS = toxic shock syndrome; UTI = urinary tract infection.

- The ***basal body temperature (BBT)*** method can be used to predict when ovulation will occur but is most effective in indicating when the fertile period has past. Ovulation is pinpointed when the BBT increases an average of 0.4–0.8°F. This upward shift usually follows a slight decrease or dip in the BBT. Studies have shown that ovulation occurs within 48 hours before—or after—the temperature increase.[11]
- The *Billings ovulation method (BOM)* (also referred to as the cervical mucous method) is based on the woman's observations of cervical mucus, which signals the beginning and the end of the fertile period, even with women who have irregular cycles. Each day, the woman touches her vaginal introitus to check the quantity and characteristics of the secretions there. For a few days after menses, cervical mucus is minimal, and the daily testing will be negative. The estrogen surge, which occurs before ovulation, increases the amount of mucus and makes it clear and elastic. Under the influence of progesterone after ovulation, the mucus thickens and the amount decreases. The fertile period consists of the "ovulation mucus" days.[8,13]
- The *calendar (or rhythm) method* is considered to be less reliable because it is based on past menstrual

cycle history, which can change in any woman because of stress, illness, or other factors. Counting the first day of menstrual bleeding as cycle day 1, women keep a record of their menstrual cycle lengths for the past 6–12 months and then record the shortest and the longest of the cycles. They then subtract 18 from the number of days in their shortest cycle, which alerts them to the likely first fertile day in the current cycle. In addition, they subtract 11 from the number of days in their longest cycle to find the likely last fertile day in the current cycle.[14] This calculation is based on the fact that the luteal phase (after ovulation) has a fixed length of about 14 days. In a woman with a short cycle of 21 days, ovulation may occur as early as cycle day 3. Table 18-2 contains examples for calculating a woman's fertile days.

- The *standard days method* is designed for women having cycles lasting 26–32 days. It was developed by scientists at Georgetown University for women wanting a simple natural method and for women living in low literacy/low health resource areas. Women are given CycleBeads®, a string of 32 colored beads representing days of the menstrual cycle. The first bead is red and represents the first day of menstrual bleeding; the next six beads are brown, representing nonfertile days preceding the ovulatory period; the next 12 beads are white, representing fertile days; and the last 13 beads are brown, again representing nonfertile days (Figure 18-1).[8,15]

Table 18-2. Calculating the Fertile Period Using the Calendar Method

If the shortest cycle has been (# of) days	The first fertile day is	If the longest cycle has been (# of) days	The last fertile day is
28[a]	10	28	17
29	11	29	18
30	12	30	19
31	13	31	20
32	14	32	21
33	15	33	22
34	16	34	23
35	17	35	24

[a]Day 1 is first day of menstrual bleeding.

- The *two-day method* uses cervical secretion monitoring as the fertility indicator. Unlike the ovulation (Billings) method, it does not involve monitoring the characteristics of the cervical mucus (color, consistency, and stretchiness). Women monitor their cervical mucus and answer two questions: "Did I notice secretions today?" and "Did I notice secretions yesterday?" The woman is considered fertile if she noticed any secretions on that day or the previous day and she should avoid intercourse. If she noticed no secretions yesterday or today (2 sequential days), the probability of pregnancy is very low.[16,17]

- The *symptothermal method* combines at least two fertility indicators and may add other fertility symptoms to detect ovulation. Experienced women may note changes in the texture, dilatation, or position of the cervix before and during ovulation. Other symptoms that the woman may monitor are abdominal or pelvic pain associated with ovulation *(Mittelschmerz)*, changes in libido, or changes in energy levels.[14,18]

- *Electronic hormonal fertility monitoring systems*, which detect luteinizing hormone in the urine (ClearPlan Fertility Monitor), specific electrolytes in the saliva (OvaCue), or visual ferning of the cervical mucus or saliva via a handheld microscope were originally introduced to the fertility market for the purpose of planning a pregnancy by identifying a woman's fertile period. The Marquette Method is a new system of NFP that uses the electronic hormonal fertility monitoring system along with other markers of fertility (e.g., changes in cervical mucus or BBT monitoring).[19] According to the U.S. Food and Drug Administration (FDA), these electronic systems cannot be marketed or sold as a contraceptive, but they may be used for fertility monitoring.[19] They are being used as an additional tool to avoid conception.[20-22]

Effectiveness

The efficacy of all of these types of family planning methods is highly dependent on a couple's motivation and consistency of use. The woman/couple must be able to accurately identify the fertile period using the method or methods of choice and, subsequently, they must be able to use a barrier method or avoid intercourse on the fertile days. Overall, the typical failure rate for the natural methods is 12% to 20%, but the range is from 3% to 22%.[10,15,17,19,23-25]

Figure 18-1. Cycle beads and how to use them.

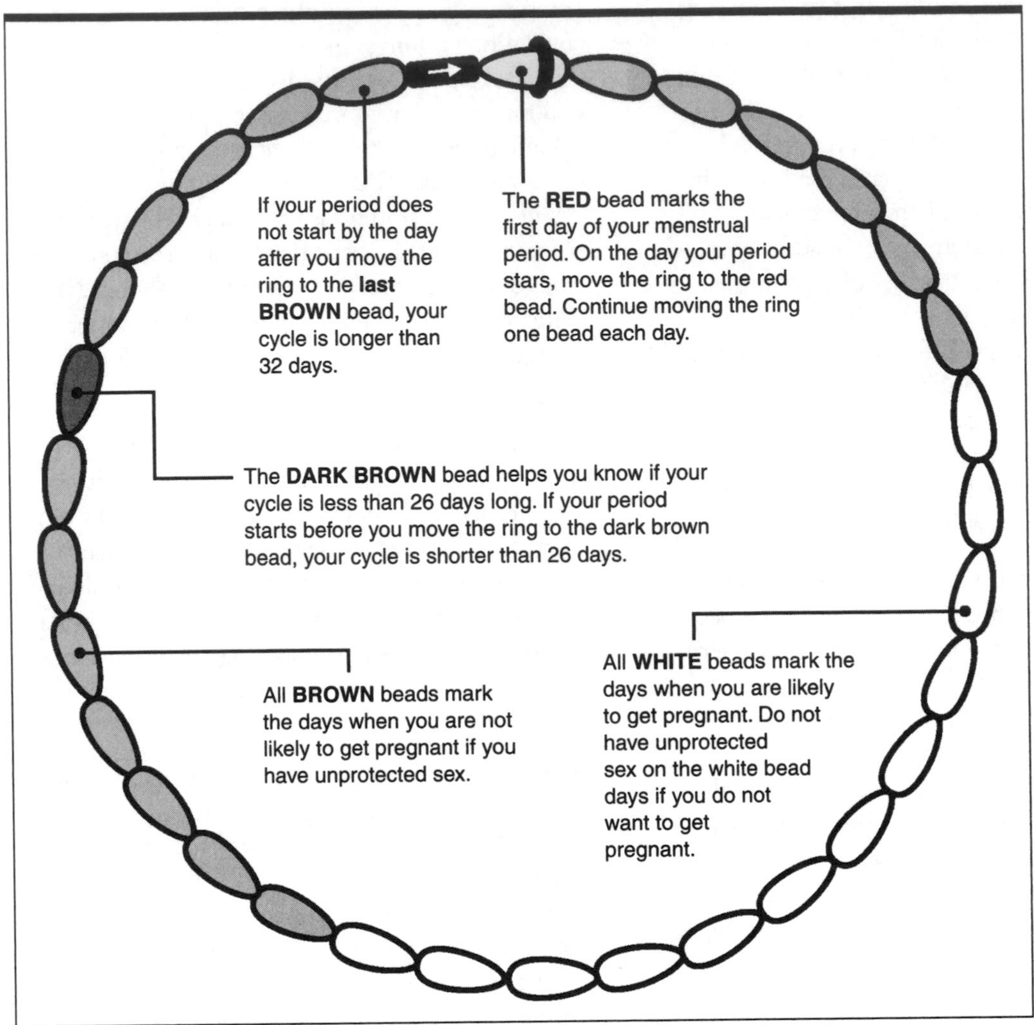

Advantages

These methods have no effect on the woman's hormone status or menstrual cycle and, in fact, have no side effects whatsoever. In addition, women and couples may benefit from having a better understanding of their reproductive physiology. Successful use by couples can result in feelings of accomplishment and working together to achieve mutual goals. With the exception of the electronic hormonal fertility monitoring systems, charting fertility signs is inexpensive, requiring only a calendar or a free fertility monitoring form, which can be downloaded from the internet at no charge. These methods may be the only ones that are acceptable because of cultural or religious beliefs. Women/couples may use these methods in reverse to plan a pregnancy.[5,8,14]

Disadvantages

None of the methods protects against STIs. For the woman, lack of the male partner's cooperation completely disrupts the use of the method. These methods may be difficult to use if the woman has recently given birth, is currently breast-feeding, has recently begun menstruating (menarche), has recently discontinued a hormonal method, or is perimenopausal.[5,8,14]

Contraindications/Precautions

FAMs and NFP are not recommended for women with irregular cycles, women who are unable to accurately interpret fertility signs and symptoms, or women who have chronic or recurrent reproductive tract infections that may affect the signs and symptoms of fertility. If a woman has a medical condition that would make pregnancy especially dangerous, natural methods would not offer high, consistent effectiveness.[5,8]

Ideal Candidates

Women with regular menstrual cycles who are willing to monitor fertility signs and symptoms on a continuing basis might do well with the natural methods, as would highly motivated and committed couples who are willing to abstain or use barrier methods at different times during the menstrual cycle.

Patient Education and Follow-up

(See Web Resources for information on Elective Female and Male Sterilization.)

Additional content available at ***www.ashp.org/womenshealth***

Patients need to know that there is a learning curve for accurately identifying the fertile period in a woman's menstrual cycle. Patients also need to know that the methods may interfere with spontaneity in sexual relations. In addition, women and couples should be instructed that preseminal fluid leaks from the penis before ejaculation. Even a small amount of preseminal fluid may contain live sperm. In-depth training of women and couples in NFP- and FAM-based methods is beyond the scope of this text.

COITUS INTERRUPTUS

Description

In this male-controlled method, the penis is withdrawn completely from the vagina before ejaculation occurs. Coitus interruptus as a contraceptive method followed the discovery that ejaculating into the vagina caused pregnancy.[25]

Effectiveness

Withdrawal before ejaculation probably confers some protection against pregnancy. The lowest expected failure rate is 4% and the typical failure rate is about 27%.[23]

Advantages

Absence of side effects and no cost are advantages of using this method. It is always available and is easy to discontinue when couples desire a pregnancy.

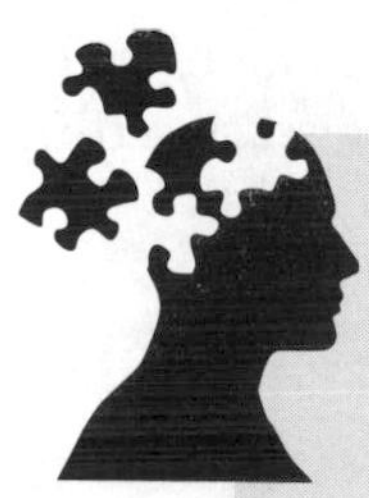

Therapeutic Challenge:

Which of the natural methods are most useful for predicting when ovulation will occur? Which method is most useful for determining that ovulation has already occurred?

Disadvantages

There is no protection from STIs, and there may be exchange of body fluids even though ejaculation does not occur. This method requires a high level of cooperation and self-control by the male partner.

Contraindications/Precautions

Like the other "natural" methods, if a woman has a medical condition that would make pregnancy dangerous, withdrawal would not offer a high level of effectiveness as a contraceptive method.

Patient Education

Withdrawal does not protect against STIs. The man must be able to sense when ejaculation is imminent and must be able to reliably withdraw his penis from his partner's vagina and ejaculate away from his partner's genitalia.

LACTATIONAL AMENORRHEA METHOD

Description

Lactation is associated with decreased fertility. All women have a period of relative infertility after giving birth. Postpartum women experience amenorrhea lasting at least 2–3 weeks, probably related to decreased gonadotropin secretion. Ovulation "causes" menstruation; therefore, ovulation usually occurs before the first episode of bleeding after a woman gives birth. In non-lactating women, menstrual bleeding usually begins 6–10 weeks postpartum. Lactating women experience a delay in the return of normal menstrual cycles related to increased prolactin from the anterior pituitary and may not have menstrual bleeding until much later. If a woman relies on the LAM, she must be breast-feeding on demand at least 5–6 times a day with 10-minute-or-more sessions or more than 65 minutes of breast-feeding per day without supplementation with other nutritional sources.[26,27] Other studies have demonstrated that the most important factors influencing pregnancy rates are the presence of amenorrhea and time since delivery.[27,28]

Effectiveness

Complete breast-feeding is associated with a <2% chance of pregnancy within the first 6 months after birth. Pregnancy rates increase to 4% to 7% by 12 months.[26,28]

Advantages

There is no cost involved, and the woman does not ingest synthetic hormones.[29]

Disadvantages

The return to menstruation and fertility is highly unpredictable, and the woman's breasts may be tender, which may decrease sexual pleasure.[28,29] The hypoestrogenic state caused by lactation may impair vaginal lubrication and result in dyspareunia.[27] Breast-feeding requires some level of privacy and continuous accessibility of mother to infant; mothers who return to work outside the home may not be able to use this method for a long period because of these factors.

Contraindications/Precautions

Women who have HIV/AIDS (acquired immunodeficiency syndrome) or who use drugs that may be harmful to the infant should not breast-feed.[30]

Ideal Candidates

Some women are highly motivated to breast-feed because of the personal and infant health benefits that breast-feeding confers, and they might be committed to using this method of contraception. Ideally, a woman should be breast-feeding exclusively or almost exclusively, her baby should be <6 months old, and her menses should not have returned.[26]

Patient Education

(See Web Resources for information on Elective Female and Male Sterilization.)

Additional content available at
www.ashp.org/womenshealth

The woman must breast-feed consistently and almost exclusively for maximum efficacy. Effectiveness decreases significantly at 6 months postpartum or when menstrual periods return, so the woman should be encouraged to begin deciding on which method of birth control she is going to use at that time.

Barrier Methods

Barrier methods include both nonprescription (patient-directed) and prescription (healthcare provider–directed) options. The male condom, the female condom, and the vaginal sponge can be obtained without consulting a physician, whereas the diaphragm, cervical cap, and vaginal shield, for proper fitting, must be prescribed. Advantages for all barrier methods include immediate effectiveness as well as immediate return to fertility for the woman.

NONPRESCRIPTION OR PATIENT-DIRECTED

Male Condom

The male condom is a sheath, most often made of latex or plastic, which is fit over the erect penis before insertion into the vagina and not removed until after ejaculation and withdrawal of the penis from the vagina. Male condoms are made by many manufacturers, available over-the-counter, and known by numerous brand names. Slang names for male condoms include prophylactics, skins, rubbers, raincoats, or umbrellas. In addition to the female condom, the male condom is the only contraceptive option that can prevent the transmission of HIV. Worldwide, the latex condom is the most often used.[31] Latex condoms are most often recommended because "natural" condoms, typically made of lamb intestines, are more porous, making them less protective against STIs. Although some marketed condoms are prelubricated with a spermicide, most healthcare providers recommend the addition of a spermicide just before intercourse; it is theorized that this method provides more even distribution of the spermicide and greater protection. Lubrication can prevent rips; however, oil-based lubricants can damage a latex condom, and they must not be used together. Plastic condoms, made of a polyurethane, are best for those (men and women) who have a latex allergy or when a woman is currently using a vaginal cream or suppository to treat an infection. Condoms made of lambskin may be considered for a partner with a latex allergy; however, these are in lower supply and, when used alone, do not protect against transmission of STIs.

Effectiveness

The failure rate for perfect use of the male condom is reported to be 2% to 3%; this rate increases to 14% to 15% with imperfect or "typical" use.

Advantages

In addition to not requiring a prescription for access, the condom is inexpensive and is a choice free from systemic side effects (barring a hypersensitivity reaction). Additionally, and perhaps most significantly from a public health viewpoint, correct use of the male condom is effective against the transmission of STIs, which makes it quite desirable for both partners.

Disadvantages

Users of the male condom must be highly motivated to avoid pregnancy and be willing to discuss birth control before the time of intimacy. Some birth control advocacy organizations define male condoms as "male-controlled" as opposed to "female-controlled," which makes them less desirable and less effective for women whose partner is unwilling to discuss or use the condom. Additionally, they are not as effective as hormonal methods.

Ideal Candidates

Male condoms and other barriers are appropriate for people who are not medically eligible or are unwilling to use hormonal methods, intrauterine contraceptives (IUCs), NFP, or sterilization. Women with low coital frequency may also make ideal users.

Appropriate Use and Patient Education/Follow-up

Ideally, both partners should be screened for latex allergy and, if present, a nonlatex condom provided.

Correct storage is the first important step for proper use. To avoid damage to the condom, the condom package must not be exposed to heat, including body heat, and therefore is best not carried in a trouser pocket or in a wallet. Once the condom is removed from the package and observed for tears, either partner can unroll the condom down on the erect penis. After orgasm and before the erection is lost, the rim of the condom is grasped and held while the penis is withdrawn, being careful to avoid spilling the semen. Condoms are not to be used more than once and are never to be used simultaneously with a female condom.[32]

Aside from proper use, the most important counseling point before using a male condom is what action a woman can take should a hole or rip be observed in the condom once it is removed and pregnancy is either unhealthy for or undesired by the woman. In the U.S., **emergency contraception** is available (see Chapter 20: Emergency Contraception) and is best discussed preemptively, while reviewing contraception options.

Female Condom

Description

The female condom is the only female-controlled barrier method that offers protection from pregnancy as well as STIs. It became available in the U.S. in 1993. The female condom is marketed in Canada, Europe, Brazil, and some African countries. The first version of the female condom was made of polyurethane and is available in the U.S., whereas a newer version is made of a nitrile polymer and is available outside the U.S. Research on a latex version is under way. The female condom works by trapping semen. It has two flexible rings, one on either end of the sheath. The smaller, inner ring, at the closed end of the condom, is placed inside the vagina to secure the sheath in place. The larger outer ring then lies over the labia. Because of this design, the female condom has been shown not only to prevent pregnancy but also reduce transmission of HIV, chlamydia, gonorrhea, and other sexually transmitted micro-organisms.[33]

Effectiveness

In a study published in 1994 and conducted in the U.S. and in Latin America, more than 300 women were asked to use a female condom as their sole method of contraception. For women in the U.S., the failure rate over 6 months of observation was 2.6%.[34] However, most publications list a failure rate of approximately 20% in the first year of typical use; this rate satisfactorily falls below 10% with perfect use. According to the 2007 edition of *Family Planning: A Global Handbook for Providers*, the pregnancy rate for perfect use is 5%.[35]

Advantages

The advantages of the female condom are numerous and include, but may not be limited to the following[36]:

- Contraceptive choice is under control of the woman.
- Neither prescription nor fitting by a healthcare provider is required, which allows for greater access.
- It is immediately effective.
- Insertion before intercourse may minimize interruption in lovemaking.
- The polyurethane material will not be damaged by heat and can transmit heat, thereby making sex more pleasurable for some.
- Water- and oil-based lubricants can be used.
- It can be used if either partner has a latex allergy.

Disadvantages

Although the female condom is available without a prescription, it is not as easily accessible as the male condom. The female condom is relatively inexpensive (usually $2 to $3 each) but does cost more than a male condom. Although insertion of the female condom can be part of lovemaking, some couples are initially displeased with the appearance of the female condom.[36] Lastly, the female condom may not be appropriate for women with physical disabilities or for those who are uncomfortable touching their vagina.

Ideal Candidates

Similar to users of the male condoms, female condoms and other barriers are appropriate for people who are not medically eligible or are unwilling to use hormonal methods, IUCs, NFP, or surgical sterilization. Women who have intercourse infrequently may also make ideal users. Individuals with an allergy to latex may also be interested candidates.

Appropriate Use and Patient Education/Follow-up

The female condom may be placed in the vagina up to 8 hours before intercourse; it may be used only once. Following proper handwashing and removal from the package, the condom is held with the open end down. The thumb and middle finger of one hand squeezes the inner ring into the shape of an oval to easily facilitate insertion of the condom into the vagina, which has been readied by the fingers of the other hand. A finger pushes the ring upward and past the pubic bone. The outer ring and part of the sheath remains outside the vagina, covering part of the labia. During intercourse, care must be taken to assure the penis is placed and stays within the sheath. After withdrawal of the penis, the female condom is removed by gently pinching together the outer ring and withdrawing the condom before the woman stands up, then the condom is appropriately discarded. To avoid damage to either, the female condom cannot be used simultaneously with a male condom. As is true for all barrier methods of birth control, counseling about emergency contraception pre-emptively is essential. Follow-up counseling would involve questions assuring proper use and consistent use, and if any dissatisfaction is reported, alternative options can be revisited (Figure 18-2).

Figure 18-2. Placement of female condom.

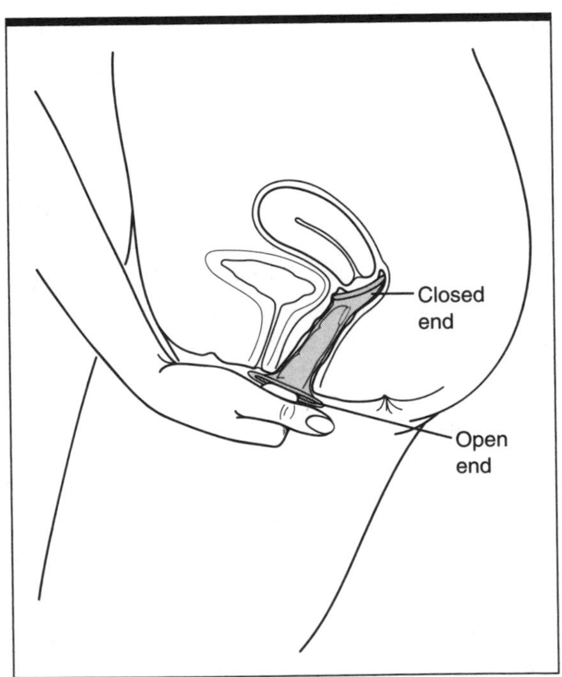

Vaginal Sponge

Description

The Today® Sponge is a single-use polyurethane sponge with a spermicide, nonoxynol-9 incorporated within it. Its marketing history is unique in that it was withdrawn from the U.S. market not because of a concern with efficacy or safety but rather because a manufacturing plant with the company that originally marketed it was reported to have an unacceptable level of bacteria in its water supply; the Today® Sponge was reintroduced in 2005 by Allendale Pharmaceuticals, Inc., and is available without a prescription for single use. Availability of the sponge has once again been challenged as it was purchased by a U.S. company in 2007 that filed for bankruptcy in the same year; the most recent acquisition of the sponge occurred in June 2008, with plans under way to increase the marketing of this contraceptive option.[37]

Effectiveness

Unlike use of male and female condoms, the failure rate of the sponge is different between parous and nulliparous women, with the difference attributed to the likely changes that occur in the cervix with pregnancy and childbirth. For 100 women who have never given birth, typical use of the sponge can result in 16 pregnancies in the first year of use, nine pregnancies if used in a perfect and consistent manner.[38] For 100 women who have been pregnant in the past, 32 women can be expected to become pregnant in the first year of typical use of the sponge, whereas 20 woman with a history of pregnancy may become pregnant in the first year with perfect use.[39]

Advantages

The contraceptive sponge uniquely offers protection against pregnancy immediately and for 24 hours after insertion; reapplication of a spermicide is not required and therefore is optional if intercourse is repeated. It is available over-the-counter, and it can be inserted up to 24 hours before intercourse, allowing greater spontaneity relative to many other barrier methods. Some women report the sponge to be less messy that other contraceptive methods, such as vaginal foams or gels.[40]

Disadvantages

The contraceptive sponge, although an attractive alternative, does not confer protection against HIV. It may not be suitable for women adverse to touching their vagina. Unique to the contraceptive sponge is a possible link to a woman's development of toxic shock syndrome (TSS). The manufacturer recommends against the use of the sponge during menses to minimize this risk. A risk of TSS associated with the contraceptive sponge has not been documented; rather, the risk is extrapolated from data reported with TSS and the prolonged use of tampons during menses.[40]

Ideal Candidates

The contraceptive sponge is a reasonable choice for nulliparous women who desire a nonhormonal method, who desire contraceptive control, who have sex infrequently, and who are without physical disabilities that would impair their ability to properly insert the sponge.

Appropriate Use and Patient Education/Follow-up

Before insertion, the sponge must be thoroughly moistened; gently adding approximately 2 tablespoons of water to the sponge facilitates insertion and activates the spermicide. Once moistened, fold the sponge in half, and place it upward into the vagina as far as the fingers can reach, with the loop facing downward. The sponge will unfold and cover the cervix. The sponge can be inserted up to 24 hours before intercourse but must be left in the vagina for a minimum of 6 hours after the last act of intercourse. Remove the sponge before 30 hours passes to minimize the risk of TSS or vaginal yeast infections. Once removed from the vagina (by placing a finger in the loop and gently pulling it downward), the sponge must be properly discarded (do not attempt to flush it down a toilet) and must not used again. A package of three typically costs less than $10.

If a woman using the sponge reports vaginal dryness during intercourse, use of a water-based lubricant can be recommended. Women must be reminded that the sponge does not protect them from STIs; additionally, women must be counseled on emergency contraception should they feel they did not follow the instructions for proper use.[38]

Spermicides

A spermicide is a chemical contraceptive; however, it is marketed in a variety of products, many of which can offer additive protection via a barrier mechanism. Nonoxynol-9 (N-9) is available in the U.S. without a prescription and as a detergent works by inhibiting the mobility and motility of sperm, thereby inhibiting their ability to fertilize ova. Detergent effects disrupting the vaginal epithelium have been proposed as the rationale for the lack of prevention of HIV transmission in high-risk patients, specifically commercial sex workers.

Effectiveness

Reported efficacy rates vary, but typical use of a spermicide, specifically N-9, when used alone, is associated with a failure rate of approximately 29% and a failure rate of 18% with correct use. When used with a barrier contraceptive, such as a condom or a diaphragm, the reported efficacy rate improves, as high as 94% with perfect use. A study was published in 2007 that compared N-9 used with a diaphragm to an acid-buffering gel used with a diaphragm. For those given the acid-buffering gel with diaphragm, the pregnancy rate for 100 women over a 6-month period was 10.1%; for those given N-9 with a diaphragm, this resulting rate was 12.3%. This difference did not reach statistical significance; rather, the researchers concluded that the acid-buffering gel was noninferior to N-9 when used with a diaphragm. The acid-buffering gel works by producing an acidic pH in the vagina, which blocks the alkalinizing action of semen (which normally eliminates vaginal acidity for hours after intercourse). Furthermore, acidifying the vagina inactivates sperm and acid-sensitive pathogens such as HIV. This acid-buffering gel is undergoing further study as a spermicidal microbiocide and, if successful, could be available as a spermicide that offers significant protection against STIs, a significant addition to the female-controlled contraceptive products available to women.[41]

Advantages

Nonoxynol-9 is available in a variety of formulations, including creams, gels, aerosol foams, vaginal tablets or suppositories, and films. Spermicides require no prescription and are widely available. With the rare exception of an allergy to N-9, these do not produce systemic side effects, are relatively easy to use, and can serve as a lubricant as well. They are safe to use when the woman is breast-feeding. With the exception of melting time of 10–15 minutes required for suppositories and films, spermicides otherwise are immediately effective.

Disadvantages

Spermicidal activity is quite short, lasting only 1–2 hours, and the product must be readily available for reapplication before each intercourse or 1–2 hours after the last application. Its use may impair spontaneity of intercourse. Its effectiveness is highly dependent on the correct and consistent use by a motivated user. Spermicides can be messy; the vaginal film tends to be less problematic. A spermicide can be irritating to the penis or the vagina because of either the active ingredient N-9 or other ingredients. Despite demonstrating antimicrobial activities in vitro, spermicides cannot be relied on to prevent STIs. Furthermore, the World Health Organization has warned that N-9 does not protect against STIs and may in fact increase a woman's risk of contracting HIV.[42] Lastly, even with perfect use, it is not as effective as other contraceptive methods.

Ideal Candidates

Similar to users of condoms and other barriers, spermicides are appropriate for people who are not medically eligible or are unwilling to use hormonal methods, IUCs, NFP, or surgical sterilization. Women who have intercourse infrequently may also make ideal users. Spermicides alone would not be recommended for use by women who have a history of STIs or who exhibit behaviors placing them at high risk for STIs.

Appropriate Use and Patient Education/Follow-up

The level of user motivation must be determined before recommendation. In general, spermicides must be applied before each act of intercourse and reapplied if intercourse does not take place in 1–2 hours. Placement of the spermicide high into the vagina is recommended, trying to assure coverage of the cervix. For creams, gels, and foams, this can be accomplished by using the plunger-type applicator that comes with the spermicide. The aerosol foam must be shaken many (e.g., 2 dozen) times before releasing into the applicator. Vaginal suppositories must be removed from the individual wrapper and can be inserted into the vagina manually or by using the applicator supplied with the suppositories. A vaginal film can be draped over the index or middle finger and inserted manually into the vagina. If the woman chooses to use the suppository or the film, she must wait 10–15 minutes after insertion before beginning intercourse. If an applicator is used, instruct the user to wash it with warm soapy water after each use.

Should vaginal or penile irritation develop, encourage the use of another type of spermicidal product. Currently, the only spermicide used in the U.S. is N-9, and if a detergent allergy is present, none of the spermicidal products may be suitable, and an alternative method of contraception will be necessary. The use of barrier methods with a spermicide is highly recommended to increase effectiveness and, in the case of condoms, to prevent the transmission of STIs.[39] As with other nonhormonal contraceptive methods, explaining the option of emergency contraception is crucial at the first and subsequent encounters with a healthcare professional.

PRESCRIPTION OR HEALTHCARE PROVIDER-DIRECTED CONTRACEPTION

Diaphragms, vaginal shields, and cervical caps are types of barrier contraceptive methods, which are available with consultation and a prescription from a healthcare provider. The primary need for consultation with a healthcare provider is to receive proper fitting of these contraceptive products as well as to receive instructions for proper use. Similar to other barrier methods, these are moderately effective in preventing pregnancy, with failure rates higher than those associated with hormonal or sterilization methods.

Diaphragm

The diaphragm, or its earlier precursors, has been used by women for decades, yet since the introduction of oral contraceptives, it is chosen <5% of the time in the U.S. among contraceptive users. The diaphragm is a dome-shaped latex cup with a flexible outer ring that is inserted manually before intercourse into the vagina to cover the cervix. The diaphragm serves as a barrier to sperm at the cervical opening. Using a spermicide with a diaphragm is typically recommended to enhance effectiveness.

Effectiveness

The effectiveness of the diaphragm is highly user dependent, meaning the user must be willing to follow proper use instructions and be motivated to use it consistently with each act of intercourse. With perfect use and with a spermicide, the effectiveness rate for a diaphragm is as high as 94%. With typical or inconsistent use, this rate drops to approximately 80%; in other words, 20 out of 100 women using the diaphragm may experience an unintended pregnancy in the first year of use.

Advantages

There are no method-related or systemic side effects with use of the diaphragm, and its use can offer protection against some STIs. Both latex and

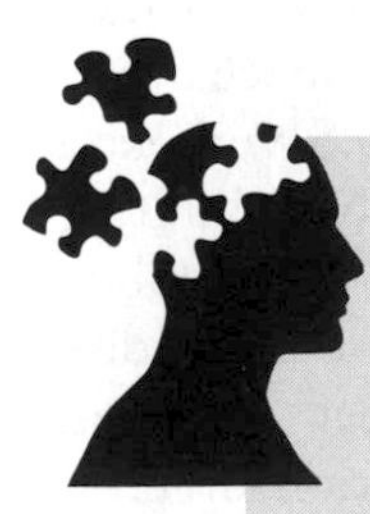

Therapeutic Challenge:

What are some of the advantages of the female condom when compared with the male condom? When compared with the diaphragm?

nonlatex silicone alternatives are available. Although use of a diaphragm cannot eliminate all risk of microbial transmission, observational and retrospective studies have shown that women who use a diaphragm or sponge with a spermicide experience up to a 65% lower rate of infection of *Neisseria gonorrhoeae* and *Trichomonas vaginalis* (compared with women who used no contraception or had a history of surgical sterilization).[43] The diaphragm is effective immediately and may be inserted into the vagina up to 6 hours before intercourse. With proper cleaning and storage, it is reusable.

Disadvantages

The diaphragm must be properly fitted by a trained healthcare provider. It must be left in place for 6 hours after last intercourse. Considering this duration of placement, the use of diaphragms has been associated with TSS; additionally, higher rates of urinary tract infections (UTIs) have been associated with women who use a diaphragm. Resizing or refitting of a diaphragm is recommended for women after pregnancy or after childbirth, if a woman has experienced a 20% change in weight, or if use is continuing 2 years after the original fitting. It is recommended that women delay using the diaphragm until a minimum of 6 weeks postpartum.[39,44]

Ideal Candidates

Women who cannot or should not use hormonal methods and who are motivated to prevent pregnancy are suitable candidates. Women who have sex with high-risk partners and want protection from STIs are appropriate candidates, as there is some evidence that diaphragms may provide protection from gonorrhea and chlamydia; however, the diaphragm should not be the only source for protection.[35] A diaphragm and spermicide can be recommended to women who desire short-term barrier contraception (e.g., those who are breast-feeding, awaiting the onset of contraception with hormonal methods, or taking an interacting drug that could diminish the effect of oral contraceptives). Women choosing to use a diaphragm should be free of genital anomalies that might cause issues with an ill-fitting diaphragm producing vaginal lesions.

Appropriate Use and Patient Education/Follow-up

Contraceptive effectiveness of the diaphragm is user dependent; therefore, counseling patients on the proper handling, use, and storage of a diaphragm is essential. The following are recommended counseling points provided to each woman:

- Discuss the effectiveness rate.
- Provide a proper fitting by a healthcare professional.
- Practice the insertion and removal of the diaphragm before leaving the healthcare provider's office. This is highly recommended.
- Emphasize use of the diaphragm with every act of intercourse.
- Empty the bladder and wash hands before inserting the diaphragm.
- Check the diaphragm for holes or rips (this can be done by holding it toward a light or filling it with water).
- Apply a water-based spermicidal lubricant to the inside of the dome (applying a small amount to the upper outside edge of the diaphragm can ease insertion).
- Squeeze the outer rim together and insert into the vagina.
- Push the diaphragm upward and toward the backbone until the rim is past the pubic bone.
- Leave the diaphragm in place for 6 hours after last intercourse and remove it soon thereafter.
- Do not leave a diaphragm in place for more than 24 hours.
- Remove the diaphragm by hooking a finger behind the upper rim, breaking the suction, and pulling downward.
- Wash the diaphragm with warm soapy water, allow to it to air-dry, and return it to its container.
- Consider emergency contraception if a woman had intercourse more than 6 hours after the last time and did not reapply spermicide or she removed the diaphragm less than 6 hours after the last intercourse.[39,44]

Cervical Cap

Smaller in size than a diaphragm, a cervical cap is a bowl-shaped device made of silicone that fits snugly over the cervix, thereby blocking entry by sperm. One cervical cap available in the U.S. is FemCap®; another type of cervical cap is Lea's Shield® and is also described as a vaginal barrier or shield. Both require a prescription, both are more effective in preventing pregnancy in nulliparous women compared with parous women (as a result in the changes in the cervix secondary to a full-term and vaginally delivered baby), and the concurrent use of spermicide is recommended for both types of caps. Both are made with latex-free silicone rubber. The major difference between the FemCap® and Lea's Shield® is the need for measurement and fitting. The FemCap® comes in three sizes and must be properly measured and fit by a trained healthcare provider. According to the manufacturer of Lea's Shield®, it is a one-size-fits-all reusable vaginal barrier contraceptive device. The device is washable and about the size of a vaginal diaphragm. It differs from a FemCap® in that it is held against the vaginal wall muscles as opposed to fitting against the cervix, the size of which varies from woman to woman. Similarly, it differs from a diaphragm, which is held in place between the pubic bone and the posterior fornix, a space that varies among women and must be properly fitted for effectiveness.[39,44]

Effectiveness

For nulliparous women, the effectiveness for both types of cervical caps is similar. With typical use, between 15–20 of 100 couples using a cervical cap with spermicide may experience an unplanned pregnancy; the rate lowers significantly to a 9% chance if the cervical cap is used correctly and consistently. For parous women who have given birth vaginally, the failure rate increases to approximately 26% for perfect use and 40% for typical use.[39]

Advantages

Similar to other nonhormonal contraceptives, the cervical caps are portable, are free from hormonal side effects, are immediately effective and reversible, and can be inserted at a time that does not interrupt intercourse.

Disadvantages

Similar to other vaginal barriers that can be left in place for several hours, women must be cautioned about TSS as well as about the increased chance for UTIs and vaginal yeast infections. Proper insertion and placement is essential for contraceptive effect, and this may be difficult to do for some women. Some women may develop irritation of the cervical tissue from the silicone rubber in the caps and by its physical pressure. Additionally, the cervical caps do not confer protection from STIs, including HIV.

Ideal Candidates

Women for whom cervical caps are acceptable contraceptive choices include those who prefer not to or should not use hormonal methods or IUCs, women who are breast-feeding, or women who have other reasons for a temporary method, such as while awaiting another method to take effect. Cervical caps can be recommended to women who have intercourse infrequently. Cervical caps are moderately expensive, starting at approximately $50. Cervical caps may last up to 2 years, but annual replacement is generally recommended.

Appropriate Use and Patient Education/Follow-up

After proper fitting for a cervical cap, it is recommended that a woman first try inserting the cervical cap while still in a healthcare provider's office or clinic, assuring that proper technique for placement is used. Instruct patients to wash their hands well and find a comfortable position before handling the devices. For the FemCap®, put ¼–1 teaspoonful of spermicide in the dome. Spread a thin layer in the dome and just up to the rim, but do not get spermicide on the rim (too much spermicide may cause the cap to slip off the cervix). Separate the labia, squeeze the rim together, and insert the cervical cap far inside the vagina, with the longer brim entering the vagina first. Use a finger to push the cap over the cervix. Insertion is easier before sexual arousal. Women can test the suction of the cap, and thereby proper placement, by gently pulling on it and feeling some resistance. Before subsequent intercourse, check the cap to determine if the proper placement is maintained; reapplication of spermicide is not required but can be recommended. The FemCap® must be left in place for 6 hours after the last intercourse but no longer than 48 hours after insertion. Removal is accomplished by using a finger to release the suction at the rim and pulling it out of the vagina; squatting or bearing down can facilitate removal. Use warm soapy water to wash the cervical cap before storing it (Figure 18-3).[44,45]

Instructions for the Lea's Shield® are similar. However, Lea's Shield® is constructed with a valve and a loop, making application of spermicide slightly different. Using less than a teaspoon of spermicide, coat the inside of the bowl around the hole, the outer part of the valve, and the front of the rim. Pinching the rim, slide the shield into the vagina with the thickest end inserted first and the valve facing down, and assuring that the loop is not sticking out of the vagina. To promote proper placement, use a finger to press on the valve a few times to release any air trapped between the shield and the cervix. After each act of intercourse, recheck the shield for placement and reapply spermicide. Lea's Shield® must remain in place for 8 hours after the last intercourse and must be removed within 48 hours after insertion.

Figure 18-3. Insertion and placement of cervical cap (FemCap®).

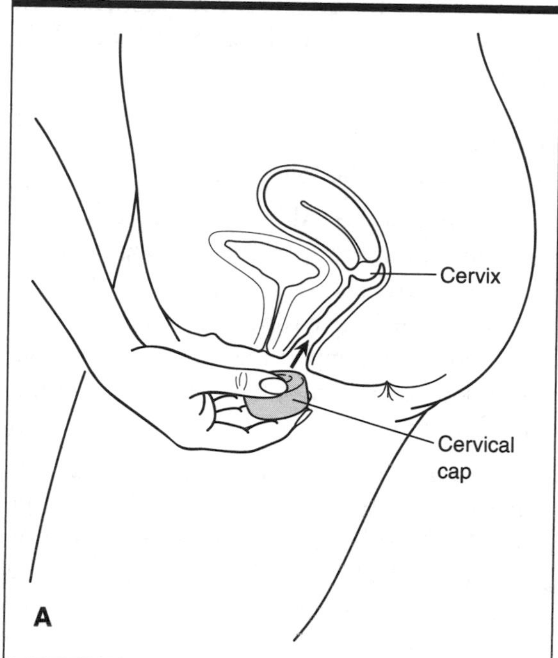

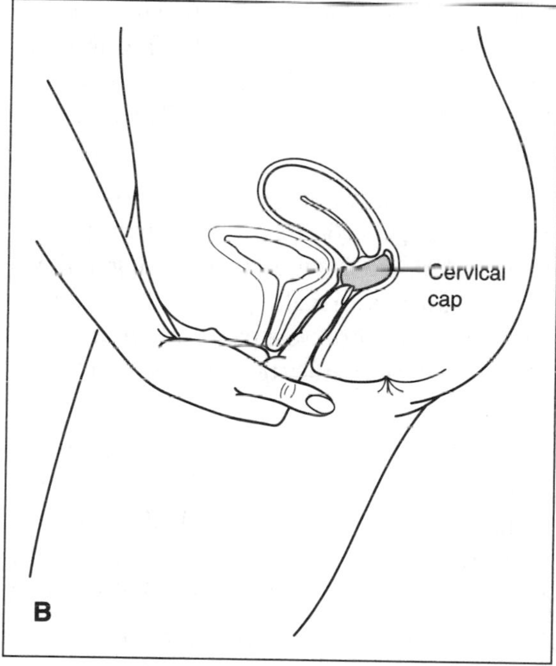

The shield may be removed either by grasping the rim with a thumb and finger and pulling it down out of the vagina or by grasping the loop with a finger, rotating the shield slightly to break suction, and pulling it down and out of the vagina.[44] Wash with warm soapy water and dry before storing it. For both cervical caps, do not douche (it could weaken the spermicide), and do not use them during menstruation (greater concern with TSS). Check regularly for holes or leaks. Each woman using a cervical cap must also be counseled about the availability and potential need for emergency contraception.

Other Nonhormonal Contraceptive Options

NONHORMONAL INTRAUTERINE CONTRACEPTIVE

IUCs offer a safe, reliable, and cost-effective alternative for contraception. Although the IUC is the most common worldwide form of contraception, the 2005 National Survey of Family Growth found that only 2% of U.S. women are users of intrauterine contraception.[46,47] Historical concerns and misconceptions regarding safety and suitability of IUCs in certain populations have limited their use in the U.S. Recent changes with an expansion in FDA indications reflect a growing recognition of the need to extend this method to more potential users.

In the U.S., the Copper T 380A (Figure 18-4) is currently the only nonhormonal intrauterine device available. This IUC is a T-shaped device of polyethylene wrapped with copper wire. It is approved for 10 continuous years. The primary mechanism of action is prevention of fertilization via disruption in tubal transport of sperm and ovum.[48] The Copper T 380A causes increases in copper ions, prostaglandins, and white blood cells in uterine and tubal fluids; these changes impair sperm and tubal functioning.[49] Secondary mechanisms include prevention of implantation with disruption of the fertilized ovum.[50]

The IUC is highly effective, with a typical-use pregnancy rate of 0.8%.[51] In addition to its efficacy as a continuous contraceptive, the Copper T 380A IUC

Figure 18-4. Copper 380 T IUC (Photo courtesy of ParaGard®).

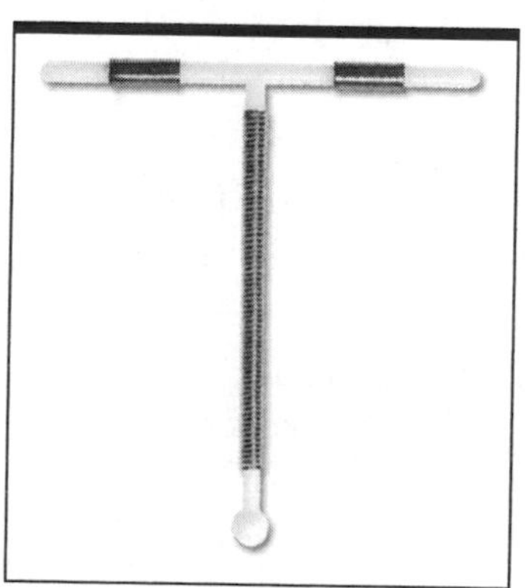

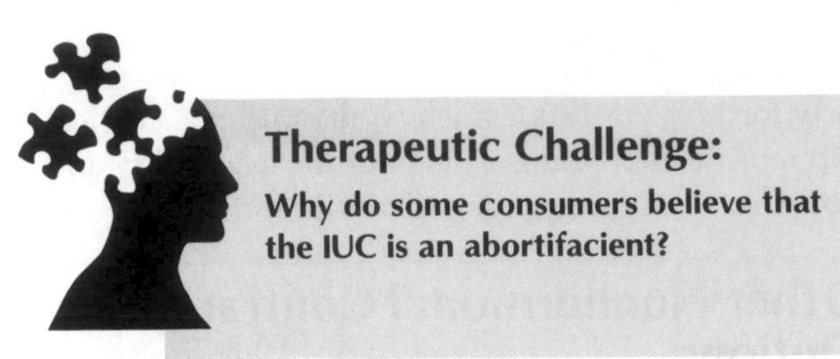

is highly effective as a postcoital contraceptive when inserted within 5 days of unprotected intercourse, with pregnancy rates <1%.[52]

Advantages

Advantages include the following:

1. *Cost-effective*—The IUC remains the most cost-effective contraceptive available. It has a relatively low initial cost, no ongoing continuation costs, and a long duration of action.[53]
2. *Safe*—Concern over safety issues has historically limited the use of the IUC in the U.S. In reality, the Copper T 380A IUC has a very high safety profile. Meta-analysis revealed that women with IUCs, following the first 20 days postinsertion, were no more likely to experience pelvic inflammatory disease (PID) than comparable nonusers.[54] Most infection-related morbidity is related to infection at the time of insertion. Other complications of insertion, such as perforation and expulsion, occur in <1% of insertions. Although there is an increased risk of ectopic pregnancy with IUC failures, pregnancies are rare; thus, the overall incidence of ectopic pregnancy is remarkably reduced.[55]
3. *Reliable*—Typical pregnancy rates are 0.8%, with failure rates lower than with oral contraceptives.[51]
4. *Not tied to coitus*—Current recommendations advise for women to check for placement of IUC before coitus. No special preparation or interruption of coital relations is required.
5. *Long-acting*—The Copper T 380A IUC may be worn continuously for 10 years. It can be removed and replaced in the same setting in patients desiring further contraception.
6. *Rapid return to fertility*—Because the Copper T 380A IUC has no hormonal action, return to fertility is immediate on removal.
7. *Private*—The IUC has the advantage of being discreet to the wearer, with no need for medication dosing or equipment.
8. *Avoids hormonal exposure*—The Copper T 380A IUC is an alternative to women who cannot or prefer not to use hormonal contraception. It has no systemic side effects and may be safely used during lactation.

Disadvantages

Disadvantages include the following:

1. *High upfront expense*—Although the IUC has a low manufacturing cost, product development and liability have increased the price of IUCs, which are cost-effective with long-term use. Furthermore, data support that IUC continuation rates are longer than those rates for users of other contraceptive types.[50]
2. *Requires medical intervention for insertion and removal*—Insertion and removal of an IUC must be done by trained medical staff under aseptic conditions. A distinct disadvantage to this method is that it cannot be self-terminated.
3. *May be associated with menstrual changes*—Women using the Copper T 380A IUC may notice an increase in menstrual bleeding and cramping initially. Overall rates of troublesome bleeding were reported in 2.9 per 100 women years of use.[56]
4. *Rare insertion complications*—Although complications are low, insertions may be complicated by perforation, expulsion, and embedding in the endometrium. Occasionally, patients may suffer a vasovagal reaction or severe pain with insertion. The risk of uterine perforation is approximately 1/1,000.[57]
5. *Potential development of PID near insertion*—By 20 days postinsertion, the risk of IUC-associated infections is similar to the PID risk of nonusers.[54] No increase in PID rates have been found in nulliparous women using the Copper T 380A IUC.[58]
6. *Limited use with some patients*—Limitations of IUC use occur in women allergic to copper, those with abnormally shaped uterine cavities, women with active or recent PID, or women at very high risk for PID. The FDA has recently removed restrictions on women, including immune deficiency, a history of ectopic pregnancy, or actinomycosis. Women with multiple sex partners have also been removed from the contraindication list.

Contraindications

Current contraindications include the following:

- Pregnancy
- Distorted uterine canal
- Genital bleeding from an unknown source
- **Wilson's disease** or copper allergy
- Active PID or current behavior suggesting a high risk for PID
- Postpartum **endometritis** or postabortion infection within 3 months
- Known or suspected uterine or cervical malignancy
- Mucopurulent cervicitis

Ideal Candidates

The ideal candidates for IUC use are women desiring continuous, long-term, reliable but reversible contraception.

Patient Education and Follow-up

Patients should be instructed to feel for the presence of strings before intercourse to assure proper placement of the device. Most patients are instructed to return in 1 month to confirm placement and review side effects. Precautions on avoidance of infections should also be given. Although extremely rare, should a patient with an IUC in place become pregnant, her physician should be notified immediately, as the IUC must be removed as soon as possible. The mnemonic PAINS has been advocated for use in counseling patients and is found in Table 18-3.[59]

SURGICAL

(See Web Resources for information on Elective Female and Male Sterilization.)

Additional content available at ***www.ashp.org/womenshealth***

Table 18-3. Counseling Points for Intrauterine Contraceptives Using the Mnemonic PAINS

P	For **p**regnancy or bleeding
A	For **a**bdominal pain
I	Exposure to **i**nfection (sexually transmitted) or discharge
N	**N**ot feeling well—fever, chills
S	**S**tring missing

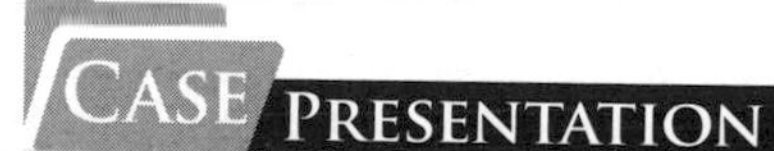

CASE PRESENTATION

Patient Case: Part 2

Assessment: K.L. has expressed interest in a long-term, reliable, reversible method of contraception that does not involve hormones because of her age and her tobacco use. She has had difficulty with adhering to the strict schedule required for oral contraception and is inconsistent with male condom use. She was dissatisfied with the use of medroxyprogesterone acetate and is concerned that it will cause her to gain weight.

Plan: K.L. is an ideal candidate for the nonhormonal IUC. If she chooses to use this method, she will be given the choice to have it inserted today (since the first day of her last menstrual period was 4 days ago) or to return to the clinic for placement of the IUC at a later time. Some healthcare providers prefer to insert the IUC during menstrual bleeding, but it can be inserted at any time during the cycle as long as there is reasonable assurance that the woman is not pregnant (modern, highly sensitive pregnancy tests are helpful).

Rationale: K.L. is not interested in a permanent birth control method (sterilization) at this time, but she is fairly certain that she does not want another pregnancy; the nonhormonal IUC will provide her with 10 years of contraception. Smokers older than age 35 should not use estrogen-containing methods of birth control; therefore, she is not a candidate for combined oral contraceptives. K.L. was dissatisfied with medroxyprogesterone acetate because of weight gain and does not want the "hassle" of using coitus-related methods, such as the male or female condom or the diaphragm. K.L. has average menstrual periods with no dysmenorrhea; rarely, the nonhormonal IUC causes menstrual changes, including heavier or more painful periods, so caution is used when a woman already has heavy or painful menstruation.

Monitoring and follow-up: Frequent monitoring of patients using an IUC is not warranted. It is recommended that the healthcare provider schedule a follow-up visit after the woman's next menstrual period. This 1-month visit should include a vaginal speculum exam to confirm that the IUC is in place and that there are no signs of infection. This visit can also be used to answer additional questions that the woman may have.

Patient education: See patient education and follow-up in IUC section above.

Summary

Nonhormonal contraceptive methods may be not only a preferred method to prevent pregnancy for a given woman but the only method, considering medical or cultural or religious needs. Sterilization methods offer high efficacy but may subject the woman to nuisance side effects or the inability to choose fertility as significant changes in her life occur. NFP methods and barrier methods convey a lower efficacy rate than sterilization or hormonal methods yet allow easier return to fertility and have limited or few side effects (aside from allergies with barriers and spermicides). However, proper instructions to couples and perfect adherence by couples are crucial to prevent unintended pregnancies. Additionally, all women are entitled to receive thorough information on effectiveness of contraceptive methods, prevention of STIs, and proper use of and access to emergency contraception. Pharmacists and healthcare providers must work with patients to ensure adherence and therapeutic success and minimize discontinuation and failure rates.

As healthcare professionals who meet professional standards and as individuals with personal values, this topic—as well as the related counseling pharmacists are asked to provide—may evoke personal conflict. That said, we acknowledge that unintended pregnancies place a tremendous emotional, social, medical, and economic burden on individuals as well as on societies. Therefore, it is imperative that pharmacists have a thorough understanding of contraceptive options, both hormonal and nonhormonal, to provide effective, nonjudgmental, and compassionate counseling for the woman and her partner seeking information. Counseling can center on identifying the cultural or religious beliefs of an individual that may be a barrier to contraceptive options and offering information that may help in overcoming these barriers.

Websites of Interest

(See Web Resources for Helpful Websites for Patient Information.)

Additional content available at
www.ashp.org/womenshealth

References

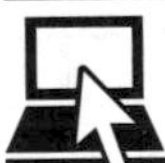

Additional content available at
www.ashp.org/womenshealth

19 Hormonal Contraception

Shareen Y. El-Ibiary, Pharm.D., BCPS; Jessica L.White, Pharm.D., BCPS

Learning Objectives

1. Compare and contrast the mechanisms of action, efficacy, dosing regimens, and reversibility of the various methods of hormonal contraception.
2. Describe the indications and contraindications in the selection of optimal and safe contraceptives for a specific patient.
3. Identify potential drug interactions and side effects with contraceptives, and design a plan to manage them appropriately.
4. Discuss the proper use of various contraceptives, and apply information about start methods and missed doses to a patient case.

Contraception, the prevention of pregnancy, has evolved through history from the time of ancient Egyptians and the Middle Ages to the present time.[1] The introduction of the first combined oral contraceptive (COC) in 1960 marked the beginning of a transition into improved female reproductive health, sex equity, quality of life for women, a sense of freedom for sexually active women, and changes in demographics regarding unplanned pregnancies. Over the last 40 years, advances in contraception have improved efficacy and minimized side effects.

Contraception is currently a worldwide issue, especially in countries where population control is important. Contraception has economic implications as well. In 2001, it was reported that about 49% of pregnancies in the U.S. were unintended; of those, 26.5% resulted in abortions.[2]

Proper use of contraception is also important, as failure rates increase with human error. In 2002, it was reported that 11.6 million women were using an oral contraceptive pill and 2 million were using injections, showing that many women are using some form of hormonal contraception.[3] Pharmacists, highly accessible healthcare providers, are starting to play a more active role in family planning. It is important for healthcare providers to tailor contraceptive agents to their patients to minimize failure rates and optimize desired outcomes.

Selecting a Contraceptive Method

The ideal contraceptive is 100% safe and effective in preventing pregnancy, easy to use, independent of timing of intercourse, affordable, reversible, and protective against sexually transmitted infections (STIs). Abstinence is the only option that meets all of these requirements. Efficacy of contraceptives is determined by how often a method prevents pregnancy based on perfect use and typical use. Both numbers are reported as percentage of pregnancies occurring in contraception users in the first year: **the perfect-use failure rate** and the **typical-use failure rate.** Perfect use assumes that the user is correctly using the contraceptive method in an ideal situation, such as taking every dose at the exact same time every day with no drug interactions or compliance issues. Typical use generally results in a higher failure rate than perfect use. The typical-use failure rate takes into account user error of the method, such as missing a dose or improperly using the method. Some contraceptive options, such as intrauterine contraceptives (IUCs), rely so little on patient compliance that they have a perfect use that is equal to that of typical use. Other medications, such as oral contraceptives, have a reported failure rate termed *typical use,* which is generally higher than the perfect-use rate (see Table 19-1 for a summary of efficacy rates).

When helping a patient to select a method of contraception, healthcare providers must take into account typical-use failure rates,

Table 19-1. Percentage of Women Experiencing an Unintended Pregnancy During the First Year of Typical Use and the First Year of Perfect Use of Contraception and the Percentage Continuing Use at the End of the First Year: United States

	% of Women Experiencing an Unintended Pregnancy During the First Year of Use		% of Women Continuing Use at 1 Year[a]
Method	Typical Use[b]	Perfect Use[c]	
Chance[d]	85	85	
Spermicides[e]	29	18	40
Periodic abstinence	25		63
Calendar		9	
Ovulation method		3	
Symptothermal[f]		2	
Postovulation		1	
Cap[g]			
Parous women	32	26	46
Nulliparous women	16	9	57
Sponge			
Parous women	32	26	46
Nulliparous women	16	9	57
Diaphragm[g]	16	6	57
Withdrawal	27	4	43
Condom[h]			
Female (reality)	21	5	49
Male	15	2	53
Pill			
Progestin only	8	0.3	68
Combined	8	0.3	68
Ring 8		0.3	68
Patch		0.3	
	8		68
Intrauterine device			
Copper T 380A	0.8	0.6	78
LNG 20	0.1	0.1	81
Depo-subQ Provera	3	0.3	
Depo-Provera	3	0.3	56
Norplant and Norplant-2	0.05	0.05	88
Female sterilization	0.5	0.5	100
Male sterilization	0.15	0.10	100

Notes: Emergency contraceptive pills: Treatment initiated within 72 hours after unprotected intercourse reduces risk of pregnancy by at least 75%.[i] Lactational amenorrhea method: A highly effective, temporary method of contraception.[j]

Source: Adapted with permission from reference 4.

[a]Among couples attempting to avoid pregnancy, the percentage who continue to use a method for 1 year.

[b]Among typical couples who initiate use of a method (not necessarily for the first time), the percentage who experience an accidental pregnancy during the first year if they do not stop use for any other reason.

[c]Among couples who initiate use of a method (not necessarily for the first time) and who use it *perfectly* (both consistently and correctly), the percentage who experience an accidental pregnancy during the first year if they do not stop use for any other reason.

[d]The percentages becoming pregnant in columns two and three are based on data from populations in which contraception is not used and from women who cease using contraception to become pregnant. Among such populations, about 89% become pregnant within 1 year. This estimate was lowered slightly (to 85%) to represent the percentages who would become pregnant within 1 year among women now relying on reversible methods of contraception if they abandoned contraception altogether.

[e]Foams, creams, gels, vaginal suppositories, and vaginal film.

[f]Cervical mucous (ovulation) method supplemented by calendar in the preovulatory and basal body temperature in the postovulatory phases.

[g]With spermicidal cream or jelly.

[h]Without spermicides.

[i]The treatment schedule is one dose within 72 hours after unprotected intercourse, and a second dose 12 hours after the first dose. The Food and Drug Administration has declared the following brands of oral contraceptives to be safe and effective for emergency contraception: Ovral (one dose is two white pills); Alesse (one dose is five pink pills); Nordette or Levlen (one dose is four light-orange pills); Lo/Ovral (one dose is four 4 white pills); Triphasil or Tri-Levlen (one dose is four yellow pills).

[j]However, to maintain effective protection against pregnancy, another method of contraception must be used as soon as menstruation resumes, the frequency or duration of breast-feeds is reduced, bottle feeds are introduced, or the baby reaches 6 months of age.

suitability for the specific medical needs of that patient, ease of use, accessibility, cost, and lifestyle factors, including cultural, religious, and political views.

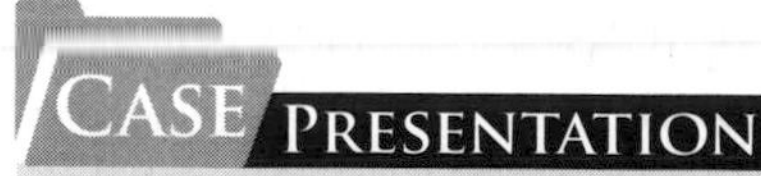

Patient Case: Part 1

K.R. is a 28-year-old woman who presents to the clinic for a yearly physical exam with her primary care physician. She seems slightly anxious and when asked, states "I just don't like getting Pap tests. I am just so uncomfortable with that area." On further discussion, K.R. reveals that she will be getting married in a few months and would like to start a regular form of birth control. She and her fiancé have been using condoms but now want something more convenient and reliable. She also states that she is worried about being able to conceive in a few years and is concerned that a hormonal contraceptive might alter her chances to have a baby. She and her fiancé would like to have children. She does not have any children and has never been pregnant. Her periods are regular, occurring about every 27 days.

HPI: Regular menses, uncomfortable touching genitalia.

PMH: Diagnosed with a major depression episode at age 26, treated with sertraline 50 mg by mouth daily for 6 months, adult onset acne age 25, seasonal allergies.

Family history: Mother—hypertension, osteoporosis; father—hypertension, stroke 1 year ago, depression.

Social history: No tobacco, occasional alcohol.

Medications: Flonase (fluticasone), uses two sprays in each nostril daily; topical sulfur 2% wash, use topically twice daily; benzoyl peroxide 2.5% cream, apply topically twice daily; Retin-A micro 0.1% apply topically twice a week as tolerated; ibuprofen 200–400 mg by mouth occasionally for headaches or menstrual cramps.

Allergies: No known drug allergies, dust, pollen.

Vitals: 5′4″, 140 lb; blood pressure 116/79 mm Hg, heart rate 76 bpm, temperature 98.6°F, respiration rate 18.

Physical exam: Normal, with the exception of mild acne.

Laboratory values: Within normal limits.

In particular, before the initiation of any hormonal contraceptive, patients should be evaluated for past and present medical history, including obstetric history and desire for future children; medication allergies; medication use, including vitamins, herbals, and over-the-counter products; an accurate sexual history focusing on number of current sexual partners; and history of STIs or pelvic inflammatory disease (PID). All of these factors are important in selecting the most appropriate hormonal contraceptive for a patient.

Combined Hormonal Contraception

Hormonal contraception uses hormones to prevent pregnancy. The most common kind of hormonal contraception is known as combined hormonal contraception. (CHC), which consists of an estrogen and a progestogen, frequently called a progestin for hormonal contraceptive agents. All CHCs have a Food and Drug Administration (FDA) indicated use for the prevention of pregnancy, a typical failure rate of approximately 8%, and a reasonable **return to fertility,** with the average being around 3 months.[4] More recently, some product combinations have been FDA labeled for acne (Estrostep, Ortho Tri-Cyclen, YAZ) and premenstrual dysphoric disorder (PMDD) (YAZ). Many of these formulations not only have the FDA indication, but are thought to help with acne and mood as well; they have just not sought out these other FDA indications.

In addition to preventing pregnancy and controlling acne and mood, CHC has many unapproved off-label uses. Most products help decrease hirsutism (abnormal male pattern hair growth in areas found on women) and acne.[5,6] The hormones help regulate the menstrual cycle, which helps many women with irregular menses to have more consistent and predictable cycles.[7] Because CHCs help control and regulate the menstrual cycle, they may also be used to help with dysmenorrhea, headaches related to menses (because some experience headaches with their menses as a result of the decrease in estrogen), pain associated with endometriosis (by helping to control the changes in the endometrial sites), bleeding associated with uterine fibroids, and, in some cases, premenstrual syndrome (PMS).[7-11] In addition, with the added hormones in CHCs, menstrual flow is usually decreased. This benefits women with menorrhagia (excessive menstrual bleeding) that is due to the hormonal effects on the thickness of the endometrial lining or those who suffer from iron-deficiency anemia.[10,11]

COMPONENTS

There are a variety of combined products available (Table 19-2 and Table 19-3). Estrogen is a key hormone in regulating the menstrual cycle. To help

Table 19-2. Selected Oral Contraceptives with Hormone Activities[86,88,120-123]

Phase Type	Brand Names	Hormone Content	Estrogen Activity	Progestin Activity	Androgen Activity	Comments
Monophasic Products with levonorgestrel	**Levlen, Levora, Nordette, Portia**	0.15 mg levonorgestrel/30 mcg EE	+	++	++	
	Seasonale (91-day pack), Seasonique (91-day pack with 10 mcg instead of placebo)					Four menstrual periods/yr
	Alesse, Aviane, Lessina, Levlite	0.1 mg levonorgestrel/20 mcg EE	+	+	+	Very low estrogen
	Lybrel (1-year formulation)	90 mcg levonorgestrel/20 mcg EE	No data	No data	No data	One menstrual period/yr
Monophasic Products with norgestimate	**Ortho-Cyclen, Sprintec**	0.25 mg norgestimate/35 mcg EE	++	+	+	
Monophasic Products with norethindrone	**Brevicon, Modicon, Necon 0.5/35, Nortrel 0.5/35**	0.5 mg norethindrone/35 mcg EE	+++	+	+	
	Ovcon-35, Femcon Fe	0.4 mg norethindrone/35 mcg EE	+++	+	+	Fe = iron tablets instead of placebo, Femcon-chewable tablet
	Necon 1/35, Norinyl 1+35, Nortrel 1/35, Ortho-Novum 1/35	1 mg norethindrone/35 mcg EE	+++	++	++	
	Ovcon-50	1 mg norethindrone/50 mcg EE	+++	++	++	High estrogen
	Necon 1/50, Norinyl 1+50, Ortho-Novum 1/50	1 mg norethindrone/50 mcg mestranol	++	++	++	High estrogen
Monophasic Products with norethindrone acetate	**Loestrin 21 1/20, Loestrin Fe 1/20, Microgestin Fe 1/20**	1 mg norethindrone acetate/20 mcg EE	+	+++	++	Fe = iron tablets instead of placebo
	Loestrin 21 1.5/30, Loestrin Fe 1.5/30, Microgestin Fe 1.5/30	1.5 mg norethindrone acetate/30 mcg EE	+	+++	+++	Fe = iron tablets instead of placebo

(*Continued on next page*)

Phase Type	Brand Names	Hormone Content	Estrogen Activity	Progestin Activity	Androgen Activity	Comments
Monophasic Products with norgestrel	**Cryselle, Lo-Ovral, Low-Ogestrel**	0.3 mg norgestrel/30 mcg EE	+	++	++	
	Ovral, Ogestrel	0.5 mg norgestrel/50 mcg EE	+++	+++	+++	
Monophasic Products with drospirenone	**Yasmin**	3 mg drospirenone/30 mcg EE	++	No data	No data	Best for acne, hirsutism, bloating (YAZ approved for acne, PMDD)
	YAZ	3 mg drospirenone/20 mcg EE	No data	No data	No data	
Monophasic Products with desogestrel	**Kariva, Mircette**	Desogestrel/EE 0.15 mg–20 mcg and EE 10 mcg	+	+++	+	Very low estrogen
	Apri, Desogen, Ortho-Cept	0.15 mg desogestrel/30 mcg EE	+++	++	+	
Monophasic Products with ethynodiol	**Demulen 1/35, Zovia 1/35E**	1 mg ethynodiol diacetate/35 mcg EE	+	+++	+	
	Demulen 1/50, Zovia 1/50E	1 mg ethynodiol diacetate/ 50 mcg EE	++	+++	+	High estrogen
Biphasic	**Necon 10/11, Ortho-Novum 10/11**	Norethindrone/EE 0.5-35/1-35 mg-mcg	+++	++	+	
Triphasic Products with desogestrel	**Cyclessa**	Desogestrel/EE 0.1-25/0.125-25/0.15-25 mg-mcg	+	+++	+	
Triphasic Products with levonorgestrel	**Enpresse, Tri-Levlen, Triphasil, Trivora**	Levonorgestrel/ EE 0.05-30/0.075-40/0.125-30 mg-mcg	++	+	+	
Triphasic Products with norethindrone	**Tri-Norinyl**	Norethindrone/EE 0.5-35/1-35/0.5-35 mg-mcg	+++	+	+	
	Necon 7/7/7, Ortho-Novum 7/7/7	Norethindrone/EE 0.5-35/0.75-35/1-35 mg-mcg	+++	++	+	
(*estrophasic)	***Estrostep 21, Estrostep Fe**	Norethindrone/EE 1-20/1-30/1-35 mg-mcg	+	+++	++	Best for women who suffer from estrogen side effects, indicated for acne, Fe = iron tablets instead of placebo

(*Continued on next page*)

Phase Type	Brand Names	Hormone Content	Estrogen Activity	Progestin Activity	Androgen Activity	Comments
Triphasic Products with norgestimate	**Ortho Tri-Cyclen Lo**	Norgestimate/EE 0.18-25/0.215-25/0.25-25 mg-mcg	+	+	+	
	Ortho Tri-Cyclen	Norgestimate/EE 0.18-35/0.215-35/0.25-35 mg-mcg	++	+	+	Approved for acne

EE = ethinyl estradiol; PMDD = premenstrual dysphoric; disorder; + = low activity; ++ = moderate activity; +++ = high activity.

Table 19-3. Classification of Estrogen Doses in Combined Hormonal Contraceptives

General Name	Amount of Estrogen	Comments
High-dose CHCs	50 mcg	Rarely used, only in special situation that require higher levels of estrogen (e.g., drug interactions)
Low-dose CHCs	30–35 mcg	Used commonly, particularly in women who have breakthrough bleeding that is due to low estrogen
Very-low-dose CHCs	20–25 mcg	Used commonly, best for women who would like to minimize exposure to estrogen or experience side effects related to estrogen

CHCs = combined hormonal contraceptives.

enhance the bioavailability of estrogens, synthetic estrogens were developed. There are two types of synthetic estrogens used in the U.S.: mestranol and, more commonly, ethinyl estradiol (EE). Mestranol is inactive but converted to EE in the liver through demethylation. Currently, only one product in the U.S. contains mestranol.

Ethinyl estradiol or estrogens in general have a variety of pharmacologic actions. It is hepatically metabolized via the CYP 3A4 isoenzyme and undergoes first-pass metabolism. It is highly bound to albumin and enters enterohepatic circulation. Estrogen helps prevent pregnancy by feedback inhibition of hormones to the pituitary gland. With the synthetic estrogens circulating in the bloodstream, follicle stimulating hormone (FSH) is not secreted (see Chapter 10: Menstrual Cycle for review of the menstrual cycle.) Without FSH, follicles in the ovary do not develop, and ovulation does not occur. At the same time, the corpus luetum is not formed and luteinizing hormone (LH) is not secreted, thus disrupting the menstrual cycle and preventing ovulation.

Estrogen has other effects on the body as well. It also increases sex-hormone binding globulin (SHBG), a hormone in the body that binds free androgens. This is one of the hypothesized reasons that most estrogen-containing hormonal contraceptive products help with acne and hirsutism.[10] Common side effects attributed to estrogen include water retention, mood changes, headache, nausea, vomiting, lack of **withdrawal bleed,** and blood clots (Table 19-4).

The progestogen component often referred to as progestin in hormonal contraceptive formulations is available as many compounds (see Table 19-2). The only natural progestogen is progesterone. However, natural progesterone has a very low oral bioavailability. To circumvent this, synthetic progestogens were invented. Progestogens, like estrogens, go through first-pass metabolism in the liver. Depending on the progestogen, some are activated to a more active form in the liver. In the U.S., there are currently 11 different synthetic compounds with varying progestational activities.

Grouped by generation, these include first generation (norethindrone, norethindrone acetate, ethynodiol diacetate, norethynodrel), second generation (levonorgestrel, norgestrel), third generation (desogestrel, norgestimate, etonogestrel, norelgestromin), and fourth generation (the spironolactone derivative drospirenone).[12] Unlike estrogens, progestogens have progestational activity as well as estrogenic and androgenic activity. Second- and third-generation

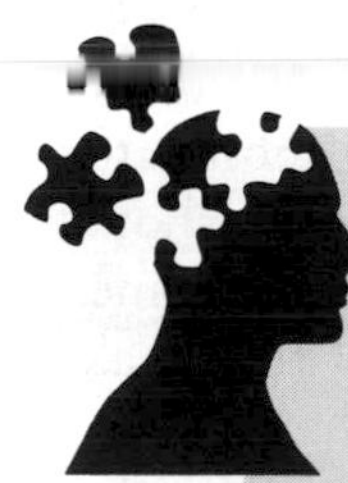

Therapeutic Challenge:

A woman comes to the pharmacy with a prescription for ethinyl estradiol 30 mcg/drospirenone 3 mg and says her dermatologist prescribed it for acne. After processing, it is found that her insurance does not cover this product but covers ethinyl estradiol 20 mcg/desogestrel 0.15 mg. What do you tell this patient in regards to her treatment of acne and selection of products?

progestogens were developed to help reduce androgenic side effects. Drospirenone is unique in that it has antiandrogenic and antimineralocorticoid properties.

Progestogens also have a variety of mechanisms that help to prevent pregnancy. Progestogens help thicken cervical mucus, making it difficult for sperm to travel; inhibit the LH surge; and cause atrophy of the endometrial lining, making the uterus an environment prohibiting implantation of a fertilized egg. Side effects of progestogens usually include mood changes, acne, weight gain, and irregular bleeding (see Table 19-4). In drospirenone-containing products, increased potassium may also be a side effect because it is similar to the potassium-sparing diuretic spironolactone.

Surprisingly, drospirenone has not been found to have a significant diuretic effect despite its similarity to spironolactone. However, because of its ability to increase potassium levels, using concurrent medications that also increase potassium—such as ACE inhibitors, potassium-sparing diuretics, and high-dose ibuprofen—should be avoided in women taking drospirenone-containing products because of the theoretical risk of interactions with drugs that have the potential to increase potassium levels.

SIDE EFFECTS

CHCs have many side effects that require counseling. The most serious include blood clots in the lungs (pulmonary embolism) and legs (deep vein thrombosis), liver changes, retinal and corneal changes, and stroke. A helpful acronym to remember when counseling is ACHES (Table 19-5), which increases patients' awareness of serious potential side effects that warrant a physician's attention.[4]

Other less severe side effects are listed (see Table 19-4). Most side effects decrease within 3 months of hormonal contraceptive use. Patients experiencing side effects other than those described in ACHES should be encouraged to try a hormonal contraceptive for at least 3 months before switching to an alternative agent.

Nausea, bleeding irregularities, mood changes, weight gain, headache, and breast tenderness are among the most commonly reported side effects in

Table 19-4. Side Effects Based on Hormone Content[120,121]

Too Much Estrogen	Not Enough Estrogen	Too Much Progestin	Not Enough Progestin
• Bloating	• Breakthrough bleeding early in cycle	• Acne[a]	• Breakthrough bleeding late in cycle
• Breast Tenderness	• Light menses	• Hirsutism[a]	• No withdrawal bleeding
• Mood changes	• Vaginal dryness	• Decrease in sex drive	• Heavy menses
• Headache	• Spotting	• Depression	
• Nausea	• No withdrawal bleeding	• Increased appetite	
• Heavy menses		• Increase in sex drive[a]	
• Fibroid growth		• Noncyclical weight gain	
• Melasma		• Less energy	
• Vision changes		• Cholestatic jaundice[a]	
• Cyclic weight gain		• Yeast infections	
		• Hair loss[a]	
		• Swelling in arms/legs[a]	

[a]Indicates androgen excess.

Table 19-5. Combination Oral Contraceptive Warning Signs[4]

Symptom	Possible Serious Side Effect
A—Abdominal Pain	Liver problem, gallbladder disease, or blood clot
C—Chest Pain (shortness of breath, coughing)	Pulmonary embolism, heart attack
H—Headache (severe headache, dizziness)	Hypertension, stroke, migraine
E—Eye Problems (seeing double, blurry vision)	Stroke or hypertension
S—Severe Leg Pain (calf or thigh)	Deep vein thrombosis

women using CHCs.[13] In one study, nausea was reported in 38% of women as the reason they quit using CHCs.[14] Nausea can generally be attributed to the estrogen component. To help alleviate nausea, a woman can take her pill at bedtime rather than in the morning. Another alternative may be to take it with food or to try another CHC with a lower estrogen strength or property.

In the same study, 33% of women reported stopping their CHC because of breakthrough bleeding.[14] Spotting or breakthrough bleeding occurs when a woman starts to have vaginal bleeding that is not at the time of her expected (or anticipated) menstrual period. Breakthrough bleeding usually requires a form of feminine napkin or tampon to absorb the amount of blood. Spotting is generally a small amount of blood that does not require a tampon or feminine napkin. Breakthrough bleeding can be attributed to deficiencies in either the progestogen or estrogen content or both, depending on when in the cycle the bleeding occurs. If bleeding occurs early in the cycle, it is likely due to estrogen deficiency; late breakthrough bleeding is usually attributed to a deficiency in progestogen. Conversely, if a withdrawal bleed does not occur while a patient is taking the placebo pills, there may be an excess of estrogen. Estrogen and progestogen work together to build the endometrium lining of the uterus. The estrogen is generally responsible for the buildup of the lining, and the progestogen maintains it. If there is not enough of estrogen, the lining will be weak, frail, and easily shed. If there is not enough progestogen to hold the lining to the uterine wall, the endometrium again will be weak and shed, resulting in breakthrough bleeding. Breakthough bleeding most often improves within 3 months of use, and women should be encouraged to continue the product; women should consider an alternative product if the breakthrough bleeding continues after 3 months of use.

Weight gain is another common side effect that concerns many women. One trial looked at the daily weights of 128 women using a low-dose COC and reported no weight gain in 52% of the women (defined as more than 2 lb from starting weight); 33% had a weight gain or loss of 5 lb or less.[15] If a woman is concerned with this issue, a low-dose estrogen and low-dose progestogen combination product is probably the best choice. Excess estrogen can lead to water retention and bloated feeling, resulting in a cyclic weight gain, whereas too much progestogen can lead to an increased appetite and noncyclic weight gain. Drospirenone has antimineralocorticoid properties that combat the effect of estrogen, resulting in less water retention and weight gain. In addition, because drospirenone has antiandrogenic properties, increases in appetite may not be as apparent. In patients experiencing weight gain or water retention, products with drospirenone may also be a good option.

Mood changes such as depression have been reported in women using CHCs. Most CHCs tend to help with mood, but for some women, CHCs may alter their mood and lead to depression. The issue is controversial, and there are no well-controlled trials to substantiate that CHCs cause depression. There are few trials that do support the use of CHCs for women suffering from PMDD or PMS.[16-19] Although many symptoms of PMDD or PMS are physical in nature and are relieved with CHCs (such as extreme bloating, menstrual cramps, and food cravings), mood changes are less well studied.

Headaches and migraines have been reported with the use of CHCs. It is thought that the sharp decrease in estrogen in the placebo week may trigger headaches in some women before or during their menstrual period.[20] Formulations that have lower estrogen content or have estrogen in place of the "nonactive" pills, such as Mircette and Seasonique, may help prevent the sharp drop in estrogen and prevent headaches. Other alternatives may include shorter placebo periods, such as 24/4 regimens, or extended-use regimens, in which menses is delayed and continuous active tablets are given. If a woman develops new onset of headaches or migraines after starting CHCs, another method of birth control should be selected and the CHC discontinued.

DRUG INTERACTIONS

CHCs are hepatically metabolized and as such may be affected by other drugs that change hepatic metabolism, and CHCs may affect the metabolism of other drugs. Because CHCs work by suppressing ovulation, it is important to maintain a certain level of hormones in the body. In particular, drugs that inhibit or induce hepatic enzymes have the most effect on CHCs (see Table 19-6). Some drugs have been shown to increase levels of CHCs.[21-24] An increase in hormone levels can result in higher risks of serious adverse effects for the patient. Estrogens in particular are substrates of cytochrome P-450 3A4 isoenzyme. Many drugs are known to affect the cytochrome p-450 3A4 isoenzyme, such as antiepileptics, HIV antiretrovirals, and St. John's wort.[25-36] Medications should be reviewed for possible interactions with CHCs. Decreased levels could decrease the efficacy of CHCs.

Antibiotics also may interfere with CHCs. Those more commonly known to induce metabolism are rifampin and rifabutin; backup birth control methods should be used during their courses. Griseofulvin, an antifungal, has been implicated in reducing serum hormone levels in various case reports.[37] Controversy exists over whether the concurrent use of broad-spectrum antibiotics interacts with the enterohepatic circulation of CHCs, resulting in decreased levels of hormones that could lead to ovulation. It is hypothesized that approximately 40% to 50% of EE is absorbed via intestinal wall or liver while the other 60% is inactivated by sulfation in the intestine. The free EE goes to the liver and is either conjugated or hydroxylated. Conjugated estrogen is then excreted into

Table 19-6. Selected Drug Interactions with Combined Hormonal Contraceptives[a]

Drugs That Increase Effect of CHCs	Drugs/Herbals That Decrease the Effect of CHCs	Drugs That *May* Decrease the Effect of CHCs (controversial)	Metabolism or Clearance Altered by CHCs
Atorvastatin	Amprenavir	Ampicillin	Acetaminophen
Atazanavir	Barbiturates	Amoxicillin	Antidepressants, tricyclic
Indinavir	Carbamazepine	Ciprofloxacin	Aspirin
	Felbamate	Clarithromycin	Benzodiazepines
	Griseofulvin	Doxycycline	Beta-blockers
	Lopinavir	Erythromycin	Caffeine
	Modafinil	Fluconazole	Corticosteroids
	Nelfinavir	Metronidazole	Cyclosporine
	Nevirapine	Minocycline	Lamotrigine
	Oxcarbazepine	Ofloxacin	Theophyllines
	Phenobarbital	Tetracycline	
	Phenytoin	Topiramate	
	Primidone		
	Rifamycins		
	Ritonavir		
	Sanquinavir		
	St. John's wort		
	Tipranavir		

CHCs = combined hormonal contraceptives.
[a]Drug list is not all inclusive. Some drug interactions may exist that are not cited in this table.

the bile and to the colon for excretion. It is thought that in the colon, bacteria hydrolyze the conjugated EE, and free EE is released in the body again.[38] Antibiotics are thought to disrupt the cycle by either killing off the bacteria in the colon, thus preventing recirculation of free estrogen, or by inducing diarrhea, in which case the gastrointestinal transit time is less. There have been two studies reporting cases of pregnancy in particular with the concurrent use of antibiotics.[38,39] More recent data suggest that broad-spectrum antibiotics do not affect CHCs and no backup contraceptive method is required.[38] The topic remains controversial. Because the consequences of an unplanned pregnancy are usually significant, the benefit of a second contraceptive method (backup method) might be worthwhile. Taking into account the risk vs. benefit, it is generally best to recommend a backup method to prevent pregnancy.

In general, when managing patients on medications that affect liver metabolism enzymes, using a CHC with a higher estrogenic strength may be recommended (e.g., 50 mcg EE formulations, excluding products with mestranol 50 mcg because it is approximately equivalent to 35 mcg of EE). Short-term use of medications may just require the use of a backup method; however, if chronically used, an alternative form of birth control (preferably nonhormonal) is probably best.

CHCs can also affect the metabolism of other drugs by competing for enzymes. Benzodiazepines are among the drugs that compete with EE, which can actually result in reducing the effect of the EE or increasing the effect the benzodiazepine.[4] In addition to competing with certain drugs for metabolism, clearance of certain drugs may be reduced when given together with CHCs. These include corticosteroids, theophylline, aspirin, and acetaminophen. An increased risk of side effects of these medications may occur, and in some cases, a dose reduction may be necessary.

When evaluating the potential for drug interactions, it is important to obtain an accurate patient medication history, including complementary and alternative medications. Drug interactions leading to a reduction in effectiveness for CHCs could have significant outcomes (e.g., pregnancy), and the potential increase in drug concentrations with other medications could lead to significant side effects or toxicity. Therefore, a careful review of concurrent medications is critical to ensure the best outcome for efficacy and safety.

CONTRAINDICATIONS

Hormonal contraception is not for everyone. It is important to note that the use of hormonal contraceptives is patient specific. The World Health Organization has classified categories of contraindications from 1 to 4, with category 4 being an absolute contraindication (Table 19-7).

RISKS

Risks with CHC products are considered to be similar, however, most studies have been conducted with oral contraceptive formulations. Because other formulations have been less studied, precautions for COCs generally apply to other formulations of CHCs as well.

Breast Cancer

There has been much controversy over whether CHCs cause breast cancer. The overall lifetime risk of breast cancer in women is reported as 12% to 13%.[40] Most research has shown that the risk of breast cancer does not increase with the use of CHCs. A meta-analysis conducted in 1996 reviewed 54 studies looking at 150,000 women with and without breast cancer.[41] The investigators reported that women taking COCs had a relative risk (RR) of 1.24 (1.15–1.33) of developing breast cancer. After discontinuing oral contraceptives for 1 to 4 years, the RR decreased to 1.16 (1.08–1.23), dropped to 1.07 (1.02–1.13) at 5–9 years, and no increase was seen after 10 years. However, this reanalysis was criticized, citing that 66% of the breast cancer cases occurred in women who were older than age 45, suggesting that age played a role rather than the hormones.[42] In 2002, a group of investigators conducted a case-control study and found no difference in RR for developing breast cancer after COC use.[43] The amount of estrogen, family history of breast cancer, age of initiation, and race were not associated with the risk of breast cancer as related to oral contraceptives.

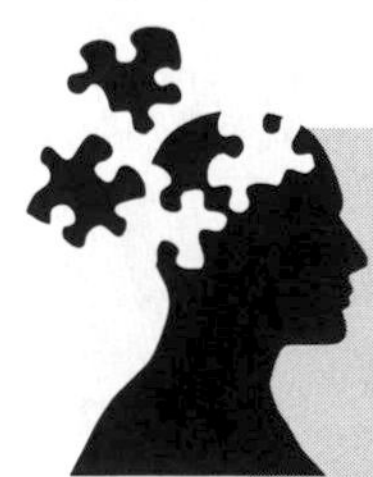

Therapeutic Challenge:

If a woman was using minocycline daily for acne and is now requesting hormonal contraception, what are some therapeutic options for this patient given the potential drug interaction?

Table 19-7. Precautions in the Provision of Combined Oral Contraceptives (COCs)

Refrain from providing COCs for women with the following diagnoses (World Health Organization category 4):

Precautions	Rationale/Discussion
Deep vein thrombosis or pulmonary embolism, or a history thereof	Estrogens promote blood clotting. Thromboembolic events related to known trauma or an intravenous needle are not necessarily a reason to avoid use of pills.
Cerebrovascular accident (stroke), coronary artery or ischemic heart disease, or a history thereof	Estrogens promote blood clotting.
Structural heart disease, complicated by pulmonary hypertension, atrial fibrillation, or history of subacute bacterial endocarditis	Estrogens promote blood clotting.
Diabetes with nephropathy, retinopathy, neuropathy, or other vascular disease; diabetes of more than 20-yr duration	Estrogens promote blood clotting.
Breast cancer	Breast cancer is a hormonally sensitive tumor. In theory, the hormones in COCs might cause some masses to grow.
Pregnancy	Current data do *not* show that hormonal contraceptives taken during pregnancy cause any significant risk of birth defects. However, hormonal contraceptives should not be given to pregnant women.
Lactation (<6 wk postpartum)	There is some theoretical concern that the neonate may be at risk because of exposure to steroid hormones during the first 6 weeks postpartum. COCs can diminish the volume of breast milk.
Liver problems: benign hepatic adenoma or liver cancer, or a history thereof; active viral hepatitis; severe cirrhosis	COCs are metabolized by the liver, and their use may adversely affect prognosis of existing disease.
Headaches, including migraine, with focal neurologic symptoms	Focal neurologic symptoms such as blurred vision, seeing flashing lights or zigzag lines, or trouble speaking or moving may be an indication of an increased risk of stroke.
Major surgery with prolonged immobilization or any surgery on the legs	Increased risk for deep vein thrombosis and pulmonary embolism is seen.
Older than 35 years and currently a heavy smoker (15 or more cigarettes a day)	Smoking increases the risk for cardiovascular disease.
Hypertension, 160+/100+ or with vascular disease	Hypertension is an important risk factor for cardiovascular disease.

Source: Reprinted with permission from reference 4.

Data from a meta-analysis conducted in 2006 showed similar results overall, but subgroup analysis showed a slight increase in the risk of breast cancer in women who used oral contraceptives before their first full-term pregnancy.[44] This study specifically looked at women younger than 50 years to account for age as a factor. Although there is no definite answer, the current thought is that oral contraceptives do not increase the risk for breast cancer. Other formulations are not that well studied.

Ovarian Cancer

CHC has been shown to have beneficial effects in decreasing the risk of ovarian cancer. Furthermore, the longer CHCs are used, the lower the risk of ovarian cancer. The lifetime risk of ovarian cancer is reported as 1.4%.[45] According to one study, the incidence of ovarian cancer decreases by 41% after 4 years of use, by 54% with 8 years of use, and by 61% with 12 years.[46] Using CHCs may also reduce ovarian cancer in those who have never had children or in those with a family history of ovarian cancer. One study showed that CHCs lowered the risk in women with a family history of ovarian cancer to a risk similar to that without the family history risk factor.[47] Similarly, another study lowered the risk for women who have not had children similar to women who have had children.[48] Data show that women who have had children tend to have a lower risk of ovarian cancer than those who have never had children.[48] Benefits of oral contraceptives can be seen within 3 months of use and continue to increase for as long as 20 years of use, but some data show that this effect may wane after 20 years.[49]

Uterine Cancer

Similar to ovarian cancer, CHCs show a benefit in decreasing the risk of endometrial cancer. The lifetime risk of endometrial cancer in women is reported to be 2.4%.[50] One study reported that COC use reduced endometrial cancer by about 50% and remained protective 15–20 years after discontinuation.[51,52] It has been suggested, however, that CHCs may exacerbate the growth of uterine fibroids (benign growths) because fibroids are affected by hormones. Studies have failed to prove this and instead have shown no risk in the development of new or increasing the size of pre-existing fibroids. Based on the available information, CHCs may be used safely in women with uterine fibroids.[53-55]

Cervical Cancer

It is debatable whether CHCs cause an increased risk of cervical cancer. Some studies have shown a slightly increased risk but have also cited confounding risk factors that influence the risk of cervical cancer, such as multiple partners, sexual intercourse at an early age, and, in particular, human papillomavirus (HPV).[56,57] HPV has been shown to increase the risk of cervical cancer, and those who are sexually active have a higher risk of contracting the virus.[58] The likely users of CHCs are those who want to prevent pregnancy and are sexually active, so it is unclear if CHCs are truly a factor in increased risk. One study suggests that the longer the use of CHCs, the higher the risk of cervical cancer increases.[59] Another study suggests that the risk of cervical cancer increases in current users, but that risk ceases after discontinuation of hormonal contraceptives for 10 years.[60]

Cardiovascular and Circulatory System

As women age, their risk of developing blood clots increases. This is more specifically known as venous thromboembolism (VTE), which can be a deep vein thrombosis (DVT), usually in the leg, or a pulmonary embolism (PE) found in the lung. Blood clots can also occur in the brain, causing vision problems. The reported incidence of VTE in women of reproductive age is considered low (approximately one case per 10,000 person-years), but increases to six cases per 10,000 years with pregnancy and three to four cases per 10,000 person-years with CHC use.[61 62] In particular, increased risks were especially seen in women with blood coagulopathies, such as factor V Leiden and protein C and S mutations. Because the risk of blood clots increases in older women and in those using CHCs, it is recommended that CHCs be used in caution in women older than 35 years or in women with known blood coagulopathies. Thrombosis has mainly been attributed to the estrogen component. However, there are some controversial data regarding second- and third-generation progestogens increasing the risk of blood clots as well. One study reported a twofold increase in nonfatal VTE for women using desogestrel or gestodene (a progestogen used in Europe) compared with women using a COC with levonorgestrel.[63] A subsequent study suggested that desogestrel-containing COCs significantly increased the risk of nonfatal VTE compared with levonorgestrel and norgestimate.[64] Both studies have been criticized for confounding variables, such as selection bias, duration of use, detection bias, smoking, age, and weight.[4] Although still controversial, in women concerned about blood clots, a COC with a second-generation progestogen may be a good choice.

Myocardial infarctions (MIs), stroke, and blood clots are considered rare in reproductive age women. There are conflicting reports about COCs increasing the risk of ischemic stroke and MI. A few studies have shown an increased risk in women who use COCs.[65-68] However, the studies also showed that these risks were much lower in women using low-dose COCs vs. older-generation COCs. One study reported an odds ratio of 1.3 for women using low-dose COCs; another study also reported that smaller doses of estrogen lowered risk as compared with higher doses.[66,67] Other studies have found no risk of MI with COC use.[69-72] Most studies consistently report, however, a much higher risk for MI and stroke in women who smoke or have hypertension. It has been reported that the number of MI and ischemic stroke cases attributable to nonsmokers and the use of oral contraceptives in women age 20–24 years is 0.4 per 100,000 person-years; 30–34 years, 0.6; and 40–44 years, 2. In contrast, for women smokers, the numbers increase to 1, 2, and 20 cases per 100,000 person-years.[12] The risk of MI and stroke in reproductive-age women remains low until around age 35.[73] Because of the combined risk of age and smoking, CHCs are not recommended for women older than 35 years who smoke more than 15 cigarettes per day; these women should select an alternate method of birth control.

In addition, estrogen has been known to increase blood pressure. Two studies showed an increase in blood pressure in women taking oral contraceptives vs. those who were not. One small, nonrandomized study showed an increase of systolic blood pressure by 8 mm Hg and diastolic blood pressure by 6 mm Hg in women using a low-dose oral contraceptive vs. no change in blood pressure for women using the copper intrauterine device.[74,75] Another small study observed a 8.33 mm Hg increase in systolic blood pressure in mildly hypertensive women using a low-dose COC compared with those who were not.[76] In addition, the risks of MI and stroke increase greatly in women older than age 40 with a history of hypertension.[12] Patients who have uncontrolled hypertension or are older than age 40 with a history of hypertension should not use CHCs.

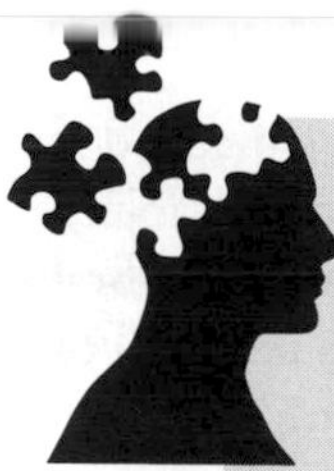

Therapeutic Challenge:

A physician is concerned about oral contraceptives causing blood clots and says she heard something about birth control pills that contain desogestrel being worse than second-generation ones. How do you handle this situation?

FORMULATIONS

Combined Oral Contraceptives

COCs come in various dose regimens: monophasic, biphasic, and triphasic. Typical doses of COCs range from 20 to 50 mcg of EE. The typical COC is 21 days of active tablet (both an estrogen and progestogen) and 7 days of placebo. Some pill packs provide only 21 active tablets with no placebo pills, and for 7 days the woman does not take any pills. Recently, 24-day active pill regimens with 4 days of placebo have been developed to decrease the length of menses and undesirable withdrawal symptoms from estrogen and progestogen. Extended regimens with the use of continuous active monophasic pills for 3 months to a year are employed. The early birth control pills were all monophasic, meaning the amount of estrogen and progestogen was consistent in the active pills. In the early 1980s, there was concern that progestogen exposure could increase the risk of hyperlipidemia. To decrease the exposure to progestogen, a triphasic formulation was developed. The triphasic formulation more closely mimics a woman's typical menstrual cycle of hormones and differs from the monophasic in that each week there are varying levels of hormones. For most triphasic formulations, the varying hormone is the progestogen, starting at a low dose the first week and gradually increasing the second and third weeks. This decreases the overall exposure to progestogens. Instead of receiving the higher dose of progestogen every day for 3 weeks, the patient is only receiving the higher dose the third week and lower doses the first 2 weeks. The risk of progestogens increasing lipids failed to be substantiated. Subsequently, a different triphasic was developed in 2001 in which the estrogen component actually varies throughout the cycle. These formulations are known as estrophasic regimens. They were developed to decrease the exposure to estrogen for those women who are sensitive to estrogenic side effects, such as water retention and nausea.

Triphasic pills were developed to decrease the side effects of COCs, but in some cases they increase side effects such as breakthrough bleeding and mood changes as a result of the varying weekly doses. Triphasic pills are the not the best choice in women with a history of breakthrough bleeding or mood changes while taking COCs. Biphasic pills are rare, and currently there is only one formulation available, which has 10 days of norethindrone 0.5 mg/EE 35 mcg for 10 days and norethindrone 1 mg/EE 35 mcg for 11 days. Instead of having three varying weeks of hormone doses, there are two phases of changing hormones in biphasic formulations. Mircette is a COC that has 2 days of placebo and 5 days of 10 mcg of EE. Mircette is classified more as a monophasic formulation, although some may classify it as a biphasic pill.

There are three methods to starting COCs: 1) Sunday-start method, 2) first-day- or same-day-start method, and 3) quick-start method. The Sunday-start method involves starting the active pills the first Sunday after menses begins. For example, if a woman begins her menses on Wednesday, she would take her first active tablet the following Sunday. It is recommended that a backup contraceptive method is used for first 7 days after starting the active tablets. The first-day-start method involves taking the first active tablet on the exact day that menses begins. For example, if a woman started her menses on Wednesday, then she would start taking the active tablets on the same day, Wednesday. It is suggested by some that with the same-day-start method, a backup birth control method is not required; however, more conservative views suggest using a backup method for 7 days. The third method, which is becoming more popular, is known as the quick-start method. This involves starting the active tablets regardless of what day the woman starts her menses. The quick-start method is predominantly done in the physician's office. It has been shown that women who start their first pill in the physician's office have a higher adherence rate than those who begin on their own.[77] A backup method should also be used for 7 days with this regimen. A more conservative approach would be to use a backup method until the next menses occurs. It is important to note that the woman will not have her menses until all active tablets have been taken, even if her menses is due in 1 week.

Proper use of COCs includes taking the pills daily, preferably at the same time. A woman can be reminded to schedule in her pill every morning (for example, after brushing her teeth) or at night before going to sleep. It is important, however, to counsel on the timing of administration, as times that women wake up or go to sleep may vary from day to day. A missed pill is considered to have occurred if a woman does not take her scheduled active pill within 24 hours of her last scheduled dose. If one active pill is missed, the woman should be instructed to take the missed pill as soon as possible, which may result in taking two pills in 1 day. No backup method is required for one CHC pill missed (for progestogen-only pills, see the progestogen-only section). If two pills are missed in week 1 or 2 of the cycle, the recommendation is to take two pills for 2 days and use a backup method for 7 days. If the two pills were missed in the third week of the cycle or more than three pills are missed any time during the cycle, a first-day starter or quick starter should begin a brand new pack that day and use a backup method for 7 days. For Sunday starters, the recommendation is to take one pill daily of the old pack while using a backup method, and then starting a new pack of pills on Sunday plus 7 days of a backup method. The reason for this is to keep the woman on her Sunday-start schedule. If placebos are missed, no backup method is necessary.

An alternative method for missed pills includes emergency contraception. If a patient has had sexual intercourse within the last 5 days, emergency contraception is a consideration. The woman should be instructed to use emergency contraception and then continue her pack of pills until the end of the pack while using a backup method for 7 days. If a woman desires to switch from one brand of COCs to another, she may begin the new pack of pills after she finishes the placebo pills in the old brand.

Chewable Oral Contraceptive Pills

In 2003, the FDA approved a new COC available in a chewable pill.[78] The product is a 21-day active, spearmint-flavored, monophasic pill formulation (norethindrone 0.4 mg and EE 35 mcg) with 7 days of iron tablets (ferrous fumerate). The pill may be swallowed whole or chewed and swallowed. If the woman chews the tablet, she should be instructed to drink an 8-ounce glass of water immediately afterward to make sure all residues in the mouth have reached the stomach.[78] The side effects, risks, and timing of administration for the chewable COC is similar to regular COCs.

Transdermal Contraceptive Patch

The transdermal contraceptive patch was in approved in 2001. The contraceptive patch is different from other CHCs in that it is applied to skin once weekly and delivers norelgestromin 0.15 mg/day and EE 20 mcg/day. The total amount of hormone content is 6.00 mg of norelgestromin and 0.75 mg of EE. The hormones pass into the skin and are metabolized by liver. Norelgestromin is converted to norgestimate in the liver.[79] The patch is a thin, adhesive square that consists of three layers. Its length is 1.75 inches, and it has a surface area of 20 cm^2.[79] In the first year of use, unintended pregnancies were reported as 1 per 100 women-years. Use in obese women has been not been recommended. Clinical trials reported that 5 out of the 15 pregnancies occurred were in women who weighed at or above 198 lb (90 kg).[79] Therefore, it has been concluded that the contraceptive patch is less effective (3% pregnancy rate vs. 0.6%) in women who weigh more than 198 lb (90 kg).

Using the patch is fairly easy, and women should be instructed to place the patch on a clean, dry, hairless skin area either on the upper arm, shoulder, buttock, or abdomen, but not on the breasts.[79] One new patch is worn each week for 3 weeks. During the fourth week, the patch is removed, and menses generally occurs. When removing the patch, it should be peeled off the skin carefully, folded together, and discarded away from pets and children (it should not be flushed in the toilet). Rotating the application site each week is important to prevent skin irritation. Women may use the patch while taking showers, swimming, exercising, or sitting in a sauna.

When initiating the contraceptive patch, without any prior use of a hormonal contraceptive, the patch should be applied either on the first day of menses or the Sunday following the start of menses.[79] The quick-start method can apply here as well. The patch is worn for 7 days and then changed on day 8, which is known as the patch-change day.[79] A backup birth control method should be used for the first 7 days of after the patch is applied. If switching from another CHC to the patch, the patch should be applied on the first day of withdrawal bleeding, and no backup method is necessary. If applied later than the first day of withdrawal bleed, then a backup birth control method is recommended for 7 days.

If the patch falls off for more than 24 hours, then a new patch should be applied. This will be considered a new cycle and a new patch-change day. Because this is considered a new cycle, a backup birth control method for 7 days is recommended.[79] Emergency contraception could be a consideration here if the woman has had unprotected intercourse in the last 5 days. The woman should be counseled that she may experience a delayed menses with new cycle of patches. If the patch falls off for <24 hours, it should be reapplied as soon as possible, and no backup birth control method is necessary.[79]

Side effects of the contraceptive patch are similar to those of COCs. Side effects commonly reported with the patch (9% to 20%) include breast symptoms, headache, application site reaction, nausea, upper respiratory infection, menstrual cramps, and abdominal pain.[79] More recently, it has been suggested that risks for VTE with the transdermal patch is higher than other CHCs, but this is controversial. Two epidemiologic studies found conflicting results. One found that the risk of VTE with patch users was similar to that of women taking COCs with 35 mcg of EE.[80] The other reported an odds ratio of 2.42 (95% confidence interval [CI], 1.07–5.46) for users of the patch compared with current COC users.[81] The pharmacokinetic profile of the contraceptive patch differs from that of COCs in that it has a higher steady-state concentration and lower peak concentrations. The area under curve (AUC) and steady state for EE from the patch is about 60% higher than that of a COC containing 35 mcg, despite the fact that the amount of EE delivered from the patch is 20 mcg/day. This could put a woman at increased risk for estrogen side effects such as VTE and may not be the best choice in women with a risk factor of VTE. Package labeling has changed over the course of the years. In 2005, the FDA requested labeling to warn of higher estrogen exposure. In 2006, labeling changed again, warning of increased hormone levels with the patch and possible increased risk of blood clots based on two studies. In 2008, the labeling changed again, stating that women concerned about blood clots should talk to their providers about alternate methods and including information from three studies.[38] Other risks, benefits, and precautions are similar to those of COCs. Drug-drug interactions are also considered to be similar to COCs; however, they are not well studied.

Compliance (adherence) and satisfaction with the contraceptive patch is high. In one study, compliance with the patch was 88.7% vs. 79.2% with the pill (p <0.001). The study particularly showed a higher compliance rate of 87.8% in women younger than 20 years vs. 67.7% with the pill.[82] For patients who have difficulty in remembering to take pills or adhering to other contraceptive methods, the contraceptive patch may be a good choice. Those who have sensitive skin, have difficulty removing the patches weekly, or who are self-conscious of the patch appearance are not good candidates for this method. The patch may be used continuously for extended regimens (see below).

Contraceptive Vaginal Ring

The contraceptive vaginal ring (NuvaRing) came onto the market in 2001. The contraceptive vaginal ring is unique in that it delivers hormones through the mucosa of the vagina. It releases etonogestrel 0.120 mg/day (progestogen) and EE 0.015 mg/day.[83] The ring is nonbiodegradable, flexible, transparent, and colorless. It is composed of ethylene vinylacetate copolymers, magnesium stearate and contains a total amount of 11.7 mg of etonogestrel and 2.7 mg of EE.[83] Its outer diameter is 54 mm, and it has a cross-sectional diameter of 4 mm. The unintended pregnancy rate with the first year of use was 1–2 per 100 women-years of use.[83]

Women should be instructed to insert the ring vaginally. It is then left in place continuously for

3 weeks at a time. For proper insertion of the ring, the woman should be instructed to squeeze the ends of the ring so that they meet and then insert it into the vagina. For ease of insertion, the woman may insert the ring while standing with one leg up, squatting, or lying down. The exact location of the ring is not important as long as it rests inside the vagina.[83] During the fourth week, the ring should be removed, and withdrawal bleeding will usually occur. The ring can also be used continuously for extended regimens (see below). Douching is not recommended with the ring use, but it may be left in place during sexual intercourse, while using a tampon, and with use of topical therapies such as antifungal creams or spermicides. Using a diaphragm concurrently with the ring is not recommended because the ring may interfere with placement of the diaphragm.

Occasionally, the ring may be expelled from the vagina, particularly when removing a tampon, or during bowel movements or severe straining. If removed or expelled, the ring should be rinsed with cool to lukewarm water and reinserted as soon as possible and within 3 hours. If the ring is left out the vagina for longer than 3 hours, a backup birth control method should be used until the ring has been in place for at least 7 days.[83] Emergency contraception could also be considered at this time if a woman had unprotected intercourse in the last 5 days.

To remove the ring, a woman can hook her index finger under the rim or grasp the ring with her index and middle finger and pull the ring out.[83] It is best to discard the ring by placing it in the foil packaging it came in and placing in the trash. The ring should not be flushed in the toilet and should be kept out the reach of children and pets.

Vaginitis, headache, upper respiratory tract infection, leukorrhea, sinusitis, weight gain, sensations of the ring, and nausea are among the most commonly reported side effects (5% to 14%).[83] Other possible side effects are similar to those of COCs.[83] Sex partners have reported sensing the ring during intercourse (~71% of men did not feel or rarely felt the ring during intercourse), but 90% of users did not cite this as a problem.[83,84] The vaginal ring is popular among those women who use it. One study looked at 1,950 women aged 18–41 years who used the contraceptive ring for 13 cycles. The study reported that 96% of users were satisfied with the ring, and 97% said they would recommend it to a friend. Women reported "not having to remember anything," and "ease of use" as top reasons for liking the contraceptive ring.[84] Compliance with the contraceptive ring is high. One study of 247 women ages 18–40 reported a compliance rate of 92.4% compared with 75.4% for contraceptive pill users.[85] Similar to the contraceptive patch, the contraceptive ring may be a good choice for women who have difficulty remembering to take pills or dislike other methods. The contraceptive ring should be avoided in women who are prone to vaginal irritation or vaginal tears, or who are uncomfortable inserting something vaginally. Risks, benefits, and precautions are similar to those of COCs. Drug-drug interactions with the ring are not that well studied but should be handled similarly to COCs.[83]

EXTENDED USE

Extended-use contraception is active hormonal contraception used for longer than the traditional 21 active days. Different FDA-approved regimens include use of active hormones for as long as 3–12 months without a hormone-free week. In 2003, the FDA approved the first extended-use contraceptive regimen, consisting of levonorgestrel 0.15 mg and EE 30 mcg available in a 91-tablet (84 active tablets and seven inert tablets) pack.[86] This extended-cycle regimen results in "four periods" per year. In 2007, the FDA approved another extended-cycle regimen (levonorgestrel 90 mcg/EE 20 mcg—Lybrel), which provides 1 year of active tablets in the form of monthly packs of 28 active tablets taken each month and results in one period per year.

These regimens, however, are associated with more breakthrough bleeding compared with the conventional 28-day cycle.[87] To combat this, another 3-month extended-use formulation was developed that contains 10 mcg of EE instead of placebo pills (Seasonique). As many as 41% of women experienced some form of irregular bleeding in the first few months of use of the 1-year regimen.[88] As with regular COCs, if breakthrough bleeding occurs, women should continue to use the regimen for at least 3 and for as long as 6 months with extended regimens. Most women reported less breakthrough bleeding with longer use.[88,89]

Extended regimens can also be used with other monophasic COCs by skipping the placebo pills of the current pack and starting active pills in a new pack. Biphasic and triphasic pills are not suitable for extended regimens because they have varying amounts of estrogen and progestogen, which may result in fluctuating hormone levels and unwanted side effects. The progestogen-only minipill has always been given in an extended regimen as an active tablet daily to maximize effectiveness.

Studies suggest that the use of the contraceptive patch and vaginal ring may also be used as extended regimens. The products would be used for 12-week periods followed by 1 week hormone free for menses. One study reported high satisfaction and reported less bleeding and spotting episodes with the contraceptive patch extended regimen.[90] Another study looked at the use of the vaginal ring for 28-day, 49-day, 91-day, and 364-day extended regimens and found that all regimens were well tolerated.[91] Bleeding and spotting, however, were reported to occur more with the longer regimens.

The extended-use regimens may be ideal in women who prefer fewer menstrual cycles or who suffer from estrogen-withdrawal side effects, such as migraines or mood swings. Other side effects are similar to regular cycle COCs. There have been concerns with extended-use regimens affecting the endometrium; however, one study showed no harmful changes to the endometrium with extended cycles.[92] Long-term side effects of the extended regimens are still being studied. Because long-term studies are not available, it may be beneficial for a woman to see her healthcare provider if breakthrough bleeding continues to verify that there are no other health issues present.

SPECIAL POPULATIONS: POSTPARTUM AND BREAST-FEEDING

CHCs should be avoided in women who are immediately postpartum and used on a case-by-case basis for those who are breast-feeding.[75] Women immediately postpartum are in a hypercoagulable state and have a higher risk of developing blood clots. Therefore, CHCs are not recommended for at least 4–6 weeks postpartum because of the estrogen component increasing the risk of blood clots.[75]

Furthermore, CHCs are generally not recommended for women who are breast-feeding. Estrogen is thought to decrease milk production, and it has been suggested that women who breast-feed should not use CHC in order to maintain adequate milk production.[93] Other reasons for not using CHCs while breast-feeding include concerns that the infant might not receive enough calories because of the decrease in milk production.[75] A systematic review concluded that there is not enough information to make a recommendation for or against use while breast-feeding.[94] It has been suggested, however, that CHCs may be started without a significant effect on milk production once milk flow is well established and adequate.[75]

Progestogen-Only Hormonal Contraception

For women with contraindications to estrogen or those desiring an alternate form of hormonal contraception, multiple forms of progestogen-only contraceptives are available. These products are FDA indicated for the prevention of pregnancy and demonstrate various levels of efficacy dependent on the dosage form and patient adherence.

Progestogens prevent pregnancy through four main mechanisms: suppression of ovulation, thickening of the cervical mucus, transformation of the endometrial lining, and alterations in tubal motility. As previously discussed, increased levels of progestogen inhibit production and secretion of FSH and LH in the anterior pituitary. This inhibition is particularly important when the midcycle surge of LH and FSH is blocked, resulting in an anovulatory state. Although progestogens are the most important hormone involved in blocking the LH surge, they do not always reliably block ovulation. The effect on the ovarian function may vary considerably depending on the dose and potency of the progestogen, with a reported 40% of traditional progestogen-only pill (POP) users continuing to ovulate.[95,96] In some women, follicular activity occurs, but the luteal function is impaired sufficiently to prevent the development of the corpus luteum. This results in an inability to maintain pregnancy. A secondary function of progestogens is to create a thick cervical mucus plug, preventing penetration of sperm into the endometrial cavity and subsequent fertilization should ovulation occur. In the presence of progestogen, the volume of cervical mucus is decreased, viscosity increased, and structure altered. Prevention of pregnancy is further augmented through progestogens inhibiting the production of progesterone receptors, resulting in an endometrium that is hostile and unsuitable for implantation because of atrophy, involution, and suppressed proliferation. Last, movement of the ovum through the fallopian tubes is slowed by progestogen.[95-98]

Progestogen-only contraceptives are associated with fewer health risks than the combined pills; however, they are not without contraindications.

In general, progestogen-based contraception should not be used in women who are or may be pregnant or who have a known or suspected carcinoma of the breast, undiagnosed abnormal vaginal bleeding, or acute liver disease, including malignant or benign liver tumors.[75,99] In addition, there are some specific contraindications for the various dosage forms of progestogen-only contraception, which will be addressed in the respective sections.

Progestogen-only contraceptives are also not without side effects. Irregular menstrual bleeding patterns are a common adverse effect and the most commonly reported reason for patient discontinuation.[100,101] Patients have also reported side effects of headache, weight gain, acne, breast pain, and dysmenorrhea.[102,103] With all progestogen-only contraception methods, formation of ovarian cysts is a possibility. Second-generation progestogens, such as levonorgestrel, vary in their adverse-effect profile as compared with the newer third generations, including desogestrel. Although irregular vaginal bleeding is not significantly different between the two categories, third generations overall have a lower incidence of adverse symptoms. Third-generation progestogens are less androgenic than second-generation progestogens, resulting in less acne, hirsutism, alterations in lipid and carbohydrate metabolism, and weight gain.[104] Some controversy exists as to whether third-generation progestogens promote a higher risk of thromboembolic events as compared with second generations.[61] In order to avoid such controversy with the arrival to the market of a novel progestogen, drospirenone (DRSP), Dinger et al. investigated whether there was a higher risk of adverse cardiovascular and other events in women taking DSRP as compared with other progestogen components. The authors of this large trial, which followed more than 58,000 women, concluded that the risk of events (cardiovascular, thromboembolic, and other) was similar between the two groups.[105]

PROGESTOGEN-ONLY PILLS

Oral progestogen-only contraception, called the *minipill,* first became available in the early 1960s.[96] The first POP was developed in response to an increasing awareness of risks associated with the estrogen component of COC, including venous thromboembolic events, metabolic changes, and clinical adverse effects. It was originally marketed to women who could not take COC because of contraindications to estrogen or lactation. Some benefits seen with POPs include reductions in symptoms such as menstruation-related migraines, cramping, breast tenderness, ovulation pains, and pain associated with endometriosis. Additionally, POPs have a relatively rapid return to fertility without the delay in ovulation seen with the longer-acting forms of progestogen.

Progestogen-only oral contraceptives are frequently used in mothers who are breast-feeding and, unlike estrogen, they have demonstrated either a positive or no effect on lactation or milk quality. Although progestogens may be measured in breast milk when taken by a lactating mother, the amounts are insufficient to cause any effects in the nursing child.[94] When used in the postpartum period, POPs may be initiated as early as 1–4 weeks following delivery in women who are not breast-feeding; however, it is generally recommended to initiate POPs 6 weeks after delivery for mothers who are nursing exclusively and at least 3 weeks after delivery for partial breast-feeding.[75,96,99]

Minipills are available in the U.S. in the forms of norethindrone (first generation) and norgestrel (second generation) in 28-day packs. They should be taken once daily at the same time each day beginning the first day of the menstrual period. They are taken continuously with no placebo pills or breaks between packs. Patients should be instructed to adhere to an accurate dosing regimen. If a woman misses her scheduled dose by 3 hours, it is considered a missed dose. The missed dose should be taken as soon as remembered, and a secondary method of contraception, such as condoms, should be used for the next 48 hours with any episode of intercourse. Emergency contraception is recommended if unprotected intercourse takes place. After that, the patient should continue with the pack, resuming the next dose at the correct time of day. If the initial pack of POPs is begun on a day other than the first day of menses, an alternate method of contraception is recommended for the first 48 hours.[96,99] Like COCs, progestogen-only products should be used cautiously in obese women, as the risk of unintended pregnancy slightly increases in women weighing more than 70 kg (154 lb).[96]

Because progestogens are metabolized by the liver, there is potential for drug interactions with other medications affected by the liver cytochrome P450 system. Inducers of the P450 enzyme system, such as primidone, carbamazepine, oxcarbazepine, topiramate, ritonavir, and St. John's wort, may decrease the efficacy of POPs.[75,96] In contrast to estrogen, levels of progestogen are not affected by broad-spectrum antibiotics that lessen enterohepatic circulation and decrease serum concentrations.[96]

Another concern with oral progestogen contraception is the increased risk for ectopic pregnancies, which is 4 per 100 pregnancies.[96] This risk is due to the reduced tubal motility that results from progestogen and contributes to its contraceptive effect, along with the fact that ovulation is not always fully suppressed. The risk of **ectopic pregnancy** from POPs is still less than in women who use no contraception.

INTRAMUSCULAR PROGESTOGEN-ONLY CONTRACEPTIVE

For patients having difficulty taking a daily dose of progestogen, depot medroxyprogesterone acetate (DMPA) is a long-acting progestogen injectable that contains 150 mg of medroxyprogesterone acetate in an aqueous microcrystalline suspension. DMPA is administered intramuscularly in the gluteal or deltoid muscle every 3 months, with the initial injection given within 5 days of the start of menstruation to ensure there is no existing pregnancy. DMPA is also marketed as a 104-mg subcutaneous injection given every 3 months and will be discussed later in this chapter.

The primary mechanism of DMPA is to inhibit the FSH and LH midcycle surge at the level of the hypothalamus and therefore prevent ovulation. In contrast to oral progestogen contraceptives, DMPA blocks ovulation reliably, often within 24 hours of a dose; it also prevents pregnancy through secondary mechanisms of thickening cervical mucus and changing the endometrium. Typically, the cervical mucus will begin to thicken within the first 24 hours following an injection but may sometimes take 3 to 7 days.[95,106] As a direct result of the inhibition of ovarian function, endometrial proliferation diminishes rapidly, resulting in a thin, atrophic endometrium, which theoretically impairs implantation. DMPA is highly effective at preventing ovulation; therefore, the chances of fertilization occurring are very low, and no current data suggest that blocking implantation is a mechanism of contraception of DMPA.[95] This fact may be important in decision making for patients who have objections to using contraception that inhibits implantation of an already fertilized ovum.

When doses are administered appropriately, pregnancy rates with DMPA are close to zero because of its consistently effective inhibition of ovulation.[98] DMPA relies minimally on the patient's ability to comply with dosing, drug absorption is independent of gastrointestinal function, and first-pass metabolism through the liver is avoided. The dosage of DMPA in each injection is sufficient that its efficacy is independent of patient weight or use of concomitant medications, and there is a 2-week grace period should a dose be delayed.[95,106] The risk of endometrial cancer is decreased by 80% after 1 year of use of DMPA. Although DMPA is indicated only for pregnancy, it has demonstrated some efficacy in multiple unapproved off-label uses because of its ability to block ovulation; these include treatment of menorrhagia and dysmenorrhea, endometriosis-associated pain, ovulatory pain, and vasomotor symptoms of menopause.[106,107]

Adverse effects specific to this injectable form include irregular bleeding, commonly during the first 3 months, or amenorrhea in more than 70% of patients by the end of 1year.[95,107] DMPA has been associated with a modest weight increase of 1–3 kg (2–7 lb), seen most commonly in women who were overweight at initiation of therapy.[95,107] Studies conducted in adolescents also revealed a lack of correlation between DMPA and weight gain in normal, healthy young women; however, adolescents who were obese (body mass index >30) had a significantly higher weight gain on average.[106] Studies have not conclusively shown whether weight gain is directly associated with DMPA.[108] A common concern with hormonal contraception is the effect on mood, which has been studied with DMPA. The majority of reports indicate a lack of causal effect between DMPA and depressed mood. Some comparisons reveal higher percentages of depression among COC users as compared with DMPA, with <2% of women followed for 1 year of DMPA therapy reporting depression.[95,107] Most studies report that DMPA does not cause depression, and a history of depression should not be considered an absolute contraindication to use of DMPA. However, because progestogens may exacerbate depression and DMPA is not easily reversible, caution may be used in patients with a history of depression.

Prolonged use of DMPA contributes to hypoestrogenism in most women, which is associated with bone loss, particularly in young women. Recent studies have investigated the relationship between DMPA use, estrogen deficiency, and bone mineral density (BMD), and the conclusions remain unclear. One small study evaluating 40 premenopausal DMPA users found that, when compared with healthy age-matched controls, use of DMPA exceeding 2 years had a significant adverse effect on BMD and bone turnover. Prolonged use worsened lumbar-spine BMD with women using DMPA for more than 5 years, demonstrating an almost 12% reduction as compared with nonusers. In this study, women using DMPA for <1 year showed no significant differences in BMD or bone turnover when compared with a control group.[109] Although decreases in BMD have been demonstrated in multiple clinical trials, no increase in the number of fractures has been observed during the 30 years that DMPA has been used as contraception.[96] However, the women who have used DMPA over the past years are just now 50–60 years old, and bone fractures occur more frequently in older populations. Information regarding the affect of DMPA on bone fracture rates in these women is yet to be determined. A meta-analysis of 10 studies concluded that the negative effects on BMD appears to be reversible following cessation of DMPA in women of all ages.[110] Another study concluded similar findings in postmenopausal women who were past users of DMPA; however, it was noted that past users had a nonsignificant trend toward lower bone densities.[111] Multiple professional organizations, including the World Health Organization, have published statements regarding DMPA and bone health. They have advised no restriction on the use of DMPA as contraception or its duration of use in women ages 18–45 years.[106] The package inserts/prescribing information for both intramuscular and subcutaneous DMPA injections bear this statement: "Women who use Depo-Provera Contraceptive Injection may lose significant BMD. Bone loss is greater with increasing duration of use and may not be completely reversible. It is unknown if use of Depo-Provera Contraceptive Injection during adolescence or early adulthood, a critical period of bone accretion, will reduce peak bone mass and increase the risk for osteoporotic fracture in later life. Depo-Provera Contraceptive Injection should be used as a long-term birth control method (e.g., longer than 2 years) only if other birth control methods of birth control are inadequate."[112]

Injectable DMPA is safe for use in the postpartum period, and because it does not contribute to thromboembolic events, it may be initiated immediately postpartum; however, package labeling, along with the American College of Obstetrics and Gynecology, advises that in lactating women, DMPA be initiated after 6 weeks postpartum.[75,99,112]

Return to fertility is delayed with the use of DMPA. Ovulation is typically suppressed for a minimum of 14 weeks following an injection. Although fertility may return in 14 weeks in some cases, on average, ovulation will not return for 5–8 months; this period may be as long as 18–22 months in some users.[96,106] For this reason, DMPA is not recommended as a form of contraceptive in any woman wishing to conceive within 1 year.[106]

When counseling on DMPA, patients should be advised to receive their dose regularly every 12 weeks. Although there is a "grace period" of up to 14 weeks, it is generally recommended that women who are more than 1 week overdue for a dose receive a pregnancy test before the next dose. Emergency contraception may also be considered. The amenorrhea caused by DMPA may be concerning to some women who are anxious about pregnancy; therefore, pharmacists should counsel patients that they may experience irregular bleeding for a short period of time, likely followed by a cessation of menstrual bleeding.

SUBCUTANEOUS PROGESTOGEN-ONLY CONTRACEPTIVE

DMPA may also be dosed as a subcutaneous injection with 104 mg injected under the skin of the anterior thigh or abdomen every 3 months. This form is indicated by the FDA for the treatment of endometriosis and for prevention of pregnancy. It is considered as effective as the intramuscular dose and also does not require dosing adjustment for obese women. Despite the lower dose of subcutaneous DMPA (104 vs. 150 mg), no pregnancies occurred among the 44% of study subjects who were overweight (26%) or obese (18%). In fact, there were no pregnancies at all in 720 women over 1 year.[113] It was thought that this formulation would allow women to administer the injection themselves; however, currently the product is still given in the providers' offices. Both intramuscular and subcutaneous DMPA injections may be given by pharmacists in the future. Some states have already piloted programs in which pharmacists provide these services, similar to immunizations.[114]

PROGESTOGEN INTRAUTERINE DEVICE

Another long-term progestogen option for contraception is the levonorgestrel-releasing intrauterine contraceptive (LNG-IUC) marketed under the trade name Mirena® IUS—S stands for system. The device consists of a 32-mm-long, T-shaped polyethylene frame surrounded by a 19-mm-long, white hormonal cylinder around the vertical stem. Within the cylinder is a combination of silicone and 52 mg of levonorgestrel. In addition to the main structure, two monofilament polyethylene threads hang from the cervix for the purposes of control and removal.[96]

The LNG-IUC is indicated for intrauterine contraception for up to 5 years; if further contraception is desired, the system should be replaced at that time. This form of contraception is recommended for women in a stable, mutually monogamous relationship who have given birth to at least one child and are without history and risks of PID and ectopic pregnancy. After placement, the IUC releases 20 mcg of LNG daily, with a progressive decrease to half that value after 5 years of use.[115]

The mechanism of action of the LNG-IUC is unique as compared with other hormonal forms of contraception, in that it does not work through inhibition of ovulation. The actual presence of a foreign body within the uterus prevents implantation and disrupts the endometrial lining. Many women suffered irregular bleeding with nonhormonal IUCs; thus, the LNG-IUC was developed to help minimize bleeding. In addition, high levels of LNG in the endometrial and uterine tissues exert a local effect by thickening the cervical mucus and altering endometrial and tubal fluids, inhibiting sperm motility. Some effect on ovulation has been observed, with studies reporting findings ranging from suppression of ovulation to ovulatory cycles with abnormal follicular growth and rupture.[96,115] When β-human chorionic gonadotropin levels are measured at the end of the menstrual cycle in women using Mirena®, the levels are very low or zero, which suggests that the IUC is successful in preventing fertilization and is not abortifacient.[96]

The LNG-IUC is contraindicated in women with current PID or a history of PID without a successful intrauterine pregnancy, women with a history of or at risk for ectopic pregnancy, women with multiple sexual partners or a single partner who is not monogamous, or those who are immunocompromised with diseases such as acquired immune deficiency syndrome (AIDS), leukemia, or intravenous drug abuse. Women with undiagnosed abnormal Pap tests; cervical, uterine, or breast carcinoma; untreated genital tract infections; or abnormal vaginal bleeding should be advised that contraception with LNG-IUC is not appropriate.[115] Insertion is considered safe for use immediately following a spontaneous or induced abortion, unless an infected abortion has occurred in the previous 3 months.[107] It may also be used beginning at 6 weeks postpartum.[115]

A study surveying more than 24,000 women using the LNG-IUC found that the main reasons for premature removal of the device were excessive bleeding and spotting, infections, and pain.[116] Although spotting is common with initial insertion of the IUC, menstrual bleeding is significantly reduced overall, a beneficial effect for women experiencing iron-deficiency anemia. Expulsion can occur with the IUC, possibly resulting in unwanted pregnancies, especially when used in nulliparous women, those with heavy menstrual bleeding, or women younger than age 20 years. There is a reported 1% to 2.5% risk of pelvic infection with IUC use, with the greatest risk present within the first 20 days following insertion of the device.[106,107]

When counseling patients on proper use of IUCs, be sure to explain the major warning signs using the pneumonic *PAINS*. Patients should be advised to seek medical care immediately when using an IUC if they have **P**eriod late; **A**bdominal pain or pain with intercourse; **I**nfection, abnormal, or odorous vaginal discharge; **N**ot feeling well, fever, chills; **S**tring (missing, shorter, longer).[4]

SUBDERMAL PROGESTOGEN IMPLANT

A new progestogen-releasing subdermal implant is available containing etonogestrel called Implanon. Implanon is a single-rod implant indicated for prevention of pregnancy up to 3 years and containing 68 mg of etonorgestrel, the active metabolite of desogestrel. It releases 60–70 mcg/day in weeks 5 to 6, then drops to 35–45 mcg/day in the first year, 30–40 mcg/day in the second year, and 25–30 mcg/day in the third year.[117] It is inserted subdermally and removed by a trained healthcare provider in an outpatient procedure.

Implanon works by maintaining a sustained release of progestogen, resulting in effective contraception with a smaller daily dose than other routes.[118] In addition to the lower doses of hormone, advantages of implants include no reliance on patient compliance and a rapid return to fertility, with ovulation occurring in more than 90% of women within 6 weeks of removal.[106] Like other progestogen contraceptives, implants suppress ovulation and thicken the cervical mucus. Progestogen levels can be detected in the serum within hours of implant insertion, and ovulation may be inhibited within the first day of use.[119]

Implanon should be placed in ovulating women sometime between days 1 and 5 of the onset of menses. If a patient is currently using oral contraceptives, DMPA, or an IUC, placement of Implanon can occur at any time without regard to menses.[106] These

CASE PRESENTATION

Patient Case: Part 2

K.R. is in need of a reliable contraceptive method with a reasonable return to fertility time. She has a history of depression and adult acne. Her family history is positive for hypertension and stroke. She is a nonsmoker and is getting married soon. She is using sulfur 2% face wash, along with benzoyl peroxide 2.5% cream and Retin-A Micro when tolerated.

Recommendation:

- Low-dose COC with lower androgenic properties, such as YAZ (ethinyl estradiol/drospirenone), Alesse (ethinyl estradiol/levonorgestrel), Yasmin (ethinyl estradiol/drospirenone), or Ortho Tri-Cyclen Lo (ethinyl estradiol/norgestimate)
- Recommend a pregnancy test, and, if negative, begin with the quick-start method. Patient is in the office now and would like to start contraception.
- Counsel patient on side effects, ACHES, and that side effects will likely lessen after 3 months if any should occur.

Rationale: Patient has a history of depression, so progestogen-only contraceptives should be avoided, such as the minipill, DMPA, etonorgestrel implant, and LNG-IUS. In particular, DMPA would not be a good option because of its irreversibility of administration and reports of serious depression. In addition, the patient desires to have children in the future and would a like quick return to fertility when desired. Again, DMPA would not be a good choice because of its delayed return to fertility. CHCs have a quick return to fertility and would be a good choice. The patient has a family history of hypertension and stroke, and therefore the contraceptive patch may not be the best choice for the patient because the patch delivers higher amounts of estrogen. The vaginal ring is a good option in this patient; however, patient is uncomfortable touching genitalia, so something inserted vaginally is not ideal. The patient also suffers from acne; a hormonal contraceptive agent with low androgenic properties may help alleviate her acne as well.

Monitoring and follow-up: Side effects of CHCs, ACHES; follow-up in 2–3 months to check blood pressure and evaluate side effects and patient satisfaction with method.

Patient education: Start today. Take one tablet by mouth at the same time daily. Talk to your doctor if you experience any of the following: abdominal pain, chest pain, headaches, eye pain or double vision, any swelling in the legs, or difficulty breathing. Take one tablet now, and use a backup method, such as condoms and spermicide, until you get your period; then discontinue the backup method if you desire. Birth control pills do not protect against STIs and HIV. If you experience nausea, take your tablet at bedtime or with food. Discuss proper protocol for missed tablets in the cycle.

guidelines are in place to better ensure that placement of an implant does not occur early in pregnancy or too late to prevent pregnancy within the first cycle of use.

Implanon is quite effective, with a typical use failure rate of 0.5%.[117] The most common reason for discontinuation of either implant was prolonged and irregular bleeding.[118] Clinical studies, however, excluded women who were 130% over their ideal body weight.[117] Therefore, use in obese women is not well studied. Adverse effects reported were similar to those of other progestogen contraceptives: swelling and irritation at site for a few days after implantation. The implant may be used as early as 4 weeks postpartum, including in lactating mothers.

Summary

A variety of hormonal contraceptive options are available. Selection of the appropriate contraceptive method is crucial for successful outcomes. Health-care providers taking into consideration factors such as accessibility, adherence, ease of use, cost, return to fertility, past medical history, and side-effect profile should be able to help tailor contraceptive methods to meet the needs of individual women. Proper education and counseling for initiation and contraceptive mishaps is also key to appropriate use and achieving optimal outcomes.

References

Additional content available at
www.ashp.org/womenshealth

20 Emergency Contraception

Don Downing, R.Ph.; Deborah A. Sturpe, Pharm.D., BCPS

Learning Objectives

1. Discuss three possible mechanisms of action by which hormonal contraception works, and identify the mechanism that is likely responsible for most of emergency contraception's activity.
2. Compare and contrast progestin-only emergency contraception to combined hormonal emergency contraception.
3. Explain how emergency contraception is provided in the U.S. under dual-label package regulations as both a prescription and nonprescription product.
4. Describe the role that healthcare providers can play in the provision of emergency contraception and follow-up services for women/men requesting it.

Emergency contraception (EC) is a **postcoital** form of contraception. When a woman recognizes that her regular contraceptive method has failed or if she has not used any method of contraception, EC can be used to prevent an **unintended pregnancy.**[1,2] In the U.S., three types of EC may be recommended. These include a combination hormone regimen containing an estrogen and progestin (often referred to as the Yuzpe method), progestin-only regimens, and the copper **intrauterine device** (IUD). A levonorgestrel-releasing intrauterine system is also available in the U.S., but this IUD is not used for EC purposes. Although the antiprogestin mifepristone (sometimes referred to as RU-486) has been studied in low doses for use as an EC agent, the drug is not available for such use in the U.S., and will not be discussed further in this chapter.

Unintended pregnancies are common in the U.S., with 1 in 20 women between the ages of 15 and 44 reporting an unintended pregnancy even with the availability of many safe contraceptive options (Chapter 18: Family Planning and Nonhormonal Contraception and Chapter 19: Hormonal Contraception).[3] The percentage of women using contraception who experience an unintended pregnancy illustrates the imperfect nature of contraceptive use in the U.S.[4] Typical use of these contraceptives results in varying rates of unintended pregnancies within 1 year of use for the following methods (% unintended pregnancy): condoms (15% male, 21% female); spermicides (29%); diaphragm (16%); oral contraceptives, Evra Patch™, and Nuva Ring™ (8%); and spermicides (29%).

The Centers for Disease Control and Prevention reports that in 2006, the birth rate of children born to women 15–19 years old rose 3% after a 14-year decline, underscoring the need for birth control education and access.[5] The health and education consequences of unintended pregnancies negatively affect the children of those pregnancies, their families, and the greater community, with approximately 50% of all unintended pregnancies in the U.S. resulting in an elective abortion. Women who have unintended pregnancies are less likely to continue their education and are 3 times as likely to become victims of interpersonal violence.[3,6] In an Oregon study with women matched for age and education, women not aware of EC were more likely to have an unintended pregnancy than those who were aware of EC.[7] Unintended pregnancies are a public health issue, and EC can play a part in ameliorating this problem. It has been estimated that when used properly, EC could prevent approximately 2 million unwanted pregnancies and 1 million abortions each year.[8]

There are many things that contribute to lack of use of highly effective contraception and contraceptive failures. Lack of patient education, lack of access to available pharmacies and clinics, existing cultural beliefs, restrictive government regulations and prescription requirements, confusing and limiting 30-day insurance coverage, nonevidence-based medical exam requirements, user or product failure of contraceptive methods, and healthcare and medication costs are common factors that increase the need for EC to be available to appropriate users.[9]

History of Emergency Contraception

EC has been used in the U.S. for more than 35 years. Canadian physician and researcher Dr. A. Albert Yuzpe first described the postcoital use of combination hormonal contraceptives containing levonorgestrel and ethinyl estradiol in the early 1970s. A levonorgestrel-only product has been available in the U.S. since 1999. EC had received little media attention and use until a progestin-only postcoital contraceptive, levonorgestrel 0.75 mg (Plan B®/OTC EC) was approved by the U.S. Food and Drug Administration (FDA) as the first over-the-counter (OTC) hormonal contraceptive available in the U.S.[10,11] EC is most effective when taken as soon as possible after unprotected sex.[12] Figure 20-1 shows how the **combined hormonal regimen** compares with the levonorgestrel regimen over 72 hours from the time of unprotected intercourse.

When Plan B® was the only dedicated OTC EC product available, it was provided to consumers without a prescription through a unique agreement made between the FDA and DuraMed Pharmaceuticals, Inc.[13] This agreement involved a program named the CARE program (Convenient Access, Responsible Education), for which DuraMed Pharmaceuticals had agreed to sell Plan B® only behind the counter to consumers eligible for OTC EC and only via a prescription for consumers ineligible for OTC EC purchasing. As part of the CARE program, pharmacists, physicians, and consumers were provided educational programs about EC, and pharmacies were monitored to ensure that they were providing Plan B® only to those eligible to receive it without a prescription.

The Plan B® product was dual labeled for OTC and prescription-only use. DuraMed filed three applications to the FDA, beginning in 2003, to make Plan B® available without a prescription. The initial filing was to make Plan B® OTC for women of all ages, but this was rejected. It was followed by a second request for OTC access by women 16 and older, which was also rejected. Finally, a third application was filed for OTC access by women 17 and older. This third application was accepted by

Figure 20-1. Pregnancy rate vs. day of administration.

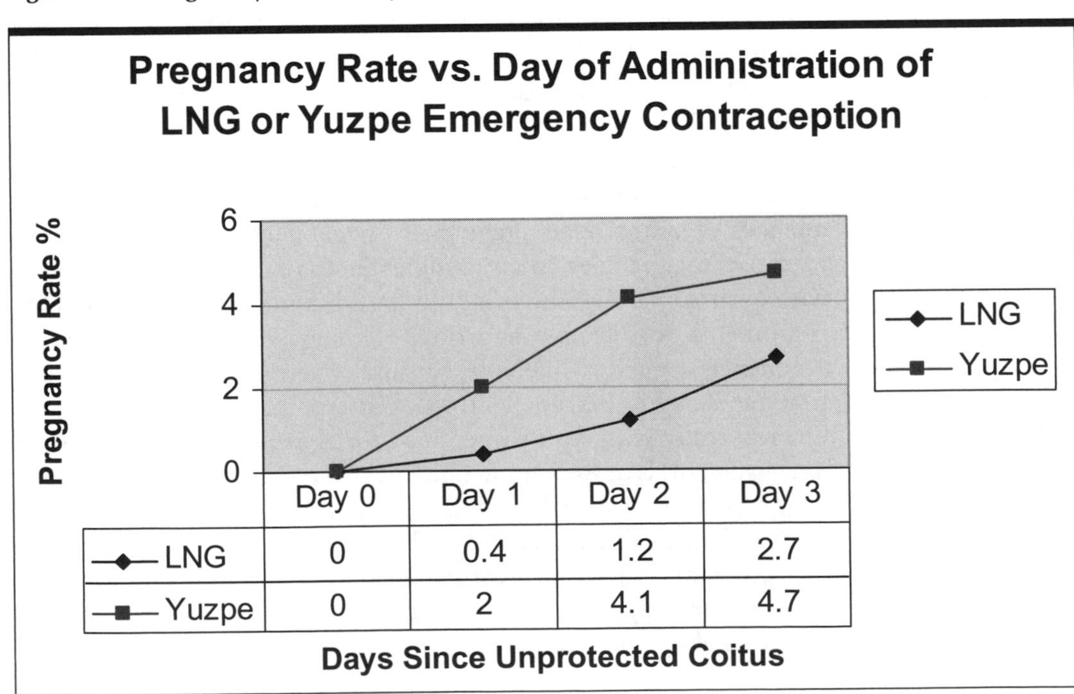

	Day 0	Day 1	Day 2	Day 3
LNG	0	0.4	1.2	2.7
Yuzpe	0	2	4.1	4.7

the FDA commissioner, but the decision was made to limit nonprescription status to women 18 and older. On March 23, 2009, the U.S. District Court for the Eastern District of New York issued a ruling that ordered the FDA to provide OTC Plan B® access to 17-year-old women within 30 days and to investigate the lifting of any age restriction. At the time of this chapter's publication, the FDA and Teva (which purchased DuraMed in December 2008) had changed the OTC Plan B® package labeling and wrote "Dear Doctor/Pharmacist" letters to inform providers of the new OTC access for women age 17 and older. Teva has now replaced the original Plan B® with Plan B® One-Step, a product that combines the original two 0.75-mg Plan B® tablets into a single dose, 1.5-mg levonorgestrel tablet. In June 2009, a new branded generic of the original Plan B® product became available as Next Choice® and thus consists of two 0.75-mg tablets of levonorgestrel. Both of these new products are available OTC for patients providing identification of age 17 or older. Currently those age 16 and younger require a prescription for these EC products.

CASE PRESENTATION

Patient Case: Part 1

J.G. is a 25-year-old sexually active woman who presents to the pharmacy today with a concern that she may be at risk of an unintended pregnancy. She's heard that there's something she can use to prevent becoming pregnant.

HPI: She indicates that she has been using oral contraceptives as her primary contraceptive and male condoms as a contraceptive backup and sexually transmitted infection preventative. Last night, after sex, her partner indicated that the condom had slipped off during sex. She realized this morning that she had missed the first 2 days of her new cycle of birth control pills. She has not had sex at any other time since her last period.

PMH: Frequent migraine headaches.

Medications: Ethinyl estradiol 20 mcg/levonorgestrel 0.1 mg (Aviane™) PO daily.

Allergies: NKDA.

Objective data: Not available.

Clinical Presentation

POSTCOITAL PRESENTATIONS

Most women currently seek EC after they realize that their contraceptive method has failed or after they have not used any contraceptive method and wish to avoid becoming pregnant. Because EC is more effective the sooner it is used after unprotected sex, it is imperative that women have access to EC at all times and that women are aware of the need to use EC as soon as possible.[14] Access to EC may be hindered by delays in contacting a pharmacist or other healthcare provider and by professional and medication costs. Studies in Washington State and California show that more than 40% of all pharmacy requests for EC occur at times when access to other healthcare providers is often very limited, such as weekends, evenings, and holidays.[15] Public and private insurance coverage for EC is also extremely variable. For example, in some states, Medicaid will cover both prescription and OTC EC, whereas in other states, neither is covered.

IMMEDIATE PROVISION OF EMERGENCY CONTRACEPTION

Women and men routinely present to community and ambulatory pharmacies and medical clinics requesting a postcoital contraceptive. They commonly ask for "the morning-after pill," Plan B®, EC, or they describe their situation and ask for assistance. Many patients self-refer, whereas others are directed to pharmacies and clinics by friends, family members, or healthcare providers. As of November 2006, and using the guidelines set forth by the FDA and the CARE program, women and men in the U.S. who are at least 18 years of age and have proper age identification have been able to acquire Plan B® without a prescription from behind the pharmacy counter. In this scenario, the ultimate user of OTC EC may or may not be the purchaser, thus the end user may not be known to the pharmacist dispensing the product. Additionally, as with all OTC products, no medical documentation or counseling is required at the time of dispensing.

OTC availability of the drug has helped to increase likelihood of quick access for women. However, if OTC EC is unavailable, either because the product itself is unavailable or the purchaser is younger than 17 years of age or doesn't have appropriate identification,

Table 20-1. Oral Contraceptives That Can Be Used for Emergency Contraception in the United States[a]

Brand	Company	First Dose[b]	Second Dose (12 hr later)	Ethinyl Estradiol per Dose (mcg)	Levonorgestrel per Dose (mg)[b]
Combined progestin and estrogen pills					
Alesse	Wyeth-Ayerst	five pink pills	five pink pills	100	0.50
Aviane	Barr/Duramed	five orange pills	five orange pills	100	0.50
Cryselle	Barr/Duramed	four white pills	four white pills	120	0.60
Enpresse	Barr/Duramed	four orange pills	four orange pills	120	0.50
Jolessa	Barr/Duramed	four pink pills	four pink pills	120	0.60
Lessina	Barr/Duramed	five pink pills	five pink pills	100	0.50
Levlen	Berlex	four light-orange pills	four light-orange pills	120	0.60
Levlite	Berlex	five pink pills	five pink pills	100	0.50
Levora	Watson	four white pills	four white pills	120	0.60
Lo/Ovral	Wyeth-Ayerst	four white pills	four white pills	120	0.60
Low-Ogestrel	Watson	four white pills	four white pills	120	0.60
Lutera	Watson	five white pills	five white pills	100	0.50
Nordette	Wyeth-Ayerst	four light-orange pills	four light-orange pills	120	0.60
Ogestrel	Watson	two white pills	two white pills	100	0.50
Ovral	Wyeth-Ayerst	two white pills	two white pills	100	0.50
Portia	Barr/Duramed	four pink pills	four pink pills	120	0.60
Quasense	Watson	four white pills	four white pills	120	0.60
Seasonale	Barr/Duramed	four pink pills	four pink pills	120	0.60
Seasonique	Barr/Duramed	four light-blue-green pills	four light-blue-green pills	120	0.60
Tri-Levlen	Berlex	four yellow pills	four yellow pills	120	0.50
Triphasil	Wyeth-Ayerst	four yellow pills	four yellow pills	120	0.50
Trivora	Watson	four pink pills	four pink pills	120	0.50

[a]Plan B® is the only dedicated product specifically marketed for EC. Alesse, Aviane, Cryselle, Enpresse, Jolessa, Lessina, Levlen, Levlite, Levora, Lo/Ovral, Low-Ogestrel, Lutera, Nordette, Ogestrel, Ovral, Portia, Quasense, Seasonale, Seasonique, Tri-Levlen, Triphasil, and Trivora have been declared safe and effective for use as EC pills by the United States Food and Drug Administration. Outside the U.S., more than 50 EC products are specifically packaged, labeled, and marketed. For example, Gedeon Richter and HRA Pharma are marketing in many countries the levonorgestrel-only products Postinor-2 and NorLevo, respectively, each consisting of a two-pill strip with each pill containing 0.75 mg levonorgestrel. Levonorgestrel-only EC pills are available either over-the-counter or from a pharmacist without having to see a healthcare provider in 43 countries.

[b]The progestin in Cryselle, Lo/Ovral, Low-Ogestrel, Ogestrel, and Ovral is norgestrel, which contains two isomers, only one of which (levonorgestrel) is bioactive; the amount of norgestrel in each tablet is twice the amount of levonorgestrel.

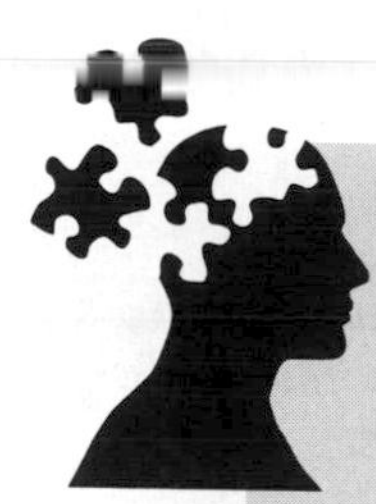

Therapeutic Challenge:

What issues should be considered when providing EC to minors, sexual assault victims, and patients with repeat requests?

then a prescription for either a "combined hormonal regimen" (Table 20-1), or another levonorgestrel-only EC product is indicated. In such cases, and in cases of a pharmacist's refusal to provide EC, a timely referral to another pharmacy or medical clinic that can provide EC or a prescription for EC is necessary to ensure that the woman has appropriate access to contraception.

It is not uncommon for EC prescriptions to allow multiple refills or for women to request EC multiple times. Women may need EC right away and desire to have additional EC available in advance of need. It may be prudent for healthcare providers to ask a woman who uses EC repeatedly if she is satisfied with her regular form of contraception and to assist the woman in obtaining a better contraceptive if appropriate. It is critical to assist women in attaining all EC that they request as they may be using EC to back up other forms of birth control or they may be victims of multiple sexual assaults (i.e., incest, rape).

Lack of knowledge regarding EC among healthcare practitioners may limit a woman's access to therapy because of reluctance of providers to recommend, prescribe, dispense, or administer therapy. Before EC was available as an OTC agent, studies suggested that prescribing rates of EC to appropriate candidates was low.[16-18] Surveys of pediatricians, family medicine physicians/residents, and pharmacists have all demonstrated that gaps exist in these practitioners' knowledge regarding EC mechanism, efficacy, timing of use, side effects, contraindications, and requirements for prescribing.[19-21] Such misperceptions may create barriers to provision of EC to women, especially if therapy is inappropriately withheld. Consequently, it is important that all healthcare providers are educated about EC so they can make informed decisions about care.

Pathophysiology

CONCEPTION AND PREGNANCY

There are a number of steps in the mechanism of conception, and only a few will be outlined here to identify processes that are interrupted with the timely use of EC. After coitus, sperm must travel through the cervix. Not all sperm travel through the cervix immediately, and millions migrate into the uterine cavity many hours after coitus. In order for ovulation to occur, a surge in the level of luteinizing hormone (LH) must occur when the dominant follicle is at the right size and level of maturity. If LH is mistimed or the surge level is blunted or totally suppressed, then fertilization is not possible.

The physiologic and legal definition of pregnancy can vary based on organizational, religious, or cultural views. For example, in their human subject guidance, the Department of Health and Human Services states that "pregnancy encompasses the period of time from implantation until delivery, while other groups define pregnancy and life as starting at conception.[22,23]

MECHANISM OF ACTION OF EMERGENCY CONTRACEPTION

The mechanism of action of EC regimens has been the subject of many studies dating back to the 1960s.[24] Proposed mechanisms of action (i.e., those listed in the Plan B® package insert) include inhibition of ovulation, inhibition of fertilization, and inhibition of implantation. However, many of the earlier studies employed combined hormonal contraceptives using various dosing regimens. More recent studies have aimed to establish the mechanism of action of short-duration EC with a particular focus on levonorgestrel-only regimens.[25-27] These studies suggest that the primary mechanism of action of levonorgestrel-only EC is the inhibition or delay of ovulation.[28]

Combined Hormonal and Progestin-only Regimens

When taken before the LH surge and before the dominant follicle approaches 18 mm in diameter, levonorgestrel has been shown to be effective in preventing follicular rupture (ovulation) (Figure 20-2).[27] By delaying ovulation, either the LH surge may be mistimed with regard to follicular maturation or ovulation is mistimed with regard to presence of viable sperm. Women taking EC who have delayed ovulation may be vulnerable to pregnancy if unprotected sex occurs again later in the woman's menstrual cycle. When taken before the start of the LH surge, levonorgestrel has also been shown to blunt or eliminate this surge, depending on the timing of the dose relative to the onset of the surge. LH surge inhibition in turn has been linked to failure of sperm to be capacitated, rendering them incapable of fertilization. Levonorgestrel has also been shown to quickly increase cervical mucus and to prevent significant numbers of sperm from passing through the cervix.[28,29] EC taken immediately after coitus has been shown to prevent the migration of later sperm by thickening cervical mucus. EC also causes the alkalinization of the uterine cavity, which causes the loss of viable sperm. Delayed consumption of EC may allow viable sperm to reach the fallopian tubes and for the fertilization process to begin.

Current FDA-approved labeling for EC includes inhibition of implantation as a possible mechanism. Although the mechanisms of interference by EC in the fertilization process itself and implantation cannot be excluded, recent studies with levonorgestrel-only EC suggest that inhibition of fertilization and postfertilization effects are much less likely than interference with ovulation. Although the precise mechanism of action of EC remains controversial, EC clearly does not interfere with a pregnancy once implantation has occurred. Ironically, progestins may increase the ability of a fertilized egg to implant and are used for this purpose in in vitro fertilization procedures.[28]

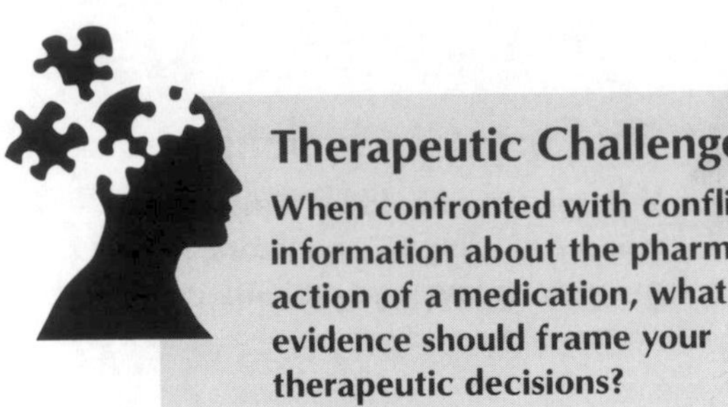

Therapeutic Challenge:

When confronted with conflicting information about the pharmacologic action of a medication, what evidence should frame your therapeutic decisions?

Copper Intrauterine Device

The copper IUD acts primarily as a spermicidal agent.[30,31] Copper ions released from the device are directly toxic to spermatozoa and create an inflammatory response within the uterus that results in additional sperm phagocytosis. Current evidence suggests that the likelihood of the copper IUD causing postfertilization effects is lower than generally acknowledged in the past, when only nonhuman studies were available; however, prevention of implantation of a fertilized egg is possible.[30] This may be more likely when the copper IUD is used for EC during the first month of insertion.[31]

Figure 20-2. Emergency contraception effectiveness throughout menstrual cycle.

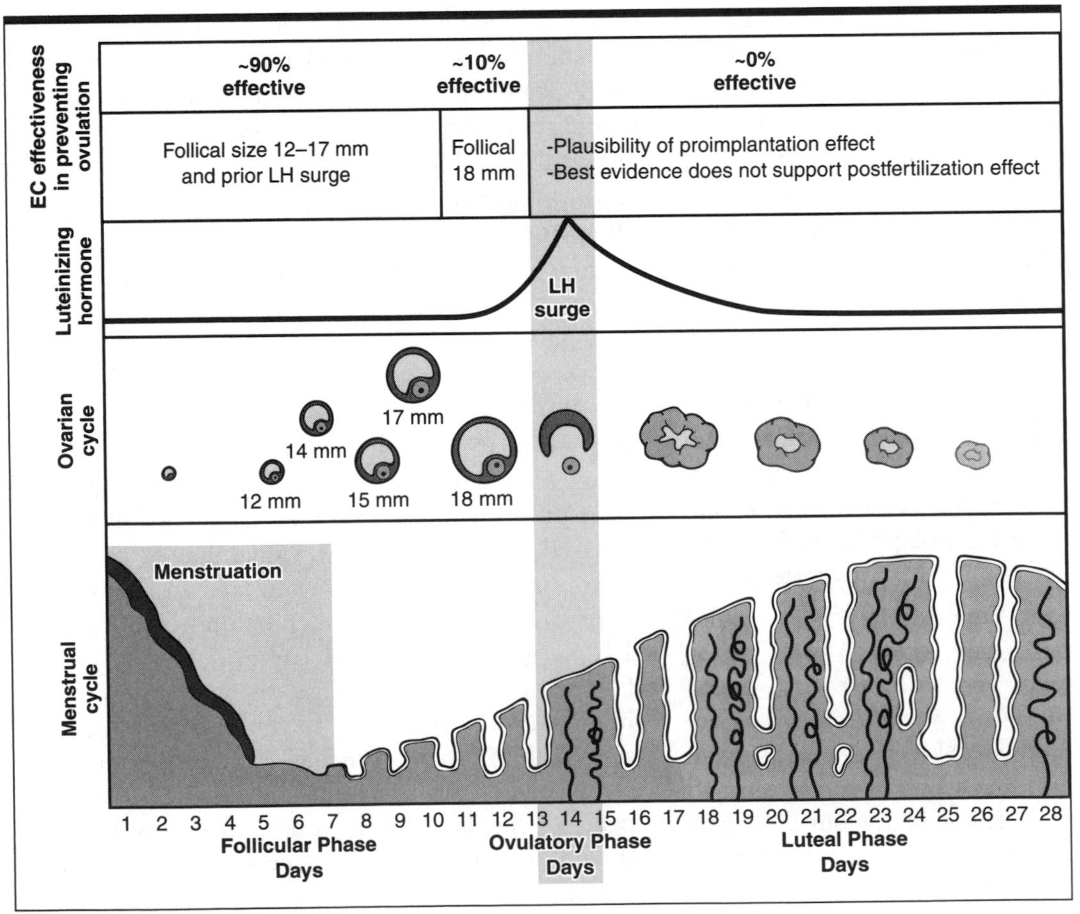

Nonsteroidal Anti-inflammatory Drugs

Nonsteroidal anti-inflammatory drugs (NSAIDs) are not currently indicated for EC use. However, interest in using NSAIDs in combination with other EC agents is a current area of research.[31] Most failures of levonorgestrel-only EC products to prevent pregnancy are thought to happen when the EC is taken after the LH surge has already occurred. Because follicular maturation and rupture are dependent on locally synthesized prostaglandins with COX-2 catalyzing the final step of prostaglandin synthesis, it has been hypothesized that NSAIDs might improve the effectiveness of hormonal EC.

Long-term Complications

There have been no long-term complications associated with EC regimens. There are no evidence-based contraindications to levonorgestrel-only EC, and combined hormonal regimens are only relatively contraindicated in women with a history of migraine headaches because of this regimen's estrogen content. Consequently, women with a history of venous thromboembolism and/or who are taking anticoagulants, who are smokers of any age, who have migraines, and who are taking seizure medications are not necessarily inappropriate candidates for EC, especially if the levonorgestrel-only option is chosen. In fact, EC for these at-risk women may prevent serious consequences of pregnancy. Pregnancy is a stated contraindication to EC, not because of known harm to the fetus or integrity of the pregnancy, but rather because there is no medical indication to take EC while pregnant.

Detection, Screening, and Diagnosis

EC is indicated in a number of situations involving unprotected intercourse. Women who are not prepared to have sex—such as in cases of rape, incest, or consumption of intoxicants—are candidates for EC use. Contraceptive or user failure of various contraceptive methods may also warrant EC. Examples include women using condoms that break or slip or who use vaginal diaphragms that develop a hole or fall out of position. Women using oral contraceptives who have missed two or more pills in a row or who start a new pack of pills 2 or more days late are candidates for EC. Women who use the Ortho Evra™ transdermal contraceptive patch may consider EC use when the patch is off the skin for more than 24 hours during a "patch-on" week, who leave the patch on more than 9 straight days, or who are more than 2 days late in putting their patch back on after the placebo week. Similarly, women using the NuvaRing™ vaginal contraceptive ring who have removed the ring for more than 3 hours during the "ring-in" weeks (accidental or purposeful), who have left the ring in more than 5 weeks in a row, or who are more than 2 days late in putting the ring in after the placebo week are candidates for EC.

Guidelines and Position Statements

The American College of Obstetricians and Gynecologists (ACOG) and American Academy of Pediatrics (AAP) have written specific guidelines or policy statements regarding use of EC.[1,33] Summary recommendations from both groups are similar and include preference for levonorgestrel-only EC because of improved efficacy and tolerability over the combined hormonal method, administration of both levonorgestrel-only pills together rather than 12 hours apart, widening the access-time window for EC administration from 72 hours after unprotected or inadequately protected intercourse to 120 hours after intercourse, and consideration for advanced provision of EC to patients. The AAP statement also addresses concerns over increased risky sexual behavior in teenage patients given access to EC by verifying that such concerns are not supported by available evidence.

ACOG and AAP, along with the American Public Health Association (APHA), have long supported increased access to EC for patients. Thus, all three organizations have strongly advocated for OTC status of levonorgestrel-only EC. The three organizations have acknowledged that the FDA decision to approve levonorgestrel-only EC as OTC for patients aged 18 and older is a "step in the right direction" but express concerns that the access barrier still exists for younger patients.[34-36] ACOG, AAP, and APHA all support expansion of OTC access to include teenage patients.

ADVANCE PROVISION OF EMERGENCY CONTRACEPTION

EC may be acquired in advance of need, and studies suggest that advance provision of EC increases the likelihood that a woman will use EC (2–4 times more frequently in five studies and no significant difference in two others) and decreases the time between the act of unprotected sex and ingestion of EC without increasing risky sexual behaviors, such as decreased condom use.[37-40] Healthcare providers should be prepared to offer EC in advance of need and be willing to dispense more than one package of product at a time. Special care should be given to informing these patients about the expiration dates on advance provided products so that patients don't mistakenly take an expired and possibly ineffective product. Although sexually active women capable of becoming pregnant should be offered EC in advance of need, women using routine forms of contraception with high failure rates (e.g., barrier methods) are ideal candidates for advance provision.

CONSCIENTIOUS OBJECTION

The issue of conscientious objection is one of national interest with regard to EC (Chapter 2: Race, Ethnic, and Religious Issues). Interestingly, a number of states have specifically cited EC when crafting language in bills designed to prevent prosecution of healthcare providers who refuse to be involved in the provision of abortions.[41] Some of these bills make an exception to this protection from prosecution if there is a medical emergency or if the refusal to provide EC results in harm to the patient. Additionally, most national pharmacy chains have developed policies that attempt to balance the rights of patients to access EC with the conscientious objection rights of pharmacy workers. National pharmacy organizations have also crafted policy statements regarding conscientious objection by a pharmacist.[42] Pharmacists also should consider any existing state standards of practice when providing EC for women who declare their need and interest in acquiring it.

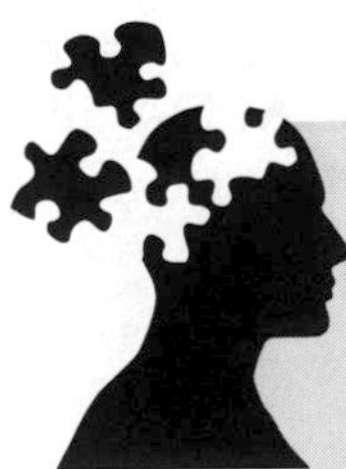

Therapeutic Challenge:

What are the laws and regulations around dispensing EC in the state or country in which you live? What is the standard of practice in providing EC in your community, state, or country?

Treatment Goals

The only treatment goal of EC is to prevent pregnancy. However, healthcare providers should be aware of the possible concurrent need for sexually transmitted infection (STI) assessment and treatment, long-term contraceptive counseling, or referral to appropriate care when rape or incest is suspected.

Pharmacologic Therapy

PROGESTIN ONLY

EC in the U.S. may refer to either the combined hormonal regimen or a levonorgestrel-only regimen, but the levonorgestrel-only regimen has been shown to be more effective and to have fewer side effects than the combined hormonal regimen.[2] Trials have shown that levonorgestrel 0.75 mg taken as soon as possible after sex and again 12 hours later can reduce the expected pregnancy rate by up to 89%. However, some more recent studies have questioned these data, and a meta-analysis of available trials showed reductions of pregnancy rates closer to 50%. None of the studies showed significant differences in pregnancy rates between groups of those provided EC in advance of need and those provided EC postcoitally.[40] These studies have shown that 64% to 79% of women with ready access to EC did not take it every time they had unprotected intercourse. Many women in these studies who falsely thought that they were not at risk of a pregnancy did not take EC and became pregnant.[40,43] In conclusion, these studies indicate that women who take EC after unprotected intercourse have approximately a 50% to 89% chance of preventing a pregnancy. Populations of women given EC in advance of need do not differ in their pregnancy rates from women without advance access, in part because of a failure in both groups to take EC each time they have unprotected sex. It is important when looking at these effectiveness studies to understand if the study is powered to look at EC effectiveness when an individual actually takes it appropriately or if the study is looking at groups of women who may or may not be taking EC after unprotected intercourse.

Although the combined hormonal regimens are routinely taken as two doses, 12 hours apart, and partially prevent a greater incidence and nausea and vomiting, considering their estrogen content, levonorgestrel has been studied as the FDA-approved, two 12-hour apart 0.75-mg dose regimen and as a recently approved single dose of 1.5 mg.[14,44] The dose can be administered either by instructing the woman to take both 0.75-mg pills of the Plan B® or Next Choice® product at one time, taking a single Plan B® One-Step tablet, or through the use of "mini pills" containing 30 mcg of levonorgestrel per tablet. The regimen consists of consuming 50 tablets at once.[45] Both regimens have been shown to be safe and equally effective, and a single dose of 1.5 mg prevents the difficulty of a patient having to take the second dose at a difficult time of the day for good adherence. Data also suggest that if traditional dosing of every 12 hours is chosen and the patient forgets to take the second pill, administration of the second dose anytime within 24 hours of the first dose is likely to result in equal efficacy.[44] The incidence of side effects are less with levonorgestrel-only regimens as compared with combined hormonal methods, with the World Health Organization study showing the incidence of nausea being 23% (vs. 51% combined hormonal) and vomiting 6% (vs. 19%). Other side effects include dizziness (11%) and fatigue (17%). Rarely do women find that they need to take an antiemetic before taking a levonorgestrel-only EC, and generally none is recommended.

COMBINED HORMONAL

All combination hormonal contraceptive products used as EC in the U.S. contain 100–120 mcg of ethinyl estradiol and 0.50–0.60 mg of levonorgestrel activity per dose and are given as a two-dose regimen taken 12 hours apart.[46] Currently available combination oral contraceptive products that can be used to provide "combined hormonal regimen" EC are shown in Table 20-1. This regimen has been shown to reduce the risk of pregnancy by up to 75% when used within 72 hours of unprotected sex.[2,8,47,48] The most common side effects of the combined hormonal regimen are nausea (51%) and vomiting (19%). Heavy menses, fatigue, and breast tenderness also occur. One randomized controlled trial that enrolled 343 women found that pretreatment with an OTC antiemetic (meclizine 50 mg) significantly reduced the incidence of nausea and vomiting associated with the combined hormonal regimen.[49] The antiemetic should be taken 30–60 minutes before taking each of the two combined hormonal regimen doses. This would mean a patient starting EC at 3:00 PM would need to take meclizine at 2:00 PM, EC at 3:00 PM, and then repeating this process at 2:00 AM and 3:00 AM. Adherence to this therapy may be difficult for most patients, but counseling a patient to start taking EC at a later time (say 10:00 PM, repeated at 10:00 AM) puts the patient at a greater risk of an unintended pregnancy because of its declining efficacy over time after unprotected sex.

A World Health Organization trial and others have shown that both combined hormonal and levonorgestrel-only EC regimens have diminishing effectiveness over time.[12] Although these studies show that effectiveness does not drop to zero after 72 hours and, in fact, EC may be somewhat effective up to 120 hours after sex, the sooner they are taken after sex, the more likely a pregnancy will be prevented.[50,51]

NONSTEROIDAL ANTI-INFLAMMATORY DRUGS

A small, pilot contraceptive efficacy study was performed in 41 women that investigated the effect of adding meloxicam, a COX-2 inhibitor, to a levonorgestrel-only EC regimen.[32] This study showed that the overall proportion of cycles with no follicular rupture or with ovulatory dysfunction increased significantly from 66% to 88% by the addition of meloxicam to levonorgestrel. Despite this apparent positive result, additional data are needed before routinely advising women to use NSAIDs in combination with EC pills.

COPPER IUD

The copper IUD, which acts through pharmacologic and mechanical mechanisms, may be used as EC if inserted within 5 days after any unprotected sexual intercourse. This time frame may be extended to 8 days if ovulation is known to have occurred more than 3 days after unprotected sex.[1,31] Unfortunately, the date of ovulation is often unknown and can only be estimated for most women. Failure rates of IUD insertion for EC is estimated to be <1%.[31] Because of the high cost of this product in the U.S. this form of EC is best reserved for patients who desire long-term continuance of contraception with the device.

Monitoring and Follow-up

Although there are no absolute requirements for monitoring or following up with women after EC use, there are a number of compelling reasons to refer women for additional care and to provide as much follow-up as reasonably possible, recognizing

Table 20-2. National Emergency Contraception Hotlines and Information Resources

Emergency Contraception Hotline: 1-888-NOT2LATE (1-888-668-2528)
Run by the Reproductive Health Technologies Project, this hotline provides prerecorded information about EC and gives the names and phone numbers of places where you can get EC. www.not-2-late.org.
National Sexual Assault Hotline: 1-800-656-HOPE (1-800-656-4673)
A 24-hour national hotline for victims of sexual abuse, operated by Rape, Abuse and Incest National Network (RAINN).
National Domestic Violence Hotline: 1-800-799-7233 /1-800-787-3224 TTY
A 24-hour national hotline for victims of domestic violence and those who are concerned about them.
Pharmacy Access Partnership: info@pharmacyaccess.org or call (510) 272-0150
Pharmacy Access Partnership was established in 1999. Its purpose is to expand consumer access to contraceptive commodities and reproductive health services in pharmacies, and to give pharmacies a stronger role in promoting community health. http://www.pharmacyaccess.org.

that most EC provided at this time is sold OTC and not necessarily sold to the ultimate consumer of the product. EC clients who are concerned that they may have been exposed to an STI or when a pharmacist recognizes that the woman may have been exposed to an STI should be prepared to make a meaningful referral to an appropriate medical provider who is geographically and financially accessible to the woman. A provider counseling a woman who repeatedly requests EC should inquire as to the woman's satisfaction with her current method of contraception, if any (other than EC), and either make a referral or, as is possible in some states, initiate ongoing contraceptive prescriptions.[52] Providers should also look for signs of abuse or coercion that might be abated by an aware and sensitive care provider. Local and national contact information for victims of sexual assault should be posted in the pharmacy (Table 20-2).

Patient Education

Ideally, healthcare providers should provide private, nonjudgmental, verbal and written information to all women and men who seek EC. One useful tool is a basic EC information handout prepared for all purchasers (Figure 20-3). Women should be counseled that EC does not prevent STIs, that if her menstrual cycle does not start within 3 weeks of taking EC she should confirm that she is not pregnant, that EC is not 100% effective, and that more effective contraceptive options should be considered if not already used or are being used suboptimally. Women using the levonorgestrel-only EC regimen should be counseled to take both pills at one time and warned about possible nausea, vomiting, and tiredness. If the combined hormonal regimen is recommended, pharmacists should counsel women to take an antiemetic before use. It is also important to remind women that future acts of intercourse are not protected against pregnancy by the current EC regimen.[1] Because EC (like all hormonal contraceptives) may potentially interfere with implantation, women taking this product should be informed of this possibility in case they have personal or religious beliefs that might preclude use of such products.

Healthcare providers should also discuss advance provision of EC with women seeking it for current postcoital use. However, many women in EC studies who had ready access to EC did not take it during the cycle in which they became pregnant; thus, it is important to also counsel women of the circumstances in which they may be at risk of an unintended pregnancy and the importance of using an ongoing form of contraception that they can adhere to or requires little or no attention to adherence (i.e., IUDs, implants).[43]

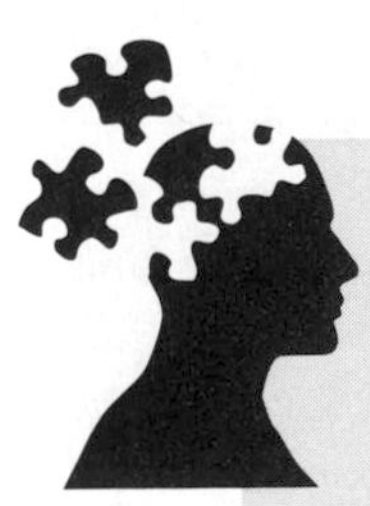

Therapeutic Challenge:

You work in the only pharmacy in town and you do not have Plan B®. How would you advise a woman who seeks EC urgently?

Figure 20-3. Emergency contraception patient instructions.

Emergency Contraception (EC)— Patient Instructions for Use

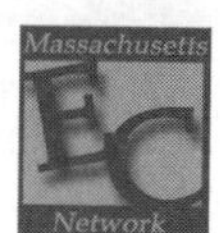

(For use if EC is provided under a standing order, as a prescription, or over-the-counter)

Instructions:

Take the first dose of Emergency Contraception (EC) as soon as possible after unprotected sex.
The medication works within the first 5 days after unprotected sex.

You have been given:

☐ Plan B

- ☐ Take 1 pill as soon as possible followed by 1 pill in 12 hours
- ☐ Take 2 pills as soon as possible

To prevent nausea, you may take ____________________.* Take this medication **1 hour before** you take the first dose of EC.

Side effects may include

- **Nausea**
  - EC makes some women feel sick to their stomach. You can take the recommended medication (see above *) 1 hour before you take the first dose of EC to prevent nausea.
- **Vomiting**
  - If you throw up more than 2 hours after taking your dose of EC, do not worry, the medicine is already in your body.
  - If you throw up less than 2 hours after taking your dose of EC, call your pharmacist. You may need to take a repeat dose.
- **Tiredness, dizziness, headache, or breast tenderness**
  - These side effects should go away within a day or two.
  - You can use an over-the-counter pain reliever like Tylenol® (acetaminophen) or Motrin®/Advil® (ibuprofen) for headache or breast tenderness. Ask your pharmacist for help.
- **Menstrual spotting** (small amount of bleeding—less than a period)
  - This should go away in a day or two.

Follow-up:

- Your next period may be a little earlier or later than usual. The flow may be heavier, lighter, or the same as usual.
- If you do not get your period within 3 weeks after taking EC, you may be pregnant. Contact your healthcare provider to get a pregnancy test.
- See your healthcare provider for an effective method of birth control and for STI/HIV testing and prevention.

(continued on back)

www.massECnetwork.org • Massachusetts Emergency Contraception Network • 41 Winter Street, Suite 65 • Boston, MA 02108-4722

(Continued on next page)

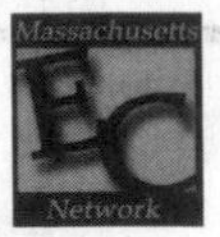

(continued from front)

- If you do not have a regular healthcare provider, ask the pharmacist for a list of providers.
- If you were raped or forced to have sex, call the Boston Area Rape Crisis Center at 1-800-841-8371 (English) or Llamanos Y Hablemos at 1-800-223-5001 (Spanish) for help.

Other information:

- If you do not want to become pregnant right now, you will need to use an effective form of birth control (like condoms, diaphragms, or oral contraceptive pills). EC does not work as well as other forms of birth control that are used before sex to prevent pregnancy.
- Taking EC before sex **will not** prevent pregnancy. EC does not prevent pregnancy from sex that happens after you take it.
- EC does not protect against sexually transmitted infections (STIs) or HIV/AIDS. Use condoms every time you have sex to protect yourself against STIs and HIV/AIDS.
- EC works best when the first dose is taken within 72 hours (3 days).
  - If you take EC within 3 days after unprotected sex, it is 75% to 89% effective at preventing a pregnancy.
  - If you take EC between 3 and 5 days after unprotected sex, it is still more than 70% effective at preventing pregnancy.
  - The sooner you take EC, the better it works.
- EC will not cause an abortion. EC is not the same thing as RU-486 (the abortion pill).
- EC will not hurt your body or your pregnancy if you took it before you knew you were pregnant.
- EC will not affect your ability to get pregnant in the future.

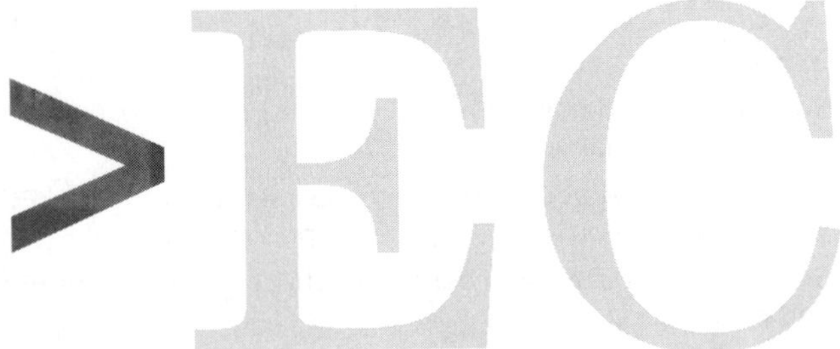

www.massECnetwork.org • Massachusetts Emergency Contraception Network • 41 Winter Street, Suite 65 • Boston, MA 02108-4722

Case Presentation

Patient Case: Part 2

Assessment: J.G. is at risk for an unintended pregnancy. She has failed to restart her next cycle of oral contraceptives in a timely manner and as such is at greater risk to ovulate this cycle. Her partner informed her that the condom protection had failed, thus exposing her to a risk of pregnancy and STIs, but by telling her about this failure, he provided her with the information needed for her to take appropriate action.

Plan: This woman is a candidate for EC having had unprotected sex within the previous 24 hours. Because levonorgestrel-only EC regimens are generally more effective and better tolerated than combined hormonal EC regimens, and especially with J.G.'s history of frequent migraine headaches, she will be offered a levonergestrel EC product that she can purchase OTC. She will be offered a single 1.5-mg dose (2 × 0.75 mg or 1 × 1.5 mg) and offered an option to purchase another package of EC to keep in advance of need. Patient will be questioned about her ability to take oral contraceptives on a daily basis and counseled on alternative contraceptives, such as the transdermal contraceptive patch, the contraceptive vaginal ring, or IUD, as they do not require daily dosing. She should be instructed to return to her medical provider for consideration of alternative contraceptive choices and for testing for STIs. She should contact her physician or to purchase an OTC pregnancy test if her next period does not begin within 3 weeks. An EC fact sheet should be given to her. Alternately, this patient could be advised to follow the instructions on her current oral contraceptive package insert regarding what to do when one or more pills are missed. She should be informed that this may be an appropriate therapeutic choice and provides a lower-cost alternative to Plan B®.

Summary

EC, although available for more than 35 years in the U.S., is still a poorly understood form of contraception and one of the least used. With this form of contraception—whether it be an IUD, one of the combined hormonal contraceptive products, or levonorgestrel—there is a potential to reduce unintended pregnancies. The misinformation and general lack of awareness of this method by providers and consumers alike has hindered its use. Pharmacists should know how to provide EC when Plan B® is out of stock or unavailable through a local pharmacy or medical clinic. Women often underestimate their risk of an unintended pregnancy, and consumer educational efforts must be undertaken by healthcare providers, advocacy groups, and governmental agencies to inform patients on their best methods of contraception and when and how to use EC effectively. Providers are encouraged to think beyond the provision of EC medications themselves and to look at systems of care that will meet all related needs, including family planning options, cost-of-care issues, sexual violence resources, insurance rules, and government regulations that make it difficult to access and take contraception effectively.

References

Additional content available at
www.ashp.org/womenshealth

SECTION FIVE

Preconception, Pregnancy, and Postpartum Care

21 Pregnancy Planning

Jennifer J. Lee, Pharm.D., BCPS, CDE; Tracy E. Thomason, Pharm.D.

Learning Objectives

1. Review the importance of pregnancy planning.
2. Educate women of childbearing age on ways to promote a healthy pregnancy.
3. Review the use of ovulation kits and pregnancy tests.
4. Explain the importance of proper diet and nutrition before conception.
5. Explore pregnancy-related complications and birth defects related to substance abuse.
6. Discuss strategies for vaccine administration during pregnancy.
7. Identify pregnancy risks associated with drugs and disease in women of childbearing age.

All women of childbearing age are candidates for receiving **preconception care** regardless of whether they are planning to conceive.[1] The American Academy of Pediatrics (AAP) and the American College of Obstetricians and Gynecologists (ACOG) recommend that all health encounters during a woman's reproductive years should include preconception care.[2] Key components include, but are not limited to, identification of preconception risks through an assessment of the woman's reproductive, family, and medical history; the family and medical history of the father; the woman's nutritional status, social concerns, and any drug or substance exposures she or the father may have; discussions regarding possible effects of pre-existing medical conditions and potential interventions; screening for infectious diseases with treatment and immunization; and discussions about environmental exposures.[1-3] Delaying discussions about preconception care until the first prenatal visit may delay targeted interventions needed to minimize poor pregnancy, fetal/infant, and maternal outcomes because detection of the pregnancy typically does not occur until the early weeks of **gestation,** when fetal organs are already developing.[1,4,5]

Adverse pregnancy outcomes from potentially preventable causes remain a prevalent health problem (i.e., unnecessary medications, untreated maternal disease, inadequate nutrition, substance abuse, vaccine-preventable diseases, infectious diseases).[3] Factors that may contribute to this include inconsistent delivery of preconception care and interventions before pregnancy, lack of physician time to provide preconception care, lack of reimbursement for these services, and lack of insurance coverage.[2,3,6,7] Furthermore, some women may have limited access to care or lack knowledge of risk factors that negatively affect maternal and fetal/infant health.[6,7] To help combat these challenges, the Centers for Disease Control and Prevention (CDC) developed national recommendations to improve health and healthcare for women before and between pregnancies (interconception care).[3] In addition, interdisciplinary approaches for pregnancy planning can help promote optimal health outcomes for the infant and mother.[1] Pharmacists are currently underutilized as pregnancy planning and counseling resources. Their accessibility to patients, close collaboration with other healthcare professionals, and knowledge of appropriate medication use during pregnancy make them ideal candidates to promote and contribute to preconception care.

Ovulation Kits and Pregnancy Tests

OVULATION KITS

Pregnancy planning involves identifying the most fertile time for conception by tracking periods of ovulation. Several methods are available to predict times of ovulation, such as luteinizing hormone

CASE PRESENTATION

Patient Case: Part 1

M.R. is a 27-year-old white woman who is a regular patient at your pharmacy. She returns this afternoon to pick up a new prescription for ibuprofen 800 mg once q 6 hr as needed for treatment of a strained muscle she obtained while playing tennis on her honeymoon. You have just finished changing her last name in her patient profile and remind her that she needs to refill her oral contraceptive next week. This statement prompts some questions from her. She and her husband are starting to think about having children. She is really worried about getting pregnant because she has been taking the pill for 6 years and she hopes to get pregnant as soon as possible if they decide to start trying. She has also heard several stories from friends concerning pregnancy that she isn't sure about. Her chief comment is: "I know there are medicines I'm supposed to take and some I'm not supposed to take when pregnant. It's just so confusing! What can I do to get ready?"

PMH: Allergic rhinitis.

Family history: Mother: hypertension; father: type 2 diabetes mellitus, hypertension, dyslipidemia.

Social history: Tobacco: denies; ethanol: occasionally 1–2 drinks on the weekends; illicit drugs: denies.

Allergies: No known drug allergies.

Medications: Levonorgestrel/ethinyl estradiol 0.15 mg/0.03 mg 1 tablet daily; ibuprofen 800 mg q 6 hr when necessary; mometasone 1 spray each nostril every morning.

Labs: Within normal limits.

(LH)-based ovulation tests, basal body temperature charting, calendar calculation, cervical mucus changes, and **mittelschmerz** (lower abdominal pain associated with ovulation).[8] Of the tests available, urinary LH prediction kits (ovulation kits) provide the greatest accuracy in predicting ovulation.[8,9] Ovulation kits were approved for home use in 1984 and detect the LH surge in urine that is present 14–48 hours before ovulation.[8,9] This LH surge signifies the final maturation of the follicle and release of the ovum.[8] Because the mature ovum can survive for approximately 24 hours and sperm can survive up to 72 hours, intercourse within 24 hours of the LH surge provides the greatest chance for pregnancy.[8]

Proper education is necessary for accurate use of ovulation kits. Patients should be counseled to read and follow all directions carefully and check the expiration date.[8] Most ovulation kits require a urine sample on a test stick with results available in minutes. Other tests may involve several steps, but this can lead to increased risk for human error.[8] Women should be counseled that early-morning urine collection is preferred, as the LH surge typically occurs early in the day and urine is most concentrated at this time. A change in color or color intensity compared with the color in the control window of the test signifies the LH surge.[8] Failure to detect an LH surge may indicate inappropriate testing time. Ovulation kits should be used 2–4 days before the estimated day of ovulation, and several months of tracking the LH surge may be necessary to predict the optimal time of sexual intercourse.[8] False positives can result from use of fertility medications, polycystic ovarian syndrome (PCOS), menopause, or pregnancy.[8]

PREGNANCY TESTS

Pregnancy tests were approved for home use in 1976; this allows for private and convenient identification of pregnancy.[8] These tests detect the presence of human chorionic gonadotropin (hCG), which is produced by the placenta when a fertilized egg implants in the uterus. hCG is detectable by home pregnancy tests within 10–12 days of fertilization; however, it may not be detected for up to 21 days in some women.[8] For most pregnancy tests, waiting to test until at least 1 week after the missed period will provide more accurate results, as concentrations of hCG will be higher.[8] Several types of pregnancy tests are available: dipstick test, collection cup test, chemical mixing test, and blood test. Tests can vary with regards to their sensitivity to detect hCG, directions for use, and response time. Tests with greater sensitivity may be able to detect pregnancy earlier than those that begin to detect hCG at 100 milli-International Units/mL.[8] First Response™ Early Result Pregnancy Tests are able to detect hCG concentrations as low as 6.5 milli-International Units/mL and are considered a reliable home pregnancy test.[8]

As with ovulation kits, proper education is necessary for accurate use of pregnancy tests. Home pregnancy testing is 99% accurate, although user error may reduce this to 50% to 75% accuracy.[8] It is important for women to read and follow all directions for the test and check the expiration date. Timing of testing for accurate results will vary based on the sensitivity of the test. Women should test early-morning urine for the most reliable results.[8] Similar to ovulation prediction kits, results of home pregnancy tests are based on a color change of the testing strip. Contaminants in urine may provide false results. For patients who get a negative result, retesting is recommended in 1 week if she has not menstruated.[8] False-negative results may occur if the test is not administered at the appropriate time after the missed period (hCG concentration too low to detect). False-positive results can be due to use of fertility medications, such as chorionic gonadotropin for injection.[8] If a home pregnancy test is positive, women should contact their primary care physician or obstetrician/gynecologist for appropriate follow-up and care.

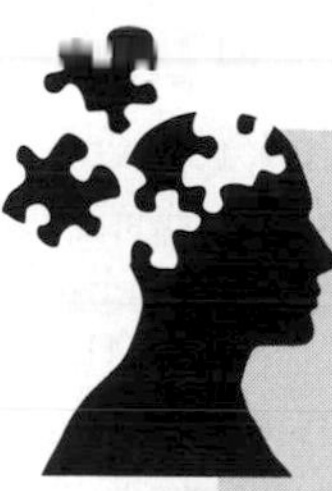

Therapeutic Challenge:

T.K. is a 31-year-old woman who would like to start trying to get pregnant. She currently consumes four to five soft drinks a day, which is equivalent to approximately 300 mg of caffeine. What do you recommend?

Preconception Nutrition

DIET

Pregnancy planning should involve assessment of nutritional habits to optimize maternal health and reduce the risk of birth defects, suboptimal fetal growth and development, and chronic health problems in offspring.[10]Appropriate weight gain, consumption of a variety of foods, and appropriate and timely vitamin and mineral supplementation are key components of a healthy lifestyle during pregnancy.[10] A healthy prepregnancy maternal weight can make conception easier and improve pregnancy outcomes. Maternal obesity can lead to increased risk for hypertension, gestational diabetes, cesarean deliveries, and complications during delivery. Children born to obese women are at increased risk for neural tube defects, **macrosomia** (newborn with excessive birth weight), low **Apgar scores,** and childhood obesity.[10] On the contrary, severe dietary restrictions can lead to nutritional deficiencies (i.e., folic acid, iron, calcium) that may negatively affect fetal development and result in increased risk for morbidity and mortality.[10] Ultimately, maintaining a healthy weight and good nutrition before, during, and after pregnancy can optimize pregnancy outcomes.[10]

Fish Intake

Consumption of long-chain omega-3 polyunsaturated fatty acids during pregnancy is critical for fetal neurodevelopment.[11] These fatty acids are necessary precursors of prostaglandins, which are incorporated into cell membranes and have other roles in the central nervous system.[12] Fish and other seafood are the major dietary source; however, concern has been raised about the potential for concomitant intake of high levels of mercury (a well-established neurotoxin).[11,13] Mercury can lead to possible birth defects and disabilities, including cerebral palsy, seizures, low birth weight, or small head circumference.[14] In addition, mercury can accumulate in the body over time and is eliminated by the body slowly.[14,15] In 2004, the U.S. Food and Drug Administration (FDA) and the Environmental Protection Agency (EPA) issued an updated advisory counseling women of childbearing age, pregnant women, nursing women, and young children to avoid consumption of fish containing high levels of mercury, such as king mackerel, shark, swordfish, and tile fish.[15] This advisory does not suggest that women of childbearing age completely eliminate fish from their diet. Because fish are a good dietary source of essential fatty acids, it is recommended that women consume up to 12 ounces per week of seafood lower in mercury content, such as shrimp, canned light tuna, salmon, pollock, and catfish. Albacore tuna steaks contain more mercury than canned light tuna, so it is recommended to limit intake to 6 ounces per week.[15]

Caffeine

Approximately 20% of adult Americans consume more than 300 mg of caffeine daily.[16] The average caffeine intake in women ages 18–34 is estimated to be 164 mg per day compared with 125 mg per day in pregnant women.[10,17] Caffeine intake among women of childbearing age and pregnant women deserves special attention as infertility, miscarriage, and low birth weight may be associated with its consumption.[10,16,18-20] Some studies have suggested a modest decrease in fertility when caffeine consumption is >250–300 mg per day.[16] Unfortunately, many studies assessing the effects of caffeine intake on pregnancy outcomes are inconsistent and difficult to assess.[18,19,21] Many studies are retrospective in nature, and data collection is based on questionnaires or interviews, which can be subject to inaccurate reporting or recall bias.[18] Furthermore, several studies include women who have known risk factors for adverse pregnancy outcomes, such as use of alcohol, tobacco, and illicit drugs.[17,18] Currently available research suggests a dose-response relationship between caffeine consumption and the risk for miscarriage.[18,19] The magnitude of this association was stronger among women without other risk factors for miscarriage.[18] Low to moderate caffeine consumption (<200–300 mg per day) has not been shown to increase rates of miscarriage.[16,18,19] Less convincing data are available regarding the association between caffeine intake and low birth weight. Because caffeine crosses the placenta, large amounts could affect the fetus. Changes in fetal heart rate and breathing patterns have been observed, and children born to mothers who consume high amounts of caffeine were more likely to experience tachycardia, tremors, and tachypnea, and spend more time awake in the days following birth.[22]

Artificial Sweeteners

Artificial sweeteners have been added to a wide variety of foods, drinks, drugs, and hygiene products.[23] The safety of artificial sweeteners has been questioned based on reports of potential carcinogenic risks.[23] However, these reports were based on data from experimental animals given high concentrations of artificial sweeteners who may have had a baseline elevated risk for cancer.[23] Since then, case-control humans studies suggest that the possible risk of cancer induced by artificial sweeteners appears negligible.[23]

Consumption of artificial sweeteners, including acesulfame-K, aspartame, saccharin, sucralose, and neotame, are considered safe for consumption during pregnancy when used within the acceptable daily intakes.[10] Early reports recommended against the consumption of saccharin in pregnant women because it can cross the placenta, remain in fetal tissues, and may be associated with bladder cancer (based on an animal study).[24] Since then, saccharin has been removed from the list of possible carcinogens.[24] The safety of acesulfame-K, aspartame, sucralose, and neotame during pregnancy has been established.[24] High doses of acesulfame-K, sucralose, and neotame do not result in change in fertility, body weight, growth, or mortality.[24] However, aspartame consumption should be used with caution in women with phenylketonuria (PKU) because elevated levels phenylalanine in the fetal circulation can lead to neurologic problems.[24]

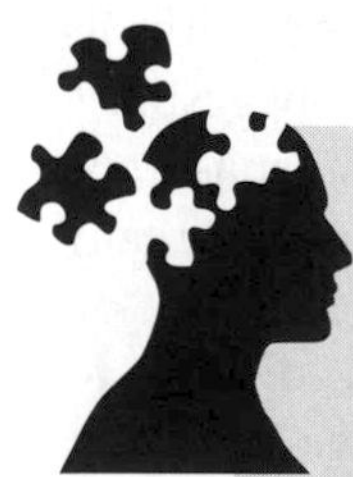

Therapeutic Challenge:

G.H. is a 28-year-old woman who is planning to have a child within the next year, but she is currently in between jobs and is not able to purchase prenatal vitamins. How would you counsel her on diet to prepare for pregnancy?

VITAMINS AND MINERALS

Aside from a well-balanced diet, supplementation with certain vitamins and minerals before conception is needed to support a healthy pregnancy. For women with poor dietary intake; those who consume little to no animal products; or those who smoke, abuse alcohol or drugs, a daily multiple vitamin and mineral supplement is recommended.[10] In some instances, timing of supplementation during the pregnancy becomes extremely important. For example, adequate intake and stores of these nutrients are necessary before conception to support fetal development, minimize risks for birth defects, and maintain healthy maternal outcomes.[25-32] Prenatal vitamins should provide adequate dosages of folic acid, iron, and calcium, so initiation before conception or as soon as possible after conception is best for mother and the developing fetus.

Folic Acid

Neural tube defects (NTDs), such as **spina bifida** and **anencephaly,** occur because of incomplete or incorrect closure of the neural tube and account for 8% of total birth defects.[25,26] Fetal formation of the neural tube and closure occurs within the first 4 weeks of embryonic development, often before a woman realizes she is pregnant.[26] Research has shown that adequate intake of folic acid decreases the incidence of NTDs by 50% to 70%.[25,27] To ensure adequate folate levels early in pregnancy, it is recommended that all women of childbearing age consume 0.4 mg of folic acid per day from fortified foods or supplementation.[25,26,27] Women who are at high risk, including those who had a previous pregnancy affected by an NTD, should consume 4 mg of folic acid per day.[25,26] In both cases, consumption should begin at least 1 month before conception and continue throughout the first trimester.[25]

In 1998, the FDA required mandatory fortification of cereal grains in an effort to decrease the incidence of NTDs. Other dietary sources of folic acid include legumes, green leafy vegetables, liver, citrus fruits and juices, and whole wheat bread.[10,25] Despite a diet rich in folate, most women of childbearing age still do not get enough folic acid to prevent NTDs.[27] A recent telephone survey conducted in women of childbearing age reported that only 19% of women knew folic acid prevented birth defects, and 33% were taking a vitamin supplement containing folic acid.[25] These data suggest the increased need for healthcare professionals, including pharmacists, to promote folic acid supplementation in all women of childbearing age.

Iron

It is estimated that <50% of women of childbearing age have adequate iron stores for pregnancy.[28] Iron is necessary throughout pregnancy to support an increase in red cell mass, expand the plasma volume, and allow for growth of the fetal-placental unit.[28,29] Low socioeconomic status, being a member of an ethnic minority, poor dietary iron intake, and blood loss related to menstruation may contribute to iron deficiency.[28] The relationship between iron deficiency early in pregnancy with preterm birth and subsequent low birth weight has been well established.[28,29] In a randomized trial, iron supplementation increased birth weight by more than 200 g and reduced preterm birth and low birth weight.[30] Women are encouraged to maintain an iron-rich diet: lean red meat, fish, poultry, dried fruits, and iron-fortified cereals.[10] The CDC recommends supplementation with 27–30 mg/day of elemental iron for pregnant women because many women have difficulty maintaining adequate iron stores for pregnancy.[10,31]

Calcium

During pregnancy, calcium plays an integral role in bone health for both the mother and fetus. For a full-term pregnancy, the fetus will require approximately 30 g of calcium, which may be absorbed from maternal bones if calcium intake is insufficient.[32] Over time, this can lead to decreased maternal bone strength and osteoporosis. Regardless of the pregnancy status, the recommended daily intake for calcium is 1,300 mg for women aged 14–18 years and 1,000 mg for women aged 19–50 years.[32] Adequate calcium intake can be attained through the diet by consumption of dairy products, leafy greens, and fortified foods.[32] If dietary calcium intake is insufficient or inconsistent, supplementation may be necessary. Multiple vitamin-mineral supplements provide 200–400 mg of calcium. Additional calcium supplementation from calcium carbonate or calcium citrate may be needed in women with poorer dietary intake. Recent data suggest that calcium supplementation may also decrease risk for pregnancy-induced hypertension and **preeclampsia,** but more research is needed before calcium is routinely recommended for this purpose.[33]

HERBAL SUPPLEMENTS

Use of herbal supplements by pregnant patients is estimated to range from 3.6% to 42%.[34] More concerning is that these agents are commonly used during the first trimester of pregnancy.[34] Few randomized, clinical trials have examined the safety and efficacy of herbal supplements and alternative therapy during pregnancy.[10] Available data suggest herbal supplements may cause miscarriage, cause preterm birth, induce uterine contractions, or cause injury to the fetus.[35] Herbal supplements of particular concern include, but are not limited to, blue cohosh, black cohosh, dong quai, goldenseal, and feverfew.[35] Until more information is available, routine use of herbal supplements during pregnancy should be avoided.

Smoking Cessation

Pregnancy planning allows women to address and treat tobacco dependence early on to avoid smoking-related pregnancy complications and long-term health consequences.[36] Preconception smoking is linked to contraception delay and primary or secondary infertility.[35] Once a pregnancy has been established, continued smoking is associated with adverse maternal and fetal outcomes.[36,37] Women who smoke are at increased risk for premature rupture of membranes, **placental abruption, placenta previa,** miscarriage, ectopic pregnancy, cancer, cardiovascular disease, and pulmonary disease.[36,37] Carbon monoxide and nicotine from smoking can decrease oxygen supply to the fetus by blocking hemoglobin's oxygen binding capacity and reducing placental blood flow.[10] This can lead to damage of the fetal brain, heart, and nervous system. Furthermore, smoking can decrease fetal birth weight by an average of 200 g and may increase risk for premature birth and fetal death. In addition, mental disabilities and possible nicotine addiction of the infant are long-term consequences of smoking during pregnancy.[10] Exposure to secondhand smoking during pregnancy also has adverse effects on the fetus, resulting in low birth weight and increased risk for intrauterine growth retardation.[10,36,37]

Despite efforts to increase awareness of the harmful effects of smoking, 11.4% of women report smoking during pregnancy.[36,37] Although smoking cessation before pregnancy will produce the greatest benefits to the fetus and mother, quitting smoking any time during pregnancy can be beneficial.[38] Therefore, it is prudent to continue to use the five A's behavioral counseling framework (ask, advise, assess, assist, arrange) throughout the duration of pregnancy.[38] Effective treatment of tobacco dependence has shown quit rates as high as 25% to 30% (see Chapter 36: Substance-Use Disorders for smoking cessation management).[36] In 2008, the U.S. Surgeon General recommended individual counseling and behavioral interventions as the first-line approach for smoking cessation during pregnancy.[38] Several FDA-approved agents are also available to assist with smoking cessation; however, it is important to keep in mind that their safety and efficacy has not been established in pregnancy, so pregnancy planning remains critical.[36]

Substance Abuse/Alcoholism

In the U.S., 90% of women who abuse illicit drugs are of childbearing age.[39] A 2002–2003 national survey found that illicit drug use among pregnant women was 4.3% compared with 10.4% in nonpregnant women of the same age group.[40] Substance abuse during pregnancy can increase fetal risk for low birth weight, small head circumference, prematurity, and other developmental problems.[10] Furthermore, substance abuse is commonly associated with other high-risk behaviors that can lead to increased risk for sexually transmitted diseases (STDs), human immunodeficiency virus (HIV) transmission, and pregnancy complications.[39]

Commonly abused substances include cocaine, marijuana, amphetamines, opioids, tobacco, and alcohol.[10,39] Cocaine is transferred across the placenta and can lead to fetal vasoconstriction.[39] Cocaine abuse during pregnancy has been associated with preterm labor, placental abruption, uterine rupture, cardiac dysrhythmias, hepatic rupture, cerebral ischemia/infarction, and death.[39] Marijuana can also be transferred directly to the fetus through the placenta.[39] Long-term follow-up studies in children exposed to marijuana prenatally have reported depressive symptoms and impairment in cognitive function.[10,39] Amphetamine use has been associated with cardiac anomalies, cleft lip and palate, biliary atresia (abnormal development of bile ducts inside or outside the liver), intrauterine growth retardation, intrauterine fetal demise, and cerebral hemorrhage.[39] Opioids can directly affect the fetus through transplacental transfer.[39] This can lead to fetal intrauterine growth restriction and symptoms of neonatal opioid withdrawl.[39] Although some of the consequences related to substance abuse are known, it is important to recognize the challenge in isolating the effects of specific substances because women who use illicit drugs are typically polysubstance abusers.[10,39]

Alcohol use among women of childbearing age remains high, with an overall incidence of 55% in women and approximately 12.4% of these women reporting binge drinking.[3,41] For women trying to conceive, moderate alcohol consumption—less than or equal to five drinks per week—can adversely affect fertility.[10,42] High rates of alcohol use also exist among women who are pregnant with an incidence of 10% and binge drinking reported in 2% of these women.[3,41]

The AAP recommends against the consumption of alcohol during pregnancy because no amount of alcohol at any stage of pregnancy is considered safe.[39,43] Complications of alcohol ingestion during pregnancy include a higher incidence of miscarriages, placental abruption, preterm deliveries, and stillbirth.[39,42] However, the effects and severity of prenatal alcohol exposures vary widely, and prevalence rates of fetal alcohol syndrome range from 0.3 to 2.0 cases per 1,000 live births.[44] Fetal alcohol syndrome refers to a variety of physical, behavioral, and cognitive abnormalities of alcohol-exposed infants. Characteristic physical anomalies include a smooth **philtrum** (flat groove in the upper lip), thin **vermillion border** (thin margin of the upper and lower lips), small **palpebral fissures** (small opening for the eyes between the eyelids), **micrognathia** (small lower jaw), cardiac defects, and eye/ear abnormalities. Children affected by this disorder may also experience growth abnormalities, mental disabilities, poor coordination, hypotonia, and attention-deficit hyperactivity disorder.[39,43,45] Because of high rates of alcohol consumption and the multitude of adverse outcomes associated with its use, pregnancy planning to prevent fetal alcohol exposure is paramount. Brief counseling, motivational interviewing, assessing readiness to change, the five A's behavioral counseling framework (ask, advise, assess, assist, arrange), and Project CHOICES are examples of preventative strategies to reduce alcohol-exposed pregnancies (see Chapter 36: Substance-Use Disorders for substance abuse management).[36,44]

Immunizations

Preconception vaccination in all women of childbearing age can provide protection to the woman and her potential fetus. Unfortunately, adult immunization rates are below national goals, which may be related to misconceptions about the safety and benefits of vaccines.[46] Insufficient maternal vaccine administration can lead to pregnancy complications and diminished immune status of the newborn infant.[47,48] For example, rubella is associated with low morbidity and mortality in pregnant women; however, maternal infection can lead to miscarriage and **congenital rubella syndrome.**[46] Measles is also associated with low maternal morbidity and mortality, but maternal infection can lead to increased risk for miscarriage and malformations.[46]

Although vaccine-associated risks to the developing fetus is theoretical, ACOG recommends preconception immunization over immunization during pregnancy.[49] Vaccine administration during pregnancy is warranted if the likelihood of disease exposure is high, when infection would pose a risk to the mother or fetus, and when the vaccine is unlikely to cause harm.[47,49] For example, influenza is associated with increased morbidity and mortality and can possibly increase abortion rates. The intramuscular influenza vaccine is an inactivated virus, and there have been no confirmed reports of the vaccine to the fetus.[49] Therefore, it is recommended that all women who are pregnant (any trimester) during the influenza season (November to March in the U.S.) get vaccinated.[47] At the time of writing, the H1N1 vaccine was not available. However, the CDC recommends that pregnant women receive the inactivated H1N1 vaccine in addition to the seasonal flu vaccine.[50]

Administration of inactivated vaccines is considered safe during pregnancy because there is no evidence of risk from vaccinating a pregnant woman.[47] Routine vaccines that are generally safe to administer during pregnancy include tetanus, diphtheria, influenza, and hepatitis B.[46] Administration of hepatitis A, meningococcal conjugate, meningococcal polysaccharide, and pneumococcal polysaccharide vaccines should be considered in women at high risk for these infections (Table 21-1).[47,51] Furthermore, additional vaccinations may be appropriate for pregnant women traveling to highly epidemic areas.[46,47]

Table 21-1. Immunizations During Pregnancy

Vaccine	Before Pregnancy	During Pregnancy	After Pregnancy	Type of Vaccine	Route
Hepatitis A	If at high risk for disease	If at high risk for disease	If at high risk for disease	Inactivated	IM
Hepatitis B	Yes, if at risk	Yes, if at risk	Yes, if at risk	Inactivated	IM
Human Papillomavirus (HPV)	Yes, if <26 yr	No, under study	Yes, if <26 yr	Inactivated	IM
Influenza-TIV, IM	Yes	Yes	Yes	Inactivated	IM
Influenza LAIV	Yes, if <49 yr and healthy	No	Yes, if <49 yr and healthy	Live	Nasal spray
MMR	Yes, avoid conception for 4 wk	No	Yes, avoid conception for 4 wk	Live	SC
Meningococcal: • polysaccharide • conjugate	If indicated	If indicated	If indicated	Inactivated Inactivated	SC IM
Pneumococcal Polysaccharide	If indicated	If indicated	If indicated	Inactivated	IM or SC
Tetanus/Diphtheria Td	Yes, Tdap preferred	If indicated	Yes, Tdap preferred	Toxid	IM
Tdap, one dose only	Yes, preferred	If high risk of pertussis	Yes, preferred	Toxoid	IM
Varicella	Yes, avoid conception for 4 wk	No	Yes, avoid conception for 4 wk	Live	SC

Source: From reference 51.

IM = intramuscular; LAIV = live attenuated influenza vaccine; MMR = mumps, measles, rubella; SC = subcutaneous; Td = tetanus, diphtheria; Tdap = tetanus, diphtheria, and pertussis; TIV = trivalent inactivated influenza vaccine.

On the contrary, live vaccines are contraindicated during pregnancy because of the theoretical risk of transmission to the fetus.[47] If a woman gets pregnant within 4 weeks of receiving a live vaccine or a pregnant woman inadvertently receives a live vaccine, she should be counseled about the theoretical risks.[47] Termination of the pregnancy is not warranted.[47] Examples of live vaccines include smallpox, measles, mumps, rubella, and varicella.[46,47,49] The smallpox vaccine can cause a rare but serious complication to the fetus called fetal vaccinia (fetal or neonatal death, premature birth) when administered to a pregnant woman.[47] Pregnant women should not come in close contact with anyone who recently (within 1 month) received the smallpox vaccine.[47]

In 2006, the CDC issued a recommendation that adults aged 19–64 should receive a Tdap (vaccine to protect against tetanus, diphtheria, pertussis) booster if they received their last Td (vaccine to protect against tetanus and diphtheria) more than 10 years earlier and have not yet received Tdap.[48] When possible, women of childbearing age should receive Tdap before becoming pregnant (intervals <10 years since the last Td are appropriate for booster protection against pertussis).[48] For women who have not previously received Tdap, a dose should be administered immediately in the postpartum period.[48] Furthermore, adults who may have close contact with an infant <12 months of age should receive Tdap to reduce the transmission of pertussis (acute, infectious coughing illness), which can lead to death.[48]

For the most up to date and accurate information regarding vaccinations during pregnancy, visit the CDC website.

Infectious Diseases: Pregnancy Complications and Fetal Risks

Management of infectious diseases during pregnancy will be covered more extensively in Chapter 25: Pregnancy and Pre-Existing Illnesses. However, early detection and treatment of a number of infections in the pregnancy planning stage offers the potential of preventing future complications from the infection and reducing fetal and maternal morbidity. Screening is paramount because many of these infections are present in asymptomatic women.

SEXUALLY TRANSMITTED DISEASES

Screening for STDs such as gonorrhea, chlamydia, syphilis, trichomoniasis, and HIV should be conducted before conception if the patient is at risk for these diseases. The treatment of several of these diseases could adversely affect the developing fetus if given during pregnancy. For example, trichomoniasis is routinely treated with metronidazole, which is potentially harmful to fetuses when administered in the first trimester of pregnancy but is less problematic if given in the second or third trimester. It is also imperative to know if a woman is infected with HIV before conception so that she can receive appropriate treatment for the disease and prevent maternal-to-fetal transmission of the virus. If left untreated during pregnancy a number of these infections could result in serious adverse fetal and maternal outcomes. Without therapy, trichomoniasis can result in premature rupture of membranes, preterm delivery, and low birth weight.[52] Gonococcal infections in pregnancy are associated with **chorioamnionitis** and preterm labor and could result in systemic neonatal infection or maternal endometritis.[53] Likewise, chlamydial infection can also increase the risk for preterm labor, low birth weight, endometriosis, and postpartum pelvic inflammatory disease.[54,55] Chlamydia infections are a cause of neonatal pneumonia and conjunctivitis.[54,55] Detection and treatment of syphilis with antibiotics before pregnancy can prevent transmission to the fetus and eliminate congenital syphilis, which, left untreated, can result in premature birth, neonatal death, and a wide variety of severe abnormalities.[56]

BACTERIAL VAGINOSIS

The U.S. Preventive Services Task Force, ACOG, and the CDC do not recommend universal screening for bacterial vaginosis.[52,57,58] However, women with a history of preterm labor may be advised that such a screening is necessary.[52,57,58]

TOXOPLASMOSIS

The low prevalence of toxoplasmosis during pregnancy does not warrant widespread screening. The screening techniques commonly used are costly and uncertain. Education of patients in prevention of this disease is the accepted approach. Currently toxoplasmosis is as commonly acquired in pregnancy through the handling of contaminated meat as it is from cat litter boxes[59]

CYTOMEGALOVIRUS

Routine testing of pregnant women for cytomegalovirus (CMV) infection is not recommended, although a simple blood test is available. Women who have already been infected with CMV in the past have little cause for concern.[60] The greatest risk to the developing fetus is if CMV infection is first acquired during or shortly before the pregnancy.[61] Groups at high risk for contracting CMV (day-care and health-care workers) should be advised that good hygiene—including frequent hand washing and avoidance of sharing utensils and glasses with young children—significantly reduces the risk for this virus.[60]

LISTERIOSIS

Pregnant women are about 20 times more likely than other healthy adults to get listeriosis, and about one third of listeriosis cases occur during pregnancy.[62-64] Infection with *Listeria* during pregnancy can result in miscarriage, stillbirth, premature labor, and health problems in the newborn.[64] Because listeriosis is usually acquired by eating foods contaminated with *Listeria* bacteria, prevention is the key. General food handling guidelines—including cooking meats thoroughly, avoiding cross-contamination, and washing raw vegetables—should be followed. In addition, women who are pregnant or are trying to become pregnant should be advised to avoid consuming undercooked hot dogs, deli meats, unpasteurized milk and milk products, and soft cheeses.[64,65]

Safe and Effective Use of Medications

The safe and effective use of medications during pregnancy is discussed in detail in Chapter 23: Drug Principles in Pregnancy and Lactation. The time of maximum vulnerability for developing fetuses is 17–57 days from fertilization or the first 10 weeks after the last menstrual period. Considering that 76% of pregnant women take at least one medication during their pregnancy, and about 59% of pregnant women taking a medication other than a vitamin or mineral supplement, the management of medication therapy in pregnant women is imperative to successful pregnancy outcomes.[66,67] The use of herbal and natural products during pregnancy is discussed earlier in this chapter in the Preconception Nutrition section. However, many women consider these products to be medications; therefore a review of their use according to the guidelines previously mentioned should also be conducted during discussion of medication use during pregnancy.

GENERAL PRINCIPLES TO MINIMIZE RISK OF BIRTH DEFECTS

A thorough medication history should be taken for all women who are considering becoming pregnant. This history should include not only questions concerning prescription and nonprescription medications, but also herbal preparations and vitamins. Prescription medications should be reduced to the lowest effective dosage or discontinued if possible. Some medications are particularly harmful to development of the fetus during the first trimester of pregnancy. Whenever possible, these medications should be suspended until after the twelfth week of pregnancy, when they can be more safely administered. In general, combination over-the-counter products should be avoided, and single-ingredient products specific to the symptom or condition present should be used. Women should also be cautioned about the use of herbal, homeopathic, and natural medications. The data concerning the safety and efficacy of these types of preparations are lacking in the general population, and experience with their use in pregnant women is even more limited. Although patients may consider these products "safer" because of their natural origin, the majority of data that is available is due to adverse effects noted in pregnant patients. Implementation of these principles in the prepregnancy period helps to ensure positive outcomes.

Rh Status

Rh blood typing and antibody screening is recommended for all pregnant women at their first prenatal visit.[68] An incompatibility between the blood of the expectant mother and the fetus can result in Rh disease. If left undetected or untreated, it can result in anemia, jaundice, brain damage, heart failure, and even death in the infant.[69] Rh disease is a concern only for women who are Rh negative.

RH DISEASE

Most individuals have Rh-positive blood, meaning they possess the Rh factor (e.g., A+).[70]An incompatibility can occur if an Rh-positive father and an Rh-negative mother conceive an Rh-positive baby. If at some point during the pregnancy, the Rh-negative mother's blood is exposed to the blood of her Rh-positive fetus, her immune system will recognize the Rh factor as foreign and produce antibodies toward it.[70] These antibodies can then traverse the placenta and cause destruction of the fetus's Rh-positive red blood cells.[70] To prevent the development of Rh antibodies (known as *sensitization*), the expectant mother can be treated with Rh immunoglobulin before exposure to the fetus's blood. Rh immunoglobulin is an antibody derived from human blood products that confers passive immunity by destroying the fetus's Rh-positive blood cells before the mother's immune system can detect them. Rh immunoglobulin injections should be administered at 28 weeks of pregnancy and again within 72 hours of delivery. Protection from Rh immunoglobulin lasts only about 12 weeks.[71]

FIRST PREGNANCY VERSUS SUBSEQUENT PREGNANCY

An Rh-negative woman must be treated during each pregnancy if she is carrying an Rh-positive fetus. It is very rare for the first Rh-positive baby of an Rh-negative woman to be affected by Rh disease. However, the first pregnancy of this nature is significant for an Rh-negative woman because she can become sensitized to the Rh-positive antigen. Each successive pregnancy with an Rh-positive fetus increases the risk of the baby developing severe Rh disease and increased chance of fetal death.[70,71] The use Rh immunoglobulin greatly diminishes that risk.

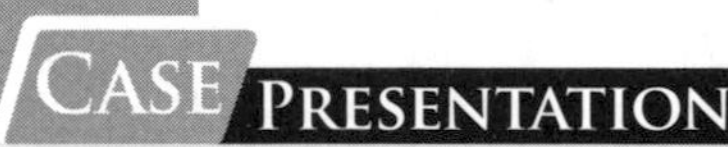

Patient Case: Part 2

Assessment: M.R. is a 27-year-old white woman of childbearing potential who is in general good health. She is a prime candidate for counseling and intervention for prepregnancy planning.

Plan: M.R. should schedule a prepregnancy counseling session at your pharmacy. Planning is important because most women are 1–2 weeks pregnant before they find out. In addition, there are steps she can take to increase her chances of conception and having a healthy pregnancy.

Patient education: The basics of conception should be reviewed with M.R. to provide the best success rate for conception when it is desired. Key points include the following:

- In general, the menstrual cycle is 28 days long, with ovulation on or about day 14.
- There is a window of opportunity to become pregnant during each menstrual cycle; once she ovulates, the ovum may only survive for 12–24 hours.
- Sperm may survive for 3–5 days after ejaculation.

M.R.'s specific concern about prolonged oral contraceptive use and difficulty in conceiving is unwarranted. Women can ovulate the next month after stopping oral contraceptives. She should be reminded that it usually takes 4–6 months to become pregnant, and infertility issues would not be addressed until after 1 year of unprotected intercourse did not result in pregnancy.

Her prescription and nonprescription medication history should be reviewed. Any potentially **teratogenic** medication should be identified and discontinued, lowered to the lowest effective dosage, or suspended until after the first trimester. The most critical period for fetal development is 17–57 days after fertilization. In particular, M.R. should be advised that ibuprofen and other nonsteroidal anti-inflammatory drugs should not be used in pregnancy, even early in the pregnancy (during the 2 weeks before she notices she missed her period). In addition, M.R. can safely continue the use of her mometasone nasal spray as needed. In review of the available laboratory data, only the low serum iron is remarkable. M.R. could begin an over-the-counter iron supplement that will deliver 30 mg of elemental iron along with a multivitamin until prescription prenatal vitamins are warranted. M.R.'s social history is unremarkable, with the exception of occasional social alcohol use. She should be counseled that there is no safe amount of alcohol that can be consumed during pregnancy, and she should abstain from its use if she suspects she is pregnant. In addition, it may be prudent to cease alcohol consumption while trying to conceive because there is some evidence that alcohol can affect rates of conception; and she may be 2 weeks pregnant before she is aware of it. Finally, evaluate M.R.'s immunization history and family history for genetic disorders. Several immunizations, particularly rubella and varicella, are recommended to be administered at least 1 month before conception. M.R. and her husband may chose not to have children if their risk for genetic disorders is particularly high, and prepregnancy screening will aid them in this decision. See Table 21-2 for a helpful prepregnancy checklist.

Summary

Preconception care as outlined in this chapter can help improve pregnancy-related outcomes in all women of childbearing age. The preponderance of unplanned pregnancies in this country make routine provision of preconception care vital to the health and welfare of the mother and fetus/infant. Discussions with healthcare providers before conception will enable women to make informed decisions about their

Table 21-2. Prepregnancy Checklist

- Discuss the physiology of ovulation and the optimal time to try conception.
- Discuss proper nutrition.
- Discuss folic acid intake preconception and during early pregnancy.
- Discuss adequate iron intake.
- Discuss risks of smoking and alcohol and drug use.
- Review the patient's immunization status.
- Review any medical problems of the patient and her partner.
- Discuss medication use while pregnant or trying to become pregnant.
- Explore family and genetic history to rule out any potential congenital conditions.
- Provide encouragement!

potential pregnancy. This counseling can also reduced adverse pregnancy outcomes from potentially preventable causes. Furthermore, the limited access to care or lack knowledge of risk factors that some women may have can be remedied through counseling from their pharmacist. Pharmacists are in a unique position to thoroughly provide pregnancy planning and counseling resources to women of childbearing potential. Their accessibility to patients and other healthcare professionals, and their knowledge of medication use during pregnancy, make them ideal candidates to promote and contribute to preconception care.

References

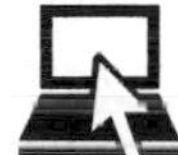

Additional content available at
www.ashp.org/womenshealth

22 Infertility

Jaou-Chen Huang, MD, FACOG; Nancy D. Ordonez, Pharm.D., BCPS

Learning Objectives

1. Distinguish primary and secondary infertility, and fertility and fecundity.
2. List the two most common causes of female infertility and the impacts of aging on fertility.
3. Be familiar with unexplained infertility and its prognosis.
4. Formulate a strategy to evaluate women with infertility.
5. Formulate nonpharmacologic and pharmacologic managements of female infertility.
6. List assisted reproductive technologies and their indications, effectiveness, and potential complications.
7. Understand the pharmacologic basis, side effects, and monitoring parameters of ovulation induction agents, such as clomiphene citrate, gonadotropins, human chorionic gonadotropin, gonadotropin-releasing hormone agonist and antagonist, lutropin alfa, and aromatase inhibitors.

Infertility is defined as the inability to have a pregnancy after 1 year of unprotected intercourse. The aforementioned pregnancy does not have to result in a live birth. Infertility affects one in six couples in the U.S.[1] In contrast, **fecundity** is the likelihood of attaining a pregnancy within a given period. Fecundity rates vary by age; under ideal circumstances with intercourse during the most fertile day of the ovulatory cycle, fecundity is up to 50% in women younger than age 25 and decreases by at least half in older women.[2] The cumulative pregnancy rate of up to 6 months of unprotected intercourse is 72% and up to 12 months is 85%.[3] The cause of infertility may be due to the male and/or female partner; this chapter will address only female infertility.

Infertility is sometimes categorized as primary or secondary. Primary infertility indicates that neither partner has attained a pregnancy in the current or prior relationship(s). Secondary infertility indicates that a pregnancy was attained in the past with the current or previous partner(s); the pregnancy does not have to result in a live birth. To some extent, this designation helps healthcare providers managing patients. When treating couples with secondary infertility, healthcare providers usually concentrate more on events after the index pregnancy to identify the cause(s) of infertility.

Epidemiology

There appears to be a decline in **fertility** in the U.S.[4] Many factors contribute to the decline, including changing roles for women, postponement of marriage, delayed childbearing age, more prevalent use of contraception, increased utilization of abortion, and a concern over deteriorating environment or limitations imposed by unfavorable economic conditions.

NORMAL FOLLICULAR DEVELOPMENT

Normal menstrual cycles last approximately 28 days. It is divided into two phases: the follicular phase and the luteal phase. During the follicular phase, the pituitary gonadotropins stimulate the growth of the follicule. The increase in follicular size is accompanied by rising levels of serum estradiol. When the size of the follicle reaches 20 mm, a sudden increase in luteinizing hormone (the LH surge) triggers the final stages of follicular development and the release of ovum (ovulation). After ovulation, the remainder of the follicle transforms to corpus luteum, which produces progesterone. Progesterone changes the endometrium and prepares it for the implantation of the embryo. In case there is no pregnancy, the corpus luteum disintegrates, followed by a drop in progesterone level and the beginning of menstruation.

CASE PRESENTATION

Patient Case: Part 1

J.S. is a 27-year-old woman who presents with no pregnancy after 14 months of unprotected intercourse and irregular periods of 3 years duration. She used birth control pills in her previous relationship 7 years earlier.

HPI: Pertinent past history include menarche at 11, menstrual cycles occur every 28 days, lasting 3–4 days with occasional menstrual cramps relieved by nonsteroidal anti-inflammatory drugs (NSAIDs). Three years ago, she began to experience irregular periods. Occasionally, she may go 3–4 months without having a period. This phenomenon occurred shortly after she started a more stressful job and gained some weight. She has intercourse 2 or 3 times a week and experiences no pain during intercourse.

Physical exam: Height: 155 cm (5′2″) and weight: 80 kg (176 lb). She has dark and thick hair on her upper lip and chin. On the back of her neck, there is acanthosis nigricans. No milk is expressed from either breast. The pelvic exam shows abundant clear mucus in the opening of the cervix (cervical os). The uterus and both ovaries are unremarkable based on bimanual examination.

Diagnostic exams: Transvaginal ultrasound shows normal uterus and slightly enlarged ovaries with approximately 10 small follicles beneath the surface, all <10 mm in diameter.

Lab test results: Luteinizing hormone (LH) 12.4 International Units/mL, follicular-stimulating hormone (FSH) 4.1 International Units/mL, testosterone 73 ng/dL, thyroid-stimulating hormone (TSH) 1.7 milli-International Units/mL, and prolactin 13 ng/mL.

AGE AND FERTILITY

After its peak in her early 20s, a woman's fertility begins to decline in her late 20s; the decline became more considerable when she reaches late 30s.[2] The causes of decreased fertility with aging are multiple: ovarian aging (the "biological clock"), gynecologic diseases such as endometriosis (which interfere with conception), hormonal changes (which decrease the fecundity), and increased likelihood of spontaneous abortions.[5] In addition to decreased fecundity, advanced age is also associated with increased spontaneous abortion (miscarriage). Many spontaneous abortions are due to chromosomal abnormalities in the fetus. The rate of spontaneous abortion is approximately 10% for a 25-year-old women; it approaches 90% when the woman is 45 or older.[6] The analysis of the Hutterites, a tribe that does not use contraception, shows 11% of women after age 34 have no additional children, compared with 33% after 40, and 87% after 45.[7] Results of donor insemination also confirm the adverse impact of aging on female fertility.[8] A recent observation on approximately 800 fertile women shows the chance of pregnancy from one single sexual intercourse on any of the 6 days before ovulation decreases with advancing age.[2] It should be mentioned that the male fertility decreases with aging. Advanced paternal age is also associated with increased spontaneous abortion.[9]

ENDOCRINE CHANGES WITH AGING

The number of oocytes contained within individual follicles reaches 6 million to 7 million at 16–20 weeks of pregnancy in a female fetus. From that point on, the female fetus continues to lose oocytes such that at the time of puberty, only 300,000 remain. Of these, approximately 400–500 oocytes are ovulated during a woman's reproductive years. Ten to fifteen years before menopause, there is an accelerated loss of oocytes. The acceleration occurs when the number of follicles containing oocytes reach ~25,000, approximately at the age of 37–38.[10] With decreasing number of follicles, women begin to experience shorter menstrual cycles and have elevated serum follicle-stimulating hormone (FSH) levels during the early follicular phase. Based on this phenomenon, serum FSH levels in early follicular phase are used to estimate the ovarian reserve. It is hoped that the information may help clinicians to predict the response to ovulation induction agents and the likelihood of treatment success. Because serum FSH levels are regulated by estradiol and inhibin produced by the remaining follicles as well as other unknown factors, predictions based on FSH levels are not always reliable.

Etiology and Pathophysiology

The etiology of female infertility can be categorized as resulting from cervical factor (<10%), uterine factor (<10%), tubal and peritoneal factor (40%), ovulatory factor (40%), and others, such as thyroid disorder. Although ovulatory, tubal and peritoneal factors are the most common causes of female infertility, the investigation of infertility is not complete until all factors, including the peritoneal factor, have been examined.

If the investigation does not reveal any cause of infertility, the couples are given the diagnosis of unexplained infertility.

MALE FACTOR

Although this chapter discusses female infertility, infertility workup without investigating the male partner is incomplete, because one third of the infertile couples has male factor. Furthermore, subjecting the woman to infertility workup involving surgical procedure (such as laparoscopy, see below) without the knowledge of the male partner is irresponsible. Semen analysis is performed on a masturbated sample collected after 3–5 days of abstinence. Based on 1992 World Health Organization (WHO) criteria, normal sperm parameters are as follows: >20 million/mL, >2 mL, >30% normal forms, >50% showing forward progression, <1 million white blood cells/mL, <20% sperm with adherent particles on Immunobead test, and <10% sperm with adherent particles on SpermMar test.[11]

CERVICAL FACTOR

The cervix is the gateway to the female pelvis. Cervical mucus functions as a gatekeeper; it forms a barrier to prevent foreign organisms from entering the pelvis but allows the entry of sperm before ovulation. Three to four days before ovulation, its quality and quantity change as a result of elevated estrogen. The mucus becomes clear and more abundant, and allows sperm to penetrate. Although the value of a postcoital test is not recognized by all healthcare providers, it does provide information on the receptivity of the cervical mucus and the survival of sperm in the female genital tract.[12] The above information is important in women receiving clomiphene citrate, because some of them develop cervical mucus that is not receptive to sperm.

OVULATORY FACTOR

Anovulation (a state of no ovulation) can have a hypothalamic, pituitary, or ovarian origin. The arcuate nucleus of the hypothalamus secretes gonadotropin-releasing hormone (GnRH) to stimulate the pituitary gland to secrete gonadotropins (FSH and LH), which stimulate the growth of antral follicles and the production of estradiol. Hypothalamic anovulation is usually associated with a low GnRH secretion and low or normal levels of LH and FSH. As a result, the antral follicles in the ovary do not develop into mature follicles, and the serum estradiol level remains low. Reversible conditions associated with hypothalamic anovulation include extensive stress, extreme weight loss because of exercise, and anorexia nervosa; an example of an irreversible condition is the Kallmann syndrome.[13,14] Conditions such as tumors or cysts of the hypothalamus and the central nervous system may or may not be reversible. It depends on the extent of permanent damages from the pressure effects. Anovulation of pituitary origin is usually associated with low or normal LH and FSH secretion; its clinical picture is similar to that of hypothalamic anovulation. Disorders of anterior pituitary causing anovulation are pituitary tumors, such as nonfunctioning adenomas or prolactinoma.[15] Reversible conditions leading to anovulation of ovarian origin may be multiple; the most common condition is **polycystic ovary syndrome (PCOS),** which is caused by disregulation of follicular maturation due to insulin resistance. The levels of gonadotropins in patients with PCOS are within the normal range, although it is common to see an LH/FSH ratio higher than 3. Irreversible anovulation of ovarian origin includes premature ovarian failure, chromosomal abnormalities, and iatrogenic causes such as chemotherapy or irradiation.[16-18] In some cases, the etiology of premature ovarian failure is unknown.

TUBAL, UTERINE, AND PERITONEAL FACTOR

The fallopian tube is the conduit of the sperm and the oocyte. Without the fallopian tubes, there is no chance of natural pregnancy. The fallopian tube can be blocked as a result of previous pelvic infection, compression from a mass (such as fibroid), or pelvic surgery. The uterine factor include conditions that change the cavity of the uterus and thus interfere with normal fertility. The peritoneal factor includes conditions that interfere with normal movement of the fallopian tube (as a result of adhesions surrounding the fallopian tube), create a barrier between the fallopian tube and the ovary (because of adhesions surrounding the ovary), or alter the pelvic environment (because of an inflammatory reaction caused by endometriosis). Therefore, a history of pelvic inflammatory disease (PID), septic abortion, ruptured appendicitis, tubal surgery, and ectopic pregnancy increases the likelihood of tubal or peritoneal factor. The incidence of subsequent tubal infertility depends on the degree of infection as well as the microorganism that causes the infection. Results from recent study are not different from those performed more than two decades ago[19,20]: 12% infertility after one PID episode caused by gonorrhea or chlamydia, 23% after two episodes, and 54% after three. In the case of tubal infection caused by tuberculosis, the risk of infertility may be as high as 60%.[21] Similarly, the incidence of tubal (ectopic) pregnancy is also increased by PID, because adhesions inside or outside the fallopian tubes may interfere with the transport of embryo. The risk of ectopic (tubal) pregnancy after PID increases by about 6.8-fold[22]; observational studies show the incidence of tubal pregnancy after PID varies from 1.8% to 10% after PID.[19,23]

Uterine factors that may play a role in infertility include anatomic and nonanatomic causes. The former includes a mass, such as fibroids, blocking the tubes or distorting the uterine cavity. The latter includes the presence of subclinical inflammation, such as chronic endometritis.

UNEXPLAINED INFERTILITY

After all tests have been performed and no pathology is found, a diagnosis of unexplained infertility is given. Approximately 10% of infertile patients will receive this diagnosis.[24] The monthly fecundity of couples with unexplained infertility is 2% to 3%. Approximately 60% of couples with unexplained infertility of <3 years duration will have a pregnancy in the next 3 years.[25,26] Therefore, for women who are younger than 30 years old, it is not an unreasonable alternative to wait for 3 years before initiating infertility workup and treatment.

Assessment of Infertile Women

HISTORY AND PHYSICAL ASSESSMENT

A thorough patient history should be taken first. The patient's menstrual history should include questions regarding painful periods as well as the regularity of menstrual cycles. A history regarding the pubertal transition should also be obtained. In addition, history of sexually transmitted disease and endocrine problems should be ascertained from the patient. Previous medical treatment that may decrease ovarian reserve (such as irradiation, chemotherapy) or surgeries that may cause pelvic adhesions should also be ascertained. Questions regarding lifestyle and whether the patient leads an active or very sedentary lifestyle, as well as the amount of stress endured, should also be obtained. The medication history should include use of prescription drugs, over-the-counter medications, herbal products, and illicit drugs. The use of caffeine, cigarettes, and alcohol should be ascertained. Questions regarding general health, pain during intercourse, and a change in hair pattern or breast discharge are also important. Changes in body weight with or without concomitant change in menstrual cycles should also be elicited.

A physical assessment of the infertile woman should include body weight, height, and a complete physical assessment with emphasis on increased hair on the upper lip, chin, around the nipple, and upper abdomen (which may indicate elevated androgen), and discharge of milk from the nipple (which may indicate hyperprolactinemia). Acanthosis nigricans, a velvety dark skin, should be looked for on the back of the neck, the arm pit, and the inner thigh. Its presence indicates insulin resistance and may be part of the PCOS manifestation. A complete gynecologic exam should be performed to assess the vagina and the cervix for infection or anomalies as well as signs of estrogen status (or lack of). The size of the uterus and ovaries are assessed by bimanual exam and confirmed by using a pelvic ultrasound.

ENDOCRINE ASSESSMENT

Endocrine evaluation of the woman includes blood tests for FSH, LH, thyroid-stimulating hormone (TSH), prolactin, and 17-hydroxy progesterone. FSH and LH are mainly to rule out premature ovarian failure or hypothalamic/pituitary anovulation (low gonadotropins). Thyroid-stimulating hormone is to rule out thyroid as the cause for anovulation: hypothyroidism itself and the associated elevated prolactin levels can cause anovulation. Prolactin may be elevated in individuals with hypothyroidism (as a result of elevated TSH and prolactin) or pituitary adenoma. The 17-hydroxy progesterone level is useful to rule out late-onset congenital adrenal hyperplasia, an inherited enzyme defect in cortisol synthesis that leads to elevated adrenal androgen and anovulation. Although a typical PCOS patient has an elevated LH/FSH ratio (3:1), FSH and LH are not required to make a diagnosis of PCOS.

TESTING THE OVARIAN RESERVE

Two tests are commonly used to assess the "reserve" of the ovary and the likelihood of treatment success. The first measures FSH on the menstrual cycle day 3. A level of >20 milli-International Units/mL is associated with poor performance with **in vitro fertilization (IVF)** and a decreased chance of spontaneous pregnancy.[27] Sometimes, the level of estradiol is also determined. An estradiol of >80 pg/mL is also associated with decreased chance of spontaneous pregnancy and reduced outcome of assisted reproductive technology (ART). The elevated estradiol level is presumably associated with a hurried recruitment of follicles in response to elevated FSH secretion. The second test is the clomiphene challenge test.[28] This test measures the change of FSH levels before and after 5 days of clomiphene citrate. The change of FSH levels reflects the degree of negative feedback on the pituitary by inhibin B and estradiol secreted by antral follicles. Clomiphene citrate (100 mg) is given menstrual cycle days 5–9, and FSH levels on cycle days 3 and 10 are compared. An increase of 26 milli-International Units/mL or more is considered as positive and is associated with increased chance of failure to achieve a pregnancy spontaneously or after treatment.

Despite the high hope promised by initial reports, both tests have low sensitivity.[29,30] Advanced age alone, even with a negative clomiphene challenge test or "normal" FSH levels, is an important factor of decreased fertility, presumably because of other oocyte conditions related to aging. On the other hand, young patients, despite slightly elevated FSH levels or positive clomiphene challenge test, may still expect good outcome, because they may produce fewer but presumably better-quality eggs. Despite these shortcomings, both tests still offer some help to healthcare providers when planning therapy.

ASSESSING THE OVARIAN FACTOR

Confirmation of ovulation is based on a biphasic basal body temperature (BBT) (see Figure 22-1), serum progesterone of >3 ng/mL, or the confirmation of a decidualized endometrial stroma in an endometrial biopsy or ovulation prediction kit, which detects the preovulatory LH surge.[31-33] Biphasic BBT is evidence of ovulation but cannot be used to predict ovulation because it is based on the thermogenic property of progesterone. Elevated

Figure 22-1. Two cycles of BBT charting. Both show biphasic patterns. (The figure is from J-C H's personal collection.)

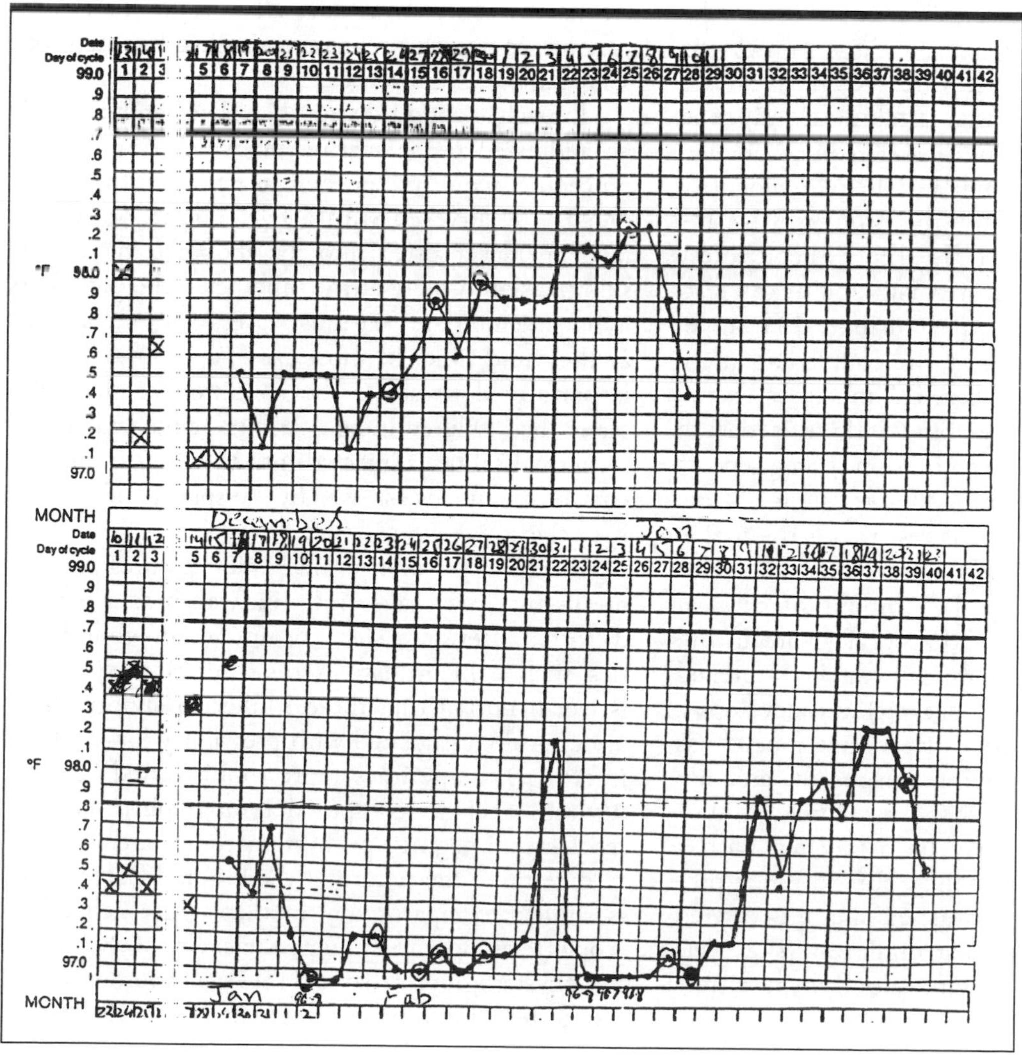

serum progesterone after ovulation "resets" the temperature set point of the hypothalamus; it raises the resting, or BBT, by 0.5°F. BBT is maintained by heat generated from our body's basal metabolism, which is reached after 4 hours of inactivity. The "resetting" of BBT, and hence the time from ovulation to elevated body temperature, may take 2–5 days. To confirm ovulation using serum progesterone, a blood sample is drawn 1 week after ovulation (menstrual cycle day 21 in a 28-day cycle or midluteal phase, i.e., 7 days after ovulation). A level of 3 ng/mL or higher is consistent with ovulation, although it is usually >10 ng/mL. Ovulation can also be confirmed based on the presence of decidualized changes of the endometrium; the sample is usually obtained 2–3 days before the anticipated period.

ASSESSING THE CERVICAL FACTOR

The extent to which cervical factor assessment contributes to the outcome of infertility workup is a controversial issue. Some believe its diagnostic and prognostic powers are limited, whereas others believe it is a useful test.[34,35] As a result, it is not used routinely by healthcare providers. Nonetheless, in some of the patients taking clomiphene citrate, the cervical mucus may become "hostile" to the sperm.[36] A postcoital test helps to identify these patients and overcome the problem with intrauterine insemination (IUI). The postcoital test is performed 2–3 days before ovulation; it can also be performed on the day after urinary LH surge. After 3–5 days of abstinence, the couple has intercourse, and the woman's cervical mucus is examined 2–8 hours after intercourse. There is debate as to the best timing of examination: Some reports suggest that a <2-hour interval gives sufficient information, whereas others suggest that a 16- to 24-hour interval provides a better assessment of sperm survival. The appearance, the amount of cervical mucus, and the quality of the cervical mucus are examined. Good cervical mucus can be stretched to 8–10 cm or more (spinnbarkeit) and develops a fern pattern when air dried. Receptive mucus has five or more sperm showing purposeful and active movement under a high-powered field (400X). A poor postcoital test may be associated with a decreased chance of pregnancy but does not preclude pregnancy.[37] IUI of washed sperm is offered to couples with a poor postcoital test. The cycle fecundity in patients receiving clomiphene citrate and IUI is approximately 20%.[38]

ASSESSING THE TUBAL, UTERINE, AND PERITONEAL FACTOR

The condition of the fallopian tube is assessed by the hysterosalpingogram (HSG) or the laparoscopy. HSG is performed 2–5 days after the end of menstruation. It is a radiologic exam. A radio-opaque contrast medium is injected via a catheter into the uterine cavity under a fluoroscopy. It fills the uterine cavity, spreads to the tubal lumen, and spills into the pelvis (see Figure 22-2). It is a dynamic study with representative still images taken for documentation purposes. HSG carries a small risk of infection (<1%) because foreign material is injected (indirectly) into the pelvis.[39] In addition to the condition of the tubes, lesions inside the uterus are revealed by HSG. They include uterine septum, submucous fibroid, and endometrial polyp. These lesions typically present as areas not filled by the contrast medium (i.e., "filling defect"). The nature of the pathology needs to be confirmed with other imaging technology or a hysteroscopy and biopsy. The mechanical "lavage" effect created by injecting the contrast medium offers some therapeutic benefits: increased pregnancy and live birth are observed after HSG procedure.[40]

The pelvic condition, on the other hand, can only be addressed by a laparoscopy, which is a surgical procedure requiring general anesthesia. The pelvic organs are surveyed with a telescope (5 or 10 mm in diameter) inserted into the abdomen via a small skin incision usually at the umbilicus. The pathology is documented and, in most cases, can be corrected at the same time. In most cases, a chromotubation is performed to assess the condition of the fallopian tubes. Diluted indigo carmine (a blue color dye) in normal saline is injected into the uterus; the patency of the tube is assessed by the spillage of dye into the pelvis.

Ultrasound reveals anatomic features of the uterus that may cause infertility, such as a mass; a distorted uterine cavity; or müllerian abnormalities, such as bicornuate uterus or uterine septum (it is worth noting that these Müllerian abnormalities are typically associated with pregnancy loss and not infertility). Sometimes more sophisticated imaging devices—such as computed tomography, magnetic resonance imaging, or hysteroscopy—are required to determine the nature of the lesion. Hysteroscopy is similar to laparoscopy in that it uses an endoscope (telescope) to evaluate the cavity of the uterus. Sonohysterography (sono-HSG) is another useful tool to reveal lesions inside the uterine cavity. Saline

Figure 22-2. (A) A normal HSG showing the dye fills both tubes and spills from the left tube. The distal ends of fallopian tubes (the ampullary or infundibular region) are slightly dilated. (B) Hydrosalpinges. Both tubes are obstructed; there was no spillage of contrast medium from either tube. (The figure is from J-C H's personal collection.)

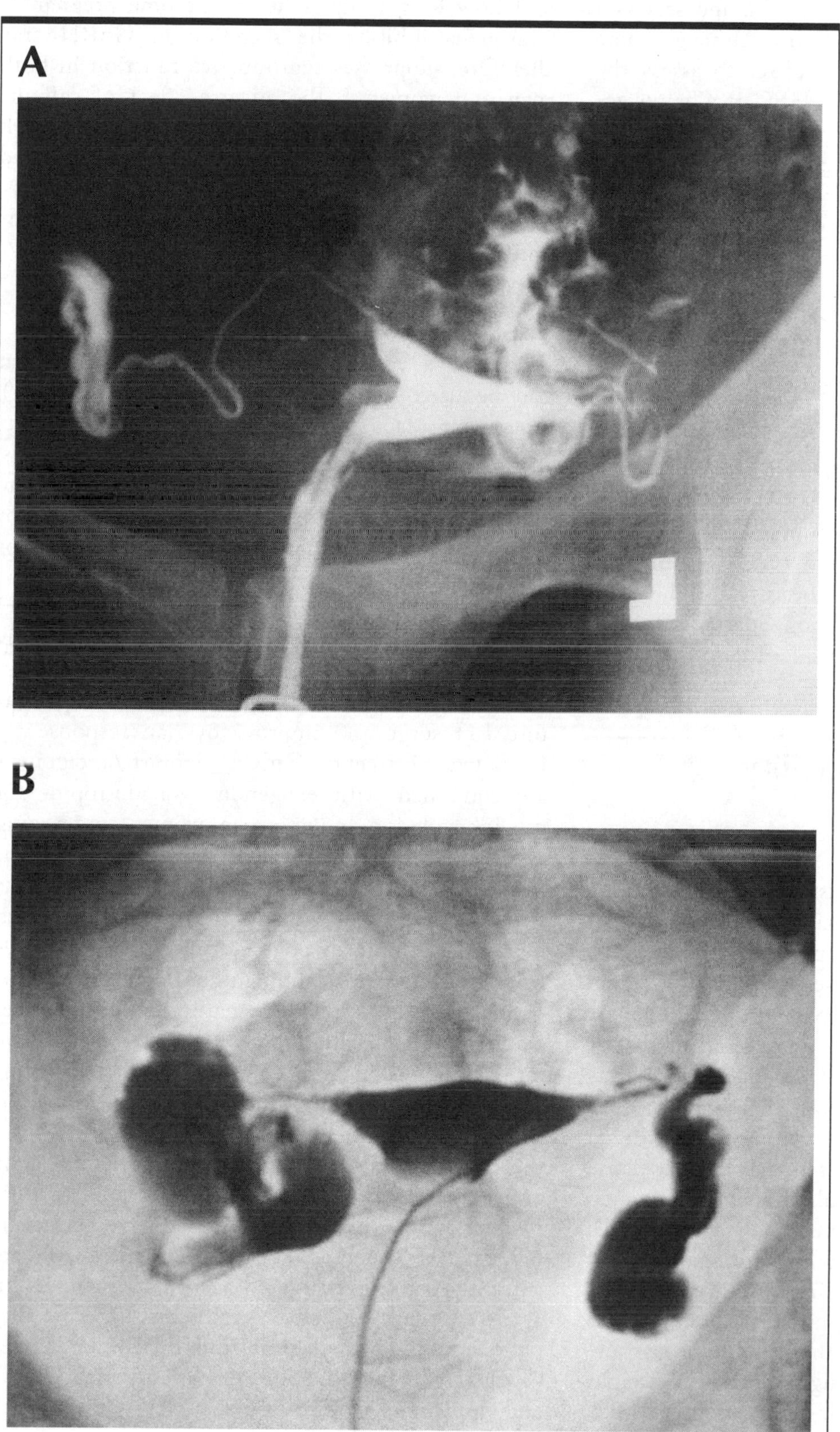

solution is injected into the uterus while a transvaginal ultrasound is performed. Intracavity lesions, such as polyps or fibroids, are easily visualized because the saline solution distends the uterine cavity, separates the opposing endometrium, and acts as a "window" for the ultrasound beam. Although some healthcare providers use sono-HSG to assess the patency of the fallopian tubes, HSG is a better accepted procedure.

In addition to confirming ovulation, endometrial biopsy helps to diagnose chronic endometritis (chronic inflammation of the endometrium), which, unlike PID, does not cause fever or abdominal pain.

ASSESSING THE MALE FACTOR

Although this chapter is limited to female infertility, treating the woman without minimum knowledge of the male partner is not the standard of care. The male partner is asked to submit semen sample for analysis. Based on 1992 WHO criteria, normal sperm parameters are >20 million/mL, >2 mL, >30% normal forms, >50% showing forward progression, <1 million white blood cells/mL, and <20% sperm with adherent particles on Immunobead test, and <10% sperm with adherent particles on SpermMar test.[11] Some healthcare providers consider these criteria too stringent.[41]

Management of Infertility

NONPHARMACOLOGIC

Lifestyle/nonpharmacologic management of infertility includes weight adjustment (either gain or loss) and cessation of smoking, alcohol, caffeine, and illicit drugs. The logical approach to reverse hypothalamic anovulation caused by stress, extreme weight loss, or anorexia nervosa is lifestyle change, such as reducing stress level, increasing weight, or decreasing exercise level.[42,43] In women with hypothalamic anovulation and a body mass index (BMI) <20, weight gain should be seriously considered as the first line of therapy as it may be associated with the resumption of ovulation and pregnancy. On the other hand, in women with a high BMI, abnormal hypothalamic GnRH secretion, pituitary LH and FSH secretion, insulin resistance, and anovulation are common.[44] Therefore, if these patients have ovulatory dysfunction, they should be encouraged to lose weight. Although ideal body weight is the ultimate goal, as little as 5% to 10% body weight loss may help to resume normal ovulation. Weight reduction is best achieved with a combination of diet and exercise. Smoking reduces the germ cells in both men and women. There is a dosage relationship between how much a woman smokes and how long it takes her to become pregnant.[45] Marijuana inhibits the secretion of GnRH and, therefore, suppresses reproductive function in both men and women.[46] The adverse affect of caffeine on fertility has not been well established, although excessive caffeine intake is associated with delayed conception.[47-49] Because infertility can cause stress, the patient should be provided with information regarding support groups such as RESOLVE (http://www.resolve.org/).

PHARMACOLOGIC

There are a variety of pharmacologic agents that can be used to treat infertility (see Table 22-1). Treatment plans are variable from different clinics and should be tailored to the patient's needs. The purpose of ovulation induction is to stimulate the development of at least one ovarian follicle, or multiple follicles in the case of superovulation or controlled ovarian hyperstimulation.[50,51] Gonadotropins, which contain either FSH alone or both FSH and LH, are injectable medications that directly act on the ovaries to induce follicular development. GnRH agonists and antagonists prevent premature LH surge and improve ovarian response.[52-54] Gonadotropins and GnRH agonists/antagonists are combined with exogenous gonadotropins for use in ovulation induction in women undergoing assisted reproductive techniques. Lutropin alfa is the only recombinant form of LH approved for use with follitropin alfa to help infertility patients with hypogonadotropic hypogonadism. Once the follicles have developed, human chorionic gonadotropin (hCG) allows follicular maturation and induces ovulation. One of the most widely used medication for ovulation induction is clomiphene citrate, a nonsteroidal oral agent that stimulates the release of gonadotropins by affecting the estrogen receptors in the hypothalamus. Clomiphene can be used alone or in conjunction with other medications to treat patients with ovulatory dysfunction. Aromatase inhibitors (AIs) such as letrozole and anastrozole are currently being investigated as ovulation induction agents. Other adjunctive treatments for infertility patients include metformin and thiazolidinediones (TZDs), which are helpful for patients with PCOS, and dopamine agonists are used for patients with hyperprolactinemia.

Table 22-1. Table of Drugs Used for Infertility Treatment

Class of Drugs	Medications
Menotropins or human menopausal gonadotropins (hMGs)	75 International Units FSH and 75 International Units LH; 150 International Units FSH and 150 International Units LH; given IM or SC
Urofollitropin	75 International Units FSH; given IM or SC
Recombinant	Follitropin alfa; 75 International Units FSH or 150 International Units; given SC Follitropin beta: 75 International Units FSH; given SC or IM
Chorionic gonadotropin (u-hCG)	10,000 units hCG; given IM
Choriogonadotropin (r-hCG)	250 mcg hCG; given SC
GnRH agonist	Leuprolide: 5 mg/mL injection; given IM Nafarelin: 2 mg/mL; intranasal spray
GnRH antagonist	Cetrorelix: 0.25 mg, 3-mg injection; given SC Ganirelix: 250 mcg/0.5-mL injection; given SC
Aromatase inhibitor	Anastrazole: Letrozole: 2.5-mg tablet; oral
Progesterone	Vaginal gel: 4%, 8% Vaginal inserts: 100 mg Vaginal suppository: compounded product Capsule: 100 mg, 200 mg; oral Injection, oil: 50 mg/mL; given IM

FSH = follicle-stimulating hormone; GnRH = gonadotropin-releasing hormone; hCG = human chorionic gonadotropin; IM = intramuscularly; LH = luteinizing hormone; SC = subcutaneously.

Clomiphene Citrate

Clomiphene citrate is a nonsteroidal estrogen agonist/antagonist that binds to and down-regulates estrogen receptors. Its antiestrogenic property at the hypothalamus leads to the inhibition of the negative feedback of estrogen, and, as a result, elevates FSH and LH secretion by the pituitary.[50,55,56] Increased levels of FSH and LH stimulate follicular growth, and LH surge occurs spontaneously to trigger ovulation. In other words, clomiphene citrate enhances the normal follicular maturation process and ovulation, but, unlike gonadotropins, does not stimulate the ovary directly.[50,52] Clomiphene citrate is most effective in women who have normal FSH and produce adequate estrogen (i.e., in women with intact hypothalamic–pituitary–ovarian axis).[50]

Clomiphene citrate is indicated for use infertility patients with ovulatory dysfunction and is available in 50-mg tablet.[57] A daily dose of 50 mg is normally given for 5 days during cycle days 5–9 after spontaneous or progestin-induced menses, although it can be initiated on cycle day 3.[55,56] There is no difference in ovulation rates, conception rate, and pregnancy outcomes if therapy is started on day 3 or day 5.[50,56,58] If ovulation is not induced in the first course of treatment, then the dose of clomiphene citrate is increased in 50-mg increments in subsequent cycles. The U.S. Food and Drug Administration (FDA) does not approve of doses >100 mg/day because there is no advantage with respect to ovulation response rate.[55,56,59,60] About 75% to 80% of pregnancies attributed to clomiphene occur within the first three ovulatory cycles.[56,59] The duration of treatment is normally limited to six ovulatory cycles.

Treatment monitoring for clomiphene citrate should include confirmation of ovulation, either by recording BBT readings or using ovulation kits that detect urinary LH surge. Another method is to measure the midluteal progesterone level.[55,56] Even though transvaginal ultrasound monitoring is not required in clomiphene citrate cycles, it may be useful in patients who have unexplained infertility or are not responding to clomiphene citrate.[55,56,60]

About 10% of women treated with clomiphene citrate experience vasomotor flushes or hot flashes as a side effect. In addition, abdominal or pelvic discomfort, ovarian enlargement, headaches, nausea, and mood swings are common side effects in <10% of patients.[57] Visual disturbances such as blurred vision, diplopia, flashes, or spots can occur in <2% of patients and may be dose related.[50,52,55] Patients who identify any signs of visual disturbance should notify the physician, and discontinuation of treatment may be indicated. Clomiphene citrate can exert antiestrogenic side effects on the cervix and the endometrium that lead to decreased quality and quantity of cervical mucus as well as reduced endometrial proliferation. It is unclear how the antiestrogen adverse effects associated with clomiphene citrate affect fecundity.[55,61] Another potential adverse effect of clomiphene is multiple births. Twin pregnancy occurs in approximately 5% of clomiphene citrate pregnancies; triplet pregnancy is 1% to 2%.[61]

For patients who are resistant to clomiphene citrate, other medications such as dexamethasone, hCG, metformin, TZDs, and gonadotropins may be used as either adjuvant or alternative therapy. Dexamethasone used in combination with clomiphene citrate to suppress adrenal androgen suppression may improve ovulation and pregnancy rates.[55,62] An addition of exogenous hCG to clomiphene citrate therapy to induce ovulation should be limited in use for patients who cannot detect urinary LH surge or are undergoing an assisted reproductive technique such as IUI.[50,55] Another option for patients unresponsive to clomiphene is the use of low-dose exogenous gonadotropins, either combined with clomiphene or alone.[55,56]

Patients with PCOS may use insulin sensitizers such as metformin and TZDs, (pioglitazone and rosiglitazone) to reduce insulin resistance. Although not approved by the FDA, metformin and TZDs have been combined with clomiphene citrate to induce ovulation in patients who do not respond to clomiphene or metformin. Metformin reduces circulating insulin levels to help normalize follicular development in PCOS women. The common dosage of metformin is between 1,500 and 2,000 mg per day, in divided doses. Common side effects of metformin are gastrointestinal tract related, such as nausea vomiting. Starting at 500 mg/day and building up the dosage gradually helps to reduce side effects. Extended-release tablets help to reduce the side effects and allow the daily dose to be taken at once. Metformin alone is inferior to clomiphene citrate in helping patients with PCOS to attain live births.[63] Although some studies involving small number of patients suggest that continuing metformin after attaining pregnancy reduces spontaneous abortions, results from multicenter randomized controlled trial studies do not support this.[63,64] The newest class of insulin sensitizer is the TZD, a synthetic peroxisome proliferator activator γ ligand. It has been used successfully to induce ovulation in patients with PCOS.[65-67]

Aromatase Inhibitors

Letrozole and anastrazole are AIs, which have reportedly been used to induce ovulation.[68,69] Both letrozole and anastrazole are oral, nonsteroidal compounds that block the enzyme aromatase, which converts androgens (androstenedione and testosterone) into estrogens. AIs lower the estrogen level, and the hypothalamus senses a hypoestrogenic state and augments the secretion of LH and FSH.[56,69] In addition, AIs may enhance follicular sensitivity to FSH stimulation because of accumulation of androgens in the ovaries.[69,70] Unlike clomiphene citrate, because aromatase inhibitors do not block estrogen receptors, the endometrium is not negatively affected.[71] Letrozole is being studied in women with PCOS either as a monotherapy or combination therapy with gonadotropins to induce ovulation.[38,72-74] Letrozole is available in a 2.5-mg tablet and is administered once daily for 5 days (cycle days 3–7 or cycle days 5–9), whereas anastrazole is available in a 1-mg tablet and is given in a similar manner. Several studies have shown that letrozole is comparable to clomiphene citrate.[51,75,76] Adverse side effects include hot flushes, nausea, vomiting, and leg cramps. Aromatase inhibitors are not approved by the FDA to induce ovulation, and there is concern regarding the safety of letrozole and the risk of congenital anomalies.[77]

Gonadotropins

Ovulation induction using exogenous gonadotropins allows the recruitment and development of multiple follicles by exposing the ovarian follicles to an increased level of FSH above the threshold to maintain follicular growth.[54,60] Gonadotropins from natural and recombinant sources are commercially available in injectable dosage forms. Menotropins or human menopausal gonadotropins (hMGs) are highly purified gonadotropins from urine of postmenopausal women containing a mixture of 1:1 ratio of FSH and LH (one vial contains 75 International Units each of LH and FSH).[54] They have been used since the 1970s. Urofollitropins are also derived from urine of postmenopausal women but contain only highly purified urinary

FSH (75 International Units of FSH). Recombinant DNA technology has led to the development of recombinant gonadotropins that contain either FSH or LH alone.[54] Follitropins such as follitropin alfa and follitropin beta contain only FSH. On the other hand, lutropin alfa contains only LH. The outcomes of ovulation induction and pregnancy using natural or recombinant gonadotropins are not different.[78,79]

The two common treatment regimens used with gonadotropins are the low-dose, step-up protocol and the step-down protocol. The use of the low-dose step-down regimen allows the FSH threshold to be reached in a gradual manner. This regimen also helps to reduce excessive ovarian stimulation.[54,60] The low-dose step-down regimen starts with initial dose of 50–75 International Units of FSH, given either intramuscularly or subcutaneously; after 7–14 days, the dose is increased in increments of 37.5 International Units at weekly intervals.[54,60] The step-down protocol begins with a dosage of 150 International Units/day of FSH until one follicle reaches ≥10 mm on ultrasound. Then the dosage is decreased in a stepwise fashion from 112.5 International Units/day to 75 International Units/day until ovulation. In a study comparing the two protocols, results showed that there was no difference in the cumulative rate of clinical gestation between the two protocols and that the step-up protocol was safer with respect to ovarian stimulation.[80]

Using gonadotropin to induce ovulation requires special careful monitoring. The serum estradiol and the sizes of the follicles need to be monitored closely so that 1) the dosage of gonadotropins can be adjusted to avoid lack of response (and no ovulation) or explosive response (and develop **ovarian hyperstimulation syndrome (OHSS)**—see below), and 2) when the follicles are mature, the final step of egg development (and its release) may be triggered by hCG, an LH surge surrogate. Besides ovarian hyperstimulation, multiple pregnancy is a complication of gonadotropin treatment. One in five pregnancies after using gonadotropin is multiple pregnancy; one third of these multiple pregnancies are triplet or more.[82] Other side effects include hot flashes, breast pain, and abdominal pain.[57]

Human Chorionic Gonadotropin

hCG is normally used with clomiphene citrate or gonadotropin to trigger ovulation. hCG shares similar chemical structure with LH and binds to LH receptors of the granulosa cells. Injection of hCG usually takes place at the end of ovulation induction to simulate a natural LH surge, which completes the final stages of follicular development (such as the resumption of meiosis II) and triggers ovulation. Available products on the market are chorionic gonadotropin (u-hCG) and choriogonadotropin alfa (r-hCG). Chorionic gonadotropin is a urinary-derived product that contains 10,000 units hCG and is given intramuscularly. Choriogonadotropin alfa is produced from recombinant technology, contains 250 mcg r-hCG, and is administered subcutaneously. Studied have shown that u-hCG and r-hCG have comparable efficacy.[83,84]

Lutropin Alfa

Lutropin alfa is a recombinant form of LH and is indicated for female patients with hypogonadotropic hypogonadism with profound LH deficiency (LH of <1.2 International Units/L). The mechanism of action is to stimulate the theca cells in the ovaries to stimulate androgen secretion, which is converted to estradiol by aromatase enzymes in the granulosa cells, and allow for follicular development.[84] This medication is approved for use with follitropin alfa and is available as an injectable product containing 75 International Units LH. It is administered subcutaneously once daily along with follitropin alfa.

Gonadotropin-Releasing Hormone Agonists

GnRH agonists are used to suppress spontaneous LH surge during ovulation induction and allow optimal duration of gonadotropin administration to maximize follicular maturation.[85] Daily GnRH agonist injection first stimulates, then down-regulates the pituitary gland by interfering with normal pulsatile GnRH secretion. As a result, during the first few days, more gonadotropins are released (the flare effect).[54] After approximately 7 days, the pituitary gland ceases to secrete gonadotropin, and down-regulation is achieved. GnRH agonists are administered with gonadotropins, and different protocols (long protocol, short or flare-up protocol, and ultrashort protocol) are used.[54]

The long protocol starts the GnRH agonist during the luteal phase of the previous cycle. Once menstruation begins, gonadotropins are administered to stimulate follicular development. This is the so-called long protocol, because the process involves two menstrual cycles. In the short or flare-up protocol, the GnRH agonist is started shortly after the menstruation begins, then the gonadotropins are initiated on cycle day 3.[54] The short protocol has been exploited to enhance ovulation induction in patients who respond poorly to gonadotropins.[54] In the ultrashort protocols, the GnRH agonists are given for 3 days and then discontinued. Several studies have demonstrated that the long protocol is more effective than the short protocol.[86-88] GnRH agonists are synthetic products available in injectable (leuprolide) and intranasal spray (nafarelin) dosage forms. Side effects associated with GnRH agonists include hot flashes, headache, mood swings, breast tenderness, and OHSS.

Gonadotropin-Releasing Hormone Antagonists

GnRH antagonists bind to GnRH receptors of the pituitary gland without invoking downstream events and thus immediately suppresses gonadotropin release. The antagonists ensure that there is no premature LH surge. As a result of this immediate suppression, the GnRH antagonists can be given during the treatment cycle. Two GnRH antagonists are available. Cetrorelix is an injectable medication available in 0.25 mg or 3 mg and administered subcutaneously. Ganirelix is available in a 0.25-mg injectable form. A single-dose and a multiple-dose regimen can be used. The single-dose approach uses 3 mg cetrorelix administered in the late follicular phase (day 7, 8, or 9) to prevent premature LH surge.[54,89] The multiple-dose regimen involves giving either 0.25 mg cetrorelix or 0.25 ganirelix daily starting on day 7 until hCG administration. GnRH antagonists may offer an alternative to GnRH agonists.[89-91]

Progesterone

Progesterone is used in women undergoing IVF cycles to supplement endogenous progesterone. Progesterone supplement comes in three different forms: 1) intramuscular injection (progesterone in oil, 50-mg intramuscular injection once daily); 2) vaginal formulation (gel 8%, inserts, and suppository); and 3) oral (tablet 100 mg or 200 mg). Progesterone is normally started the day after oocytes are retrieved and discontinued between 8 and 10 weeks of pregnancy (from the last menstrual period), despite that fact that the placenta takes over the role of the ovary to support the pregnancy at 8 weeks (from the last menstrual period).[52,92] Adverse side effects include breakthrough bleeding, breast tenderness, and galactorrhea.[57]

Pharmacologic Agents to Treat Hyperprolactinemia

In patients with hyperprolactinemia, elevated prolactin decreases GnRH pulse frequency, which decreases FSH and LH release from the pituitary.[93,94] Bromocriptine, a dopamine agonist, normalizes prolactin level and restores normal FSH and LH secretion. The main side effects of bromocriptine are nausea, vomiting, and orthostatic hypertension. Caution should be taken in patients taking antihypertensive medications. To minimize these side effects, bromocriptine is usually started at 1.25 mg at bedtime, increased to twice a day after 1 week, then to 2.5 mg twice daily over the next 2 weeks as necessary to achieve reduction in prolactin levels. Normal ovulation usually resumes in 4 weeks. Patients can become resistant to bromocriptine therapy.[94] Cabergoline is an ergot-derived dopamine agonist that can be used for hyperprolactinemia. It is available in a 0.5-mg tablet, and, because of its long half-life, the dosing is reduced to twice-weekly or weekly basis.[94]

Assisted Reproductive Techniques

INTRAUTERINE INSEMINATION

IUI involves delivering washed sperm into the uterine cavity via a soft catheter. The washing process reduces the volume and removes dead sperm and unwanted material from the semen. In randomized control clinical trials, IUI enhanced the cycle fecundity in couples with unexplained infertility.[95] Occasionally, unwashed semen samples are used for intracervical insemination, which is less effective in enhancing cycle fecundity.[95]

IN VITRO FERTILIZATION

IVF was originally developed as a technique for treatment of tubal factor infertility but now is considered appropriate for many other indications. In IVF, eggs are retrieved from the ovaries and fertilized in vitro. The embryos are transferred back to the uterus a few days later. Under ultrasound guidance,

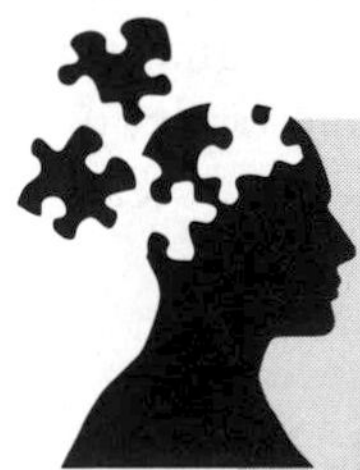

Therapeutic Challenge:

A young couple underwent IVF and had five good embryos. The infertility specialist transfers three embryos, and two grow into two healthy babies, one boy and one girl. At the time of embryo transfer, this couple inquires about the options for the remaining two embryos.

the follicles are punctured, and the oocytes are collected into tubes that are connected to the needle. The eggs are then fertilized by the sperm in a Petri dish. The fertilized eggs are cultured 3–5 days before being transferred to the uterus through the cervix. The first successful IVF was performed in 1978 in a woman who had tubal factor infertility. It has since been used in women with unexplained infertility, severe pelvic adhesion disease, endometriosis, male factor infertility, and partners with genetic diseases (with the help of preimplantation genetic diagnosis to select unaffected embryos). As of 2005, slightly more than 1% of the babies born in the U.S. are IVF babies. The successful rate of IVF depends on the age of the female patient. Based on the most recent data (2005), approximately 40% of women 35 years of age or younger are expected to have a live birth after one IVF cycle, and increasing age of the woman is associated with a decline in live birth rate (http://www.cdc.gov/art). Although IVF is overall a safe procedure, a small but statistically significant increase in birth defects have been reported in IVF children compared with their naturally conceived counterparts.[96]

Most of the ART procedures performed today are IVF. Gamete intrafallopian transfer (GIFT) and zygote intrafallopian transfer (ZIFT) are rarely used nowadays. The former involves transferring eggs and sperm into the fallopian tube and allowing fertilization to take place in vivo. The latter involves transferring fertilized eggs or early-stage embryos to the fallopian tubes. Neither procedure offers better outcome than conventional IVF, although GIFT may be more appealing to couples whose religious beliefs favor natural fertilization.[97]

INTRACYTOPLASMIC SPERM INJECTION

Intracytoplasmic sperm injection (ICSI) involves injecting single sperm into the cytoplasm of an egg. The procedure requires a microscope equipped with micromanipulators and a fine needle to deliver the sperm. ICSI overcomes the problem associated with severe male factor infertility—the sperm count or activity is too low such that natural fertilization in IVF is not likely to occur. The fertilization rate after ICSI is similar to that of IVF (~60% to 70%). ICSI may transfer defective genes associated with male infertility, such as abnormal Y chromosome or cystic fibrosis gene mutation to the offspring. In addition, children born after ICSI have twice as high the risk of major birth defects as naturally conceived counterparts.[98]

ASSISTED REPRODUCTIVE TECHNOLOGY IN OLDER COUPLES

The experience with donor oocyte programs supports the notion that age-related decline in women is primarily due to aging oocytes rather than to the aging of the endometrium/uterus. With donor eggs, a pregnancy rate of 40% to 50% per cycle can be achieved in patients older than 40, and a cumulative pregnancy rate per patient can reach 90% with four or more cycles.[100] It is worth mentioning that the rate of miscarriage or spontaneous abortion in older women receiving oocytes from donors aged 20–24 years was about 14%; this is in contrast to 44.5% when the donors were older than age 35.[100]

SURGERY TO INDUCE OVULATION IN POLYCYSTIC OVARY SYNDROME PATIENTS

In women who do not respond to clomiphene citrate and insulin sensitizer(s) ("clomiphene resistant"), gonadotropins are used to induce ovulation. Occasionally, surgery to the ovaries is performed instead of using gonadotropin. The first such surgery, reported by Stein and Leventhal, involved opening the abdomen and removing a wedge of ovarian stroma, which produces testosterone. Nowadays, the procedure is performed via laparoscopy. Instead of wedge resection, electrocauterization, CO_2 laser "drilling," multiple punch biopsies, and photocoagulation are performed with the same goal of removing the testosterone-producing ovarian stroma. After the surgery, there is a transient (~6–12 months) hormonal change, which results in spontaneous ovulation.[101] A recent Cochrane review showed that there is no difference between gonadotropin and ovarian "drilling" in live birth rates and pregnancy rates.[102] Although these procedures are relatively easy to perform and appear not to carry major complications, most healthcare providers prefer to use gonadotropin because the benefit of surgery lasts only 6–12 months, and adhesion, which further complicates the treatment, forms in 15% to 20% of patients.[103]

Complications of Infertility Treatment

OVARIAN HYPERSTIMULATION SYNDROME

OHSS is a rare but severe complication of ovulation induction.[104] It is mainly seen in patients receiving gonadotropin (with or without IVF). The clinical presentation of severe OHSS consists of enlarged ovaries, ascites, hydrothorax, decreased urine output, and hemoconcentration and hypercoagulability. OHSS causes life-threatening complications, such as kidney failure, thrombosis, and stroke. One of the mediators of OHSS is vascular endothelial growth factor (VEGF), which is secreted by luteinized follicles.[105] Elevated VEGF levels lead to leaky blood vessels and fluid accumulation in the third space. OHSS usually occurs in patients with a high level of estradiol (>2,000 pg/mL) and multiple follicles in the ovary. If the hCG is withheld, OHSS can be avoided, because granulosa cells are not luteinized. Supportive therapy is the only treatment, which may include infusing albumin to hold free water in the intravascular space. OHSS resolves spontaneously. In women who become pregnant in the same cycle, OHSS may take longer to resolve (~8 weeks from the last menstrual period).

MULTIPLE BIRTHS

Multiple births are one of the complications of fertility treatment. It involves both the mother and the offspring. Five to eight percent of pregnancies from clomiphene therapy are multiple pregnancy (mostly twins).[61] Twenty-five percent of pregnancies after gonadotropin ovulation induction and approximately 35% of IVF pregnancies (http://apps.nccd.cdc.gov/ART2005/nation05.asp) are multiple pregnancies.[81] High-order multiple pregnancies—triplets or more—represent 11% of the IVF multiple pregnancy in the above survey. Multiple pregnancy (especially triplet or higher) is associated with higher mortality and morbidity in mother and child. Hypertension, diabetes, and preterm labor are more likely to happen in women carrying multiple gestations than single gestation. Premature babies are more likely to have developmental problems and long-term sequelae, such as learning disabilities and brain dysfunction. It is hoped that the recent trend to transfer fewer embryos may reduce the incidence of multiple pregnancies.[106]

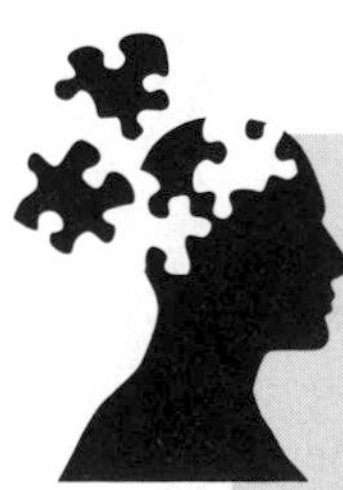

Therapeutic Challenge:

A 34-year-old woman with family history of two first-degree relatives with ovarian cancer presents to your clinic requesting options for infertility treatment. Is clomiphene citrate an appropriate treatment option?

CASE PRESENTATION

Patient Case: Part 2

Patient assessment: The clinical presentation consists of obesity, irregular periods (anovulation), hyperandrogenism, and infertility. J.S.'s past history does not include risk factors for tubal or peritoneal factor. Physical exam shows the feature of hyperandrogenism and a normal pelvic exam. The pelvic ultrasound shows the ovaries have typical PCOS features. The blood test rules out other causes of anovulation, such as thyroid and pituitary problems. The LH/FSH ratio is 3:1.

Treatment plan: The first-line ovulation induction agent is clomiphene citrate. Should clomiphene citrate fail to result in pregnancy, the second-line agent is gonadotropins or laparoscopic ovarian surgery (such as ovarian frilling). The use of gonadotropins is associated with increased chances for multiple pregnancy and, therefore, intensive monitoring of ovarian response is required. Laparoscopic ovarian surgery is usually effective in <50% of women, and additional ovulation induction medication may be required under these circumstances. Overall, ovulation induction using clomiphene and gonadotropins is highly effective with a cumulative singleton live birth rate of 72%. The third-line treatment is IVF. More patient-tailored approaches should be developed for ovulation induction to avoid OHSS.

The treatment plan for our patient is, therefore, outlined as follows: J.S.'s partner is asked to submit semen sample for analysis. J.S. has a counseling session to discuss nonpharmacologic intervention/lifestyle changes.

Patient education: J.S. is educated about the importance of weight reduction and exercise. She is informed that weight loss is likely to enhance the effects of treatment and that as little as 5% weight loss (8 lb) may be sufficient to restore her menstrual pattern and ovulation. An exercise and diet program is then initiated.

Patient monitoring: After 3 months, progress is evaluated and, if necessary, ovulation induction with clomiphene citrate is started. Once ovulation is documented by midluteal phase progesterone, a postcoital test will be performed to assess the sperm/mucus interaction. If the postcoital test is satisfactory, the patient will be given an additional three cycles of clomiphene citrate. If it is unsatisfactory, IUI (using husband's washed sperm) may be used to bypass the cervix. In either case, if J.S. is not pregnant after four trials, assessment of tubal, uterine, and peritoneal factor will be achieved by a laparoscopy with concomitant chromotubation and hysteroscopy. After the evaluation, J.S. will receive gonadotropin to induce ovulation in combination with IUI using her husband's sperm. If she does not attain pregnancy after three attempts, IVF will be offered.

CANCER RISK

The relationship between ovulation induction (or fertility treatment as a whole) and ovarian cancer remains controversial.[107] Those in favor of this view believe that because oral contraceptive pills, which inhibit ovulation, reduces ovarian cancer risks, fertility treatment, which induces ovulation, may increase ovarian cancer risks.[107] Individual reports, mostly case control studies, are limited by their short follow-up. There is no prospective, randomized controlled trial. Available data suggest that infertility in nulliparous women is associated with a slightly higher risk of ovarian cancer than in their parous counterparts and that ovarian stimulation with fertility drugs does not increase the risk.[107,108]

Summary

Infertility due to ovulation dysfunction responds favorably to medical treatment. It is expected that 50% of patients receiving clomiphene citrate become ovulatory, 30% become pregnant, and 25% have a live birth.[61] The cumulative live birth rate after receiving clomiphene citrate or gonadotropin is 72%.[60] Because most patients become pregnant within three cycles, a new treatment modality should be considered while a patient is receiving her third treatment cycle.

References

Additional content available at
www.ashp.org/womenshealth

23 Drug Principles in Pregnancy and Lactation

Pamela D. Berens, MD; Thomas W. Hale, R.Ph., Ph.D.

Learning Objectives

1. Discuss the principle of drug transfer across the placenta to the fetus.
2. Describe the principles of drug transfer into breast milk and subsequent factors affecting drug transfer to the infant.
3. Compare and contrast the classification of drugs during pregnancy and lactation.
4. Understand how to use resources for information regarding drug effects during pregnancy and lactation.

The use of medications in pregnant and breast-feeding women has risen significantly over the last few decades, and it is estimated that between 40% and 90% of pregnant women take at least one medication during pregnancy.[1,2] The increased frequency of medications used during pregnancy is likely the result of more extensive clinical experience and the perception of a clearer safety profile for many therapeutics.

Although the majority of these medications are prescribed by the patient's physician, many mothers still use over-the-counter medications, often without seeking medical advice. Even more often, women may consume some medication before the realization that they are pregnant.[3] Most recent information available from the Pregnancy Risk Assessment Monitoring System (PRAMS) from 2004 indicates that only 30% of women reported seeking advice from a healthcare provider regarding preparation for a healthy pregnancy and infant.[4]

Information from one population-based study conducted during 1998–2002 found that although the prevalence of medication use decreased from 72% before pregnancy to 56% during pregnancy, it returned to 78% in the postpartum period.[5] The most commonly used medications during pregnancy in this population included antibiotics (75%), oral contraceptives (45%), and nonsteroidal anti-inflammatory drugs (NSAIDs; 17%). In the postpartum period, the most commonly used medications were NSAIDs (56%), oral contraceptives (53%), and antidepressants (13%). Another study has indicated that antiemetics, tranquilizers, antihistamines, and diuretics are additional frequently used medications in pregnancy.[6]

Ultimately, the use of medications during pregnancy and lactation involves a level of complexity not usually encountered by most healthcare providers when prescribing drugs. Contrary to the most typical situation, in which a healthcare provider's risk/benefit analysis involves only the patient, pharmacotherapeutics involving pregnant and lactating women must take into account both the patient (i.e., the mother) and the potential impact on the fetus or newborn. The range of possibilities include 1) teratogenicity associated with either dose or timing of the drug exposure, 2) untoward pharmacologic effect, and 3) loss of efficacy for the mother because of increased volume of distribution or increased clearance secondary to the presence of additional compartments and clearance mechanisms via the fetus. The fetus may or may not receive benefit from treatment and may be subject to untoward side effects or experience overt toxicity secondary to the mother's medication use. Thus, a risk-vs.-benefit assessment is almost always required, and both the health of the mother and her infant must be individually evaluated with respect to the medication chosen.

Because there are few data collected during the development of new drugs with regard to the pharmacodynamics or toxicity in pregnant and breast-feeding women, data are often anecdotal or derived from investigator-initiated studies. This situation is neither surprising nor easily corrected as there is a considerable amount of difficulty and potential risk associated with the testing of new drugs in pregnant and lactating women.

Prior experience has revealed some currently available medications are significantly hazardous to the fetus or the breast-feeding infant, and healthcare providers attempt to avoid their use. However, most drugs cross the placenta to some degree and still have the potential to produce yet unknown untoward effects in the infant. This still occurs today despite more extensive knowledge in this area. In breast-feeding mothers, the teratogenic risk is removed, but the risk of clinically untoward or toxic effects in the infant remains. Fortunately, the placenta and the human breast prevent or diminish the entry of some drugs and chemicals into their compartments, likely mitigating the relative number of medications that are truly hazardous to a fetus or a breast-feeding infant. This chapter will discuss the entry of medications into these two compartments: the placenta and fetus, and the human breast-milk compartment.

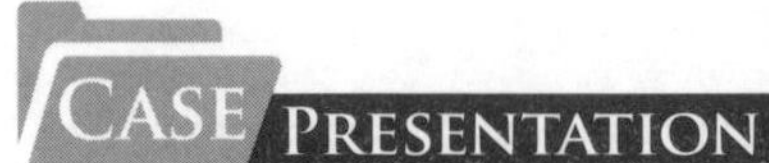

CASE PRESENTATION

Patient Case: Part 1

A patient and her husband are seeking preconceptual care as they are planning to pursue pregnancy in the upcoming months. They are interested in your recommendations for her management during her upcoming pregnancy and advice regarding breast-feeding after her delivery.

HPI: The patient is a 26-year-old woman who has never previously been pregnant. Currently she has no symptoms to report and on review of body systems voices no concerns.

PMH: Her past medical history is significant only for a history of rheumatic fever as a child. Because of the consequences of this, she subsequently underwent valve replacement with a mechanical heart valve. She is followed by a cardiologist who has already evaluated her cardiac function, and she has received clearance from her cardiologist to pursue pregnancy. She has no alterations in her daily activities related to her heart. She has no other significant medical or surgical history.

Family history: Her family history is unremarkable for inherited diseases or history of cardiac anomalies.

Medications: Her current medications include only prenatal vitamins, which she has begun in anticipation of pregnancy and warfarin. She has no known drug allergies.

Physical exam: On examination, her pulse is 82, blood pressure is 112/78, respiratory rate is 16, and she is afebrile. Her remaining physical exam is unremarkable, excluding findings consistent with a mechanical heart valve. Records from her cardiologist include a recent cardiac echocardiography report that reveals a normal ejection fraction indicating normal cardiac function.

Pregnancy

MATERNAL-FETAL UNIT

The maternal-fetal unit is a fragile but exquisitely sophisticated system in which the placenta acts as the primary demarcation between the fetal circulation and maternal circulation. The major functions of the placenta are to provide a structure for complete exchange of nutrients, to facilitate gas transfer from mother to fetus, to assist in removal of carbon dioxide and other waste products from the fetal circulation, and to produce hormones. At the same time, the placenta offers a significant barrier from exchange of maternal proteins, blood, and other components that are predominantly excluded from the fetal circulation. Thus, the placenta provides a unique transfer function through the exchange of those substances required by the fetus while it provides a barrier between the maternal and fetal circulation to protect the fetus from unwanted xenobiotics in the maternal circulation. The placenta also plays a major role in the synthesis of hormones, peptides, and steroids required for sustaining pregnancy.

But the placenta only partially impedes the transfer of xenobiotics to the fetus. Nearly all drugs will enter the placental compartment by passive diffusion to some degree, although their ability to do so is greatly moderated by their physiochemistry. Some drugs are actually pumped across the placental barrier by a series of active transporters located in the fetal or maternal sides of the trophoblastic layers.[7]

PLACENTAL ANATOMY AND PHYSIOLOGY

All mammals have placentas, but they various enormously in anatomy and occur in three structural types:

1) hemochorial (rat, rabbit, guinea pig), 2) endotheliochorial (cat, dog), and 3) epitheliochorial (sheep, pig, horse).[8] Because the structural integrity of these three types of placenta varies enormously, the study of drug transport between species is different as well. Thus, drug studies with these various species are hard to interpret with regards to humans. The human placenta is closest to the hemochorial type, in which fetal tissue is in direct contact with maternal blood, although it still varies significantly from that of the others in this group (rat, rabbit, and mouse).

The human placenta is a discoid organ of approximately 3 cm in thickness and 20 cm in diameter, and it weighs approximately 500 g at term.[8] It is composed of 20–40 small compartments called cotyledons, which ultimately function as the respiratory/vascular unit of the placenta.[9] Each cotyledon has a villus tree formed of fetal tissue. The villus tree consists of a central fetal capillary, villus stroma, and an outer fetal trophoblastic layer that is in direct contact with maternal blood.

The placenta is formed from trophoblastic tissue. The extravillous trophoblast invades and secures the developing placenta to the decidua of the uterus. Early in pregnancy, the cytotrophoblast forms a continuous layer, but in later pregnancy, the cytotrophoblast component of the placenta is much less prominent. The syncytiotrophoblast covers much of the surface area of the term placenta, and cellular turnover occurs as a result of apoptosis of cells. The rate of turnover is affected by complicating pregnancy conditions, such as fetal growth restriction and gestational hypertensive disorders, in which the turnover is accelerated compared with normal pregnancies.[10] The syncytiotrophoblast is also responsible for placental transport of various materials, nutrient exchange, and production of human placental lactogen and human chorionic somatomammotropin. The maternal surface of the syncytiotrophoblast is covered by microvilli, which then directly contact the intervillous spaces filled with maternal blood.[9] Pregnancies complicated by high altitude have an increase in capillary loops and trophoblastic surface area for increased exchange, whereas those complicated by growth restriction have abnormal higher-resistance vascular development.[11] The placenta is divided into a fetal portion (chorion frondosum) and a maternal portion (decidua basalis) and at term is divided into cotyledons by decidua septa.

The maternal and fetal circulations are essentially separated. The thickness of the placental barrier between these circulations decreases after 16 weeks of gestation. The distance between circulations varies from as much as 10 μm in early pregnancy to as little as 1–2 μm later on. In addition, the average exchange area of the placenta ranges from 3.4 m^2 at 28 weeks gestation to 12.6 m^2 at term.[12]

Maternal blood does not actually perfuse the placenta for the first 10 weeks of gestation. Thus, the transfer of nutrients, amino acids, and xenobiotics must passively diffuse from maternal tissues to fetal tissues up until 10 weeks when the placenta and cotyledons are present.

DRUG TRANSPORT AND DIFFUSION INTO THE PLACENTAL UNIT

The transplacental transfer of drugs and other substances is known to involve passive diffusion, active transfer, facilitated diffusion, phagocytosis, and pinocytosis.[13] The passive diffusion of drugs is the primary route of membrane transport identified in mammalian tissues. Active, carrier-mediated transport systems are increasingly being identified.[7] Phagocytosis and pinocytosis as mechanisms of drug transport are simply too slow to account for significant transport of drug to the fetus.

Drug properties that affect transport to the fetus include such issues as molecular weight, lipid solubility, and polarity. Just as is the case with most other compartments, the placenta resembles a lipid-bilayer membrane structure. Drugs must diffuse through this lipid bilayer (trophoblastic cells) before entering the fetal circulation. Medications that are small in molecular weight (<500 Da), are highly lipid soluble, and have limited polarity are more likely to passively diffuse through these bilayer membranes. Larger molecular weight drugs, such as the heparin preparations (3,000–15,000 Da), simply fail to enter the fetal circulation because of size limitations.[14] Lipid soluble drugs, particularly those that enter the central nervous system (CNS), transfer readily into the fetal circulation. This is particularly true for the selective serotonin reuptake inhibitor (SSRI) drugs, which basically attain fetal levels equivalent to the maternal plasma.

Although the transfer in various body compartments may be controlled to some degree by protein binding, maternal and even fetal plasma albumin levels change significantly during gestation, thus affecting the maternal/fetal ratio of drugs throughout gestation. Indeed, predicting protein binding during pregnancy is all but impossible. Even some disease processes, such as pre-eclampsia or excessive fluid hydration, may reduce maternal protein binding and thus alter fetal drug levels.

A number of drugs have been found to bind to placental tissue, which then accumulates various drugs and acts as a depot of the fetal supply of this drug. However, the transfer to the fetus is highly dependent on the affinity of the drug for the syncytiotrophoblast. In the case of buprenorphine, most of this drug was selectively sequestered in the placenta tissues, reducing its fetal levels.[15]

Active transport of medications across the placenta by protein "pumps" is poorly understood. Active transport can occur against a concentration gradient and requires expenditure of energy, as this is a carrier-mediated process. In the case of methods of transfer using a carrier, it is possible for this carrier to become saturated, and thus the transport may become rate limited based on carrier capacity. Molecules that usually use this transport carrier may be affected because of competitive inhibition or displacement from the carrier system. Transplacental drug transfer typically increases during the third trimester owing to an increase in blood flow, increase in placental surface area, and thinning of the placental barrier.

Many investigators have examined the active transport of amino acids, glucose, and vitamins, but studies of drug transport are few. Active transporters are located on the apical surface of the syncytiotrophoblast in the fetal circulation to transport drugs back into the maternal circulation, or on the basal syncytiotrophoblast surface to pump drugs from the maternal to the fetal circulation.

P-glycoprotein is an efflux pump that moves substrates from the intracellular to the extracellular compartment. It is expressed in the trophoblast, with greater expression earlier in pregnancy. This may be important in protecting the developing fetus from toxins. Many different transport proteins have been identified in the human placenta.[16] In addition to efflux transporters, which would move medications away from the fetal compartment, there are also influx transporters, which may facilitate transfer of drugs toward the fetus or embryo. Transporters may also be important for the movement of endogenous compounds and drugs, which compete for these transporters, and may then affect the normal transport of these compounds. Readers are directed to a recent reviews by Ganapathy and colleagues or Myllynen and colleagues for a more detailed description of active transport processes in the placenta.[16-18]

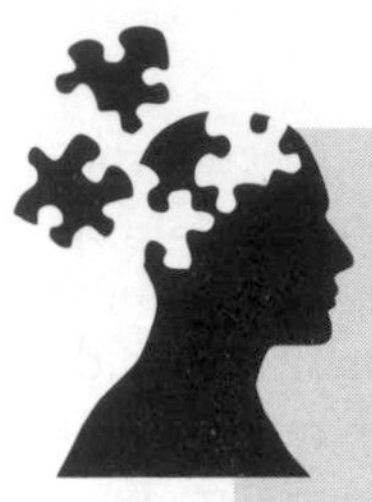

Therapeutic Challenge:

What is the optimal approach to counseling a pregnant woman about her exposure to a known teratogenic agent?

DRUG USE DURING PREGNANCY

Pregnancy is traditionally dated from the first day of the last menstrual period. This is referred to as menstrual age. The embryonic age refers to the age of the fetus itself, and this age differs from menstrual age in that embryonic age is 2 weeks younger. Typically, ovulation occurs approximately 14 days after the start of the preceding menses; thus, the menstrual age will be 4 weeks when the embryonic age is 2 weeks. When assessing medication effects, it is important that an accurate timing of exposure is considered, if possible, as there potentially differing effects of the same medication exposure at different times during gestation.

Studies of the epidemiology of drug use during pregnancy suggest that an increasing number of drugs are used during pregnancy. Indeed, some studies suggest that pregnant women use an average of 4.7 drugs.[6] Analgesics, antacids, antiemetics, antibiotics, tranquilizers, antihistamines, and diuretics are the most widely used medications in pregnant women. Because of the well-known complications of diabetes, depression, asthma, anemia, hypertension, maternal heart disease, and seizure disorders, virtually all of these syndromes are routinely treated during pregnancy.

Malformations result from a disturbance in the normal developmental process and may be the result of numerous but different influences. Major causes of malformations include genetic alterations, accounting for approximately 20% to 25%; environmental factors (such as environmental exposures, medications, maternal illnesses, or infections), accounting for approximately 10%; and unknown causes, accounting for the remaining percentage. The number of malformations believed to be caused by maternal medications specifically is quite small, likely accounting for 1% or less.[19] The prevalence of major birth defects is 3% to 5% of liveborn infants, but is higher when stillborn and aborted infants are also considered.[20-22]

In addition to potentially causing malformations, however, medications can potentially result in other fetal effects that may not present or be associated with the exposure until long after the exposure has occurred. These effects can present as abnormalities of cellular growth, which can result in growth restriction, abnormal neural development, abnormalities in vascular flow, and, rarely, carcinogenesis. In addition, there is potential for neonatal drug withdrawal from certain chronically administered medications that cross to the fetus during gestation. This is commonly reported in women who consume opioids or SSRIs during pregnancy.

Exposure to a **teratogen** early in development (typically the first 2 weeks after conception) may result in sufficient cellular disruption as to prove lethal or, in some instances, have no effect at all (all or none). If significant cellular disruption occurs, a spontaneous abortion may result. If the disruption is less severe, the other undifferentiated cells replace the damaged cells, and the pregnancy continues with little or no effect.

The period of organogenesis occurs after this brief initial period and continues through approximately 10 weeks of menstrual age (days 18–40 after conception). This is referred to as the embryonic period. This interval is most critical regarding teratogenic exposure. The end-organ toxicologic results are reflected in the organ systems that are undergoing most developmental changes during that period.[23] Miscarriage can continue to occur during the embryonic period because of changes resulting from a teratogenic exposure. Some malformations may still occur outside of this period.

Exposures that occur after the embryonic period typically result in changes in cellular growth rather than a teratogenic effect. This is referred to as the fetal period. Although the more common fetal effect of an exposure during this time is a growth effect, other potential fetal effects can include damage to a structure or system that formed initially normally during embryogenesis, which then subsequently results in a fetal malformation. Coumarin derivatives are an example of this effect in that hemorrhagic events can then result in apparent CNS and ophthalmologic malformations.[24] Another potential fetal effect occurring later in pregnancy is stillbirth.

In addition to the more acute effects of medication exposure during pregnancy, latent effects can present after delivery. Latent effects may include growth and development changes that present remote from the medication exposure or subsequent neonatal effects. Potential neonatal effects include metabolic or functional alterations, such as hypotension, hypoglycemia, or oliguria. A rare but clinically significant potential adverse effect can include neonatal withdrawal from a medication.

The timing of the exposure, the total amount and dosage of medication taken, and the duration of the exposure all may lead to differences in a toxicologic event on the developing child. Additionally, there is a threshold amount of exposure for most medications below which an effect is unlikely. The difficulty is that this threshold amount is frequently unknown in humans. Animal study information may be the basis of our attempts to determine this threshold. In the absence of studies in humans, teratogenicity information from animal studies that suggests a threshold of less than 10-fold higher than the therapeutic dosage in humans warrants concern that the drug may have potential teratogenic effects. Conversely, animal information at 100 times the human therapeutic dosage that fails to suggest a teratogenic effect is reassuring that the drug is unlikely to be teratogenic in humans. There is significant concern, however, that animal study information is not optimal at assessing potential for human injury. The limitations to all currently available methods of medication testing will be reviewed later.

Counseling the patient based on the timing of the exposure to the particular medication during the pregnancy and the information available on potential effects to the developing child requires care in presenting the information to the patient and her family. The use of a specialist or genetic counselor may be indicated, depending on the practice situation. It is important to remember the potential for feelings of guilt in the patient and also to take account of the patient's cultural and moral beliefs. In addition to good counseling, other technology is available that may be of benefit for the healthcare provider in attempting to investigate the risk for potential malformations. For instance, testing for alpha-fetoprotein may be useful in situations in which exposures are linked to neural tube effects. Similarly, ultrasound may help to identify neural tube defects, limb abnormalities, clefting, and other structural defects. Fetal echocardiography would be indicated when the exposure has been linked to cardiovascular structural defects in the fetus.

PHYSIOLOGIC ALTERATIONS DURING PREGNANCY

There are many physiologic alterations during pregnancy that may also affect the absorption, distribution, metabolism, and elimination of medications. These changes often begin early in pregnancy and may not return to basal levels until after an often variable duration of time during the puerperium. Depending on the physiologic alteration, typically nonpregnant physiology may resume between 2 and 8 weeks postpartum, although some alterations may persist throughout lactation. These alterations also have the potential to affect drug metabolism in the nursing mother.

Maternal plasma volume increases early in pregnancy beginning at approximately 4 weeks. The plasma volume peaks at 4,700–5,200 mL at approximately 32 weeks of gestation, which reflects an additional 1,200–1,600 mL of volume compared with their nonpregnant counterparts.[25-27] The expansion of plasma volume is even greater in pregnancies with multiple gestations. There is also an increase in red blood cell count, but this is exceeded by the increase in total blood volume and thus results in a dilutional anemia of pregnancy. Pregnancies complicated by eclampsia and fetal growth restriction have been shown to experience a smaller increase in blood volume expansion than normal pregnancies.[28] Serum albumin decreases from the second trimester onward, resulting in levels that are approximately 70% to 80% of normal values at delivery. Mean albumin concentrations in the nonpregnant woman are 4.2 g/dL compared with 3.6 g/dL during the second trimester of pregnancy.[29] Despite the lowered albumin caused by an increased blood volume, there are minimal changes in total protein. Changes in protein binding that occur during pregnancy, coupled with the increase in plasma volume, can alter the apparent volume of distribution of drugs. Drugs measured with total plasma concentrations may underestimate unbound or active plasma concentrations. Serum colloid osmotic pressure is reduced by approximately 14% at term.

Maternal cardiac output is also increased during pregnancy by 30% to 50%.[30-32] This increase also begins as early as 5 weeks of gestation, with 50% of the increase occurring by 8 weeks. This involves both an increase in stroke volume and an increase in heart rate, which is approximately 20% higher during pregnancy (with further increase during labor). Blood pressure decreases secondary to a decrease in systemic vascular resistance. There is an approximately 9% decrease in blood pressure by 9 weeks. The normal nadir in blood pressure occurs at 28 weeks of gestation, after which blood pressure gradually increases to normal levels at term. During the third trimester of pregnancy, blood pressure may be altered based on maternal positioning that is due to vena caval compression by the gravid uterus, with lowest blood pressures obtained in the left lateral recumbent position. Again, the increase in cardiac output is greater in mothers experiencing multiple gestations.

Regional blood flow is altered during pregnancy. There is an increase in blood flow to the uterus accounting for approximately 20% of cardiac output. An increase in renal blood flow occurs, although this is reduced in the supine position. There is increased blood flow to the skin and breasts, whereas there is a decrease in splanchnic blood flow and blood flow to skeletal muscle. Hepatic blood flow accounts for 24% to 27% of cardiac output during pregnancy but increases to 37% of blood flow 10–12 weeks postpartum.[33]

Hepatic clearance of drugs is dependent on multiple factors, many of which are altered by pregnancy. Protein binding, enzymatic activity, and blood flow are all changed. Pregnancy has been found to increase the activity of multiple cytochrome P450 enzymes.[34] Increases in CYP 3A4, CYP 2D6, CYP 2C09, and CYP 2AG have been noted. There have also been increases in other enzymes, such as uridine diphosphate glucuronosyltransferase UGT 1A4 and UGT 2B7. Conversely, decreased activity of CPY 1A2 and CYP 2C19 have been reported. These alterations can have substantial effects on drug metabolism during pregnancy.

Kidney function is also altered by pregnancy, with an increase in glomerular filtration rate (GFR) of 50% during the first trimester and continued increase over baseline during pregnancy, although there is some decrease in GFR during the last month of pregnancy.[35] There is an 80% increase in effective renal plasma flow in the second trimester, which then also decreases in the third trimester. Serum creatinine is reduced as pregnancy progresses. Glomerular filtration rate then returns to baseline levels by 8–12 weeks postpartum.

Maternal weight is increased during pregnancy and the puerperium. The recommended weight gain during pregnancy varies according to prepregnant body mass index (BMI).[36] Average weight

Table 23-1. Increase in Body Water and Fat Based on BMI (14–37 weeks of pregnancy)

BMI Category	Weight Gain (kg)	Water Gain (L)	Fat Gain (kg)
Underweight <19.8 kg/m²	12.6 +/− 4.4	6.1 +/− 2.4	4.8 +/− 3.8
Normal Weight 19.8–26 kg/m²	12.2 +/− 4.0	7.0 +/− 2.7	3.9 +/− 3.7
Overweight 26–29 kg/m²	11.0 +/− 4.6	7.8 +/− 3.5	2.8 +/− 5.4
Obese >29 kg/m²	8.7 +/− 5.6[b]	7.3 +/− 2.9	0.2 +/− 5.-0[a]

Source: Reference 37.
BMI = body mass index.
[a]$p < 0.05$ ANOVA.

gain in the first trimester varies between 1 and 3.5 kg (2–8 lb). During the second and third trimesters, usual weight gain is linear, with an average of approximately 0.75 lb per week for women with an appropriate prepregnant BMI. Maternal weight gain reflects a gain in water weight as well as fat gain (Table 23-1).[37] Postpartum weight retention is common. Postpartum weight loss during the 6 months after delivery varies between 0.8 kg/mo for affluent populations and 0.1 kg/mo for underprivileged populations. Body fat also varies during the puerperium, with a decrease from approximately 28% at 1 month to 26% at 4 months. Change in fat mass was found to be greater in lactating women compared with those not breast-feeding during the 3–6 months after delivery. Studies also vary by population between 0.4 and 3.8 kg long-term weight retention results from pregnancy. Women who gained more weight than recommended during pregnancy are also more likely to retain a larger amount of weight 5 years after delivery (6.5 kg for those gaining recommended weight verses 8.4 kg for those exceeding Institute of Medicine recommendations).[38,39] Women who breast-feed beyond 12 weeks and participate in aerobic exercise are less likely to retain weight. Accurate information regarding the patient's current weight and time since delivery may provide for more predictable drug dosing.

Other physiologic alterations occur that may also have an impact on drug metabolism in certain situations. Respiratory changes include a compensated respiratory alkalosis during pregnancy, with a decrease in $PaCO_2$ and an average maternal pH of 7.44. There is also an increase in respiratory tidal volume and oxygen consumption. The diaphragm is superiorly displaced by the gravid uterus as pregnancy progresses. Tidal volume is increased by 30% to 40%, but residual capacity is decreased 20% to 25%. Gastrointestinal changes include decreased gastric acidity and decreased gastric motility, resulting in an increase in gut transit time especially during the third trimester. There is delayed gastric emptying during labor. All of these physiologic alterations may affect drug absorption. Immune alterations occur, with a decrease in cellular immune response and an increase in humoral immune response. Normal white blood cell (WBC) count during pregnancy varies between 8,000 and 8,500/mm³, but this may increase dramatically during labor. By 1 week postpartum, the WBC count has returned to normal levels. Carbohydrate metabolism is altered during pregnancy, with a fasting hypoglycemia and postprandial hyperglycemia. There is also a relative hyperinsulinemia.

Delivery results in blood loss. The average blood loss is commonly estimated at 500 cc for a vaginal delivery and 1 L for cesarean delivery. Immediately after delivery, there is an increase in cardiac output, a shift of blood from the uterus to the intravascular space, loss of vena caval compression, and mobilization of extravascular fluid. A postpartum diuresis subsequently occurs, with approximately 3 kg of weight loss occurring between days 2 and 5 after delivery.

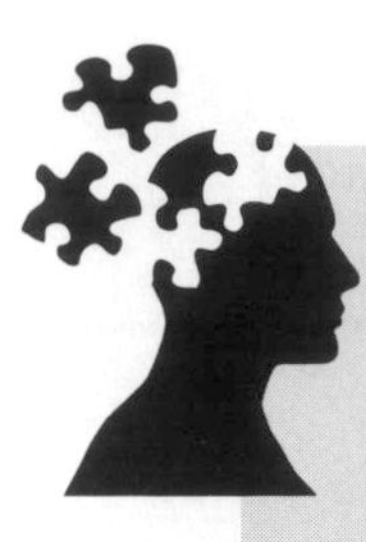

Therapeutic Challenge:

To what extent does the fetus have the capacity to conjugate or metabolize xenobiotics, and what impact does this have on drug levels in mother and infant?

FETAL PHYSIOLOGY

The direct effect of a drug on the fetus is dependent on the concentration of the drug in the fetal circulation. Ultimately, however, the major determinate of fetal blood drug concentration is actually the concentration in the maternal circulation.[40] As maternal blood levels of drugs rise, so do levels in the fetus. This results in a multiple compartment model that is inadequately understood for most drug exposures.

For drugs that do cross into the fetal compartment, fetal physiology can further alter the potential drug effect. Whereas maternal albumin is decreased during pregnancy, the fetal production of albumin increases through gestation. This may result in concentration differences as pregnancy progresses. Unbound concentrations of drug cross the placenta, after which the drug may become protein bound in the fetus. Fetal pH is slightly more acidic than the maternal pH. This can result in weak bases being more likely to cross to the fetus. These drugs can be more ionized in the fetal circulation, and this can result in "ion trapping." Drugs that are absorbed from oral or gastrointestinal exposure and that are excreted by the fetal kidney into the amniotic fluid have the potential to be recirculated as the fetus swallows amniotic fluid.

TERATOGENIC DRUGS

The study of teratogenicity is vast and is beyond the scope of this review. However, there are only a few drugs documented to be human teratogens: ethanol, isotretinoin, warfarin derivatives, valproic acid, thalidomide, angiotensin-converting enzyme (ACE) inhibitors, and folate antagonists (methotrexate). Timing of exposure is of paramount importance when considering teratogenic potential. Many drugs may or may not cause untoward effects on the fetus if they are administered at times that are not hazardous. For instance, the classic teratogen, thalidomide, may not induce changes in the fetus if it is not administered from days 34–50 of pregnancy. The ACE inhibitors are quite hazardous to renal development, but only during the 2nd and 3rd trimester. So timing of medication exposure is of paramount import. Most, but not all, teratogens have very specific intervals within which they are hazardous, and when administered outside this time frame, they may have few or no effects on the fetus.

Lactation

The American Academy of Pediatrics (AAP) and the World Health Organization (WHO) recommend exclusive breast-feeding for the first 6 months of life, with continued breast-feeding through the first year or two of life. An age of weaning is not typically stipulated; rather, breast-feeding is encouraged as long as mutually desired.

Providing accurate information regarding medications for the nursing mother requires that the healthcare provider have details regarding the infant and the specific clinical condition of the mother. A detailed history involving both the mother and infant is warranted to provide adequate medication information for the nursing dyad (Table 23-2). If the

Table 23-2. Some Important Considerations When Evaluating Medication History During Lactation

Mother	Infant
Which medication?	What is the age and weight of the infant?
What is the indication for the medication?	Was the infant born full term or prematurely?
Are safer alternatives or alternatives with more safety information regarding lactation available?	What other health concerns, if any, does the infant have (i.e., episodes of apnea and bradycardia, glucose 6 phosphate dehydrogenase deficiency, hyperbilirubinemia, others)?
What is the dose of the medication and planned duration of therapy?	What percentage of the infant's diet is composed of breast milk?

infant is taking medications, there is potential for drug:drug interactions between infant medications and maternal medications that pass through into breast milk. Premature infants may warrant special consideration. Often care providers focus on primarily caring for either the infant or the mother, and the involved care provider may not have adequate information about the other component of the nursing couple.

ALVEOLAR ANATOMY

Human milk is a complex mixture composed of thousands of substances, including living cells such as macrophages, leukocytes, stem cells, and other cellular species and proteins, peptides, lipids, and cytokines. These components are dispersed in several compartments: an aqueous phase containing water-soluble components; colloidal dispersions of proteins (casein); oil-in-water emulsions of triglyceride-rich fat globules; and living cells (e.g., macrophages, lymphocytes, leukocytes).

During pregnancy, the human breast undergoes a massive change that includes the migration of ductal tissues from the nipple through the naive breast thoracic fat pads and connective tissue to form a tree-like structure within the adipose tissue of the breast. The forming ducts canalize themselves through the fat pads primarily during the first and second trimester. Each duct ends in a series of grapelike clusters of alveoli that are lined by alveolar epithelium (lactocytes), which actually synthesize milk.[41] The breast increases in size and weight from roughly 200 g nonpregnant to 400–600 g near term and 600–800 g during lactation. Blood flow to the breast increases as well.

The marked proliferation of ductal and alveolar epithelium is largely dependent on elevated levels of prolactin, estrogen, and progesterone. Because only 10–15 ducts terminate at the nipple, the breast is therefore subdivided into unique and individual lobuloalveolar clusters, each drained by an individual ductal system. The alveolar apparatus in each cluster is lined with a single layer of polarized epithelial cells (lactocytes) that synthesize milk de novo.[42] A specialized connective tissue stroma surrounds each alveolus and supports this structure. Surrounding and atop this structure is a basketlike layer of specialized smooth muscle or "myoepithelial" cells that contain specialized receptors for oxytocin. Milk is thus forced down into the ductal system by release of oxytocin from the mother's pituitary during breast-feeding. This is termed the *milk ejection* or *letdown*.

Although many of the principles of drug entry into the fetus are somewhat similar to that of breast milk, the systems are uniquely different. Drugs not only enter the milk compartment, but they also maintain an equilibrium with the maternal plasma compartment, going into the milk compartment and then exiting as a function of the maternal plasma levels of the drug. Also, each time an infant breast-feeds, the compartment is more or less completely emptied of drug, and new transport of the drug is required subsequently. Second and most important, during pregnancy, the mother handles the elimination of drugs from both the maternal circulation and the fetal compartment. Postpartum, the infant then must metabolically handle elimination of drugs absorbed via milk. Thus the clinical effect of the drug is determined by the infant's ability to metabolize, sequester, or eliminate ingested medications. Not all infants can do this effectively, particularly premature infants.

PASSAGE OF DRUGS ACROSS ALVEOLAR EPITHELIUM

During the initial stage of lactation, in particular the first 48 hours postpartum, the alveolar apparatus is underdeveloped, with large gaps between the lactocytes. Virtually anything in the maternal plasma compartment may enter this premature milk called colostrum. This includes many cells (e.g., macrophages, stem cells, lymphocytes, T-cells), large-molecular-weight proteins (IgG, IgM, IgA), and all the electrolytes present in the maternal plasma compartment. Fortunately, the volume of colostrum created is low, seldom exceeding 30–60 mL/day the first 2–3 days. Soon thereafter, related to the delivery of the placenta and with falling levels of progesterone and estrogen, the lactocytes begin to grow and form tight cell-to-cell junctions. At this point, the milk compartment is relatively tight, and drug transport then falls under the laws of pharmacology that govern all drug entry into remote compartments. Drugs must be lipid soluble, low in molecular weight, and relatively nonpolar to enter the milk compartment.

Drug Classification

MOLECULAR WEIGHT OF THE DRUG

Drugs with large molecular weights transfer poorly into breast milk. Typically, medications with a molecular weight <300 Da transfer easily into milk.

This feature is similar to placental drug transfer. A medication such as lithium, with no protein binding and a molecular weight of 6.94 Da, readily transfers into milk.[43] Small-molecular-weight, lipid-soluble drugs include the amphetamine family and other CNS active drugs. Conversely, drugs with large molecular weights (>5,000 Da), such as peptides or proteins (heparin, low-molecular-weight heparin, immunoglobulins) are virtually excluded from the mature alveolar compartment. Some will inevitably enter milk through open gaps or pores, but the clinical dose is virtually nothing. In addition, most peptides or proteins will simply be digested by trypsin and other enzymes in the gastrointestinal tract of the infant. It is known that some milk proteins, peptides, and immunoglobulins such as IgA do enter milk and do so in large concentrations. This is due to specific transport systems that exist on the alveolar surfaces. Such transport processes include insulin, IGF-1, prolactin, and many others. Without such a transport process, other proteins are virtually excluded from the milk compartment.

LIPID SOLUBILITY OF THE DRUG

The lipophilicity of a drug is measured by its partition ratio (P) between the highly lipophilic solvent octanol and water. Thus, drugs with high lipid solubility readily pass through lipid bilayers such as the lactocytes. As such, the degree of lipophilicity of a drug clearly controls its entry into the milk compartment. Once there, the drug easily disperses into the lipid content of the milk. The lipid content of milk is high, ranging from 10% in hindmilk to 2% to 3% in foremilk, and thus many lipid soluble drugs can become sequestered to some degree in the lipid content of milk. The best way to remember this is that if the drug enters the CNS, it will probably easily enter the milk compartment as well.

Fat content of mature human milk increases during each episode of milk expression. The terms *foremilk* and *hindmilk* refer to milk obtained either from toward the beginning (fore) or end (hind) of an expression. Hindmilk contains more fat and calories and less water than foremilk. Arbitrarily, foremilk is typically described as that produced within the first 3–5 minutes of the feeding.[44]

MATERNAL PLASMA LEVELS OF DRUGS

The amount of drug that is available to transfer into the maternal milk is related to the maternal plasma level of the medication. Drugs or drug dosages that result in low plasma levels in the mother will generally produce lower levels in milk. Medications such as inhaled beta agonists or inhaled steroids used for the treatment of asthma often result in extremely low maternal plasma levels and incredibly low levels in milk as well. Thus, medications that fail to produce significant maternal plasma levels also fail to produce clinically relevant levels in milk.

PROTEIN BINDING

As during pregnancy, drugs that are highly protein bound (e.g., warfarin) are not typically available for transfer into milk. Therefore, drugs with high protein binding generally fail to produce significant levels in human milk as well.

The more lipid soluble the drug, the easier it is for it to diffuse into the milk compartment. This again is similar to lipid-soluble medications transferring more easily across the placenta. Human milk has a pH of approximately 7.2, somewhat lower than plasma. Those drugs with a high pKa become more polarized and hence are sequestered in milk. Thus, drugs that have a low molecular weight, low protein binding, high pKa, and high lipid solubility and are nonionized are more likely to enter the milk compartment. This is quite similar to the placenta.

BIOAVAILABILITY OF DRUGS IN MOTHERS AND INFANT

The bioavailability of a drug is largely dependent on the method of administration. In breast-fed infants, the method of administration is oral, following ingestion of the milk. One of the most important factors concerning the clinical efficacy of breast milk–administered medications is obviously that they require oral absorption. Many medications prescribed to the mother are not orally absorbed by the infant. Drugs administered orally are absorbed directly into the portal circulation and then pass through the liver before entering the general circulation. Although it is true that an infant's cytochrome P450 systems are not fully functional, the liver of the infant is still able to sequester drugs and prevent their entry into the general circulation. One of the most important determinations of clinical efficacy of breast-milk drugs is that many of them are not bioavailable. In those instances, the drug may produce changes in gut flora (such as with antibiotics) or simply pass out of the infant without being absorbed. Thus, we consider that drugs that are not orally bioavailable in an infant are relatively safe to use in breast-feeding mothers.

MILK/PLASMA RATIO

The transfer of medications from the maternal plasma compartment to the milk is often reported as the milk to plasma ratio (M/P ratio). This can be based on information from a particular time point relative to dosing or may be the result of accumulated data points over the dosing interval, using area under the curve (AUC) estimates. A drug that transfers equally into milk from the plasma compartment will have an M/P ratio of 1.0 (ethanol), whereas a drug that is concentrated in milk will have an M/P ratio >1.0 (lithium). The vast majority of drugs have M/P ratios of <1.0. The M/P ratio can only be used to measure milk levels when the maternal plasma level is known, and this is rare. Overall, the M/P ratio should not be used, as it may not realistically reflect the clinical dosage of the drug. In most cases, the M/P ratio has a limited role in assessing drug safety in breast-feeding mothers because in the majority of cases, we simply do not know the maternal plasma level of the drug.

RELATIVE INFANT DOSE

The most useful determinant for assessing drug safety in breast-feeding is the relative infant dose (RID). This calculation provides a standardized means of referencing infant exposure to maternal exposure on a dose/weight basis. Relative infant dose is calculated by dividing the infant's dose (in milk) in mg/kg/day by the maternal dose in mg/kg/day. In essence, this provides the percentage of the maternal dose that reaches the infant via milk. This percentage is then interpreted using a notional safe "level of concern" of 10%. In 1996, Bennett suggested a cutoff value of 10% of RID be used as a notional safety level for drugs in breast milk.[45] This level is now regularly accepted as reasonable. Although this range of 10% is useful, it should only be used following a close evaluation of the infant, taking into account the infant's age and ability to handle and excrete drugs, and, most particularly, the toxicity of the drug itself (Table 23-3).

Relative Infant Dose

$$\text{RID (\%)} = \frac{\text{Absolute Infant Dose (mg/kg/day) via milk}}{\text{Maternal Dose (mg/kg/day)}}$$

Table 23-3. Commonly Used Medications in Breast-feeding Mothers and Their Relative Infant Dose

Drug	RID%	Comment	References
Analgesics			
Acetaminophen	1–2.8	Compatible	46
Celecoxib, rofecoxib	0.2, 0.3	Compatible	47, 48
Naproxen	2.0, 2.8	Compatible, but only short course; bleeding reported	49, 50
Codeine	0.6, 1.2	Compatible, but use with caution; apnea reported	51, 52
Hydrocodone		Compatible; some sedation, observed for apnea, sedation	53
Morphine	0.4–3.4	Compatible in normal doses; observe for sedation, constipation; caution	54–56
Antibiotics			
Amoxicillin	0.9	Compatible; observe for changes in gut flora	57
Cephalexin	0.5	Compatible; observe for changes in gut flora	57
Dicloxacillin	1	Compatible; observe for changes in gut flora	58
Azithromycin	5.8	Compatible; observe for changes in gut flora	59
Doxycycline	4, 6	Compatible for short-term use (<3 wk)	60, 61
Metronidazole	10.5–13	Compatible; may produce metallic taste in milk	62–64

(Continued on next page)

Drug	RID%	Comment	References
Antidepressants/Antipsychotics			
Citalopram	0.7–7.3	Compatible, but less so than escitalopram	65–67
Fluoxetine	2.6–6.5	Compatible; some reports of withdrawal	68–70
Paroxetine	1.1–1.4	Compatible, but no longer preferred in many patients	71–73
Sertraline	0.3–0.9	Compatible; ideal; no adverse effects reported	74–77
Anticonvulsants			
Lamotrigine	22.8	Compatible, although levels high, but no untoward effects yet noted; monitor plasma levels	78–80
Valproic acid	0.68	Compatible	81–83
Carbamazepine	4.4	Compatible	84
Escitalopram	5.3	Compatible, but studied in few patients	92

Source: Adapted with permission from reference 53.

RID = relative infant dose.

RISK-BENEFIT ANALYSIS

The breast-fed infant generally has nothing to gain from exposure to drugs via the mother's milk. Methods for reducing or avoiding infant exposure should always be entertained. Mothers should only expose themselves to medications when they are absolutely indicated and should avoid herbal and even high-dose vitamin products that are not specifically indicated.

If maternal drug treatment is specifically indicated, then drugs that enter milk poorly should be preferentially used. At present we have a significant body of information on drug levels in breast milk, and this should be used. Unfortunately, the current prescribing information on nearly all drugs is inaccurate and should never be used to make a breast-feeding decision. Numerous medications are quite safe to use in breast-feeding mothers, and there is always a preferred choice available to treat virtually any syndrome. The healthcare provider must always take into consideration that breast-feeding is incredibly important to the health of the newborn infant, as this has been repeatedly documented in numerous studies.

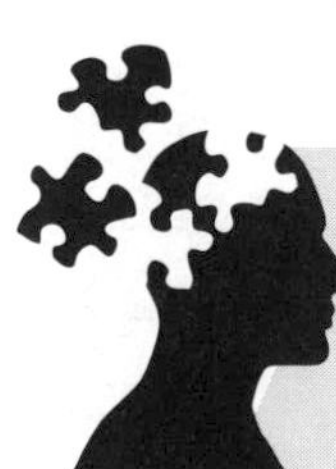

Therapeutic Challenge:

Consider possible approaches to prospective drug investigation during pregnancy and lactation. What information from other research would be needed, and what findings from these studies would be sufficiently reassuring to ethically proceed with prospective study of the medication in pregnant and breast-feeding women?

Study Model Limitations and Resources for Information

As previously mentioned, there are limitations to all currently available methods of studying medications during pregnancy. Animal models give some information, but because of placental differences among species, information gained from animal research may not be optimally reflective of human experience. Other methods of study include information from pregnant women themselves. Outside of the ethical considerations that this entails, there are potential differences throughout gestation that may provide different results related to exposure to the same medication. Often, medications are studied during labor and cord blood levels compared with maternal levels. This does provide some information regarding placental transfer, but, again, may not be reliable for extrapolating to first-trimester use of the same medication. Population surveys and pregnancy registries are other commonly used methods to attempt to document medication safety during pregnancy. This type of information, though useful, has certain limitations. One significant limitation is that rare adverse outcomes may not be realized until after exposure of a large number of pregnant women to the offending agent. An additional limitation is the potential for recall bias: Those women with adverse outcomes may apply increased scrutiny to their history to remember an exposure that those women without the adversity may not remember. This may apply to exposures to commonly used over-the-counter products as well.

Other methods for medication research during pregnancy include the use of placental perfusion models. This allows for determination of cord/maternal serum drug levels and also accounts for the potential influence of placental metabolism. The extrapolation of these data to the in vivo use of medications may vary.

Ideally, study of drugs during pregnancy and lactation is needed. Difficulty with recruitment and an increase in dropout rate in these populations may be expected. Currently the U.S. Food and Drug Administration (FDA) does not require drug manufacturers to study the use of their medications during pregnancy or lactation.

Several reliable resources for information are available that provide information during pregnancy, some of which are listed in the following section. *The Physicians' Desk Reference (PDR)* has information regarding drug characteristics that may assist the healthcare provider when more detailed information regarding the drug during pregnancy is not available.

PREGNANCY RESOURCES

- REPROTOX. Washington, DC: Reproductive Toxicology Center, Columbia Hospital for Women Medical Center.
- TERIS and Shepard's Catalog of Teratogenic Agents (teratogen information system). Seattle, WA.
- Briggs, Freeman, Yaffe, eds. *Drugs in Pregnancy and Lactation.* 7th ed. Baltimore, MD: Lippincott Williams & Wilkins; 2005.

The previously used FDA categories during pregnancy have limitations but remain somewhat useful in guiding medication use during pregnancy. These categories are not an equally weighted scale of safety, but rather are devised to reveal the type of scientific study available and are an attempted assessment of risk vs. benefit for the use of the particular medicine

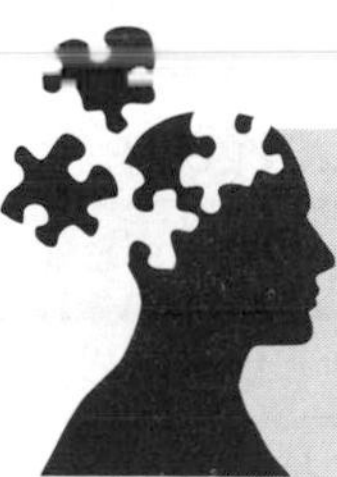

Therapeutic Challenge:

When a medication with potential adverse fetal effects has been required during pregnancy for the health of the mother and she desires to breast-feed after delivery, how do we provide optimal information for her regarding further potential infant exposure to the medication from breast-feeding based on the currently available research? How do we best weigh the risk of potential continued infant exposure to small amounts of medication from breast milk to the risk of not breast-feeding for the infant?

(Table 23-4). Future revisions to the current method of evaluating drug safety during pregnancy and lactation are anticipated.

BREASTFEEDING RESOURCES

Resources regarding drug safety in lactation are also available. Some of the pregnancy resources include limited information regarding lactation; lactation-specific resources may provide more information.

- Hale TW. *Medications and Mothers' Milk.* 13th ed. Amarillo, TX: Hale Publishing LP; 2008.
- American Academy of Pediatrics Committee on Drugs. Transfer of drugs and other chemicals in human milk. *Pediatrics.* 2001;108(3):776-789.
- Lawrence R. *Breastfeeding: A Guide for the Medical Professional.* 6th ed. St. Louis, MO: Mosby; 2006.
- National Library of Medicine. LactMed database. Available at http://toxnet.nlm.nih.gov.

Similar to pregnancy categories attempting to provide information regarding the amount of available research on drugs during pregnancy, a lactational risk category schema has also been devised. One approach is use of the five-point scale to determine lactational risk categories similar to the drug safety categories for pregnancy (Table 23-5). The AAP categorizes the reviewed drugs into the following categories: 1) cytotoxic, 2) drugs of abuse with adverse effects, 3) radioactive compounds,

Table 23-4. Hale's Lactation Risk Category

L1 SAFEST	Drug that has been taken by a large number of breast-feeding mothers without any observed increase in adverse effects in the infant. Controlled studies in breast-feeding women fail to demonstrate a risk to the infant, and the possibility of harm to the breast-feeding infant is remote; or the product is not orally bioavailable in an infant.
L2 SAFER	Drug that has been studied in a limited number of breast-feeding women without an increase in adverse effects in the infant and/or the evidence that a demonstrated risk that is likely to follow use of this medication in a breast-feeding woman is remote.
L3 MODERATELY SAFE	There are no controlled studies in breast-feeding women, but the risk of untoward effects to a breast-fed infant is possible; or controlled studies show only minimal nonthreatening adverse effects. Drugs should be given only if the potential benefit justifies the potential risk to the infant.
L4 POSSIBLY HAZARDOUS	There is positive evidence of risk to a breast-fed infant or to breast-milk production, but the benefits from use in breast-feeding mothers may be acceptable despite the risk to the infant (e.g., if the drug is needed in a life-threatening situation or for a serious disease for which safer drugs cannot be used or are ineffective).
L5 CONTRAINDICATED	Studies in breast-feeding mothers have demonstrated that there is significant and documented risk to the infant based on human experience, or it is a medication that has a high risk of causing significant damage to an infant. The risk of using the drug in breast-feeding women clearly outweighs any possible benefit from breast-feeding. The drug is contraindicated in women who are breast-feeding an infant.

Source: Used with permission from reference 53.

4) drugs whose effects are unknown but "may be of concern," 5) drugs that should be used "with caution," and 6) drugs that are generally "compatible with lactation." Many medications have not been reviewed by the AAP. Again, the PDR typically provides little specific information regarding lactation but may be of use in situations in which the healthcare provider is researching basic characteristics such as molecular weight and protein binding.

Table 23-5. Relative Risk of Teratogenicity of Various Drugs and Their Timing During Gestation

Drug	Teratogenic Timing (day)[a]	Relative Risk	Effect	References
Ethanol	Conception and first 2 mo but later as well	High (30% to 40% alcoholic mothers)	Fetal alcohol syndrome: cognitive deficit, hyperactivity, craniofacial abnormalities, low birth weight, cardiac and renogenital anomalies, hemangiomas; neonatal alcohol withdrawal if used heavily at term	19
Cigarette	Throughout	High (15% increase in preterm birth, 25% increase in abruption)	Miscarriage, low birth weight, preterm birth, placenta previa, placental abruption, neonatal complications	85
Isotretinoin	14–35	23% to 28%	Malformations of CNS, craniofacial defects, cardiovascular defects, thymic defects, limb reduction defects; multiple anomalies reported; abnormal intellectual development	3, 24, 86

(Continued on next page)

Drug	Teratogenic Timing (day)[a]	Relative Risk	Effect	References
Warfarin	28–77, but later risks as well	10% to 25%	Fetal warfarin syndrome: nasal hypoplasia, hydrocephaly, CNS defects, microcephaly, mental retardation, stippled epiphyses, ophthalmologic anomalies; growth restriction; miscarriage, stillbirth	3, 24, 86
Valproic acid	31–44	High	Neural tube defects (1% to 2%), cardiovascular defects, fetal valproate syndrome with facial and limb anomalies; growth restriction, hepatotoxicity, neonatal withdrawal	3, 24, 86
Lamotrigine	1st trimester	Low if present	No specific syndrome reported (sample size of early exposures is limited)	86, 87
Carbamazepine	1st trimester	1% 10%	Neural tube defects; craniofacial abnormalities, minor limb defects, fingernail hypoplasia, developmental delay	3, 24, 86
Phenytoin	1st trimester and throughout	10%	Fetal hydantoin syndrome: microcephaly, growth retardation, craniofacial abnormalities, hypoplasia of nails, limb defects; tumors; hemorrhage at birth; dependent on epoxide formation	3, 24, 86
Thalidomide	34–50	High (20% to 50%)	Phocomelia (absence of the long bones from the upper and lower limbs), cardiovascular defects, CNS defects, genitourinary and gastrointestinal defects	3, 24
ACE inhibitors	2nd and 3rd trimester	High	Oligohydramnios, neonatal anuria, congenital hypocalvaria, renal anomalies, nephrotoxicity, and perinatal renal failure; growth restriction, prematurity, neonatal hypotension	3, 86
Methotrexate	56–70 and throughout	High	Methotrexate embryopathy: decreased ossification of calvarium, craniofacial abnormalities, hydrocephaly, mental retardation, growth restriction, limb abnormalities; newborn myelosuppression	86
SSRIs	Throughout	2% to 3%	Cardiac malformations such as atrial septal defects (paroxetine) but risk appears low (1st trimester); disruption in neurobehavior and neonatal withdrawal (3rd trimester)	3, 19, 88, 89
Antipsychotics	Throughout	Low if present	No increase in malformations with most of these drugs; transient effects in neonates exposed in late gestation of hypotension and extrapyramidal tract symptoms	90
Diethylstilbestrol	1st trimester and throughout	High	Müllerian tract anomalies (both upper and lower), cervical and vaginal clear cell adenocarcinoma	24, 91

ACE = angiotensin-converting enzyme; CNS = central nervous system; SSRI = selective serotonin reuptake inhibitors.

[a]Timing is approximate and may vary according to individual drug. Timing is listed as menstrual day.

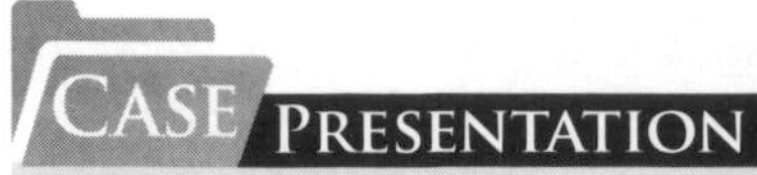

Patient Case: Part 2

Assessment: The patient with a mechanical heart valve planning pregnancy may wish to consider an alternative anticoagulant with her physician before pursuing pregnancy. This involves an assessment of risk and benefit to both herself and the developing embryo and fetus should conception occur.

Treatment plan: This discussion involves a great deal of complexity. All different agents used for anticoagulation continue to provide the pregnant woman with an increased risk of bleeding. This risk can be significant both to maternal health (e.g., increased risk of hemorrhage should the woman experience an ectopic pregnancy or miscarriage) and to the health of the developing pregnancy (e.g., subchorionic hemorrhage or placental abruption). This risk is, however, usually small when compared with the risk to maternal health related to not continuing anticoagulation of some type when a mechanical valve is in place.

Warfarin is an anticoagulant frequently used outside of pregnancy because of the ease of oral administration. Warfarin has a relatively low molecular weight and easily crosses the placenta. It is known for potential teratogenic effects with first-trimester exposure, potentially resulting in fetal warfarin syndrome. Heparin (and low-molecular-weight heparins) are much larger in molecular weight and do not appear to readily cross the placenta. These agents are not orally administered.

Patient education: When planning pregnancy, it would be advisable to change the patient from the warfarin she is currently taking to a heparin anticoagulant to avoid the potential teratogenic exposure related to warfarin, although potential for bleeding complications exists with all anticoagulants. All anticoagulant medications also have varying implications specific to the time of delivery and anesthetic choices for delivery.

Patient monitoring: During breast-feeding, maternal anticoagulation with warfarin, heparin, or low-molecular-weight heparin would all be relatively safe alternatives for the full-term healthy infant. Warfarin has the added patient convenience that it is orally dosed. Warfarin is highly protein bound in the maternal circulation and, because of this, very little is transferred into human milk. Limited information from the study of nursing infants suggests that the drug was undetectable in infant plasma. Warfarin is also rendered ineffective by the administration of vitamin K, which is routinely given at birth. Consideration of the numerous potential drug and food interactions with warfarin should be kept in mind. Additional information can be gained by evaluating the infant for any effect on bleeding with laboratory testing if concern remains. Heparin and low-molecular-weight heparins are not orally absorbed and would therefore not be available to the nursing infant. In addition, the large molecular weight would make transfer of these drugs into human milk unlikely.

Summary

From the above information, it is apparent that the understanding of the potential impact of many medications on the developing pregnancy and nursing infant is currently insufficient. Thus far, the vast majority of information has been collected from experience regarding medications that have been used and the subsequent outcome related to the exposure. Development of a more accurate preclinical model for evaluation of drug exposure during pregnancy is warranted. Prospective research could then follow regarding drug metabolism in the pregnant and nursing population. An improved understanding of the relationship between maternal and infant exposure to medications would provide a more enlightened understanding of risk and benefit analysis. The development of research protocols to evaluate and address the intricate and dynamic relationship between the mother and the developing embryo, fetus, neonate, and subsequent nursing infant are being heavily encouraged both at the healthcare provider and FDA and National Institutes of Health level.

References

Additional content available at ***www.ashp.org/womenshealth***

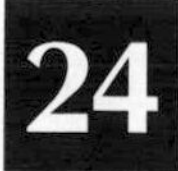

24 Conditions Associated with Pregnancy

Patricia Rozek Wigle, Pharm.D., BCPS; Karissa Y. Kim, Pharm.D., CACP, BCPS

Learning Objectives

1. Discuss the pathophysiology of nausea and vomiting, gastroesophageal reflux disease, constipation, insomnia, and thromboembolism of pregnancy.
2. Compare and contrast medications used for the treatment of nausea and vomiting, constipation, diarrhea, gastroesophageal reflux disease, venous thromboembolism, and cough and cold during pregnancy.
3. List antibiotics that can be safely used to treat infectious diarrhea during pregnancy.
4. Formulate a comprehensive clinical plan, including nonpharmacologic and pharmacologic therapy for a pregnant woman with nausea and vomiting, gastroesophageal reflux disease, and venous thromboembolism.

During the 40 weeks of pregnancy, there are common conditions—including nausea and vomiting, gastrointestinal reflux, changes in bowel function, insomnia, infections, and **thromboembolism**—that have unique management during pregnancy because of the limited, if any, information on drug safety during pregnancy. The principles of drug safety in pregnancy are discussed in depth in Chapter 23: Drug Principles in Pregnancy and Lactation. In this chapter, the focus will be to review the management of symptoms associated with these conditions and discuss any potential impact on the mother or developing fetus. Unfortunately, often in the absence of formal clinical data, management recommendations are conservative, primarily nonpharmacologic interventions, which then proceed to pharmacologic interventions until resolution of symptoms.

Common Gastrointestinal Disorders During Pregnancy

NAUSEA AND VOMITING IN PREGNANCY/ HYPEREMESIS GRAVIDARUM

Nausea and vomiting is a common occurrence in pregnancy. The duration and severity of these symptoms vary from one individual to another. In the worst scenario, nausea and vomiting can progress to a condition called **hyperemesis gravidarum,** a condition in which persistent vomiting can result in weight loss, electrolyte disturbances, and fluid loss.[1]

Epidemiology

It is estimated that up to 80% of women will experience nausea and/or vomiting during pregnancy (NVP). Typically, this condition will resolve after the first trimester, but in some women, it can persist throughout the entire pregnancy.[2] It was estimated that 25% of employed women requested time off from work because of these symptoms.[3] Approximately 0.5% to 2% of pregnant women will present with hyperemesis gravidarum, which is the most common reason for hospitalization in early pregnancy.[4]

Clinical Presentation

Nausea and vomiting are two separate symptoms that may exist together. Although nausea and vomiting during pregnancy is often referred to as *morning sickness,* this term may not be an accurate descriptor because nausea may occur throughout the day.

Nausea and vomiting during pregnancy may affect both mother and fetus. Nausea and vomiting may interfere with the pregnant woman's ability to have restful sleep, which can affect her mood, ability to work, and her overall weight.[5] In the extreme case, such as with hyperemesis gravidarum, the persistent NVP can represent a

CASE PRESENTATION

Patient Case: Part 1

B.H. is a 28-year-old woman who presents to the pharmacy. She states, "I need something to help me stop this nauseous feeling."

HPI: B.H. describes the nauseated feeling as being strongest in the morning, and it reappears periodically throughout the day. She denies fever, weight loss, dehydration, abdominal discomfort, and vomiting. She is currently 5 weeks pregnant.

PMH: She has no active medical conditions. She has a history of one miscarriage (2003).

Family history: Noncontributory.

Social history: Denies alcohol use. Quit smoking 3 months ago, along with her husband, in preparation for conception. She works as an elementary school teacher and has missed 2 days of work this week because of her nausea.

Medications: B.H. takes a prenatal vitamin daily and has not tried any interventions to control her nausea.

Allergies: NKDA.

Laboratory values: Within normal limits.

Physical exam: Weight 66.8 kg; Height: 160 cm; Temp 37.6° C; BP110/76 mm Hg (seated); P 84 (seated); BP 116/70 mm Hg (standing); P 88 (standing).

Assessment: Nausea—likely etiology is pregnancy-related nausea.

risk to both the mother and the fetus because of the potential for dehydration and electrolyte abnormalities. Some studies have suggested a benefit to nausea and vomiting in reducing the miscarriage rate. Nausea and vomiting in the first trimester has been associated with lower miscarriage rates (OR 0.36; 95% CI, 0.2–0.42).[6-8]

Pathophysiology

The pathophysiology of NVP is unclear, but several hypotheses have been proposed. A higher level of human chorionic gonadotropin (hCG) secretion is believed to be a key causative factor for the symptoms of NVP because there is a temporal relationship between peak hCG levels and symptoms.[9] Additionally, hCG stimulates the thyroid gland in pregnancy, and the resultant transient hyperthyroidism could cause nausea and vomiting.[4,10] Another hypothesis is that nausea and vomiting result in lower energy intake, which leads to lower levels of anabolic hormones and insulin. This reduction in hormone levels and maternal undernutrition would result in compensatory growth of the developing fetus.[11] A final hypothesis proposes the emetogenic potential of estrogen. As estradiol levels rise in pregnancy, nausea and vomiting symptoms increase, whereas symptoms decrease with decreasing estradiol levels.[4]

In addition to hormonal changes, there are possible risk factors for NVP. Other potential risk factors include a predisposition to motion sickness, a history of migraine headaches, psychologic predisposition, a diet high in fat before conception, maternal age at conception, genetics, and a history of nausea with combined oral contraceptives.[4,9] Conversely, vitamins, which may contain vitamin B_6, have been shown to have a protective effect against NVP.[4,12,13]

Diagnosis

The time of day when symptoms occur and the trimester can be clues as to whether the pregnant patient is presenting with NVP. However, the patient should be interviewed further to determine whether another cause for the nausea and vomiting is present. Other medical conditions that can present with nausea and vomiting that should be ruled out include, but are not limited to, gastroparesis, appendicitis, gastrointestinal obstructions, migraine headaches, and vestibular lesions.[4,14]

Treatment

The goals of treatment are to minimize signs and symptoms, decrease complications that may occur because of progressive nausea and vomiting, and treat hyperemesis gravidarum to minimize adverse effects on the mother and fetus. See Figure 24-1.

Nonpharmacologic Therapy

The initial recommendation for the management of NVP is to use nonpharmacologic treatments. Avoiding triggers—such as smells, foods, and motion—as much as possible should be advocated.[9] Small, low-fat meals and drinking chilled or tart beverages may also be beneficial.[15] The use of acupressure for the treatment of NVP has shown mixed results and a strong placebo effect.[4,16-18] However, it may be a reasonable adjunct therapy as this option has not been associated with adverse effects.[19]

Pharmacologic Therapy

Vitamin B. Vitamin B_6 or pyridoxine was formerly combined with doxylamine and dicyclomine to form the product Bendectin®. This product was voluntarily withdrawn from the market in 1984 after several false allegations that the drug was teratogenic.[9,20,21]

Figure 24-1. Algorithm for treatment of nausea and vomiting during pregnancy.[34]

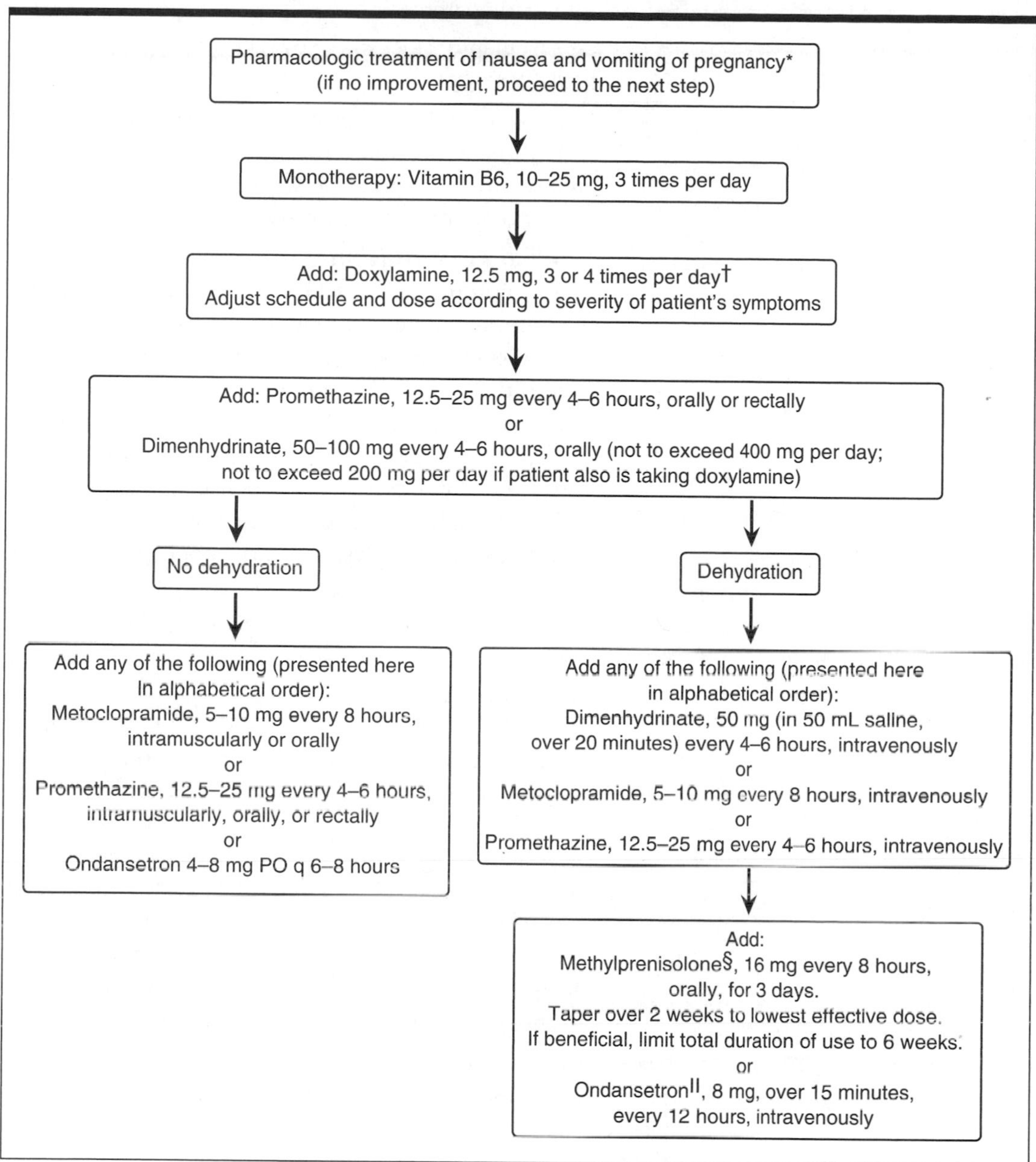

*This algorithm assumes other causes of nausea and vomiting have been ruled out. At any step, consider parenteral nutrition if dehydration or persistent weight loss is noted. Alternative therapies may be added at any time during the sequence depending on patient acceptance and clinician familiarity; consider acupressure with wrist bands or acustimulation or ginger capsules, 250 mg 4 times daily.

†In the United States, doxylamine is available as the active ingredient in some over-the-counter sleep aids; one half of a scored 25-mg tablet can be used to provide a 12.5-mg dose of doxylamine.

‡Thiamine, intravenously, 100 mg daily for 2–3 days (followed by intravenous multivitamins), is recommended for every woman who requires intravenous hydration and has vomited for more than 3 weeks. No study has compared different fluid replacements for nausea and vomiting of pregnancy.

§Corticosteroids appear to increase risk for oral clefts in the first 10 weeks of gestation.

||Safety, particularly in the first trimester of pregnancy, not yet determined; less effect on nausea.

Vitamin B_6, at dosages ranging from 10–25 mg 3 times daily, has been shown to be effective in reducing nausea and retching. The results on vomiting are conflicting.[20,22] Congenital abnormalities and pregnancy complications were not seen in these studies. Antihistamine use in pregnancy will be discussed in the section on the treatment of the common cold later in this chapter.

Ginger. Ginger has been studied in several trials, but data from randomized, controlled trials are limited. Like vitamin B_6, it has been shown to decrease nausea and retching but has had conflicting results with reduction of vomiting episodes.[22-25] Belching and heartburn were seen more frequently with ginger.[22,24] A confounding variable to some ginger trials is the concurrent use of other antiemetics during the course of the trial.[22,25] The most often studied dosage for ginger for the treatment of NVP is 250 mg 4 times daily.[26]

Phenothiazines. Promethazine is a first-line choice if nonprescription interventions have failed.[4] It can be given by various routes of administration and is therefore beneficial regardless of patient hydration status. It has not been associated with major malformations when used in the first trimester.[4,15,27] Sedation has been noted to occur with promethazine at rates similar to ondansetron.[28]

Metoclopramide. Metoclopramide dose for metoclopramide to 5–10 mg 3 times daily. As needed is listed as an option after the patient has failed better studied and less side effect–inducing medications.[4,15,29] A small, retrospective study by the Euromap study group did not find an association between the use of metoclopramide and preterm delivery, low birth weight, or malformations.[30] These findings were supported by a study by Berkovitch and colleagues.[31]

Ondansetron. Safety data for the use of common ondansetron regimens of 4–8 mg every 8 hours (intravenously or by mouth) in pregnant women is limited. One prospective study of 176 women who had taken ondansetron in their first trimester showed no statistically significant differences in miscarriages, stillbirths, therapeutic abortions, major malformations, or birth weights with ondansetron use. Six patients in the ondansetron group, three patients in the antiemetic treatment group, and three patients in the control group had major malformations (p = 0.57).[2] Ondansetron has been compared with promethazine for the treatment of nausea in a nonpregnant population and for hyperemesis gravidarum.[32] Given the difference in cost and lack of additive efficacy found in this small trial, ondansetron should not be recommended for first-line therapy at this time.[4,28]

Corticosteroids. Methylprednisolone 16 mg orally every 8 hours for 3 days is another option for patients who have signs and symptoms of dehydration and have failed other standard treatments.[4] There has been an association between methylprednisolone use in the first trimester and cleft palate.[4] Thus, it should be avoided in the first trimester and used only in cases of hyperemesis.

HEARTBURN AND GASTROESOPHAGEAL REFLUX DISEASE

Many women develop **gastroesophageal reflux disease** (GERD) and heartburn during pregnancy. It occurs in an estimated 30% to 50% of pregnant women, but the incidence may be as high as 80%.[33]

Clinical Presentation

The symptoms of GERD during pregnancy do not differ from the general population. The predominant symptom is heartburn, but regurgitation also occurs frequently.[33,34] GERD and heartburn can occur at any time during pregnancy but is generally worse during the last trimester.[35,36] Because GERD during pregnancy usually resolves after delivery, complications such as esophagitis and stricture are rare.[33] Alarm symptoms, such as dysphagia, odynophagia, bleeding, weight loss, or anemia, suggest complicated disease. When these symptoms are present, urgent diagnostic evaluation is recommended.[37]

Pathophysiology

The pathogenesis of GERD during pregnancy is multifactorial and not completely understood. However, reduced lower esophageal sphincter (LES) pressure plays an important role in the pathogenesis. During pregnancy, progesterone levels increase and reduce resting LES pressures.[33,38,39] Abnormal gastric emptying or delayed small bowel transit may also contribute to the development of heartburn during pregnancy. Finally, the role of increased abdominal pressure resulting from an enlarging uterus is controversial.[33,40,41]

Diagnosis

The American College of Gastroenterologists published updated guidelines for the diagnosis and

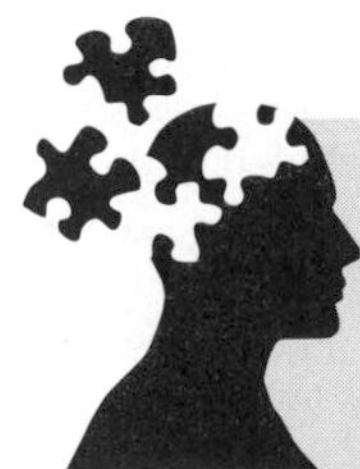

Therapeutic Challenge:

G.H. has struggled with weight gain during her pregnancy. The first 13 weeks she was so nauseated, she was not very interested in food. She did okay for a few months, but now G.H. is in week 24 and finds that eating causes quite a bit of pain and discomfort, so she has been eating less and not gaining weight. The ob/gyn is very concerned about the impact on fetal development. How would you intervene?

treatment of GERD.[37] The initial diagnosis of GERD in pregnancy can be reliably made based on clinical history. If uncomplicated GERD symptoms are controlled with empirical therapy, no further diagnostic workup is necessary.[37,42] The procedure of choice to evaluate severe reflux symptoms or complications is upper gastrointestinal endoscopy, which can be performed safely in pregnant women.[33,37] Barium radiographs are not recommended because of radiation exposure to the fetus. Ambulatory pH monitoring can also be performed safety but is rarely necessary.[33,42]

Treatment

The goals of treatment are to control symptoms and prevent or resolve significant complications, prevent recurrence of symptoms, and tailor treatment to meet patient needs.[34] Moreover, treatment should be safe for the expectant mother and fetus.

Nonpharmacologic Therapy

Lifestyle and dietary modification is the preferred and safest first step of GERD treatment and may be adequate to control symptoms in women with mild symptoms. Dietary modifications include avoiding foods and beverages that increase heartburn symptoms, such as fried and fatty foods, spicy and heavily seasoned foods, orange juice and tomato juice (highly acidic citrus products), alcoholic drinks, caffeinated or carbonated beverages (e.g., coffee), chocolate, and peppermint and spearmint. Additional measures, such as eating small well-balanced meals, avoiding smoking, and raising the head of the bed 6–8 inches may provide further relief.[34,41,42] Chewing gum stimulates salivary glands, which can help neutralize acid and may help with symptoms.

Pharmacologic Therapy

Antacids. Data on the safety of antacids on the fetus are sparse. Antacid use has not been shown to be unsafe, but there have been no controlled studies.[43] Although there are few safety data on antacids, magnesium-, calcium-, or aluminum-containing antacids are considered safe during pregnancy.[34,44] Antacids provide fast relief and can be taken as needed or as rescue therapy for breakthrough symptoms.[33,34] Calcium-containing antacids may be preferred because they provide an additional source of calcium, which may help prevent hypertension and preeclampsia.[34] High doses of aluminum-containing antacids may increase aluminum levels and cause fetal harm.[33,34,45,46]

Histamine-2 Receptor Antagonists. Histamine-2 receptor antagonists (H_2RA) are effective for treating GERD. For pregnant women with refractory symptoms despite lifestyle modification and antacid use, H_2RA may be an alternative. All H_2RAs are U.S. Food and Drug Administration (FDA) pregnancy category B. Both cimetidine and ranitidine have been used during pregnancy over the last 30 years, but some prefer ranitidine because of more available data specifically in pregnant women.[33,35,47] The safety and efficacy of other H_2RAs during pregnancy have not been evaluated in prospective, randomized studies specifically; regardless, the general consensus is that cimetidine and possibly famotidine are safe.[33,34]

Proton-Pump Inhibitors. Proton-pump inhibitors (PPIs) are recommended in pregnant women with complicated GERD, refractory to other therapies.[33,34] Retrospective and prospective cohort studies suggest that usual dosages of omeprazole and other PPIs during the first trimester of pregnancy are not a major teratogenic risk in humans and are safe to use during pregnancy (Table 24-1).[48-52] Some healthcare providers consider omeprazole the drug of choice, although it is FDA pregnancy category C, because it is the oldest agent in this pharmacologic class and has more fetal safety data.[53]

Other Agents. Sucralfate is not absorbed systemically and has been studied in one randomized-controlled study during pregnancy. More patients treated with sucralfate had complete remission of symptoms compared with dietary and lifestyle modification. Metoclopramide increases LES pressure, improves esophageal acid clearance, and promotes gastric emptying. It is considered safe to use during pregnancy.[54] Because more effective therapies are available, the use of metoclopramide is reserved for NVP.

CONSTIPATION

Constipation is another common problem during pregnancy. Pregnant women may newly develop constipation or chronic constipation may worsen during pregnancy.[55] The reported prevalence is approximately 11% to 38%.[56]

Clinical Presentation

Constipation symptoms include straining, feelings of incomplete evacuation, and changes in stool frequency and/or consistency. Patients may report pain, straining, and decreased frequency of stools. More worrisome symptoms include rectal bleeding, severe abdominal pain, weight loss, anorexia, or tenesmus.[34]

Pathophysiology

Constipation can develop during pregnancy due to numerous factors. Changes in diet, the ingestion of constipating medications such as iron, decreased

Table 24-1. Pharmacologic Agents for Treating Common Conditions Associated with Pregnancy

Drug	FDA Pregnancy Category	Recommendations for Pregnancy
	Medications for Nausea and Vomiting	
Antihistamines[a]—Avoid in last 2 weeks of gestation		
Promethazine	C	Compatible
Doxylamine	A	Compatible
Dimenhydrinate	B	Compatible
Diphenhydramine	B	Compatible
Antidopaminergic Agents		
Metoclopramide	B	Compatible
Other		
Trimethobenzamide	C	Low risk Adverse events limit its use
Ondansetron	B	Animal data suggest low risk
Ginger	C	Compatible
Pyridoxine/Vitamin B_6	A/C	Compatible
	Medications for GERD	
Antacids		
Aluminum-based antacids	None	Most low risk: minimal absorption
Calcium-based antacids	None	Most low risk: minimal absorption
Magnesium-based antacids	None	Most low risk: minimal absorption
Sodium bicarbonate	None	Not safe: alkalosis
Histamine-2 Receptor Antagonists		
Cimetidine	B	Controlled data: low risk
Famotidine	B	Limited human data: low risk in animals
Nizatidine	B	Limited human data: low risk in animals
Ranitidine	B	Low risk
Proton-Pump Inhibitors		
Esomeprazole	B	Limited data: low risk
Lansoprazole	B	Limited data: low risk
Omeprazole	C	Embryonic and fetal toxicity reported, but large data sets suggest low risk
Pantoprazole	B	Limited data: low risk
Rabeprazole	B	Limited data: low risk
Other		
Sucralfate	B	Low risk

(*Continued on next page*)

Drug	FDA Pregnancy Category	Recommendations for Pregnancy
	Medications for Diarrhea	
Antibiotics		
Amoxicillin/clavulanic acid	B	Low risk
Ampicillin	B	Low risk
Ciprofloxacin (all quinolones)	C	Potential toxicity to cartilage: avoid
Diphenoxylate/Atropine	C	Teratogenic in animals: no human data
Doxycycline	D	Contraindicated: teratogenic
Metronidazole	B	Low risk: avoid in first trimester
Rifaxamin	C	Animal teratogen: no human data
Tetracycline	D	Teratogenic
Trimethoprim-sulfamethoxazole	C/D (near term)	Teratogenic
Vancomycin	C	Low risk
Antidiarrheals		
Bismuth subsalicylate	C	Not safe: teratogenicity
Loperamide	B	Low risk: possible cardiovascular defects
	Medications for Constipation	
Laxatives and Stool Softeners		
Bisacodyl	C	Low risk in short-term use
Castor oil	X	Avoid
Docusate	C	Compatible
Lactulose	B	No human studies
Lubiprostone	C	No human studies: fetal loss in animals
Magnesium citrate	B	Avoid long-term use: hypermagnesemia, hyperphosphatemia, dehydration
Methylcellulose	None	
Mineral oil	C	Avoid: neonatal coagulopathy and hemorrhage
Polycarbophil	C	
Polyethylene glycol	C	First-choice laxative in pregnancy
Psyllium	C	
Senna	C	Low risk in short-term use
Sodium phosphate		Avoid long-term use: hypermagnesemia, hyperphosphatemia, dehydration

(*Continued on next page*)

Drug	FDA Pregnancy Category	Recommendations for Pregnancy
Medication for Common Cold and Allergic Rhinitis		
Topical Decongestants		
Oxymetazoline Xylometazoline	C	Limited human data: no relevant animal data
Oral Decongestants		
Pseudoephedrine	C	Limited human data: no relevant animal data Avoid in 1st trimester
Oral Antihistamines[a]		
Cetirizine	B	Limited human data: animal data suggest low risk
Chlorpheniramine	B	Compatible
Diphenhydramine	B	Compatible
Loratadine	B	Limited human data: animal data suggest low risk
Ophthalmic Antihistamines		
Ketotifen Levocabastine Olopatadine	C	No information
Topical Corticosteroids		
Budesonide	B	Compatible—maternal benefit > fetal risk
Other		
Cromolyn	B	Compatible
Medications for Sleep Disorders		
Diphenhydramine	B	Compatible Avoid use in last 2 weeks of gestation
Zolpidem/Zolpidem CR	B/C[b]	Limited human data: animal data suggest low risk

Source: Adapted from references 1, 4, 5, 27, 46, 73, and 77.

CR = controlled release; FDA = U.S. Food and Drug Administration; GERD = gastroesophageal reflux disease.

[a]There has been an association between retrolental fibroplasia in premature infants and antihistamine exposure in the last 2 weeks of pregnancy.

[b]Zolpidem is a pregnancy category B; however, the Ambien CR formulation is a pregnancy category C medication.

physical activity, or mechanical factors may cause constipation.[57] Moreover, constipation may develop as a result of hormonal changes (i.e., elevated levels of progesterone) during pregnancy.[55] Progesterone decreases smooth muscle contractility and slows gastrointestinal transit and may inhibit motilin, which also affects gastrointestinal transit time.[58,59] Other predisposing factors for constipation include an enlarging **gravid** uterus.[55]

Diagnosis

The diagnostic criteria suggested by experts include low frequency of stools (<3 stools per week), hard stools, and/or difficulties on evacuation.[34,60]

Treatment

The goals of treating constipation are to provide effective symptom relief with interventions that are safe for the mother and fetus. No formal guidelines on treating constipation during pregnancy have been developed; however, one option for a treatment algorithm is shown in Figure 24-2.[34]

Nonpharmacologic Therapy

Lifestyle modification is the preferred and safest initial treatment for constipation. Dietary changes that may relieve constipation are increasing dietary fiber, increasing liquid intake, and avoiding constipating foods (e.g., cabbage, bananas, carrots, and cheese).[61]

Figure 24-2. Chronic constipation treatment guidelines.[34]

[a]Stimulant laxatives (e.g., senna) should be used with caution during pregnancy.

[b]Saline osmotics may induce diarrhea in neonates.

[c]Current data suggest lactulose is not as efficacious as other first-line laxative options.

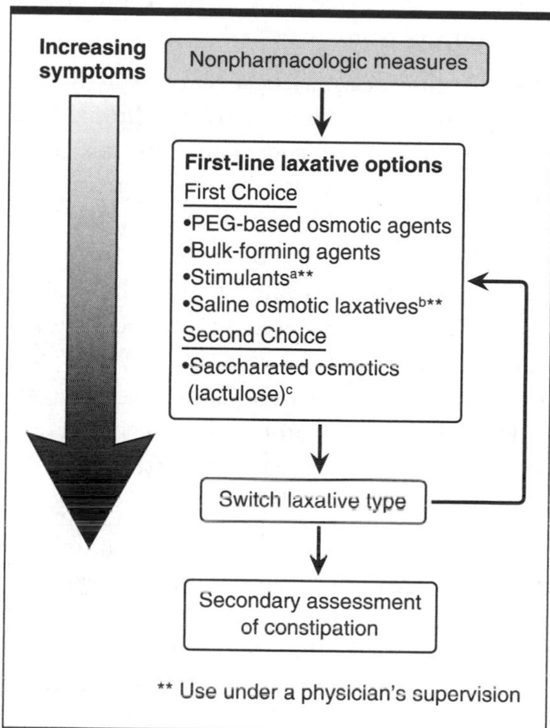

Increased fluids work best as a treatment for constipation in patients who are dehydrated.[58] Regular exercise and avoiding or minimizing stress may also help with constipation. Medications that can cause constipation should be avoided, if possible.

Pharmacologic Therapy

Many therapies are available to treat constipation (Table 24-1).

Osmotic Laxatives. Osmotic laxatives include polyethylene glycol–based osmotic laxative, lactulose, and saline osmotics (e.g., magnesium or sodium salts). Owing to its safety and efficacy, the American Gastroenterological Association (AGA) recommends polyethylene glycol as the laxative of choice during pregnancy.[46] Lactulose may be an alternative, but there are no human data on its safety during pregnancy. Saline osmotic laxatives provide fast relief but are unsuitable for long-term use. Magnesium-containing laxatives can cause hypermagnesemia, which can be fatal, and sodium phosphate can cause acute and severe elevations in phosphorus. Mineral oil should be avoided because it can decrease vitamin absorption and may increase bleeding risk with chronic use. Castor oil should not be used during pregnancy because it may be associated with induction of labor and can cause nausea.[34,46,55]

Bulk-Forming Laxatives. Three common bulk-forming laxatives are methylcellulose, polycarbophil, and psyllium. Although most bulk-forming laxatives are pregnancy category C, their use during pregnancy is acceptable because they have a good safety profile and minimal systemic absorption. Long-term use should be limited to women with uncomplicated constipation, and these agents should be avoided in patients with fecal impaction or existing bowel obstruction.[34]

Stimulant Laxatives. Senna and bisacodyl, two stimulant laxatives, are low risk with short-term use, although both are pregnancy category C. Senna has not been shown to be teratogenic in animals or humans.[27,58,62] Stimulant laxatives can be used when other therapies have failed and under the guidance of a physician, but long-term use should be avoided.[34]

Other Agents. Docusate sodium is a pregnancy category C medication but undergoes minimal systemic absorption and has not been associated with congenital defects. Many prenatal vitamins contain docusate to prevent constipation, and it is considered low risk during pregnancy.[46] The safety and efficacy of lubiprostone during pregnancy is unknown. It is a pregnancy category C and should be avoided until additional safety data are available.[63]

DIARRHEA

Diarrhea may also occur during pregnancy, but the exact prevalence is unknown.[55,64] Frequent bowel movements were reported in 34% of women during pregnancy in one study.[65]

Clinical Presentation

Diarrhea is described as loose, watery stools or more than three bowel movements in one day.[66] Acute diarrhea is usually self-limiting and resolves without specific treatment. Acute diarrhea may also present with abrupt onset of nausea, vomiting, abdominal pain, headache, fever, chills, and malaise.[59]

Pathophysiology

Acute diarrhea during pregnancy is commonly due to viral, bacterial, or parasitic infection.[55,64] Approximately 80% of acute episodes of diarrhea are due to viral infection, with rotavirus and Norwalk virus being the most frequent causes. Common bacterial pathogens include *Campylobacter*, *Shigella*, *Escherichia coli*, and *Salmonella*. Noninfectious etiologies of diarrhea include medications, food intolerances, food poisoning, and sugar substitutes, such as sorbitol and mannitol. Moreover, women may develop diarrhea during pregnancy because of pre-existing conditions, such as irritable bowel disease and inflammatory bowel disease.[55,59] Increased prostaglandins during pregnancy in theory may also cause diarrhea.[59]

Diagnosis

Acute episodes of diarrhea during pregnancy are usually mild and self-limiting and do not warrant extensive diagnostic evaluation. If diarrhea is profuse and leads to dehydration, if fever exceeds 38.3° C, if stools are grossly bloody, or if the illness persists for more than 48 hours without improvement, detailed diagnostic evaluation is necessary.[55] Tests to determine the etiology of diarrhea include stool collection for bacterial culture, stool analysis for ova and parasites, histologic examination for fecal leukocytes, and stool assay for *Clostridium difficile* toxin. Careful flexible sigmoidoscopy may be needed to rule out other disorders if conservative treatment does not resolve symptoms.[59]

Treatment

The goals of treatment are to relieve symptoms without harming the fetus or mother.

Nonpharmacologic Treatment

Conservative measures, such as rehydration of fluids and electrolytes, are the first step of therapy. All cases of diarrhea can initially be treated with oral replacement therapy (ORT) using decaffeinated beverages and juices. Sorbitol-containing ORTs may worsen diarrhea and should be avoided. Advise women to minimize or avoid caffeine, alcohol, and sugary beverages because these products may worsen pre-existing diarrhea.[55,67] The World Health Organization recommends a solution made of 1 L water, 1 teaspoon of salt, and 8 teaspoons of sugar for high-volume diarrhea.[55] As bowel function returns to baseline, semisolid and low-fiber foods can gradually be reintroduced.

Pharmacologic Treatment

Opiates and Opiate Derivatives. Loperamide is pregnancy category B. Although its use in pregnancy has not been associated with major malformations, one study showed there may be an association between loperamide use and fetal cardiac malformation.[27,68] Diphenoxylate with atropine is teratogenic is animals, and malformations have been observed in infants with first-trimester exposure. The AGA does not advocate the use of loperamide or diphenoxylate with atropine because of potential risk.[46]

Codeine and paregoric (camphorated opium tincture) are other opioids used to treat diarrhea in nonpregnant patients. The pregnancy risk of paregoric has not been classified, and codeine is pregnancy category C. The AGA does not mention the use of these agents during pregnancy.[46]

Antibiotics. Antibiotics may be necessary if there is an infectious etiology for diarrhea. Ampicillin, azithromycin, and vancomycin are considered low-risk drugs during pregnancy. Metronidazole is also a low-risk drug with short-term use after the first trimester.[46,55,59]

Some antibiotics should be avoided in pregnancy. Quinolones are associated with arthropathies in children and cartilage defects in animal studies and should be avoided, if possible. Doxycycline, tetracycline, and trimethoprim/sulfamethoxazole are teratogenic and are contraindicated in pregnancy. Rifaxamin has been associated with birth defects in animals, but there are no data in humans.[46,55,59]

Other Agents. Although adsorbents, bismuth subsalicylate, and loperamide are available over-the-counter for the management of diarrhea, limited efficacy and safety data in pregnancy make these products inappropriate options for self-treatment of diarrhea in pregnant patients.

SUMMARY

Nausea and vomiting, GERD, constipation, and diarrhea are common gastrointestinal problems during pregnancy. Nonpharmacologic interventions are preferred initially; however, drug therapy may be necessary in many cases. When choosing drug therapy, the efficacy and safety for mother and fetus should be considered.

Common Cold and Allergic Rhinitis

The treatment of a pregnant woman with respiratory symptoms takes into consideration risks to both the mother and the fetus and the risks of not treating the patient. For allergic rhinitis, the treatment arsenal contains some of the same medications that would be used for a nonpregnant individual. Similarly, a pregnant patient can receive the inactivated influenza vaccine if she has no contraindications. However, treating common cold symptoms is much different. Because the symptoms associated with a common cold are self-limiting and not life-threatening, there is a heavier emphasis on nonpharmacologic therapy throughout pregnancy, especially in the first trimester.

Epidemiology

The prevalence of perennial rhinitis and seasonal allergic rhinitis is between 1% to 18% and 1% to 40%, respectively.[69] Comparable to other pre-existing medical conditions, the symptoms of allergic rhinitis can improve, worsen, or remain the same during the course of any given pregnancy. It is estimated that allergy symptoms will increase in as many as 30% of pregnant women.[70,71]

Clinical Presentation

The symptoms of allergic rhinitis and the common cold during pregnancy are equivalent to those of nonpregnant individuals. For both conditions, the patient may present with clear rhinorrhea, nasal congestion, sneezing, fatigue, cough, and itching of the nose and eyes. Symptoms can affect both mother and fetus. The symptoms of allergic rhinitis and the common cold may affect the woman's quality of life, interrupting her normal sleep cycle as well as causing discomfort. The lack of appropriate treatment may lead to exacerbation of underlying asthma or sinus problems. One retrospective study linked snoring to an increased risk of fetal growth retardation.[72]

Pathophysiology

Hormonal changes and an increase in the blood volume of a pregnant woman can augment nasal vascular growth, which can lead to an increase in nasal congestion.[70] These hormonal changes can result in a condition known as rhinitis of pregnancy. This condition is confined to the period of gestation, and women exhibit marked congestion during the course of the pregnancy, with resolution typically occurring shortly after delivery.[71]

Diagnosis

Diagnosis is based on presence of common symptoms, such as nasal congestion, headache, sinus pressure, cough, or fever. The symptoms of allergic rhinitis and the common cold could be the result of a viral infection.

Treatment

The goals of treatment are to decrease symptoms, improve or preserve patient functional status, and prevent complications of untreated allergic rhinitis or common cold on the patient's other medical conditions.

Nonpharmacologic Therapy

Hand washing and antiseptic gels may decrease virus transmission. Allergic rhinitis symptoms may be minimized by avoiding triggers such as smoke, staying indoors on high-risk days, buying an air filter, and avoiding allergens when possible.

Pharmacologic Therapy

Antihistamines, cromolyn, and decongestants are used for the treatment of both the common cold and allergic rhinitis. Immunotherapy is an important treatment for allergic rhinitis that can be continued into pregnancy only if initiated before pregnancy.[73] It is generally not recommended to start this therapy during pregnancy because of the potential risk for anaphylaxis.[69,71,73] Similar to their nonpregnant counterparts, select intranasal corticosteroids can be used for allergic rhinitis. Acetaminophen can be given to women suffering common cold symptoms and for muscle aches and low-grade fever because there are potential adverse events with nonsteroidal anti-inflammatory drugs during pregnancy. Owing to the potential complications associated with influenza, the American College of Obstetricians and Gynecologists (ACOG) recommends vaccination. Women who are pregnant or will become pregnant during influenza season should receive the inactivated influenza vaccine.[74] Several ophthalmic antihistamines are available with and without a prescription, but there are no controlled clinical trials of these medications in pregnant women.

Antihistamines. When an antihistamine is necessary during pregnancy, chlorpheniramine is recommended.[73] The relative safety of these products in pregnancy has been reported in the data from the Collaborative Perinatal Project and the Michigan Medicaid recipient study.[27,73,75,76]

Loratadine or cetirizine are the second-generation antihistamines of choice.[77] In one study, patients exposed to loratadine (n = 210), other antihistamines (n = 267), and matched controls (n = 929) were evaluated. There were no differences in stillbirths, major or minor anomalies, or preterm deliveries, but a statistically significant difference in miscarriages was noted between loratadine and the other antihistamine group. It is unknown if the statistically significant difference in gestational age and maternal age between these two groups may have contributed to this outcome.[76] In a second study, loratadine was not associated with malformations.[78] There have been reports of hypospadias with loratadine, but confounding factors may not have been controlled for in these trials.[79] There are some reassuring safety data for cetirizine.[80]

Decongestants. Pseudoephedrine is the oral decongestant of choice during pregnancy.[77] There has been an association between the use of pseudoephedrine alone and in combination and an increased risk of **gastroschisis,** but one study did not show an increased risk of gastroschisis for the single entity pseudoephedrine product.[81] Phenylephrine has been associated with malformations in the animal model and should not be used in pregnant women.[27,75,82]

Cough Suppressants/Expectorants. The American College of Chest Physicians (ACCP) does not recommend the use of nonprescription cough suppressants and expectorants for the treatment of cough that is due to the common cold.[83] Birth defects with dextromethorphan have been reported in the chick embryo model but not in humans.[84,85] Guaifenesin has been associated with inguinal hernias.[27,86]

Other Agents. Nonprescription saline nasal sprays can be used for either condition. Cromolyn nasal spray has some safety data in pregnancy.[71,87] Intranasal cromolyn can be used for allergic rhinitis, but its use for common cold treatment is limited because of a delayed onset of action. Intranasal steroids have a low risk of systemic effect when used at recommended dosages.[77] Intranasal budesonide is pregnancy category B and has not been associated with an increased risk of malformation in limited study data.[88] The American College of Allergy, Asthma, and Immunology notes this medication may be relatively safe for pregnant women.[89]

SUMMARY

Allergic rhinitis symptoms can worsen or improve with pregnancy. Many of the therapeutic options available for nonpregnant patients can also be used in pregnant patients. Cromolyn nasal spray, chlorpheniramine, and pseudoephedrine can be used to address common symptoms. Similarly, these medications can be used for the treatment of the common cold. Because of the self-limiting nature of the common cold, the use of medication in the first trimester is not recommended. The influenza vaccine is recommended for patients who are pregnant or will be pregnant during influenza season.

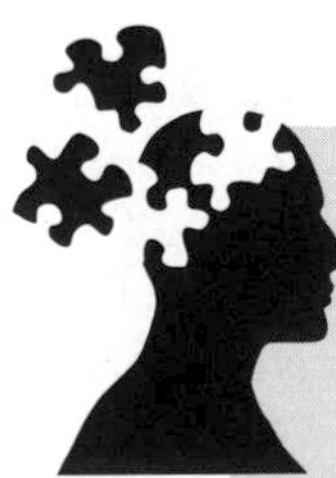

Therapeutic Challenge:

R.H. is entering her 20th week of pregnancy and presents for her routine monthly follow-up appointment with a chief symptom of "disruptive" sleep patterns: She is exhausted/falling asleep all day yet cannot sleep all night.

Insomnia

It would be inaccurate to define sleep disorders of pregnancy only in terms of insomnia. Many changes in sleep patterns can occur in pregnancy. This may be due to hormonal changes or to physiologic changes that occur during the course of a normal pregnancy.

Epidemiology

Changes in sleep patterns occur in pregnancy with a higher prevalence as the pregnancy progresses. It is estimated that as many as 90% of women will experience a disturbance in their normal sleep habits and behaviors by the third trimester.[90]

Clinical Presentation

The growing fetus can cause increased sleep disturbance during pregnancy. Frequent awakenings and decreased sleep efficiency have been observed in sleep studies performed in pregnant women.[90] There was a correlation between disrupted sleep during pregnancy and labor length, as well as the need for delivery by cesarean section.[91] Changes in breathing patterns for pregnant patients may result in hypoxemia. Depending on the severity of the hypoxemia, intrauterine growth restriction might occur.[92]

Pathophysiology

The menstrual cycle and pregnancy are both marked by changes in the production of various hormones and steroids, such as estradiol, progesterone, prolactin, melatonin, and cortisol.[90] Estradiol, as well as cortisol, may have a negative impact on rapid eye movement (REM) sleep.[92] It is hypothesized that the effect of progesterone on the upper airways may alter breathing patterns during sleep and may stimulate non-REM sleep.[90,92] Oxytocin increases at night; thus, uterine activity does as well. This may lead to insomnia in some pregnant women.[92] Additional contributing factors are increased urination and increasing size, leading to difficulty becoming comfortable.

There are no clear-cut risk factors for determining the severity and type of sleep disruption seen in pregnancy. It is hypothesized that the incidence of restless legs syndrome increases during gestation, especially for women who do not consume adequate amounts of folate.[90,93] Understandably, the presence of restless legs syndrome can affect the patient's sleep habits.

Diagnosis

The initial evaluation should include a complete sleep history. A complete sleep history should include when the sleep disturbance began, what the change is, how often it occurs, and its severity. Prior or current history of anxiety, depression, or acute stressors should be evaluated. Several medications have been associated with insomnia, including corticosteroids and bupropion. Medical conditions that may cause sleep disturbances, such as nocturnal asthma, should be treated before treating insomnia. A sleep diary with documentation of stressors, duration of sleep, restfulness of sleep, and medications consumed will provide the healthcare provider with information regarding the possible causes of the patient's sleep disturbance.

Treatment

The goals of treatment are to restore normal sleep habits, minimize effects of sleep disturbance on patient's level of functionality and quality of life, and minimize risk to the growing fetus by reserving pharmacologic therapy for those who fail nonpharmacologic interventions.

Nonpharmacologic Therapy

Some nonpharmacologic interventions are available for women suffering from sleep disorders in pregnancy. If the patient has additional symptoms—such as heartburn, nausea, or nocturia, which may increase nighttime awakenings—these symptoms should first be treated appropriately.[90,93] Back pain may also increase wakefulness and should be treated with acetaminophen or by the use of pregnancy pillows.[92] Sleep hygiene, relaxation therapy, and stimulus control can be recommended.[92] Stimulus control involves using the bed only for sleep and not spending >20 minutes in bed while awake and unable to sleep. Avoiding caffeine and exercise before bedtime may also be helpful.

Pharmacologic Therapy

The treatment of insomnia and associated sleep disturbances in pregnancy is different than for their nonpregnant counterparts. Benzodiazepines, as a class, are generally avoided because of the possible risk to the developing fetus. Most benzodiazepines are pregnancy category D, with temazepam being pregnancy category X. Antidepressants, even sedating ones, are not recommended unless the patient has concurrent depression. It should be kept in mind that certain sedating antidepressants, such as tricyclic antidepressants, should be avoided in pregnancy. Although diphenhydramine may make the patient feel sleepy, it may not improve sleep quality. Avoid diphenhydramine products containing analgesic medications to minimize exposure of unnecessary medication.

Eszopiclone, zaleplon, and ramelteon are pregnancy category C. Eszopiclone is an isomer of zopiclone. Zopiclone did not have an increased risk of major malformations, but the sample size of the studied populations was very small.[94,95] There are no published human studies evaluating eszopiclone, zaleplon, or ramelteon.

Zolpidem can be used for the short-term treatment of insomnia in adult patients (recommended duration of treatment 7–10 days). Primarily in animal data, it has not been shown to be teratogenic at elevated dosages.[96] Information about its use in pregnant women is very limited. In one case report of a pregnant patient with substantial zolpidem use, it was found the medication did cross the placenta, but the infant did not exhibit signs of withdrawal after delivery.[97] This medication should be used only when absolutely necessary because of its minimal safety data in pregnant patients.

SUMMARY

Several sleep disturbances occur in pregnancy. These conditions occur with varying frequency, depending on trimester, and have multiple potential causes. It is important to determine the presence of sleep disturbances and recommend nonpharmacologic interventions. If these recommendations fail or if symptoms increase in frequency or severity, the patient should be referred to see a physician for evaluation.

Thromboembolism during Pregnancy

Pregnancy and the **puerperium** are risk factors for venous thromboembolism (VTE). Women may develop **deep vein thrombosis** (DVT) and **pulmonary embolism** (PE), which are two manifestations of VTE. Pregnant women are approximately 4–5 times more likely to develop VTE than women who are not pregnant.[98,99] During 1991–1999, the leading cause of pregnancy-related death (i.e., 20%) was **embolism.**[100] New data suggest that VTE can occur at any time during pregnancy and the postpartum period. The greatest risk of PE occurs in the postpartum period.[101]

Clinical Presentation

The symptoms of VTE do not differ in pregnant women. Patients experience pain and tenderness, heaviness or discomfort in the leg, edema, discoloration of the skin, and increased leg circumference (2 cm difference between the normal and affected leg).[101] Some of these symptoms, such as edema, are common to pregnancy in general. If edema is asymmetric, DVT is often suspected. Up to 90% of DVTs occur in the left leg because the gravid uterus compresses the left iliac vein.[101-103] Symptoms of PE include dyspnea, pleuritic chest pain, apprehension, cough, syncope, and hemoptysis. Associated signs include tachypnea and tachycardia.[101]

Pathophysiology

Virchow's triad (venous stasis, vascular injury, and/or hypercoagulability) describes conditions that may predispose to thrombotic disorders. During pregnancy, all elements of Virchow's triad are present. Venous stasis in the lower extremities occurs because of compression of the inferior venal cava and pelvic veins by the enlarging uterus, and deep vein capacitance increases secondary to increased circulating levels of estrogen.[104] Endothelial damage occurs at vaginal delivery or following cesarean delivery and contributes to the increased risk of VTE.

Alterations in the proteins of the coagulation system, fibrinolytic system, and natural anticoagulation system occur during pregnancy and puerperium. Although these changes probably evolved to protect women from hemorrhage at childbirth, they may increase the risk of VTE.[104,105] Clotting factors I, VII, VIII, IX, and X are increased and levels peak at term, and there is an overall increase in thrombin generation.[105] Levels of protein S, a physiologic anticoagulant, decline significantly during pregnancy, whereas fibrinolytic activity is decreased because of increased levels of plasminogen activator inhibitors. These changes result in increased propensity to form clots, decreased anticoagulant properties, and decreased fibrinolysis.[104,105]

Inherited thrombophilias have emerged as important risk factors for pregnancy-related VTE.[106,107] Approximately 30% to 50% of pregnant women with VTE have an inherited thrombophila.[102,108] The factor V Leiden mutation has been associated with increased VTE risk during pregnancy.[109] Other inherited thrombophilic conditions include prothrombin gene 20210A mutation, antithrombin deficiency, protein C deficiency, and protein S deficiency.[106,108] The antiphospholipid syndrome has been shown to increase adverse pregnancy outcomes, such as VTE and miscarriage.[108]

Other important risk factors for pregnancy-related VTE include previous history, family history of VTE during pregnancy, age 35 or greater, smoking, black race, obesity, delivery by cesarean section, immobilization, and parity (>4).[103,110-113]

Diagnosis

Recommendations for diagnosing VTE during pregnancy are largely empirical.[114] Elevated D-dimer levels may indicate VTE, but during pregnancy, there is a progressive increase of D-dimer levels. Therefore, elevated D-dimer levels alone should not be considered diagnostic of VTE during pregnancy.[115] Noninvasive tests used to diagnose DVT include compression ultrasonography and duplex Doppler ultrasonography. Venography or magnetic resonance imaging may be considered in patients with persistent symptoms despite negative noninvasive tests results when there is a high index of suspicion for DVT.[114,116,117] Tests for evaluation of PE include D-dimer, arterial blood gas measurement, chest radiograph, electrocardiogram, ventilation–perfusion (V/Q) scanning, helical computed tomography (CT) scan, compression ultrasonography of lower extremities, and pulmonary angiography. Both V/Q scanning and helical CT poses negligible fetal radiation exposure and are useful noninvasive modalities for the detection of PE.[99,114,116] Pulmonary angiography remains the gold standard, but its invasive nature limits its widespread use.

Detection, Screening, and Diagnosis Guidelines and Position Statements

The ACOG developed a practice bulletin on thromboembolism during pregnancy.[99] The 8th ACCP Conference on Antithrombotic and Thrombolytic Therapy also provides guidelines for the treatment and prevention of VTE during pregnancy.

Treatment

The goals of treatment of acute VTE are to alleviate the signs and symptoms, prevent pulmonary embolism in those with DVT, prevent death, prevent recurrence of thromboembolic event, and prevent long-term complications, such as the post-thrombotic syndrome.

Nonpharmacologic Therapy

Nonpharmacologic therapy includes placement of an inferior vena caval filter or surgical removal of thrombus. Patients may undergo inferior vena caval filter placement if anticoagulants are contraindicated or the clot propagates despite adequate anticoagulation. Retrievable filters may reduce some of the complications associated with permanent filters.[118] Surgical intervention, such as thrombectomy, can be considered in emergent cases only.[116] Elastic compression stocking may be used during pregnancy.[119]

Pharmacologic Therapy

Both the ACCP guidelines and ACOG recommend the use of intravenous unfractionated heparin (UFH), subcutaneous UFH, or low-molecular-weight heparin (LMWH) to treat acute thromboembolism during pregnancy. Heparins, either low molecular weight or unfractionated, do not cross the placenta and are considered safe for the fetus.[120,121]

Low-Molecular-Weight Heparins. Low-molecular-weight heparins are the heparin of choice for the treatment of acute VTE during pregnancy.[116,121] Weight-adjusted full-dose LMWH is recommended.[121] Low-molecular-weight heparin is preferred over UFH because there may be less bone loss, a lower risk of heparin-induced thrombocytopenia, and possibly fewer bleeding complications. Numerous studies suggest that LMWH is safe and effective in pregnancy-related VTE.[122,123] The observed rates of bleeding and adverse fetal outcomes with LMWH did not differ from UFH in pregnant women.[102,123]

Pregnancy may alter the pharmacokinetics of LMWH. As the pregnancy progresses and the woman gains weight, the volume of distribution and half-life changes.[124,125] The dosage of LMWH can be adjusted in proportion with the change in weight to accommodate these changes. It is also recommended to monitor anti-factor Xa levels, usually 4 hours after injection. Low-molecular-weight heparin dosages can then be modified to achieve anti-Xa levels of 0.6–1.0 units/mL with twice daily dosing or 1–2 units/mL with daily dosing of LMWH.[121]

Unfractionated Heparin. Unfractionated heparin is a second-line agent owing to the higher incidence of osteoporosis (approximately 2%) and heparin-induced thrombocytopenia.[102,120] If the decision is made to use UFH given subcutaneously, midlevel aPTT measurements (i.e., 6 hours after dose) should be checked at least monthly, and dosages should be adjusted to maintain adequate aPTT values 1.5–2.5 times the average laboratory control value.

Coumarin Derivatives. Coumarin derivatives are considered relatively contraindicated during pregnancy, although the FDA pregnancy category is X. These drugs cross the placenta and have been associated with **embryopathy,** especially during weeks 6–12 of gestation. Mental retardation, cleft lip and palate, optic atrophy, nasal hypoplasia, and stippling of bone have been reported. The use of warfarin close to term may result in the delivery of an anticoagulated fetus. For these reasons, warfarin is absolutely contraindicated between 6 and 12 weeks of gestation and close to term, but the risks associated with warfarin during the remainder of pregnancy have been considered smaller. Because warfarin may cause serious complications, it should be avoided in the acute treatment of VTE during pregnancy as safer alternatives are available. Warfarin may be safely used in the postpartum period if chronic anticoagulation is necessary.[102,121]

Other Agents. Fondaparinux is a selective anti-Xa inhibitor. Placental transfer of fondaparinux was not observed in an in vitro human model, but it was reported to have minor transplacental passage in vivo.[126-128] For patients who have hypersensitivity skin reactions to heparins or danaparoid- or heparin-induced thrombocytopenia, case reports suggest the feasibility of using fondaparinux in pregnant patients for prophylaxis of VTE.[129-132] Other anticoagulants are not recommended. Neither argatroban nor bivalirudin have been studied in pregnant women. Lepirudin and other hirudins cross placenta in rats and have not been evaluated during pregnancy.[121]

Anticoagulation Management in the Intrapartum and Postpartum Period. Anticoagulant therapy must be managed appropriately around delivery to minimize maternal and fetal risk. Recommendations for managing anticoagulation at the time of delivery are based on expert opinion. One strategy is to schedule induction after 37 weeks of gestation. Women can be instructed to stop LMWH 12 hours before planned induction or cesarean section when prophylactic doses of LMWH are used, or 24 hours before if therapeutic doses of LMWH are used. If spontaneous labor occurs in women receiving UFH, heparin must be stopped. Careful monitoring of aPTT is required when they go into labor. Protamine may be used as an antidote if the aPTT is markedly prolonged. For patients who are considered very high risk, patients can be switched to intravenous UFH, which can be discontinued 4–6 hours before expected time of delivery. Another option is to convert from LMWH to UFH at 36–37 weeks of gestation or sooner. The rationale for converting to UFH is to take advantage its shorter half-life and to reduce the possibility spinal or epidural hematoma if labor occurs unexpectedly.[111]

Restarting anticoagulation with LMWH or UFH may be considered 6-12 hours after uncomplicated delivery, 12 hours after epidural removal, or 24 hours after cesarean delivery if hemostasis is established.[108,111,121] In the postpartum period, warfarin is started concurrently with heparin.[108] Heparin should be continued until a therapeutic International Normalized Ratio of 2–3 is achieved. For women who have had a thrombotic event during the current pregnancy, she should remain on warfarin for at least 6 weeks postpartum (for a minimum total duration of therapy of 6 months), although a longer duration may be necessary. For women on lifelong anticoagulation, warfarin will be continued indefinitely. Warfarin passes minimally into breast milk and is not a contraindication to breastfeeding.[111,121]

Thromboprophylaxis during Pregnancy. Some women may be candidates for thromboprophylaxis during pregnancy. However, there are no randomized data to guide healthcare providers, and recommendations are largely based on retrospective studies and expert opinion.[112,116,133] When the decision is made in favor of thromboprophylaxis, it should be initiated soon after conception. If ovulation induction is planned, thromboprophylaxis should begin when induction therapy is initiated.[111]

SUMMARY

The risk of venous thromboembolism is increased during pregnancy, and VTE is a significant cause of maternal morbidity and mortality. Patients at risk for developing VTE because of previous history or thrombophilia should received thromboprophylaxis antepartum and postpartum. Although both UFH and LMWH are effective, LMWHs are associated with fewer adverse effects and have emerged as the drugs of choice.

CASE PRESENTATION

Patient Case: Part 2

Treatment Plan:

1) Recommend nonpharmacologic interventions for B.H. Advise her to change positions slowly when awakening. She may eat bland food or sip a chilled or tart beverage before getting out of bed. Saltine crackers and ginger ale have antidotal evidence, and these may be helpful interventions. Advise her to eat small meals that are low in fat and can pass more easily through her stomach.
2) Advise her to continue her prenatal vitamin tablets daily.
3) Recommend vitamin B_6 25 mg 3 times daily. Follow up with her in 5–7 days because most clinical trials were of limited duration to assess for efficacy and adverse events.

Patient education: Reassure B.H. about the usual duration of nausea and that she may have nausea resolution within the next several weeks. Advise her to inform her physician if any of the warning symptoms occur (e.g., signs/symptoms of dehydration, severe abdominal pain). Review the nonpharmacologic interventions to also implement, such as eating small frequent meals 5–6 times a day and avoiding any "trigger foods."

Summary

Pregnancy is a time of extraordinary change for a woman, both physiologically and psychologically. In all the common conditions discussed in this chapter, nonpharmacologic interventions are preferred as the primary intervention. However, if symptoms do not improve, often drug therapy options will be indicated. When choosing drug therapy, the efficacy and safety for mother and fetus should be considered. If these recommendations fail or symptoms increase in frequency or severity, the patient should be encouraged to communicate with her physician for evaluation and alternative approaches for management.

References

Additional content available at ***www.ashp.org/womenshealth***

25 Pregnancy and Pre-existing Illnesses

Jeanne Hawkins VanTyle, Pharm.D., MS; Trisha LaPointe, Pharm.D., BCPS

Learning Objectives

1. Describe the potential effects of prepregnancy chronic health conditions on pregnancy, including an evaluation of preconception readiness and the potential risks for mother and fetus when pregnancy occurs.
2. Compare and contrast the considerations for the use of drug vs. nondrug therapies in the treatment of a pregnant patient with asthma, seizure disorders, hypertension, and diabetes.
3. Evaluate the risk vs. benefit for appropriate management of chronic conditions during pregnancy in both mother and fetus.
4. List and discuss appropriate monitoring parameters for pregnant patients with asthma, seizure disorders, hypertension, and diabetes.

This chapter summarizes experience and recommendations for drugs used to treat women with medical disorders existing before pregnancy. Because these conditions are diagnosed before pregnancy, this chapter will not discuss the pathology or diagnosis of the conditions and refers the reader to the respective clinical chapter in Section 6 of this text. With more women pursuing postsecondary and college education, today's mother is likely to be older and more likely to have concurrent disease conditions. In 1970, the average age for a first-time mother was about 21. Today she is more likely to be 25–29 years old.[1] Furthermore, the birth rate among older women is getting higher, with women older than 35 represent more than 12% of **primagravidas** in married women.[1] In general, chronic diseases occur more frequently with pregnancy in older patients. Older women may be more likely to have pre-existing asthma, diabetes, hypertension, seizures, or other chronic conditions requiring daily treatment with medications. Chronic medical conditions can contribute to the complexity pregnancy.

Many pregnant women have chronic medical conditions—such as asthma, high blood pressure, depression, or diabetes—that require them to continue taking drugs they were on before pregnancy. Today women take an average of three to five drugs during pregnancy. As a woman's body changes throughout her pregnancy, it may affect the dosage she needs of a particular drug. In addition, pre-existing diseases may get worsen during pregnancy, altering drug treatment requirements. The question to be asked in this patient population is: How does the disease affect pregnancy, and how does pregnancy affect the disease? This will guide the course of treatment for the chronic conditions in pregnancy. Another consideration for management of chronic conditions is that a woman will often need to take medications while she is breast-feeding, potentially exposing her child to the effects of these medications. The safety and use of medications while breast-feeding will be discussed in Chapter 29: Postpartum Care.

Asthma

In the U.S., asthma is a prevalent common chronic disease affecting approximately 4% to 9% of all pregnancies.[2] As seen in many conditions that exist concurrently with pregnancy, approximately one third remain similar to pregnancy, one third worsen, and one third improve.[3] Asthma is reported to be undertreated during pregnancy. Suboptimal asthma control presents significant risk to the outcome of pregnancy.[4-7] Pregnancy complications may arise as a result of the asthma or the drug therapy. Asthma may complicate pregnancies and has the potential to affect the health of the fetus and the mother. It is potentially the most common serious medical problem to complicate pregnancy. Poor asthma control and severity before pregnancy is associated with an increased risk of hypertension during pregnancy and intrauterine growth retardation.[8,9] The 2004 National Asthma Education and Prevention Program reports "inadequate control of asthma is a greater risk to the fetus than asthma medications are."[10] Asthma medications, including inhaled corticosteroids (ICSs), inhaled short acting beta-2 agonists, and inhaled long-acting beta-2 agonists, have become established as safe during pregnancy.

CASE PRESENTATION

Patient Case: Part 1

J.H. is 34 years old and will be having her first baby in approximately 8 weeks. She has come to your pharmacy for more than 5 years. She requests a refill of a prescription for albuterol inhaler.

HPI: In her medication profile, you notice that she filled a prescription for an albuterol inhaler earlier this month. While checking the refill history over the last year, you see that an albuterol inhaler prescription has been filled approximately every 6 months. There is a prescription for a fluticasone-salmeterol 250 mcg/50 mcg for inhalation (Advair Diskus) that has not been filled since J.H. learned that she was pregnant. She is experiencing some chest tightness and shortness of breath at least three nights a week but attributes this to the pregnancy. While entering the order for J.H.'s albuterol inhaler, you casually ask if she needs a refill of her Advair Diskus. She indicates to you it did not seem like the Advair Diskus helped as much as much as the albuterol to control her asthma, and she does not want to be on any medication that could hurt the baby.

PMH: J.H. has had asthma since age of 10; otherwise, she is in good health.

Family history: Noncontributory.

Social history: J.H. denies any use of alcohol or tobacco during her pregnancy.

Allergies: None.

Medications: Albuterol 90 mcg/actuation inhaler: two puffs every 6 hours as needed for shortness of breath; prenatal multivitamin with iron: one capsule daily.

Labs: Not available.

Diagnostics: Not available.

Patient assessment: J.H. is having worsening chronic asthma symptoms that have been untreated during her pregnancy.

EFFECTS OF PREGNANCY ON ASTHMA

Asthma has been associated with maternal morbidity, including worsening of the asthma and increased hospitalization for exacerbations. All pregnant patients need to be monitored by peak expiratory flow rate (PERF) and forced expiratory volume in 1 second (FEV_1) testing during pregnancy. Exacerbations are most likely to occur between 24 and 36 weeks of pregnancy.[11] In a prospective study, respiratory viral infections were the most common precipitants of exacerbations of asthma during pregnancy (34%), followed by nonadherence to inhaled corticosteroid medications, occurring in 34% compared with 29% of patients, respectively.[12]

As pregnancy progresses, the diaphragm is raised, which reduces lung capacities. Chronic maternal hypoxia should be avoided at all costs. Classification of asthma severity has important clinical implications on asthma morbidity. Failure to classify severity of asthma may result in suboptimal outcomes. In prospective clinical trials, low birth weight was more common in women with daily symptoms of moderate asthma than in women without asthma.[13]

In an evaluation of more than 37,000 pregnancies in women with asthma and compared with other pregnancies in their database of 243,000 pregnancies in women without asthma, results reported that women with asthma have similar reproductive risks compared with women without asthma in the general population with respect to placental insufficiency, placenta previa, preeclampsia, gestational diabetes, and thyroid disorders.[13] The risk of miscarriage, depression, or cesarean section increased moderately in women with more severe asthma and previous asthma exacerbations.[13] Hence, the data support that well-controlled asthma is associated with better pregnancy outcomes.

MANAGEMENT OF ASTHMA DURING PREGNANCY GUIDELINES

There are two primary guidelines available to assist in the management of asthma symptoms during pregnancy. The first from National Institutes of Health–National Heart, Lung and Blood Institute was released in 2004, which was similar to the guidelines from the American College of Obstetricians and Gynecologists (ACOG) published in 2008.[10,14]

TREATMENT OF ASTHMA IN PREGNANCY

Goals

The ultimate goal of therapy for asthma in pregnancy is first to deliver a healthy baby as well as to maintain adequate oxygenation of the fetus by preventing hypoxic episodes in the mother. In addition, in the mother the goal is to achieve minimal or no chronic symptoms during the day or night, with no periods of exacerbation, night-time awakenings, or limitations of activities. In the process of achieving normal or near-normal pulmonary function, the goal is to limit use of short-acting beta-2 agonists to minimize adverse effects from asthma medications. Obstetric care should include monitoring of asthma status during prenatal visits.[14]

Asthma treatment in pregnancy is organized around four components of management, including assessment, management of aggravating factors, patient education, and pharmacologic treatment interventions.[10,14] Initial assessment and routine monitoring of asthma should include objective measures of pulmonary function, such as measure of peak flow with spirometry, throughout pregnancy because the course of asthma will change during pregnancy. As much as possible, patients should limit exposure to aggravating factors, such as allergens or environmental irritants that are known to contribute to the severity of their asthma symptoms. Although dealing with chronic conditions, a review of patient education to ensure that patients know exactly how to monitor and manage their asthma is merited. Finally, a stepwise approach to pharmacologic therapy while recognizing special considerations in pregnancy is recommended (Table 25-1).

Management of Acute Asthma in Pregnancy

It is important to intervene rapidly and closely monitor maternal and fetal well-being during an acute asthma attack. The patient should be monitored closely to maintain oxygen saturation >95% and avoid pCO_2 ≥40 mm Hg. Hypotension can be prevented with positioning, hydration, and treatment. To achieve optimal blood return, place the woman in a left lateral position. Provide ample hydration with intravenous fluids if oral intake is not adequate. If intravenous hydration required, then isotonic saline at 125 mL/hr is the desired fluid.

Management of Chronic Asthma in Pregnancy

Mild Intermittent Therapy

In general, no daily medication is needed. Albuterol is the preferred short-acting beta-2 agonist because it has an excellent safety profile and the greatest amount of data related to safety during pregnancy of any currently available inhaled beta-2 agonist.[10] The use of beta-2 agonists in approximately 1,800 women reported no significant relationship with adverse pregnancy outcomes.[15]

Mild Persistent Asthma

Similar to nonpregnant patients, ICSs are the most important and effective controller medications and the first-line recommended therapy in pregnancy.[10,14] ICSs are the cornerstone of treatment for asthma regardless of severity. It has been shown that ICSs

Table 25-1. Medical Management of Asthma in Pregnancy

Classification	Preferred Treatment in Pregnancy	Alternative
Mild intermittent asthma	No daily medications Inhaled albuterol as needed	None
Mild persistent asthma	Low-dose inhaled corticosteroid	Cromolyn, leukotriene receptor antagonist, or low-dose theophylline (serum level 5–12 mcg/mL)
Moderate persistent asthma	Low-dose inhaled corticosteroid and salmeterol OR (when needed) medium-dose inhaled corticosteroid and salmeterol	Low-dose inhaled or medium-dose inhaled corticosteroid and salmeterol AND either leukotriene receptor antagonist or low-dose theophylline (serum level 5–12 mcg/mL)
Severe persistent asthma	High-dose inhaled corticosteroid and salmeterol and (if needed) oral corticosteroid	High-dose inhaled corticosteroid and theophylline (serum level 5–12 mcg/mL) and (if needed) oral corticosteroid

during the first trimester of pregnancy, regardless of the dosage, was not significantly associated with an increase in the risk of all congenital malformations. In fact, moderate dosages of ICS taken during the first trimester were associated with about a 60% reduction in the risk of all congenital malformations compared with no ICS.[16]

Dosages were reported as beclomethasone-CFC equivalents in mcg/day as low (1–500 mcg/day), moderate (500–1,000 mcg/day), and high (>1,000 mcg/day). They are safe in pregnancy, and systematic reviews have shown that they are not associated with fetal malformations or perinatal morbidity. This is based on the strong effectiveness data in nonpregnant women as well as effectiveness and safety data in pregnant women that show no increased risk of adverse perinatal outcomes.[16] Budesonide is the preferred ICS because there are more data available on using budesonide in pregnant women than are available on other ICSs.[17] There are no data indicating that the other ICSs are unsafe during pregnancy. In spite of the fact that many studies in pregnancy have studied budesonide, the usual recommendation is that the corticosteroid that was used successfully before pregnancy should be continued through childbirth.

Other potential agents for management of mild persistent asthma include cromolyn, leukotriene receptor modifiers, and theophylline. These are considered alternative but not preferred therapies. In the OTIS (Organization of Teratology Information Specialists) Asthma Medications in Pregnancy Study, 96 women took leukotriene antagonists sometime during pregnancy.[18] The National Asthma Education and Prevention Program (NAEPP) expert panel does not recommend leukotriene modifiers during pregnancy. Leukotriene modifiers currently include compounds available for use orally. Montelukast and zafirlukast are leukotriene receptor modifiers, and zileuton is a 5-lipooxygenase pathway inhibitor.

Theophylline is an alternative treatment for mild persistent asthma. Theophylline has demonstrated clinical effectiveness and has many years of experience with pregnant women. At recommended dosages (to a serum concentration of 5–12 mcg/mL), theophylline is an alternative to the preferred treatment of a low-dose ICS for pregnant patients with mild, persistent asthma.[10,19] The main advantage of theophylline is the long duration of action with sustained-release products, in the range of 8–12 hours. This is useful in the treatment of nocturnal asthma.

Moderate Persistent Asthma

The two treatment options are either a combination of a low-dose ICS and a long-acting beta-2 agonist (LABA) or an increased dosage of the ICS and a LABA. In trials of nonpregnant adults, it has been shown that LABA added to ICS results in a greater effect than simply increasing the dosage of the ICS. Two long-acting inhaled beta-2 agents are available: salmeterol and formoterol. There are more data on salmeterol than on formoterol in pregnancy. Limited data in pregnancy describe the effectiveness of combination therapy of ICS and LABA in pregnancy. Few data exist on LABAs used alone or in combination with ICSs in pregnant women. Higher dosages of salmeterol and formoterol have been associated with fetal malformations in animals, but current data in women do not indicate cause for concern.

Severe Persistent Asthma

If additional medication is required after assessing patient adherence with medications, then ICSs should be increased to maximal dosages and a LABA added if the patient is not already receiving it. The use of budesonide is preferred. If further action to manage asthma symptoms is needed, then the addition of systemic corticosteroids is warranted.[10] Oral corticosteroid use, especially during the first trimester of pregnancy, is associated with an increased risk for isolated cleft lip with or without cleft palate. The risk of cleft lip in the general population is 0.1%, and the risk in pregnant women on oral corticosteroids is 0.3%. However, very few pregnant women who had oral steroid–dependent asthma were included in the studies, and aspects of the study—such as length of use, timing and dosage at time of exposure—were not well described. The available data make it difficult to separate the effects of the oral corticosteroids on these outcomes from the effects of severe or uncontrolled asthma. It is known that prednisone is inactivated at 90% by the placenta, which serves to limit the fetal exposure to the active drug and the risk of fetal withdrawal.

Allergic Rhinitis

Allergic rhinitis is often associated with asthma. It is more frequently observed in pregnancy. Intranasal corticosteroids are the most effective medications for the management of allergic rhinitis and have a low risk of systemic effects when used in recommended dosages.[10] Montelukast can be used for the treatment of allergic rhinitis, but minimal data are available on the use of leukotriene receptor modifiers in pregnancy. The current second-generation antihistamines of choice are loratidine or cetirizine. Systemic decongestants used in the first trimester are associated with small increases in risk of fetal gastroschisis and intestinal **atresia,** and the risk should be considered.[20]

In general, topical decongestants like oxymetazoline should be considered before the use of oral decongestants. Many women will have nasal congestion in the last 4–6 weeks of pregnancy because of estrogen that is produced during pregnancy, which tends to inhibit acetylcholinesterase activity and leads to edema of the nasal mucosa with resultant congestion. This congestion of late pregnancy will clear a few days after delivery. Intermittent use of the topical agents can be considered. In cases when a cough suppressant is required, there are data to support the safety of dextromethorphan in pregnancy.[21]

MONITORING AND FOLLOW-UP

Lung function should be monitored as in the nonpregnant state with PEFR and FEV_1. A monitoring plan for red, yellow, and green zones with appropriate patient education should be developed. Effective patient education and self-management are essential to enhance asthma control during pregnancy. Approximately two thirds of pregnant women experience a change in asthma control during pregnancy.

Many elements of asthma monitoring are the same as in nonpregnant women, but some elements should be emphasized in the pregnant patient. Emphasize dangers of self-treatment with over-the-counter (OTC) drugs without physician approval. Many OTC cold remedies contain agents (sympathomimetics) that may interfere with or enhance the actions of inhaled bronchodilators. Most complications of asthma during pregnancy are from undermedication; thus, the goal is to emphasize the importance and safety of therapy.

PATIENT EDUCATION

Patient education should focus on the importance and safety of the medication to the fetus and to the mother. Make sure patients understand the potential harm to the fetus and increased risk to themselves with undertreatment or unnecessary delays in seeking additional care. It is beneficial to review the warning signs that indicate they should go to the emergency department. Finally, to avoid confusion, the use of written guidelines for managing an exacerbation and for prudently using the emergency department is recommended.

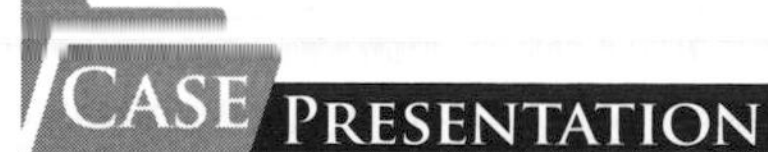

PRESENTATION

Patient Case: Part 2

Recognizing that J.H.'s night-time symptoms and increased albuterol use may be related to her pregnancy, you encourage her to tell her obstetrician about the night-time symptoms and her need for albuterol. She indicates that she will think about it and leaves your pharmacy with her albuterol refill. One week later, J.H. returns to your pharmacy with a prescription for budesonide 90 mcg with directions of 1 puff twice daily.

Patient education: To reduce barriers of compliance, patient should be counseled on proper inhalation technique. Emphasize the importance of using the inhaler 2 times daily to control lung inflammation to help maintain asthma control for health and quality of life, as well as for normal fetal maturation. Assure the patient that budesonide is the preferred inhaled corticosteroid because of the reassuring safety data, and it is considered the agent of choice when an inhaled corticosteroid needs to be initiated during pregnancy.

Patient monitoring: Review with J.H. the signs and symptoms of worsening asthma and a plan for the management of an acute exacerbation, including when to go to the emergency department if needed.

SUMMARY

The NAEPP report states that "inadequate control of asthma is a greater risk to the fetus than asthma medications are"; this is consistent with the current literature and the consensus guidelines. There is risk to both mother and fetus with undertreatment of asthma in pregnancy. Asthma medications, particularly those inhaled, are established as safe and effective in pregnancy.[22] It is important for healthcare providers to be sure that the patient has time to ask questions and understands the importance of adherence with her individual asthma plan.

Diabetes

Pregnant women with diabetes continue to present management problems for healthcare providers involved in their care. If a woman with diabetes can achieve normoglycemia, then the metabolic environment in which the fetus develops should result in a near-normal pregnancy outcome. Today, maternal mortality is rare, in contrast to a <50% chance of survival before the advent of insulin in the 1920s. Fetal and neonatal morbidity and mortality remains much higher than in the general population. The goal for the management of diabetes in a pregnant woman is to achieve outcomes similar to those in women without diabetes. Morbidity in the neonate associated with diabetes includes macrosomia, congenital malformations, and unexplained fetal death.[23] Keys in the management of pregnancy complicated by pregnancy include a balance of diet, exercise, and medications.

EPIDEMIOLOGY AND INCIDENCE IN WOMEN

Women who are known to have diabetes before pregnancy are often referred to as having established diabetes or pregestational diabetes. Nearly 4% of pregnant women in the U.S. have diabetes. Of those, 88% have gestational diabetes, and 12% have pre-existing diabetes. Of those developing gestational diabetes, approximately 50% will develop type 2 diabetes later in life.[24] This chapter will deal with the issues surrounding pregnancy in women with pre-existing diabetes. Management of gestational diabetes is discussed in Chapter 24: Conditions Associated with Pregnancy.

IMPORTANCE OF DIABETES MANAGEMENT DURING PREGNANCY

The importance of maternal glucose control before and during pregnancy cannot be understated. Ideally, women with known diabetes should be in good control before conception. Diabetes can result in a variety of metabolic imbalances, such as hyperglycemia, hypoglycemia, ketonemia, and hypoxia, which can be associated with adverse fetal outcomes. The incidence of congenital anomalies in infants of women with diabetes is increased over that of the general population.

Poorly controlled diabetes before conception and during the first trimester of pregnancy can cause major birth defects in 5% to 10% of pregnancies and spontaneous abortions in 15% to 20% of pregnancies. Poorly controlled diabetes during the second and third trimesters of pregnancy can result in excessively large babies, posing a risk to both mother and child.

Prepregnancy counseling of women with diabetes is optimal to assist in the prevention of complications in the mother and to assist in the prevention of congenital anomalies. It is important that all women, but especially women with diabetes, take folic acid early in gestation. Ideally, all women of childbearing potential would take a daily vitamin supplement with folic acid, but especially a woman with diabetes planning a pregnancy.

Major congenital anomalies are the leading cause of perinatal mortality in pregnancies complicated by diabetes mellitus. Generally, glycemic control during the preconception period and in the early phases of gestation determines the risk of fetal congenital malformations. It is estimated that 6% to 12% of infants of mothers with diabetes will have an anomaly; most notable are neural tube defects and congenital heart disease.[25] Patients at the highest risk for complications from diabetes in pregnancy include those with pre-existing vasculopathies, those with poor glucose control, those with a previous stillbirth, and patients with noncompliance issue history. Poor glucose control during the critical weeks of organogenesis, 5–8 weeks after the last menstrual period, is thought to be the key etiologic factor.[25,26] Early studies demonstrated that hemoglobin A1C of 8.0% was associated with a fetal malformation rate of 3.4%. However, hemoglobin A1C >9.5% was associated with a fetal malformation rate approaching 22%. Clinical studies have also shown that poor preconception control is associated with an increased rate of spontaneous abortion.

HYPERGLYCEMIA DURING PREGNANCY

The plasma glucose concentration of the fetus follows that of the mother, with the mother's glucose concentration about 10 mg/dL (0.5 mmol/L) higher than the fetus. With an increase in maternal glucose concentrations, the maternal-fetal difference increases until the system of facilitated diffusion appears to be saturated at a maternal value of about 100 to 230 mg/dL (11–13 mmol/L). After this, despite considerable increases in the maternal glucose, it is not reflected in the fetus further. This phenomenon can be viewed as a protective mechanism for the fetus to avoid the damaging effects of severe hyperglycemia.[27]

Insulin appears in the fetal circulation as early as 10–12 weeks of gestation. Fetal insulin concentrations appear to be elevated in response to maternal elevated glucose. There is agreement that insulin does not cross the placenta at physiologic concentrations. In utero effects on the fetal pancreas may have profound long-term effects on the fetus, especially with respect to later likelihood to develop impaired glucose tolerance and type 2 diabetes.[27] Pedersen proposed that the fetal hyperglycemia resulting from maternal hyperglycemia stimulates fetal pancreatic beta-cell hypertrophy, resulting in fetal hyperinsulinemia.[28]

Management of Hyperglycemia

Maternal insulin requirements generally increase throughout pregnancy. On average, insulin needs increase by about 0.7–1 unit/kg/day as pregnancy progresses.[29] Unlike oral hypoglycemic agents, insulin does not cross the placenta, and it is considered the drug of choice for management of hyperglycemia in pregnancy. Insulin has a molecular weight of approximately 5,700 and is limited in its movement into the fetus. Average daily insulin requirements are likely to increase twofold because of hormones produced by the placenta. Cortisol, estrogen, progesterone, prolactin, placental growth hormone, and human placental lactogen have been shown to contribute to insulin resistance and reduced sensitivity to insulin action.[30] Human placental lactogen is a polypeptide placental hormone with a function similar to that of human growth hormone. It acts to modify the metabolic state of the mother during pregnancy to facilitate the energy needs of the fetus. Human placental lactogen is an anti-insulin. It is produced only during pregnancy. In addition, tumor necrosis factor–alpha and leptin have been implicated as contributing to the insulin resistance as well.[31]

GUIDELINES AND POSITION STATEMENTS

Both ACOG and the American Diabetes Association developed and have published current guidelines for the management of pre-existing diabetes during pregnancy that would be helpful tool for the reader to use in daily practice.[30,32,33]

PRECONCEPTION CARE

Preconception planning can help a woman have better outcomes. Some patients may need assessment and treatment of retinopathy, neuropathy, or nephropathy to be ready for pregnancy.[33] First, it is important to focus on blood glucose control. It is important to stabilize the blood glucose and achieve euglycemia even months before the pregnancy. Because the period of organogenesis occurs days 21 to 56, it is important that the patient plan the pregnancy and test for evidence of implantation so as to prevent congenital malformations that occur before the seventh week of gestation (Table 25-2). If the blood glucose levels are well controlled beginning before pregnancy, the risk of these complications falls to almost the same as general population risk.

TREATMENT AND GOALS

The treatment goals for pregnant women with diabetes are similar to the nonpregnant population. First and foremost, achieve normalization of blood glucose (defined as a fasting glucose ≤95 mg/dL; premeal values of 100 mg/dL or less, 1-hour postprandial levels of 140 mg/dL or less, and 2-hour postprandial levels of 120 mg/dL or less.[31] Manage diabetes appropriately to avoid extreme fluctuations in insulin and plasma glucose concentrations and especially avoid severe hypoglycemia. The ultimate success of treatment can be measure by achieving a glycosylated hemoglobin A1C concentration of no higher than 6%.

Table 25-2. Summary of the Increased Risk of Fetal Abnormalities Associated with Uncontrolled Diabetes

Fetal Abnormality	Increase Risk Compared with General Population
Congenital heart defects	5 times average incidence
Renal abnormalities	5 times average incidence
Situs inversus	84 times average incidence
Dextrocardia, anal/ rectal atresia	5 times average incidence
Neural tube defects	10 times average incidence
Anencephaly	5 times average incidence
Caudal regression	300 times average incidence

Nonpharmacologic Therapy

Similar to the nonpregnant patient with diabetes, the focus on blood glucose control by dietary management and exercise is preferred. Ideally, women with diabetes will meet with a dietitian before pregnancy to customize a plan. Morning sickness with nausea and vomiting can further complicate issues. Patients may need a plan to deal with the alteration of carbohydrates in diet and plans to cover lost carbohydrates

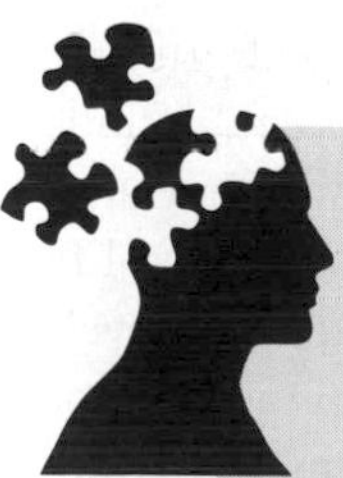

Therapeutic Challenge:

K.J. is a 37-year-old woman with insulin-dependent type 1 diabetes that has been well controlled for 15 years. However, she comes to you for advice on how to manage her glucose levels with all the "pregnancy cravings" she has been having for chocolate and ice cream.

in the event of vomiting. To fill any possible nutritional gaps, a prenatal vitamin is recommended even 3–6 months before pregnancy. It is recommended that women receive at least 1 mg of folic acid during this critical time. For women who find the prenatal vitamins too large to swallow and risk not taking them, a multivitamin contains approximately 400 mcg or folic acid. OTC folic acid tablets are available in 400- and 800-mcg sizes. Women could also take a children's chewable with iron and a separate folic acid tablet.

It is important for the patient to continue to include physical activity in the daily routine. The patient should talk with her care provider about exercise and determine if there are any limitations.

It is hard to decide when diet and exercise have failed and drug therapy should be initiated. Most authorities agree that drug therapy should be initiated when 1-hour postprandial levels are ≥140 mg/dL or when 2-hour postprandial glucose levels are ≥120 mg/dL.

Pharmacologic Therapy

The objective of diabetic control in pregnancy is to maintain normoglycemia at all times. The typical approach to glycemic control in pregnant women with diabetes is dietary control, with the additional of insulin when diet alone is not sufficient. New agents, such as the insulin analogs and oral hypoglycemic agents, have altered the management of diabetes in pregnancy.

Insulin Regimens

To achieve euglycemia throughout the 24 hours, both short-acting insulin and longer-acting insulin are required. Typically, three doses of short-acting insulin are given before meals combined with one dose of long-acting insulin at night.

Over the past five decades, perinatal outcome in pregnancies complicated by diabetes mellitus has improved dramatically, in large part because of better maternal glycemic control. Self–blood glucose monitoring in combination insulin treatment, including the use of newer insulin analogs and insulin pump therapy, has dramatically improved glucose control in most pregnancies complicated by diabetes. In developing an insulin regimen, careful attention must be paid to both basal and prandial insulin needs. Every effort must be made to avoid hypoglycemia and prevent ketoacidosis.[34] A team approach—including the physician, patient, diabetes nurse educator, pharmacist, nutritionist, and social worker—is ideal.

In a retrospective study comparing the pregnancy outcomes using basal insulin glargine or NPH insulin in T1DM, pregnancy outcomes were compared in 30 T1DM women with 43 healthy pregnant control women. All patients with T1DM were treated with conventional basal-bolus insulin therapy with either aspart or lispro insulin at the three main meals, plus glargine or NPH insulin at bedtime. Fifteen of the 30 T1DM women received glargine and 15 received NPH insulin. Metabolic status of all women was evaluated with 2-hour postprandial blood glucose and Hb_{A1c} at 3-month intervals. Fetal measurement included head circumference, abdomen circumference, and femoral length evaluated by ultrasound at the second and third trimesters. Neonates were classified at birth according to the fetal growth curves for the requisite population. No significant difference was observed between the glargine-treated group and the NPH-treated group with regard to pregravidic hypertension, third-trimester pre-eclampsia, material complications, and their progression during pregnancy (diabetic hypoglycemia and/or micro- or macroalbuminuria).[35]

Material and neonatal outcomes were compared in diabetic pregnancies treated with either insulin glargine or NPH insulin by retrospective chart review of 52 patients with diabetes. Twenty-seven of the 52 patients with diabetes were treated with insulin glargine. Glycemic control was similar in women who used NPH insulin and insulin glargine as determined by Hb_{A1C} levels and mean blood sugar values. There were no differences in mode of delivery, average birth weight, or neonatal outcomes. Thus insulin glargine and NPH insulin appear to be equally effective in the management of diabetes in pregnancy.[36]

The risk of maternal and fetal complications, including fetal congenital abnormalities, in pregnant women with diabetes mellitus is related to the level of glycemic control in early pregnancy. Consequently, it is recommended that patients attempt to achieve strict metabolic targets (i.e., Hb_{A1c} of 4.0% to 6.0%). In an effort to comparatively evaluate insulin aspart vs. human insulin, 322 pregnant women with T1DM in a basal-bolus protocol using NPH insulin for basal therapy were randomized to receive either insulin aspart or human insulin for the bolus portion of their insulin regimen. Results of the study indicated that insulin aspart is as effective and well tolerated as human insulin. Eighty percent of the study participants in both groups achieved an Hb_{A1c} of <6.5%, and in the second trimester, insulin aspart was associated with a lowered postprandial blood glucose and a reduced risk of hypoglycemia, suggesting that it may offer advantages over human insulin in this patient population.[37]

Oral Hypoglycemic Agents

There are several oral hypoglycemia agents acting through diverse mechanisms of action that are available to treat patients with diabetes. When the patient is pregnant, some of these agents may need careful examination and consideration for alteration of therapy. Women on oral medications for type 2 diabetes need to review their medications and may need to be switched to insulin. Oral hypoglycemic agents have fewer data to support their use in pregnancy and should not be used if compliance with insulin injections can be achieved. Patients with type 2 diabetes on oral agents are typically converted to insulin, although some recent studies reported in literature are examining the roles of oral agents in the treatment of the pregnant women with diabetes.

Glyburide has been studied in pregnancy since reports in 2000 endorsed the use of the glyburide as an alternative to therapy with insulin during pregnancy.[38] Intensified therapy, in comparison with the conventional approach used for women with gestational diabetes, resulted in pregnancy outcomes comparable to the general population in a large prospective study.[39] Intensified therapy is an approach to achieving established levels of glycemic control using memory-based self-monitoring of blood glucose, dietary regulation with a low carbohydrate diet plan, strict criteria for initiation of pharmacologic therapy, and an interdisciplinary team to insure patient education and adherence.[40]

MONITORING AND FOLLOW-UP

It is important for the patient to carefully monitor for hypoglycemia, hyperglycemia, and ketonemia/ketonuria. **Diabetic ketoacidosis** can endanger the lives of both the mother and the fetus. Dietary compliance can be monitored by regular weighing of the woman combined with blood glucose concentration observations. Patients should continue daily self-monitoring of glucose (fasting and postprandial) to achieve normal glycemia without evidence of hypo- and hyperglycemia, and the Hb_{A1c} concentration should be measured every 4–6 weeks, with a goal being a normal value <6%. During the second and third trimesters, close monitoring is recommended to avoid blood glucose fluctuations associated with insulin resistance seen in response to placental hormones.

LABOR AND DELIVERY ISSUES SPECIFIC TO DIABETES

Insulin requirements during labor also require close monitoring. Typically, insulin requirements decrease during labor, partly as a result of the energy use and partly as a result of the mother's fasting state. An insulin infusion during labor and delivery allows the mother's care to be individualized. The insulin resistance of pregnancy resolves within hours after delivery.

Labor is a form of exercise, and it necessitates an eightfold increase in glucose substrate to prevent maternal hypoglycemia and ketosis. Likewise, maternal hyperglycemia should be avoided because it can result in neonatal hypoglycemia.

PATIENT EDUCATION

A study examined health literacy in pregnant women with diabetes and found approximately one fourth of the patients in their study had low functional health literacy. These patients were more likely to have an unplanned pregnancy, to have discussed pregnancy beforehand with their physician, or to have taken folic acid.[41] This underscores the need for all members of the healthcare team to take extra time with these patients to ensure their understanding and adherence to the recommendations for diabetic care.

Patient education key points include that prenatal care is of vital importance in women with diabetes. During pregnancy, a woman with diabetes often needs more frequent monitoring: blood glucose; urine/blood tests to check for anemia or kidney problems; ultrasound to check the growth and development of the fetus; electronic fetal monitoring to detect signs of problems the fetus may be having late in pregnancy. To monitor the well-being of the fetus, the patient may be asked to keep a kick count to check for fetal activity.

Seizure Disorders

Pregnancy in women with epilepsy is associated with worse outcomes than those pregnancies in healthy women.[42] Babies exposed to antiepileptic drugs (AEDs) have a 1.8- to fourfold increased risk of congenital abnormalities. Pregnancy is complicated by the seizure disorder itself. During pregnancy, women can have an increase in seizure activity, and the use of antiepileptics can pose a significant risk of fetal abnormalities. Maternal seizures during pregnancy increase the risk of fetal bradycardia, reduced placental blood flow, and decreases in fetal oxygen supply.[43] Complications of AED use in pregnancy have been documented for years in the literature and include fetal anomalies, spontaneous abortions, stillbirths, placental defects, abruption, preterm labor, pre-eclampsia, and hemorrhage.[44] Overall, the major abnormalities seen with the use of AEDs in pregnancy are heart and neural tube defects, cleft palate, and urogenital abnormalities.[45] The reality is that it is necessary to continue to treat epilepsy during pregnancy and to gather information on the use of these drugs on fetal outcomes.

CHALLENGES OF ANTIEPILEPTIC DRUG USE IN PREGNANCY

Physiologic changes that occur during pregnancy complicate the pharmacokinetics of the antiepileptic medications. Pharmacokinetic changes—such as increased volume of distribution, along with increases in hepatic metabolism and renal clearance and a decrease in gastric emptying—lead to decreased drug levels. During pregnancy there is a decrease in serum albumin, resulting in freer drug (nonprotein bound); therefore, it may not be at levels sufficient for treatment or may increase the risk of adverse effects. These changes are a particular concern with medications that are highly protein bound or have a narrow therapeutic window, such as phenytoin.[46]

TREATMENT AND GOALS

The overall goal for treating epilepsy in pregnancy is to deliver a healthy baby and to keep the mother seizure free, as well as to decrease the risk of congenital abnormalities from the use of therapeutic agents in pregnancy.

Nonpharmacologic Therapy

The treatment of epilepsy requires management with drug therapy. The only nonpharmacologic treatment available is the ketogenic diet, which is more widely studied in the pediatric population. Its use is reserved for seizures that have not been successfully managed by drug therapy such as Lennox-Gastaut. The diet consists of high fat, low carbohydrates. Theoretically, this diet would not support the nutritional needs of pregnancy.

Pharmacologic Therapy

According to the American Academy of Neurology, the indication for epilepsy management during pregnancy is to use monotherapy.[42] The choice of the exact medication can be controversial, but the drug of choice should be the drug that controls the patient's seizure disorder.

Phenytoin is most commonly used in the management of primary and secondary tonic-clonic seizures. There is a substantial amount of literature to support that phenytoin is associated with fetal abnormalities. Fetal hydantoin syndrome is a condition that is characterized by significant craniofacial abnormalities, limb abnormalities, hypoplasia of the fingernails, congenital heart problems, developmental delays, and growth retardation. Phenytoin has also been associated with neural tube defects and oral clefts.[47,48] There are many theories as to the exact mechanism in which phenytoin causes birth defects. One theory describes the inhibition that phenytoin has on the potassium channels that results in hypoxia and deoxygenation of the fetus.[49] The hypoxic episode in fetus has been linked to the possibility of developing cleft palate.[50] Both ACOG and the American Academy of Pediatrics recommend the discontinuation of the phenytoin in pregnancy because of these significant birth defects.[42,69]

Carbamazepine exposure had been shown to increase the risk of major malformation from 2.7% to 6.7%.[51] Carbamazepine has been associated with an increased risk of neural tube defects, cardiovascular defects, and urinary tract defects. The literature supports that carbamazepine is associated with several physical abnormalities, such as hypoplasia of the nose, anal atresia, ambiguous genitalia, congenital heart disease, cleft lip, hypoplasia of the nails, and spina bifida.[52,53] Infants exposed to carbamazepine have a 24-fold increase in cleft palate development. A series of four cases of infants exposed to carbamazepine in utero developed unilateral multicystic dysplastic kidney.[51] The exact mechanism at which carbamazepine causes defect is not well understood, but it is hypothesized that carbamazepine catabolism reduces the epoxide hydrolyase that is required for the detoxification of epoxides and free radicals; this therefore produces oxidative stress, and the free radicals have a direct toxic action.[51]

Valproic acid has several case reports indicating that it is also associated with several physical abnormalities, such as fetal neural tube defects, spina bifida, and cardiac defects. Based on data from the North AED Pregnancy Registry, valproic acid exposure is associated with a 10.7 % increase in the risk major malformations.[54] An increased incidence of neural tube defects was apparent when women were exposed to the valproic acid during the first trimester.[55-57] A prospective study confirmed that valproic acid exposure during pregnancy significantly increases the risk for the development of major malformations, particularly spina bifida and hypospadias.[58]

The North American AED Pregnancy Registry has documented cases that indicate that prenatal exposure to phenobarbital significantly increases the risk of fetal abnormalities by 6.5%.[59] Phenobarbital has been associated with a three- to fourfold increase of several physical abnormalities, such as heart and facial defects, particularly when used during organogenesis.[60,61]

According to findings of the International Pregnancy Registry, birth defects observed with lamotrigine use were similar to that of the normal average. In a study of 414 first-trimester pregnancies with exposure to lamotrigine (as monotherapy), there was a 2.9% incidence of birth defects.[62] Recent findings confirmed that there is a significant risk of oral cleft palates in lamotrigine-exposed infants with a frequency of 1:405 or 2.5/1,000 compared to 0.37/1,000 in the comparison group.[63,64]

Available data are limited with the use of the topiramate in pregnancy. Animal studies have documented fetal abnormalities. One case report noted an infant born to a mother using topiramate as monotherapy. The infant was born with some abnormities, such as growth deficiency, hirsutism, a third fontanelle, and short nose with anteverted nares.[64,65] Information of the teratogenic potential of many of the agents used to manage seizures is limited and primarily reported as case reports only. For example, in a case report involving 26 mothers and infants that were exposed to zonisamide during pregnancy, there was one case of a voluntary abortion and one case a septal defect.[67] In another series of cases describing minimal events from the use of tiagabine in pregnancy, one abnormality of the lip was described out of 22 exposures during pregnancy.[67] Finally, in a three patient case series conducted of women who were exposed to monotherapy levetiracetam during pregnancy, all the pregnancies were normal and resulted in infants with no notable abnormalities.[68] At 6 months, there were no developmental, cognitive, or medical problems observed.[68]

GUIDELINES FOR TREATMENT

Below are the guidelines according to the American Academy of Neurology. The American Academy of Neurology, ACOG, and the International League against Epilepsy suggest the following guidelines in conjunction with the monotherapy to prevent the possible adverse effects of using antiepileptic medications during pregnancy.[69,70] First, optimize a treatment regimen before conception, using the most effective drug based on symptoms/seizure type at the lowest effective dosage. The antiepileptic drug dosage should be based on the nonprotein bound (free) concentration when possible. Provide folic acid supplementation at a dosage of 0.4–4 mg per day before conception and throughout gestation. Last, provide the pregnant woman with vitamin K, 10 mg per day, during the last month of gestation because of the potential for neonatal hemorrhage.

PATIENT MONITORING AND FOLLOW-UP

Monitor the antiepileptic drug levels, including the nonprotein-bound levels at each trimester, before delivery, and 4–8 weeks after delivery. Typically, the physiologic changes noted in pregnancy that may interfere with drug levels return to prepregnancy status in about 4–5 weeks. Postpartum drug levels should be monitored and dosages adjusted as needed. Offer prenatal testing with anatomic ultrasound and maternal serum alpha-fetoprotein at 15–20 weeks of gestation.

The North American AED Pregnancy Registry has been developed to help determine the safety of AEDs in pregnancy.[60] The registry is maintained at Massachusetts General Hospital in Boston. Pregnant women currently taking an AED for seizure control or mood disorders are encouraged to participate. Women enroll themselves by calling the registry's toll-free number as soon as possible once pregnancy is confirmed. There are three patient interviews that occur: the first at the first phone call, the second at 7 months of gestation, the third after the baby is born.

PATIENT EDUCATION

It is important to educate the patient on the risk of AED use in pregnancy with respect to fetal harm. In this discussion, healthcare providers should stress the need for prenatal vitamin use, particularly increased folic acid supplementation. Throughout pregnancy, serum drug levels will need to be followed closely, and fetal ultrasounds will be useful to assess any impact on development.

SUMMARY

The management of seizure disorders in pregnancy requires a practitioner to evaluate risk vs. benefit. The disorder itself, particularly if the pregnant woman has a seizure, is a risk for birth defects. Studies have confirmed that 54% to 67% of patients have unchanged seizure control during pregnancy, whereas 15% to 32% experience the onset of more frequent seizure, therefore reinforcing the need for AED use in the pregnancy.[71] The use of AEDs is also a concern. Drug registries have been established to further investigate medications being used in pregnancy, and it is hoped they will provide practitioners and patients with further guidance in evaluating risks and benefits.

Hypertension

Pre-existing hypertension in pregnancy is commonly called chronic hypertension. Hypertension during pregnancy can complicate the pregnancy by 10%.[72] Hypertension is a concern during pregnancy because it has been shown to increase the morbidity and mortality of the mother and infant. Chronic hypertension is defined per the seventh report of the Joint of the National Committee on Prevention, Detection, Evaluation, and Treatment of High Blood Pressure as a blood pressure reading of ≥140/90 mm Hg before pregnancy or before the 20th week of gestation.[73]

Based on population-based data, chronic hypertension complicates about 1% of pregnancies. Prevalence appears to be dependent on race and age. Black women having a higher incidence of developing pre-eclampsia because of the higher incidence of chronic hypertension at baseline. In women ages 30–39, underlying chronic hypertension was documented in 22.3% of black women compared to 4.6% of white women. Underlying chronic hypertension appears to be more prevalent in women older than 35 years. Overweight women (body mass index ≥35) are at higher risk of having chronic hypertension.[74]

Ninety percent of chronic hypertension is considered to be primary. The remainder is associated with secondary causes, such as renal parenchymal disease and endocrine disorders. It is estimated that 20% to 25% of women with chronic hypertension will go on to develop pre-eclampsia.[73] The management of pre-eclampsia will be discussed in Chapter 24: Conditions Associated with Pregnancy.

COMPLICATIONS WITH PREGNANCY

Chronic hypertension complicates pregnancy by interfering with maternal health and also fetal development. In the U.S. between 1991 and 1999, hypertension during pregnancy accounted for 15.7% maternal mortality. Diastolic blood pressure ≥110 mm Hg has been shown to increase placental abruption and cause fetal growth retardation. In most serious cases, high blood pressure can lead to maternal seizures as well as target organ damage, which can lead to decrease fetal oxygen and fetal intrauterine death. Studies have documented an increase and perinatal mortality of 2–4 times the general population.[75,76] One study evaluated 337 pregnancies in which the women had documented chronic hypertension. The results showed of perinatal mortality rate of the mother to be 45 per 1,000, compared with a rate of 12 per 1,000 in the general population.[75]

Pregnancy itself can complicate hypertension. During pregnancy, it is well known that blood volume increases, therefore increasing the demand on the heart. Blood pressure is decreased during pregnancy, particularly in the first trimester, which can complicate diagnosis. Normal blood pressures in pregnancy are considered to be the prepregnancy normal for the patient.[77]

GUIDELINES AND POSITION STATEMENTS

Initiation of therapy recommendations varies among several different organizations. There appears to be consensus between ACOG and the Joint National Committee on Prevention, Detection, Evaluation, and Treatment of High Blood Pressure.

TREATMENT AND GOALS

Pharmacologic treatments for chronic hypertension should be used with the goal of decreasing hypertension to decrease both maternal and fetal complications. A goal blood pressure in pregnant women is <140/90 mm Hg. The choice of hypertensive therapy should be based on fetal safety. Nonpharmacologic therapy should include lifestyle modifications, such as weight reduction before pregnancy, exercise, and smoking cessation.

Nonpharmacologic Therapy

Pregnant women with stage 1 hypertension are not candidates for pharmacologic treatment. This is based on the low possibility for serious cardiac effects in this population and also that blood pressure lowers during the first trimester. Diet should be adjusted to include low sodium (<2.4 g/day). Weight loss even in overweight patients should not be attempted during pregnancy. Aerobic exercise is not recommended because of the possibility that strenuous exercise might result in decreased fetal oxygen supply and the possibility of developing pre-eclampsia. Home blood pressure monitoring should be encouraged.[73,76] Pharmacologic therapy should be started in pregnant women when blood pressures reach 150–160 mm Hg systolic or 100–110 mm Hg diastolic.[73]

Pharmacologic Therapy

In hypertension, treatment begins with agents that have a long record of safety and efficacy. A central-acting antihypertensive, methyldopa, is the drug of choice in the management of chronic hypertension in pregnancy. Methyldopa treats blood pressure while maintaining sufficient uteroplacental blood flow.[78] There is strong evidence to support the efficacy and safety of methyldopa use in pregnancy. A study that evaluated a small number of infants for 7.5 years after birth found no adverse effects in the children exposed to methyldopa.[78]

Use calcium channel blockers (CCBs) in pregnancy has limited supportive data. Magee and colleagues conducted a multicenter cohort study evaluating CCB exposure in the first trimester and found no significant adverse effects.[79]

Data are limited on the use of beta-blockers because many of the studies use beta-blocker/alpha-blocker combinations. Some beta-blockers can be used with caution in early pregnancy. A study indicated that atenolol use in early pregnancy may cause growth restriction.[80] However, labetalol, which is a combined beta- and alpha-blocker, has been used in pregnancy, particularly in pre-eclampsia.[80]

Use of diuretics in pregnancy is controversial. There are no specific data to discourage their use in pregnancy. The concern with diuretic use is that pharmacologically, this class decreases blood volume. In pregnancy, blood volume needs to increase to prevent the potential to develop pre-eclampsia and cause fetal harm, in which low blood volume is a known cause. Again, this relationship has not been documented in the literature and is only based on theory. Because of the potential interactions and the potential for fetal harm, the diuretics are typically not used in pregnancy.[81]

The angiotensin-converting enzyme (ACE) inhibitors are considered to be pregnancy category D for the whole pregnancy. Until 2008, the U.S. Food and Drug Administration (FDA) considered ACE inhibitors to be category C for the first trimester and category D for the second and third. Angiotensin-converting enzyme inhibitors should not be considered for therapy during pregnancy. In a 2006 cohort study of more than 29,500 infants born between 1985 and 2000, more than 200 infants had exposure to ACE inhibitors in the first trimester only.[82] The risk ratio for birth defects for this group was 2.71 as compared with infants who had no exposure to antihypertensive medications. Subsequent to this study, the FDA issued an alert and public health advisory and, in 2008, proposed ACE inhibitors as high risk for the entire pregnancy.

Angiotensin-converting enzyme inhibitors have been noted to cause significant fetal malformations, including fetal growth restriction, oligohydramnios, limb deformities, neonatal renal failure, and fetal death. The majority of reports of major malformations occur during exposure to the ACE inhibitor in the second or third trimesters.[83,84] The exact mechanism for these malformations is unknown. One hypothesis describes a potential mechanism in which the ACE inhibitors lower fetal blood pressure and cause renal complications in the infant, speculating that the lower uterine pressures on the fetal head may explain the occurrence of oligohydramnios.[85] Although there is no evidence at this time that the angiotensin receptor blockers causing these effects, the possibility should not be ruled out.[86]

MONITORING AND FOLLOW-UP

During pregnancy, patients should monitor blood pressure at home to follow trends. In high-risk patients, monitoring for pre-eclampsia—including blood pressure, proteinuria, and liver enzymes AST and ALT—should occur frequently because early detection of pre-eclampsia is the best mode of treatment.

PATIENT EDUCATION

Similar to nonpregnant hypertensive patients, it is recommended that patients understand how to monitor blood pressure readings at home. Recommend that patients avoid excessive sodium intake (<2,000 mg/day) and eat a healthy diet by eating fewer processed foods and avoiding salt at the table. Although obesity can be a contributing factor, healthcare providers should recommend that pregnant patients not try to lose weight; patients should eat well and gain usual pregnancy weight. Finally, remind pregnant patients to continue to exercise throughout pregnancy with activities such as low-impact aerobics, swimming, and prenatal yoga.

SUMMARY

Women who have a history of hypertension should have preconception counseling and care, including stabilizing their blood pressure before pregnancy. During pregnancy, dietary modifications should be encouraged, especially with respect to sodium content in the diet, not weight loss. Strenuous and aerobic exercise is not supported. Patients who have prehypertension or stage 1 hypertension are not candidates for treatment. Stage 2 hypertension requires intervention to prevent serious fetal adverse effects. The drug of choice in chronic hypertension is methyldopa because of strong evidence and experience. Second-line therapy would include a combination alpha/beta blocker, such as labetalol. Third-line therapy would include beta-blockers or CCBs.[73]

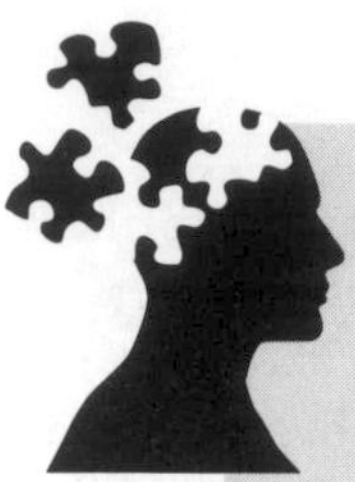

Therapeutic Challenge:

L.M. is 34 years old and in the 14th week of her pregnancy. She stopped all her antidepressants when she discovered she was pregnant because she doesn't want to "drug" her baby. Today she feels great but admits she has frequent "bad moments" throughout her week, especially when she starts to plan for the arrival of this baby. Is it okay for her to continue not taking her antidepressants?

Depression

A women's estimated lifetime risk of depression is 10% to 25%, with the highest incidence in the childbearing years.[87] Depression is known to develop during pregnancy in 9% to 14% of women.[87,88] Among women who are treated with depression who become pregnant, the risk of treatment vs. relapse of depression is a concern. Untreated depression has been shown to lead to poor weight gain in the mother (even weight loss) during pregnancy and poor nutrition intake, therefore resulting in preterm births and low-birth-weight infants.[89] In the past, it was thought that pregnancy provided some form of protection or remission from depression, but recent data have refuted that theory. Of women who discontinued therapy about the time of conception, 68% experienced a relapse in their depressive symptoms during pregnancy; 50% of these cases occurred during the first trimester, and by the second trimester, 90% had a relapse.[90] There are significant data to support that this risk of relapse is similar in nonpregnant patients, with a one-in-three chance of relapse within 6 months following discontinuation of therapy.[91]

Major depression activates the hypothalamus pituitary adrenal axis, which results in release of hormones—most notably adrenocorticotropin and β-endorphin, which have been associated with low birth weight and prematurity in infants.[92] Animal studies have confirmed that stress in pregnancy can lead to hypoxia, low birth weight in the offspring, and miscarriage.[93]

Since the early 1990s, more data have become available regarding the use of the most common antidepressants: tricyclic antidepressants (TCAs) and selective serotonin reuptake inhibitors (SSRIs). The risk vs. the benefit of treatment of depression during pregnancy has to be considered on a case-by-case basis.[94] Recommendations from ACOG are that treatment of depression be individualized and decisions be made for each specific patient.[95]

TREATMENT AND GOALS

Goals for the treatment of depression in pregnancy are to deliver a healthy baby, to control depression symptoms, and to not have the patient harm herself or the baby. Treatment options should minimize both congenital abnormalities in the infant as well as withdrawal symptoms in the baby after delivery.

Nonpharmacologic Therapy

Nonpharmacologic therapy for the treatment of depression, such as psychotherapy, may not be sufficient. The treatment of depression often requires medication to ensure that the maternal symptoms are under control.

Pharmacologic Therapy

Selective Serotonin Reuptake Inhibitors

SSRIs (fluoxetine, paroxetine, sertraline, citalopram, escitalopram, fluvoxamine) are known to be effective in the management of depression and are most commonly recommended based on their efficacy and general safety profile. Original data demonstrated that the SSRIs appeared to be safe in pregnancy, and no known risk was associated with their use.[89,96] Recent data conflict with this, indicating that SSRIs are associated with birth defects, persistent pulmonary hypertension, and neonatal behavioral syndrome. In early 2006, the FDA received evidence to support that paroxetine exposure during pregnancy resulted in cardiac malformations. This resulted in an FDA pregnancy category change of paroxetine to FDA category D.[97] The evidence that prompted this change was based on two different pregnancy registry databases. The Swedish National registry indicated that women taking paroxetine in the first trimester had a twofold increased risk of giving birth to an infant with a cardiac defect as compared with infants not exposed. The cardiac defects are described as atrial and ventricular septal defects. The impact of this defect on the infants ranges from a defect that required surgical repair to those that resolved spontaneously.[97] Shortly thereafter, a second report based on data from the U.S. insurance claim database indicated that women who were exposed to paroxetine in the first trimester had a 50% increased chance of giving birth to an infant with a cardiac defect compared with those exposed to another antidepressant agent.[97] Aside from the evidence of paroxetine, there are currently no data to support that other SSRI exposure results in cardiac defects.

Neonatal abstinence syndrome (NAS) is another potential complication associated with exposure to SSRIs during pregnancy. NAS is a condition in which an infant exposed to agents in utero develops symptoms beginning at birth that could appear up to 3 weeks of age. The symptoms are consistent with symptoms seen in patients that abruptly stop a medication. Data suggest that SSRIs and the serotonin-norepinephrine reuptake inhibitors (SNRIs) venlafaxine and duloxetine are associated with the development of NAS. Neonatal symptoms on birth that are seen in infants that were exposed to SSRIs include tremors/jitteriness, poor feeding, irritability, and respiratory depression.[98] NAS is most commonly seen in late pregnancy and in third-trimester exposure to SSRIs or SNRIs. In 18 cases of SSRI/SNRI exposure in utero, the overall risk of developing NAS was 30%.[98] Fluoxetine and paroxetine were the most common exposures noted, with paroxetine making up 61%.[98] Another study that described 60 cases of infants exposed to paroxetine, fluoxetine, citalopram, sertraline, or venlafaxine in utero and the development of NAS revealed a 30% chance of infants exposed developing NAS.[99] The World Health Organization Collaborating Center for International Drug Monitoring has also confirmed the risk of NAS from SSRI exposure in utero, indicating a higher incidence with paroxetine and fluoxetine use. The exact mechanism as to how SSRIs induce NAS is not well understood because of the limited understanding of neonatal psychopharmacology, but it is clear that the symptoms are similar to those seen in adult abrupt discontinuation of SSRIs.[98,99] When fetal blood levels of the SSRIs and their metabolites were evaluated, 86.8% of antidepressant levels were detected in umbilical cord blood.[100] Overall, this study found that the fetal drug concentrations are usually much lower than maternal drug concentrations. The lowest fetal serum concentrations are seen with sertraline and paroxetine exposure, and the highest concentrations are seen in citalopram and fluoxetine exposure. This study concluded that maternal use of SSRI in late pregnancy does not lead to any additional accumulation of the agents in the fetal blood.[100] However, it is unclear whether there is a correlation between fetal blood concentration of a particular SSRI and the occurrence of NAS. In newborns with defective cytochrome P450 (CYP) 2D6, metabolism of paroxetine is poor, which increases the risk of developing NAS. 2D6 is the enzyme system responsible for the metabolism of paroxetine.[101]

All the data indicate that SSRIs and the occurrence of NAS are associated with exposures that occur in late pregnancy. To reduce the risk of NAS, it is recommended that the SSRI be tapered to discontinuation starting 2 weeks before the due date. The agent can be restarted after delivery. There is no strong evidence to support a benefit, and caution should be used based on each patient.[98]

Recent data have suggested the development of persistent primary pulmonary hypertension (PPPH) in the newborn with the use of SSRIs. There are several theories on the mechanism of how SSRIs can cause PPPH. The first theory describes the fact that antidepressants, including the SSRIs, accumulate in the lung. The vasoconstriction properties of the SSRI, along with its mitogenic and comitogenic effects on the pulmonary smooth muscle, lead to increased pulmonary vascular resistance.[102,103] The second theory proposed is that the SSRIs inhibit nitric oxide production; this has been observed following fluoxetine exposure in utero.[104,105] In a study of 377 women who gave birth to newborns with PPPH and 836 control women, there were 14 newborns with PPPH who were exposed to an SSRI in the first 20 weeks of pregnancy, an odds ratio of 6.1—meaning that 1 in 100 infants exposed to an SSRI will develop PPPH.[102] Data are still limited and not strong enough to fully support the risk of SSRIs and the risk of PPPH.

Tricyclic Antidepressants

In several comparative studies looking at adverse fetal outcome in TCAs vs. SSRIs, no significant difference between the classes is found. A meta-analysis that looked at 414 cases of TCA exposure found no significant difference in congenital malformations when compared with controls.[106] In a prospective study that evaluated the long-term effects seen in infants exposed to TCA in utero—such as IQ, language, and behavior between ages of 15 and 71 months—no significant differences were found in those exposed to TCA vs. those not exposed.[107]

MONITORING AND FOLLOW-UP

Patients should be followed regularly to assess the severity or occurrence of new depression symptoms. In addition, ultrasound should be performed between 18 and 20 weeks of gestation to ensure normal fetal development.

PATIENT EDUCATION

Healthcare providers should stress the importance of medication therapy to limit symptoms of depression to all patients, but especially during pregnancy. Urge patients to report suicidal thoughts or thoughts of hurting the baby immediately to their healthcare provider. As always, encourage psychotherapy in addition to the pharmacotherapy interventions.

SUMMARY

Untreated depression poses a risk to a fetus. Several studies have indicated that untreated depression can lead to spontaneous abortions, increase uterine artery resistance, and increase the mother's risk of developing postpartum depression.[108] Infants born to depressed mothers tend to be born prematurely and at lower weights than infants born to nondepressed mothers. Overall, the major treatments show no major congenital abnormalities. The American Psychiatric Association recommends that treatment of depression be top priority. The American College of Obstetricians and Gynecologists agrees that depression needs to be treated and recommends the use of SSRIs (with the exception of paroxetine), given the known efficacy of SSRIs in the management of depression and the known safety information in their use in pregnancy. The North American Antiepileptic Drug Registry should help in this endeavor.[109]

Chapter Summary

It can be quite a challenge to review drug therapy for chronic medical conditions in pregnancy. Most women with chronic diseases have concerns for their fetus and want to do all that is possible to make conditions favorable. Chronic disease may make it necessary to continue therapy for the condition, although a medication change or dosage change is commonly needed. Because more than 50% of all pregnancies are unplanned, it is important to do a thorough review of all drugs as soon as the pregnancy is confirmed to minimize risks for teratogenic or embryonic toxic effects. Pharmacists and healthcare providers need to be alert to indications that a woman may be pregnant and indicate pregnancy in the patient profile records to prevent problems. Such indications may be as subtle as a woman on an ACE inhibitor who now presents a prescription for a prenatal vitamin. Such alertness to detail will be of great help to the patient and provide immeasurable reward to the healthcare providers.

References

Additional content available at
www.ashp.org/womenshealth

26 High-Risk Pregnancies

Kirk D. Ramin, MD; Timothy S. Tracy, Ph.D.

Learning Objectives

1. Discuss the increased maternal and fetal risks associated with multiple gestation and its management.
2. Explain what characteristics and behaviors increase the risk for gestational diabetes, and describe the methods of managing gestational diabetes.
3. Describe the diagnostic criteria and appropriate management of pre-eclampsia.
4. Compare and contrast the most appropriate management and timing of treatment (pharmacologic, radiologic, and surgical) for cancer being diagnosed during pregnancy.

Pregnancy and childbirth are expected to be times of great joy and happiness for the expectant mother and her loved ones. The development of effective contraception has allowed women the choice to delay pregnancy. Unfortunately, with advancing maternal age at the time of first pregnancy, increases in infertility, diabetes, and hypertension occur. Modern pharmacologic therapy manages many of these complications so that pregnancy can be a success.

Marked improvement in infertility therapy has resulted in significant increases in the rates of multiple births. These resulting pregnancies have more than doubled the rates of maternal hospitalization, bed rest, cesarean delivery, **pre-eclampsia,** and blood loss. In addition, the worldwide obesity epidemic has had major ramifications for the mother and child. Marked increases in gestational diabetes have been observed with increasing maternal weight and age. Not only are the infants of gestational diabetes larger, they also suffer short- and long-term metabolic consequences. Furthermore, the mother has long-term increases in risk of adult onset diabetes, and cardiovascular diseases are just beginning to be recognized and understood. Pre-eclampsia remains one of the most common causes of maternal deaths. Recognition and appropriate management of pre-eclampsia can all but prevent these losses. The diagnosis of cancer during pregnancy often invokes denial, fear, and anger in both the patient and her caregivers. Concerns for maternal mortality, as well as fetal harm from diagnostic and therapeutic interventions, permeate pregnancy. Fortunately, most diagnostic and therapeutic procedures can be carried out with relative safety during gestation after the first trimester.

Multiple Gestations

The incidence of multiple gestations has continued to increase, primarily because of increased use of assisted reproductive technology (ART). In the U.S., the increased use of ART has resulted in a 66% increase in twins and a 500% increase in **higher-order multiples** compared with the incidence in 1980.[1] Although multiple gestations account for approximately 3% of all live births, they carry a disproportionate burden of neonatal morbidity and mortality, primarily as a result of preterm birth. This risk increases proportionally as the number of fetuses increases. Other than ART, factors that influence the rate of multiple gestations include maternal race, parity, family history, and maternal age.

Multiple gestations most commonly result from the concomitant fertilization of two or more ova by individual sperm, resulting in fraternal (dizygotic) gestations. Each gestation arises from a distinct zygote. Less commonly, identical gestations may arise from a single fertilized ovum that divides into two or more identical or

CASE PRESENTATION

Patient Case: Part 1

M.J. is a 34-year-old, primigravid woman who presents at 10 weeks with nausea, vomiting, and a 5-lb weight loss.

HPI: M.J. has a 3-year history of infertility. She underwent ovulation induction to conceive this current pregnancy.

PMH: Negative for diabetes, gastroesophageal reflux disease, or thyroid disease.

Family history: Her family history is significant for her mother and maternal aunt having adult-onset diabetes mellitus.

Allergies: She denies any known drug allergies.

Medications: Over-the-counter prenatal vitamins.

Physical exam: Temp = 37°C; BP 110/70; HR 69; otherwise unremarkable.

Laboratory values: Within normal limits.

Diagnostic tests: Office ultrasound reveals a twin gestation with a thin intervening membrane.

Assessment: Her physician informs her that this is possibly a monochorionic twin pregnancy, which explains her nausea and vomiting. She also informs M.J. that there is a risk for twin-to-twin transfusion syndrome, and she will need serial ultrasound examinations to assess fetal well-being.

monozygotic gestations. When the single fertilized ovum divides will determine which type of identical monozygotic gestation results (Table 26-1).

PHYSIOLOGIC ALTERATIONS IN MOTHER WITH MULTIPLES VS. SINGLETONS

The physiologic alterations associated with multiple gestations are essentially an exaggerated response of the physiologic changes observed in a singleton gestation. These alterations begin early in the first trimester, although the timing in which they may become perceptible is variable.

Nausea and vomiting during pregnancy, often referred to as "morning sickness," is a common symptom of early pregnancy and may be more severe in multiple gestations. This may be related to the increased placental mass and the increased quantity of human chorionic gonadotropin present in the maternal serum of women carrying multiple gestations. Management of nausea and vomiting pregnancy is discussed in detail in Chapter 21: Pregnancy Planning.

The gastrointestinal system also undergoes other changes that may be hormonally regulated. There is decreased lower esophageal sphincter tone, likely a result of progesterone effect on smooth muscle tone. There is also delayed gastric emptying, which, combined with the latter change, may cause symptoms of gastroesophageal reflux. This also increases the risk for aspiration of gastric contents if consciousness is compromised, such as during induction of general anesthesia. Alkaline phosphatase levels are also normally increased, usually because of placental production. Serum estrogen may induce increases in serum cholesterol profile; therefore, hypercholesterolemia cannot be accurately diagnosed during pregnancy.

The gravida also experiences cardiovascular changes in the first trimester that are due to pregnancy. There is a marked increase in blood volume (50% to 65% in twin gestations), but only approximately a 25% increase in red cell mass, which results in a dilutional anemia. There are also increases in cardiac output (approximately 50% in twin gestations). These changes increase even more as the number of fetuses increases.

NUTRITIONAL REQUIREMENTS

The recommended weight gain in twin gestations is 35–40 lb, assuming a normal body mass index (BMI) before pregnancy.[2] The recommended weight gain changes depending on the initial BMI, with overweight and obese gravidas recommended to gain less than those with normal BMI. The converse is true for underweight gravidas. The recommended diet is 35 kcal/kg for a patient with a normal BMI, compared with a singleton pregnancy, in which the recommendation is approximately 30 kcal/kg for normal BMI. Included in dietary counseling is a general recommendation of at least 1mg of folic acid and 60 mg iron daily.[3]

FETAL RISKS AND THERAPY

The risk for both congenital and chromosomal anomalies increase directly as the number of fetuses increase, with twin and higher-order multiples carrying an increased incidence of these anomalies compared with singleton gestations.

The majority of twin gestations deliver preterm (before 37 completed weeks of gestation). Preterm delivery is most commonly caused by either spontaneous preterm labor or preterm premature rupture of membranes and is the primary cause of increased morbidity and mortality in multiple gestations.

Table 26-1. Timing of Zygote Division in Monozygotic Twins and Resulting Types of Twins

Timing of Division	Type of Twin	Placental and Fetal Membrane Characteristics
Day 1–3	Dichorionic/diamniotic	Two separate placentas with two chorions and two amnions
Day 4–8	Monochorionic/diamniotic	Single fused placenta with single chorion and two amnions
Day 8–13	Monochorionic/monoamniotic	Single fused placenta with single amniotic sac, no intervening membrane
>Day 13	Conjoined twins	Fused placenta with fused twins

Growth restriction may also occur in multiple gestations. This is defined as an estimated fetal weight less than the 10th percentile for gestational age. Discordant growth, with a difference of >20% between the larger and smaller fetus, may also occur. The latter may be associated with twin-to-twin transfusion syndrome (TTTS), fetuses discordant for a chromosomal anomaly or genetic syndrome, fetal infection, or inequity in fetal placentation. This can also be due to discordant structural abnormalities.

Twin-to-Twin Transfusion Syndrome

TTTS is a condition unique to monochorionic, diamniotic gestations in which there are imbalanced vascular connections between the two fetuses within the commonly shared placenta. In this syndrome, one fetus receives an increased proportion of blood (recipient) at the expense of the other fetus (donor). The donor fetus may be growth restricted and severely anemic, whereas the recipient fetus may be plethoric with an excessive amount of amniotic fluid. Both fetuses are at risk for heart failure, neurologic compromise, and intrauterine fetal demise because of their compromised cardiac status. TTTS affects 10% to 15% of all monochorionic, diamniotic gestations. It can be diagnosed on ultrasound based on the findings of monochorionic, diamniotic gestation with oligohydramnios (maximum vertical pocket of amniotic fluid <2 cm) in one twin with polyhydramnios (maximum vertical pocket of >8 cm) in the other twin.

Diagnosis and Screening in Multiples

Ultrasound has become a mainstay in the management of multiple gestations. The ability of ultrasound to discern the chorionicity of placentation allows the care provider to select out the monochorionic multiples that are at risk for TTTS. Indicators on ultrasound include the visual documentation of separate placentas, measurement of the intervening membrane, and the visualization of the "twin peak" sign.[4] If these findings are present, then dichorionic placentation can be presumed. This knowledge allows the care provider the ability to offer selective fetal reduction in cases complicated by lethal anomalies in a cotwin or for higher-order multiple gestations to reduce the preterm delivery risk. Selective fetal reduction using potassium chloride injection in monochorionic twins carries a risk of injury or loss to the remaining cotwin because of placental vascular communications. Using ultrasound guidance, a 22-gauge spinal needle is inserted into the fetal thorax, and 2–3 mEq of potassium chloride is injected. This approach is associated with fair success rate; in 200 with multiples, 181 delivered a viable infant.[5] Appropriate counseling and support needs to be provided to mother and family to work through all the challenges associated with the decision for selective reduction in serious health-risk situations.

Treatment Interventions for Twin-to-Twin Transfusion Syndrome

Pharmacologic Treatment Options

Indomethacin has been used with mixed success in an attempt to reduce urine production by the recipient twin to thus reduce the amniotic fluid volume. Indomethacin induces premature closure of the fetal ductus arteriosus, reducing fetal systemic cardiac output. The development of fetoscopic-directed laser therapy with improved outcomes has led to the demise of indomethacin for this condition.

Nonpharmacologic Treatment Options

The mode of treatment used most definitively is laser ablation of the communicating vessels. Laser therapy, aimed at selectively coagulating the aberrant vascular communications between the donor and recipient fetuses, has been demonstrated to increase perinatal survival with a lower incidence of neurologic complications when compared with the procedure of amnioreduction, but this has not been the case in a smaller, more recently reported trial.[6,7] The former procedure involves the use of an endoscopic laser that is inserted into the amniotic cavity, which allows for direct visualization and coagulation of the abnormal vascular anastomoses. The latter procedure involves removing the excessive fluid surrounding the fetus with polyhydramnios. The mechanism through which the procedure acts is not certain, but many speculate that the decrease in pressure in the amniotic sac of the twin with polyhydramnios aids in restoration of normal blood flow.

Umbilical cord ablation, in which the umbilical cord of one fetus is interrupted, generally is not used in cases of TTTS, unless one twin exhibits an anomaly or severe hydrops with impending death. This procedure is associated with a high incidence of obstetric complications, most commonly preterm delivery or preterm premature rupture of membranes.

Intrapartum Management

Multiple gestations pose unique management considerations at the time of delivery. There is no consensus and insufficient evidence to determine the optimal route of delivery for twin gestations or higher-order multiple gestations. The decision regarding route of delivery is usually based on fetal presentation at time of delivery. Certainly, other obstetric indications for cesarean delivery would influence route of delivery. In clinical practice, the majority of triplets and higher-order multiples are delivered by cesarean section.

The **perinatal mortality** rate has been observed to increase after 38 weeks and after 35 weeks for twin and triplet gestations, respectively.[8] Many practitioners will choose to deliver multiple gestations at these thresholds, although there are no data from randomized controlled trials to support this practice. Intrapartum management also includes increased risk for postpartum hemorrhage that is due to atony and its management.

MATERNAL RISKS WITH MULTIPLE GESTATIONS

Pre-eclampsia is more common in multiple gestations, with the incidence directly proportional to the number of fetuses. Rates of pre-eclampsia with multiples have been reported to be as high as 8% with twins, 10% with triplets, and 12% with quadruplets, whereas the rate of pre-eclampsia in singleton gestations is estimated to be approximately 5% to 8%.[9,10] This increased risk is compounded by the fact that when pre-eclampsia does occur in a multiple gestation pregnancy, it is more likely to occur earlier in the gestation and be more severe or atypical in presentation.[11-13] The management principles of pre-eclampsia and other hypertensive disorders of pregnancy are generally the same as with singleton gestations.

Prevention of Preterm Labor

Tocolytic therapy for preterm labor should be used with caution in patients with multiple gestations, as these patients are at a higher risk for complications associated with tocolytics, particularly pulmonary edema. Although bed rest is used by many practitioners as a modality for treatment of preterm labor, it has not been demonstrated to be an effective form of prevention of preterm labor. Only one randomized controlled trial exists testing the efficacy of bed rest in singleton gestations as a treatment vs. either no intervention or placebo. In this study, which included 1,266 women, there was no evidence that either hospital or home bed rest prevented preterm labor. There are also negative effects associated with bed rest, including the overall cost from job loss, loss of productivity, hospital costs associated with hospital bed rest, muscle wasting, bone loss, and the risk of deep vein thrombosis from the thrombogenic state of pregnancy compounded with venous stasis. There have been no randomized controlled trials comparing bed rest with no intervention in multiple gestations.

Other risks among women with multiple gestations include increased incidence of spontaneous miscarriage, aneuploidy, gestational diabetes, maternal anemia, and postpartum hemorrhage (see Chapter 24: Conditions Associated with Pregnancy, Chapter 25: Pregnancy and Pre-existing Illnesses, Chapter 27: Prenatal Diagnosis, and Chapter 28: Labor and Delivery).

Gestational Diabetes

Gestational diabetes (GD) is defined as carbohydrate intolerance that is first diagnosed during pregnancy. GD complicates approximately 2% to 5% of all pregnancies in the U.S.[14] Its diagnosis does not preclude the possibility of underlying, pregestational carbohydrate intolerance. The rate of GD diagnosed in pregnancy was the same as the rate of undiagnosed glucose intolerance in nonpregnant women between 20 and 44 years of age.[15]

DIAGNOSTIC SCREENING

There is no consensus regarding the use of either selective vs. universal screening for GD during pregnancy. The American Diabetes Association has identified low-risk characteristics for GD and has stated that if the gravida possesses these characteristics, they need not be screened during pregnancy. These characteristics include the following: <25 years of age, normal body weight (BMI ≤25), no first-degree relative with diabetes mellitus (DM), not a member of an ethnic group that is at high risk for DM type 2, and no personal history of impaired glucose metabolism or history of poor obstetric outcome typically associated with GD. Examples of at risk ethnic groups include women of Hispanic, African, Native American, Pacific Islander, or Southeast Asian heritage. However, in most clinical practices, the majority of patients will not meet all of the above criteria. Thus, a policy of universal screening for GD is commonly used.

Screening for GD is generally performed between 24 and 28 weeks of gestation.[16] This is composed of a 50-g oral glucose load followed by a measurement of plasma glucose post 1 hour.[17] A glucose level ≥130–140 mg/dL indicates a positive screening test and necessitates further evaluation. By using the lower threshold for screening, the detection rate for GD is approximately 90%, but with approximately a 25% false-positive rate. The higher threshold of 140 mg/dL decreases the false-positive test rate to approximately 15%, but also decreases the detection rate to 80%. If the threshold for the screening test is met, a diagnostic test is then indicated, which is a 100-g oral glucose load taken after an overnight fast followed by glucose plasma levels at 1, 2, and 3 hours postglucose ingestion. Two values that meet or exceed cutoff values are diagnostic of GD. Two sets of cutoff values are currently used: either the National Diabetes Data Group cutoff values of a fasting of <105 mg/dL, or postingestion levels of 190 g/dL, 165 mg/dL, or 145 mg/dL at 1, 2, and 3 hours, respectively; or fasting of <95 mg/dL and postingestion levels of 180 mg/dL, 155 mg/dL, and 140 mg/dL at 1, 2, and 3 hours, respectively.[18,19]

Risk Factors

Patients at high risk for GD, such as those with obesity or a strong family history of type 2 DM should be tested at the first prenatal visit.[17] If this initial test is negative, the screening test should again be performed at the usual time of 24–28 weeks.

Drug Induced

Beta-agonists, such as terbutaline, used for the treatment of preterm labor have been associated with increases in blood glucose levels, increased insulin levels, and reduced insulin sensitivity, although one study has reported no change in glucose levels.[20-24] This increase in glucose levels and insulin secretions is thought to be due to stimulation of beta-receptors in the pancreas. Certainly, one must carefully monitor glucose levels in women with GD and also those experiencing preterm labor.

The use of steroid preparations has also been associated with increases in blood glucose and thus must be used with caution in women with GD. It is well established that glucocorticoids raise blood glucose levels by stimulating the liver to produce more glucose from amino acids and glycerol, and activating lipolysis.[25] Phenytoin is occasionally used for seizure prophylaxis in pregnant women, and it too has been associated with increased glucose concentrations that are due to inhibition of insulin secretion.[25] Occasionally used in pregnancy, beta-blockers can have a converse effect on blood sugar through a reduction in blood glucose and masking signs of hypoglycemia. However, short-term studies have not demonstrated a significant effect on blood glucose when beta-blockers are administered during pregnancy.[26,27]

With respect to herbal preparations, several have been purported to exert effects on blood glucose; however, none have formally been evaluated the safety or efficacy in the pregnant patient population. For example, *Panax ginseng* has been reported to lower hemoglobin A1C levels and blood glucose in patients with type II diabetes.[28] In normal subjects, *Ginkgo biloba* has been demonstrated to increase the fasting plasma insulin area under the curve (AUC) following a glucose tolerance test. However, in noninsulin-dependent patients with diabetes, *Ginkgo biloba* therapy reduced the plasma insulin AUC after an oral glucose tolerance test.[29] As suggested above, this becomes particularly problematic if the patient chooses to self-medicate without consulting the physician. In general, use of any herbal supplements is not recommended during pregnancy without consulting with the physician.

MANAGEMENT OF GESTATIONAL DIABETES

Nonpharmacologic Interventions

Once the diagnosis of GD has been made, the primary therapy is dietary modifications. The dietary recommendations include caloric modification to approximately 30 kcal/kg/day (for normal body weight, based on prepregnancy body weight), with the majority of the dietary intake composed of complex carbohydrates (30% to 40%) and the remainder composed of protein (20%) and fats (35% to 40 %).[30] All patients should receive dietary education regarding modifications in intake and instructions on monitoring the prescribed dietary intake. In addition, 30 minutes of exercise has been recommended per day.[31] Specifically, brisk walking or seated arm exercises for 10 minutes after each meal daily is appropriate. Interestingly, mild exercise on a stationary bike has been shown to increases glucose tolerance better than moderate levels of exercise.[32]

Patient Monitoring After Initial Nonpharmacologic Interventions

Once dietary and exercise therapies have been implemented, glucose monitoring should be concomitantly initiated. Capillary blood glucose can easily be monitored using a glucometer, which requires minimal patient training. Patients are instructed to check capillary blood glucose multiple times a day, which is typically composed of a fasting and 1- or 2-hour postprandial levels after each meal. The goal for fasting levels is <95 mg/dL, 1-hour postprandial levels <140 mg/dL, and 2-hour postprandial levels <120 mg/dL. Patients may continue on dietary and exercise modifications alone if the majority of their glucose levels are within the goal range. However, if >50% of their levels exceed the levels stated above despite adherence to dietary and exercise regimens, further intervention is warranted.

Pharmacologic Agents

Insulin

Insulin is typically the first line of therapy used once the previously mentioned therapies have failed (Table 26-2).[33,34] The insulin regimen typically is calculated based on the patient's gestational age and body weight in kilograms. In the first trimester, the starting dosage is 0.7–0.8 units/kg/day, whereas 0.8–1.0 units/kg/day is used in the second trimester and 1.0–1.2 units/kg/day in the third trimester. These calculations are used to determine the total insulin dosage per day. The dosage is then further subdivided to two thirds to be administered in the morning before the first meal and the remaining third to be administered in the evening. The morning dose is administered as two-thirds (intermediate-acting) NPH and one-third short-acting Regular, and the evening dose administered at half (intermediate-acting) NPH and one-half short-acting Regular. Modifications on the dosage of insulin can then be made depending on the glucose measurements reported.

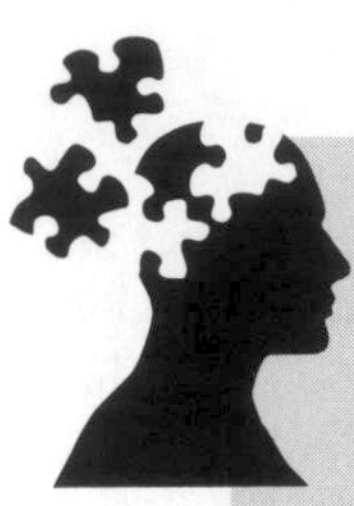

Therapeutic Challenge:

G.S. is a 36-year-old in her 28th week of pregnancy who has failed diet and exercise interventions to control her glucose levels. Her physician recommends insulin, but she has enormous fear of needles and refuses to self-administer daily injections. What are her alternative therapeutic options?

Oral Hypoglycemic Agents

Oral hypoglycemic agents, specifically glyburide and metformin, are increasing in utilization during pregnancy for the management of GD. Glyburide is a second-generation sulfonylurea previously thought not to cross the placenta; emerging data have confirmed that it does, but implications on fetus are unknown. However, glyburide has been demonstrated to be comparable to insulin in management of GD.[35] The starting dosage is typically 2.5 mg twice a day, which can be increased as needed, depending on the parameters described above. Once the maximum dosage of 10 mg twice a day has been reached, and if glycemic control has not been reached, insulin therapy should be initiated. Metformin is an alternative agent that can also be used safely during pregnancy. It is currently unknown if it crosses the placenta, but it has demonstrated safety in limited human case reports and cohort studies.

MATERNAL AND PLACENTAL COMPLICATIONS

Patients diagnosed with GD are at higher risk to develop hypertensive disorders of pregnancy.[36] In addition, there is also an increased risk for delivery by cesarean section because of marked increases in the number of fetuses that are large for gestational age. Last, women with persistently elevated glucose values suffer higher rates of stillbirth, which is thought to be due to osmotically induced fetal umbilical cord vessel vasospasm.

FETAL AND NEONATAL COMPLICATIONS

If adequate glucose control is not established, there are a variety of potential fetal complications associated with GD. There appears to be an approximately

Table 26-2. Gestational Diabetes Mellitus (Failed Diet)

Drug	Action	Comment
Neutral Protamine Hagedorn (NPH)	2–4 hr, peak 6–12 hr, duration 10–16 hr	Most commonly used
Regular insulin	50–60 min, peak 2–3 hr, duration 3–6 hr	Most commonly used
Lispro	5–15 min, duration <5 hr, peak 30–90 min	Lower postprandial glucose concentration; improved hemoglobin A1C, reduced hypoglycemia[a]
Insulin aspart	10–20 min, peak 1–3 hr, duration 3.5 hr	Lower postprandial; less hypoglycemia; safety similar to regular insulin[33]
Insulin glulisine	10–15 min, peak 0.5–1.5 hr, duration <3 hr	Reduced A1C values; reduced postprandial variability; no known clinical trials in pregnancy[33]
Insulin glargine	1–4 hr, minimal peak, during 24 hr	No reported malformations[34]
Insulin detemir	1–4 hr minimal peak, up to 24 hr	No known pregnancy trials[34]

12% risk of fetal **macrosomia** in pregnancies complicated by GD.[36] This increased risk of fetal macrosomia increases the risk of operative delivery, shoulder dystocia, and birth trauma. The neonates also have an increased risk for hyperbilirubinemia and hypoglycemia that could be profound. Stillbirth (as mentioned above) seems to be increased only in those gravidas with persistently elevated glucose values. Risks to the neonates of women with pregestational diabetes also include congenital abnormalities such as cardiac defects, spina bifida, and caudal regression. Stillbirth typically occurs in pregestational diabetes and uncontrolled GD.

MATERNAL MANAGEMENT AND FOLLOW-UP POSTPARTUM

Women diagnosed with GD are at risk for development of DM type 2. The American Diabetes Association recommends that all women diagnosed with GD be evaluated for persistent glucose intolerance at 6–8 weeks postpartum. Patients should undergo a 75-g oral glucose challenge with assessment of a 2-hour postingestion venous glucose or fasting glucose levels. The diagnosis of DM is made if the fasting meets or exceeds 126 mg/dL or the 2-hour postingestion level meets or exceeds 200 mg/dL. The glucose tolerance test will also help to identify women with impaired glucose tolerance without overt diabetes, and this may help for counseling in future pregnancies.

Patients should also be encouraged to continue dietary and lifestyle modifications postpartum, particularly if they are overweight. It may be prudent to evaluate patients with a history of GD before a subsequent pregnancy, particularly if they are at high risk for development of type 2 DM.

Pre-eclampsia

Hypertensive disease affects between 12% and 22% of all pregnancies, with one third to one half of these cases due to pre-existing (chronic) disease.[37-39] Although the exact incidence of pre-eclampsia is unknown, it has been reported to complicate between 5% and 8% of all gestations, depending on populations studied and definitions used.[39,40] Hypertensive disease is third only to embolism and hemorrhage as a leading cause of pregnancy-related maternal deaths.[41]

ETIOLOGY

The etiology of pre-eclampsia remains unknown. The presence of chorionic villi in certain women instigates vasospasm, hypertension, and serious organ dysfunction, especially of the placenta, kidneys, liver, and sometimes brain.[42] Nulliparity, familial history, diabetes, multiple gestations, extremes of age, pre-existing hypertension, vascular renal disease, hydatidiform mole, and fetal hydrops have all been associated with an increased risk of pregnancy-induced hypertension.[43-44]

The immunologic theory finds support in the observation that pregnancy-induced hypertension is most commonly a disease of first pregnancy, increased in multiparas with a new spouse or undergoing donor insemination, and more common in immunocompromised women.[45] It has been observed that the daughters of mothers with **eclampsia** were at higher risk than were the daughters-in-law for this disorder in a single recessive gene fashion; however, a multifactorial inheritance could not be ruled out.[44-46]

Abnormalities of placentation develop early in gestation before the onset of clinical disease. Excessive placentation, as seen in multiple gestations or molar pregnancies, or pathology of the walls of the uterine spiral arteries has repeatedly been documented in cases of pregnancy-induced hypertension.[46] Investigations centering on the etiology of vessel wall pathology have found that the trophoblastic cells fail to attenuate or ablate the vessel wall musculoelastic layer during development. This failure is most likely a result of an immunologically induced error in cell surface receptors of the trophoblast. The affected vessels, usually the terminal segments of the uterine spiral arteries, are incapable of vasodilation, which results in decreased placental blood flow.

Risk Factors

In those patients exhibiting hypertension, one clearly must avoid vasoconstricting medications, such as decongestants. These agents can serve to increase blood pressure and thus potentially worsen the condition. The principal ingredient in decongestant products today is pseudoephedrine. More likely to be self-administered by the patient following over-the-counter purchase, rather than by prescription, these products represent a readily available and seemingly innocuous (to the patient) source of medication that could increase blood pressure and worsen pre-eclampsia. Few herbal products have been associated with increases in blood pressure, with the exception of ephedrine- and synephrine (*Citrus aurantium*)-containing products.

Diagnosis

Pre-eclampsia is a pregnancy-specific syndrome diagnosed with new-onset hypertension (blood pressure ≥140/90) and new onset proteinuria (≥1+ random urine or ≥300 mg 24-hour urine collection) that occurs after 20 weeks of gestation and resolves following delivery.[47] In this same report, it is recommended that the diagnosis be made on a 24-hour urine collection or a timed collection corrected for creatinine excretion because of the discrepancy seen with random urine protein determinations. The distinction of mild and severe pre-eclampsia is no longer made; rather, the following increases the certainty of the pre-eclampsia syndrome: systolic blood pressure (BP) >160 mm Hg, diastolic BP >110 mm Hg, 2 g or more of protein in 24 hours, serum creatinine ≥1.2 mg/dL, platelet count <100,000 cells/mm and/or elevated lactic acid dehydrogenase (microangiopathic hemolytic anemia), elevated hepatic enzymes (ALT or AST), and persistent headache, visual disturbances, or epigastric pain.[47,48] HELLP is the acronymn for (hemolysis, elevated liver enzymes, low platelet count) syndrome.[42,49] Eclampsia is diagnosed when generalized nonclonic convulsions occur in gravid women with pregnancy-induced hypertension or pregnancy-aggravated hypertension.

It has been demonstrated that Doppler wave velocity measurements of uterine arterial flow can be used to screen patients for pre-eclampsia as early as 18 weeks of gestation.[50] This reduction in maternal uterine blood supply to the developing fetus is underscored by the fact that women destined to develop pre-eclampsia demonstrated lower plasma levels of placental growth factor than normotensive controls.[51] Others have suggested that this reduced ability to provide adequate perfusion to the fetus may provide lifelong protection against the development of cancer among women who previously experienced pre-eclampsia.[52]

ORGANIC SYSTEM IMPACT OF PRE-ECLAMPSIA

In normal pregnancy, a marked rise in cardiac output and fall in systemic vascular resistance occurs to accommodate the growing conceptus. Women suffering from severe pre-eclampsia have remarkable elevations in both pulmonary and systemic vascular resistances, as well as hyperdynamic left ventricular function.[53] In these women, overzealous hydration, concomitant infection, decreased **oncotic** draw, and increased pulmonary capillary permeability can lead to potentially fatal pulmonary edema.[53]

Significant laboratory abnormalities occur in pre-eclampsic patients. Microangiopathic hemolysis is severe in women with pre-eclampsia as is evident by the appearance of schizocytes, spherocytes, and reticulocytes.[54,55] In approximately 5% of women with severe pre-eclampsia, oliguria can be seen most commonly as a result of acute tubular necrosis and is associated strongly with postpartum hemorrhage or placental abruption.[56] The reduction in glomerular filtration rate with pre-eclampsia leads to rises in serum creatinine and uric acid levels. Elevations of serum creatinine with severe pre-eclampsia may rise to 3 mg/dL.[42] In addition, elevation in serum hepatic transaminase levels is often observed in women with eclampsia, hemolysis, and thrombocytopenia.[57]

Cerebral hemorrhage, transient cortical blindness, and coma are all rare but significant central nervous system (CNS) complications associated with pre-eclampsia.[58-61] Transient blindness may occur without seizures and may persist up to 8 days with complete resolution being the norm.[60] Coma is extremely rare, but when it occurs in the setting of pre-eclampsia/eclampsia, it is a harbinger of a poor prognosis. Coma occurs with severe hypertension and is thought to be caused by intracerebral hemorrhage or severe generalized cerebral edema.

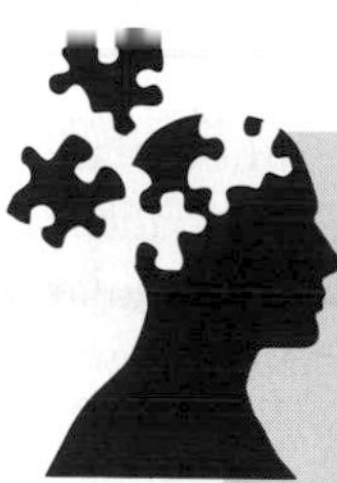

Therapeutic Challenge:

F.G. is 28-year-woman who would like to have a third child. She has suffered pre-eclampsia in both her previous pregnancies. In the last pregnancy, she experienced transient blindness. Is it safe for her to try for a third pregnancy?

Fetal Outcomes

The development of pre-eclampsia heralds marked increases in risk to the unborn child of premature delivery, placental abruption, placental insufficiency, and death. Fetal growth restriction is seen in higher rates in women who develop pre-eclampsia and correlates with reduced overall survival.[62] Once the diagnosis of pre-eclampsia is made, tests of fetal well-being (ultrasound for growth, biophysical profiles, or fetal heart rate monitoring) are recommended until delivery.

Pharmacologic Management

Antihypertension medications are usually reserved for use in the acute management of women with severe pre-eclampsia, defined as systolic blood pressures of ≥160 mm Hg and diastolic blood pressures of 110 mmHg and greater.[63-64] The goal of this therapy is to safely reduce the blood pressures to a level that maintains fetal perfusion and maternal cardiac output, and has minimal fatal adverse effects.[64] Although a number of agents are used to treat hypertension in pregnancy, angiotensin-converting enzyme inhibitors are not recommended for treatment of chronic hypertension during pregnancy, especially during the second and third trimesters, because they have been associated with fetal renal dysgenesis or death. Angiotensin-converting enzyme inhibitors have also been found to be deleterious in the first trimester. Because of their similar mechanism of action, angiotensin II blockers should also be avoided during pregnancy.

Hydralazine has been a mainstay for this purpose for more than five decades.[63] Hydralazine is typically given as a 5- or 10-mg initial intravenous bolus and repeated every 20–30 minutes based on therapeutic response.[64-65] Blood pressures are monitored typically every 5 minutes. Dosage is repeated every 20–30 minutes until "safe" blood pressures are obtained.

Labetalol intravenously administered has also been used with good efficacy for this same purpose. Typically it is administered as 20-mg bolus with a doubling of repeat dosages every 10 minutes to 80 mg (i.e., 20 mg, 40 mg, and 80 mg). Maximum dosages vary from 220 mg to 300 mg.[64-65]

Sodium nitroprusside infusions are of concern, with potential fetal cyanide toxicity with more than 4 hours of use. Use of nifedipine in the presence of magnesium sulfate seizure prophylaxis is worrisome for reduced maternal cardiac output and hypotension.

The role of diuretics in the management of acute severe hypertension is limited. Most appropriate use is for those women who develop pulmonary edema and not for the acute management of severe hypertension. For this, initial doses of 5 mg or 10 mg intravenous furosemide with careful monitoring of fetal heart rate and maternal urinary output response are recommended. Hypotencion and development of an ominous fetal heart rate tracing has been known to occur. Dose may be repeated until an appropriate response is reached. Although once the mainstay at many institutions, diuretics no longer have a role in pre-eclampsia prevention or management except in those women who have congestive heart failure and pulmonary edema. Diuretics are still used in women with chronic hypertension who are taking them before becoming pregnant. Spironolactone is typically avoided early in pregnancy because of its virilizing effects on the fetus.

Magnesium sulfate given as an intravenous loading dose followed by either intravenous infusion or intramuscular doses for 24 hours is used for the prevention of seizures in pre-eclampsia. This regimen includes a magnesium 4-g loading dose followed by maintenance infusion of 1 g/hr for 24 hours. As an alternative to the intravenous the route, the intramuscular route of administration of magnesium sulfate has the benefit of achieving uniform therapeutic serum levels.[42,66] Following a 3-g intravascular and a 10-g intramuscular load, the average peak level at

60 minutes is 4.5 mEq/L.[67] Furthermore, 4 hours after this load, cumulative renal excretion approaches 50%. The major disadvantage of the intramuscular route is maternal discomfort, abscess, hematoma, and nerve damage locally. Intravascular magnesium sulfate therapeutic regimens have varied widely in the suggested rates of infusion. Most protocols include a 4-g intravascular load followed by either 1–3 g/hr maintenance.[68,69] Management of magnesium sulfate therapy when used in patients with compromised renal function with magnesium toxicity is summarized in Table 26-3.

LONG-TERM CONSEQUENCES OF UNCONTROLLED PRE-ECLAMPSIA

Although eclampsia in a primiparous woman is not a harbinger of chronic hypertension, when eclampsia occurs in a multiparous woman, her fate is markedly worse, with a threefold increase in expected deaths; almost 80% of these deaths are related to chronic hypertension.[67,70-72] The long-term follow-up of 1,070 women with a history of pre-eclampsia documented an increased relative risk of death among those with pre-eclampsia of 2.1 (1.8–2.5).[73] Other studies have demonstrated a consistent reduction in survival among women with pre-eclampsia and preterm birth compared with those who did not suffer pre-eclampsia and preterm birth.[74] These women with cardiovascular disease had a remarkable eightfold higher risk of death. This has led many to propose rigorous follow-up of women suffering pre-eclampsia and aggressive management of their blood pressure and cardiovascular health to improve their long-term survival. Many universities are establishing clinical trials to assess if quality of life and longevity can be improved. It will take considerable effort to complete proposed intervention trials.

Cancer in Pregnancy

Cancer is second only to accidents as a leading cause of the death among reproductive-age women, accounting for almost one fifth of those deaths.[75] Slightly more than 4,500 cases of malignancy occurred among 4.8 million women (1/1,000) with live births in California from 1991 to 1999.[76] More than two thirds of these were cancers of the breast, cervix, thyroid, malignant melanoma, and Hodgkin's lymphoma. Two out of three occurred in the postpartum period, with minimal impact on perinatal outcome. It is estimated that 1 in 650 adults will be long-term cancer survivors.[77]

RISKS TO FETUS

Making the decision to perform operative procedures during pregnancy creates anxiety and fear among patients as well as providers. Background rates for spontaneous abortion are approximately 10% to 15% and rise markedly with advancing maternal age.[78] Almost 10% of 12,000 cases of women having non-obstetric surgery in the first trimester suffered loss.[79] Maternal deaths, fetal birth defects and diminished developmental outcomes were not increased in this series. This clearly demonstrated that improved

Table 26-3. Monitoring Magnesium Sulfate Therapy

Hourly Assessments	
Patellar reflexes	Present
Respirations	≥12/min
Urine output	≥100 mL/4 hr
Toxicity	
Absence patellar reflexes	10 mEq/L
Respiratory arrest	12 mEq/L
Cardiac conduction abnormalities	15 mEq/L
Decreased Renal Function	**Monitor Levels q 4 h**
Creatinine clearance >50 mL/min	4-g load and ½ maintenance dosage or 1 g/hr
Anuric (renal dialysis)	4-g load only

diagnostic accuracy will result in less overall surgeries and thus improved pregnancy outcomes.

Still, each of the common diagnostic techniques (magnetic resonance imaging [MRI], computed tomography [CT], x-ray, and ultrasound) invokes special concern with both the expectant parents and care providers. Because both MRI and ultrasound do not involve ionizing radiation, they have not been "associated with known adverse fetal effects."[80] Concern with potential radiofrequency pulse hearing effects and acoustic noise have been raised.[81] Current data reveal no known adverse fetal effects with magnetic field strengths of ≤1.5T.[82]

Both CT and x-ray involve ionizing radiation, and these carry considerable risk to the fetus. This risk is two pronged with radiation-induced teratogenesis and carcogenesis.[83] Ionizing radiation leads to cell death and changes in nuclear DNA. These adverse effects lead to morphologic abnormalities as well as carcinogenic changes.[83,84] Cell death results in loss of the conceptus during the embryonic period. Commonly, this has been referred to as the "all or none" phenomenon.[80] Teratogenic effects include microcephaly, intrauterine growth restriction, and poor mental development.[80] These adverse effects are thought not to occur with radiation exposures <5 rad.[85] It has been estimated that 1–2 rad exposure to the fetus results in one child in 1,000 developing leukemia.[80] Mental retardation is thought not to occur unless exposure exceeds 20–40 rads.[86] Radioactive iodine-based contrast agents cross the placenta and have the potential to eliminate or reduce fetal thyroid function. Technetium Tc99^{m} agents appear to be much safer if imaging is required in pregnancy.[87]

Radiation

Radiotherapy is used widely in the management of nonpregnant individuals therapeutically and palliatively. Both therapeutic and palliative radiation for abdominopelvic malignancies during pregnancy are contraindicated.[88] Radiation doses are often 1,000-fold the level seen with diagnostic procedures.[89] Therapy for malignancies outside the abdomen and pelvis can still be performed with appropriate shielding of the maternal abdomen and pelvis with minimal fetal exposure.[89,90] As with diagnostic radiologic procedures, first-trimester exposures can lead to congenital malformations or loss, especially before 8 completed weeks of gestation.[91] After 8 completed weeks until 25 weeks, the CNS alone appears to be sensitive to radiation exposure of 0.1 Gy or more.[92] After 25 completed weeks, fetal effects are minimal.[90]

The approach to radiotherapy during gestation like that of chemotherapy involves knowledge of fetal gestational age. First-trimester exposure is contraindicated and dosage dependent, as was discussed earlier with diagnostic radiation exposure. Likewise, in the second and third trimesters, calculations of fetal dosages before implementation of therapy can be made such that parents may make an informed decision.[89] Radiation may increase childhood cancers by as much as 40%, or three to four cases per 1,000 children.[89,90] Maternal risks of chemotherapy and radiotherapy are not different than seen in nonpregnant individuals. Exceptions include risk of metritis, septic abortions, and peripartum hemorrhage as consequences of both immunosuppression and myelosuppression.

Chemotherapeutic Agents

The diagnosis of a cancer during pregnancy is devastating news to expectant parents. Not only does the mother have to cope with her own potential mortality, she also must deal with marked increased risks of fetal malformation, fetal loss, and preterm delivery. In a series of 23 gravid women with ovarian cancer, 17 (73.9%) were stage I and achieved complete remission.[93] Among six women with advanced disease, five died. Sixteen babies survived without apparent complications, and two were lost as a result of prematurity. These authors concluded that chemotherapy can be used in the second and third trimesters with little risk to the fetus. Chemotherapy in the first trimester is contraindicated because of high abortion and malformation rates.[89,92-95]

The use of these agents in the second and third trimesters is associated with increases in preterm birth (5%), fetal death (6%), intrauterine growth restriction (7%), myelosuppression (4%), and potential adverse central nervous system effects to the unborn child.[89,93,95-97] Concerns for myelosuppression in the fetus have led to recommendation of discontinuing, if possible, chemotherapy 2–4 weeks before delivery.[89,98] Breast-feeding is not recommended when undergoing chemotherapy.[93,95,96,98]

There are no known pharmacokinetic studies for chemotherapeutic agents in pregnancy. In theory, chemotherapeutic agents are of a low molecular weight and have easy transplacental access to the fetus and increased renal and hepatic clearance, and dilute out in the increased maternal plasma volume of pregnancy.[89] In general, platinum and alkylating agents are favored over the antimetabolites, as they appear to be less teratogenic.

Case Presentation

Patient Case: Part 2

Diagnosis: Ultrasound examination confirms TTTS.

Treatment plan: After extensive discussion of all her options, M.J. opts for laser ablation of the communicating vessels.

Patient monitoring: Serial ultrasounds will be employed to monitor the safety and development of the growing fetuses. Mother and family appropriate counseling and support to handle the situation and prepare for potential complications and outcomes.

Patient education: M.J. needs to understand that in TTTS, one fetus receives an increased proportion of blood, developing stronger at the expense of the other fetus and leading to potential growth restriction and anemia. Despite interventions, both fetuses could be at risk for heart failure, neurologic compromise, and intrauterine fetal demise because of their compromised cardiac status.

Summary

Pregnancy for most women is a period filled with worry and concern for the welfare of their unborn child. Medical and surgical disorders that complicate pregnancy only serve to heighten the level of anxiety that is normally seen. Pregnancy in and of itself is a relative high-risk period for women because of increased risks for hemorrhage, surgical intervention (cesarean delivery), and thrombotic events. The individual whose pregnancy is complicated by multiple gestation is placed at a marked increase of risk for preterm birth, poor fetal growth, and fetal loss. These same women have a higher risk for the development of GD while pregnant. Knowledge of the physiologic alterations affecting pregnancy will aid those assisting in the care of these high-risk women. Medication dosing is often difficult during pregnancy, as few trials exist that establish the pharmacokinetics of most medications in pregnancy. The diagnosis of cancer in pregnancy can be devastating. Concerns for her unborn child, potential for her own mortality, and potential inability to have future offspring can be devastating. There currently are no standards of care for the treatment of cancer during pregnancy, and treatment plans need to be created based on clinical judgment and the desires of mother and family. There are continual research efforts to improve the knowledge and treatment options for management of GD, preeclampsia, and cancer to improve overall outcomes for mother and child.

References

Additional content available at ***www.ashp.org/womenshealth***

27

Prenatal Diagnosis

Tiki Bakhshi, MD; Andrea L. Coffee, Pharm.D., BCPS, MBA; Joan M. Mastrobattista, MD

Learning Objectives

1. Describe prenatal diagnostic testing options.
2. Describe the difference between screening methods and invasive diagnostic techniques.
3. Discuss the 2007 ACOG recommendations for offering prenatal diagnostic testing.
4. Become familiar with literature regarding pregnancy outcomes associated with prenatal fetal testing.

Prenatal diagnosis is a broad term and involves the detection of chromosomal or structural fetal abnormalities before birth. This has become an integral part of prenatal care offered to all pregnant women. It is important to understand that making the diagnosis of a chromosomal or structural problem before delivery is a multistep process. Typically, this involves identification of risk factors, discussion of first- and **second-trimester screening** tests, targeted ultrasound, genetic counseling, discussion of the option of diagnostic tests, and patient follow-up.

Screening and Diagnostic Tests

Screening tests are becoming more common in obstetrics. Screening involves the use of tests, exams, or procedures to assist in the presumptive diagnosis of patients with unrecognized disease. Screening tests are used to help identify individuals who are more likely to have disease from those who are less likely to have disease. These tests are usually applied to a low-risk population. Individuals identified by a positive screening test or an abnormal screening test normally undergo further diagnostic testing to see if they truly have the disease or the diagnosis being investigated.[1]

There are several properties that are important principles of a good screening test. The disease or medical condition should be a serious medical problem. The natural history of the disease should be known, and there should be an early period or stage that may be identified through testing. The test should be able to be applied to a large low-risk population, and it should be suitable and effective. Standard policies and procedures should be in place to determine which patients should be referred for further diagnostic testing. Access to health-care facilities for further diagnostic testing and treatment should be available. The screening test itself should be easy to perform, quick, inexpensive, safe, and have good sensitivity and specificity.[1]

The sensitivity of a screening test is described as the ability of a test to correctly identify those who have the disease. Specificity, on the other hand, is the ability of a test to correctly identify the absence of disease. Diagnostic tests are performed on individuals who have a positive screening test and seem more likely to have the disease.[1]

POTENTIAL RESULTS OF A SCREENING TEST

A true-positive result is when the screening test indicates the presence of disease and the patient truly has the disease. A true-negative result is obtained when the test result is negative for disease and the patient is truly unaffected. A false-positive result occurs when the screening test is positive but the individual is disease free. A false-negative result occurs when the screening test is negative for disease and the individual actually has the disease.[1]

INDICATIONS FOR INVASIVE FETAL TESTING

The use of genetic screening tests and diagnostic tests for the detection of chromosomal or structural abnormalities should be discussed with each patient during her pregnancy. Imperative in this discussion is an explanation of the different options along with their detection rates, advantages, disadvantages, and limitations. Pregnancy options can be discussed in the event that a congenital abnormality is detected. Some women decline prenatal diagnostic testing or screening. Prenatal diagnosis may not change the course of their pregnancy, and undergoing a screening test with a false-positive rate of 5% can produce unwanted stress and anxiety. However, for women who desire genetic screening, the choice of which screening test to perform depends on gestational age, availability of testing in their locale, and patient preference.

Classically, indications for invasive testing included women of advanced maternal age (AMA)—women age 35 or older at the time of delivery. In addition to AMA, other indications for invasive testing include a major structural fetal abnormality detected by ultrasound (such as a cardiac defect or a neural tube defect), a prior child with a chromosome abnormality (e.g., Down syndrome), or certain genetic conditions, such as sickle cell disease.

Recently, there has been a dramatic paradigm shift in the indications for invasive fetal testing. In January 2007, the American College of Obstetricians and Gynecologists (ACOG) released revised guidelines for prenatal screening for chromosomal abnormalities.[2] These guidelines suggest that all pregnant women should be offered prenatal diagnostic testing. According to these new guidelines, maternal age alone should no longer be used as a cutoff or a threshold for deciding whom to offer invasive testing. These updated recommendations emphasize the importance of counseling all woman regarding their risk of having a fetus with a chromosomal abnormality; the difference between screening tests and diagnostic tests; the testing methods that are available (based on gestational age and the availability in the community); the risk of pregnancy loss or miscarriage following invasive fetal testing; and the limitations of using a screening test, such as the detection rate and the false-positive rate.[3] In practice, most physicians counsel patients based on their age-related risk, results of serum screening tests, and abnormal ultrasound findings to identify women at highest risk who should be offered invasive testing.

PRENATAL DIAGNOSTIC TESTING

The purpose of prenatal diagnosis is to assist women in making informed decisions regarding the detection of fetal chromosomal or structural abnormalities. This begins with some form of screening for **aneuploidy**—conditions that involve an extra chromosome or missing chromosome. Examples of aneuploidy that are routinely screened for include Down syndrome (an extra chromosome 21), trisomy 18 (an extra chromosome number 18), and trisomy 13 (an extra chromosome number 13). After a first- or second-trimester screening test is performed, patients are informed of their risk of having a child with a chromosomal abnormality. Women with a positive screening test, or trisomy 18 for Down syndrome, are generally offered both an ultrasound and a diagnostic test, such as **chorionic villus sampling (CVS)** or amniocentesis. Diagnostic tests are invasive and carry a risk of complications.[2]

Women with a negative screening test are informed that they are not an increased risk of having a fetus with a chromosomal abnormality. Patients must then weigh their calculated risk of having a fetus with a chromosomal abnormality with the risk of having a fetal loss or miscarriage following invasive fetal testing and their desire for prenatal diagnosis. Regardless of the results of the screening test, it is important to emphasize that only invasive fetal testing, which obtains fetal cells for chromosomal analysis, can identify a karyotypic abnormality.[2]

BACKGROUND

Prenatal screening for fetal abnormalities was first used to identify patients at increased risk of having a child with open neural tube defects (ONTD).[4] Physicians realized that most neural tube defects occur in individuals with no prior family history of such an abnormality(<5%). This led to the search for a marker to identify women at increased risk for having a child with an ONTD. The first serum analyte identified was **maternal serum alpha-fetoprotein (MSAFP).** Investigators found that elevated levels of MSAFP were associated with an increased incidence of ONTD.[5]

In 1984, the modern era of Down syndrome screening began, and investigators noted that low levels of MSAFP were associated with an increased risk of Down syndrome.[5] In the 1990s, additional serum proteins were identified as markers: **human chorionic gonadotropin (hCG) unconjugated estriol (uE$_3$)**, and **inhibin A.**

hCG begins to increase in the maternal serum following successful implantation of the embryo into the uterine lining. Increased levels of hCG in the fetal serum are seen in women carrying a fetus with Down syndrome. uE_3, which is produced by the placenta, is associated with Down syndrome when levels in the maternal serum are about 25% lower than in women with a normal pregnancy.[6] These three proteins—MSAFP, hCG, and uE_3—constitute the triple screen. Although the detection rate of the triple screen is only about 70% with a screen-positive rate of 5%, this new screening test changed obstetric practice.[2] Offering the triple screen to all pregnant women between 15 and 20 weeks of gestation became the standard of care.

As more women were screened for Down syndrome, the limitations of the triple screen were noticed on a large scale. The 70% detection rate resulted in some women having a negative screening test but who gave birth to a child with Down syndrome. In addition, the 5% screen-positive rate caused unnecessary anxiety in some women, prompting some to undergo an amniocentesis, which was normal. The search for other analytes and screening modalities that were more sensitive and specific began to intensify.

The next serum marker identified, inhibin A (INHA), is produced by the corpus luteum early in pregnancy. At about 8 weeks, the placenta takes over its production. Increased levels of INHA have been noted in the maternal serum of pregnant women carrying a fetus with Down syndrome. Adding INHA to the analytes in the triple screen improved the detection rate for Down syndrome. This new combination of four analytes—the quadruple screen or quad screen—has an 80% detection rate with a 5% false-positive rate.[6]

The most recent advance in prenatal screening has been the development and implementation of first-trimester screening. First-trimester screening uses levels of **pregnancy-associated plasma protein A (PAPP-A)** and **free or total β-hCG** in the maternal serum along with a measurement of the fluid collection at the back of the fetal neck. Maternal age, weight, and ethnicity are combined to calculate an individual's risk of carrying a fetus with Down syndrome or trisomy 18. Patients can now have prenatal screening performed as early as the first trimester.[2,6]

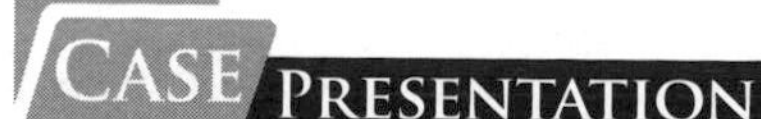

CASE PRESENTATION

Patient Case: Part 1

A 36-year-old woman presents to her obstetrician at 12 weeks of gestation to ask questions and discuss concerns about the health of her baby.

HPI: She is concerned because her cousin recently delivered a baby with Down syndrome. The patient is counseled regarding different options for screening and elects to undergo first-trimester screening.

Physical exam: Within normal limits.

Medications: Prenatal vitamin with omega 3.

Allergies: Codeine.

Lab results: Serum analytes were sent and the results return 1 week later. They show that her risk of having a child with Down syndrome is 1 in 89.

Diagnostics: An ultrasound is performed that revealed a single intrauterine gestation with a thickened nuchal fold.

Patient assessment: The assessment of this patient is that she is of advanced maternal age with a positive screening test for Down syndrome.

Serum Screening

It is important to emphasize that screening tests have limitations. They are designed to identify women at increased risk that may benefit from invasive testing. The quad screen, with a detection rate of 80%, will give false-negative results to some women who are carrying a fetus with Down syndrome. A normal screening test does not guarantee a normal fetus at delivery. In addition, the false-positive or screen-positive rate of 5% will result in some women having invasive testing, even though the fetus they are carrying is genetically normal.

FIRST-TRIMESTER SERUM SCREENING/NUCHAL TRANSLUCENCY

Background Literature

First-trimester screening was developed in the United Kingdom in the late 1990s and was tested in several large population-based studies in the U.S. over the last few years.[2] As prenatal screening for chromosomal abnormalities became the standard of care in the 1990s, the potential benefits of a first-trimester screening test became apparent.

How the Test Is Performed

First-trimester screening uses an ultrasound measurement of the **nuchal translucency (NT)** and the levels of PAPP-A and free or total β-hCG present in the maternal serum to calculate the patient's risk of having a baby with Down syndrome or trisomy 18. Nicolaides and colleagues and Sniders and colleagues studied more than 100,000 pregnant women and found first-trimester screening to be valuable.[7,8]

Interpretation of Test Results

First-trimester screening provides the patient with a risk estimate of having a child with Down syndrome or trisomy 18. This risk adjustment is based on her age, level of serum proteins, and the NT measurement. This first-trimester screening risk calculation will be compared with known laboratory standards. Women with abnormal first-trimester screening tests are offered invasive testing such as CVS or amniocentesis.

Risks and Potential Benefits

First-trimester screening allows women earlier prenatal diagnosis. Those with an abnormal result may be referred for CVS. This allows time for decision making early in the pregnancy. If a pregnancy interruption is desired, the maternal mortality rate following first-trimester termination is significantly lower than in the second trimester.[9] For women with twins or higher-order multiple gestations, first-trimester screening may be the preferred method of screening due to the incorporation of the ultrasound component. Maternal serum screening has lower sensitivity in multiple gestations because the maternal serum will contain protein levels from both the normal and the aneuploid fetus. This may mask the results or give a false-negative result.[2]

Detection Rate for Down Syndrome and Trisomy 18

First-trimester screening using the NT, PAPP-A, and free or total β-hCG has a Down syndrome detection rate of 87% when performed at 11 weeks, 85% when performed at 12 weeks, and 82% when performed at 13 weeks.[10] The detection rate is superior to both the triple and quad screens, with results available in the first trimester. The detection rate for trisomy 18 is 90% for all women, with a 5% false-positive rate.[11] The screen-positive rate for first trimester testing is 5%. For women older than the age of 35, the detection rate is 90%, but the screen-positive rate increases to 16% to 22%. The screen-positive rate for trisomy 18 is 5%, regardless of maternal age.[12]

SECOND-TRIMESTER SERUM SCREENING

Interpretation of Test Results

The second-trimester screening tests, triple screen or quad screen, yield a risk assessment for Down syndrome, trisomy 18, and ONTDs. The screening test is considered positive if the calculated risk is greater than 1 in 270, which is the value of a 35-year-old in the midgestation.[6]

There is a characteristic pattern of the serum protein levels in the triple screen that are suspicious for Down syndrome. The serum analytes are measured in multiples of the median. The pattern of a low MSAFP, a high hCG, and low uE_3 are seen in fetuses affected with Down syndrome.[3] When interpreting the triple-screen results for trisomy 18, all of the serum analyte levels are decreased. When using the quad screen, INHA, the fourth serum analyte, is elevated in fetuses with Down syndrome. In trisomy 18, the level of INHA does not contribute to the detection rate.[13]

The second-trimester serum tests will also give a risk estimate for ONTDs based on the MSAFP level. In ONTDs, the level of MSAFP is elevated because cerebral spinal fluid leaks into the amniotic fluid cavity and then crosses into the maternal bloodstream.[14]

A targeted ultrasound is indicated for patients who have an elevated MSAFP. The differential diagnosis of an elevated MSAFP includes an ONTD, incorrect gestational age, fetal demise, multiple gestation, alloimmunization, and other fetal anomalies (e.g., a gastroschisis, omphalocele, or cystic hygroma). Ultrasound is useful to narrow the differential diagnosis as it can verify gestational age, identify a fetal demise or multiple gestations, and identify additional fetal anomalies such as a gastroschisis or omphalocele. If no obvious explanation for the elevated MSAFP is noted on ultrasound, amniocentesis should be considered. A fetus with an ONTD may also leak **acetylcholinesterase (AchE)** into the amniotic fluid. If an amniocentesis is performed, the amniotic fluid should be sent for both AFP and AchE for confirmation.[3]

Second-trimester serum screening is noninvasive and is offered between 15 and 20 weeks of gestation, when most women have initiated prenatal care. The detection rate for Down syndrome when using the triple screen is 70% with a 5% screen-positive rate; with the quad screen, the detection rate is 80% with a 5% screen-positive rate (Table 27-1).[2]

Targeted Ultrasound

Targeted ultrasound performed between 18 and 22 weeks of gestation may be used as a noninvasive screening tool to detect fetal abnormalities. Major fetal abnormalities and soft ultrasound markers may

Table 27-1. Screening Tests for Down Syndrome and Detection Rates

Trimester	Screening test	Detection Rate (%)	False Positive (%)
First trimester	NT measurement	64–70	5
	NT measurement, PAPP-A, free β-hCG	82–87	5
Second trimester			
	Triple screen (MSAFP, hCG, uE_3)	69	5
	Quad screen (MSAFP, hCG, uE_3, inhibin-A)	81	5
First and second trimester			
	Integrated (NT, PAPP-A, quad screen)	94–96	5
	Serum integrated (PAPP-A, quad screen)	85–88	5

Source: Reference 10.

NT = nuchal translucency; PAPP-A = pregnancy-associated plasma protein A; hCG = human chorionic gonadotropin; MSAFP = maternal serum alpha-fetoprotein; uE_3 = unconjugated estriol.

be identified. Additional markers for fetal aneuploidy are under investigation. In 2001, an association was noted between the absence of a nasal bone on ultrasound at 10–12 weeks and fetuses diagnosed with Down syndrome. The orginal report described an 82% detection rate with an 8.3% false-positive rate.[15] Even more encourging, when the absence of the nasal bone was combined with first-trimester NT measurement, the Down syndrome detection rate was 92%, with a false-positive rate of 3.5%.[16]

Not all researchers have been able to replicate these detection rates, and assessment of the nasal bone at 10–12 weeks is difficult, even for experienced sonographers. However, assessment of the nasal bone has the potential to improve Down syndrome screening if it can be reliably integrated into existing screening protocols.

EVALUATION FOR STRUCTURAL ANOMALIES AND GROWTH DELAY

Ultrasound has a role not only in screening and detection of fetal anomalies, but in pregnancy management as well. Many structural and chromosomal abnormalities are associated with intrauterine growth restriction and will require ongoing assessments of fetal growth by ultrasound. In addition, antepartum fetal testing may be instituted in the third trimester for fetal surveillance, which uses ultrasound as part of the testing scheme.

Chorionic Villus Sampling

BACKGROUND LITERATURE

CVS is a diagnostic test performed under direct ultrasound guidance that may be performed in the first trimester between 10 and 13 completed weeks. Placental tissue for chromosomal analysis is obtained. Rhesus-negative patients should receive RhD-immune globulin (Rhogam) after the procedure.[17]

RISK OF LOSS

When CVS is performed between 10 and 13 completed weeks by an experienced operator, the risk of fetal loss is similar to that of amniocentesis performed between 16 and 20 weeks.[18] Large trials performed in both the U.S. and Canada showed that the fetal loss rate following CVS was not statistically different than following amniocentesis.[19]

BENEFITS OF THE TEST

CVS can provide information about chromosomal abnormalities in the first trimester. For women carrying multiple gestations, particularly higher-order multiples, CVS may be used to detect aneuploidy in one or more of the fetuses. Some consider selective fetal reduction, and CVS may serve as an adjunct to identifying fetuses with karyotypic abnormalities.

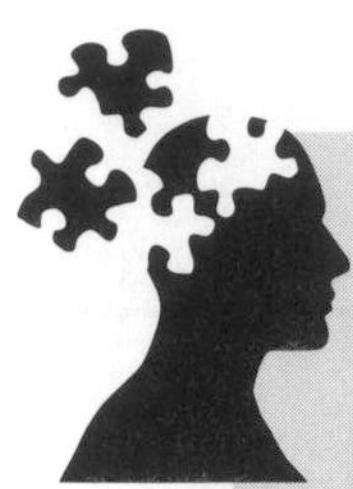

Therapeutic Challenge:

P.H. is a 42-year-old woman who, after trying to get pregnant for 8 years and after three miscarriages, has finally reached the 12th week of her pregnancy. She is relieved and very excited that this should be a successful pregnancy. At her monthly checkup, her obstetrician recommends a genetic amniocentesis, considering her history of miscarriages and advanced maternal age. P.H. is very concerned about the risk of loss of the pregnancy. How would you counsel, and what would you recommend to P.H.?

One limitation of CVS, in comparison with amniocentesis, is that it does not provide a risk assessment for ONTDs. Therefore, women who undergo CVS should have an MSAFP level drawn between 15 and 20 weeks and/or a targeted ultrasound evaluation performed at 20 weeks to assess for spinal abnormalities.[3]

CONFINED PLACENTAL MOSAICISM

When the fetal cells from CVS are analyzed, sometimes two different cells lines are identified. Confined placental mosaicism occurs when the fetal cell line is intact but there is more than one cell line detected in the placenta. When mosaicism is confined to the placenta, the risk of fetal abnormalities is low, and follow-up amniocentesis may be offered for confirmation.[20]

Genetic Amniocentesis

BACKGROUND

Amniocentesis is an invasive test that involves sampling the amniotic fluid. The procedure was first described in the 1950s and has made an enormous impact on prenatal diagnosis.[21,22] When amniocentesis is performed at 15–20 weeks of gestation (traditional) for the purposes of chromosomal analysis, it is described as genetic amniocentesis. Amniocentesis may also be performed in the third trimester for the purpose of documenting fetal lung maturity.

During the procedure, a 20- or 22-gauge spinal needle is advanced into the uterine cavity under direct ultrasound guidance. Twenty to 30 mL of amniotic fluid are withdrawn, which contain fetal cells. Fetal amniocytes are grown in tissue culture and then the chromosomes are evaluated. The karyotype will detect the number of chromosomes and the presence or absence of large deletions or translocations. This information can be used to diagnose Down syndrome, trisomy 18, trisomy 13, other forms of aneuploidy, and fetal sex. Rhesus-negative women should receive RhD-immune globulin after the procedure.[6]

Prenatal fluorescence in situ hybridization is a rapid test that can evaluate chromosomes 13, 18, 21, X, and Y. This test may be requested at the time of the amniocentesis and performed using the amniotic fluid obtained. The results are typically available within 24–48 hours, and the full karyotype takes approximately 10–14 days. This test can detect trisomies 13, 18, 21, and abnormalities in the sex chromosomes.

GESTATIONAL AGE

Amniocentesis is typically performed between 15 and 20 weeks of gestation. Early amniocentesis is performed between 13 and 15 weeks. Early amniocentesis is technically more difficult to perform because of possible membrane tenting, has a higher risk of leakage of amniotic fluid, and is associated with an increased risk of club foot.[18] Given the higher rate of fetal loss and complications, early amniocenteses are usually not performed. In most cases, women either elect for a CVS between 10 and 13 completed weeks or wait to have a traditional amniocentesis at 15 weeks.

RISK OF LOSS

The procedure-related risk of fetal loss following amniocentesis performed at 15–20 weeks of gestation is classically reported to be 1 in 200.[23] More recent publications have estimated the loss rate to be 1 in 300 to 1 in 500 or less.[2,24]

BENEFITS OF THE TEST

Traditional amniocentesis has an excellent safety record with a low procedure-related loss rate. The procedure is available to women initiating care in the late first or early second trimester.[6] Because amniocentesis is a diagnostic test, it provides the parents with the knowledge of whether their child has a major chromosome abnormality before birth. The results of a normal amniocentesis provide reassurance to the parents and the physicians taking care of them. When an amniocentesis identifies a chromosomal abnormality, such as Down syndrome or trisomy 18, it allows the patient to know early enough to make an informed decision regarding the pregnancy. Additionally, this allows the patient and the obstetrician, neonatologist, anesthesiologist, and nurses involved in her care time to make a plan for delivery and neonatal care after birth.

Fetal Blood Sampling

BACKGROUND

Fetal blood sampling (FBS) is an invasive fetal test performed under direct ultrasound guidance in the second or third trimester (Figure 27-1). FBS involves advancing a spinal needle directly into the umbilical vein or hepatic vein to obtain fetal blood.[25] Fetal blood may be sent for a rapid fetal karyotype or may be sent to determine fetal blood type, hemoglobin, hematocrit, platelet count, and for bacterial, viral, or parasitic studies if fetal infection is suspected.[26]

RISK OF LOSS

The procedure-related risk of fetal loss after FBS has been reported by ACOG and others to be <2%.[3,17] It is important to remember that the underlying disease process can influence the individual loss rate. A fetus that is severely anemic and requiring transfusion is at a higher risk of fetal loss. Additional complications associated with FBS include bleeding from the umbilical cord, umbilical cord hematoma formation, and fetal distress requiring emergent delivery.

FBS allows direct access of the fetal blood for diagnosis and intrauterine fetal therapy. In the presence of oligohydramnios or other limitations to amniocentesis, an FBS may be warranted.[17]

Figure 27-1. Fetal blood sampling.

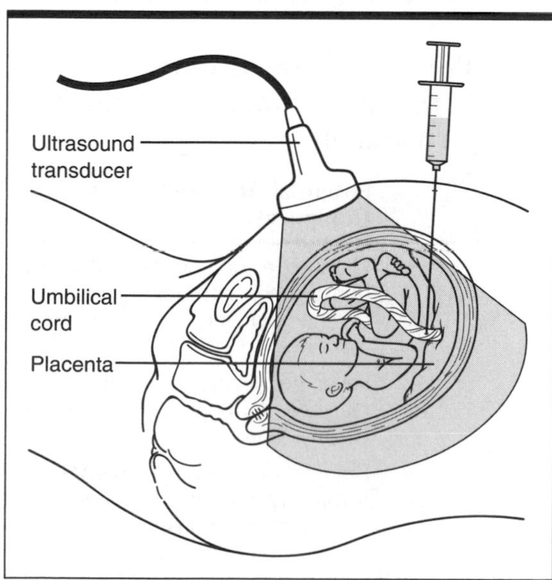

INDICATIONS FOR TESTING

Some indications for FBS include suspected fetal anemia due to alloimmunization or infection and suspected fetal karyotypic abnormality after a major fetal anomaly is identified by ultrasound. FBS requires a team approach, and this procedure is usually performed in tertiary care facilities.

Noninvasive Prenatal Diagnosis Using Fetal Cells in the Maternal Circulation

Given the risks of invasive testing for prenatal diagnosis, noninvasive methods have been pursued for many years. One promising new discovery was the detection of fetal DNA in maternal blood. This fetal DNA exists as free nucleic acids that have been released from fetal cells and are in the maternal circulation. Fetal nucleic acids have been recovered as early as the fifth week of pregnancy, but they are most often present by 7 weeks gestation.[11] These cells are present throughout pregnancy but decrease rapidly following delivery and seem to be absent within 48 hours.[27]

Clinical application of this technology is promising but has had to overcome some challenges. The quantity of fetal cells in the maternal circulation is relatively small, with only approximately 20 fetal cells present in about 20 mL of maternal blood. This low quantity of fetal cells requires the application of molecular techniques to isolate the fetal cells, amplify them, and distinguish them reliably from other sources of nucleic acids.

The United Kingdom has implemented the use of free fetal DNA for prenatal diagnosis to assist with early diagnosis of fetal sex, fetal Rh D typing, and detection of single gene disorders. The U.K. experience has shown that the use of free fetal DNA to detect fetal sex is 98% accurate when performed at or beyond 7 weeks of gestation. This early identification has resulted in a decrease in the need for invasive testing using CVS or amniocentesis for X-linked conditions by about 45%.[28]

For women with a history of hemolytic disease of the newborn and RhD antibodies, free fetal DNA can test for the fetal RhD status. If the fetal cells do not contain the RhD antigen, then the patient does not require further monitoring during her pregnancy.[29]

The future application of free fetal DNA for noninvasive prenatal diagnosis will require improvements in current techniques for extraction, enrichment, and amplification of fetal DNA in maternal blood. Advances in technology in proteonomics and genetics may lead to the use of free fetal DNA for earlier noninvasive diagnosis of fetal aneuploidy.

Genetic Counseling

Genetic counseling is an integral part of prenatal diagnosis that may help identify a family history of a heritable problem or genetic syndrome. Genetic counselors explain the meaning of the various screening tests and review information patients may gain from invasive testing. Counselors have the psychosocial training to deal with patient anxiety, grief, and loss. Post-test counseling is an important aspect of genetic counseling. Test results may be explained and risk of recurrence discussed. Some couples may benefit from a referral to a pediatric medical geneticist for certain conditions diagnosed prenatally. Many women experience significant grief reactions after learning of abnormal results and may be referred for psychiatric or psychological counseling.

Medical Termination

Medical termination might be considered in pregnancies when mother or fetus has a life-threatening medical condition. Women with significant medical problems should have a discussion of the potential risks to her life of continuing the pregnancy with her care provider. Couples may also consider pregnancy interruption for lethal fetal conditions. Appropriate counseling and support needs to be provided to mother and family to work through all of the challenges associated with the decision for medical termination in these serious health-risk situations. For some women, this event might be traumatic and may require long-term mental health support and counseling

Prenatal diagnosis may be performed by CVS at 10–13 weeks or amniocentesis at 15–20 weeks of gestation. Thus, patients who are diagnosed with a fetal anomaly and in whom medical termination of pregnancy is considered would be counseled regarding medical and surgical options in the late first trimester or the mid-second trimester.

There are different methods of medical termination of pregnancy available to the patient. In general, medical termination in the first trimester is associated with fewer complications, has a lower risk of maternal mortality, and provides more patient privacy (Table 27-2).[9] Pharmacologic intervention is an option in the first trimester with misoprostol (prostaglandin E_1) or surgically by suction dilation and curettage (D&C). Misoprostol, given in a dose 800 mcg vaginally and repeated in 24 hours for up to three doses, is an effective method of medical termination of pregnancy with a success rate of 88%.[30] Suction D&C, when performed by an experienced obstetrician, may be safely completed with a low risk of complications in the first trimester (Table 27-2).

Second-trimester medical termination of pregnancy is more difficult as the fetus is larger and the fetal skeleton and cranium are more developed. Pharmacologic termination may be performed using misoprostol or high-dose oxytocin in the second trimester. Many different regimens of misoprostol are used with different dosages and frequency of administration. One effective regimen is misoprostol 600 mcg vaginally, followed by 400 mcg every 6 hours.[31] This regimen achieved delivery in 95% of patients within 24 hours. Oxytocin may also be used for second-trimester termination and is very effective. However, the dose of oxytocin required is higher than the dose used for normal labor at term. This is likely due to the lower number of oxytocin receptors present on the uterus at this stage of pregnancy. One such regimen uses 50 units of oxytocin in 500 mL of normal saline, which is infused over 3 hours. Over the next hour, no oxytocin is infused, and the patient is allowed time for diuresis. Then the process is repeated with 100 units of oxytocin mixed in 500 mL

Table 27-2. Potential Complications Associated with Interventions for Medical Pregnancy Termination

Intervention	Potential Adverse Effects/ Complications
Surgical (suction dilation and curettage [D&C])	Uterine perforation, cervical injury, hemorrhage, intestinal injury, retained placenta, infection, febrile reaction
Misoprostol	Fever, headache, abdominal pain, diarrhea, lethargy, nausea, vertigo, uterine rupture
Oxytocin	Bradycardia, headache, hematoma, hypertension/hypotension, hyponatremia, nausea/vomiting, seizures, uterine rupture

of normal saline infused over 3 hours, followed by a 1 hour rest period. This cycle repeats, and the dose of oxytocin is increased in increments of 50 units, up to a maximum of 300 units of oxytocin mixed into 500 mL of normal saline. This regimen is extremely effective with an 80% to 90% success rate.[32] Each of these medical interventions require admission to labor and delivery and supervision by an obstetrician and skilled nursing personnel.

Surgical options in the second trimester include dilation and evacuation (D&E) and hysterotomy. A D&E requires an obstetrician with experience and training in performing this procedure, and specialized instruments are needed to extract the fetus and the placenta. The risks of surgical management by D&E, when performed after 14 or 15 weeks of gestation, are higher than that of a suction D&C that is performed in the first trimester and include complications such as uterine perforation, bleeding, cervical laceration, infection, or retained products (Table 27-2).[33] Hysterotomy (laparotomy and incision in the uterus to remove the fetus) is a less-utilized option as it is a major surgical procedure and generally is performed only in very rare circumstances.

Case Presentation

Patient Case: Part 2

CVS will allow prenatal diagnosis to be completed in the first trimester, rather than waiting for an amniocentesis to be performed at 15 weeks with the final results coming back in the mid-second trimester.

Treatment plan: The plan is to perform CVS for prenatal diagnosis. The patient will be able to know definitively if this unborn child has Down syndrome. CVS will allow prenatal diagnosis to be completed in the first trimester.

Patient monitoring: Baseline ultrasound before initiating testing, fetal heart rate evaluation during procedure, and rest postprocedure would be recommended (redundent).

Patient education: She is told that these procedures have risks, including the possibility of miscarriage or fetal loss following the procedure. The patient does not want to put this pregnancy at risk, but she is unsure if she can go through the rest of the pregnancy without knowing the answer. She wants to find out so she can prepare appropriately for birth of her child. Based on test results, appropriate counseling and resources should be provided to mother and family to prepare for raising a child with Down syndrome.

Summary

Prenatal diagnosis involves the detection of a chromosomal or structural abnormality in the fetus before birth. Prenatal diagnosis assists women in making informed decisions regarding their pregnancy options. All pregnant women should be offered screening for chromosomal and structural abnormalities. Invasive diagnostic testing is available to women regardless of maternal age. Because invasive testing has risks to the pregnancy, screening tests, ultrasound, and maternal age are used to identify patients at increased risk and that are most likely to benefit from invasive testing. Procedures used for prenatal diagnosis include CVS, amniocentesis, or FBS. CVS is a diagnostic test to detect chromosomal abnormalities that may be performed in the first trimester between 10 and 13 completed weeks while amniocentesis is perfsormed between 15 and 20 weeks. FBS allows direct access to the fetal blood for diagnosis and intrauterine fetal therapy. These procedures used for invasive testing have risks to the patient and the pregnancy. Consequently, they should be performed by obstetricians or maternal-fetal medicine specialists with specific training and expertise in this area. The use of free fetal DNA in maternal blood is an emerging technology. The use of this test may provide prenatal diagnosis by examining the maternal blood. This noninvasive method of prenatal diagnosis has several promising potential applications in upcoming years. Improved scientific techniques and methods for extraction, amplification, and molecular testing are needed for widespread use.

Genetic counseling is an integral part of prenatal diagnosis and should be provided to patients to help them understand the different options for screening tests and diagnostic tests, as well as their risks and limitations. Pregnancy medical termination may be considered by some women who become pregnant and have life-threatening pre-existing medical conditions or lethal fetal conditions.

References

Additional content available at ***www.ashp.org/womenshealth***

28 Labor and Delivery

Carla Ann Martinez, MD; Julie J. Kelsey, Pharm.D.; Mildred M. Ramirez, MD

Learning Objectives

1. Describe criteria used for the diagnosis of preterm labor, labor, and abnormal labor. Explain the physiology of labor and the pathophysiology of preterm labor.
2. Understand appropriate pharmacologic and nonpharmacologic therapies in the management of labor and induction of labor.
3. Compare and contrast commonly used tocolytics for the treatment of preterm labor.
4. Define common causes and treatments for postpartum hemorrhage.

Labor is the physiologic process by which the fetus and placenta are expelled from the uterus. Labor is defined as the presence of uterine contractions of sufficient intensity, frequency, and duration to bring about demonstrable **effacement** (thinning) and dilatation of the cervix.[1] It involves a complex interaction of maternal, fetal, and placental signals. These complicated endocrine, paracrine, and autocrine mechanisms have been shown to be different among different species. In humans, all of the mechanisms responsible for labor have not been completely elucidated, but the timing of delivery appears to be determined by the placenta and the expression of the corticotropin-releasing hormone gene.[2-4]

Parturition, or giving birth, has been divided into four cervical and uterine phases corresponding to the physiologic changes that occur during pregnancy.[5,6] Although the uterus and cervix are part of the same organ, they respond differently during pregnancy. The uterus transitions from a state of relative quiescence, or rest, to activation of the **myometrium** in preparation for labor, followed by the actual process of labor and eventually recovery.[5] The cervix performs its transformation early in pregnancy, beginning with softening in the first month, and slowly progresses to **cervical ripening** during the last few weeks of the pregnancy. This is followed by dilatation during labor and concludes with repair and remodeling during the postpartum period while the uterus is undergoing involution.[6,7]

This chapter will examine the physiology of labor and the appropriate pharmacologic and nonpharmacologic therapies in the management of labor and induction of labor. In addition, the pathophysiology of **preterm labor** will be reviewed, including discussion of the commonly used tocolytics for the treatment of preterm labor. Finally, the common causes and treatments for postpartum hemorrhage will be defined.

Pathophysiology

PHYSIOLOGY OF LABOR

Comprehensive analyses of each of the individual pathways reviewing the process of labor have been described in detail elsewhere.[5,6,8,9] Below is a brief overview of each of the phases of parturition to better understand the pharmacologic treatments involved in labor and delivery.

Parturition has been divided into four cervical and uterine phases corresponding to the physiologic changes that occur during pregnancy (Table 28-1).[5,6] Phase 0 (quiescence) is a tranquil state for uterine smooth muscle and a time of cervical integrity. This phase constitutes 95% of the pregnant state.[5] The uterine smooth muscles

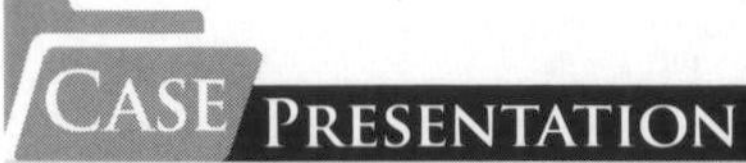

Presentation

Patient Case: Part 1

T.K., a healthy 28-year-old **primigravid,** is currently at 40 weeks of gestation based on excellent dating criteria. She is now at her due date and questions her obstetrician about the possibility of induction of labor.

HPI: Her prenatal course has been unremarkable. She reports good fetal movement and denies regular contractions, vaginal bleeding, or leakage of amniotic fluid.

Lab results: Within normal limits.

Medications: None.

Physical exam: On examination, the fetus is vertex (head down in the pelvis) by **Leopold's maneuver.** Her cervix is dilated 2 cm, 50% effaced, and the presenting part is at −2 station. The cervix is midposition and soft. Her Bishop score is 6.

may contract during this phase, but they do not normally produce cervical dilatation. The uterine activity is of low frequency and poorly coordinated contractures, often referred to as Braxton Hicks contractions or false labor.[5]

The cervix and uterus must progress through a transition of being reasonably unyielding and quiescent to one of activation in preparation for labor. Phase 1 (activation) includes a time of increased inflammatory cell infiltration, increase in hyaluronic acid, and a decrease in dermatan sulfate, resulting in degradation of collagen in the uterine cervix.[10,11] Mechanical methods and pharmacologic agents, such as prostaglandins E_2 (PGE_2) and E1 (PGE_1), are used clinically to induce these changes and will be discussed later in this chapter.

The smooth muscle of the myometrium undergoes changes related to its contractility. There is an up-regulation of contraction-associated proteins, an increase in myometrial oxytocin receptors, and myometrial gap junction proteins, including connexin 43.[2,12] The myometrial tissue is excitable and transitions from poorly coordinated, relatively painless, uterine contractures of low frequency to coordinated uterine contractions of high frequency and high amplitude in the myometrial smooth muscle.[13] Once this change has occurred, the myometrium can now respond to stimulation (Phase 2) and is responsive to endogenous and exogenous agonists.[12] It is during this period that a well-formed lower uterine segment (inferior aspect of the uterus adjacent to the cervix) is developed. The patient may report that the baby has "dropped," a phenomenon also referred to as lightening, as a result of the fetal head descending into the pelvis.

Phase 2 (stimulation) is equivalent to active labor, in which uterine contractions lead to progressive cervical dilatation and delivery of the fetus and placenta. Clinically, phase 2 is divided into three stages. The first stage comprises regular uterine contractions that produce cervical effacement and dilatation. It is completed when the cervix is fully dilated, corresponding to approximately 10 cm. The second stage begins when the cervix is completely dilated and ends with delivery of the fetus. The third and final stage commences immediately after the delivery of the fetus and ends with the delivery of the placenta. Uterotonins, prostaglandins (PGs), and oxytocin stimulate the activated myometrial smooth muscle, while increased numbers of leukocytes in the cervix correlate with the extent of cervical dilation during labor.[6] Stimulation of the myometrium by uterotonins can occur through endogenous or exogenous routes to

Table 28-1. Phases of Parturition

	Phase 0	Phase 1	Phase 2	Phase 3
Uterine	Quiescence	Activation	Stimulation	Involution
Cervical	Softening	Ripening	Dilatation	Repair
	↑ Initiation of Parturition			↑ Parturition
			Active labor (3 stages)	

Source: Based on references 5 and 6.

produce regular contractions. Oxytocin is produced by the posterior pituitary and, when insufficient, can be given intravenously to augment labor or overcome labor **dystocia.** Dystocia is defined as a difficult labor and is characterized by an abnormally slow progress of labor.[14]

The final phase, phase 3, is uterine involution and is primarily mediated by oxytocin. Immediately following the delivery of the fetus and placenta, the uterus maintains a relatively contracted state that results in compression of large uterine vessels and prevents postpartum hemorrhage. The uterus continues to contract and retract, resulting in involution and a return of the uterus to its nonpregnant state within the pelvis.[14]

DYSFUNCTIONAL LABOR

When labor is abnormal, it can result in preterm labor, dystocia, or **post-term pregnancy.** Preterm labor will be discussed separately. Dystocia is the result of abnormalities that can be classified into three simple categories: powers, passenger, and passage. Abnormalities of powers can be the result of inadequate or uncoordinated uterine contractions that fail to efface or dilate the cervix, or inadequate maternal expulsive efforts to effect delivery of the fetus. Abnormalities of the passenger relate to the position, presentation (i.e., cephalic or breech), or size of the fetus resulting in slow labor. Passage refers to the maternal bony pelvis and soft tissues that can impede the progress of labor.

Dystocia is diagnosed when slower-than-normal cervical dilation or lack of descent of the fetal head or both are encountered. The rate of dilation and descent are based on studies by Friedman.[15] He studied the progress of labor and descent of the fetus through the maternal pelvis against time and plotted it graphically. What resulted was the characteristic sigmoid pattern representing the labor curve that is still clinically used today. Using this graph and the defined minimal normal rate of change and descent of the fetus, one can follow the progress of labor. When a patient begins to fall below the minimal normal rate of change or descent, dystocia can be diagnosed and treated. Treatment, if appropriate, consists of augmentation, or stimulating uterine contractions, as spontaneous contractions have failed to result in progressive cervical dilatation or descent of the fetus.[1] At this point, intravenous oxytocin may be used to produce contractions of sufficient frequency and amplitude in an attempt to further cervical change. In other cases, treatment may consist of an operative intervention. Modern-day obstetrics have questioned whether the validity of the Friedman definitions of labor protraction and arrest may be too stringent for modern-day use.[16]

POST-TERM PREGNANCY

Post-term pregnancy as defined by the American College of Obstetricians and Gynecologists (ACOG) refers to a pregnancy that has extended to or beyond 42 weeks of gestation (294 days from the last menstrual period).[17] Post-term pregnancy is associated with significant risk to the fetus, as well as the mother. The fetus is at risk for uteroplacental insufficiency, meconium aspiration, and increased perinatal death, and the mother is at risk for labor dystocia and cesarean delivery.[17] Factors involved in the management of post-term pregnancy are accurate gestation dating, appropriate surveillance of the fetus, and evaluation of the condition of the cervix. Induction of labor may be undertaken for fetal or maternal indications, or can be considered when the cervix appears "favorable" in a low-risk pregnancy without other indications for delivery.

The condition of the cervix is based on physical exam and quantified by a method describe by Bishop in 1964.[7] The elements of the Bishop score consist of cervical dilatation, effacement, station, cervical consistency, and cervical position. Cervical dilatation describes the gradual opening of the cervical os during labor to allow the fetus to leave the uterus, whereas effacement is an estimation of thickness of the cervix. The station is the relationship in centimeters between the presenting part of the fetus and the level of the ischial spines of the mother. The consistency of the cervix is determined by palpation and is firm, medium, or soft. Finally, as the cervix prepares for labor, the position of the cervix moves from posterior to midanterior to anterior. The importance of determining the condition of the cervix, or the "favorability," helps to predict the success of labor induction. The probability of vaginal delivery after labor induction is similar to that after spontaneous labor if the total Bishop's score is >8.[18] Induction of labor will be discussed in more detail below.

PRETERM LABOR

Preterm labor, by definition, consists of regular contractions associated with cervical change before the completion of 37 weeks of gestation.[19] The preterm birth rate continues to rise annually in the U.S., with the last reported preterm birth rate at

12.7% in 2005, up 20% from 1990.[20] Preterm birth is one of the leading causes of infant morbidity and mortality. It accounts for nearly one half of all congenital neurologic defects and more than two thirds of infant deaths.[21]

Causes of preterm birth fall into three general categories: 1) iatrogenic, in which there is a complication of pregnancy (e.g., preeclampsia or fetal distress, which requires obstetric intervention); 2) premature rupture of the fetal membranes with or without infection; and 3) idiopathic preterm labor. Like term labor, several theoretical mechanisms of preterm labor have been described, as the etiology of preterm labor has also not been elucidated.[5,22-24] Possible pathways include intrauterine inflammation or infection, uterine overdistention, and early fetal endocrine activation. Presently, there are no effective diagnostic indicators of preterm birth, nor are there effective treatments for this condition. The diagnosis is often based on clinical impression alone and can often be imprecise, with up to 50% of women who present in preterm labor delivering at term.[25]

Screening and Diagnosis of Preterm Labor

A patient's past history of previous preterm delivery may be the most important risk factor for future preterm delivery. Up to 30% of women with a prior history of preterm delivery will deliver preterm in a subsequent pregnancy. Risk-scoring systems have been evaluated but unfortunately have not been validated in other populations. Furthermore, up to 40% of deliveries will be in nulliparous women who therefore will not have a history of preterm delivery. Other markers ascertaining risks have been evaluated in an attempt to accurately identify women at risk of preterm delivery.

CERVICAL LENGTH

The relationship of a short cervix with increased risk of preterm delivery is undisputable.[26] In low-risk populations, the risk for preterm delivery increases with decreasing cervical length. In patients with prior preterm delivery, cervical length measured between 14 and 18 weeks has a sensitivity of 69%, specificity of 80%, and positive predictive value of 55% for delivery <35 weeks of gestation.[27] Unfortunately, interventions to reduce the risk of preterm delivery when a short cervix is identified on routine sonogram, such as **cervical cerclage** (surgical suturing of the cervix), have not proven to be effective.

FETAL FIBRONECTIN

Fetal fibronectin is a glycoprotein secreted by the fetal membranes that is found in the choriodecidual junction. When detected in the cervicovaginal secretions, it is associated with increased risk of preterm labor and delivery.[28] The fetal fibronectin test is considered positive if measured at a level of ≥50 ng/mL. When evaluated in low-risk women screened at 2-week intervals between 22 and 30 weeks, the sensitivity of fetal fibronectin is 63% to predict a delivery <28 weeks with a specificity of 96% to 98%. In contrast, the positive predictive value for <37 weeks is only 36%.[29] The utility of fetal fibronectin is its high negative predictive value, identifying women at low risk of preterm delivery and possibly reducing costly interventions.

AMNIOCENTESIS

Amniocentesis is a technique used to withdraw amniotic fluid from the amniotic sac using a needle inserted through the woman's abdominal wall. The procedure is performed under sonographic visualization to avoid the risk of fetal trauma and umbilical cord puncture. In some cases, evaluation of amniotic fluid by amniocentesis can be performed to ascertain the risk of infection in patients with preterm labor or premature rupture of membranes. Determination of decreased glucose and identification of bacteria, white blood cells, interleukin 6 and 8, or a positive bacterial culture of the amniotic fluid can identify women with an intrauterine infection, indicating the need for delivery.

Amniocentesis may also be performed to determine fetal lung maturity before induction of labor or cesarean delivery when delivery is indicated before 39 weeks of gestation or the patient's dating criteria is uncertain. Again, the procedure is performed under sonographic visualization to avoid the risk of fetal trauma and umbilical cord puncture. Fetal lung maturity may be determined via a number of measurements, including lecithin/sphingomyelin ratio, phosphatidylglycerol, fluorescence polarization, or lamellar body counts.[30]

In summary, amniocentesis can assist the obstetrician in determining when delivery may be indicated as in the case of an intra-amniotic infection either in the setting of preterm labor or premature rupture of membranes. In addition, amniocentesis assists in evaluation of the status of fetal lung maturation in patients who experience complications during pregnancy and in determining the timing of delivery.

Guidelines and Position Statements

INDUCTION OF LABOR

The goal of an induction of labor is to stimulate contractions before onset of labor to achieve a vaginal delivery. An induction of labor can be either elective or medically indicated, and the benefits of labor induction must be weighed against the potential maternal or fetal risks associated with this procedure. Elective indications supported by ACOG include logistic reasons, such as the risk of rapid labor or the patient lives a long distance from the hospital, or psychosocial indications.[18] In this setting, ACOG recommends fetal lung maturity be established before the induction of labor.[18] In contrast, an induction of labor is medically indicated when the benefits to either the mother or the fetus outweigh those of continuing the pregnancy.

ACOG provides practice guidelines of maternal or fetal conditions that may be indications for induction of labor. Some examples include maternal medical conditions (e.g., diabetes mellitus, renal disease, chronic pulmonary disease, and chronic hypertension), fetal compromise, preeclampsia, and fetal demise.[18] In these settings, fetal lung maturity does not need to be established before the induction.

Contraindications to labor induction are the same as those that preclude a spontaneous labor and a vaginal delivery. Examples of these may include placenta previa (when the placenta is implanted over the cervical canal), the fetus is in **transverse lie,** and previous classical cesarean delivery.

STEROID ADMINISTRATION FOR FETAL LUNG MATURITY

In 1994, the National Institute of Child Health and Human Development convened a consensus development conference on the effect of corticosteroids for fetal maturation on perinatal outcomes. Data were presented by 19 experts in the fields of neonatology, obstetrics, and pharmacology. At the end of the conference, a consensus statement was issued, recommending a single course of corticosteroids to all pregnant women between 24 and 34 weeks of gestation who are at risk of preterm delivery within 7 days.[31] A second conference was reconvened in 2000 to address the issue of repeat courses of corticosteroids. They concluded that repeat courses of corticosteroids should not be routinely used, supporting their original recommendations.[32] These conclusions were supported by ACOG in 2002 and reaffirmed in 2005.[33] The Cochrane Database of Systemic Reviews recently reviewed 21 studies comparing antenatal corticosteroids with placebo or no treatment given to women at risk for preterm birth because of preterm labor, premature rupture of the membranes, or elective preterm delivery.[34] They continue to support a single course of antenatal corticosteroids for women at risk of preterm birth, with few exceptions.[34] Two new randomized trials comparing single vs. repeated doses of antenatal corticosteroids have confirmed the improved outcome (reduction in mechanical respiratory support and need for surfactant administration (MFMU) and respiratory distress syndrome and serious neonatal morbidity (ACTORDS) with repeated doses of corticosteroids when compared with a single course. Findings of lower birth weight and smaller head circumference raised concerns about the long-term neurologic outcomes of these infants. A 2-year follow-up evaluating infant neurodevelopment and anthropometric measurements found that infants exposed to repeated doses of corticosteroids did not differ in physical or neurocognitive measurements. Of concern was a nonsignificant trend in the rate of cerebral palsy.[35] In contrast, the ACTORDS trial 2-year follow-up only identified increase in attention problems in the children exposed to multiple doses of corticosteroids.[36] The recommendations for administration of multiple doses of corticosteroid for women at risk of preterm delivery differ. The optimal dosing of corticosteroids continues to be debated. The administration of corticosteroids to women experiencing preterm labor is discussed later in this chapter.

Primary Prevention

Progesterone is a naturally occurring progestin that is secreted by the corpus luteum and is the prototype of the progestins. The progestins elicit several physiologic changes that relate to the maintenance of pregnancy and preparation for delivery. Progesterone relaxes the pregnant myometrial smooth muscle blocking the action of oxytocin and inhibits the formation of gap junctions. Withdrawal of progesterone is pivotal in initiation of parturition in many mammalian species. It is therefore not surprising that progesterone administration has been evaluated as a intervention for reduction of miscarriages and preterm delivery.

Resurgence in the interest in the use of progesterone was initiated by a meta-analysis of control trials using 17-alphahydroxyprogesterone caproate (17P).[37] The vehicle used to deliver 17P was castor oil, which is stable at room temperature. Although there was no evidence to support the use of 17P for the prevention of miscarriage, it appeared there was a reduction in the preterm delivery rate. The 17P injection is not commercially available and may only be obtained via specialty compounding pharmacies and distributors.[38]

More recently, the National Institute of Child Health and Human Development–Maternal-Fetal Medicine Network published a multicenter trial in which women with a history of prior preterm delivery were randomized to receive weekly intramuscular injections of 250 mg 17P or placebo from 16 to 36 weeks of gestation.[38] Although treatment with 17P reduced the relative risk of preterm delivery by 34%, the mean difference in gestational age at delivery was 1 week (95% CI 0.3, 1.5), and no net survival benefit was demonstrated. Concern has been raised regarding the applicability of these data, as the preterm birth rate in the placebo arm was considerably higher than that reported in other Maternal Fetal Medicine Unit Network trials.

Other studies have confirmed similar reductions in preterm birth using daily 100-mg vaginal progesterone suppository in women considered to be high risk for preterm delivery.[39] The use of vaginal progesterone has also been shown to reduce the risk of preterm delivery in women with a diagnosis of short cervix on routine sonogram at 20–25 weeks of gestation.[40]

Induction of Labor

NONPHARMACOLOGIC THERAPIES

Amniotomy

Artificial rupture of the membranes, or amniotomy, is a low-cost intervention for induction or augmentation of labor (pharmacologic or surgical interventions to help stimulate contractions and increase the progression of a previously dysfunctional labor). If used alone, it has been associated with a long interval before the onset of regular contractions. Amniotomy is sometimes used when the cervix is favorable. At present, there is insufficient evidence to support its use as the only agent for the induction of labor.[41] When used in combination with oxytocin, the induction to delivery time is shorter when compared with amniotomy alone.[42] Risks associated to amniotomy may include increased risk of chorioamnionitis, prolapse of the umbilical cord, and increased frequency of umbilical cord compression. Amniotomy is contraindicated in patients who are HIV (human immunodeficiency virus) positive.[41]

Hygroscopic Cervical Dilators

Hygroscopic cervical dilators (DILAPAN-S™) (FEMA International, J.C.E.C. Co, Kendall Park, New Jersey) and osmotic dilators (*Laminaria japonicum*) are two of the mechanical dilation methods. The hygroscopic dilators are hydrophilic rods made from a proprietary AQUACRYL drawing fluid from the cervical tissue that cause expansion of the rod, producing cervical softening and dilation. *Laminaria japonicum* are made from the stems of the brown seaweed, which are cut, shaped, dried, and sterilized. The presumed mechanism of action is similar to the hygroscopic dilators: attracting fluid and causing cervical expansion. Compared with *Laminaria japonicum*, the hygroscopic dilators are associated with decreased time to achieve complete dilation (10.8 hours vs. 14.7 hours). In addition, a reduction in the number of devices per patients was reported in the same study.[43] Infection has been described with the use of these agents. Other potential risks include entrapment, breakage, and retraction of the device into the uterus.

Foley Catheter with and Without Extra-amniotic Saline Infusion

The French Foley balloon, extra-amniotic saline infusion (EASI), and the double balloon device (Atad Ripener Device) are effective mechanical cervical dilators.[44] Multiple studies have shown their efficacy. When compared with PGs, they are associated with decreased costs. Other benefits include stability at room temperature and a reduced risk of **hyperstimulation.**[44,45] When compared with oxytocin, mechanical methods are associated with decreased cesarean delivery rate.[44] Possible risks associated with the Foley catheter include the risk of bleeding in patients with undiagnosed low-lying placenta, rupture of membranes, febrile morbidity, and displacement of the presenting part.[46]

Other inexpensive induction methods include membrane stripping and unilateral nipple stimulation. Membrane stripping, or sweeping of the membranes, is a common obstetric practice. Membrane stripping is accomplished by inserting a finger between the membranes of the bag of water and the wall of the uterus to loosen the membranes from the wall. The postulated mechanism of action is thought to be mediated by increased phospholipase A_2 activity and an increase in prostaglandin F_{2a} levels. Reduction in the incidence of induction of labor has been reported.[47] Complications associated with membrane stripping may include bleeding from an undiagnosed placenta previa and accidental amniotomy. The safety of membrane stripping in women with positive group B streptococcus colonization has not been determined. Nipple stimulation is a natural nonmedical method for labor induction. A systematic review of the literature found a significant reduction of women not in labor at 72 hours when low-risk women with favorable cervix nipple stimulation were compared with no intervention. Additional benefit with breast stimulation was a reduction in the risk of postpartum hemorrhage.[48]

PHARMACOLOGIC THERAPIES: INDUCTION OF LABOR/CERVICAL RIPENING AGENTS

Dinoprostone

Dinoprostone, also known as PGE_2, has been used for cervical ripening in numerous forms. Commercially, it is available as a removable, extended release 10-mg vaginal insert (Cervidil®) that releases 0.3 mg/hr for up to 12 hours dosed one time, or as an intracervical gel (Prepidil®) that contains 0.5 mg dinoprostone/dose given every 6 hours for a maximum of three doses in 24 hours.[49,50] Vaginal suppositories (Prostin E_2) have also been used to extemporaneously compound intravaginal gels, although this is no longer routinely done given the availability of commercial products.

Side effects associated with dinoprostone include hypotension, headache, nausea, vomiting, diarrhea, uterine hyperstimulation, with or without fetal heart rate abnormalities, uterine rupture, fever, and back pain. A case series has been published describing three women who experienced anaphylaxis following intracervical administration of dinoprostone.[51]

Dinoprostone has been studied in all forms against each other, oxytocin, misoprostol, and nonpharmacologic methods. A study comparing intravaginal and intracervical dinoprostone in women with an unfavorable cervix at term determined that the intravaginal preparation was more effective at causing cervical ripening and inducing labor than the intracervical compound in two studies.[52,53] The incidence of uterine hyperstimulation appears to be less with the intracervical route.[54] Intracervical dinoprostone has been studied against intracervical Foley catheters alone and along with EASI. An Indian study found more advanced cervical ripening and a shorter intervention to delivery time in the Foley catheter group than the dinoprostone arm.[55] However, in comparing dinoprostone with a Foley catheter or oral misoprostol, all three methods were found to be equally efficacious in inducing labor.[56]

Misoprostol

Misoprostol is a PGE_1 analog that is approved only for prevention of nonsteroidal anti-inflammatory drug (NSAID)-induced gastric ulcers. However, it has been well studied in the obstetric population for pregnancy termination along with mifepristone, and for cervical ripening and labor induction. Misoprostol is used and is effective both orally and vaginally. Misoprostol is significantly less expensive than all forms of dinoprostone, it can be conveniently and easily dosed orally, and it is stable at room temperature, making it potentially a better choice for countries around the globe.

Side effects with misoprostol include diarrhea, abdominal pain, headache, nausea, vomiting, fever, uterine hyperstimulation with or without fetal heart rate abnormalities, and uterine perforation or rupture.[57] There are numerous case reports of uterine rupture with and without a prior uterine incision; therefore, monitoring is essential in all cases. Caution should be used when PGs are given to patients with asthma, hypertension, renal or hepatic disease, cardiovascular disease, seizure disorders, or diabetes.

Misoprostol effectiveness has been compared with placebo, different routes of administration, dosages, and oxytocin. In two studies in which it was compared with placebo, oral misoprostol at doses of 50 mcg and 100 mcg have been shown to be more effective for labor induction after term premature rupture of the membranes.[58,59] The second study compared doses of 50 mcg and 100 mcg with placebo and found no difference between the doses between the treatment groups. Two women in the higher-dose group had uterine hyperstimulation. The multiparous women included in the study did not respond as well to the 50-mcg dose as the primiparas.[59]

Oral misoprostol compared with vaginal misoprostol indicates that vaginal misoprostol may be more effective in producing delivery within 24 hours. Vaginal misoprostol is approximately 3 times more bioavailable than the oral route, leading to reduced requirements.[60] Lower doses of oral misoprostol (50 mcg) require more supplementation of oxytocin than doses of 100 mcg or 200 mcg. The vaginal route tends to cause higher rates of hyperstimulation but less meconium-stained amniotic fluid than the oral route.[61]

Vaginal misoprostol, 50 mcg, was found to be equivalent, with similar induction to delivery times to a low-dose oxytocin infusion (see oxytocin section) in women presenting with ruptured membranes at term.[62] Both groups had similar rates of uterine hyperstimulation. Misoprostol vaginally in doses of 25 mcg and 50 mcg have been compared with one another. The 50-mcg dose yields shorter induction-to-delivery times but causes more hyperstimulation than 25-mcg doses.[63] The dosing interval has also been studied extensively, although there is no consensus as to whether it should be every 3, 4, or 6 hours. In 2002, the U.S. Food and Drug Administration (FDA) approved a new label on the use of misoprostol for cervical ripening and induction of labor. However, it does not stipulate dosing, its safety, or its efficacy. ACOG Practice Bulletin No. 10 concludes that misoprostol at 25 mcg at 3–6 hours is effective for cervical ripening and induction of labor. Higher doses, 50 mcg every 6 hours, may be appropriate in certain situations. Misoprostol is contraindicated in patients with a previous cesarean delivery because of the increased risk of uterine rupture.[18]

Oxytocin

Oxytocin is a nonapeptide hormone secreted from the posterior pituitary. It is normally secreted in a pulsatile manner during labor, increasing in frequency as parturition nears. Oxytocin receptors are located primarily in the fundus of the uterus and increase in number throughout gestation. Activation of these receptors also increases prostaglandin synthesis, another substance known to cause uterine contractions.[64]

Oxytocin is very similar to antidiuretic hormone in amino acid sequence. Excessive doses of oxytocin can lead to water intoxication and hyponatremia, especially when it is mixed in intravenous solutions containing no electrolytes. Oxytocin should always be diluted in normal saline or lactated Ringer solution to prevent hyponatremia from occurring. Other adverse effects of oxytocin include hypotension when given by rapid intravenous injection and uterine tachysystole or hyperstimulation. Management of tachystole usually involves discontinuation of the oxytocin infusion and administration of a tocolytic agent, such as the betamimetic terbutaline, if needed.

Oxytocin can be mixed as a 10-units/L standard infusion, although more concentrated infusions can be made for fluid-restricted patients. Oxytocin in a concentration of 200 units/L has been studied for immediate use after compounding.[65] Oxytocin infusions are dosed in milliunits/min and can be divided into low-dose and high-dose protocols. Low-dose protocols typically start at an infusion rate of 1–2 milliunits/min and increase by 1–2 milliunits/min every 15–60 minutes. High-dose protocols instead start at 4–6 milliunits/min and increase by the same every 15–30 minutes. Maximum doses of oxytocin rarely exceed 40 milliunits/min. Traditionally, high-dose protocols have involved more intense nursing and monitoring but show a faster induction to delivery time and lower cesarean section rates over low-dose protocols. A more recent publication suggests that the total labor length may be shorted with high-dose protocols, but the cesarean section rate does not appear to differ.[66] Intravenously infused oxytocin has a half-life of approximately 3 minutes.[14] ACOG supports the use of either low- or high-dose protocols when proper precautions are met. Oxytocin is infused to titrate a dose to effect, and each woman's response to the dose may be different and therefore can not be predicted. High-dose protocols are associated with more tachystole and may be used in multiparous women.[1]

The Institute of Safe Medication Practices (ISMP) considers oxytocin a high-alert medication. Oxytocin, dosed incorrectly, can cause significant harm to the mother and fetus, including fetal demise. Oxytocin requires safeguards to reduce the risk of administration errors. Potential ways to reduce these risks would be to limit access to oxytocin infusions, using auxiliary labels, standardized concentrations and ordering, and additional checks from other automated or independent resources.[67]

TOCOLYTICS FOR PRETERM LABOR

Magnesium Sulfate

Despite a lack of data supporting efficacy, magnesium sulfate is utilized as first-line therapy in many institutions for the treatment of preterm labor. Magnesium inhibits myometrial contractions by inhibiting the influx of calcium into cells. It can be given intramuscularly, but most commonly it is administered as a continuous intravenous infusion. Generally, magnesium is started as a loading dose of 6 g over 15–30 minutes and followed by a continuous infusion of 2–4 g/hr. Contraction frequency should

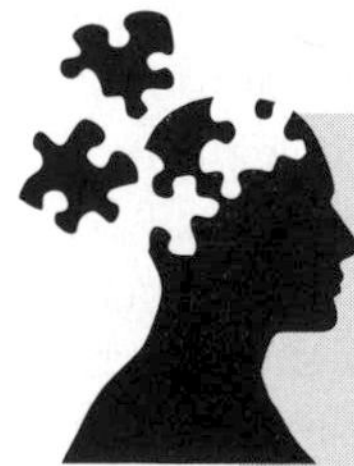

Therapeutic Challenge:

R.G., a 19-year-old G3P0201, presents to clinic for obstetric care. She is currently 18 weeks of gestation. Her past medical history is significant for two prior preterm deliveries at 28 and 23 weeks of gestation. The plan of care is discussed with the patient, and she inquires if there are any interventions available that could reduce her risk of preterm delivery.

guide the upward or downward dosing titration of magnesium. The goal is to achieve less than six contractions/hr.[68]

Magnesium side effects are extensive for both the woman and fetus. Common adverse reactions include a general feeling of warmth, flushing, diaphoresis, blurred vision, nausea, weakness, and slurred speech. Difficulty in retaining and comprehending information, chest tightness, and pulmonary edema have also been reported. Fetal/neonatal complications of magnesium therapy include decreased fetal heart rate variability on cardiotocography, loss of muscle tone at birth ("floppy infant"), poor suckling, and respiratory depression of the neonate. Long-term magnesium use has lead to case reports of bone demineralization in the newborn as well as osteoporosis in the mother.[69,70]

Magnesium is eliminated exclusively through the kidneys. It is imperative to monitor urine output for women on this therapy. Women with underlying renal impairment should have either a smaller loading dose if given at all or a decreased rate of the continuous infusion. Anuric women should receive only a loading dose with no maintenance infusion.[71] Magnesium serum levels >8 mg/dL can cause a loss of deep tendon reflexes, electrocardiograph changes, weakness, hypotension, respiratory depression, asystole, coma, and death. The ISMP considers magnesium sulfate to be a high-alert medication.[67] There are significant risks to the mother with magnesium overdoses. Practices that may help reduce this risk include standardizing dosing by using protocols, performing a double check with an independent resource, monitoring the patient frequently, and having calcium gluconate readily available when a woman is receiving magnesium sulfate.

Recently, the efficacy of magnesium and its potential harmful effects has raised the question as to whether magnesium should be used at all for tocolysis.[72] Large clinical trials and a Cochrane data review have not shown a benefit of magnesium over no treatment, placebo, or other tocolytic agents (Table 28-2).[73,74] Some studies have shown harm to the fetus or neonate from exposure to magnesium, especially when standard dosing regimens have been used.[72] However, others have not shown adverse

Table 28-2. Tocolytic Agents

	Side Effects		
Agent	**Maternal**	**Fetal or Neonatal**	**Contraindications**
β-Adrenergic-receptor agonists	Tachycardia, chest pain, palpitations, atrial fibrillation, shortness of breath, pulmonary edema, hypotension, apprehension, restlessness, emesis, headache, tremulousness, hallucinations, insomnia, hyperglycemia, hyperinsulinemia, hypokalemia, lactic acidosis or ketoacidosis	Tachycardia	Maternal cardiac disease, poorly controlled diabetes mellitus
Magnesium sulfate	Flushing, diaphoresis, nausea, loss of deep tendon reflexes (at doses of 10 mEq/L = 12 mg/dL), respiratory depression (>10 mEq/L), respiratory paralysis and arrest (≥12 mEq/L)	Loss of heart rate variability on cardiotocography, loss of muscle tone at birth ("floppy infant"), poor suckling, and respiratory depression of the neonate	Myasthenia gravis
Calcium-channel blockers	Dizziness, flushing, hypotension, headaches, nausea, hepatotoxicity, myocardial infarction		Hypotension, preload-dependent maternal cardiac disease
Cyclo-oxygenase inhibitors	Gastritis, gastrointestinal bleeding, potential platelet dysfunction	In utero (premature) closure of ductus arteriosus, necrotizing enterocolitis, intraventricular hemorrhage, oligohydramnios	Platelet dysfunction or bleeding disorder, hepatic or renal dysfunction, gastrointestinal or ulcerative disease, asthma

effects to the fetus, neonatal, or infant.[73] Until further randomized clinical trials are available, the general consensus is to discontinue the use of magnesium for preterm labor.[72,74]

Addendum

More recently, magnesium's neuroprotectant effect on the fetus has been recognized and this may become the primary use for this agent in women at less than 32 weeks of gestation. Several trials performed in the U.S. and worldwide have shown a decrease in the rate of substantial gross motor dysfunction and cerebral palsy in infants who were exposed to magnesium prior to delivery.[109] The number needed to treat to prevent one case of cerebral palsy appears to be 63, with an even lower number when only very early gestational ages are involved (<28 weeks). The studies reviewed were very heterogeneous, leading many more questions than answers as far as how to dose the agent, the correct duration, and whether one exposure is enough or does the therapy need to be given immediately before delivery.

Beta-Adrenergic Receptor Agonists

Beta agonists work by increasing levels of cyclic adenosine monophosphate (cAMP), ultimately lowering levels of intracellular calcium and preventing activation of contractile proteins. Ritodrine was the first and only agent to be approved for the treatment of preterm labor. The oral formulation was removed from the market in 1995 voluntarily after a large study failed to find overall improvement in perinatal morbidity and mortality or preterm delivery rates. Today, terbutaline is the most common agent in this class, and it will be the only agent discussed.

Terbutaline can be given orally, typically at dosages of 5 mg every 4–6 hours, subcutaneously at doses of 0.25 mg, or intravenously at doses of 0.125 mg. Subcutaneously, it can be initially dosed every 20–30 minutes for up to four doses. If successful, it can be continued every 3–4 hours until uterine quiescence is achieved for 24 hours. Doses should be held if the maternal heart rate exceeds 130 beats/min. Subcutaneous terbutaline is occasionally administered continuously via an infusion pump with a basal rate, scheduled boluses, and rescue boluses. Scheduled bolus doses can occur every 2–4 hours and are scheduled according to when the woman is having the most contractions. Side effects of terbutaline include tachycardia, chest pain, palpitations, shortness of breath, hypotension, apprehension, restlessness, emesis, headache, tremulousness, hallucinations, and insomnia. The incidence of side effects with subcutaneous terbutaline occur in approximately 15% of patients, with the most frequently reported severe reaction being pulmonary edema.[75] Atrial fibrillation has also been reported.[76] It can also induce metabolic changes, such as hyperglycemia, hyperinsulinemia, hypokalemia, and lactic or ketoacidosis. There is a higher rate of tachyphylaxis associated with terbutaline given orally over other routes.

The Cochrane Database of Systematic Reviews reported that all beta-agonist randomized trials, including ritodrine, showed that fewer women delivered within 48 hours after starting therapy when compared with no treatment.[77] However, this meta-analysis did not show a reduction of preterm deliveries (<37 weeks). Only two trials used terbutaline, and both compared it with ritodrine. Despite the fact that the beta agonists can prolong pregnancy, they do not reduce the perinatal morbidity and mortality associated with preterm delivery.[74]

Subcutaneous terbutaline has been studied in women with recurrent preterm labor. The first large study followed women with twins who were treated first with oral terbutaline, followed by subcutaneous terbutaline when oral therapy failed. Pregnancy was prolonged by an average of 7.6 weeks over the reported 5 weeks reported for placebo.[78] A smaller, case-control study evaluated women who received a subcutaneous terbutaline infusion after successful tocolysis using magnesium sulfate.[79] Significantly, more women in their control group delivered before 32 weeks as compared with more than half of the terbutaline group delivering after 37 weeks. This evidence suggests that use of subcutaneous terbutaline therapy may be helpful in prolonging pregnancies in women at high risk for preterm delivery, such as in the case of twins or recurrent preterm labor. Other larger trials have not shown benefit to using terbutaline infusions.[80]

Calcium Channel Antagonists

Nifedipine is the only calcium channel antagonist to be studied for preterm labor. It works directly on calcium channels, blocking calcium entry through the cell membrane, which inhibits activation of contractile proteins. Nifedipine can be given as sole tocolytic therapy or as maintenance therapy following intravenous magnesium. Caution should be exercised when using nifedipine in close proximity to magnesium, as significant hypotension, other major cardiac effects, and neuromuscular blockade can occur.[74]

Nifedipine can be used at an initial loading dose of 10 mg every 15–30 minutes for up to 40 mg followed by 10 mg or 20 mg every 4–6 hours. Some studies have used sublingual therapy, which has since been banned. Sublingual nifedipine has been shown to cause significant hypotension, which has led to fetal distress, myocardial infarction, and death.[81] If used for maintenance therapy, nifedipine should be started following the discontinuation of magnesium sulfate to reduce the risk associated with double tocolysis. Nifedipine and magnesium sulfate both are calcium antagonists, which can lead to an increased hypotensive effect.[82] Side effects of nifedipine are generally mild and include dizziness, flushing, hypotension, headaches, nausea, hepatotoxicity, and myocardial infarction. Symptoms can be exacerbated with cytochrome P450 3A4 inhibitors.

A recent publication compared nifedipine with magnesium sulfate.[68] The authors found little differences between the groups, although more women receiving magnesium delivered after 48 hours, and their infants had longer durations of stay in the neonatal intensive care unit. Of those women who were successful with nifedipine tocolysis, the duration to uterine quiescence was shorter, and there were significantly fewer mild and major side effects than with the magnesium group.[83]

Nonsteroidal Anti-inflammatory Drugs

NSAIDs, such as indomethacin and sulindac, have been studied for the inhibition of preterm labor, although not as extensively as other agents. The NSAIDs are known inhibitors of cyclo-oxygenase (COX). There are two COX isoforms: COX-1, which is present in myometrial tissue, decidua, and fetal membranes; and COX-2, which is also present in these tissues, but the amount increases significantly in women who are in labor, either preterm or term.[74] NSAIDs are nonspecific inhibitors of both COX-1 and COX-2 and hence have been studied for the treatment of preterm labor.

Indomethacin is often loaded with a dose of 50–100 mg followed by 25 mg orally every 6 hours. Side effects of indomethacin and other NSAIDs include gastritis, gastrointestinal bleeding, and potential platelet dysfunction. The more important side effects occur in the fetus and neonate. Premature closure of the ductus arteriosus, necrotizing enterocolitis, intraventricular hemorrhage, and oligohydramnios are all reported side effects of the agents. A study of 124 women using indomethacin for prolonged periods, though, suggests that these effects are less common than previously thought.[84] They did not find any connection between duration of therapy and constriction of the ductus arteriosus or oligohydramnios. Most healthcare providers still use a maximum duration of 48–72 hours of therapy and restrict use to gestational ages <32 weeks because of these concerns.

Of the NSAIDs studied, indomethacin has been shown to increase pregnancy duration and reduce preterm births.[73] A recently published meta-analysis included 10 trials, of which three were compared with a placebo arm, and there was reduction of preterm birth <37 weeks with a relative risk of 0.21 (CI, 0.07–0.62). Unfortunately, no difference was reported in perinatal mortality, respiratory distress, or intraventricular hemorrhage.[85] Sulindac was thought to be less problematic, because it must be metabolized to become an active drug. It was believed that only the prodrug could cross the placenta and was not metabolized by the fetus; this is now known to be incorrect. Sulindac was studied against placebo as maintenance therapy following magnesium sulfate tocolysis. The overall response was equal in the two groups, with similar rates of women delivering after 34 weeks of gestation.[86]

The selective COX-2 inhibitors celecoxib and rofecoxib have both been studied. Celecoxib 100 mg orally every12 hours was compared with indomethacin for the initial treatment of preterm labor. Either therapy was given for 48 hours or until delivery.[87] Close attention was paid to ductal velocity, which increased significantly with indomethacin, indicating ductus arteriosus constriction, and amniotic fluid index during the study period. A significant decrease in amniotic fluid volume from baseline was seen with both groups at 48 hours. However, the fluid had reaccumulated by 72 hours. There were no other differences between the two groups. Rofecoxib, which has now been removed from the U.S. market, was compared with magnesium tocolysis.[88] This much-larger study found a similar rate of success between the two groups, with more side effects in the women treated with magnesium.

Additional Agents

Other tocolytic agents being evaluated include oxytocin receptor antagonist and nitric oxide donors. Several oxytocin receptor antagonists have been studied, but by far the most studied is atosiban. In a recent meta-analysis of six trials comparing atosiban vs. placebo or with other tocolytic agents, atosiban did not reduce the incidence of preterm birth or improve neonatal outcomes when compared with placebo, was associated with lower birth weight, and was associated with an increase in infant death in the first year of life.[89,90] Given the negative associations with atosiban, the FDA has not approved its use for the prevention of preterm labor.

Nitric oxide donors, with the prototype being nitroglycerin, have been evaluated as possible tocolytic agents. The basis of nitric oxide donors use comes from observations in animals; human data have been contradictory, therefore making its clinical use controversial.[91] The Cochrane Database of Systematic Reviews found that nitroglycerin offered no delay in delivery or improvement in neonatal outcomes when compared with placebo, no treatment, or other tocolytics and is not routinely used in obstetrics today.[91]

INDUCTION OF FETAL LUNG MATURITY: ANTENATAL CORTICOSTEROIDS

Betamethasone and dexamethasone are both potent corticosteroids used to accelerate fetal lung maturation in women experiencing preterm labor before 34 weeks of gestation. Corticosteroids are thought to stimulate lung maturation by affecting type II pneumocytes, ultimately increasing the production of surfactant and increasing lung compliance and lung volume.[92] Betamethasone is dosed at 12 mg intramuscularly every 24 hours for two doses, whereas dexamethasone is given in 6-mg doses every 12 hours for four doses. In an attempt to hasten dosing when delivery seems imminent, some healthcare providers have dosed betamethasone in 12-hour increments instead. A retrospective review evaluated the outcomes of neonates born to women who delivered before 48 hours after receiving their initial betamethasone dose.[93] There were no differences between the neonates who delivered within 24 or 48 hours, even when mothers only received one dose of betamethasone.

Corticosteroids have been shown to reduce the incidence of neonatal demise, respiratory distress syndrome, and intraventricular hemorrhage.[94] This therapy has been determined to lessen the need for respiratory support, lower the total time on a ventilator, reduce the need for oxygen, and require less surfactant treatment. When women delivered before 24 hours, there was no reduction in respiratory distress syndrome or intraventricular hemorrhage as compared with those who delivered within 48 hours after the first dose.[94] There may be differences in outcomes between betamethasone and dexamethasone.[95] Trends toward a decrease in intraventricular hemorrhage, retinopathy of prematurity, and neonatal deaths have been seen with betamethasone compared with dexamethasone. However, both were effective in reducing the risk of respiratory distress syndrome and severe intraventricular hemorrhages. Hence, betamethasone is the preferred corticosteroid, if available, with dexamethasone as an acceptable alternative.

Many early trials seem to indicate that the benefit of corticosteroids on respiratory distress syndrome does not last beyond 7 days after the first dose, leading to a practice of weekly dosing.[94] This has been all but abandoned, as animal data began to show decreased birth weights, brain sizes, and increased adrenocortical activity.[96] In humans, decreased head circumferences and lower birth weights have been seen in patients receiving multiple courses of steroids (two or more).[95] Neonates had a higher risk of infection if they received multiple courses of steroids following premature rupture of the membranes. At this time, multiple courses are not recommended for routine preterm labor. However, extenuating circumstances, such as extreme prematurity at first course (<26 weeks), may justify repeating corticosteroids in some cases.

Complications of Labor and Delivery

Following the delivery of the fetus, complications can be encountered in the mother. Postpartum hemorrhage describes the excessive bleeding that is sometimes encountered and can follow a vaginal or cesarean delivery. Traditional definitions of postpartum hemorrhage have defined the amount of blood lost following a vaginal delivery as 500 mL or more and 1,000 mL or more following cesarean delivery. Identifying the cause of the bleeding is paramount in deciding the optimal treatment.

NONPHARMACOLOGIC THERAPIES

The most common cause of postpartum hemorrhage is uterine atony, or failure of the uterus to contract properly following delivery. The initial approach to the management of a patient with uterine atony is to begin with fundal massage. This consists of manual stimulation to the fundus of the uterus through the patient's relaxed abdomen muscles. If this does not result in uterine contraction, one can also perform a bimanual uterine compression by massaging the posterior aspect of the uterus with a hand on the abdomen while a fist placed in the vagina massages the anterior uterine aspect.[14] If these measures do not control the hemorrhage, pharmacologic therapy must be employed. Typically, if simple fundal massage does not control the bleeding, uterotonics will be requested, and while waiting for them to arrive, the attendant can perform a bimanual uterine compression.

UTEROTONICS FOR POSTPARTUM HEMORRHAGE

Oxytocin

Traditionally, oxytocin has been used either in the active management of the third stage of labor or given routinely following delivery of the placenta for prevention of postpartum hemorrhage in conjunction with effective uterine massage. It is considered the first-line agent in treating uterine atony. Oxytocin is most often added to intravenous fluids, 20 units in 1,000 mL of lactated Ringer or normal saline at approximately over 1 hour (333 milliunits of oxytocin/min).[14] Oxytocin may also be given intramuscularly or intramyometrially at a dose of 10 units. There are no postpartum contraindications for the use of oxytocin, but oxytocin should never be given as an undiluted bolus, as dangerous hypotension or cardiac arrhythmias may occur.[14] When compared with no treatment, oxytocin has clear benefits, leading to fewer postpartum hemorrhages <500 mL, and reducing the need for further oxytocic treatments.[97] There may also be an increased rate of manual removal of the placenta following delivery when oxytocin is not used along with other active management strategies, such as gentle umbilical cord traction.

Methylergonovine

Methylergonovine, or methylergometrine, is an ergot alkaloid used for the prevention and treatment of postpartum hemorrhage as a second- or third-line agent. Ergots directly stimulate the uterine muscles, increasing contractile strength. It is normally given in 0.2-mg doses intravenously or intramuscularly, including directly into the myometrium, repeated in 2- to 4-hour intervals if needed. It may also be followed by oral therapy of 0.2 mg every 6 hours for at least 24 hours following to extend the contractile effect. The intramuscular route should be used rather than the intravenous route, as it can result in dangerous hypertension and cerebrovascular accidents. It is contraindicated in patients with hypertension, especially preeclampsia. It should be used with caution in patients with heart disease, sepsis, and hepatic or renal dysfunction. It has also been known to cause myocardial ischemia and infarction in some patients.[98] Side effects that can occur with methylergonovine include abdominal cramping, nausea, vomiting, diarrhea, diaphoresis, headache, dizziness, and bradycardia or tachycardia.

Methylergonovine has been compared with both oxytocin and misoprostol for the third stage of labor. In comparison to 5 units oxytocin, dosed either at the delivery of the baby or placenta in a bolus or infusion fashion, methylergonovine 0.2 mg dosed in the same fashion was not as effective at preventing postpartum hemorrhage.[99] This result was significant only when examining the bolus dose of oxytocin immediately following delivery of the fetus. When studied against 600 mcg oral misoprostol, methylergonovine was shown to be just as effective but less convenient in dosing because of the injectable nature of the agent.[100]

Carboprost

Carboprost is 15-methyl $PGF_{2\alpha}$, a prostaglandin analogue that is used for second- or third-line pharmacologic therapy in controlling postpartum hemorrhage. It can be given intramuscularly or directly into the wall of the uterus, intramyometrially, at a dose of 250 mcg. Doses can be repeated every 15–90 minutes. It is contraindicated in patients with active cardiac, pulmonary (including asthma), hepatic, or renal disease. However, it can be given to women who are hypertensive. Side effects of carboprost include nausea, vomiting, diarrhea, cramping, and backache.

Rectal misoprostol was compared with intramuscular carboprost in a study of 120 women from India.[101] Women received either 400 mcg misoprostol or 125 mcg carboprost immediately following delivery. Oxytocin was administered only if the estimated blood loss was 500 mL or greater. There was the need for further therapy in more women in the misoprostol group when compared with carboprost, but this did not reach statistical significance. Side effects were primarily gastrointestinal, affecting the carboprost group most notably. The authors concluded that these therapies were comparable for active management of the third stage of labor.

Misoprostol

Misoprostol has been used for prevention and treatment of postpartum hemorrhage and may be a first-line agent in developing countries, where storage, cost, and route of administration are important issues. Misoprostol has been used orally, sublingually, vaginally, and rectally at doses ranging from 400 mcg to 1,000 mcg. A pharmacokinetic study in early pregnancy evaluating three routes of administration found the sublingual route to provide the highest peak concentration, the oral and sublingual route affording similar times to peak concentrations, and the vaginal route provided the longest duration, although with a similar AUC (area under the curve) to oral therapy.[102] The rectal route is similar to the vaginal route, although the peak is significantly lower than with either the oral or vaginal route.[103] During the third stage of labor, small amounts of misoprostol can be seen in the serum at <10 minutes with both oral and rectal misoprostol, although the peak occurs on average at 18 minutes with oral therapy and at 40 minutes with rectal.[104] The rectal route leads to higher doses for a longer period, which may help prevent recurrent hemorrhage; however, the faster time to peak with oral therapy may be preferable in emergent situations. The vaginal route in the treatment of postpartum hemorrhage is not very feasible, with blood loss likely washing away the drug before absorption can occur.

Misoprostol has been compared against oxytocin for both prevention and treatment of postpartum hemorrhage. Oral misoprostol at a dose of 400 mcg compared with 5 units of oxytocin within 1 minute of delivery yielded more misoprostol women requiring oxytocin, but there was no significant difference in total drop in hematocrit associated with either group.[105] The same dose given sublingually was compared with 20 units of oxytocin as an intravenous infusion in cesarean section patients. The groups were comparable in results, although significantly more side effects, such as shivering, pyrexia, and a metallic taste, occurred in the misoprostol group, like the previous study.[106] However, in large meta-analyses, misoprostol seems to be associated with higher blood losses at delivery (>500 mL), but not severe hemorrhages (>1,000 mL), when compared with traditional oxytocics. Oral misoprostol consistently produces more side effects than other routes of administration, such as nausea, vomiting, diarrhea, shivering, severe shivering, and pyrexia.[107] A subanalysis of studies comparing rectal with other methods of misoprostol administration found that rectal administration was associated with a higher use of other oxytocics.[108] This may be due to the later peak associated with rectal dosing and other agents used before misoprostol's therapeutic effect taking place.

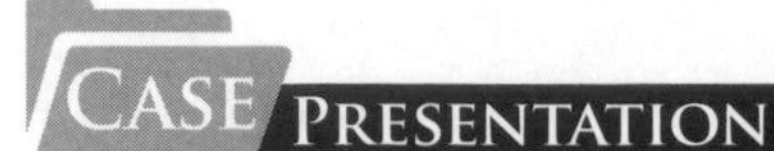

Patient Case: Part 2

Assessment: T.K.'s obstetrician discusses the risks associated with an elective induction of labor.

Treatment plan: After further consideration, T.K. opted to delay induction for another week and wait for spontaneous labor.

Patient education: T.K. needs to be counseled on all the signs and symptoms of early labor. She will need additional support as her gestational period exceeds 40 weeks.

Patient monitoring: Once weekly pelvic exam until delivery.

Summary

Many physiologic changes occur during the pregnancy. The uterus and the cervix must undergo a transition from quiescence with retention of the fetus to expulsion of a fetus at term. Extreme variations in the timing of labor may increase maternal and fetal morbidity. In this chapter, we have discussed the pharmacologic interventions currently available to delay preterm delivery, accelerate fetal lung maturation when delivery is inevitable, assist with elective induction of labor at term, or prevent postpartum hemorrhage immediately after birth. The goal of interventions in modern obstetrics is to decrease maternal, fetal, and neonatal morbidity and mortality. Much work remains to be explored in this field.

References

Additional content available at
www.ashp.org/womenshealth

29 Postpartum Care

Charlie C. Kilpatrick, MD; Manju Monga, MD

Learning Objectives

1. Understand the normal physiologic adaptations to the postpartum period, including changes to the uterus, cardiovascular system, and urinary tract.
2. Describe complications associated with breast-feeding and treatment methods for them, both pharmacologic and nonpharmacologic.
3. Compare and contrast appropriate antihypertensive medications commonly used in the postpartum period for persistent hypertension.
4. Discuss birth control options, postpartum initiation of birth control, and the effects of these on breast milk production.
5. Distinguish between the normal and abnormal postpartum psychological reactions, and explain how to identify postpartum depression.

The 6 weeks after the delivery of an infant has been referred to as the puerperium. Postpartum women will undergo a number of physical and emotional changes. There are also medical problems that are unique to this period. This chapter will review the management of women postdelivery as the body begins to recover from pregnancy.

Clinical Presentation

The postpartum period is classically defined as the 6 weeks that follow the delivery of the infant. It is also referred to as the puerperium, derived from the Latin *puer,* meaning "child," and *pario,* meaning "to bring forth." Significant physical changes take place during this time.

At term, the human uterus can weigh as much as 1,100 g and impinge on the inferior border of the rib cage.[1] Within 24–48 hours of delivery, the uterus involutes to the level of the umbilicus because of constriction of the myometrial cells. Its size returns to the prepregnant state in approximately 8 weeks. In an ultrasound study by Mulic-Lutvica et al., the uterus in its greatest A/P diameter was approximately 9 cm on the day of delivery and decreased to 3–4 cm by day 56.[2] This was also accomplished with a rotation of the uterus around the internal os by 100–180 degrees. The rapid involution of the uterus decreases blood flow to the placental site, limiting bleeding at the time of delivery. The involution of the placental site with subsequent regeneration of implantation site endometrium typically takes 6 weeks, and the postpartum bleeding pattern mirrors this regenerative process.[3] At its zenith, uterine blood flow is 400–600 mL/min, with a decrease noted immediately postpartum. Using pulsatility index to look at uterine blood flow, Tekay and Jouppilla were able to demonstrate a significant increase in uterine vascular resistance by day 2 postpartum.[4]

An enormous increase in cardiac output is seen in the postpartum period. Three factors account for this increase: autotransfusion of uteroplacental blood, release of the venocaval obstruction by the gravid uterus, and mobilization of extravascular fluid.[5] The return of cardiac output, stroke volume, and systemic vascular resistance to prepregnant values may take longer than first postulated.[6]

The renal system does return to its prepregnant state by 6 weeks, with a return to normal of renal plasma flow, creatinine clearance, and glomerular filtration rate.[7] The actual size of the kidney and collection system may take longer to return to prepregnant values.

At the 6-week postpartum visit, women should be asked a number of questions. The amount of bleeding, or lochia, at this point should be minimal. Initially after delivery, the bleeding is bright red and referred to as lochia rubra, which can last 3–4 days. This is composed of mainly blood and decidual cells. For the next 2–3 weeks, the lochia becomes pale and watery and is referred to as lochia serosa,

Case Presentation

Patient Case: Part 1

A 19-year-old Hispanic woman, pregnant for the first time, presented to the hospital at term reporting a headache. She said that the headache started that morning and was unrelieved with Tylenol. She had no history of headaches and no significant past medical history.

HPI: Six weeks ago, she was admitted to the hospital and underwent a long induction after it was discovered that she had **severe pre-eclampsia.** She developed intra-amniotic infection, delivered vaginally, and was treated for **endomyometritis.** She went home on postpartum day 3 and presents now for her first postpartum visit. She is tearful and reports having had little sleep lately. She is frustrated, feels overwhelmed with having to take care of the infant, and feels she is doing "nothing right."

PMH: Unremarkable.

Family history: She had no family history of headaches. Her mother had been diagnosed with depression, for which she takes a medicine she obtained from Mexico, and her father has hypertension. She is unsure of the medical history of her siblings.

Social history: She is unemployed, and recently came to America from Mexico to live with the father of the baby. She is not married, and this has caused her family much anxiety. She is living with a cousin because she has had some difficulty with her partner. Living conditions are not ideal, and there are six people living in a two-bedroom apartment.

Medications: She takes no medications and has no known drug allergies.

Lab results: Within normal limits.

Physical exam: On physical exam, she is normotensive, afebrile, and not tachycardic. She is alert and oriented times three, but has a sad disposition and is tearful. Before beginning the physical exam, she tells you that she has had a rough postpartum course. She has not been sleeping well, even when the infant is asleep. Her interest in daily activities is minimal, and she is very tired. She has moved in with the father of the infant, and his parents are helping with childcare issues. She says she has been breast-feeding, but initially she had difficulty with milk production and then developed an infection. She even has a picture of what her breast looked like. You look at the picture and make out the redness around the areola and how this seems to spread along the medial breast tissue (Figure 29-1). She went to the emergency room because her breast was red, swollen, and tender, and she was having fevers. She was given antibiotics, and the infection, which she was told was called **mastitis,** went away. She was going to bottle-feed, but she has run out of the formula that was given to her and cannot afford any more, so she is breast-feeding again. On physical exam, her lung and cardiac exam is within normal limits, her abdomen is nontender, and her breast exam is without evidence of infection, with normal-appearing breasts. Vaginal exam shows normal external female genitalia, parous introitus, and well-healed laceration on the perineum; bimanual exam reveals that the uterus is of normal size, and no adnexal masses are palpated.

followed by a yellowish-white lochia alba. This usually lasts about 40 days and is often shorter in the parous woman.[8]

Breast-feeding is another question to address at this visit. Breast-feeding has been shown to provide numerous short- and long-term advantages to the infant compared with bottle-feeding. Gastrointestinal growth and function is promoted by breast-feeding. Also, the incidence of acute illness is lower in the breast-fed infant when compared with the bottle-fed infant, likely because of the immunoglobulins and other antimicrobial components contained in breast milk.[9] Long-term advantages include associations between children breast-fed and a decreased incidence of obesity and childhood cancer.[10,11] There is also some association between breast-fed infants and future cognitive development, but these studies are not as definitive.

Figure 29-1. Picture of mastitis revealing redness around the areola and medial breast tissue.

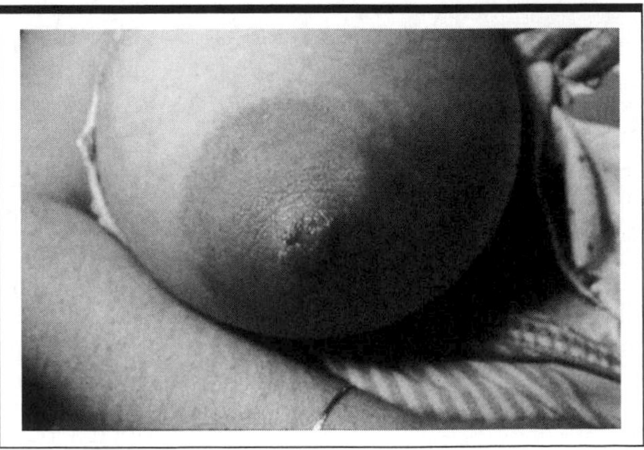

There are numerous maternal benefits from breast-feeding, including quicker weight loss postpartum, more rapid subinvolution of the uterus, and partial protection against pregnancy. Breast-feeding is less expensive than formula and promotes bonding between mother and infant. Breast-feeding leads to a high prolactin levels, which cause a negative feedback on the gonadotropin-releasing–hormone pulse generator in the hypothalamus, thereby inhibiting ovulation. Regular breast-feeding (every 4 hours during the day and 6 hours at night, without the use of formula supplementation) within the first 6 months of delivery can provide a natural form of birth control. Kennedy and Visness, in a review of 346 women, were able to show that consistent breast-feeding without supplementation for the first 6 months postpartum was associated with a life table pregnancy rate of 0.7/100 women.[12] With supplementation, the pregnancy rate was similar to other typical modern contraceptive use at 6 and 12 months.[12] The consistent use of breast-feeding, especially in the early postpartum, should be encouraged to all mothers. Breast-feeding complications can occur and should be recognized.

Engorgement of the breasts is not uncommon and usually resolves with correct feeding, full emptying of the breast, and antiinflammatories. In a Cochrane review, Snowden and colleagues found serrapeptase and bromelain/trypsin complex to be efficacious in alleviating pain.[13] Little data exist on the concentration of these medications in breast milk. The long-term effect of these medications on growth and development in the newborn is unknown. There is usually some tissue edema associated with engorgement, so the use of warm compress can sometimes worsen the condition. Sometimes a plugged duct can cause pain and even be confused with infection. A warm shower may promote letdown and even unclog the duct. If there is no relief within 48–72 hours, then physician consultation should be sought.

Mastitis is infection of the breast tissue. Symptoms are similar to a plugged duct, with the addition of fever and erythema to the tissue. Treatment consists of fully emptying the affected breast, antiinflammatories (as mentioned above), and antibiotics (dicloxacillin 500 mg 4 times a day for 10–14 days).[14] If complete emptying is not assured with feeding, breast pumping after feeding to ensure complete emptying may help. Some women are under the impression that feeding from the affected breast is harmful to the infant, but it actually facilitates resolution of the infection. If the symptoms do not improve or worsen, admission to the hospital for parenteral antibiotics may be necessary, and a thorough exam to exclude an abscess should be undertaken.

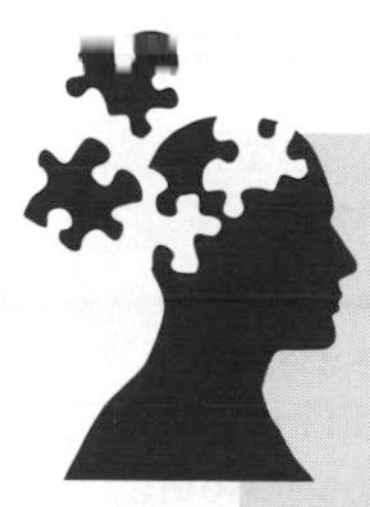

Therapeutic Challenge:

Devise a study to look at the effects of oral contraceptive pills on breast milk production and venous thromboembolism. What would be your end points? What other factors would you consider?

Consistent breast-feeding in the postpartum period is not always feasible, especially for the working mother, so other forms of contraception should be addressed, ideally before discharge from the hospital.

Contraceptive options are numerous. In the breast-feeding woman, nonhormonal contraceptive options including condoms, copper intrauterine devices, and other barrier methods. Permanent sterilization should be considered. These forms of contraception have no effect on the quality or quantity of breast-milk production. When choosing hormonal contraception methods, progesterone-only contraception, such as depot medroxyprogesterone acetate injection and progestin-only tablets, does not decrease breast-milk quantity or quality.[15] The new etonogestrel implant, Implanon, is similar with regards to breast-milk production. There are two theoretical concerns in regards to progesterone-only contraceptive methods. Immediately postpartum, the progesterone level declines, which is thought to be necessary to initiate lactation. Administration of progesterone during this time may affect the initiation of lactation. Also, exposure to high levels of progesterone, especially injectable medroxyprogesterone acetate, when the newborn has little ability to break down these products, has prompted others to wait to initiate these medications until at least 3 weeks postpartum.

The quantity of breast-milk production in combination pill users vs. progesterone users is less, although in this study, there was no effect on the infant's weight regardless of the amount of breast milk produced.[15] Also, there is the concern of increasing the risk of venous thromboembolism at a time when the risk is already high because estrogen in the combination pill increases thrombogenic factors. Neither of these two concerns has been addressed

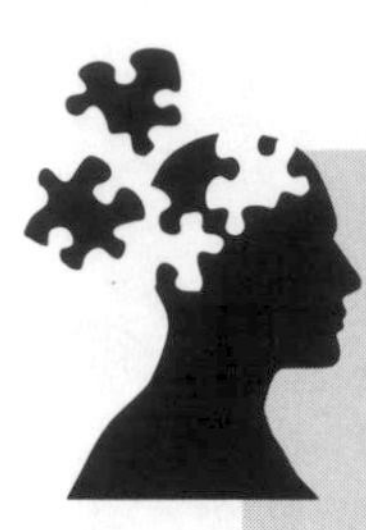

Therapeutic Challenge:

What antihypertensive medications should be begun in those patients with persistent hypertension in the postpartum period? How long should they be continued?

in a randomized controlled trial.[16] Combination oral contraceptive pills also cause a slight increase in blood pressure. Those patients with gestational hypertension or pre-eclampsia in the antenatal period should have their blood pressure checked to ensure they are normotensive before initiating combination oral contraceptive pills.

Currently, the American College of Obstetricians and Gynecologists recommends waiting 2–3 weeks for oral progesterone-containing contraception and 6 weeks to resume combination oral contraceptive pills or injectable depot medroxyprogesterone acetate.[17] Individualized care should be taken, as some women have little access to healthcare. Balanced with the theoretical concerns presented above, administering progestational agents before discharge from the hospital may be the only way to ensure a reliable form of contraception in these women.

Postpartum Depression

Vegetative signs of postpartum blues are difficulty sleeping, crying, and frustration. These symptoms do not appear in every woman, and there are no conclusive data to explain them. Some have theorized that these symptoms are from the abrupt withdrawal of progesterone that occurs postpartum.[18] Usually these symptoms will abate by 2 weeks postpartum, but if they continue or get worse, the patient may be depressed. The prevalence of postpartum depression is similar to that of depression in the nonpregnant state: 5% to 6%.[19] This systematic review by Gavin and colleagues pointed out that their results must be interpreted with caution, as the confidence intervals were large, the heterogeneity within individual studies was small, and the tools used to diagnose depression varied. They also admitted that their estimation of the prevalence of postpartum depression was lower than in other studies because they used stringent diagnostic criteria rather than self-report scores.[19] Attention must be paid to factors that may put the patient at greater risk for depression in the postpartum period. Risk factors for postpartum depression are listed in Table 29-1.

PATHOPHYSIOLOGY

The underlying pathophysiology behind postpartum depression is similar to depression in the nonpregnant state. Also, there is interplay of genetic susceptibility, hormonal changes, and stressful life events. Because the underlying cause of postpartum depression is not well understood, it is important to be aware of risk factors and the signs and symptoms used to make the diagnosis.

DIAGNOSIS

The diagnosis of postpartum depression is similar to diagnosis in the nonpregnant state, with the realization that some of the signs and symptoms are similar in a normal postpartum woman. Insomnia, frustration, and crying are all normal behavior in the immediate postpartum period. It is when these symptoms begin to fill the entire day or carry on longer than should be expected that concern is warranted. Other symptoms that may be more specifically linked to postpartum depression are the following: excessive weight loss, complete lack of energy or appetite, intense feelings of guilt or anger, anxiety or panic attacks, and poor maternal/infant bonding. Andersson and colleagues followed more than 200 women during and after pregnancy and found fatigue or loss of energy and diminished interest in daily activities to be the two most common symptoms of postpartum depression.[20] Before more recent research, there were some who believed that the incidence of depression was greater in the postpartum period, possibly linked to the sudden change in hormone levels. This could be true in a

Table 29-1. Risk Factors for Postpartum Depression

- Personal history of depression and/or anxiety
- Depression and/or anxiety during pregnancy
- Stressful life events
- Poor social support
- Marital strife
- Low socioeconomic status

subset of women.[21] The onset of the disease in the postpartum state is most common within the first 3 months postpartum, and the postpartum state itself does not lend itself to an increase in the diagnosis compared with the antenatal state.[22,23] In this cohort, the diagnosis of depression was more common during pregnancy than the postpartum period.

PRIMARY PREVENTION

Prevention of postpartum depression should be considered in those with a prior history of postpartum depression or depression in the nonpregnant state. These women should be seen sooner after delivery, at 2 weeks, and screened for the disease.[24] Use of the Edinburgh Postnatal Depression Score (EPDS) is a good screening tool for evaluating women in the postpartum period at risk for depression and has been validated.[25] Little success in preventing postpartum depression has been made. Intensive counseling by a mental health professional may improve depressive symptoms and decrease the rate of depression, but hasn't had great success. Cognitive behavioral treatment, aimed at reducing symptoms by targeting and modifying negative patterns of thinking and behavior, was recently evaluated in a randomized controlled trial. Its success, measured by a decrease in EPDS scores, was not proven when compared with an information booklet.[26] Pharmacologic interventions aimed at preventing postpartum depression have been equally unsuccessful and lacking in number. In a prospective fashion, Wisner and colleagues evaluated 22 women with a history of postpartum depression and randomized them to placebo vs. sertraline for the 17 weeks that followed childbirth.[27] Only one of the sertraline-treated women had a relapse compared with four in the placebo, so there could be some promise in pharmacotherapy, but obviously larger numbers are needed to make a recommendation currently.

TREATMENT GOALS

Goals of treatment are to improve maternal/infant bonding, prevent marital strife (which can be a consequence or risk factor for postpartum depression), prevent infanticide and suicide in the mother, and improve maternal functional ability. Infants of mothers with postpartum depression are more likely to have behavioral and cognitive problems. Improving the mood of the mother may positively affect each of these problems.

Nonpharmacologic Treatment

Psychosocial therapy for the treatment of postpartum depression has shown good results, especially in women with mild symptoms. O'Hara et al., in a randomized controlled trial, showed 12 weeks of interpersonal therapy improved depression self-assessment scores, but there was little change or measure of maternal/infant bonding and marital relationship.[28] Other nonpharmacologic interventions are group therapy and cognitive behavioral therapy. In a review of 15 trials with 7,900 women, Dennis could not pinpoint an intervention that reduced the number of women diagnosed with postpartum depression.[29] There was some evidence to support the use of intense postpartum support by trained individuals in reducing the symptoms of depression. Most of the success has come with pharmacologic therapy.

Pharmacologic Therapy

Pharmacologic therapy should be considered in those patients with more than minor depression symptoms and in those who fail to respond to nonpharmacologic therapy. In the non–breast-feeding woman, the medication choices used to treat postpartum depression are similar to the nonpregnant state and are based on a number of factors, including previous response to a particular antidepressant, interactions with other medications, and the side-effect profile of the medication in light of her symptomatology.

Based on all the available literature on breast-feeding and the use of selective serotonin reuptake inhibitors (SSRIs), all of the SSRIs are excreted into the breast milk at some level. Sertraline and fluvoxamine seem to have the lowest excretion rates, with paroxetine somewhat higher, and citalopram and fluoxetine the highest.[30] There are no long-term studies to discuss the effect of these medications on the future growth and development of the infant. In these cases, monitoring the infant to look for signs/symptoms of adverse medication reactions is crucial.

Other medications, such as venlafaxine or duloxetin (a serotonin/norepinephrine reuptake inhibitor), have had little study in the literature, with only case series in the former and nothing concerning the latter. Bupropion (a dopamine reuptake inhibitor) levels were studied in breast milk and infant plasma, and high levels in the breast and low levels in the plasma found.[31] Tricyclic antidepressants are usually used in postpartum depression in those women refractory to SSRIs or if they have documented previous favorable

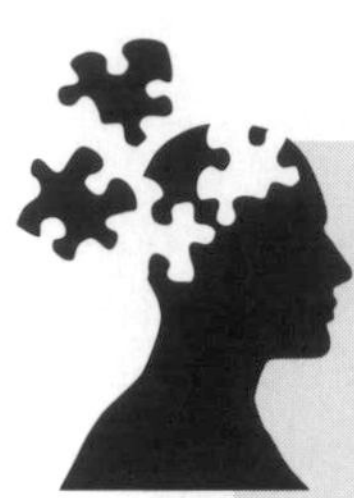

Therapeutic Challenge:

What SSRI would you give a woman with newly diagnosed postpartum depression who is currently breast-feeding? A woman with postpartum depression, previously treated successfully with fluoxetine, presents concerned about breast-feeding and taking her SSRI. What would you advise her?

response to them. Little information in the literature exists to provide recommendations concerning long-term effects on growth and behavior.

MONITORING AND FOLLOW-UP

Monitoring of the patient after medications have been started is crucial and should be undertaken by a trained professional. Follow-up intervals are based on the symptoms and overall well-being of the patient. In general, after beginning medication, the patient should be seen within 2 weeks and from there based on the progress of the individual. Frequent visits and even hospitalization may be necessary in severe cases.

PATIENT EDUCATION

Patients should be counseled on what to expect after starting medications in relation to their disease course and the side-effect profile of the medication. In general, improvement should be seen between 2 and 6 weeks. If no improvement is manifested by this time, then another agent is warranted, and referral to a psychiatrist to help in this decision should be made. During this time, it is important to provide the woman with a reliable form of birth control to prevent pregnancy.

Summary

The puerperium is a time of incredible change for a woman, both physiologically and psychologically. The benefits of breast-feeding to mom and the new infant should be discussed before delivery and precautions given for potential complications. Persistent hypertension in the postpartum state is not uncommon, with little good literature available to provide guidance. Better studies are needed on this subject to determine the best treatment options. There are a plethora of birth control options available, and the choice should be tailored to each individual's needs,

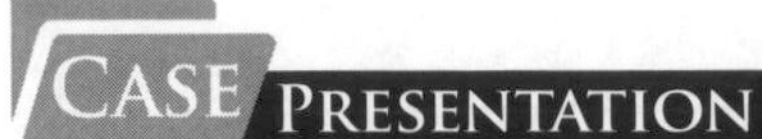

Case Presentation

Patient Case: Part 2

Assessment: After the exam, you talk to the patient in your office. She does not have the infant with her; her mother-in-law is watching him. You ask her whether she is glad that her mother-in-law is watching the infant, and she is, as she gets really frustrated at home while trying to feed and care for the baby. You ask her about her sleeping, and she admits that she has been sleeping very little since delivery, even when the infant is sleeping and the house is quiet. She has not been eating well, has lost weight, and tells you that she doesn't like the taste of the food. After hearing all of this, you are concerned that she is depressed.

Patient education: When you begin to tell her that she is depressed, she begins to cry. She tells you that her mother was depressed when she was young. You try to reassure her by explaining that it is a disease much like any other disease, and there is no reason to feel ashamed. You explain that postpartum depression is common and that she is not alone. You consider using nonpharmacologic therapy, but her symptoms seem to be too severe, and you are worried that she would not be able to attend all of the counseling sessions.

Treatment plan: In discussion with her, you decide to begin a medication that will improve her mood and initially decide on an SSRI. Selective serotonin reuptake inhibitors have been well studied in the treatment of depression and have a low side-effect profile compared with other medications.[32] She is concerned about breast-feeding with the use of the medication, and you reassure her that you are choosing a medication with the lowest breast milk excretion ratio.

Plan is for her to take sertraline 25 mg PO every morning, to increase the dosage by 25 mg increments every 2–3 days as tolerated. Your goal is to increase to a dosage of 100 mg a day, with a maximum of 200 mg a day. You counsel her that it may cause some insomnia, so you give her a prescription for some trazodone 25 mg to be taken at night to help sleep. You also counsel her that there is little evidence on long-term effects of these medications on growth and development of the child, but their excretion in breast milk is low. She is reluctant to begin the medicine at first, but you convince her that her symptoms should improve.

Patient monitoring: In 2 weeks, she returns and she feels somewhat better. She brought the infant with her, and she admits that she has been sleeping and eating better. She reports occasional episodes of tearfulness but not as much as before, and you encourage her to continue the medication. She does report that she was a little jittery at first, but that has subsided. She inquires as to how long she should take the medication, and you let her know that 9 months of therapy would be ideal. You also let her know that she should begin to see a psychiatrist to follow up with her and let her know that continuing to take the medication on a consistent basis is the key.

Because it has been longer than 6 weeks, you discuss with her the need for a form of contraception and, after a lengthy discussion, decide on oral contraceptive pills. You let her know when to begin them, and she seems reassured that she has made the right choice and will see the psychiatrist you recommend.

taking into account her desire for future childbearing and whether she is currently breast-feeding. Postpartum depression can affect maternal/infant bonding, and awareness of symptoms and risk factors for its development is crucial.

References

Additional content available at
www.ashp.org/womenshealth

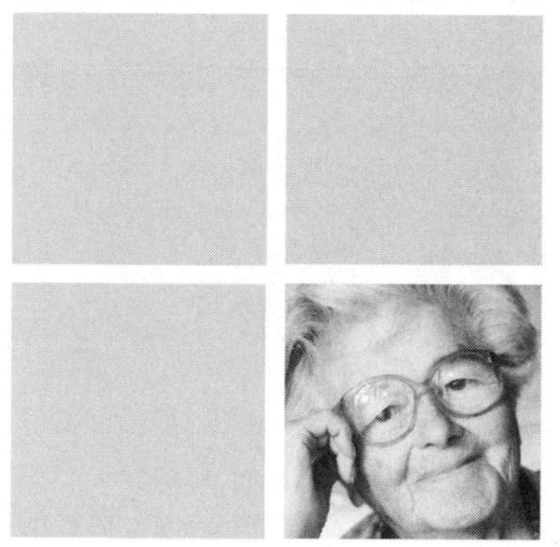

SECTION SIX

Selected Conditions in Women

30 Cardiovascular Disease

Anne L. Hume, Pharm.D., FCCP, BCPS; Lisa B. Cohen, Pharm.D., CDE

Learning Objectives

1. Describe sex disparities in the prevention and treatment of cardiovascular diseases.
2. Assess the potential effects of estrogens alone or in combination with a progestin on the cardiovascular system and on major risk factors for cardiovascular disease.
3. Compare the major clinical trials of hormone therapy on cardiovascular outcomes, and resolve the disparate findings from observational studies and the Women's Health Initiative.
4. Educate health professionals and postmenopausal women regarding the potential cardiovascular effects of hormone therapy using an evidence-based approach.
5. Assess the overall cardiovascular risk status of women, and identify issues with standard assessment instruments.
6. Demonstrate an understanding of the management of major cardiovascular risk factors for the primary and secondary prevention of cardiovascular disease in women, and develop an appropriate treatment plan.
7. Identify potential differences in the pathophysiology, clinical presentation, and management of coronary heart disease, heart failure, and atrial fibrillation in women as compared with men.
8. Discuss common adverse drug events involving the cardiovascular system in women.

One in every three adult women in the U.S. has cardiovascular disease.[1] In 2004, an estimated 460,000 women died from cardiovascular diseases, including **coronary heart disease,** stroke, and heart failure. By comparison, breast cancer killed approximately 40,500 women in the same year.[1] Although 42 million American women have cardiovascular disease, many more are at risk because of increasing rates of obesity, diabetes mellitus, and physical inactivity. Black women are at high risk of cardiovascular disease, and their death rates from coronary heart disease are almost 30% greater than those of white women.[1] These staggering numbers emphasize the need for effective strategies for the prevention and treatment of cardiovascular disease in women. This chapter covers four areas, including sex disparities and research issues; estrogen, cardiovascular system, and hormone therapy; evaluation and management of major cardiovascular risk factors; and evaluation and treatment of common cardiovascular diseases in women.

Sex Disparities

Between 1980 and 2000, the age-adjusted death rate from coronary heart disease declined for both men and women. For women, the death rate decreased from 263.3 to 134.4 deaths per 100,000, whereas among men, the rate dropped from 542.9 to 266.8 deaths per 100,000.[2] Further advances in decreasing death rates in women are dependent on appropriate assessment and management of risk factors as well as aggressive treatment of established cardiovascular disease.

Studies have shown that women do not receive high-quality care, ranging from cholesterol screening and adherence to the recommendations of the National Cholesterol Education Program (NCEP) to the use of coronary angiography and angioplasty.[3-5] Although research has focused primarily on sex disparities in the management of cardiovascular disease in the inpatient setting, reports from large managed care organizations have demonstrated that sex disparities also exist in the ambulatory management of women who have cardiovascular disease or who are at significant risk of cardiovascular disease.[6,7] One study of managed care plans demonstrated that women were less likely than men to achieve a low-density lipoprotein (LDL) cholesterol goal of <100 mg/dL, with the largest disparity among women with coexisting diabetes and cardiovascular disease.[7]

Sex disparities in the management of heart failure have been identified with women with systolic heart failure less likely to receive anticoagulation for concomitant atrial fibrillation, education on heart failure management, and implantable cardioverter defibrillator than

Case Presentation

Patient Case: Part 1

R.F. is a 51-year-old black woman who is in clinic today. Her concerns are focused on her increasing difficulty in sleeping. She reports awakening in the middle of the night and being soaking wet. She has tried a few of her husband's sleeping pills (zolpidem 10 mg) but without relief of her difficulty in sleeping. She tells you that she's confused about estrogen and other hormones, but her older sister's severe hot flashes and sleeping problems were cured by hormones.

PMH: Chronic obstructive pulmonary disease × 5 years, hypertension × 7 years, dyslipidemia × 2 years, diet-controlled type 2 diabetes × 1 year, severe gastroesophageal reflux disease (GERD), hypothyroidism, depression, G5/P4, a history of a deep venous thrombosis (DVT) following the birth of her last child 11 years ago.

PSH: Hysterectomy at age 43.

Family history: Father died of cancer at age 63, mother had diabetes and died of myocardial infarction at age 53; an aunt developed breast cancer at age 63; several aunts have sustained hip fractures.

Social history: Married for 30 years; two daughters and two sons are alive and well; cigarette smoking 1PPD × 35 years; occasional glass of wine.

Medications: Amlodipine 10 mg daily, albuterol inhaler one puff twice daily, salmeterol/fluticasone 50/250 mcg inhaler twice daily, recent addition of niacin (Niaspan®) 500 mg daily, levothyroxine 0.2 mg daily, omeprazole 40 mg twice daily, vitamin E 400 International Units daily, and desipramine 25 mg at bedtime.

Allergies: NKDA.

Review of systems: Difficulty in sleeping through the night; frequent awakenings of feeling hot and sweaty; GERD symptoms are frequent.

Vitals: 5'3", 185 lb; BP 145/91; HR 77; Temp 98°F; RR 16.

Physical exam: Normal, with R.F. fanning herself and asking if anyone else is "really hot" today.

Laboratory values: Significant findings include fasting plasma glucose 128 mg/dL, total cholesterol 215 mg/dL, LDL 149 mg/dL, HDL 30 mg/dL, TG 180 mg/dL, serum creatinine 0.7 mg/dL, A1C 7.7%.

men.[8] The use of angiotensin-converting enzyme (ACE) inhibitors, angiotensin receptor blockers (ARBs), beta-blockers, and aldosterone antagonists was similar between men and women.[8] Results from the Acute Decompensated Heart Failure National Registry (ADHERE) indicate that women had similar use of intravenous diuretics and in-hospital mortality rates but were less likely to receive vasoactive therapy and procedure treatments.[6]

Fewer women are also offered revascularization after admission for an acute myocardial infarction. Only 20% of women compared with 32% of men were offered this intervention in one study.[9] Several factors contribute to this finding in that women were less likely to be referred to a hospital capable of revascularization.[10] Women are also less likely to receive beta-blocker therapy after a myocardial infarction.[7] Disparities in the use of cardiac ablation for atrial fibrillation and implantable cardioverter-defibrillators for the prevention of sudden cardiac death have also been reported.[11,12]

The causes of these disparities are multifactorial. In a study of 300 primary care physicians, 100 cardiologists, and 100 gynecologists, intermediate-risk women were perceived to be at lower cardiovascular risk than men even when their calculated Framingham risk scores were similar. The gynecologists provided primary care services to approximately 67% of their patients, yet they believed they were unprepared to address the risk of heart disease in women.[13] Gynecologists also recommended antioxidant vitamins to prevent cardiovascular disease, contrary to national guidelines.[13]

Women's own perception of their cardiovascular health may contribute to their undertreatment. The Health Belief Model proposes that patients will seek treatment for an illness if they perceive that they will have negative consequences if they do not search for a solution to their problem.[14] Women may not seek treatment because of a perception of a decreased severity of their illness. In one study of **acute coronary syndrome,** women had an increased symptom burden, lower physical functioning because of cardiac disease, and a lower health status compared with men. However, women rated their cardiovascular disease as less severe than the men enrolled in the study.[15] The American Heart Association's program, Go Red for Women, may be useful in changing women's beliefs about individual risks, as well as those of their primary care providers.[16]

Sex-Related Issues in Cardiovascular Research

The conduct and dissemination of high-quality research is the foundation of evidence-based practice. The best example of research challenging traditional beliefs to improve the care of women is the Women's Health Initiative (WHI).[17,18] Before this study and the Heart and Estrogen/progestin Replacement Study (HERS), an accepted "truth" was that estrogen therapy alone or in combination with a progestin prevented coronary heart disease in women.[19,20] Only after the release of findings from HERS and WHI did healthcare providers question the true value of estrogen therapy for the **primary** and **secondary prevention** of cardiovascular disease in postmenopausal women.

The inclusion of women into research funded by the National Institutes of Health (NIH) has been required since 1986, unless a clear reason exists to exclude them. An analysis of large federally funded cardiovascular studies conducted between 1965 and 1998 reported that the number of women participating has increased over time.[21] This has been due to the funding of studies such as WHI, which only included women. When these studies are excluded, the enrollment of women into cardiovascular studies has remained unchanged, at about 38% of the study samples. The enrollment of women into studies of heart failure has continued to be about 25% and focused on left ventricular dysfunction (systolic heart failure), which is less common among women.[21] A recent follow up of this prior analysis identified that the enrollment of women into phase 3 and 4 clinical trials of cardiovascular disease funded by the National Heart, Lung, and Blood Institute (NHLBI) remains low, despite concerted efforts during the recruitment period.[22] Approximately 27% of the NHLBI-funded study samples consisted of women compared with an estimated 53% of people with cardiovascular disease actually being women.[22]

Adequate numbers of women must be included in clinical trials to ensure that results may be applied to the broader population and that there is sufficient power to analyze results by sex. Finding the balance between a homogenous study sample to identify the efficacy of an intervention and one that includes diverse individuals at risk of a given disease is difficult. Traditionally, fewer women have been enrolled in studies, in part because cardiovascular diseases are less common in women than in men of a similar age.

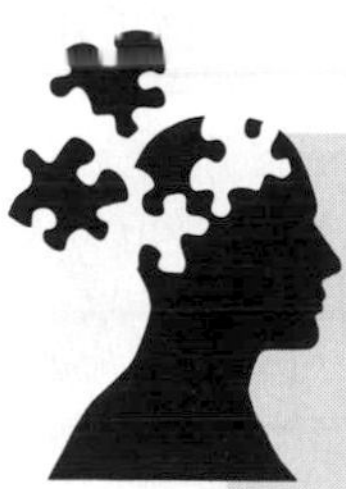

Therapeutic Challenge:

What are unique challenges in recruiting women into clinical trials of cardiovascular disease? Should funding agencies require enrollment of sufficient numbers of women into clinical trials to establish valid sex-specific recommendations regarding drug therapy? Should peer-reviewed journals require sex-specific analyses of all cardiovascular research studies that include both men and women?

Women are older than men when they are diagnosed with cardiovascular disease and have more comorbid illnesses, such as diabetes. Advanced age and comorbid conditions are common reasons for exclusion from randomized clinical trials, resulting in insufficient numbers of female participants.[23]

Although women must be included into NIH-funded studies, publication of sex-specific data is not required. An analysis of 628 cardiovascular studies published in major journals in 2004 reported that only 153 presented sex-specific results. The NIH-funded studies reported sex-specific results in 51% of studies as compared with 22% of studies not funded by the government.[24] When sex-specific findings are presented, women may be reported as failing to achieve a benefit from the intervention. This finding may also be due to insufficient power to detect a difference rather than a true differential response. Subgroup and post hoc analyses should be interpreted with caution, as the benefit from randomization may have been lost unless the separate analyses were preplanned.

Estrogen and Cardiovascular System

Men and women differ in many respects to the cardiovascular system. In general, women have smaller hearts, most likely the result of their smaller body size, and a higher resting heart rate.[25] The stroke volume may be slightly smaller; however, with the increased heart rate, the actual cardiac index is similar between men and women.[25] The length of the cardiac cycle is shorter in women and may vary throughout the menstrual cycle. Girls and boys have similar QT interval lengths until puberty, when women begin to develop longer rate-corrected QT intervals that are due to slower cardiac repolarization.[26] The lumen of coronary arteries in women may be smaller, although wide variability exists. Collateral circulation may be less in women than in men.[25] Blood pressure has been reported to vary during the menstrual cycle in women of reproductive age and was the highest with the beginning of the follicular phase in one small study.[27]

ESTROGEN RECEPTORS

Estrogens have complex effects on the heart and the vasculature. Estrogen causes rapid vasodilation mediated through several mechanisms. Calcium-activated potassium channels are stimulated in vascular smooth muscle cells, and nitric oxide synthetase is released by endothelial cells.[28,29] Estrogen also has longer-term effects that are mediated through activation of one or both estrogen receptors (ER-α and ER-β). Both receptors are present in many tissues and serve as transcription factors. When estrogen and growth factors bind to these receptors, gene expression is altered. Growth factors bind to the receptors when local estrogen concentrations are low, as in postmenopausal women. Many coactivator and corepressor proteins are involved in the processes controlling gene expression.[28,29] Vascular smooth muscle cells, endothelial cells, and myocardial cells contain ER-α (and ER-β) in both men and women. The ERs activate multiple genes responsible for regulating vascular tone and the response to vascular injury and atherosclerosis. The effects on vasodilation may be through gene-mediated effects on formation of prostacyclin synthetase and nitric oxide synthetase. Estrogens increase endothelial cell growth after vascular injury, potentially by increasing the release of vascular endothelial growth factor.[30] In vitro, estradiol has been shown to inhibit the **apoptosis** of cultured endothelial cells. Smooth muscle proliferation may be inhibited, as well as many other effects.[31] In summary, estrogen protects the vasculature by inhibiting the growth of vascular smooth muscle cells and stimulating the regrowth of endothelial cells, especially after injury.

The effects of estrogen on the vasculature may differ in younger women in the menopause transition compared with older women who have pre-existing atherosclerosis. In younger women, estrogen's effects to induce **matrix metalloproteinases** may maintain the size of the vessel lumen in early atherosclerosis.[28,29] The development of atherosclerosis after the menopause may potentially be slowed by improving normal endothelial function and the lipid profile. In older postmenopausal women who already have atherosclerosis, the increased activity of matrix metalloproteinases may result in degradation of extracellular matrix and erosion of an existing plaque. This may result in rupture of the plaque and an acute thrombotic event, such as a myocardial infarction.[28,29] Research has increasingly focused on the finding that ER-α and ER-β polymorphisms exist, and the presence of specific variants of ER-α may contribute to the disparate cardiovascular responses to estrogens.[29,30]

OTHER PHYSIOLOGIC EFFECTS

Blood Pressure

Systolic and diastolic blood pressures increase in women as they age, especially after 50 years. This effect may be due to the estrogen deficiency that occurs after the menopausal transition. Although the synthetic estrogens in oral contraceptives may increase blood pressure in women of reproductive age, estrogen therapy has had varied effects on blood pressure in postmenopausal women. In WHI, systolic blood pressure was increased by only 1 mm Hg with estrogen therapy alone or in combination with medroxyprogesterone and is not clinically important. Diastolic blood pressures were unchanged.[17,18] Data from the Baltimore Longitudinal Study on Aging, an observational study, indicated that postmenopausal women taking hormone therapy for more than 10 years had only a 7.6 mm Hg increase in systolic blood pressure compared with an 18.7 mm Hg increase among similar women not taking hormones.[32]

Lipoprotein Concentrations

Lipid and lipoprotein concentrations may change during the menopausal transition. Total and LDL cholesterol concentrations rise, whereas the cardioprotective high-density lipoprotein (HDL) concentrations may decline. Estrogens have multiple effects on lipid and lipoprotein concentrations that depend on the specific compound, dosage, and route of administration. Transdermal estrogen formulations have fewer effects of lipid and lipoprotein concentrations. The addition of progestins may influence the lipid effects of estrogens, depending on their degree of androgenicity with the more androgenic agents decreasing HDL cholesterol concentrations.[33]

Low-Density Lipoprotein Cholesterol

Oral estrogens generally decrease LDL cholesterol concentrations by up-regulating apolipoprotein B-100 receptors. Conjugated equine estrogens 0.625 mg daily alone or combined with medroxyprogesterone decreased LDL cholesterol by 12% in WHI.[17,18] Similar to other lipoproteins, LDL contains different subfractions. Estrogens may decrease the larger particle LDL subfractions because of an increased clearance rate of these particles from the plasma; the amount of the potentially more atherogenic, small, dense LDL subfraction is unchanged.[34]

High-Density Lipoprotein Cholesterol

Oral estrogens generally increase HDL cholesterol concentrations by decreasing its metabolism by hepatic lipase and increasing the synthesis of **apolipoprotein A1**. Oral conjugated equine estrogens 0.625 mg daily increased HDL cholesterol by 14% in women in WHI.[18] In comparison, the concomitant use of medroxyprogesterone with conjugated equine estrogens increased HDL cholesterol concentrations by only 7.3%.[17]

Triglycerides

Oral conjugated equine estrogens may increase triglyceride concentrations primarily through increased synthesis of very-low-density lipoproteins. In WHI, triglyceride concentrations increased by 22% with estrogen alone, and by 6.9% over placebo when combined with medroxyprogesterone.[17] Transdermal formulations of estrogens do not significantly affect triglyceride concentrations.

Hemostasis and Thrombosis

Oral estrogens and progestins such as gestodene have multiple effects on the coagulation and fibrinolytic systems. These actions depend on the specific compound, dosage, and route of administration. Oral estrogens, through their effects on the liver, may produce small increases in factor VII and XII, whereas protein C, protein S, and antithrombin III concentrations are decreased. Plasminogen activator inhibitor-1 (the major inhibitor of tissue-type plasminogen activator) and fibrinogen may also be decreased by oral estrogens.[29] Oral estrogens may also reduce platelet aggregation. Transdermal estrogen products generally have less effect on the coagulation system.[35] A case-control study of women using oral and transdermal estrogen products reported the risk for venous thromboembolism was 4.2 (95% CI, 1.5–11.6) and 0.9 (95% CI, 0.4 –2.1), respectively, compared with nonusers.[35] When oral estrogens are first initiated, the procoagulant effects may predominate. In HERS, thromboembolic events, including DVT, were more common in women taking hormone therapy during the first 2 years of the study and declined thereafter.[19]

The risk of venous thromboembolism is also increased with the use of combined oral contraceptives, especially products containing desogestrel or gestodene. The risk of thromboembolism with these progestins is 2- to 2.5-fold greater than with levonorgestrel.[35,36] The presence of hypercoagulable states, such as **factor V Leiden deficiency** and prothrombin G20210A mutation, exponentially increase the risk of thromboembolic events with oral contraceptives.[35-37] The risk of thromboembolism with estrogen therapy is also two- to threefold greater than placebo.[18,35-39] Factor V Leiden deficiency also increases the risk of thromboembolism with estrogen therapy.[36,37] Although micronized progesterone does not increase the risk of thromboembolism, the evidence with medroxyprogesterone is conflicting, with some data indicating an increased risk when used in combination with estrogen therapy.[35,36,38] Although clinical trials have demonstrated a two- to fourfold increased risk of thromboembolism with estrogen therapy alone or with a progestin, the actual absolute risk for such an event should be considered. The reported risk translates into an increase in the number of thromboembolic events from 34 events annually per 10,000 women using estrogen therapy alone vs. 16 events per 10,000 women not using estrogen therapy.[37,39]

Therapeutic Challenge:

Why do transdermal estrogen products have fewer effects on lipid and lipoprotein concentrations? What are the major types of progestins, and how do they differ in their effects on lipid and lipoprotein concentrations?

Hormone Therapy

At the beginning of the 21st century, one out of almost every two postmenopausal women was receiving hormone therapy.[40] Usage grew rapidly in the 1980s as observational studies suggested a 40% reduction in the risk of coronary heart disease among women using estrogen therapy. During the 1990s, estrogen therapy alone or in combination with a progestin was an accepted option for the primary and secondary prevention of coronary heart disease in women. The therapy was included in clinical guidelines, such as the 1993 second report of the NCEP and the 1995 American Heart Association scientific statement on preventing coronary heart disease.[41,42] In 1998, beliefs began to change with the publication of HERS, a secondary prevention trial, and the first major clinical trial of hormone therapy.

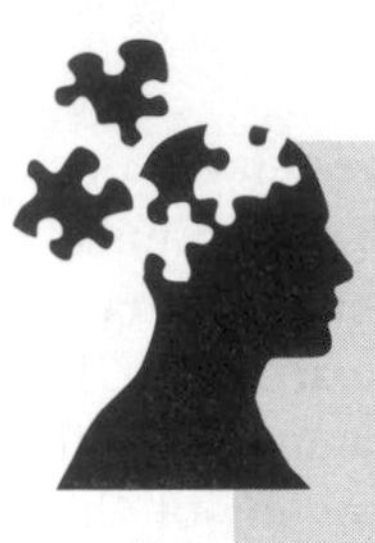

Therapeutic Challenge:

Women's Health Initiative used a global index to assess overall risks and benefits. What were the different components evaluated in this global index, and what were the outcomes for each component?

MAJOR CLINICAL TRIALS

Heart and Estrogen/Progestin Replacement Study

The HERS enrolled 2,760 postmenopausal women with a mean age of 66.7 years and documented coronary heart disease.[19] Hormone therapy consisting of conjugated equine estrogens 0.625 mg and medroxyprogesterone 2.5 mg daily did not have a significant benefit on coronary heart disease, despite women having an 11% decrease in LDL cholesterol and a 10% increase in HDL cholesterol concentrations compared with placebo. Data suggested that coronary heart disease events were declining at the end of the study. In an open-label follow-up study of the women in HERS, the expected decrease in coronary heart disease did not occur.[20]

Women's Health Initiative

Beginning in 1993, the Women's Health Initiative enrolled more than 162,000 postmenopausal women between the ages of 50 and 79 years into clinical trials and an observational study.[17] The WHI study was designed to be a primary prevention study. One clinical trial evaluated the risks and benefits of hormone therapy in 16,608 women without coronary heart disease. The active treatment included conjugated equine estrogens 0.625 mg plus medroxyprogesterone 2.5 mg daily in women who had an intact uterus.[17] Another WHI study of 10,739 women used conjugated equine estrogens 0.625 mg daily in women who had undergone a hysterectomy.[18] Nonfatal myocardial infarction and death that was due to coronary heart disease was the primary outcome measure, and the development of invasive breast cancer was the primary adverse outcome.

The WHI study of combination hormone therapy in women who had an intact uterus was terminated early when the predetermined limit for invasive breast cancer was reached and the global index indicated that risks exceeded benefits. The hazard ratio for coronary heart disease was 1.29 (95% CI, 1.02–1.63) and for stroke was 1.41 (95% CI, 1.07–1.85). These findings represented an additional seven coronary heart disease events and eight strokes per 10,000 person-years associated with the use of hormone therapy. The risk of coronary heart disease was highest in the first year of the study.[43] The estrogen-alone study did not demonstrate a reduction in coronary heart disease.[18] The risk for stroke was increased and represented an additional 12 strokes per 10,000 person-years.

A secondary analysis of WHI evaluated whether trends in the effect of estrogen therapy on coronary heart disease, stroke, total mortality, and global index differed according to age and years since menopause.[44] Data were analyzed by age (50–59 years, 60–69 years, and 70–79 years) and by the time since menopause (<10 years, 10–20 years, >20 years). Women between 50 and 59 years of age did not exhibit an increase in the risk of coronary heart disease or stroke with hormone therapy. Total mortality was actually reduced with hormone therapy compared with placebo in the 50–59 age group, whereas women in the oldest age group did not exhibit this benefit. Women who were <10 years since menopause also had lower risk of coronary heart disease compared with women taking the placebo. Women who were postmenopausal for 20 or more years had a higher risk of coronary heart disease, and the risk was primarily limited to a subgroup of older women with moderate-to-severe vasomotor symptoms. The risk of stroke did not vary based on the number of years since menopause.[44] Of note, more recent data from the WHI clinical trials, along with findings from the WHI observational study, has questioned this "timing" hypothesis for estrogen use.[95,96]

The use of hormone therapy declined rapidly after the release of findings from WHI as the study was widely discussed in the media because of its early termination.[40] Because WHI included healthy women without coronary heart disease, many considered the study to be more applicable to middle-aged and older American women than HERS. Many women discontinued hormone therapy without a clear understanding of the major findings and frequently overestimated the actual risks.

Women's International Study of Long Duration Oestrogen After Menopause

The Women's International Study of Long Duration after Menopause (WISDOM) study is the most recent trial reporting the effects of hormone therapy on cardiovascular outcomes.[45] Before WISDOM was terminated because of the findings of WHI, 5,700 out of the intended 22,000 women had been enrolled and had a mean age of 63. Women were approximately 14 years after menopause, and the median duration of therapy was 11.9 months. Women randomized to hormone therapy had a higher rate of cardiovascular disease and venous thromboembolic disease. Although the findings of WISDOM and WHI were similar, the risk of venous thromboembolism was greater in WISDOM, whereas the risk of cardiovascular disease was lower than in the first year of WHI.

Women's Estrogen for Stroke Trial

Similar to coronary heart disease, early observational studies suggested that estrogen therapy was associated with a decreased risk of stroke in postmenopausal women. The Women's Estrogen for Stroke Trial (WEST) was a randomized double-blind study that evaluated whether oral estradiol in a dosage of 1 mg daily reduced the risk of recurrent ischemic stroke or death in women who had experienced a stroke or transient ischemic attack. Among the 664 women enrolled, 99 strokes or deaths occurred in the women in the estradiol group and 93 in the placebo group.[47] The risk of fatal stroke was significantly higher among women taking estradiol compared with the placebo group.[47] A meta-analysis of 28 studies that included WHI similarly reported an increase in total and more serious ischemic strokes.[48]

Observational vs. Clinical Trials: Why Did the Results Differ?

Since the initial publication of HERS and WHI, investigators have searched for explanations for the discrepancies between observational and clinical studies of hormone therapy. Table 30-1 summarizes the factors potentially contributing to the identified differences.[49,50]

Table 30-1. Possible Explanations for Findings from Major Hormone Therapy Studies

Clinical Trials

- Conjugated equine estrogens used instead of natural estradiol?
- Medroxyprogesterone used instead of natural progesterone?
- Inappropriate dosages and drug regimens used?
- Study population too old
  - In WHI, approximately two thirds of women were >60 years of age, and 21% were >70 years of age
  - Older women may have had subclinical atherosclerosis
- Statistical issues, including differential unblinding due to uterine bleeding
- Decision of the Data Safety Monitoring Board to terminate the study early

Observational Trials

- Overestimated potential benefit due to confounding and compliance biases
- Hormone users were healthier and better educated, had a higher income, and were more adherent to preventive measures than nonusers in cohort studies
- Inadequate controlling for baseline demographic differences
- Inadequate capture of early acute events such as DVT that result in quick discontinuation
  - Women misclassified as nonusers, potentially inflating baseline risk of coronary heart disease among nonusers and overestimating the benefits from hormones among users
- Age from menopause
  - Observational studies include women taking hormone therapy within several years of menopause compared with WHI

DVT = deep venous thrombosis; WHI = Women's Health Initiative.

Source: From references 49–50.

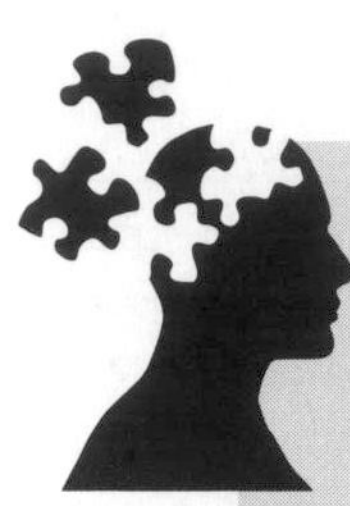

Therapeutic Challenge:

How should the potential cardiovascular risks with hormone therapy be explained to middle-aged women who are in the menopausal transition and interested in using hormones for moderate to severe vasomotor symptoms? How should women be assessed for their potential use of hormone therapy for this purpose?

RECOMMENDATIONS

The major clinical trials and guidelines from professional organizations provide evidence for making decisions about hormone therapy in postmenopausal women. Both the North American Menopause Society (NAMS) and the International Menopause Society (IMS) stress that hormone therapy should not be used for secondary prevention of coronary heart disease in postmenopausal women.[51,52] In addition, cardiovascular risk factors should be aggressively managed with proven therapies for primary prevention. Both organizations indicate the need for further research on the potential role of hormone therapy for primary prevention in younger women who are perimenopausal.[51,52]

In addition to the NAMS and IMS position statements, the American College of Cardiology/American Heart Association (AHA) guidelines on the management of patients with non-ST-elevation myocardial infarction (NSTEMI) also reviewed the available evidence with hormone therapy.[53] The guidelines state that hormone therapy should not be used for secondary prevention in women following NSTEMI. Women taking hormones at the time of the cardiovascular event should discontinue therapy, especially while they are at bed rest. The 2007 AHA guidelines on prevention of cardiovascular disease in women also specifically recommend against the use of hormone therapy for primary and secondary prevention.[54]

In summary, the use of hormone therapy by postmenopausal women has declined significantly as the true risks and benefits emerged as a result of studies such as HERS and WHI. Perhaps the most important lesson learned is that the findings from observational studies, no matter how strong and consistent, are never a substitute for evidence from a well-conducted large clinical trial. The estrogen saga has highlighted the problems with relying on surrogate markers such as improvements in LDL cholesterol concentrations instead of end points such as reductions in the risk of myocardial infarction. Finally, the estrogen saga has also advanced our understanding of the complex interactions of hormones, aging, genetics, and the cardiovascular system of women throughout the life cycle.

Prevention of Cardiovascular Disease

Recent evidence has demonstrated continued declines in the death rate that are due to coronary heart disease both in men and women.[2,55] Although the death rate from coronary heart disease also decreased by 5.4% among women 35–54 years of age between 1980 and 1989, the decline was only 1.2% between 1990 and 1999, and began to increase between 2000 and 2002.[55] Most importantly, concern exists that the death rate may continue to increase given the increasing prevalence of diabetes and obesity among middle-aged women.[55]

Effective prevention strategies require recognition of the diverse causes of cardiovascular diseases. These factors include inflammation, endothelial dysfunction, and thrombosis, among many others. Certain conditions unique to women, such as polycystic ovary syndrome (PCOS) may also increase their risk of cardiovascular disease (Chapter 16: Polycystic Ovary Syndrome). In addition, the use of hormonal contraceptives has been associated with the development of cardiovascular disease in women of reproductive age (Chapter 19: Hormonal Contraception).

CARDIOVASCULAR DISEASE RISKS UNIQUE TO WOMEN

Maternal-Placental Syndromes

Maternal-placental syndromes include infarction of the placenta, **abruption of the placenta**, **preeclampsia**, and hypertensive disorders of pregnancy (Chapter 26: High-Risk Pregnancies). These syndromes are more common in women who have obesity, diabetes, hyperlipidemia, and hypertension before the pregnancy. The Cardiovascular Health after Maternal Placental Syndromes (CHAMPS) study examined whether maternal-placental syndromes increased the risk of premature vascular disease in women.[56] This study was a retrospective population-based cohort of more than 75,000 women with a history of maternal-placental syndromes. The primary outcome was combined cardiovascular disease, including hospitalization for peripheral vascular disease, coronary or cerebrovascular disease, or revascularization. A history of maternal-placental syndromes doubled the woman's risk of developing premature cardiovascular disease.[56]

Another retrospective cohort study reported that women who had developed pre-eclampsia, eclampsia, and gestational hypertension had higher risk of having hypertension later in life.[57] More than 40% of women in the pre-eclampsia, eclampsia, or gestational hypertension groups had hypertension compared with 26.7% in the control group.[58] The incidence of ischemic heart disease and stroke was also higher in women who had pre-eclampsia, eclampsia, or gestational hypertension.[57]

Turner's Syndrome

Turner's syndrome is a genetic disorder in which a woman has only one functional X chromosome instead of the usual two. Women with Turner's syndrome have higher rates of hypertension and cardiovascular disease, as well as a higher mortality rate due to cardiovascular complications such as dissection of the aorta compared with women without this disorder.[59,60] Insulin resistance and elevated LDL cholesterol concentrations with reduced HDL cholesterol concentrations contribute to the development of coronary artery disease.[59] These women frequently have congenital heart defects, such as **coarctation of the aorta** and bicuspid aortic valve dysfunction. As growth hormone is a common treatment in this condition, a woman's blood pressure and echocardiogram should be closely monitored to prevent cardiac complications.[60]

TRADITIONAL CARDIOVASCULAR RISK FACTORS

The management of risk factors for cardiovascular disease, specifically for preventing coronary heart disease and heart failure, requires a comprehensive approach in both men and women. This approach should emphasize a thorough assessment and reduction in overall cardiovascular risk rather than focusing solely on blood pressure measurements or serum glucose concentrations. Table 30-2 lists selected considerations with the use of drug therapy in women for the prevention and treatment of cardiovascular disease.

Table 30-2. Summary of Cardiovascular Pharmacotherapy Considerations in Women

Antiarrhythmic agents	Increased risk of torsades de pointes with ibutilide in women as compared with men; QT prolongation with ibutilide may be more pronounced during first half of menstrual cycle
ACE inhibitors	Risk of cough may be increased in women
	ACE inhibitors did not significantly reduce total mortality from systolic heart failure
	ACE inhibitors use in women and men post-MI with left ventricular dysfunction had a 20% reduction in risk of death and hospitalizations
	ACE inhibitors are considered to be high risk during pregnancy (category C first trimester and category D second and third trimester and should be avoided)
ARBs	Risk of cardiovascular deaths was not reduced in women with systolic heart failure taking ARB, candesartan; but there was a reduced risk of hospitalizations
	ARB are considered to be high risk during pregnancy (category C first trimester and category D second and third trimester and should be avoided)
Beta-blockers	Use of metoprolol after myocardial infarction showed similar reduction of cardiovascular death in both men and women
Digoxin	Women receiving digoxin had an all-cause mortality rate of 33.1% vs. 28.9% receiving placebo potentially due to increase in digoxin toxicity vs. an effect that may be unique to women
Diuretics	
Thiazide	Use may be associated with a decreased risk of osteoporosis; hyponatremia from thiazides may be more common in older women than in men
Loop agents	Use may be associated with an increased risk of osteoporosis
Spironolactone	May cause menstrual irregularity, postmenopausal bleeding, breast tenderness, hirsutism, deepened voice, amenorrhea

(Continued on next page)

Table 30-2. Summary of Cardiovascular Pharmacotherapy Considerations in Women (*Continued*)

Niacin	May worsen vasomotor symptoms if rapid-release formulation used Niacin is pregnancy category C when used in pharmacologic dosages
Statins	May have increased risk of myopathy likely due to advanced age, smaller body size, and/or multiple interacting medications Statins are classified as pregnancy category X and should not be used during pregnancy
Glycoprotein IIb/IIIa	Women are at a higher risk of excessive dosing and a 72% increased likelihood of bleeding with inhibitors excessive dosages
Omega-3 fatty acids	Higher intake was associated with a decrease death of coronary heart disease as compared with women with limited intake

ACE = angiotensin-converting enzyme; ARBs = angiotensin receptor blockers; MI = myocardial infarction.

The 2007 AHA guidelines for the prevention of cardiovascular disease in women include three risk categories.[54] High-risk women include those who have established coronary heart disease, cerebrovascular disease, peripheral vascular disease, abdominal aortic aneurysm, diabetes mellitus, or end-stage kidney disease. In addition, high-risk women are those with a 10-year Framingham risk score >20%. A second category are women who have one or more major risk factors, such as cigarette smoking, or who have evidence of subclinical cardiovascular disease, metabolic syndrome, or poor exercise capacity on treadmill testing. The third category includes women who have a Framingham risk score of <10% and a healthy lifestyle with no risk factors. Interventions to reduce cardiovascular risk include both lifestyle and pharmacologic approaches. The 2007 AHA guidelines for the prevention of cardiovascular disease in women (and the evidence supporting the recommendation) are summarized in Tables 30-3 and 30-4.[54]

Traditional cardiovascular risk factors have included smoking, obesity, diabetes, hypertension, sedentary lifestyle, elevated total and LDL cholesterol concentrations, low HDL cholesterol concentrations, and advanced age, among others.[61] Diabetes, obesity, and dyslipidemias may be more important for women than for men.[61] These risk factors, as well as hypertension, are discussed in the following paragraphs.

Diabetes Mellitus

An estimated 10 million adult American women have diabetes and another 24 million may have prediabetes.[1] Women with diabetes have a 50% increased relative risk of cardiovascular disease than men with diabetes.[24,62] The risk of death that is due to coronary heart disease is greater in women with diabetes than

Table 30-3. Classification and Levels of Evidence for the 2007 American Heart Association Recommendations for Cardiovascular Disease Prevention in Women

Classification	Strength of Recommendation
Class I	Intervention is useful and effective
Class IIa	Weight of evidence/opinion is in favor of usefulness/efficacy
Class IIb	Usefulness/efficacy is less well established by evidence/opinion
Class III	Intervention is not useful/effective and may be harmful
Level of Evidence	
A	Sufficient evidence from multiple randomized trials
B	Limited evidence from single randomized trial or other nonrandomized studies
C	Based on expert opinion, case studies, or standard of care

Source: Reproduced with permission from reference 54.

Table 30-4. Guidelines for Prevention of Cardiovascular Disease in Women: Clinical Recommendations

Lifestyle interventions

Cigarette smoking

Women should not smoke and should avoid environmental tobacco smoke; provide counseling, nicotine replacement, and other pharmacotherapy as indicated in conjunction with a behavioral program or formal smoking cessation program (Class I, Level B)

Physical activity

Women should accumulate a minimum of 30 min of moderate-intensity physical activity (e.g., brisk walking) on most, and preferably all, days of the week (Class I, Level B); women who need to lose weight or sustain weight loss should accumulate a minimum of 60–90 min of moderate-intensity physical activity (e.g., brisk walking) on most, and preferably all, days of the week (Class I, Level C)

Rehabilitation

A comprehensive risk-reduction regimen, such as cardiovascular or stroke rehabilitation or a physician-guided home- or community-based exercise training program, should be recommended to women with a recent acute coronary syndrome or coronary intervention, new-onset or chronic angina, recent cerebrovascular event, peripheral arterial disease (Class I, Level A), or current/prior symptoms of heart failure and an LVEF <40% (Class I, Level B)

Dietary intake

Women should consume a diet rich in fruits and vegetables; choose whole-grain, high-fiber foods, consume fish, especially oily fish[a] at least twice a week; limit intake of saturated fat to <10% of energy, and, if possible, to <7%; cholesterol <300 mg/dL; alcohol intake to no more than 1 drink/day,[b] and sodium intake to <2.3 g/day (approximately 1 tsp salt); consumption of trans-fatty acids should be as low as possible (e.g., <1% of energy) (Class I, Level B)

Weight maintenance/reduction

Women should maintain or lose weight through an appropriate balance of physical activity, caloric intake, and formal behavioral programs when indicated to maintain a BMI between 18.5 and 24.9 kg/m^2 and a waist circumference ≤35 in (Class I, Level B)

Omega-3 fatty acids

As an adjunct to diet, omega-3 fatty acids in capsule form (approximately 850–1,000 mg of EPA and DHA) may be considered in women with CHD, and higher doses (2–4 g) may be used for treatment of women with high triglyceride levels (Class IIb, Level B)

Depression

Consider screening women with CHD for depression and refer/treat when indicated (Class IIa, Level B)

Major risk factor interventions

Blood pressure—optimal level and lifestyle

Encourage an optimal blood pressure of <120/80 mm Hg through lifestyle approaches, such as weight control, increased physical activity, alcohol moderation, sodium restriction, and increased consumption of fresh fruits, vegetables, low-fat dairy products (Class I, Level B)

Blood pressure—pharmacotherapy

Pharmacotherapy is indicated when blood pressure is ≥140/90 or at an even lower blood pressure in the setting of chronic kidney disease or diabetes (≥130/80 mm Hg); thiazide diuretics should be part of the drug regimen for most patients unless contraindicated or if there are compelling indications for other agents in specific vascular diseases; initial treatment of high-risk women[c] should be with beta-blockers and/or ACE inhibitors/ARBs, with addition of other drugs, such as thiazides, as needed to achieve goal blood pressure (Class I, Level A)

(*Continued on next page*)

Table 30-4. Guidelines for Prevention of Cardiovascular Disease in Women: Clinical Recommendations (*Continued*)

Lipid and lipoprotein level—optimal levels and lifestyle

The following levels of lipids and lipoproteins in women should be encouraged through lifestyle approaches; LDL-C <100 mg/dL, HDL-C >50 mg/dL, triglycerides <150 mg/dL, and non-HDL-C (total cholesterol minus HDL cholesterol) <130 mg/dL (Class I, Level B); if a woman is at high risk[c] or has hypercholesterolemia, intake of saturated fat should be <7% and cholesterol intake <200 mg/dL) (Class I, Level B)

Lipids—pharmacotherapy for LDL lowering, high-risk women

Utilize LDL-C–lowering drug therapy simultaneously with lifestyle therapy in women with CHD to achieve an LDL-C <100 mg/dL (Class I, Level A) and similarly in women with atherosclerotic CVD or diabetes mellitus or 10-year absolute risk >20% (Class I, Level B); a reduction to <70 mg/dL is reasonable in very-high-risk women[d] with CHD and may require an LDL-lowering drug combination (Class IIa, Level B)

Lipids—pharmacotherapy for LDL lowering, other at-risk women

Utilize LDL-C–lowering therapy if LDL-C level is ≥130 mg/dL with lifestyle therapy and there are multiple risk factors and 10-year absolute risk 10% to 20% (Class I, Level B); use LDL-C–lowering therapy if LDL-C level is ≥160 mg/dL with lifestyle therapy and there are multiple risk factors even if 10-year absolute risk <10% (Class I, Level B)

Utilize LDL-C–lowering therapy if LDL-C level is ≥190 mg/dL regardless of the presence or absence of other risk factors or CVD on lifestyle therapy (Class I, Level B)

Lipids—pharmacotherapy for low HDL or elevated non-HDL, high-risk women

Utilize niacin[e] or fibrate therapy when HDL-C is low or non-HDL-C is elevated in high-risk women after LDL-C goal is reached (Class IIa, Level B)

Lipids—pharmacotherapy for low HDL or elevated non-HDL, other at-risk women

Consider niacin[e] or fibrate therapy when HDL-C is low or non-HDL-C is elevated after LDL-C goal is reached in women with multiple risk factors and a 10-year absolute risk of 10% to 20% (Class IIb, Level B)

Diabetes mellitus

Lifestyle and pharmacotherapy should be used as indicated in women with diabetes (Class I, Level B) to achieve an A1C <7% if this can be accomplished without significant hypoglycemia (Class I, Level C)

Preventive drug interventions

Aspirin, high risk

Aspirin therapy (75–325 mg/day)[f] should be used in high-risk[c] women unless contraindicated (Class I, Level A); if a high-risk[c] woman is intolerant of aspirin therapy, clopidogrel should be substituted (Class I, Level B)

Aspirin—other at-risk or healthy women

In women ≥65 years old, consider aspirin therapy (81 mg daily or 100 mg every other day) if blood pressure is controlled and benefit for ischemic stroke and MI prevention is likely to outweigh the risk of gastrointestinal bleeding and hemorrhagic stroke (Class IIa, Level B) and in women <65 years old when benefit for ischemic stroke prevention is likely to outweigh adverse effects of therapy (Class IIb, Level B)

Beta-blockers

Beta-blockers should be used indefinitely in all women after MI, acute coronary syndrome, or left ventricular dysfunction with or without heart failure symptoms, unless contraindicated (Class I, Level A)

ACE inhibitors/ARBs

ACE inhibitors should be used (unless contraindicated) in women after MI, and in those with clinical evidence of heart failure or an LVEF ≤40% or with diabetes mellitus who are intolerant of ACE inhibitors, ARBs should be used instead (Class I, Level B)

(*Continued on next page*)

Table 30-4. Guidelines for Prevention of Cardiovascular Disease in Women: Clinical Recommendations (*Continued*)

Aldosterone blockade
Use aldosterone blockade after MI in women who do not have significant renal dysfunction or hyperkalemia who are already receiving therapeutic dosages of an ACE inhibitor and beta-blocker and have LVEF ≤40% with symptomatic heart failure (Class I, Level B)

Source: Adapted with permission from reference 54.

LVEF = left ventricular ejection fraction; BMI = body mass index; EPA = eicosapentaenoic acid; DHA = docosahexaenoic acid; CHD = coronary heart disease; ACE = angiotensin-converting enzyme; ARB = angiotensin receptor blocker; LDL-C = low-density lipoprotein cholesterol; HDL-C = high-density lipoprotein cholesterol; CVD = cardiovascular disease; MI = myocardial infarction.

[a]Pregnant and lactating women should avoid eating fish potentially high in methylmercury (e.g., shark, swordfish, king mackerel, or tilefish), should eat up to 12 oz/wk of a variety of fish and shellfish low in mercury, and check the Environmental Protection Agency and the U.S. Food and Drug Administration's websites for updates and local advisories about the safety of local catch.

[b]A drink equivalent is equal to a 12-oz bottle of beer, a 5-oz glass of wine, or a 1.5-oz shot of 80-proof spirit.

[c]Criteria for high risk include established CHD, cerebrovascular disease, peripheral arterial disease, abdominal aortic aneurysm, end-stage or chronic renal disease, diabetes mellitus, and 10-year Framingham risk >20%.

[d]Criteria for very high risk include established CVD plus any of the following: multiple major risk factors, severe and poorly controlled risk factors, and diabetes mellitus.

[e]Dietary supplement niacin should not be used as a substitute for prescription niacin.

[f]After percutaneous intervention with stent placement or coronary artery bypass grafting within previous year and in women with noncoronary forms of CVD, use current guideline for aspirin and clopidogrel.

in men with diabetes, although the risk of nonfatal myocardial infarction is similar.[24] Women with diabetes have more cardiovascular risk factors overall than women of the same age who do not have diabetes. This difference is not present in men with and without diabetes (Chapter 25: Pregnancy and Pre-existing Illnesses discusses the pharmacotherapy of diabetes mellitus in women).[24] In the United Kingdom Prospective Diabetes Study (UKPDS) part 73, patients were evaluated on the incidence of hypoglycemia when treated with diet, sulfonylureas, metformin, or insulin. Hypoglycemia occurred more commonly in women (3.0% vs. 2.2%) than in men.[63] Women with type 2 diabetes were more likely than men to lose weight with diet, whether or not they were taking metformin.[64] Insulin sensitizers, such as thiazolidinediones and metformin, decrease insulin resistance, improve symptoms of PCOS, and improve arterial stiffness.[65]

Obesity

An estimated 36 million adult American women have a **body mass index (BMI)** >30 kg/m^2, and a total of 68 million are overweight with a BMI >25 kg/m^2. Women who are obese have a higher incidence of developing cardiovascular disease than are similar men. Among women, the risk of developing cardiovascular disease increased when the waist-to-hip ratio increased, regardless of their BMI.[66] The waist-to-hip ratio and the risk of developing cardiovascular disease were significant only in men at a normal weight.[66] FDA-approved drug therapy includes sibutramine, orlistat, and phentermine with other drugs soon to be approved (see Chapter 32: Overweight and Obesity). A meta-analysis evaluated studies of at least 1 year in duration with two- thirds to three quarters of the study samples being women.[67] Orlistat decreased the incidence of diabetes and improved blood pressure, LDL cholesterol concentrations, and glucose control in individuals with diabetes. Sibutramine raised blood pressure and decreased HDL cholesterol concentrations.[67]

Dyslipidemias

An estimated 55 million adult American women have a total cholesterol concentration of at least 200 mg/dL or higher, and 38.6 million have an LDL cholesterol of 130 mg/dL or higher.[1] In addition, 12.3 million women have an HDL cholesterol concentration of <50 mg/dL.[1] As HDL cholesterol concentrations may slightly decline in postmenopausal women, triglyceride and LDL cholesterol concentrations rise. Concentrations of LDL cholesterol may increase because of down-regulation of LDL receptors in the liver and resulting decreased clearance during the menopausal transition. Low HDL cholesterol concentrations may be a more important risk factor for cardiovascular disease in older women than elevated LDL cholesterol concentrations.[61] High concentrations of HDL cholesterol, however, do not necessarily

Table 30-5. Summary of Major Statin Studies for Primary and Secondary Prevention of Coronary Heart Disease

Study	# Patients	% Women	Intervention	Benefit in Women
Primary				
WOSCOP[71]	6,595	----	Pravastatin 40 mg/day	N/A
AF/TexCAPS[72]	6,605	15%	Lovastatin 20–40 mg	Subgroup analysis in women showed a benefit and may have been better in women than men
ALLHAT-LLT[73]	10,355	49%	Pravastatin 40 mg/day	No benefit on all-cause mortality or CHD in full cohort potentially due to only 16.7% decrease in LDL-cholesterol
ASCOT-LLA[74]	10,305	18%	Atorvastatin 10 mg	Lack of significant benefit of primary end point of nonfatal MI and fatal CHD in women
Secondary				
4S[75,76]	4,444	19%	Simvastatin 20–40 mg	Benefit in women in secondary end point of preventing major coronary events; subgroup of women too small to detect effect on primary end point of mortality
CARE[77,78]	4,159	14%	Pravastatin 40 mg	Reduced primary end point of fatal and nonfatal MI by 43% and 57%, respectively, and reduced secondary end points of necessitating invasive cardiac procedures; also, the benefit was seen early in treatment, within 6–12 mo
LIPID[79]	9,014	17%	Pravastatin 40 mg	Women had an equivalent lower risk of developing a major coronary event in patients with a history of previous MI or unstable angina; the lower risk was more visible in patients with diabetes, but a substudy of women with diabetes in this trial was underpowered
MIRACL[80]	3,086	35%	Atorvastatin 80 mg/day	Differences in men vs. women were not shown; may not have enough power to examine differences; ischemic events within the first 16 weeks were reduced by atorvastatin 80 mg in patients with acute coronary syndrome
PROVE-IT[81]	4,162	22%	Atorvastatin 80 mg vs. pravastatin 40 mg	Similar benefit in men and women of reducing death and coronary events in patients with acute coronary syndrome taking high-dose atorvastatin vs. pravastatin
HPS[82]	20,536	25%	Simvastatin 40 mg	Women and men had same effect of a reduction of vascular events in high-risk individuals with varying levels of cholesterol
A to Z[83]	4,497	25%	Simvastatin 40/80 mg vs. placebo/simvastatin 20 mg	No difference noted between men and women, although the trial showed a trend toward early initiation of intensive statin therapy, but no significant effect on primary composite end point of death, MI, or readmission for ACS
CARDS[84]	2,838	32%	Atorvastatin 10 mg	In patients with lower cholesterol levels, both men and women had a reduced risk of first cardiovascular events and stroke in patients with type 2 diabetes

(*Continued on next page*)

Study	# Patients	% Women	Intervention	Benefit in Women
AVERT[85]	341	16%	Atorvastatin vs. percutaneous coronary revascularization	There were small, but significant baseline differences in numbers of men vs. women; lower incidence of ischemic events in both men and women, but did not reach significance
TNT[86]	10,001	19%	Atorvastatin 10 mg vs. atorvastatin 80 mg	Primary outcome of relative risk reduction of 80 mg vs. 10 mg for major cardiovascular events; no significant differences in women as compared with men

WOSCOP = West of Scotland Coronary Prevention Study; AF/TexCAPS = Air Force/Texas Coronary Atherosclerosis Prevention Study; ALLHAT-LLT = Antihypertensive Agent and Lipid Lowering Heart Attack Trial; CHD = coronary heart disease; LDL = low-density lipoprotein; ASCOT-LLA = Anglo-Scandinavian Cardiac Outcomes Trial-Lipid Lowering Arm; MI = myocardial infarction; 4S = Scandinavian Simvastatin Survival Study; CARE = Cholesterol and Recurrent Events; LIPID = Long-term Intervention with Pravastatin in Ischemic Disease; MIRACL = Myocardial Ischemia Reduction with Aggressive Cholesterol Lowering; ACS = acute coronary syndrome; PROVE-IT = Pravastatin or Atorvastatin Evaluation and Infection Therapy; HPS = Heart Protection Study; A to Z = Aggrastat to Zocor; CARDS = Collaborative Atorvastatin Diabetes Study; AVERT = Atorvastatin Versus Revascularization Treatment; TNT = Treating to New Targets.

predict cardiovascular protection.[68] **Lp(a)** is a strong predictor of stroke, all-cause mortality, and cardiovascular death in elderly men, but not women.[69]

Table 30-4 lists the goal lipid values for women. Of note, reducing LDL cholesterol concentrations to <70 mg/dL is recommended for women with coronary heart disease who are at very high risk. A woman is considered to be at very high risk if established coronary heart disease is present and she multiple major risk factors, severe and poorly controlled risk factors, or diabetes mellitus. Lowering the LDL cholesterol concentration is the primary lipid goal, with reduction of the non-HDL cholesterol concentration (total cholesterol minus the HDL cholesterol) as a secondary goal.

The NCEP III recommendations for the management of dyslipidemias are similar in men and women.[70] Statins remain the primary therapy of hypercholesterolemia, with fibrates, niacin, and drugs such as colesevelam used concomitantly, depending on the specific lipid abnormality present. A unique consideration in the management of dyslipidemias (with the potential exception of hypertriglyceridemia) in women is that treatment is usually discontinued during pregnancy. Statins are classified as pregnancy category X and should not be used during pregnancy, as cholesterol synthesis is needed for the developing fetus. Niacin is pregnancy category C when used in pharmacologic dosages, whereas cholestyramine, colestipol, and colesevelam are pregnancy category B because they are not systemically absorbed.

Most studies of statins for primary and secondary prevention have included women, although they may constitute only 20% of the study sample. In women with established coronary heart disease, lipid-lowering therapy reduced the risk of death from coronary heart disease by 26%, nonfatal myocardial infarction by 36%, and major cardiovascular events by 26%.[74] The effects of lipid-lowering therapy on total mortality in women are not known.[74] Table 30-5 summarizes the major statin studies for primary and secondary prevention. A meta-analysis of data from 14 randomized trial reported that statin therapy decreased the likelihood of coronary events in women (OR 0.82; 95% CI, 0.73–0.93).[87]

Hypertension

An estimated 39 million adult American women have hypertension with a blood pressure of at least 140/90 mm Hg.[1] Many more women have prehypertension, which has been defined as a systolic blood pressure between 120 and 139 mm Hg or a diastolic blood pressure between 80 and 89 mm Hg. Recently, the presence of prehypertension has been linked to a significant increase in the risk of myocardial infarction, stroke, heart failure, and cardiovascular death in a large substudy of the Women's Health Initiative.[88]

The seventh report of the Joint National Committee (JNC) and the 2007 AHA hypertension guideline do not provide sex-specific recommendations regarding the management of hypertension in women.[89,90] The JNC only briefly discusses hypertension in women, acknowledging that oral contraceptives may increase blood pressure; the report also recommends vasodilators and beta-blockers, including labetalol, as preferred antihypertensive drug therapy during pregnancy.[89] In a recent review of hypertension in women, female patients were identified as having a higher incidence of left ventricular hypertrophy and heart failure with preserved ejection fraction.[91]

The treatment of hypertension should include the use of nonpharmacologic therapies whenever possible. Dietary modification, such as the Dietary Approaches to Stop Hypertension (DASH) diet, may reduce systolic blood pressure by 3–7 mm Hg.[92,93] The DASH diet includes increased intake of fruits and vegetables, as well as whole grains and lean sources of protein. Women respond similarly to men in terms of their blood pressure response with this diet.[92] Aerobic exercise, weight reduction, and moderation of alcohol intake may be appropriate as well.

The first-line antihypertensive agents include thiazide diuretics, beta-blockers, ACE inhibitors (or ARBs), and calcium channel blockers.[54,89,90] The selection of drug therapy should be tailored to concomitant conditions and compelling conditions such as heart failure, if present.[54,89,90] In individuals with stable angina, unstable angina/NSTEMI and ST-elevation myocardial infarction (STEMI), beta-blockers (if the patient is hemodynamically stable) and ACE inhibitors (or ARBs) are generally preferred.[90] In women with hypertension and diabetes, the use of an ACE inhibitor or ARB is usually preferred over other antihypertensive therapy. The most important point is that many women will require lifestyle interventions as well as the use of multiple antihypertensive agents, titrated to optimal dosages, to achieve the desired blood pressure goal. Clinicians should recognize that there may be special considerations in choosing between medications for hypertension (Table 30-2).[95,96]

Although the benefits from antihypertensive therapy in men are well established from many clinical trials, the outcomes from treatment in women are influenced by age and race.[94] In black women of any age, antihypertensive therapy reduced the risk of fatal and nonfatal cerebrovascular events by 53% and fatal and nonfatal cardiovascular events by 45%.[94] All-cause mortality in black women with hypertension was reduced by 34%. In white women 55 years of age and older, antihypertensive therapy reduced the risk of fatal and nonfatal cerebrovascular events by 38% and fatal and nonfatal cardiovascular events by 25%. Treatment of white women between the ages of 34 and 54 did not show a significant benefit in these outcomes in clinical trials.

Therapeutic Challenge:

What are possible explanations for the reported lack of benefit on cardiovascular outcomes from antihypertensive therapy in younger white women with stage 1 hypertension?

Two major studies have differed in their reported outcomes from antihypertensive therapy in women. The 6-year Antihypertensive and Lipid-Lowering Treatment to Prevent Heart Attack Trial (ALLHAT) study compared chlorthalidone, amlodipine, and lisinopril in 33,357 participants who were 55 years of age and older with hypertension and at least one other risk factor for coronary heart disease. (Doxazosin was originally another arm of the study, but this treatment was discontinued early because of an increased risk of hospitalization for heart failure.) The ALLHAT study sample was unique in that almost one third was black, 47% were women, and 36% had diabetes. The major outcomes studied were similar with all three drugs in both men and women.[97] In the Second Australian National Blood Pressure Study Group, thiazides were compared with ACE inhibitors in 6,083 older adults who were at lower risk of cardiovascular disease than participants in ALLHAT. The rate of combined cardiovascular events was lower with the ACE inhibitor compared with the diuretic, but only in men.[98] The potential reasons for these differences may be related to the baseline difference in cardiovascular risk, especially among women in the two studies, with women in ALLHAT at a much higher risk of cardiovascular disease.

Emerging Risk Factors

In addition to the traditional risk factors for cardiovascular diseases, interest has increased in novel or emerging risk factors such as **homocysteine** and selected biomarkers. Inflammatory markers—including tumor necrosis factor, interleukin-6, and **C-reactive protein** (CRP)—may be important in predicting coronary heart disease risk for both men and women.[99] CRP was evaluated prospectively in the Women's Health Study. Increasing baseline quartiles for CRP were a strong marker for an increased risk of cardiovascular events.[100] Recently in the Justification for the Use of Statins in Prevention: an Intervention Trial Evaluating Rosuvastatin (JUPITER) study, men and women with elevated concentrations of CRP and desirable LDL cholesterol values actually demonstrated a reduction in major cardiovascular events.[101] Both men and women responded to the use of rosuvastatin to reduce CRP values. Although promising, the use of CRP especially as a treatment target remains controversial. In clinical practice, high-sensitivity CRP concentrations are used primarily for men and women who are considered to be at intermediate risk for cardiovascular disease and not as part of a routine assessment of cardiovascular risk.

Another emerging potential risk factor for cardiovascular disease may be depression (Chapter 34: Mental Health). For many years, depression has been identified as a common comorbid condition in both men and women with cardiovascular disease. The presence of depression frequently complicates the optimal management because of its effects on adherence to treatment plans. Recently, the AHA issued a guideline that identified depression as potentially contributing to the development of cardiovascular disease.[102]

ASSESSING OVERALL CARDIOVASCULAR RISK

Prediction Models

Framingham Heart Study

The Framingham Heart Study began in 1948 and has advanced the understanding of many cardiovascular diseases and their associated risk factors.[103] This study has been one of the few longitudinal studies to include women from its inception. The Framingham risk scoring system for men and women is based on data from the ongoing longitudinal study. Although the Framingham models differ slightly, points are assigned generally based on age group, total (or LDL) cholesterol (according to age), smoking status (according to age), HDL cholesterol, diabetes, and systolic blood pressure (according to treatment status).[104] Patients are classified into categories such as high risk (>20% risk of a major cardiovascular event in the next 10 years), moderately high risk (10% to 20% risk), and moderate risk (<10% risk).

Although useful, the Framingham risk score may be less accurate for women. Most women will not score high enough into an intermediate or high-risk range until they are 70 years old and, as a result, may not be offered effective prevention strategies. Many women may warrant drug therapy according to the NCEP guidelines but may be low-risk according to the Framingham risk score. Other groups, such as Native American women, need adjustments to their risk scores to adequately predict cardiovascular events using the Framingham equations.[105]

Reynolds Risk Score

The Reynolds Risk Score is a new validated risk score that developed a more effective way to categorize women in the appropriate cardiovascular risk group.[106] This cardiovascular risk score uses smoking status, age, systolic blood pressure, total cholesterol, HDL cholesterol, high-sensitivity CRP, and family history of early heart disease to evaluate overall cardiovascular risk for women. This scoring system has reclassified about 40% to 50% intermediate-risk women into either higher or lower risk categories and may be valuable for evaluating women at intermediate cardiovascular risk.[106] One limitation of this tool is that it has been studied primarily in white women, so its potential applicability to women from different ethnic and racial groups is unclear.

Women's Ischemia Syndrome Evaluation

The Women's Ischemia Syndrome Evaluation (WISE) investigation has been an ongoing cohort study of 936 women referred for diagnostic coronary angiography. The purpose of the study is to assess the diagnostic reliability of cardiovascular testing in women as well as the symptoms of cardiovascular disease in women and the effects of menopausal status and reproductive hormones.[107] The WISE study group has identified concerns regarding hypertension among younger women and emphasized the need for stronger preventative efforts in women of reproductive age who have hypertension. Preliminary analyses have indicated that many women with coronary artery disease do not have the "typical" anginal symptoms.[107]

OTHER CARDIOVASCULAR DISEASE PREVENTION STRATEGIES

Aspirin

Table 30-4 outlines the appropriate usage of aspirin for the prevention of cardiovascular disease in women. Aspirin, or alternatively, clopidogrel, should be used in women at high risk of a cardiovascular event. For women 65 years of age or older who are at lower risk or those who are healthy, the potential risks and benefits of aspirin should be carefully weighed before starting the antiplatelet agent.

Primary Prevention

The Women's Health Study evaluated almost 40,000 women 45 years or older taking aspirin 100 mg every other day compared with placebo.[108] Women were monitored for more than 10 years for a primary end point of nonfatal stroke, nonfatal myocardial infarction, or death from any cardiovascular disease. The risk of ischemic stroke was decreased by 17%; however, the primary end point of a reduction in nonfatal myocardial infarction or all-cause cardiovascular mortality was not achieved.[108] A subgroup analysis of women 65 years of age and older at randomization demonstrated a 26% reduction in the major cardiovascular events, a 30% reduction in ischemic stroke, and a 34% reduction in myocardial infarction.[108] A sex-specific meta-analysis of six studies, including the Physician's Health Study (men) and the Women's Health Study, evaluated the risks and benefits with aspirin. The composite end point of cardiovascular events included nonfatal myocardial infarction, nonfatal stroke, and cardiovascular mortality. Among women, the benefit was from a reduction in the risk of ischemic stroke, whereas that for men was from a reduction in myocardial infarction.[109] Recently, the U.S. Preventive Services Task Force recommended the use of aspirin for primary prevention among women 55–79 years of age, when the potential reduction in ischemic strokes would offset the risk of gastrointestinal bleeding.[110] This guideline acknowledged that the potential risks and benefits in women age of 80 and older is unknown.[110]

Secondary Prevention

Aspirin in dosages ranging from 75 mg to 325 mg daily reduces the risk of myocardial infarction, stroke, and cardiovascular death by 20% to 25% in women with documented coronary heart disease or at high risk of coronary heart disease.[111,112] In a meta-analysis of the effects of sex on aspirin in primary and secondary prevention of myocardial infarction, trials consisting primarily of men showed a larger risk reduction of nonfatal myocardial infarction (RR = 0.62; 95% CI, 0.54–0.71) compared with trials that were composed predominantly of women (RR = 0.87; 95% CI, 0.71–1.06).[113]

Aspirin Resistance

Aspirin resistance has been proposed to be an underlying mechanism for the development of thrombotic events despite the consistent use of appropriate dosages of aspirin. Women may be at increased risk of aspirin resistance, but the evidence is contradictory, as women with coronary artery disease tend to be older and have more concomitant diseases than men.[113] Interpatient variability in the response to aspirin occurs, and subgroups of patients such as those with diabetes or who are obese may require higher dosages.[112] Although the bioavailability of aspirin may be greater in women and the clearance of the drug slower, one report has indicated that the platelets of women are more reactive at baseline.[114,115] Most importantly, platelets may be activated through mechanisms that are independent of those blocked by aspirin and other antiplatelet agents.[116] Genetic differences between individuals may also contribute to the varying effects of aspirin on platelet aggregation.[117]

Antioxidant Vitamins

In the past, antioxidant vitamins—including vitamins C, E, and beta-carotene—have been recommended for preventing cardiovascular disease. The recommendation had been based on observational studies of dietary patterns and cardiovascular disease.[118] The proposed benefit from antioxidants was based on their activity as free-radical scavengers that limit the effects of oxidation, including lipid peroxidation and damage to the endothelium. The Women's Antioxidant Cardiovascular Study reported that vitamin C 500 mg daily, vitamin E 600 International Units every other day, and beta-carotene 50 mg every other day did not reduce the risk of cardiovascular events in high-risk women. The 8,171 participants had a self-reported history of cardiovascular disease or at least three risk factors for cardiovascular disease. The combined primary end point was myocardial infarction, stroke, coronary revascularization, or cardiovascular death. Secondary end points were the individual components of the primary outcome measure.[119] A recent meta-analysis evaluated the effects of antioxidants on mortality in primary and secondary prevention studies (of diseases not limited to cardiovascular conditions). A potential increase in all-cause mortality was reported with beta-carotene and vitamin E.[120]

Recent outcomes from the Women's Health Study showed that women taking natural source vitamin E 600 International Units on alternate days vs. placebo for 10 years had a decreased risk of venous thromboembolism. Before initiation of vitamin E, women were tested for factor V Leiden deficiency and prothrombin mutations. Women who had no history of venous thromboembolism had a 27% reduction (relative hazard, 0.73; 95% CI, 0.57–0.94), whereas women with factor V Leiden deficiency or a prothrombin mutation had a 49% reduction (relative hazard, 0.51; 95% CI, 0.30–0.87) with vitamin E supplementation.[121]

Folic Acid and B vitamins

Supplementation with folic acid and other B vitamins has been proposed to reduce homocysteine concentrations and potentially to lower the risk of cardiovascular events. Because of small numbers of women enrolled in many trials, the specific effect in women was unknown. Studies such as the Norwegian Vitamin Trial (Norvit) and the Heart Outcomes Prevention Outcome (HOPE-2) have not demonstrated reductions in cardiovascular events from folic acid alone or in combination with B vitamins.[122,123] Most recently, the effects of folic acid 2.5 mg, vitamin B_6 50 mg, and vitamin B_{12} (in a single pill) or placebo daily were evaluated in 5,442 female health professionals aged 42 years and older with cardiovascular disease or three or more cardiovascular risk factors. The outcome measure was a composite of myocardial infarction, stroke, coronary revascularization, or cardiovascular disease mortality. Patients were treated for 7.3 years. The composite outcome was similar between the two groups (226.9/10,000 person-years vs. 219.2/10,000 person-years for the active vs. placebo group).[124] As a result, the use of folic acid alone or in combination with B vitamins should not be routinely recommended.

Omega-3 Fatty Acids

Omega-3 fatty acids either from dietary sources such as fish or from supplements have potential protective effects against cardiovascular disease, although many observational studies and clinical trials have included relatively few women.[125] In the **Nurses Health Study,** women with the highest intake of omega-3 fatty acids either from diet or dietary supplements had a 34% decrease in deaths that were due to coronary heart disease compared with women with limited intake.[126]

One caution with ingesting fish or dietary supplements made from oily fish is the potential for mercury ingestion if the woman is pregnant. However, this is unlikely to be a significant concern as oxidized mercury is water soluble and would not be expected to accumulate in fish oils. In addition, the production of fish oil supplements include multiple purification processes.[127] The availability of a prescription omega-3 fatty acid preparation makes this less of a concern as the product undergoes a multistep purification process.

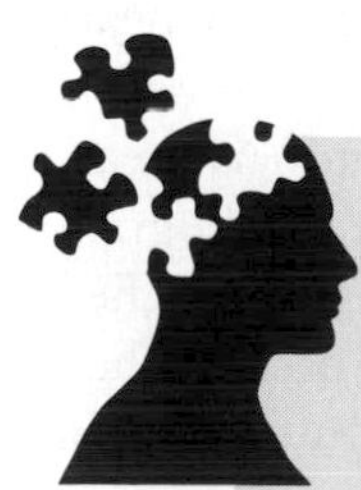

Therapeutic Challenge:

Why do many studies of primary or secondary prevention of cardiovascular disease use combined end points? What are the limitations of using these complex combined end points?

CASE PRESENTATION

Patient Case: Part 2

Assessment and plan: This patient has five potentially modifiable risk factors for cardiovascular disease and a Framingham risk score of 14%. Counseling efforts should emphasize the multiple ways for her to reduce her overall cardiovascular risk. She should be encouraged to set priorities and personal goals.

Obesity: This patient has a BMI of 32.8 kg/m^2. Lifestyle changes should be strongly encouraged as she may have improvements in her diabetes, hypertension, and dyslipidemia with weight loss. She should be counseled regarding portion sizes and the use of lean meats, as well as fruits and vegetables. A referral to a nutritionist is also indicated for dietary management.

Smoking cessation: Although not addressed in this chapter, her potential interest in smoking cessation should be assessed. Smoking cessation has many cardiovascular and noncardiovascular health benefits; her HDL cholesterol concentration may also improve. The 2008 guidelines on smoking cessation have identified that women may have unique barriers to smoking cessation, including greater concerns about weight gain; little sex-specific research on smoking cessation in women is available.[128] Counseling and pharmacotherapy with a nicotine replacement product, bupropion or varenicline, may be appropriate, although because of her history of depression, varenicline may not be the preferred therapy.

Hypertension: Her goal blood pressure is <130/80 mm Hg secondary to her diagnosis of diabetes. It is inadequately controlled with the low-dose amlodipine. An ACE inhibitor should be added to her regimen for renal protection secondary to type 2 diabetes and aggressive management of her hypertension, along with other antihypertensive agents as necessary, to attain her goal blood pressure.

Type 2 diabetes: Metformin should be initiated for glucose control and may produce a slight weight loss as well. Optimal glucose control may improve her lipid profile. Niacin may cause elevations in blood glucose, but may not necessarily warrant discontinuation of the medication at this time.

Dyslipidemia: Continue niacin, as it increases HDL cholesterol concentrations when used in relatively low dosages. Add a statin such as atorvastatin 20 mg daily for her dyslipidemia. Finally, she should be counseled regarding the lack of efficacy and potential

(*Continued on next page*)

harm associated with the use of vitamin E. This antioxidant vitamin is not appropriate for prevention of coronary heart disease. She should be counseled to discontinue the vitamin E supplement and instead to use low-dose aspirin for cardioprotection because she is classified as being at high risk of coronary heart disease because of her diabetes.

Vasomotor symptoms: Although the patient is interested in hormone therapy and is early in the menopausal transition, other therapies should be used for her vasomotor symptoms, especially because she has a history of a DVT after a pregnancy. Options include nonpharmacologic measures, as well as potentially the use of venlafaxine (although this might further increase her blood pressure).

Gastroesophageal reflux disease: Her symptoms of severe GERD are poorly responsive to high dosages of omeprazole. This condition should be investigated further to ensure that these symptoms are not actually due to myocardial ischemia.

Prevention of osteoporosis: Because she is in the menopausal transition, her risk factors for osteoporosis should be assessed. Her use of omeprazole and high dosages of levothyroxine should be reevaluated. An assessment of her thyroid functioning should be performed to ensure she is not now hyperthyroid, as this might increase her risk of osteoporosis.

Adherence and education: A thorough medication history is needed to assess her understanding and adherence with her drug regimen, because she has been borrowing her husband's medications.

Treatment of Cardiovascular Disease

CORONARY HEART DISEASE

An estimated 7.2 million adult American women have coronary heart disease (also known as coronary artery disease), including 3 million who have had a myocardial infarction. Almost 220,000 women died from coronary heart disease in 2004.[1] Acute coronary syndromes (ACSs), the result of coronary heart disease, are characterized by myocardial ischemia and include unstable angina, NSTEMI, and STEMI. In the majority of cases of ACS, the erosion or rupture of an existing atherosclerotic plaque begins a series of events, including platelet aggregation, which ultimately results in thrombus formation.

Clinical Presentation

Sex-related differences exist in the clinical presentation of ACSs. Women are more likely than men to present with unstable angina and are less likely to have STEMI. Women frequently have "atypical" symptoms, including shortness of breath, weakness, and fatigue, as well as syncope, indigestion, nausea, and vomiting on presentation.[53] These may be easily overlooked if physicians are focused on more "typical" symptoms of chest pressure, "tightness" or "heaviness," as well as diaphoresis and pain radiating down the left arm. Prodromal symptoms, especially in black women, include unusual fatigue, anxiety, and sleep disturbances. The sex-specific differences in clinical presentation are most apparent in younger and middle-aged women than in older women.

Diagnostic Issues

Women and men have similar frequency of ST segment changes, but women tend to have T-wave inversion more commonly.[53] The serum **troponin** and creatine kinase-MB concentrations are less likely to be elevated in women than in men.[53] Elevated troponin concentrations indicate similar increase in the risk of death in both men and women. The risk of nonfatal myocardial infarction associated with an elevated troponin concentration is greater in women than in men.[24] Women may be more likely to have elevated CRP and **B-type natriuretic peptide** (BNP) concentrations.[53]

Data from a meta-analysis of eight major treatment studies of non-ST-elevation ACS reported that women were significantly less likely to have obstructive coronary artery disease on angiography than men.[129] The value of other diagnostic tests for coronary heart disease, such as an exercise electrocardiogram and thallium stress testing, has been questioned, and evidence suggests that their accuracy in women may be low. The Agency for Healthcare Research and Quality funded two comprehensive reports to review the available evidence on the diagnosis, prevention, and treatment of coronary heart disease in women and identified that the accuracy of exercise echocardiogram to diagnose coronary heart disease is higher than exercise electrocardiogram and thallium in women. The report also identified that coronary calcium scores are only useful when the value is 0, as it likely rules out atherosclerosis in women.[130] (Calcium is deposited in response to inflammation and is present in larger plaques, although not necessarily the plaques most likely to rupture and cause acute myocardial infarction.)

Pharmacotherapy

The treatment of ACS and adherence to the recommendations of the American College of Cardiology and the AHA has improved over the previous years. Early mortality from ACS is higher in women, as are complications from procedures and pharmacotherapy. When women are treated intensively with a reperfusion strategy using primary percutaneous coronary interventions and standard pharmacotherapy, their 1-year mortality is similar to that of men, despite having a higher risk of complications.[131] The recent meta-analysis reported that high-risk women with non-ST-elevation ACS received a comparable benefit from aggressive interventions (invasive diagnostic procedure with the intent to perform revascularization) as did men in terms of the composite end point of death, myocardial infarction, or hospitalization with ACS. Women at lower risk, such as those who did not have elevated troponin concentrations, did not have a similar benefit and may actually have an increased risk of death or myocardial infarction with invasive strategies for non-ST-elevation ACS.[53,129] A conservative strategy of medical management is followed by invasive approach when medical therapy fails to relieve anginal symptoms or when evidence of ischemia is present.

The management of STEMI is focused on initiating reperfusion therapy either with fibrinolysis or primary percutaneous coronary intervention within 12 hours of the onset of symptoms in appropriate candidates. In the Global Use of Strategies to Open Occluded Arteries in Acute Coronary Syndromes (GUSTO), women had a 30-day death rate of 9.8% vs. 4.4% for men. Female sex was an independent risk factor for bleeding from fibrinolytic agents alone or in combination with glycoprotein IIb/IIIa inhibitors, such as tirofiban, eptifibatide, and abciximab in STEMI.[132]

Women with non-ST segment ACS also have a higher risk of bleeding whether or not they are given glycoprotein IIb/IIIa inhibitors, even in appropriate dosages.[133] When women do receive these drugs, they are at higher risk of excessive dosing and a 72% increased likelihood of bleeding with excessive dosages.[134] Appropriate dosing of these drugs may lessen the risk of bleeding, especially in patients with concomitant kidney impairment. Women have been reported to be at increased risk of bleeding from other antithrombotic agents, and evidence suggests that this adverse effect may be independent of body size.[132]

Antiplatelet agents should be used in patients with unstable angina/NSTEMI. For individuals who are treated medically without stenting, aspirin in a dosage of 75–162 mg daily should be used indefinitely. For patients treated with bare-metal **stents,** aspirin 162–325 mg daily is prescribed for at least 1 month and continued at 75–162 mg daily indefinitely. In patients who receive drug-eluting stents, aspirin 162–325 mg/day should be prescribed for at least 3 months with sirolimus-eluting stents and 6 months with paclitaxel-eluting stents. Then aspirin is continued indefinitely at 75–162 mg/day. Clopidogrel in a dosage of 75 mg daily should be prescribed for at least 1 month and is recommended for 1 year in both types of drug-eluting stents.[53]

Benefits from other standard therapies following myocardial infarction remain inadequately studied in women. A meta-analysis of five major studies demonstrated a similar reduction in cardiovascular death among men and women with the use of metoprolol after myocardial infarction.[134] Studies using ACE inhibitors have had varying findings. In a study of the use of ACE inhibitors after myocardial infarction with left ventricular dysfunction, both men and women had 20% reduction in the risk of death and in hospitalization that was due to myocardial infarction or heart failure.[135] The Heart Outcomes Prevention Study reported a similar reduction in death as a result of coronary heart disease among men and women, with women having a 20% reduction in combined end point of myocardial infarction, stroke, or cardiovascular mortality.[136] The risk for myocardial infarction was 10% lower in women.

HEART FAILURE

An estimated 2.6 million adult American women have heart failure with an estimated 35,200 deaths that were due to the disease in 2004.[1] Women have a lower mortality rate from heart failure than men in observational studies, but in the Studies of Left Ventricular Dysfunction (SOLVD), they had a higher 1-year mortality rate. B-type natriuretic peptide concentrations may differ in their significance between women and men. Women who have BNP concentrations >500 pg/mL had a 5.1-fold increase in mortality compared with a 1.8-fold increase risk of mortality in men with similar BNP measurements.[137]

Research Issues

Research in heart failure has resulted in major advances in its management and significant reductions in morbidity and mortality. Unfortunately, clinical trials of heart failure have had the lowest enrollment of women compared with studies of other cardiovascular diseases. The primary reason is that most studies have focused on systolic heart failure, in which coronary heart disease is a common etiology and the **left ventricular ejection fraction** (LVEF) is impaired. Systolic heart failure is more common in middle-aged men. Diastolic heart failure with preserved LVEF is more common in women in whom the cause of the heart failure is systolic hypertension and not ischemic cardiovascular disease. One theory to explain this difference in heart failure is that women may have an adaptive response to increased pressure on the left ventricle from systolic hypertension, which results in the development of concentric hypertrophy. Systolic function is preserved in women, but eventually diastolic failure develops.

Pharmacotherapy

The 2006 guidelines of the Heart Failure Society of America (HFSA) recommends diuretic treatment with loop diuretics—such as furosemide, bumetanide, and torsemide—when clinical evidence of volume overload is present in patients with heart failure and preserved LVEF.[138] Therapy with either an ACE inhibitor or ARB is also recommended in these patients, especially if symptomatic cardiovascular disease (or diabetes plus an additional risk factor) is present.[138] Beta-blockers are recommended if prior myocardial infarction, hypertension, or atrial fibrillation requiring rate control is also present. (Diltiazem or verapamil are recommended for rate control if the beta-blocker is not tolerated.)[138]

Limited data are available on the use of ACE inhibitors and ARBs in diastolic, as well as systolic, heart failure in women. In the Candesartan in Heart Failure-Assessment of Reduction in Morbidity and Mortality (CHARM) preserved study, which included many women, the ARB did not reduce the risk of cardiovascular deaths compared with placebo.[139] A reduced risk of hospitalization was reported with candesartan. A review of 30 studies of systolic heart failure reported that total mortality (and total mortality plus hospitalization for heart failure) was not significantly reduced in women taking ACE inhibitors.[140]

The value of beta-blockers for treating diastolic heart failure in women remains unclear. An analysis of the Metoprolol Extended-Release Randomized Intervention Trial in Heart Failure (MERIT-HF) study reported that women with impaired LVEF (systolic dysfunction) had a 21% reduction in all-cause mortality and all-cause hospitalizations. In addition, hospitalizations that were due to worsening heart failure were reduced by 42% among women taking metoprolol.[141] A systematic review from the two Cardiac Insufficiency Bisoprolol Studies (I and II) demonstrated a 30% reduction in the risk of death in women with ejection fraction <40%.[142]

The role of digoxin in heart failure was evaluated in the Digitalis Investigation Group (DIG) study, which enrolled 6,800 patients with systolic heart failure. A post hoc analysis reported that women receiving digoxin had an all-cause mortality rate of 33.1% vs. 28.9% receiving placebo.[143] Serum digoxin concentrations were not routinely obtained in the DIG trial, so the increased risk of death may reflect digoxin toxicity rather than unique adverse effects in women. (Other authors have suggested that women may have fewer sodium pumps and that this may contribute to the observed results.[24]) A retrospective study identified that the excess risk of mortality was only apparent when serum digoxin concentrations were >1.2 ng/mL.[144] Women had higher digoxin concentrations than did men in this study.[144] Caution should be used in interpreting the findings given the subanalyses and the small number of women in the subgroups.

ATRIAL FIBRILLATION

Atrial fibrillation is a **supraventricular tachyarrhythmia** and is the most common arrhythmia in women older than 80 years of age. Symptoms frequently include palpitations, lightheadedness, confusion, chest pain, and shortness of breath. Atrial fibrillation can be either chronic or paroxysmal in nature and can result in ischemic stroke and heart failure. Women may be at a higher risk of thromboembolism from atrial fibrillation regardless of their use of warfarin.[145,146] The primary goals in the management of atrial fibrillation are prevention of thromboembolism (and subsequent ischemic stroke), rate control, and correction of the rhythm disturbance.[147]

Pharmacotherapy

The treatment of atrial fibrillation includes the use of antithrombotic agents such as warfarin and aspirin (preferred for individuals at low risk of stroke). Drugs to control the heart rate include beta-blockers, **nondihydropyridine calcium channel blockers,** and digoxin. For most individuals with persistent atrial fibrillation, the use of a beta-blocker, such as metoprolol, or a calcium channel blocker, such as verapamil or diltiazem, is preferred for rate control. Antiarrhythmic agents, such as amiodarone and propafenone, may also be used for maintenance of normal sinus rhythm. **Electrocardioversion** and **radiofrequency ablation** may also be used in the treatment of atrial fibrillation.

Antithrombotic therapy with warfarin to achieve an International Normalized Ratio (INR) of 2 to 3 is recommended for all individuals unless contraindications or lone atrial fibrillation is present.[147] Warfarin is of benefit in treating atrial fibrillation in both women and men, with women having a similar rate of major bleeding from the drug.[146]

Traditionally, rhythm control was considered the preferred approach to the management of atrial fibrillation until several studies demonstrated that rate control was not inferior to rhythm control.[147] In the Atrial Fibrillation Follow-up Investigation of Rhythm Management (AFFIRM), 4,060 patients with a mean age of 69.7 years were randomized to either rhythm or rate control. The rhythm control group included class IA and IC antiarrhythmics agents, as well as sotalol, amiodarone, and dofetilide. The rate control group used a beta-blocker, a nondihydropyridine calcium channel blocker, and digitalis, either alone or in combination. Approximately 40% of the study participants were women. In both men and women, a nonsignificant trend toward an increased risk of death in the rhythm control group existed over the rate control group.[148]

In the Rate Control vs. Electrical Cardioversion (RACE) study, 522 patients, including 192 women with recurrent atrial fibrillation, were randomized to rate or rhythm control. Rate control used a beta-blocker, a nondihydropyridine calcium channel blocker, and/or digitalis.[149] The participants in the rhythm control group received electrocardioversion followed by antiarrhythmic drug therapy with amiodarone, sotalol, or class IC agents such as propafenone. The mean age of women was 71 years, whereas the mean age of men was 67 years of age. Women randomized to rhythm control had a greater risk of developing heart failure, thromboembolic complications, and adverse effects from antiarrhythmic drug therapy compared with women in the rate control group.[149] The adverse effects from antiarrhythmic therapy in the RACE study was due to bradyarrhythmias and not to **torsades de pointes.** This difference between rate and rhythm control was not evident among men in the study. Rate control should strongly be considered in women with persistent atrial fibrillation, and current guidelines recommend rate control at least initially, especially for older adults.[147,149]

Adverse Drug Events

INTERPRETING SEX-RELATED ADVERSE DRUG EVENTS

Women may also exhibit differences in the risk of adverse drug effects. These include sex-related differences from cardiovascular drugs such as statins (e.g., myopathy), diuretics (e.g., hyponatremia), and spironolactone (e.g., menstrual irregularities).[150] In addition, cardiovascular adverse effects from noncardiac drugs may be more common in women compared with men. Important points in evaluating any purported sex-related difference in adverse effects are whether the observed difference is due to women receiving a proportionally higher dosage simply because of their smaller body size. Also, consideration should be given to whether the sex-related difference is related more to the older age of women when they have cardiovascular disease rather than a true sex-related difference.

The underlying prevalence of the disease and resulting increased likelihood of drug exposure in women vs. men should also be considered. As an example, fenfluramine (in combination with phentermine) and dexfenfluramine were withdrawn from the U.S. market after their association with the development of valvular heart disease, primarily aortic and mitral regurgitation.[151] Most of the patients with valvular heart disease from these drugs were women, and this likely reflects the common usage patterns of anorexic agents in younger women rather than a true sex-related difference. In addition, many case reports of heart failure with drugs such as infliximab have been women and again may reflect the higher prevalence of diseases such as rheumatoid arthritis in women than men. The use of bisphosphonates have been proposed to increase the risk of atrial fibrillation and flutter, although a population-based case-control study of bisphosphonate use in women found no evidence of an increase risk of atrial fibrillation or atrial flutter.[152]

TORSADES DE POINTES

Female sex has been identified consistently as a risk factor for the development of torsades de pointes.[153] Many drugs have been associated with this arrhythmia, including ibutilide, dofetilide, quinidine, amiodarone, selected macrolide, and quinolone antibiotics.[153] In one study, patients who were taking ibutilide and subsequently developed torsades de pointes, 5.6% were women compared with 3% men.[154]

Table 30-6. Cardiovascular Effects from Chemotherapeutic Medications

Effect	Medication
Hypertension	alemtuzumab, anastrozole, bendamustine, bevacizumab, bicalutamide, bortezomib, busulfan, capecitabine, carboplatin, cetuximab, cisplatin, denileukin diftitox, docetaxel, exemestane, gemtuzumab ozogamicin, goserelin, letrozole, nilotinib, nilutamide, paclitaxel, pemetrexed, pentostatin, porfimer, rituximab, sorafenib, sunitinib, teniposide, trastuzumab, vinblastine, vincristine, vinorelbine
Myocardial ischemia and infarction	bevacizumab, bleomycin, cisplatin, dasatinib, denileukin diftitox, docetaxel, capecitabine, erlotinib, estramustine, fludarabine, fluorouracil, ibritumomab tiuxetan, idarubicin, irinotecan, ixabepilone, letrozole, paclitaxel, rituximab, sorafenib, toremifene, trastuzumab, vinblastine, vinorelbine
Heart failure	alemtuzumab, bevacizumab, bortezomib, cisplatin, dasatinib, fluorouracil, cyclophosphamide, trastuzumab, capecitabine, daunorubicin, docetaxel, doxorubicin, epirubicin, estramustine, idarubicin, imatinib, lapatinib, letrozole, mitomycin, mitoxantrone, porfimer, rituximab, sunitinib, toremifene
Arrhythmias	denileukin diftitox, anthracyclines, taxanes, and antimetabolites such as fluorouracil
Venous thromboembolic disease	tamoxifen, bevacizumab, denileukin diftitox, epirubicin, estramustine, fluorouracil, letrozole, oxaliplatin, paclitaxel, pemetrexed, sunitinib

A single-dose study with ibutilide also suggested that QT prolongation with ibutilide may be greatest in the first half of the menstrual cycle.[155] Pharmacokinetic drug interactions involving the use of inhibitors of cytochrome 3A4 frequently are major contributing factors to its development. Pharmacists should carefully monitor for these types of pharmacokinetic interactions, especially in women taking multiple medications that have been strongly associated with the development of torsades de pointes.

CARDIOVASCULAR INJURY WITH CANCER TREATMENT

Although cardiovascular disease is much more common among women, breast cancer is the disease that American women dread. The dose-related anthracycline-induced left ventricular heart failure is well recognized, and many of the newer advances in the treatment of breast cancer are also associated with at least short-term cardiovascular injury. Table 30-6 lists selected chemotherapy associated with hypertension, myocardial ischemia or infarction, heart failure, arrhythmias, and venous thromboembolic disease.[145] When combined with radiation and aggressive treatment to cure, older women clearly have an increased risk for cardiovascular disease as a result of the multiple adverse cardiac effects.

Summary

Almost 500,000 American women die of cardiovascular disease, including coronary heart disease, stroke, and heart failure. Despite advances in the management of cardiac diseases, sex disparities in the prevention and treatment of cardiovascular diseases continue to exist. Enrollment of women into many studies of cardiovascular disease has remained largely unchanged except for single-sex studies, such as the Women's Health Initiative. Aggressive management of overall risk factors as well as of cardiovascular diseases is essential to improve the cardiac care of women.

References

Additional content available at ***www.ashp.org/womenshealth***

31 Nutrition and Eating Disorders

Kimberly Braxton Lloyd, Pharm.D.; Connie Kraus, Pharm.D., BCPS

Learning Objectives

1. Discuss the importance of proper nutrition for the maintenance of optimal health and wellness.
2. Outline important counseling points for patients concerning nutrition and exercise habits to promote health and wellness.
3. Describe screening tools and resources used for evaluation of weight status.
4. Describe the criteria used for the diagnosis of eating disorders such as anorexia nervosa, bulimia nervosa, and binge-eating disorders.
5. Explain the pathophysiology of disordered eating.
6. Review nonpharmacologic interventions for the management of eating disorders.
7. Compare and contrast the pharmacotherapy for eating disorders.
8. Formulate a clinical plan for the nonpharmacologic and pharmacologic management of patients with disordered eating patterns.

Good nutrition is vital for health. It is a fundamental component of growth and development among children and disease prevention among adults. Unfortunately, many adolescent girls and adult women develop disordered eating patterns that often lead to underweight, drastic weight fluctuations, or obesity. Failure to maintain healthy eating and exercise patterns can result in numerous health problems. Underweight can be associated with health complications such as hormone disorders, osteoporosis, electrolyte abnormalities, seizures, and heart disease.[1] Overweight and obesity can lead to complications such as diabetes, cardiovascular disease, osteoarthritis, sleep apnea, gallbladder disease, gastroesophageal reflux disease, and various cancers.[2] In the U.S., weight-related morbidity and mortality is a major concern, so nutrition is a public health focus. Healthy People 2010 encourages healthcare providers to promote healthy nutrition and exercise patterns among their patients.[3] Establishing healthy eating and exercise patterns is vital to effectively managing all patterns of disordered eating and preventing the possible weight-related complications associated with being underweight or overweight.

Nutrition and Healthy Weight Status

Disordered eating patterns are very common, especially among women. Therefore, healthcare providers should be prepared to evaluate a patient's weight status to screen for the need for weight gain or loss.[4] This allows the healthcare provider to provide counseling on weight changes that may be required to decrease the risk of weight-related complications. Then, the healthcare provider can provide counseling on how to achieve and maintain an appropriate weight through implementation of healthy nutrition and exercise patterns. Healthcare providers can also reinforce healthy nutrition and exercise behaviors, and provide positive feedback to patients. Healthcare providers should prepare for this role by staying abreast of guidelines. Providers who are familiar with current dietary recommendations for health maintenance are more prepared to recognize and respond to aberrant eating patterns of their patients that might lead to health complications. This familiarity also provides the foundation for the provider to initiate a dialogue with the patient. Often a frank discussion about the importance of healthy eating habits is necessary to capture a patient's attention and initiate behavioral change. These discussions might begin to shift the patient's attention from focusing on a number on a scale to instead focusing on healthy nutrition and exercise behaviors. Guidelines are published by government agencies to assist the healthcare provider in this role.[4-7]

EVALUATION OF WEIGHT AND BODY COMPOSITION ANALYSIS

There are many methods of evaluating whether a person's weight and percent body fat are within a healthy range. However, many of these technologies are expensive and not readily available to healthcare providers and consumers. Therefore, the National Institutes of Health (NIH) has recommended using the body mass index (BMI) and the **waist circumference** (WC) as surrogate markers to predict a patient's weight-related health risks.[4] The first step in calculating a BMI is obtaining an accurate height and weight measurement.[8] To measure a patient's height, the healthcare provider needs a large ruler mounted to a wall (without baseboards) in a room that has a level floor or an adjustable rod measuring stick (or stadiometer). Shoes, outer clothing, and hats should be removed. Also, if the patient has a ponytail or other hair style that adds height, it should be taken down for the evaluation. The patient should stand upright with shoulders level, hands to the sides, feet flat, and thighs and heels together. Head, shoulders, and buttocks should be pressed against the wall or measurement device, and eyes and ears should be aligned for correct head position. The patient should take a deep breath and hold it during the measurement. The headpiece should be lowered until it contacts the crown of the head, and then the height can be recorded to the nearest 0.125 inches (0.1 cm).

After an accurate height is obtained, the patient should be weighed on a digital or balance-beam platform scale. The scale should be placed on a firm, noncarpeted floor. The weight should be recorded to the nearest 0.25 pounds or kilograms. Once these data are collected, the BMI can be calculated by taking the weight in kilograms divided by the height in meters squared (kg/m^2) or weight in pounds multiplied by 703 divided by height in inches squared (lb/in^2). The BMI is a good indicator of adiposity in most cases.[4] However, BMI might overestimate adiposity in patients who are athletic, muscular, or fluid overloaded and might underestimate adiposity in patients who have experienced muscle atrophy (e.g., advanced age, paralysis). Therefore, the NIH recommends measurement of WC to evaluate abdominal fat and use of these data in conjunction with BMI to evaluate a patient's weight-related health risks. The process for measuring an accurate WC is depicted in Figure 31-1. The desired WC is <35 inches in women and <40 inches in men. A patient who has a BMI of 25.0 kg/m^2 or greater and a WC greater than the sex-specific threshold is at risk of having increased abdominal adiposity and visceral fat stores. This increases the risk of weight-related health complications such as type 2 diabetes and coronary artery disease.

Figure 31-1. Measurement of waist circumference.
To measure waist circumference, locate the upper hip bone and the top of the right iliac crest. Place a measuring tape in a horizontal plane around the abdomen at the level of the iliac crest. Before reading the tape measure, ensure that the tape is snug but does not compress the skin and is parallel to the floor. The measurement is made at the end of a normal expiration. Desirable waist circumference in adults: male ≤40 inches; female ≤35 inches.
Source: Modified from reference 5.

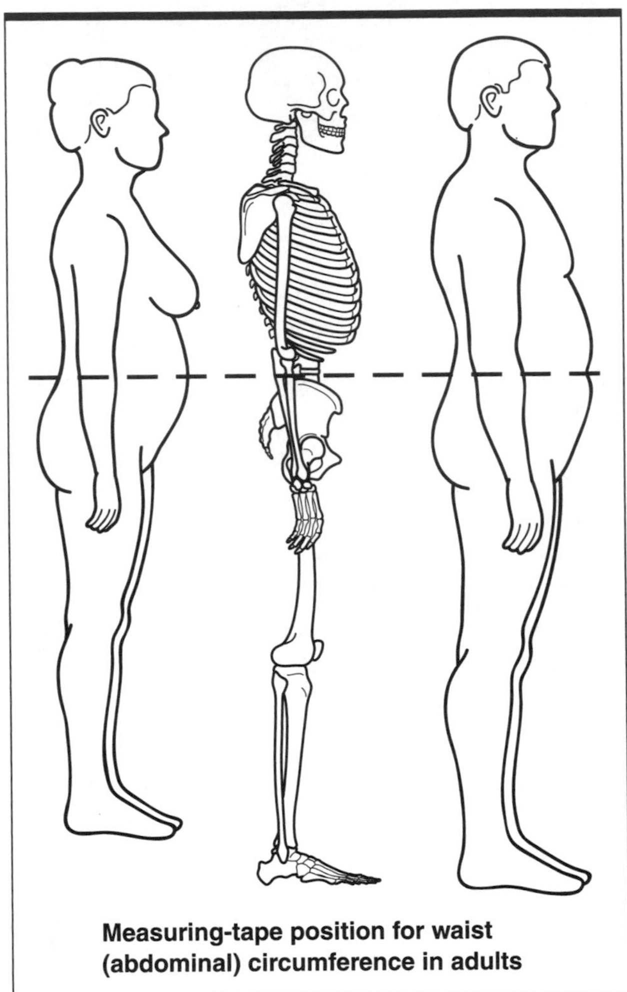

These assessments are simple and straightforward and require minimal equipment.[4] A healthcare provider can conduct these screenings with a ruler, measuring tape, and scale. There are other methods of evaluating body composition.[9-11] The gold standards are underwater weighing technologies and **dual energy x-ray absorptiometry.** These methods give excellent estimates of percent body fat and lean muscle mass. However, they are very expensive, and access to these technologies is limited. Other more accessible methods include anthropometrics (e.g., skin-fold pinch) and **bioelectrical impedance analysis** (BIA). Both of these methods are often conducted in physical education classes, community exercise facilities, healthcare clinics, and other venues. There are professional and consumer versions of weight and body composition scales available that use BIA technology to estimate body composition and provide feedback on the total body weight, percent body fat, fat weight, fat-free weight (lean body weight), and total body water. These readings can help monitor changes in fat weight. Monitoring fat weight is more informative for patients who are making lifestyle changes to decrease body fat. Increases in lean body weight caused by gains in lean muscle mass that are due to increased exercise or increases of total body water that is due to fluid retention can be detected. Changes in lean body mass can mask true changes in fat weight, and this can be discouraging for patients who are closely monitoring their weight during a weight-loss attempt. One thing that must be remembered is that BIA measures the impedance of electricity conducted through body tissues and uses this reading to estimate body fat.[12] Therefore, any factor that might affect hydration status might affect the accuracy of the BIA body composition results. Studies have shown that when using BIA, it is very important to accurately measure the patient's height and weight and standardize conditions in relation to previous exercise, dietary intake, body positioning, and skin temperature with each reading. Consistency in these variables improves the accuracy of the readings. The typical error on total body water and lean body weight using BIA is 2% to 4%.

GUIDELINES AND/OR POSITION STATEMENTS

There are several guidelines that provide direction for patient weight assessment and information on healthy nutrition and exercise practices[4-7]:

- Department of Health and Human Services (DHHS) Office of Disease Prevention and Health Promotion and United States Department of Agriculture (USDA). Dietary Guidelines for Americans, 2005. [6] These guidelines outline healthy dietary behaviors for people 2 years of age and older. These guidelines are used for the development of federal educational programs on nutrition.
- USDA Center for Nutrition Policy and Promotion. Steps to a Healthier You: the Food Guide Pyramid.[7] This website provides tools to assist consumers in developing individualized nutrition plans.
- National Institutes of Health. Clinical Guidelines on the Identification, Evaluation, and Treatment of Overweight and Obesity in Adults: The Evidence Report.[4] These evidence-based guidelines were developed by the National Heart, Lung, and Blood Institute in cooperation with the National Institute of Diabetes and Digestive and Kidney Diseases. This reference provides an overview of the appropriate evaluation and management of the overweight or obese patient.
- National Institutes of Health. The Practical Guide: Identification, Evaluation, and Treatment of Overweight and Obesity in Adults.[5] This publication provides practical tools for the healthcare provider to use in practice.

PREVENTION: HEALTHY NUTRITION AND EXERCISE BEHAVIORS

The NIH guidelines on the identification, evaluation, and treatment of overweight and obesity emphasize the importance of maintaining weight within a healthy range for age, height, and sex.[4] This should be accomplished by balancing the number of kilocalories consumed through food and beverages with the number of kilocalories expended throughout the day (kilocalories in = kilocalories out).[4] Daily energy requirements vary from person to person and are a function of their basal metabolic rate, activities of daily living, and additional exercise.[13] These energy requirements vary depending on the patient's sex, age, height, and weight. These concepts will be discussed in more detail in the chapter on overweight and obesity.

Nutrient Selection

When selecting the diet, all calories are not created equal. The NIH guidelines recommend that individuals choose nutrient-dense foods that are rich in vitamins and minerals.[4-7] For a person who requires an average 2,000-kcal daily diet, it is recommended that he or she consumes at least two servings of fruit and three servings of vegetables a day. Fruits and vegetables are high-fiber carbohydrates that are nutrient rich. Many are filled with antioxidants, vitamins, and minerals that are essential for health. On average, fruits and vegetables have lower calories per serving and are satisfying. They are considered a nutrition "bargain." Individuals should also limit high-fat foods such as fried foods, oily or greasy foods, high-fat meats, full-fat dairy, and butter. The amount of saturated fats (fats that are solid at room temperature, such as bacon grease, shortening, and butter) and trans fats (fats used to extend shelf life of prepared foods) should be limited. People should select healthy unsaturated fats rich in omega-3 and omega-6 fatty acids, such as oily fish, olive and vegetable oils, and nuts. Refined carbohydrates and sugar should be limited. Instead, fiber-rich carbohydrates, such as fruit, vegetables, and whole grains, are suggested. The goal fiber intake is at least 25 g of fiber/day. When selecting carbohydrates, it is recommended to select whole-grain pasta, brown rice, corn tortillas, high-fiber cereals, high-fiber breads, and other whole-grain starches. It is also recommended to limit dietary sodium to <2,300 mg of sodium/day (equivalent to 1 teaspoon of salt); ingest 1,000–1,500 mg of elemental calcium from diet and supplements in divided servings not to exceed 500 mg at one time for maximum absorption; and eat a balanced diet to get trace minerals. The National Osteoporosis Foundation recommends that individuals younger than age 50 years get 400–800 International Units of vitamin D/day, and people age 50 and older target 800–1,000 International Units/day.[14] Excessive alcohol and caffeine intake should be avoided.

Behaviors to Improve Healthy Nutrition

To become nutrition savvy, it is necessary to improve awareness and knowledge of nutrition basics.[4-7,15] It is important to pay attention to portion sizes, measure foods and drinks, read nutrition labels, and avoid overeating. When patients are beginning to learn more about healthy nutrition and are first altering their eating habits to obtain healthier nutrition habits, it is often helpful to measure foods and maintain a nutrition diary to monitor intake.

There are a number of recommendations, tricks, and tools for patients to use when changing behaviors to achieve a healthy diet.[15] For instance, when eating out, simple things such as asking for nutritional information for items on the menu, sharing an entrée with a friend, and asking for a to-go box can help decrease the tendency to overeat. At home, small changes—such as serving meals on smaller plates and avoiding distractions, such as the television, during mealtime—can improve nutrition habits. Also, when trying to modify unhealthy behaviors, it is often a good idea to develop a support network. Friends and family can have fun cooking together, sharing meals, trading recipes, and exercising together. Emphasizing the importance of nutrition and exercise goals within the family also helps teach children in the household good habits that will help them maintain healthy habits for a lifetime.

Increased Activities of Daily Living

Americans should also focus on increasing their activities of daily living and just moving more throughout the day.[4-7] Even simple efforts to overcome a sedentary lifestyle—such as walking to appointments, taking the stairs, parking further away, and playing with kids—can have a significant impact on weight maintenance and overall health. A tool called a pedometer can be purchased to wear on the belt to count the number of steps one takes per day.[16] The goal for good health should be to walk 10,000 steps per day. The pedometer can provide objective data concerning a person's daily activity level.

Increased Daily Exercise

In addition to increased activities, formal exercise is very important.[4-7] Americans should engage in at least 150 minutes of aerobic exercise per week.[4] It is important for people to select an activity they enjoy and can incorporate into their life to make it easier to accomplish this goal. Best results are obtained with a combination of aerobic, resistance, and flexibility exercises. Weight-bearing activities and resistance training activities are important for bone health.[14]

SEX DIFFERENCES

Research has shown that there are sex differences in the resting energy expenditure between men and women because differences in muscle mass between sexes.[17] In general, men have a higher lean body weight and, therefore, basal metabolic rate (kcal/day) when compared with women. In fact, one of the most frequently used equations to estimate basal metabolic rate (BMR), the Harrison Benedict Equation, has a different equation for men vs. women[18]:

For women: $BMR = 655 + (4.35 \times \text{weight in pounds}) + (4.7 \times \text{height in inches}) - (4.7 \times \text{age in years})$

For men: $BMR = 66 + (6.23 \times \text{weight in pounds}) + (12.7 \times \text{height in inches}) - (6.8 \times \text{age in years})$

Therefore, when comparing the energy requirements for a man and woman who are the same age, height, and weight, the man often requires more calories for weight maintenance than the woman because of the increased amount of lean body mass when compared with women. For instance, using the Harris Benedict equation, a man who is 32 years of age, 68 inches tall, and weighs 160 pounds has an estimated BMR of 1,709 kcal/day. A woman who is the exact age, height, and weight has an estimated BMR of 1,520 kcal/day. Other factors that have a significant impact on energy requirements are age and adiposity.[17]

NUTRITION SUMMARY

Healthcare providers should assist their patients in identifying their weight-related health risks and nutritional goals.[4-7] This includes evaluating their height, weight, BMI, WC, and body composition. Using these data, an ideal weight range can be established and a plan developed to obtain or maintain one's weight within these targets. Healthy nutrition should be emphasized as the foundation for a healthy lifestyle to avoid weight-related health complications or aid the recovery from eating disorders.

Eating Disorders

Although diagnostic criteria may point to unique features of various eating disorders, it is more likely that they are part of a spectrum.[19] Eating disorders are more common among women. Girls and women diagnosed with disordered eating may fluctuate between **anorexia nervosa, bulimia nervosa, binge-eating disorder,** and other atypical eating patterns. Therefore, patients who experience problems with disordered eating can be underweight, normal, or overweight and may even experience wide weight fluctuations. Resumption of healthy nutrition is fundamental to recovery.[20] Some individuals with disordered eating may have comorbid mental health conditions, such as anxiety, depression, and body dysmorphic disorder. A full discussion of these conditions can be found in Chapter 34: Mental Health.

ANOREXIA NERVOSA

(See Web Resources for Patient Case: Anorexia Nervosa.)

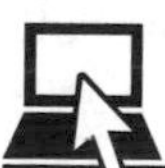

Additional content available at ***www.ashp.org/womenshealth***

Anorexia nervosa often begins in adolescence and is characterized by an exaggerated drive for thinness, focusing on dieting and, in some cases, other interventions (e.g., excessive exercise, purging) resulting in sustained low weight.[21] Altered body image, fear of weight gain, and a continued desire to lose weight are common features of this disorder.

Anorexia nervosa is most commonly seen in Western societies, affecting primarily white women (90%), especially from higher social classes.[19] The prevalence is estimated to be 0.7% among teenaged girls, and the lifetime risk among women is believed to be 0.3% to 1%.[21]

Clinical Presentation

Women with anorexia nervosa overevaluate the shape and size of their body.[19] They engage in a sustained and focused pursuit of weight loss and, therefore, generally succeed at achieving very low weight. Some women with anorexia nervosa overexercise. There are two subtypes of anorexia nervosa: 1) restricting (withholding nutrients only), and 2) purging (self-induced vomiting or use of laxatives or diuretics).[20] Depression (50% to 75% of patients), anxiety disorders (>60%), mood swings, loss of concentration and sexual desire, and obsessive behaviors (>40%) may be comorbid conditions.[19,21,22] As weight decreases, these symptoms may worsen and often improve with weight gain.

Common signs and symptoms associated with anorexia nervosa may include orthostatic hypotension, bradycardia, hair loss, impaired menstrual function, and loss of subcutaneous adipose tissue.[21] Serum electrolyte and thyroid function may be affected.

Pathophysiology

Little is known about the causes of anorexia nervosa.[19] Anorexia nervosa appears to be related to genetic, family, and social factors.[22] Eating disorders tend to run in families with linkages to anorexia nervosa and obsessive and perfectionist traits, but there is uncertainty about the extent of the genetic contribution.[19] Research literature suggests alterations in serotonergic and dopaminergic function.[23] Other risk factors—such as sexual abuse, poor parenting, having received criticism regarding weight, or occupational or recreational pressure to be slim—may contribute.[19] Perfectionism is often found as a premorbid characteristic.

Long-term Complications

Complications from anorexia nervosa may affect a large number of organ systems.[21] With prolonged and severe cases of anorexia nervosa, there is an increased risk of osteopenia, osteoporosis, and fracture.[19] Younger patients with anorexia may have shorter stature as adults and may also be more at risk for stress fractures.[21] Loss of gray matter during long periods of food refusal may cause reduction of cognitive function. Anorexia nervosa may also have an effect on future fertility, with a higher rate of miscarriage and lower-birth-weight infants. Most women with anorexia nervosa recover partially or completely, but 5% die of the condition and for 20%, the condition may be chronic.[22] Women with purging anorexia nervosa and substance abuse are at higher risk for premature death.[21] Starvation and purging-related arrhythmias are the most common medical causes for death. Likelihood of recovery is inversely related to severity of weight loss and presence of other psychiatric disorders. Fifty to 70% of adolescents, however, do recover and regain health over 5–7 years. Outcomes for adults with anorexia are not as promising, with only 25% to 50% of those hospitalized reaching recovery.

Diagnosis of Anorexia Nervosa

The diagnosis of anorexia nervosa is based on a history of overvaluation of thinness, food restriction, excessive exercise, and other possible behaviors (e.g., purging).[21] Additionally, diagnostic criteria, such as the *Diagnostic and Statistical Manual of Mental Disorders, 4th edition, (DSM-IV),* assist in establishing the diagnosis. The key diagnostic element from this tool is the refusal to maintain body weight at or above a minimal normal weight (≥85% of expected weight) for age and height.[20,21,24] Other features include 1) intense fear of gaining weight or being fat, even though underweight; 2) distorted view of body weight or shape, self-evaluation focused on weight or shape, or denial of seriousness of current low weight; and 3) amenorrhea (absence of three consecutive periods).[21] It is unnecessary to rule out other medical causes of weight loss if these criteria are met. Subthreshold anorexia nervosa (missing one element, such as amenorrhea) is common.[20] Indeed, many authorities have become more flexible with regard to the weight criteria needing to be below 85% of normal body weight and the duration of amenorrhea of more than 3 months for making the diagnosis.[21]

In addition, a careful assessment of symptoms, behaviors, and mental status is also important.[25] Height and weight history, exercise patterns, determination of restrictive vs. purging practices, attitudes about gaining weight, and evaluation of other potential comorbid mental health disorders should be evaluated. Additionally, family history of psychiatric disorders or eating disorders should be determined.

The physical exam includes vital signs, height and weight (including calculation of BMI), cardiovascular and peripheral vascular system evaluation, skin exam, and examination for self-injuries.[25] A psychiatric evaluation—including evaluation of suicidal ideation and plans—is important to ensure patient safety.

Guidelines and Position Statements

1. ***American Academy of Pediatrics Committee on Sports Medicine and Fitness.*** Promotion of Healthy Weight Control Practices in Young Athletes.[26] This guideline identifies unhealthy weight control practices for young athletes and provides information regarding healthy methods of weight loss and gain. Additionally, the guideline provides information that healthcare professionals may use in counseling athletes, parents, school administrators, and athletic coaches.
2. ***Management of Eating Disorders.***[24] This guideline is based on a systematic review of the literature assessing the efficacy of treatment for anorexia nervosa, bulimia nervosa, and binge-eating disorder. This guideline also addresses harms associated with treatments, factors associated with treatment efficacy/outcomes, and the possible influence of sociodemographic characteristics on treatment outcomes.
3. ***American Psychiatric Association: Treatment of Patients with Eating Disorders, 3rd ed.***[25] This evidence-based guideline provides treatment of eating disorders, including psychiatric management and selection of a treatment site and choice of specific treatments for anorexia nervosa, bulimia nervosa, and eating disorder not otherwise specified.
4. ***Position of the American Dietetic Association: Nutrition Intervention in the Treatment of Anorexia Nervosa, Bulimia Nervosa, and Other Eating Disorders.***[20] This position statement emphasizes the need for nutritional interventions, including nutritional counseling, as an important component of the interdisciplinary approach to the care of patients with anorexia nervosa, bulimia nervosa, and other eating disorders.

Primary Prevention

The Eating Disorders Awareness Prevention and Education Act of 2003 recognized the prevalence of eating disorders in school-aged children and need for education.[20] Two resources for healthy eating directed at women and girls include *Girl Power* (http://www.girlpower.gov/) and *BodyWise* (http://www.4women.gov/owh/programs/girl.cfm) (Office on Women's Health of the U.S. DHHS).

Treatment Goals

The goals of treatment of anorexia nervosa include 1) restoring a healthy weight (e.g., a weight that permits return of menses and ovulation); 2) treating complications; 3) enhancing the patient's cooperation and participation in restoring eating patterns; 4) providing education related to healthy eating and nutrition; 5) assisting patients with evaluating and changing dysfunctional thoughts, conflicts, and feelings; 6) treating comorbid psychiatric conditions; 7) engaging family support and providing appropriate counseling; and 8) preventing relapse.[25]

Treatment of anorexia nervosa is complex and requires expertise of a variety of healthcare professionals.[20,25] There is little evidence to support the use of inpatient vs. outpatient settings.[27] Treatment outcomes among adolescents are generally good but may be less successful in adults.

Nonpharmacologic Treatment

Nutritional Treatment

Refeeding is a necessary component of treatment but is of limited value without other interventions.[22] Some evidence suggests that a lenient approach to nutritional intervention may be preferable to a strict approach, and nasogastric feeding is rarely required.

Nutritional goals include restoration of a healthy weight and normalization of eating patterns.[20] Nutrient intake should be gradually increased. A baseline level of 30–40 kcal/kg/day (actual weight) (1,000–1,200 kcal/day) may be titrated to achieve weight gain of 0.5–1.0 lb/wk for outpatients. During the weight-gain phase, some patients may require up to 70–100 kcal/kg/day.[25] Restoration of weight is also important for reducing risk of osteoporosis.[20] Elemental calcium 1,500 mg/day and vitamin D 400 International Units/day may prevent bone demineralization in patients with deficiencies.

Although weight restoration is generally accomplished in the outpatient setting, there may be occasions during which inpatient care is necessary.[27] Criteria include risk of suicide, unfavorable home situation, and failure of previous attempts. Additionally, severe malnourishment (e.g., <70% of healthy body weight), electrolyte imbalance, infection, hypoglycemia, or significant comorbid conditions may also warrant hospitalization.[20,22] For hospitalized patients, a weight gain of 2–3 lb/wk is targeted.[25] If life-preserving nutrition is needed, continuous nasogastric feeding is recommended.

Physical activity prescriptions should reflect the patient's cardiac function and bone mineral density.[25] When weight is restored, physical activity should be used to promote fitness rather than caloric expenditure.

Psychotherapy

Goals of psychotherapeutic interventions include promoting 1) understanding of and cooperation with nutritional and physical rehabilitation; 2) understanding and change with respect to behaviors and attitudes toward the eating disorder; 3) improvement in interpersonal skills and social function; and 4) ability to address comorbid psychiatric conditions that may reinforce the eating disorder.[25]

A systematic review of 32 studies regarding treatment of anorexia nervosa included 18 behavioral intervention trials, including cognitive, supportive, family, individual, group, and dynamic therapy. Therapeutic warming was also used in one trial.[24] Of the 11 behavioral treatment trials that were rated as good or fair, four were studies of adolescents (mean age 14–15), six included persons 18 years of age and older, and one combined groups. Three trials used **cognitive behavioral therapy** (CBT). CBT targets exploring, identifying, and modifying beliefs, behaviors, and assumptions that cause disturbed emotions (see Web Resources for more information on Cognitive Behavioral Therapy).[28]

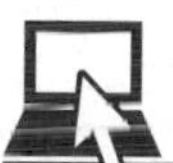

Additional content available at ***www.ashp.org/womenshealth***

CBT is often patient and situation specific, and addresses the particular needs of the individual. Patients are often asked to monitor, reflect, and journal on the thoughts, feelings, and circumstances associated with the disordered eating. The therapist is then able to discuss, analyze, and reframe the patient's thoughts and actions to address triggers and inappropriate responses. The patient can then be challenged to respond differently in the future. CBT can be adapted for group therapy and has even been used in self-help manuals, software, and other resources.

In one trial (described within the systematic review) that followed inpatient weight restoration of adults with anorexia nervosa, CBT significantly reduced risk of relapse and increased positive outcomes compared with nutritional education.[24] However, of those receiving CBT who had positive outcomes, a large number were also using antidepressants. It is not known if CBT is helpful during the acute stages of the illness, while the patient is still underweight. Another study showed nonspecific supportive treatment to be more effective than CBT or interpersonal psychotherapy in the acute stages. Family therapy sessions worked well in one study of adolescents with short duration of illness, but three studies in adult patients with longer duration of illness did not show a benefit. Two studies of CBT failed to show benefit for weight, eating, or mood outcomes. No well-designed studies combining psychotherapy and pharmacotherapy were identified in this systematic review.

Pharmacologic Treatment

Selective Serotonin Reuptake Inhibitors

The literature on pharmacotherapeutic treatments for anorexia is limited (Table 31-1).[29] Of 32 trials in a systematic review, two medication trials were viewed as good and six as fair. Most trials had small sample sizes.

Two of the trials in this systematic review described use of the selective serotonin reuptake inhibitor (SSRI) fluoxetine. One studied 31 inpatient women, ages 16–45 years, who had returned to at least 65% of their ideal body weight. The mean BMI at the time of randomization was 15 mg/m^2. Patients were randomized to receive placebo or fluoxetine 60 mg daily. Psychotherapy was continued. There was no difference between the groups in terms of weight gain, psychological features of anorexia nervosa, anxiety, or depression. A similar outcome occurred in another study of 39 people randomized to placebo or fluoxetine titrated to 60 mg/day over the 52 weeks of the study. At the time of randomization, subjects were at 76% to 100% average body weight. Psychological therapy was permitted. Again, there was no difference between the groups in terms of eating, biomarker measures, or psychological measures.

Fluoxetine has also been studied as a treatment to prevent relapse in patients who have regained weight. A randomized, double-blind, placebo-controlled trial evaluated the effectiveness of fluoxetine in patients who had regained weight to a minimum BMI of 19.[30] Forty-nine subjects received fluoxetine and 44 received placebo over 52 weeks. Fluoxetine was started at 20 mg/day and titrated to 60 mg/day during the first week. The dosage of 60 mg/day was then maintained but could be decreased based on side effects or increased to 80 mg/day at the discretion of the investigator. The main outcome measures were recovery and time to relapse. There was no significant difference between the two groups in time to relapse (hazard ratio 1.2; 95% CI, 0.65–2.01; $p = 0.64$).

Despite the lack of evidence for efficacy in treating anorexia nervosa, SSRIs may be used in conjunction with psychotherapy in patients with comorbid depression, anxiety, or obsessive compulsive symptoms.[25]

Other Antidepressants

Bupropion should not be used in patients with anorexia nervosa because of increased risk for seizures.[25] Tricyclic antidepressants and monoamine oxidase inhibitors may pose risks for adverse reactions in this population.[25]

Second-Generation Antipsychotics

Second-generation antipsychotics such as olanzapine, quetiapine, and risperidone have been use in case series and individual cases with some success in situations in which patients have strong resistance to gaining weight, severe obsessions, or delusional thinking.[25] A systematic review of the efficacy/toxicity of olanzapine for treatment of anorexia nervosa assembled data from 22 case reports, two open-label trials (n = 35), a randomized, controlled trial (n = 15), and two retrospective studies (n = 32).[31] Most subjects successfully gained weight and had improvements in psychological symptoms when using dosages of 2.5–15 mg daily. Limitations include small sample sizes, open-label designs, and low completion rates.

Vitamin and Mineral Supplementation

Calcium and vitamin D are recommended if deficiencies are likely due to dietary intake and exposure to sunlight, respectively.[25] Zinc supplementation has been reported to improve weight gain in some people. Multivitamin and mineral supplements may be used to complement increased dietary intake of foods, but weakly designed trials have not demonstrated specific value in treatment of symptoms of anorexia nervosa.[25]

Hormone and Bisphosphonate Therapy

No good evidence supports the efficacy of hormone therapy for improving bone mineral density in female patients with anorexia nervosa.[25] In a randomized, placebo-controlled trial, women with anorexia nervosa received an oral contraceptive containing norgestimate/ethinyl estradiol (n = 53; mean BMI = 17.9 km/m^2) or placebo (n = 59; mean BMI = 17.6 kg/m^2) for 13 cycles.[32] Dual energy x-ray absorptiometry scans of the lumbosacral spine were obtained at baseline and at the sixth and thirteenth cycle. At the end of the thirteenth cycle, there was no significant difference between the groups in increase in bone mineral density at the spine or hip. There is also no indication for use of alendronate for prevention of bone demineralization.[25]

Table 31-1. Benefits and Risks of Pharmacotherapy for Eating Disorders[61]

Medication (Dosages Studied)	Eating Disorders Studied	Efficacy Data	Possible Adverse Effects	Pregnancy Category	Contraindications and Cautions
Antidepressants					
Antidepressants may worsen depression or increase suicidal ideation, especially among children and adolescents. It is important to screen for suicidal ideation before starting therapy and to slowly and cautiously initiate therapy in severe major depression or bipolar disorder. Patients should be closely monitored. Do not discontinue therapy abruptly.					
Desipramine	BN BED	Efficacy data available for BN and BED	Postural hypotension, syncope, arrhythmias, QT interval prolongation, palpitations, rash, syndrome of inappropriate antidiuretic hormone, weight gain, xerostomia, anticholinergic effects, sedation, lethargy, psychosis, headache, confusion, memory impairment, paresthesias, seizures, photosensitivity, gastroesophageal reflux disease, sexual dysfunction	C	• Contraindicated during acute recovery phase of acute myocardial infarction • Do not initiate in a patient who has used a monoamine oxidase inhibitor within 14 days • Use with caution in patients with cardiovascular disease, seizure history, hyperthyroidism, and renal insufficiency • Cross-reactivity with other dibenzodiazepines may occur • Trazodone has been associated with priapism; surgical intervention may be required • Do not initiate in a patient who has used a monoamine oxidase inhibitor in the past 14 days; never use concomitantly; and wait 5 wk (fluoxetine) or 2 wk (fluvoxamine, sertraline, and citalopram) after the discontinuation of the SSRI before starting any of these agents • Increased risk of bleeding (especially of gastrointestinal tract) when used with nonsteroidal anti-inflammatory drugs, aspirin, and other medications that affect bleeding • Use with caution with other serotonergic medications because of an increased risk of serotonin syndrome • Fluoxetine should never be used within 5 wk (before or after) of or thioridazine or mesoridazine • Sertraline oral concentrate
Imipramine	BED			D	
Trazodone	BN	Most AN studies failed to show efficacy of SSRI therapy; however, it may benefit patients with depression, anxiety, or obsessive-compulsive symptoms		C	
Fluoxetine (Dosage = 60 mg daily)	AN BN BED			C	
Fluvoxamine (Dosage = 50–300 mg daily; average studied = 182 mg daily)	BN BED			C	
Sertraline (Dosage = 50–100 mg daily)	BED		Trazodone has lower anticholinergic effects than desipramine and imipramine	C	
Citalopram (Dosage = 20–60 mg daily)	BED	SSRIs are most effective for BN when combined with CBT SSRIs have shown efficacy for BED	Nausea, vomiting, diarrhea, appetite changes, weight gain or loss, insomnia, somnolence, disrupted sleep, weakness, fatigue, headache, anxiety, emotional changes, nervousness, sexual dysfunction, rash, sweating, allergic reactions, vasculitis, hyponatremia, syndrome of inappropriate antidiuretic hormone	C	
Antipsychotics					
Olanzapine (Dosage = 2.5–15 mg daily)	AN	Overall, limited evidence for efficacy; may be useful in patients with strong resistance to weight gain, severe obsessions, and delusional thinking	Sedation; anticholinergic adverse effects; extrapyramidal symptoms; adverse effects such as akathisia, dystonia, tardive dyskinesia, weight gain, metabolic changes, diabetes mellitus, headache	C	Contraindicated in patients with severe central nervous system depression, coma, bone marrow suppression, blood dyscrasias, or severe hepatic disease
Quetiapine				C	Moderate to high sedation; use in caution in patients with central nervous system disorders, such as Alzheimer's and Parkinson's disease; use with caution in breast cancer or other prolactin-dependent tumors
Risperidone				C	

(Continued on next page)

Medication (Dosages Studied)	Eating Disorders Studied	Efficacy Data	Possible Adverse Effects	Pregnancy Category	Contraindications and Cautions
Anticonvulsants					
Topiramate (Average Dosage = 100 mg/day)	BN BED	Decreases anxiety and promotes weight loss	Xerostomia, paresthesia, fatigue, somnolence, difficulty concentrating, attention deficit, confusion, depression, memory loss, vision changes, dyspepsia, abdominal pain	C	Use cautiously in patients with hepatic or renal impairment
Zonisamide	BED	Decreased binge eating, weight loss, BED clinical severity, but significant study attrition	Headache, agitation, mood changes, fatigue, memory changes, difficulty concentrating, schizophrenic behaviors, seizures, weight loss, nausea, abdominal pain, taste changes, paresthesia, weakness	C	Contraindicated in patients with sulfonamide allergy
Weight Loss Medications					
Sibutramine (Dosage = 15 mg daily)	BED	For BED, showed decreased binge episodes, improved depression scores, and weight loss	Headache, insomnia, anorexia, xerostomia, constipation, rhinitis, tachycardia, palpitations, chest pain, nervousness, anxiety, depression, emotional changes, dyspepsia, gastritis	C	Contraindicated in patients with AN and in patients who have taken a monoamine oxidase inhibitor within 2 wk of initiating sibutramine therapy; use with caution in patients with hypertension and cardiovascular disease; do not use if hypertension is uncontrolled or poorly controlled; do not use concurrently with serotonergic agents
Orlistat (Dosage = 120 mg TID before meals)	BED	Possible weight loss when combined with CBT, but weight loss not sustained at 2-mo follow-up evaluation	Headache, abdominal pain/cramping, flatulence, diarrhea, oily stools, increased defecation, fecal urgency, fecal incontinence, nausea, vomiting, fat soluble vitamin deficiency, back pain, upper-respiratory infections, fatigue, anxiety	B	Contraindicated in patients with chronic malabsorption syndromes and with cholestasis

AN = anorexia nervosa; BN = bulimia nervosa; BED = binge-eating disorder; CBT = cognitive behavior therapy; SSRI = selective serotonin reuptake inhibitor; TID = 3 times a day.

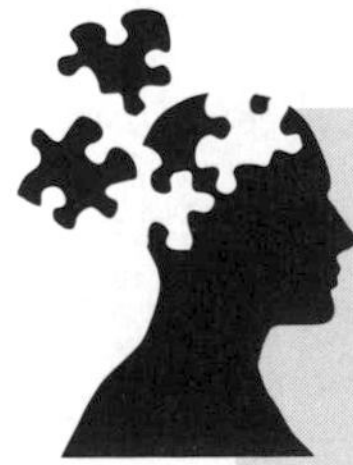

Therapeutic Challenge:

What vitamin and mineral supplementation is recommended in patients with anorexia nervosa to prevent health complications?

Monitoring and Follow-up

Eating disorder symptoms and behaviors should be frequently monitored.[25] Patients may be at risk for suicide because of the eating disorder and/or some treatments, so screening is critical. It is important to monitor the patient's general medical condition,

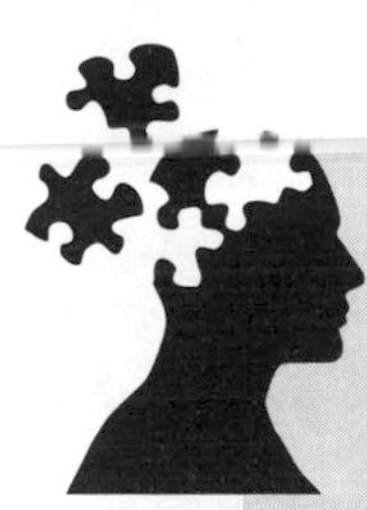

Therapeutic Challenge:

Are any pharmacotherapeutic interventions helpful for the prevention of bone demineralization in young women with anorexia nervosa?

including weight, blood pressure, pulse, and other cardiovascular parameters at frequent intervals (e.g., weekly initially).[21,25] Dental exams are important for patients with purging behaviors. Bone mineral density should be obtained if patient has been without menses for >6 months. Growth and sexual development should be monitored in younger patients.

Second-generation antipsychotics require monitoring for extrapyramidal effects and akathisias, especially in highly debilitated patients.[25] It is also important to monitor for insulin resistance, lipid abnormalities, and prolonged QT intervals in patients using these medications.

Patient Education

A fundamental component of psychiatric care is the provision of educational materials, including self-help literature.[25] Even though self-help literature has not been well studied in patients with anorexia nervosa, it has been proven to be of benefit for patient with other eating disorders.[33] Information about community-based resources and online materials may be provided. If appropriate, family education may also be provided.

Dietitians should develop the nutrition component of the treatment plan and work with the patient to assist in understanding and implementation of the nutritional prescription.[20] Ideally, the dietitian will have contact with the patient throughout the course of therapy.

Sex Differences

The incidence of anorexia nervosa in women is estimated at 19/100,000 per year vs. 2/100,000 in men.[19] It is most common in adolescents, with an estimated prevalence of 0.7% in teenage girls.

Summary

The literature on pharmacotherapeutic and behavioral treatment for adults with anorexia nervosa is sparse and inconclusive.[29] Use of medications alone to treat anorexia nervosa is inappropriate. CBT may be beneficial in reducing relapse rates for adults with anorexia nervosa once weight is restored. Family therapy may be beneficial in adolescents with anorexia nervosa of short duration but does not appear effective in adults. There is a lack of well-designed trials evaluating combination of psychological and medication therapies.

BULIMIA NERVOSA

Up to 25% of patients with bulimia nervosa initially meet criteria for anorexia nervosa, but recurrent episodes of binge eating interrupt dietary restriction.[27] A common feature of patients with bulimia nervosa is a sense of loss of control. Like anorexia, bulimia nervosa is most commonly seen in Western societies, in white people, and primarily in women. Unlike anorexia nervosa, it has a more even distribution among social classes and is more often seen in young adults as opposed to adolescents. It is the most common eating disorder among athletes (overall prevalence of eating disorders in this population estimated at 10% to 20%).[20] The prevalence of bulimia nervosa is 1% of young women.[34]

Clinical Presentation

In patients with bulimia nervosa, attempts to control shape and weight are countered by binge-eating episodes accompanied by a sense of loss of control.[27] Methods to lose weight may include self-induced vomiting; excess exercise; use of ipecac, diuretics, or laxatives; or fasting.[20] Even with purging, most patients with bulimia retain an average of 1,200 kcal, so most are of normal weight.[20,35] If patients induce vomiting, electrolyte disturbances and dental erosions may be present.[27] Laxatives may increase loss of water but do not affect absorption of nutrients.[20] Ipecac, when used chronically, may have adverse effects on the heart. Because of the distress associated with loss of control, patients with bulimia nervosa may be more likely to seek treatment.[27] Physical abnormalities are generally minor. After 10 years, 50% of people with bulimia nervosa will recover, one third will partially recover, and 10% to 20% will remain symptomatic.[34]

Pathophysiology

As is the case with anorexia nervosa, bulimia nervosa appears to have a genetic influence.[27] Serotonergic systems are believed to play a role.[35] Other risk factors may include early menses, parental obesity, parental alcoholism, receiving negative comments about weight by family members, childhood obesity, low self-esteem, difficulty with coping and feeling alone.[20,27]

CASE PRESENTATION

Patient Case: Part 1

D.S. is a 25-year-old woman who presents for a well-woman exam. She states she is somewhat fatigued, but otherwise describes herself as being in good health. She has occasionally missed a menstrual period (one or two per year) over the past 3 years; she believes this is due to stress. She also states that she is frustrated with her current weight and would like advice about weight-loss strategies. On further discussion, she admits that her weight struggle is compounded by episodes of binge eating (e.g., eating a quart of ice cream or large bag of candy or nuts without stopping), which makes her feel guilty. She also shared that she often self-induces vomiting after eating large quantities of food. These episodes of overeating and purging occur several times a week and have been present for the past year.

PMH: Patient began menstruation at age 11 years. She states that she struggled with obesity as a child, but was able to diet during middle school to achieve weight reduction. Patient shared there was a period during college when she drank excessive amounts of alcohol almost every weekend during parties with her friends. She states she only occasionally uses alcohol now.

Family history: Older sister—had anorexia nervosa during adolescence, but is now in good health. Father—age 55 years with type 2 diabetes and hypertension. Mother—age 50 years also had an eating disorder as an adolescent, but is now slightly overweight. No other health conditions.

Social history: Patient works as a laboratory technician. She drinks two or three alcohol-containing beverages per week and does not use tobacco products. She is not sexually active.

Medications: Multivitamin once daily.

Allergies: NKDA.

Vitals: Height 5′6″, weight 135 lb; BMI 21.8; ideal body weight 130 lb.

Physical exam: BP 110/70 Left Arm Sitting (LAS), HR 55 bpm, loss of tooth enamel noted, patient appears to have "chubby cheeks" likely associated with salivary gland irritation from induction of vomiting, three fingers of right hand also show evidence of skin breakdown.

Laboratory values: Complete metabolic panel values all within normal limits, but the serum potassium was low/normal (3.5 mEq/L).

Long-term Complications

Loss of tooth enamel, dental carries, swelling of the salivary glands, and erosions on the dorsum of the hands may occur with self-induced vomiting.[35] Frequent vomiting may also result in esophageal tears and dyspepsia. Abuse of laxatives may cause severe constipation. Self-induced vomiting may also create disturbances in fluid and electrolytes. Both abuse of diuretics and self-induced vomiting may result in metabolic alkalosis. Low potassium levels occur in 5% of patients. Unlike anorexia nervosa, patients with bulimia nervosa generally have normal bone mineral density. Menstrual irregularity may occur in patients with active bulimia nervosa, but future fertility is generally unaffected in women who recover.

Diagnosis of Bulimia Nervosa

Criteria for diagnosis of bulimia nervosa (e.g., *DSM-IV*) include the following features: 1) recurrent episodes of binge eating consisting of eating within a 2-hour period more food than most people would consume and sensing a loss of control during the eating episode; 2) recurrent inappropriate behavior to compensate for eating, such as misuse of laxatives, enemas, fasting, excessive exercise, or self-induced vomiting; 3) cycles of bingeing and compensatory behavior occurring at least twice weekly for 3 months; 4) self-value strongly based on body shape and weight; and 5) anorexia nervosa determined to not be a current problem.[24] Two types of bulimia nervosa are described. The purging type includes compensatory behaviors like self-induced vomiting or misuse of laxatives or other medications. The nonpurging form consists of behaviors such as fasting or excessive exercise.

Guidelines and Position Statements

See anorexia nervosa guidelines and position statements summarized above.[20,24-26] These guidelines also discuss bulimia nervosa.

Primary Prevention

The Eating Disorders Awareness Prevention and Education Act of 2003 recognized the prevalence of eating disorders in school-aged children and need for education.[20] The American Academy of Pediatrics has also published guidelines for the promotion of healthy weight-control practices in young athletes.[26] These guidelines stress the importance of healthy diet and careful assessment of weight and eating patterns in young athletes.

Treatment Goals

Treatment goals for bulimia nervosa include 1) reducing or eliminating bingeing/purging; 2) treating physical complications; 3) enhancing patient motivation to participate in treatment and restore healthy eating; 4) providing education about nutrition and health eating; 5) assisting patients to re-evaluate and change core dysfunctional thoughts, conflicts, feelings, and attitudes; 6) treating comorbid psychiatric conditions (mood disorders, impulse regulation, self-esteem, behavior); 7) encouraging family support and counseling as possible; and 8) preventing relapse.[25]

Nonpharmacologic Treatment

Nutritional Treatment

An important intervention is to work with the patient to develop a structured meal plan.[25] Nutritional intake assessments should be conducted for all patients, including those of normal weight. Adequate intake of nutrients is an important step for reducing cycles of restriction and bingeing.

In a randomized, prospective trial, 85 college women with full or subthreshold bulimia nervosa were assigned to the Healthy Weight Program (n = 43) or to a wait list (n = 42).[36] The Healthy Weight Program provides tools for reaching a healthy weight. The intervention emphasizes an organized approach to calorie restriction, which differs from conventional approaches. Small groups of six to eight subjects each participated in six sessions. Sessions were held weekly for the first 4 weeks, then every other week until completion. Those in the intervention group had modest weight loss and significant decrease in bulimic symptoms that continued through 3 months of follow-up.

Psychotherapy

CBT has been shown to be the single most effective intervention in treating acute bulimia nervosa.[25] CBT provides rapid remission of eating symptoms, but when other psychodynamic and psychological interventions are added to CBT, long-term effects may be enhanced.

A Cochrane review evaluated outcomes of studies of various types of psychotherapy for adults with nonpurging bulimia nervosa, binge-eating disorder, and other bulimia-type disorders.[37] Studies with dropout rates exceeding 50% were omitted (excluding studies with high dropout rates may skew results to overemphasize positive outcomes). CBT and CBT-BN (a type of treatment specific to bulimia nervosa) were found to be effective in treatment with subjects with bulimia nervosa when administered in group sessions or on an individual basis. CBT is associated with a greater probability of remission and decrease of vomiting and binge eating than interpersonal therapy when administered on an individual basis. Both treatment modalities have shown significant efficacy when offered in group settings.[38] CBT is more effective than either nutritional counseling or support groups alone.

A variety of self-help programs have been effective for patients with bulimia nervosa.[25,38] Use of structured CBT manuals also appears to be useful.[37]

Light Therapy

An 8-week trial with 220 subjects evaluated the effectiveness of 10,000-lux white light vs. 50-lux red light for treatment of bulimia nervosa.[38] Those receiving white-light treatment had significantly fewer binge eating episodes than the control group.

Pharmacologic Treatment

Antidepressant Therapy

Antidepressants are an effective component of treatment for bulimia nervosa.[25] Antidepressant medications appear to have an antibulimic effect, promoting a decline in frequency of binge/purge cycles and improvement in mood.[19] Antidepressants may also benefit patients with comorbid conditions, such as depression, obsessions, anxiety, or impulse disorders.[25] Therapy with antidepressants alone does not appear to be as effective as CBT, but the combination of antidepressants with psychotherapy may result in greater rates of improvement.[19,25]

Fluoxetine. Fluoxetine is the most widely studied medication for treatment of bulimia nervosa and has Food and Drug Administration (FDA) approval for this indication.[25] A systematic review of 47 studies addressing treatment efficacy for bulimia nervosa revealed 12 trials of medications that met inclusion criteria (total n = 1,430).[38] Six of these trials evaluated fluoxetine vs. placebo (n = 1,091). Most trials using fluoxetine 60 mg/day (8–16 weeks in duration) demonstrated significant decrease in binge eating and purging; studies using 20 mg/day showed less efficacy. Some studies also reported improvements in food preoccupation, restraint, concerns about weight, and body satisfaction. One study using 60 mg/day over 52 weeks also demonstrated significantly lower rates of relapse (33%) vs. placebo (51%). Dropout rates in trials varied from 0% to 83%. Common side effects included asthenia, nausea, sexual dysfunction, dizziness, tremor, sweating, urinary frequency, rhinitis, and insomnia.

Other Antidepressants. Fluvoxamine (average dosage 182 mg/day) was compared with placebo in one trial lasting 19 weeks posthospital discharge (n = 72).[38] Lower rates of bingeing, vomiting and depression scores were reported, but dropout rate was high (51%) relative to placebo (14%). Trazodone 400 mg daily vs. placebo (n = 46) and desipramine 200–300 mg/day vs. placebo (n = 78) were studied over 6-week periods in two separate trials. Both agents significantly decreased binge eating and vomiting. Subjects using desipramine also had improved scores on tests of attitudes regarding eating and perception of body and reported improvements in depression and anxiety, whereas those using trazodone also demonstrated a decreased fear of eating. In both studies, however, there was no significant difference between treatment and placebo groups in abstinence from bingeing and purging. A small, 8-week trial (n = 36) with the monoamine oxidase inhibitor brofaromine (not available in the U.S.) vs. placebo did not demonstrate differences in binge eating or psychologic behaviors, but it did significantly reduce vomiting. Side effects included dizziness, sleep difficulties, and nausea. Currently, tricyclic antidepressants and monoamine oxidase inhibitors are not recommended as initial treatment for bulimia nervosa.[25]

Other Agents

Topiramate (mean dosage 100 mg/day) was evaluated in a 10-week trial vs. placebo in 68 subjects with bulimia nervosa.[38] There was a significantly greater decrease in binge/purge days, drive for thinness, body dissatisfaction, and scores on an eating attitudes test. However, abstinence rates for bingeing and purging between the two arms were not significantly different. Topiramate also appeared to reduce anxiety and promoted weight loss.

Ondansetron vs. placebo was evaluated in a 4-week trial including 26 subjects.[38] The medication was self-administered when the urge to binge or vomit occurred. Ondansetron use was associated with significantly decreased frequency of bingeing and purging and demonstration of bulimic behaviors and increased normal consumption of meals.

Combined Pharmacotherapy and Psychotherapy

A systematic review of 47 studies revealed six combination studies (n = 1,895) of medication plus behavioral therapy.[38] Two trials were rated good, the others fair.

Fluoxetine and Cognitive Behavioral Therapy

Three trials (n = 258) studied the efficacy of combined CBT and fluoxetine.[38] One trial comparing fluoxetine 60 mg daily to fluoxetine 60 mg daily plus CBT to CBT demonstrated that combined therapy or CBT alone led to greater decreases in bingeing and vomiting episodes than fluoxetine, although all three treatments improved core bulimic symptoms. Another study looked at the effectiveness of adding a CBT-oriented self-help manual to fluoxetine treatment. The self-help materials alone did not appear to enhance the fluoxetine effect. Another similarly designed study similarly did not find self-help material to have an independent effect on improving outcomes.

Other Medications and Cognitive Behavioral Therapy

A trial of CBT plus desipramine vs. desipramine vs. CBT (n = 71) over 16-week vs. 24-week periods showed superior efficacy for combined treatment in decreasing bingeing and purging.[38] Abstinence rates, however, were not different between groups. Follow-up at 1 year also favored combined therapy and CBT. An additional five-group trial comparing 1) CBT plus antidepressants (all patients started with desipramine and transitioned to fluoxetine if no response); 2) CBT plus placebo; 3) supportive therapy plus antidepressants; 4) supportive therapy plus placebo; and 5) antidepressants alone showed that CBT was superior to supportive therapy, and behavioral interventions plus medication were superior to behavioral interventions alone in improving a number of parameters.

Monitoring and Follow-up

Eating disorder symptoms and behaviors should be frequently monitored.[25] Patients may be at risk for suicide because of the eating disorder and/or some treatments, so screening is critical. It is important to also monitor the patient's general medical condition, including weight, blood pressure, pulse, and other cardiovascular parameters at frequent intervals (e.g., weekly initially).[21,25] Dental exams are important for

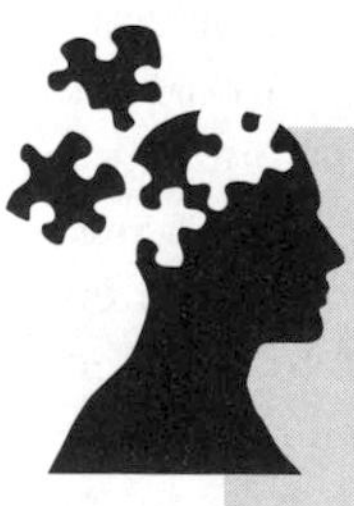

Therapeutic Challenge:

What concerns may exist for young adults using SSRIs for treatment of bulimia?

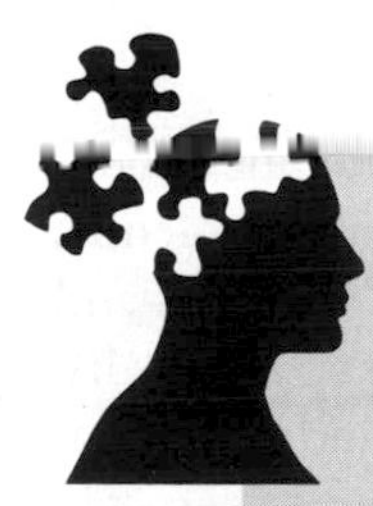

Therapeutic Challenge:

What is known about bulimia nervosa prevalence and effective pharmacotherapy for bulimia in women of different racial and ethnic groups?

patients with purging behaviors. Bone mineral density should be obtained if patient has been without menses for >6 months. Growth and sexual development should be monitored in younger patients.

Patient Education

Nutritional education stresses the importance of a healthy eating, physical and psychological effects of starvation, misconceptions about weight, nutrient requirements and metabolism, and adverse effects related to purging.[20] Patients need to learn how to develop a regular eating pattern (three meals a day with snacks) and become reacquainted with cues related to hunger and feeling full. Additionally, patients should learn to self-monitor by keeping a food diary, evaluating the record, and discovering reasons for weight fluctuations.

Cognitive behavioral and other types of self-help materials are available and may be used to supplement other psychotherapeutic and pharmacologic interventions.[25]

Sex Differences

Approximately 90% of people with bulimia nervosa are women.[34] Prevalence is 1% in women and 0.1% in men across the U.S. and Western Europe.[38]

Summary

There is good evidence for a beneficial effect of fluoxetine 60 mg daily in the treatment of bulimia nervosa.[38] Other medications (e.g., other antidepressants, topiramate) may be beneficial, but research evidence is limited. CBT has strong evidence for a beneficial and rapid effect. There are fewer studies of combined medication with psychotherapy, but preliminary results appear promising.

CASE PRESENTATION

Patient Case: Part 2

Assessment: D.S. has bulimia nervosa, purging type, based on her frequent binge-eating episodes followed by self-induced vomiting. Her weight and laboratory findings are all within the normal range.

Recommendation:

1. Referral to psychiatrist (or other mental health provider) for evaluation and plan. There is strong evidence for effectiveness of CBT when delivered in a group setting or individually. Provide patient with information about self-help materials and community resources.
2. Referral to registered dietitian for nutritional assessment and to assist patient in creating and implementing a nutritional plan. Dietitian to provide ongoing care and dietary monitoring.
3. Consider use of fluoxetine 60 mg daily if delays exist in accessing mental health services, if psychotherapy is not effective, or if other comorbid conditions (e.g., depression, anxiety) may benefit from treatment with an SSRI. Monitor patient for efficacy and side effects (including suicidal ideation/plan).
4. Schedule frequent, regular visits with primary care provider to coordinate and follow progress.
5. Referral to dentist for evaluation of tooth enamel and possible dental carries.

Rationale: Bulimia nervosa, like other eating disorders, requires coordinated care from a number of healthcare providers, including psychiatrists, dietitians, primary care providers, pharmacists, and dentists. Psychiatric, dietary, and pharmacologic treatments have demonstrated efficacy in treatment of this condition.

Patient education: Creation of a structured meal plan with the assistance of a dietitian reduces binge and purge cycles. Self-help materials may also complement psychotherapy. Medications used to treat bulimia nervosa require monitoring for safety and efficacy.

BINGE-EATING DISORDER

(See Web Resources for Patient Case: Binge-Eating Disorder.)

Additional content available at
www.ashp.org/womenshealth

Everyone tends to overeat from time to time, but this is a serious problem for a subset of Americans. These individuals suffer from a condition of disordered eating called binge-eating disorder (BED).[39,40] The issue of whether to include BED as an eating disorder has met controversy and debate in the psychiatric community over the years, but it is now recognized as a subset of "eating disorders not otherwise specified" (EDNOS), and there is a body of research on this topic.[24,41] It is currently estimated that 0.7% to 3.0% of the U.S. population—or more than 4 million Americans—have BED, making it the most common eating disorder.[24,39,40] It is estimated that as many as 10% to 15% of people who are overweight or mildly obese who attempt to lose weight on their own using various commercial diet plans have BED, especially if they experience wide fluctuations in weight through yo-yo dieting.[40] It is more common among individuals who are obese, affecting 5% to 8% of obese Americans.[24] Unfortunately, data on the epidemiology of BED are limited, but it does appear that the demographic profile of BED is broader than that observed with bulimia nervosa and more equally distributed between populations.[24,42] Binge-eating disorder appears to be more prevalent in women, affecting three women for every two men.[40]

Clinical Presentation

Patients with BED often eat abnormally large amounts of food within a very short amount of time, even if they do not feel hungry.[24] This occurs at least 2 days per week for months at a time. In contrast to bulimia, patients with BED do not compensate for the excessive calories ingested and tend to gain weight because their calories ingested exceed their caloric demands. Therefore, they may be overweight or obese or experience wide fluctuations in weight.[24,43] Many individuals with BED will be embarrassed about their lack of control during a binge and will eat in private. These feelings may lead to chronic anxiety, depression, sleep disorders, and even suicidal thoughts. Overall, patients with BED might have low self-esteem, be socially withdrawn, and may develop major depression.

Pathophysiology

The pathophysiology of BED is not well understood, and the etiology of binge eating is most likely complex and multifactorial.[44] Many of the causes of binge eating disorders are common between bulimia and BED.[24] It appears that women who are subjected to negative comments concerning their eating habits, weight, size, or shape during childhood are at increased risk of bingeing in adulthood. Also, women with BED appear to have an increased likelihood of other adverse childhood experiences, a family history of depression in parents, and a personal risk of depression. There might also be a connection between BED and level of perceived stress.[44] Although there has been no genetic marker identified for BED, it has been observed to aggregate in families up to 41% of the time.[24] This connection is being explored in research evaluating the genetics of obesity.

Long-term Complications

Because BED can lead to overweight and obesity, the patient is at risk of long-term, weight-related medical complications.[24] These might include type 2 diabetes mellitus, high blood pressure, dyslipidemia, coronary artery disease, obesity-related cancers, and gallbladder disease.[4] Also, BED is associated with possible psychological morbidity, including social withdrawal, anxiety, major depression, and even suicidal ideation.[24] It can adversely affect a patient's health-related quality of life.

Diagnosis of Binge-Eating Disorder

The *DSM-IV* criteria for binge-eating disorder (307.50) define bingeing very similarly to bulimia nervosa.[24] A binge is characterized by 1) ingesting a large amount of food during a discrete amount of time (such as a 2-hour period) that is much larger than what most people would eat in a similar time frame under similar conditions; and 2) experiencing the sense of lack of control during this eating episode. Binge-eating disorder is also associated with three (or more) of five possible criteria that include 1) eating faster than normal; 2) eating so much that discomfort develops; 3) eating excessively even when not hungry; 4) eating in private because of embarrassment about the amount of food ingested; or 5) feeling disgusted, depressed, or guilty about overeating patterns. To be defined as BED, the individual must binge 2 or more days per week for 6 months. In contrast to bulimia nervosa, BED is not associated with any compensatory interventions to avoid weight gain, such as purging, fasting, excessive exercise, diuretic use, or laxative abuse. Also, based on the diagnostic criteria, BED cannot occur exclusively during the clinical course of other eating disorders such as anorexia or bulimia nervosa.

Guidelines and Position Statements

See the guidelines and position statements summarized in the anorexia nervosa section above.[4,5,20,24-26] These guidelines also discuss EDNOS. Also, see the guidelines and position statements summarized in the healthy nutrition section. These guidelines provide direction for the management of overweight and obesity, which is a common sequelae of BED.

Primary Prevention

Parents, coaches, teachers, and other role models in a child's life contribute significantly to a child's self-confidence and positive body image. It is important that these role models help a child develop healthy eating and exercise habits early in life that might prevent disordered eating as the child ages. The foundations of healthy nutrition that were discussed in the previous section should be emphasized.[4-7] Individuals should be taught to avoid severe calorie restriction, extreme food limitations, skipping meals, or fasting that might lead to excessive hunger and subsequent bingeing. Healthcare providers should closely monitor pediatric and adult height and weight and watch for fluctuations, and carefully screen for evidence of bingeing.[45] If bingeing is occurring, an early intervention may be effective in helping the patient institute healthy behaviors before they become problematic. The practice guidelines identified above are designed to help healthcare providers make these interventions.

Treatment Goals

The primary treatment goal for BED is for the patient to institute normal eating patterns and avoid binges.[24,39,46] The patient should match caloric intake with caloric demand to stabilize weight. The patient should institute healthy nutrition habits with a well-balanced diet rich in nutrients. If the patient is overweight or obese, the patient should create a calorie deficit of 500–1,000 kcal/day to achieve a slow steady weight loss of 1–2 lb/wk by following healthy nutrition and exercise practices that were previously discussed.[4-7]

Nonpharmacologic Treatment

A number of nonpharmacologic interventions have been explored for the management of BED. One of the most important interventions is psychotherapy with a psychologist or psychiatrist to explore the emotions that might trigger, cause, or exacerbate the bingeing behavior. One type of psychotherapy that is evidence based and effective is CBT.[25,28,39]

Also, because of the increased risk of overweight and obesity associated with BED, diet and exercise are very important for managing the disorder.[4-7] Patients might explore resources for self-help to improve nutrition and lose weight or might pursue commercial weight loss programs. Healthcare professionals can also assist patients with weight management. In some cases, if the patient is morbidly obese with health risks, weight loss surgery might be considered.[47] Overweight and obesity interventions are discussed further in Chapter 32: Overweight and Obesity.

Pharmacologic Therapy

The efficacy and safety of several pharmacotherapy drug classes have been evaluated for the management of BED.[24,39] These include tricyclic antidepressants, second-generation antidepressants, anticonvulsants, and appetite suppressants. These therapies have been studied with and without adjuvant therapies such as CBT, group therapy, psychotherapy, and weight management counseling and interventions. Results of studies have varied, but several agents show evidence of efficacy and safety. Most BED studies conducted to date have enrolled primarily women and have lacked ethnic diversity with mostly white subjects. Therefore, further research in expanded populations is required to fully elucidate the role of these therapies in the management of BED.

Tricyclic Antidepressants

Both desipramine and imipramine have shown promise in clinical trials for the management of BED. As early as 1990, desipramine was studied to evaluate its effect on the management of nonpurging bulimia (now classified as BED).[48] This was a small (n = 23), double-blind, randomized, controlled 12-week study. The frequency of binge episodes decreased 63% in the treatment group and increased by 16% in the placebo group. After 12 weeks, 60% of the treatment group, but only 15% of the placebo group, abstained from binge eating. The women who received desipramine reported significantly more dietary restraint and less hunger. These preliminary findings suggest that the therapeutic effects of desipramine established in the treatment of purging bulimia nervosa may extend to BED.

Imipramine has also been evaluated for the management of BED in one small (n = 31) double-blind, placebo-controlled 8-week study.[39,49] In this trial, low-dose imipramine (25 mg 3 times a day) helped overweight and obese BED patients lose weight (average = 2.2 kg) and maintain their weight loss over a 32-week observation period, whereas the placebo group experienced weight gain. The imipramine group also had a statistically significant decline in the depression score and a decline in binge episodes during the trial (7.1 episodes per week at baseline to 2.8 episodes per week with treatment). Imipramine was well tolerated during the trial, and dropout was low and similar between groups (6% to 7%).

Another study evaluated the role of desipramine in the management of binge eating. This study randomly assigned patients to receive one of three interventions: 1) 9 months of weight loss therapy alone; 2) 3 months of CBT followed by 6 months of weight loss therapy; or 3) 3 months of CBT followed by 6 months of weight loss therapy combined with pharmacotherapy (desipramine, dosage = 300 mg/day). Results showed CBT to be beneficial at 12 weeks but not later in the study. The greatest weight loss was observed at 3 months in the desipramine group (–4.8 kg), and this weight loss was maintained.

The results of these studies indicate that both desipramine and imipramine are promising pharmacotherapy options for obtaining and maintaining weight loss among patients with BED. Further study is warranted to evaluate the efficacy and safety of these agents.

Selective Serotonin Reuptake Inhibitors

Fluoxetine. Fluoxetine has been studied as monotherapy and in combination with other medications and interventions for the management of BED.[39,51] One study evaluated fluoxetine monotherapy in a flexible-dose titration (average dosage = 71.3 mg/day). In this study, fluoxetine significantly decreased binge frequency, BED severity, and healthcare provider–rated depression score. Patients in both arms of the study gained weight, but the fluoxetine group gained less weight than placebo. However, there was significant dropout in this study—57% fluoxetine and 23% placebo—which is a significant limitation of this trial and should be considered when interpreting these data during pharmacotherapy selection.

Fluoxetine has also been studied in conjunction with CBT.[39] In one double-blind, placebo-controlled trial, fluoxetine +/– CBT was compared with placebo +/– CBT.[52] This study showed that there was no difference between the CBT group with or without fluoxetine and that both CBT groups were better than fluoxetine therapy alone. Weight loss did not differ across groups and was very modest. Therefore, this trial showed that CBT is an effective treatment for the behavioral and psychological sequelae of BED but did not have an effect on obesity.[52] A similar study evaluated the impact of CBT and fluoxetine as adjuncts to group behavioral therapy for BED. Fluoxetine was associated with an improvement in symptoms of depression but did not improve binge frequency, abstinence, or weight.[53]

Fluvoxamine. There have been two studies that have evaluated fluvoxamine monotherapy for BED.[39] The first study was 9 weeks and evaluated fluvoxamine (50–300 mg/day) vs. placebo.[54] The treatment group experienced a decrease in the rate of binge-eating episodes, but the remission rate did not differ between groups. The rate of improvement in BED severity and reduction in BMI was also greater in the treatment group. However, final BMI and follow-up was not reported. There was no change in depressive symptoms observed. A similar 12-week trial of fluvoxamine (average dosage = 239 mg/day) showed no difference between treatment and placebo on the frequency of binges, self-reported depression, or weight change.[55]

Sertraline. There have been two studies that have evaluated the role of sertraline for the management of BED. One was a 6-week study, and the next extended the observation period to 24 weeks.[39] The first trial showed that sertraline significantly decreased the rate of binges, severity of illness, and weight over placebo but did not lead to disease remission or improvement in depression scores.[56] Follow-up data were not provided. The dropout rate was high in both groups (28% sertraline and 19% placebo). The 24-week trial was an open-label study that investigated the use of sertraline in BED.[57] A therapeutic benefit of sertraline was observed after 8 weeks of therapy with a decrease in the score on the binge-eating scale and weight loss that was sustained until the end of the study. However, because of the lack of blinding, the impact of the "placebo effect" is unknown. The results of these two trials suggest that more randomized controlled trials should be conducted to explore the role of sertraline in the management of BED.

Citalopram. Two separate 6-week trials have evaluated the role of citalopram (40–60 mg/day) for the management of BED, and the results were very similar to other SSRIs.[39,58] There was an observed decrease in the rate of binging, but no remission of the disease. Also, there was a greater weight loss in the treatment group (–2.7 kg) vs. a gain in the placebo. The citalopram group showed a greater reduction in healthcare provider–rated assessment of obsession, compulsion, severity of illness, and depressive symptoms. However, the final outcomes were similar between groups. Dropout was high in both arms of the study.

Overall, when evaluating the SSRIs, fluoxetine has been studied the most both as monotherapy and in combination with CBT, but several SSRIs have been evaluated as monotherapy for BED management.[39] Although results of the studies vary slightly, overall the data suggest that SSRIs decrease the rate of binges and BED disease severity but do not result in disease remission. Several therapies decrease the symptoms of depression, and SSRIs might be good treatment options for patients experiencing these symptoms. There are currently no head-to-head trials that compare the safety and efficacy of the SSRIs for the management of BED or compare SSRI with tricyclic antidepressants for management of these disorders. Therefore, the selection of a treatment option should be based on patient-specific considerations, such as history of efficacy and safety with past use of antidepressants, comorbid conditions that might influence product selection (e.g., avoidance of tricyclic antidepressants with cardiovascular disease or benign prostatic hypertrophy), compliance issues (dosing frequency), patient concerns about adverse effects (e.g., insomnia, sexual dysfunction), and formulary issues.

Anticonvulsants

Topiramate is an anticonvulsant that has been associated with decreased appetite and weight loss when used in the management of epilepsy. Therefore, its potential for the management of obesity associated with BED has been considered.[59] This has led to studies to evaluate topiramate for the management of BED.[39] One 14-week study evaluated topiramate (average dosage = 212 mg/day) with placebo and found that the treatment group experienced an improvement in the rate of change in binge episodes, number of binge days per week, and severity of illness.[60] There was no change in depression scores. Topiramate was associated with a statistically and clinically significant weight loss (–5.9 kg). However, there was a high rate of dropout in both groups (47% in topiramate and 39% in placebo).

The most common adverse effects associated with topiramate therapy are central nervous system effects, such as paresthesia, fatigue, somnolence, difficulty concentrating, attention deficit, confusion, depression, and memory problems.[61] Topiramate also has an increased risk of metabolic acidosis.

Zonisamide has also been evaluated for BED in a 16-week, randomized, controlled flexible-dose trial.[39,62] The treatment group had a greater rate of reduction of binge-eating frequency, body weight, BMI, and clinical-severity scale. There was significant attrition in both arms. Zonisamide is contraindicated for use in patients with a sulfonamide allergy.[61]

Weight-Loss Medications

Sibutramine (15 mg/day) has been shown effective in one small (n = 60) randomized controlled clinical trial.[39,63] The treatment group experienced decreased binge episodes per week, depression scores, and significant weight loss (–7.4 kg). The placebo group gained weight. However, abstinence rates and long-term outcomes were not reported. Dropout was high in each arm.

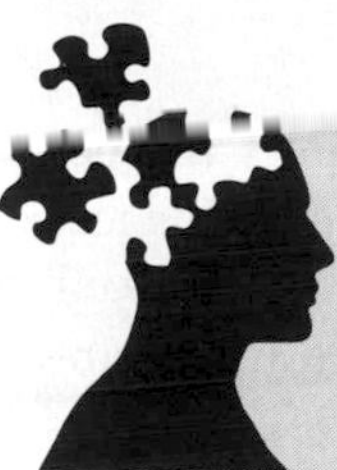

Therapeutic Challenge:

If pharmacotherapy is initiated for binge-eating disorder, how long should it be continued?

Another study looked at the use of orlistat (120 mg 3 times a day before meals) in combination with CBT and found that the active group lost more weight, but this weight loss was not maintained at the 2-month follow-up visit.[39]

Monitoring and Follow-up

Patients should be seen frequently for follow-up when being treated for BED.[4-7,20,24-26] On these visits, the healthcare provider should collect information concerning the frequency of binges, review the patient's nutrition and exercise diary, measure weight and perform body-composition analysis, and monitor for weight-related complications. The safety of any prescribed therapy should also be closely monitored based on the anticipated adverse effects of the medication.

Patient Education

Patients should be educated on the health risks associated with overweight and obesity and the importance of behavioral change to avoid these potential sequelae.[4-7,20,24-26] They should be educated on the importance of routine health exams to screen for these potential complications. Guidance should be provided on healthy nutrition and exercise habits, and patient referral to a dietician and/or exercise physiologist might be necessary for further training. Strategies for behavioral modification should be suggested, such as maintaining a food and exercise journal, measuring portions, and increasing daily activities. Patients should also receive counseling on any pharmacologic therapy recommended for the treatment of BED.

Sex Differences

Binge-eating disorder is more equally distributed between women and men than other eating disorders, but some reports estimate that it occurs 1.5 times more often in women than in men (three women for every two men).[40]

Summary

Binge-eating disorder is associated with overweight and obesity and increased risk of weight-related morbidity and mortality.[20,24,25,39] Therefore, it is important that healthcare providers screen for BED and provide treatment when appropriate. Nonpharmacologic interventions are very important to address the behavior, but there are a growing number of evidence-based pharmacotherapy treatment options as well. Currently, the antidepressants imipramine and desipramine have shown good results for BED. The SSRIs all have shown success in decreasing the rate of binge episodes and other markers of disease control but do not result in disease remission. Tricyclic antidepressants and SSRIs might be very beneficial in patients with symptoms of depression. The anticonvulsants topiramate and zonisamide have shown some efficacy for the management of this disorder. The appetite suppressant sibutramine has shown a significant weight loss and improvement in BED control. However, because of the current lack of controlled, head-to-head trials comparing these treatment options, product selection must be based on patient-specific characteristics.

Chapter Summary

Because of the sensitive nature of eating disorders and secretive behaviors often associated with them, many women do not seek medical help.[20] Thus, the true prevalence may not be known. No best-practice models exist for prevention of eating disorders, but nutrition messages should stress a health-centered approach rather than a weight-centered approach. Research regarding optimal treatments has been challenging because of the resistance to treatment sometimes seen with patients with eating disorders, especially anorexia nervosa.[29] Because of this resistance to behavior change, dropout rates from trials are often high, adding to the difficulty in providing evidence-based recommendations. For some eating disorders, pharmacologic therapy and psychotherapy have evidence for benefit.

Healthy nutrition is fundamental to the treatment of disordered eating. It is also remains fundamental to promotion of health and prevention of a variety of other health disorders.

References

Additional content available at
www.ashp.org/womenshealth

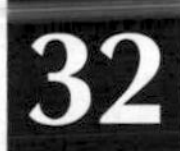

32 Overweight and Obesity

Judy T. Chen, Pharm.D., BCPS, CDE; Amy Heck Sheehan, Pharm.D.; Martha Stassinos, Pharm.D.; Karim Anton Calis, Pharm.D., MPH, FASHP, FCCP

Learning Objectives

1. Explain the epidemiologic impact of overweight and obesity in women.
2. Evaluate clinical presentations and long-term risks associated with obesity.
3. Discuss the pathophysiologic abnormalities pertinent to the development of obesity in women.
4. Describe criteria used for the diagnosis and management of overweight and obesity.
5. Formulate nonpharmacologic therapies for women with overweight and obesity.
6. Formulate a comprehensive pharmacotherapy plan for women with overweight and obesity based on patient-specific factors.
7. Discuss the role of bariatric surgery for women with extreme obesity.
8. List the monitoring parameters necessary to assess therapeutic outcomes and adverse effects in women.

The worldwide obesity epidemic is a pervasive public health challenge affecting millions of women in both developed and developing countries.[1] Approximately 61.4% of women aged 20 years or older living in the U.S. can be categorized as either overweight (body mass index [BMI] $\geq$25 kg/m^2) or obese (BMI $\geq$30 kg/m^2).[2] Although overweight is more common among men than women, 39.4% vs. 27.4%, respectively, the prevalence of obesity and extreme obesity (BMI $\geq$40 kg/m^2) is higher among women, 34% and 7.3%, compared with 31.7% and 3% in men.[2] This sex difference is more pronounced among racial and ethnic minority women, school-aged children, and adolescents. It is currently estimated that approximately 54% of black women are obese compared with 42% of Mexican-American women and 30% of non-Hispanic white women.[3] Furthermore, women of lower socioeconomic class are more commonly affected by obesity compared with men.[2] Of particular concern is the growing prevalence of overweight among young girls ages 2–19, which will further compound the magnitude of obesity comorbidities observed in the current generation of obese adults.[2] Reducing the prevalence of obesity is one of the national health objectives for Healthy People 2010.[4]

Clinical Presentation

Premenopausal women tend to accumulate excess body fat in the subcutaneous tissues, predominately in the gluteal and femoral regions, which redistributes more viscerally after menopause.[5] In contrast, men concentrate a higher portion of their body fat in the visceral adipose tissue throughout their lifetime.[6] Overweight and obesity are central constituents of the metabolic syndrome, characterized by multiple risk factors, such as abdominal obesity, atherogenic dyslipidemia, elevated blood pressure, insulin resistance, and systemic inflammation, which often are asymptomatic.[7] The constellation of these risk factors further contributes to elevated risks of developing cardiovascular disease and type 2 diabetes.[7] Women with abdominal obesity often present with insulin resistance, low high-density lipoprotein cholesterol (HDL-C), elevated triglyceride concentrations, high apolipoprotein B, elevated small atherogenic low-density lipoprotein (LDL) particles, and hypertension.[7] Higher prevalence of type 2 diabetes and coronary heart disease (CHD) are observed among obese women.[8] Furthermore, a myriad of comorbidities—such as stroke, degenerative joint diseases requiring knee and hip replacements, chronic kidney disease, **sleep apnea**, asthma, hepatic **steatosis**, **cholelithiasis**, psoriasis, urinary incontinence, menstrual irregularities, **infertility**, and physical disabilities—have been correlated with excess body fat.[9-19] A recent national survey found obesity and extreme obesity among women has been associated with

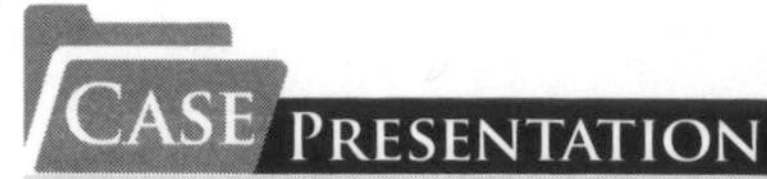

Patient Case: Part 1

J.C. is a 47-year-old mixed-race (black and Korean) woman who presents to the bariatric surgical center for Roux-en-Y gastric bypass.

HPI: Patient has been obese since childhood and became extremely obese soon after pregnancy. She has dieted on and off since her teen years with nonprescription and prescription weight-loss therapies and has joined self-help weight-loss groups. She has successfully lost weight many times in various amounts up to 23 kg but always regained it "with extra." To qualify for surgery, she has been attending a medically supervised weight-management clinic, where she is evaluated weekly by a physician, and attends behavior-modification and nutrition classes. She uses the clinic's prepackaged meal substitutes that provide her a very-low-calorie diet. Her starting weight was 126.4 kg. She lost 18.2 kg over the last year and has regained 3.2 kg.

PMH: Hysterectomy at age 44 for menorrhagia attributed to fibroids; severe hot flashes and sleep disturbance starting 1 year after hysterectomy, requiring estrogen therapy; type 2 diabetes, hypertension, and hyperlipidemia; all three conditions diagnosed 4 years ago; milk intolerance; intermittent low back pain; and bilateral knee pain.

Family history: Mother—diabetes and obesity; father—hypertension, death from stroke at age 62.

Social history: Lifetime nonsmoker; rarely drinks alcohol; back and knee pain cause great difficulty for her to exercise by walking or use a stationary bicycle. She is a divorced mother of one daughter.

Medications:

estradiol patch 0.1 mg applied twice weekly
hydrochlorothiazide 12.5 mg every morning
lisinopril 20 mg every morning
glipizide-metformin 5–500 mg, two tablets twice daily with meals
simvastatin 40 mg every evening
ibuprofen 600 mg 3 times daily as needed
acetaminophen 1,000 mg as needed for aches and pains
multivitamin one tablet daily
aspirin enteric coated 81 mg every morning with food
calcium carbonate 500 mg twice daily with meals
lactase one to two tablets as needed with dairy products
denied using any herbals or dietary supplements

Allergies: Penicillin.

Vitals: 5'4", 111.4 kg (245 lb), BMI 42 kg/m^2, BP 132/75 mmHg, HR 68 bpm, Temp 98.6°F, RR 20 breaths/min.

Physical exam: Obese woman with some dark pigmented areas on back of neck and buttocks, bilateral mild edema of lower extremities.

Laboratory values: Significant findings include HbA_{1c} of 8.5%, fasting glucose 224 mg/dL, total cholesterol 235 mg/dL, TG 160 mg/dL, HDL-C 50 mg/dL, LDL-C 105 mg/dL, serum creatinine 0.9 mg/dL. Thyroid panels were within normal limits.

comorbid psychiatric disorders, such as atypical major depressive episodes in bipolar I disorder, specific phobia, and antisocial and avoidant personality disorders.[20]

Pathophysiology

CAUSES OF OBESITY

The pathogenesis of obesity is a complex and multifactorial process. Energy balance follows the laws of thermodynamics, with fat stored being the remainder of energy intake less expenditure. Several factors may contribute to weight gain in women, including environmental influences, genetic predisposition, fluctuations in sex hormones, psychosocial factors, medications, and certain medical conditions.[21-23] In general, no single factor is thought to be responsible for the development of obesity; rather, a combination of several factors contributes to weight gain. However, women do have a higher percentage of total body fat and an increased risk of obesity and extreme obesity when compared with men.[23]

The increasing incidence of obesity over the last several decades is thought to be partially attributed to the modern environment, in which there is an increased availability of calorie-dense foods in combination with declining physical activity.[22] Obesity has also been postulated to be a consequence of genetic success, in that human evolution has allowed fat storage as a means of surviving famine.[21] Genetic influences appear to affect the location on the body where fat is stored and to what degree, as well as feeding behavior. Twin studies conducted in women indicate that genetic influences may describe up to 80% of the variation in BMI over time.[24,25] In addition, numerous genetic defects have been described that may predispose particular individuals to weight gain.[26] Although research regarding potential sex differences for these genetic defects is ongoing, at least one genetic polymorphism associated with obesity has been found in women and not in men.[27] Women also have higher circulating concentrations of leptin, a hormone secreted by adipose tissue that regulates body weight.[28]

Adults commonly gain weight as they age, and epidemiologic studies have shown that the prevalence of overweight in women increases from ages 20 to 60 years.[29] Sex-hormone fluctuations associated with pregnancy and menopause have been implicated as contributing to the risk of weight gain over time in women.[23] For example, obesity may result from failure to lose the excess weight gained during pregnancy. Weight loss following pregnancy can be influenced by several factors, including the amount of excess weight gained during pregnancy, caloric intake, physical activity, lactation status, and the amount of time that elapses between pregnancies. Weight gain is common in women during the perimenopausal period, accompanied by a shift in body fat distribution.[5]

Medical conditions, such as anxiety, Cushing's disease, depression, hypothyroidism, and schizophrenia, and certain medications, including corticosteroids, antipsychotics, antidepressants, and antiepileptics, may also contribute to weight gain.[30] Social factors, such as economic status[2] and the weight status of an individual's peer group, also play a role.[31] Finally, the likelihood of persistence of obesity from childhood into adulthood increases with age.[21] Therefore, an increased prevalence of overweight and obesity in adolescent girls can be expected to carry over into adult women.

LONG-TERM COMPLICATIONS

The long-term complications of obesity are significant, making it the second most common factor contributing to preventable death in the U.S.[32] The Nurses' Health Study followed more than 115,000 middle-aged women for approximately 8 years and documented a direct relationship between body weight and all-cause mortality.[33] Obesity is a primary risk factor for the development of hypertension, dyslipidemia, type 2 diabetes, stroke, and CHD and contributes to the development of several other conditions in women, including gall bladder disease, degenerative joint disease, nonalcoholic fatty liver disease, metabolic syndrome, sleep apnea, polycystic ovarian syndrome, menstrual irregularities, stress incontinence, pregnancy complications, infertility, and cancers.[34-36] Cardiovascular disease, a consequence of the most common obesity-related comorbidities (i.e., hypertension, hyperlipidemia, and type 2 diabetes), is the number-one cause of death in women.[37] Accumulation of body fat in the abdominal region associated with a range of metabolic disorders—including elevated fasting blood glucose, elevated serum triglycerides, decreased HDL cholesterol, and hypertension—is commonly referred to as metabolic syndrome.[36] Women with metabolic syndrome have an increased risk of cardiovascular morbidity and mortality, regardless of BMI.[38] Extreme obesity has been shown to reduce average life expectancy by 9 years in women and 12 years in men.[39] Furthermore, obese women experience an increased risk of certain types of cancers, such as leukemia, postmenopausal breast cancer, endometrial cancer, renal cancer, and colorectal cancer.[40-44] A plethora of evidence emphasizes that obesity is associated with significant morbidity and mortality. Moreover, living in a culture in which female thinness is considered physically desirable and attractive, women who are obese often experience tremendous psychological distress resulting from social discrimination and stigmatization.[45] Consequently, many young obese women also suffer from depression, body images distress, eating disorders, and self-esteem difficulties.[16]

Detection and Diagnosis

DEFINITION

Obesity is defined as an accumulation of excess body fat to an extent that adversely affects health. Because it is often difficult to assess body-fat composition directly, BMI is the preferred method to measure total body fat in clinical practice.[19] BMI is expressed by dividing weight in kilograms by height in meters squared to calculate weight adjusted for height. A high BMI generally correlates with an increased percentage of total body fat and conveys increased morbidity and mortality.[19] According to clinical guidelines established by the National Institutes of Health (NIH), a healthy weight for adults is defined as BMI (kg/m^2) between 18.5 and 24.9, overweight as BMI $\geq$25 and obesity as BMI $\geq$30 (Table 32-1).[19] Extreme obesity, defined as BMI $\geq$40 kg/m^2, is a subgroup often associated with life-threatening comorbidities. These risk-based definitions are derived from mortality and morbidity outcomes observed in epidemiologic studies.[19]

DIAGNOSIS

Simple anthropometric measurements with height and weight can be use to calculate BMI and diagnose the severity of excess body fat. However, it is

Table 32-1. Classification of Overweight and Obesity by BMI, Waist Circumference, and Associated Disease Risk[a]

Classification	BMI (kg/m²)	Disease Risk[a] Relative to Normal Weight and Waist Circumference	
		Men ≤40 in (≤102 cm) Women ≤35 in (≤88 cm)	Men >40 in (>102 cm) Women >35 in (>88 cm)
Normal[b]	18.5–24.9	----	----
Overweight	25.0–29.9	Increased	High
Obesity	30.0–34.9	High	Very high
	35.0–39.9	Very high	Very high
Extreme obesity	≥40	Extremely high	Extremely high

Source: Adapted from reference 19.
BMI = body mass index, calculated by dividing weight (in kilograms) by height (in meters) squared. To convert from nonmetric measurements (pounds/inches²), multiply the quotient by a factor of 704.5.
[a]Disease risk for type 2 diabetes, hypertension, and cardiovascular disease.
[b]Increased waist circumference can also be a marker for increased risk even in women of normal weight.

important to note that interpretation of BMI may vary based on sex, age, and other factors. At the same BMI, women tend to have a higher percentage of body fat compared with men because of their lower muscle and bone mass.[2] Gradually, as fat distribution changes with age, an elderly patient will also have a higher percentage of body fat compared with a younger adult of the same BMI. In the presence of edema, high muscularity, muscle wasting, or for adults shorter than 5 feet, BMI may present with less validity, and clinical judgments must be used.[19]

In addition to BMI, measurement of waist circumference provides added predictive value to assess a woman's visceral fat distribution, the degree of obesity, and identify overall risks for adults with BMI between 25 and 34.9 kg/m².[19] Visceral obesity is more prevalent in women than in men with CHD.[47] A greater waist circumference is associated with more atherogenic fat and reduced insulin sensitivity, and appears to be a stronger predictor of type 2 diabetes in women than in men.[8,19] A woman with a waist circumference of >99 cm (35 inches) is also at a higher risk for developing dyslipidemia, hypertension, and CHD.[8,19] Therefore, diagnosis of obesity should consist of evaluation of BMI, waist circumference, and overall medical risk (Table 32-2).[19] Extensive evaluation is warranted in women with extreme obesity and those who suffer from abnormal fat distribution or experience sudden weight gain.

Obesity Management Guidelines

The growing epidemic concern of obesity in the U.S. led to the U.S. Preventive Services Task Force recommendation to screen all adults for obesity in clinical practice.[48] An initial step is to evaluate a woman's risk factors and other obesity-related conditions (Table 32-2).[19] Management guidelines established by the NIH recommend initiating weight-loss interventions for overweight (BMI 25–29.9 kg/m²) adults and/or those with an elevated waist circumference in the presence of at least two concomitant risk factors, such as hypertension, obstructive sleep apnea, dyslipidemia, CHD, or type 2 diabetes.[19] In the absence of these identifiable risk factors, weight-loss intervention is indicated for all obese adults with a BMI of at least 30 kg/m².[19] Healthcare providers should offer intensive counseling with behavioral interventions to encourage consistent weight loss in obese adults.[48] Benefits of weight loss have been well documented with favorably influencing overall cardiovascular risks, decreasing triglycerides and increasing HDL-C, decreasing blood pressure, decreasing glycosylated hemoglobin A_{1c} (HbA_{1c}), decreasing severity of sleep apnea, reducing pain associated with degenerative joint disease, and improving gynecologic symptoms.[19] A safe and realistic weight reduction is recommended at the rate of approximately 0.5–0.9 kg (1–2 lb) per week, with

Table 32-2. Risk Factors for Obesity Related Morbidity and Mortality[a]

Very High Absolute Risk[b]
Established coronary heart disease
History of myocardial infarction
History of angina pectoris (stable or unstable)
History of coronary artery surgery
History of coronary artery procedure (e.g., angioplasty)
Presence of other atherosclerotic diseases
Peripheral arterial disease
Abdominal aortic aneurysm
Symptomatic carotid artery disease
Type 2 diabetes
Sleep apnea
High Absolute Risk[c,d]
Cigarette smoking
Hypertension
LDL cholesterol >160 mg/dL (or 130–159 mg/dL with ≥ two other risk factors)
HDL cholesterol <35 mg/dL
Impaired fasting glucose
Family history of premature cardiovascular disease
Male ≥45 years of age
Female ≥55 years of age (or postmenopausal)
Other Contributing Risk Factors
Serum triglycerides >200 mg/dL
Physical inactivity

Source: Adapted from reference 19.
HDL = high-density lipoprotein; LDL = low-density lipoprotein.
[a]Patients with a body mass index (BMI) >30 kg/m^2, OR ([BMI 25–29.9 kg/m^2 OR waist circumference >88 cm or >102 cm] AND ≥ two risk factors) should undergo weight-loss therapy.
[b]Indicates need for aggressive cholesterol-lowering therapy in addition to weight loss.
[c]Patients with three or more of these risk factors are at a high absolute risk or obesity-related disorders.
[d]Presence of three or more risk factors indicates need for increased intensity of cholesterol-lowering therapy and blood pressure management in addition to weight loss.

an initial target to decrease baseline weight by 10% over 6 months.[19] Once this initial target is achieved, a further weight-loss goal of 10% can be attempted if indicated. The majority of overweight and obese women often set unrealistic goals, expecting to lose approximately 30% of their initial body weight, so it is important to emphasize that even moderate weight reduction of as little as 5% can significantly decrease obesity-related chronic diseases.[49-51] Rapid weight loss over a short period is likely to be associated with greater weight regain and nutritional deficiencies. For women who have failed to achieve or maintain their initial weight loss goal after 6 months of lifestyle modification with a reduced-calorie diet, appropriate physical activity, and behavior therapy, pharmacotherapy can be considered as an adjunct to lifestyle modifications in adults with BMI of at least 30 kg/m^2 in the absence of obesity-related medical conditions, or BMI of at least 27 kg/m^2 with at least two concomitant risk factors.[19] Bariatric surgery should be reserved for adults presenting with a BMI of at least 40 kg/m^2 without comorbid conditions or at least 35 kg/m^2 with significant risk factors suffering from complications of obesity.[19,39] These criteria are endorsed by a number of organizations, both in the U.S. and abroad.[52] In addition, requirements for bariatric surgery include failure of medical weight control efforts and absence of medical or psychological contraindications.[53] Individuals who are considering surgical intervention should understand the risks and benefits of the procedure, and must have consistent motivation to comply with postsurgical behavior modification to ensure long-term weight loss.[54] More conservative criteria (BMI ≥50 kg/m^2 or BMI ≥40 kg/m^2 with severe medical comorbidities) are recommended for adolescents considering surgical intervention because of concerns for potential lifelong complications and monitoring requirements.[55] Despite potential weight gain associated with smoking cessation, smokers, regardless of baseline weight, should be encouraged to stop smoking.[19] Patients who undergo bariatric surgery should discontinue smoking at least 6 months before surgery.[53] Regardless of the treatment strategy chosen, appropriate lifestyle modifications, including low-caloric diet, adequate physical activity, and behavioral therapy, are the cornerstones of obesity management and must be well integrated within the various treatment options to maximize and sustain their benefits.[19] Figure 32-1 depicts an evidenced-based algorithm for the treatment of obesity.[51]

Figure 32-1. Evidence-based medicine.

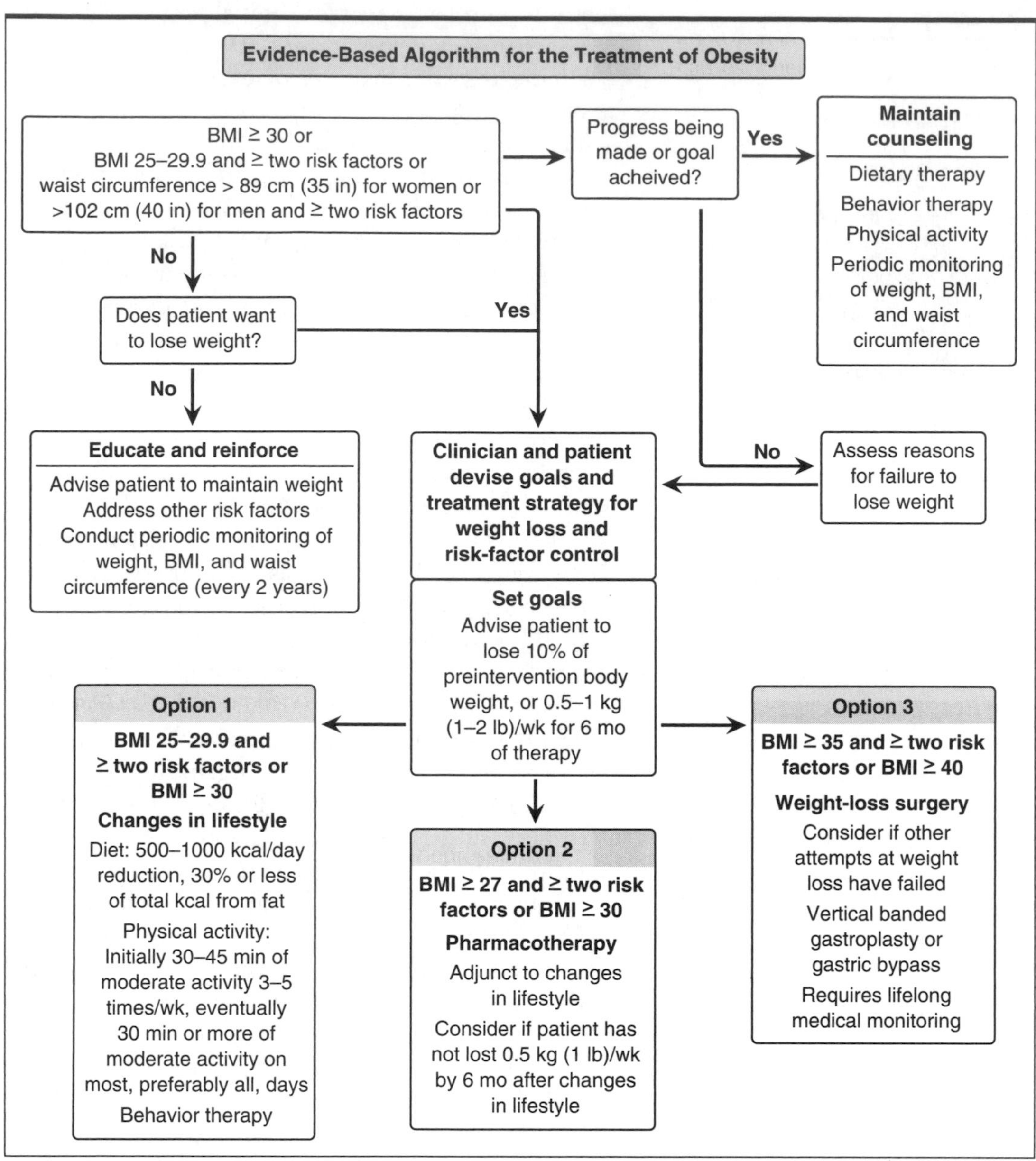

Source: Reprinted with permission from reference 51 (Massachusetts Medical Society, all rights reserved).
BMI = body mass index.

Primary Prevention

Energy imbalance, triggered by sedentary lifestyle and excessive caloric intake, is the foremost modifiable cause of obesity. Primary prevention is the key strategy to reduce and manage the obesity epidemic. The 2005 Dietary Guidelines for Americans established a framework of evidence-based recommendations to prevent chronic diseases through health promotion.[56] Gradual weight gain can be prevented by consumption of balanced nutrition while reducing daily caloric intake by 50–100 kcal and engaging up to 60 minutes of moderate- to vigorous-intensity physical activity daily.[56] Reduction of caloric intake can be made through prudent selection of food preferences to limit intake of saturated and *trans* fats, cholesterol, sugar, and alcohol while increasing intake of nutrient-dense foods and dietary fiber within the caloric requirements.[56] Moderate or vigorous physical activity, such as hiking, walking, dancing, running, or swimming, are all appropriate strategies to enhance energy expenditure to prevent excessive caloric imbalance that results in weight gain over time.[56]

Treatment

TREATMENT GOALS

The primary treatment goals for obesity and extreme obesity are to reduce weight long term, improve obesity-related comorbidities, and prevent weight regain. The initial goal of weight-loss therapy is to reduce body weight by approximately 10% from baseline over 6 months.[19] The preferred approach is gradual and consistent decreases in weight, a goal that is beneficial, attainable, and maintainable.

NONPHARMACOLOGIC TREATMENTS

The recommended nonpharmacologic treatment for obesity is a reduced-calorie diet in combination with increased physical activity and behavioral modification. Current treatment guidelines recommend a low-calorie diet (LCD) consisting of approximately 800–1,200 kcal per day.[19] Patients should be instructed to follow the Step I Diet outlined by the Third Report of the Expert Panel on the Detection, Evaluation, and Treatment of High Blood Cholesterol in Adults (ATP III).[57] Very-low-calorie diets, composed of 250 to 800 kcal/day, are generally not recommended, as safety concerns exist and long-term weight loss is not significantly different than that achieved with an LCD.[19,58] Low-carbohydrate, high-protein diets may be an option for selected patients. Comparisons of these diets to the conventional LCD have reported similar weight-loss efficacy after 1 year of treatment.[59,60] The combination of LCD and increased physical activity can enhance weight loss and improve cardiovascular risk factors. The recommended goal for physical activity in healthy individuals ages 18–65 years is a minimum of 30 minutes or more of moderate-intensity exercise on 5 days each week or vigorous-intensity exercise for a minimum of 20 minutes on 3 days each week.[61] Finally, behavior-modification strategies should be used in combination with diet and exercise to help enhance weight loss. The primary goal of behavioral modification is to recognize and ultimately change the behaviors that are associated with overeating and decreased physical activity.

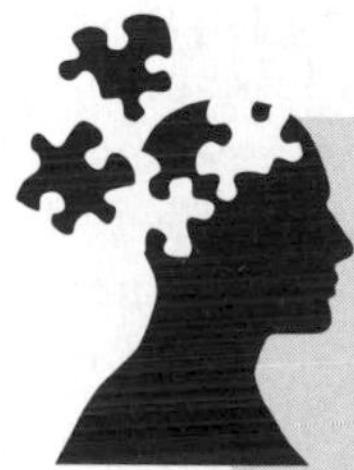

Therapeutic Challenge:

What are the long-term safety concerns associated with various popular diets, such as Atkins, Mediterranean, South Beach, or Zone?

PHARMACOLOGIC TREATMENTS

Pharmacologic interventions may be considered as part of the treatment plan for women unable to achieve adequate weight loss with diet, increased physical activity, and behavioral modifications. The majority of evidence from clinical trials supporting the efficacy of weight-loss interventions are derived from moderate to very obese white women.[48] A recent meta-analysis has shown that regardless of weight loss efficacy, treatment with weight-loss medication can help ameliorate depression, whereas both weight loss and treatment can especially improve self-esteem among obese women.[62] Selection of the appropriate anti-obesity therapy should be carefully considered based on patient characteristics and adequate safety and efficacy profiles of each agent. The Food and Drug Administration (FDA)–approved pharmacologic treatment options for long-term management of obesity are listed in Table 32-3.

Sympathomimetic Agents

Sympathomimetic agents suppress appetite by releasing norepinephrine in the nucleus of the hypothalamus. The only over-the-counter agent approved in this class, phenylpropanolamine, was widely used as an appetite suppressant and a decongestant but was withdrawn from the market because of subsequent concerns of hemorrhagic stroke in women.[63] Efficacy and safety data for phentermine, diethylpropion, benzphetamine, and phendimetrazine are mainly generated from short-term clinical trials, with the longest trial lasting only 36 weeks.[64] Phentermine is the most widely prescribed sympathomimetic for short-term weight loss. Previous treatment of phentermine in combination with a serotonin-releasing agent, fenfluramine or dexfenfluramine, contributed to the undesirable adverse effects of valvular heart diseases and pulmonary hypertension, which consequently led to the withdrawal of fenfluramine and dexfenfluramine from the market in 1997.[63] Although independent use of phentermine has not been associated with valvular heart diseases, expected adverse effects of sympathomimetics include nervousness, insomnia, constipation, euphoria, tachycardia, and hypertension.[51] Use of these agents is therefore contraindicated in women with underlying cardiovascular diseases. Furthermore, because these products lack sufficient long-term evaluation and possess the potential for abuse, their utilities in the treatment of obesity are not approved beyond 12 weeks.[64] This is inconsistent with current

Table 32-3. FDA-Approved Long-term Pharmacologic Treatments for Overweight and Obesity

Generic Name	Brand Name	Mechanism of Action	Effective Dosage	Side Effects	Pregnancy Category
Sibutramine	Meridia®	NE, 5HT reuptake inhibitor	10–15 mg once daily	Hypertension, tachycardia, headache, insomnia, dry mouth, constipation, anorexia	C
Orlistat	Xenical™	Lipase inhibitor	120 mg 3 times daily with meals[a]	Nausea, steatorrhea, oily spotting, oily evacuation, increase defecation, fecal urgency and incontinence, malabsorption	B
	Alli™	Lipase inhibitor	60 mg 3 times daily with meals[a]	Similar, but incidence of GI distress may be less with reduced strength[b]	B

FDA = U.S. Food and Drug Administration; GI = gastrointestinal; NE = norepinephrine; 5HT = serotonin.
[a]Dose should be administered within 1 hour of digesting a meal. Dose may be omitted if a meal is missed or lacks fat content.
[b]Approved for over-the-counter use in the U.S.

treatment guidelines, which recommend long-term management.[19]

Sibutramine

Introduced in 1997, sibutramine (Meridia®) was the first FDA-approved appetite suppressant for the long-term management of obesity. Originally developed as an antidepressant with dual mechanisms involving inhibition of norepinephrine and serotonin reuptake, sibutramine was subsequently discovered to be an effective weight-loss agent through promoting early satiety, reducing hunger, and increasing energy expenditure. Additionally, sibutramine may also exert sympathetic activity and stimulate thermogenesis to produce weight loss in obese women.[65] The initial starting dosage of sibutramine is 10 mg/day, which offers the convenience of once-daily dosing. In general, a reduction of at least 1.8 kg (4 lb) can be expected within the first 4 weeks of initial therapy when used in combination with the recommended diet and lifestyle modifications. Initial response to sibutramine is highly predictive of its long-term efficacy.[66] Therefore, if a patient fails to achieve adequate weight loss after 4 weeks of initial therapy, a higher dosage (15 mg/day) may be used, as sibutramine appears to have a dose-dependent response, or the therapy may be discontinued.[66,67] Because sibutramine promotes satiety, women treated with sibutramine may experience the most success when the drug is used in conjunction with a dietary program that emphasizes portion control during meals.[68] Results from a meta-analysis (selected studies included 56% to 80% women) reported that a 4.5 kg (10 lb) greater weight loss was observed with sibutramine therapy (10–15 mg/day) when compared with placebo as an adjunct to lifestyle modification in trials lasting 1 year.[69] The efficacy of sibutramine is greatly enhanced with a group comprehensive program consisting of diet, exercise, and behavioral therapy to achieve an overall average weight loss of 12.1 kg (26.6 lb) after 1 year of therapy, compared with reduction of 5 kg (11 lb) in the sibutramine-alone group.[70] Weight reduction with sibutramine was reported to be similar among healthy obese adults and individuals with type 2 diabetes, hypertension, and hyperlipidemia.[69]

The long-term efficacy of sibutramine has been evaluated for up to 2 years in the Sibutramine Trial of Obesity Reduction and Maintenance (STORM) study, which was a randomized, double-blind, placebo-controlled trial evaluating more than 600 obese patients, 82.3% of whom were women.[67] At year 2, sibutramine-treated patients achieved significantly more weight loss compared with the placebo-treated patients, 10.2 kg (22.4 lb) and 4.7 kg (10.3 lb), respectively. Furthermore, a higher percentage of patients treated with sibutramine (average dosage 13.5 mg/day) was able to maintain at least 80% of their original weight loss compared with the placebo-treated group (43% vs. 16%, $p < 0.001$). A proportional decrease in triglycerides, very-low-density lipoprotein (vLDL) cholesterol, insulin C-peptides, and uric acid were also noted with weight loss among the sibutramine-treated group. Of note, women treated with sibutramine experienced a 20.9% increase in HDL-C over the 2-year period compared with 19.9% observed in men and 12.4% observed in placebo. The long-term benefits on HDL-C were independent of sibutramine-induced weight loss.

Additionally, sibutramine was shown to significantly improve quality of life in a trial comprised of 83% women.[71] However, discontinuation of therapy is associated with regain of up to 55% of weight lost after 18 months.[67] Although sibutramine has demonstrated moderate weight-loss effect, its long-term morbidity and mortality data in high-risk overweight and obese adults still have to await results from the SCOUT (Sibutramine Cardiovascular OUTcomes) trial expected in 2010.[72]

Even though sibutramine has not been associated with valvular heart diseases or pulmonary hypertension, normotensive individuals treated with sibutramine have demonstrated a dose-dependent increase in blood pressure and pulse.[66,73] At 1 year, the mean increases over placebo were approximately 4.6 mmHg for systolic blood pressure, 2.8 mmHg for diastolic blood pressure, and 5.9 beats per minute for pulse.[69] Dangerous increases in blood pressure (≥15 mmHg for systolic blood pressure and ≥10 mmHg for diastolic blood pressure) and pulse (≥10 beats per minute) have been consistently observed in some patients.[66] With these potential cardiovascular concerns, sibutramine should be avoided in women with uncontrolled blood pressure or a history of coronary artery disease, heart failure, arrhythmias, or stroke.[66] Therefore, it is prudent to monitor blood pressure and pulse before initiation of therapy and periodically monitor associated cardiovascular changes in patients receiving sibutramine therapy. Women who experience a clinically significant increase in blood pressure will require a dosage reduction or discontinuation of therapy.[66] Other common adverse effects of sibutramine include dry mouth, headache, anorexia, constipation, and insomnia.[66] Because increases in serotonin level have been associated with dose-dependent sexual dysfunction in those treated with selective serotonin reuptake inhibitors, a similar hypothetical concern was postulated with use of sibutramine. Nevertheless, findings among overweight and obese women suggested sibutramine did not induce sexual dysfunction, but in fact positively affected their sexual function, which paralleled the extent of weight reduction observed over an 8-week period.[74]

Sibutramine is a cytochrome P450 (CYP450) 3A4 isoenzyme substrate; therefore, caution should be applied when sibutramine is used in combination with other medications metabolized through the CYP450 3A4 isoenzyme system, or other serotonergic or noradrenergic agents, or monoamine oxidase inhibitors.[66] For patients using oral contraceptives, a change in birth control method is not required as sibutramine has not shown to alter suppression of ovulation when administered in conjunction with oral contraceptives.[66] Women of childbearing potential should ensure adequate contraception while receiving sibutramine therapy because pregnancy complications, such as hypertensive disorders and spontaneous abortion, have been reported after sibutramine exposure during the first and second trimesters.[66,75,76] Exposure of sibutramine on the developing fetus is not adequately known.[75] Sibutramine is currently classified as pregnancy category C; thus, use of therapy should be considered only if the potential benefits justify any potential risks to the fetus.[66] Furthermore, because of limited available data, use of sibutramine is not recommended for mothers who wish to breast-feed.[66]

Orlistat

Orlistat is a reversible gastric and pancreatic lipase inhibitor that uniquely targets the lumen of the gastrointestinal tract to reduce dietary fat absorption.[77] Undigested triglycerides are eventually excreted in the feces.[78] Because of its unique mechanism of action, orlistat should be administered within 1 hour of ingesting each fat-containing meal. If a meal is missed or lacks fat content, the dose may be omitted.[77] At the recommended prescription-strength dosage, 120 mg 3 times daily, up to approximately 30% of dietary fat absorption may be inhibited.[78] The half-strength (Alli™) over-the-counter formulation is the only FDA-approved nonprescription therapy to facilitate weight reduction in overweight adults.

The efficacy of orlistat (120 mg 3 times daily) has been collectively evaluated in a meta-analysis consisting of 29 controlled clinical trials comprised of 73% women.[79] Total weight loss observed with orlistat at 6 months was approximately 5.4 kg (11.9 lb). At the end of the first year of therapy, adults treated with orlistat achieved an average total weight loss of 8.1 kg (17.8 lb); this was 2.9 kg (6.4 lb) greater than those who received placebo.[79] Although most weight loss occurred rapidly (within the first 3 months), peak weight reduction with orlistat generally was evident by the first year followed by a gradual weight regain.[77,80] Benefits of modest weight reduction with orlistat have also been demonstrated in obese adolescents, patients with type 2 diabetes, and those with metabolic syndrome.[77] The over-the-counter dosage of orlistat (60 mg 3 times daily) has been reported to achieve approximately 4.2% weight loss with short-term use in overweight individuals.[81]

Weight loss after 4 months of therapy averaged 3.1 kg (6.8 lb) compared with 1.9 kg (4.2 lb) with diet alone. This additional 1.2 kg (2.6 lb) reduction with treatment was demonstrated to be statistically significant.[81]

Treatment with orlistat offers additional advantages beyond weight reduction. Significant improvement in cardiac risk factors, such as reducing blood pressure, waist circumference, and total and LDL cholesterols, has been demonstrated after orlistat therapy.[77,82] Furthermore, small improvements in glycemic control, such as reduction in HbA_{1c}, fasting plasma glucose, and postprandial glucose levels, were also evident after orlistat treatment.[77] Reduction of triglycerides and oxidative stress markers, such as C-reactive protein, tumor necrosis factor α, insulin-like growth factor, and adipokines, were also reported in obese women after orlistat treatment combined with hypocaloric diet.[83]

Long-term outcomes of orlistat have been assessed in the XENDOS (XENical in the prevention of Diabetes in Obese Subjects) trial, which was a randomized, double-blind, placebo-controlled 4-year trial enrolling more than 1,600 obese adults with normal or impaired glucose tolerance; 55% of the study participants were women.[80] Results from XENDOS demonstrated that a significantly higher percentage of adults who received orlistat treatment were able to maintain ≥10% weight loss compared with those who received placebo at end of the fourth year (41% vs. 20.8%). The total weight reduction maintained by year 4 was 5.8 kg (12.8 lb) with orlistat therapy compared with 3 kg (6.6 lb) with placebo (p <0.001). Despite the modest weight change, adults who received orlistat had a significant 37.3% reduction in overall incidence of type 2 diabetes compared with placebo; this risk reduction was greater for adults with impaired glucose tolerance at baseline.[80,84] It is important to emphasize that all reported benefits of orlistat therapy were observed in conjunction with hypocaloric diets plus lifestyle modifications.

The adverse effect profile associated with orlistat is predominantly gastrointestinal in nature, reflected by its mechanism of action. Transient adverse effects such as nausea, soft stool, episodes of oily spotting, oily evacuation, **steatorrhea,** increased defecation, and fecal urgency/incontinence were commonly recognized in clinical trials, varying from mild to moderate in severity.[77] Patients receiving orlistat experienced greater than a threefold increase in diarrhea and flatulence.[79] Although these side effects generally resolve with continued treatment, some patients may be embarrassed or unable to tolerate these symptoms, thereby compromising adherence to therapy. The incidence of gastrointestinal symptoms appears to be less with the 60-mg dose.[81] Nevertheless, adverse gastrointestinal distress increases with consumption of high-fat meals (>30% total calories from fat). Thus, it is important to educate all patients to evenly distribute their daily intake of fats, carbohydrates, and proteins over three main meals to minimize gastrointestinal adverse events.[78] Additionally, women should be advised to supplement with a daily multivitamin, administered 2 hours before or 2 hours after a dose of orlistat to prevent possible nutrient deficiencies due to partial malabsorption of fat-soluble vitamins (particularly vitamins E and D) and β–carotene.[77] Previous concerns of increased breast cancer risk among women treated with orlistat were alleviated after an extensive retrospective analysis concluded most reported cases of breast cancer were antedated before initiation of orlistat.[85,86] Furthermore, the drug's negligible systemic absorption (<1%) makes this casual association even less plausible. Although orlistat has not been shown to alter suppression of ovulation by oral contraceptives, women who experience severe diarrhea with orlistat should be cautioned that the bioavailability of their oral contraceptives may be reduced, and alternative backup methods are needed.[77] Although orlistat is categorized as pregnancy category B, well-controlled human studies in pregnant women are still lacking. Therefore, the manufacturer does not recommend orlistat be continued during pregnancy or breast-feeding.[78]

Combination Therapy

Short-term efficacy of combination therapy (sibutramine 15 mg/day plus orlistat 120 mg 3 times daily) has been assessed in a randomized controlled trial among 89 normotensive obese women com-

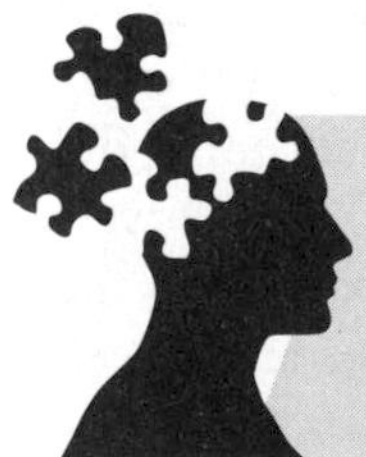

Therapeutic Challenge:

Long-term weight maintenance data beyond 2 years for sibutramine and 4 years for orlistat are limited. What is the optimal duration of treatment for each of the anti-obesity medications for management of weight loss? Should obesity be managed with long-term pharmacotherapy similar to other chronic diseases?

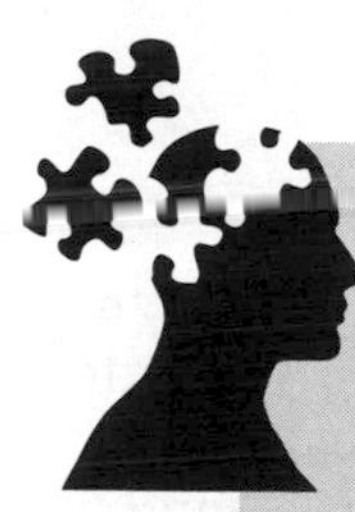

Therapeutic Challenge:

Does use of anti-obesity medication reduce the long-term morbidity and mortality associated with overweight and obesity?

pared with sibutramine alone (15 mg/day) or orlistat alone (120 mg 3 times daily) in conjunction with diet modification.[87] Results at 6 months suggested sibutramine alone and combination therapy promoted significantly greater weight reduction than orlistat alone. Mean percent weight reduction observed among women who received combination therapy was 10.6%, compared with 10.2% among sibutramine alone and 5.5% among orlistat alone. However, the addition of orlistat to sibutramine did not achieve further weight reduction than women who received sibutramine monotherapy.

Dietary Supplements and Alternative Therapies

The increasing prevalence of obesity has led to the growing popularity of dietary supplements as a strategy to promote loss weight. More women than men pursue use of weight-loss dietary supplements, with the highest use among women ages 18–34 years.[88] A 2007 survey of U.S. adults found that approximately 20.6% of women reported ever using a weight-loss supplement, and 11.3% of women reported they had used one in the past year.[88] Alternative therapies commonly promoted for weight loss include, but are not limited to, chitosan, ginseng, hoodia, glucomannan, guarana (caffeine), spirulina (blue-green algae), chromium picolinate, garcinia (hydroxycitric acid), pyruvate, ephedra (*ma-huang*), and bitter orange (*Citrus aurantium*). These therapies are commonly perceived as an appealing alternative to diet, behavioral, and lifestyle modifications because patients often misinterpret dietary supplements as "natural" and assume they offer safety assurance. Almost 74% of respondents who admitted to using weight-loss supplements consumed supplements containing stimulants, including ephedra, caffeine, and/or bitter orange.[88] Sale of dietary supplements containing ephedra was prohibited by the FDA in 2004 because of serious safety concerns, including seizures, strokes, and deaths.[89] Consequently, numerous popular "ephedra-free" dietary weight-loss products marketed are now substituted or reformulated to include bitter orange. One of the active constituents found in bitter orange is *m*-synephrine (or phenylephrine), a sympathomimetic amine that is structurally related to ephedrine and possesses potential to cause adverse cardiovascular effects as ephedrine alkaloids.[90] Similar to other weight-loss dietary supplements, bitter orange lacks adequate clinical data and quality control, and has not undergone rigorous testing for safety and efficacy; therefore, its evidence remains inconclusive.[90-93] Of note, some nationwide products marketed as dietary supplements have been found to contain potentially harmful, undeclared ingredients that can be very dangerous when consumed. Therefore, it is crucial for healthcare professionals to strongly advise patients against use of dietary supplements as part of a weight-loss regimen until sound scientific data of these supplements are firmly established with minimal safety concerns.

Monitoring and Follow-up

Adherence to drug therapy in conjunction with diet, lifestyle modifications, and scheduled follow-up visits are crucial to the efficacy of an overall weight-management plan. A recent survey found only approximately 56% of patients are adherent to drug therapy, and most nonadherence occurred within the first 3 months of treatment.[94] For many, efforts to maintain the weight lost is more challenging than losing the initial weight. Weight regain after nonadherence can be significant: 5.2 kg (11.4 lb) for orlistat and 6.1 kg (13.4 lb) for sibutramine after about 9 months of nonadherence.[94] Close monitoring is recommended within the first 6 months of therapy. Weight changes should be recorded weekly at home and routinely every 4 weeks during follow-up visits. Additionally, potential adverse effects of drug therapy should be assessed regularly and any obstacles affecting therapy adherence should be identified. Understanding patients' difficulties in achieving adherence and continual assessment of patients' progress are essential to ensuring success of the overall treatment plan.

Patient Education

- Set realistic weight-loss goals, with an aim to achieve 0.5–0.9 kg (1–2 lb) per week with an initial target to decrease baseline weight by 10% over 6 months. Even moderate weight loss—as little as 5%—can decrease cardiovascular risk factors associated with obesity.
- Only use FDA-approved therapy. Alternative and dietary supplements have not undergone stringent safety and efficacy review and can be dangerous.

- Drug therapy for weight loss should never be used alone. The efficacy of drug therapy is only successful when used in combination with diet, lifestyle, and behavioral modification.
- Weight-loss maintenance cannot be expected to continue after drug therapy discontinuation unless lifestyle changes are permanently implemented as part of daily life.
- Educate patient regarding specific adverse effects associated with weight-loss therapy.

BARIATRIC SURGICAL TREATMENTS

Obesity can be largely refractory to diet and pharmacologic interventions. Although many women attempt weight loss with diet and exercise, long-term weight loss is not commonly sustained. The National Institutes of Health report that 95% of people who are morbidly obese will regain the weight lost (nonsurgically) within 1 year.[52] Bariatric surgery is the only durable option for weight loss in most people who have this chronic disease.[95,96] With the growing number of individuals with extreme obesity, increased media coverage of bariatric surgery with its potentially positive outcomes, higher consumer demand, and more insurance coverage from third-party payers for these procedures, the number of bariatric surgeries is expected to increase substantially.[97]

Definitions of Surgical Procedures

Surgical weight-loss procedures have been performed for decades, starting with the jejunal bypass done in the 1970s, various versions of gastric bypass developed in the 1980s, and banded gastroplasty in the 1980s and 1990s. Evolution of the procedures has gone from open to laparoscopic surgery. The most common weight-loss surgery currently performed in the U.S. is the Roux-en-Y variation of the gastric bypass. An increasing number of procedures employing adjustable gastric banding is being performed. The vertical sleeve gastrectomy, in which most of the stomach is removed, requires less operative time and has no surgical **anastomosis.** It was originally developed as part of a two-stage surgical approach for patients with extreme BMI (>50 kg/m^2). This surgery—designed to decrease excess weight by 25% and improve safety to allow more extensive gastric bypass—is now being performed on patients with less extreme BMI as well because of its effectiveness.[95] Table 32-4 illustrates the different weight-loss surgical procedures.[54]

Outcomes of Surgical Weight-Loss Procedures

It is important to note that bariatric surgery is the only treatment for obesity that has been shown to reduce long-term mortality.[98,99] More than 3 times as many women than men had bariatric surgery in the U.S. between 1990 and 2003.[95,96] This may be a reflection of adverse social consequences of obesity affecting women more than men, in addition to other social factors, including willingness to seek self-care. Loss of excess weight varies, depending on the type of surgery performed, ranging between 50% and 70%. A large meta-analysis found that patients undergoing a variety of surgeries experienced mean overall excess weight loss of 61% over 2 years.[95] Excess weight loss was 47.5% for gastric banding, 61.6% for gastric bypass, 68.2% for gastroplasty, and 70.1% for biliopancreatic diversion or duodenal switch. Long-term mortality can be improved as much as 29% to 40% after bariatric surgery, as shown in a comparison of two severely obese groups primarily made up of women.[98,99] Bariatric surgery can be curative for many patients with diabetes. Blood glucose abnormalities resolved in as many as three quarters of patients who underwent malabsorptive procedures and in as many as half of patients who underwent gastric banding alone.[96] It is speculated that change in gut hormone mediator milieu plays a role. Hypertension is improved in proportion to amount of weight loss. Hyperlipidemia was greatly improved and obstructive sleep apnea resolved in 80% of patients.[96] Weight loss in women, which is greater after surgery than with lifestyle changes alone, is linearly associated with a decline in C-reactive protein.[100]

Complications can be divided into those that occur in conjunction with surgery and immediately postsurgically, and those that are delayed or long-term in nature. Immediate postsurgical complications include leaks at anastomotic sites and along internal staple lines, wound infections, and pulmonary embolism.[101] Late complications include bowel obstruction, incisional hernias, stenosis, and symptomatic ulcers at surgically involved areas.[101] Long-term complications may include electrolyte imbalance, constipation, **dumping syndrome,** difficulty of transit of certain foods through the esophagus or modified stomach area, and other motility disorders.[102] Some patients experience malnutrition with the potential for anemia and bone loss.[103]

Table 32-4. Common Surgical Procedures for Weight Loss

Restrictive (stomach only)		Restrictive and Malabsorptive (stomach and intestine)	
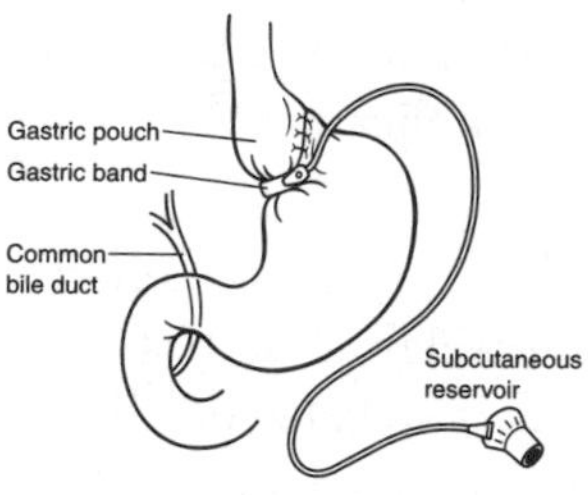 Gastric pouch, Gastric band, Common bile duct, Subcutaneous reservoir	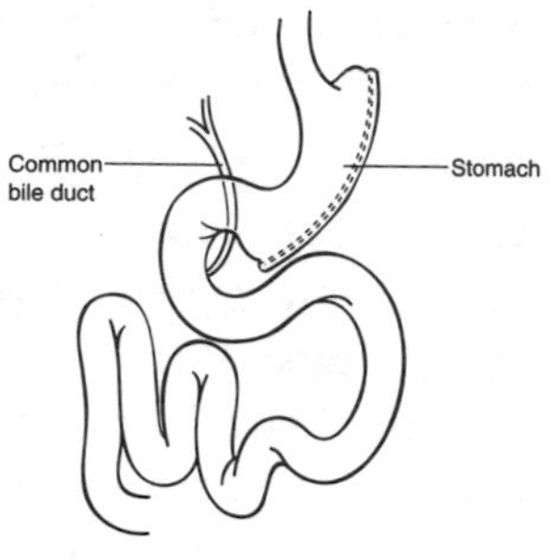 Common bile duct, Stomach	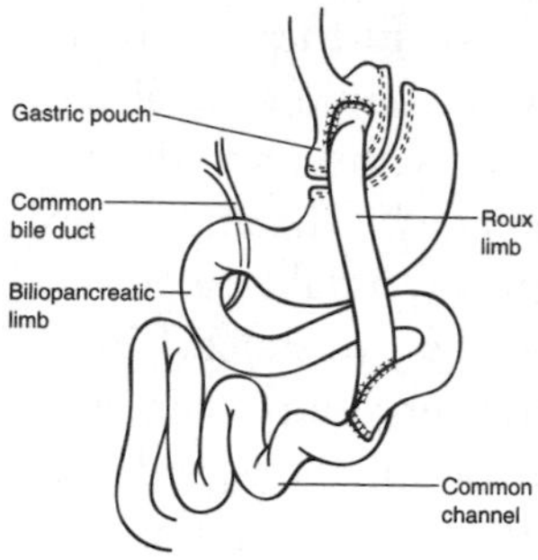 Gastric pouch, Common bile duct, Roux limb, Biliopancreatic limb, Common channel	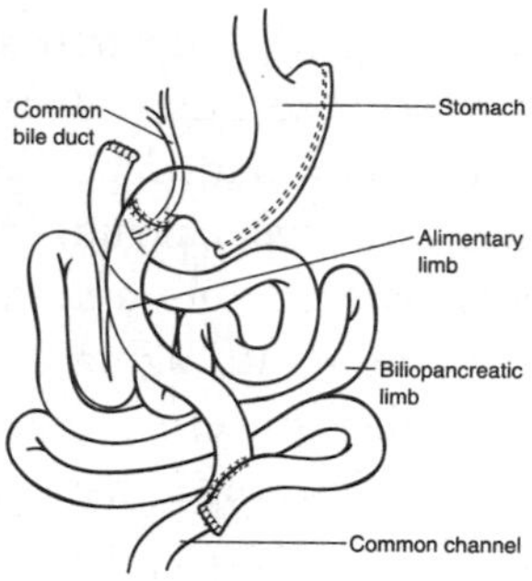 Common bile duct, Stomach, Alimentary limb, Biliopancreatic limb, Common channel
Laparoscopic adjustable gastric banding	Sleeve gastrectomy	Roux-en-Y gastric bypass	Biliopancreatic diversion/duodenal switch
Initial Stomach Pouch Volume			
1–2 oz	2–3 oz	1 oz	4–5 oz
Characteristics that Contribute to Weight Loss			
- Restricts volume and type of food - Delayed emptying, sensation of fullness - No dumping or malabsorption	- Restricts volume of food - No dumping or malabsorption	- Restricts volume of food - Dumping syndrome when sugar or fats are eaten - Mild malabsorption	- Restricts volume of food - Diarrhea and bloating when fats are eaten - Moderate malabsorption
Percent of Excess Weight Loss at 2 and 10 Years			
60% and unknown (longer follow-up needed)	60% to 70% and unknown (longer follow-up needed)	70% and <50%	80% and more
Lifetime Nutritional Supplements Required			
- Multivitamin - Calcium/vitamin D	- Multivitamin - Calcium/vitamin D	- Multivitamin - Calcium/vitamin D - B_{12} - Folate	- Multivitamin - Calcium - Fat soluble vitamins A, D, E, K
		Iron (in menstruating women)	

Source: Figure illustrations obtained from reference 54 (Massachusetts Medical Society, all rights reserved). Bariatric surgery for morbid obesity. *N Engl J Med.* 2007;356:2176-2183. Massachusetts Medical Society. All rights reserved.

General Considerations After Bariatric Surgery

Deficiency in vitamins and minerals is a concern as a result of both restrictive and malabsorptive surgeries, with the degree of deficiency potential depending on the type of surgical procedure (Table 32-4).[54] Lifelong calcium supplementation is recommended in all bariatric surgery patients. Depending on the type of surgery performed, bypass patients require supplementation of fat-soluble vitamins (A, D, E, K), as well as vitamin B_{12} and folate. Supplementation with vitamin B_{12} needs to be administered sublingually, nasally, or by injection because the oral formulation will not be adequately absorbed due to decreased acid secretion and availability of intrinsic factor with bypass surgery. Iron supplementation is recommended in all women who are menstruating.[54,104] Absorption for both calcium and iron are pH dependent. Proton-pump inhibitors are prescribed postsurgically for varying periods and with removal of much of the stomach; stomach acidity may be permanently impaired and can further contribute to altered absorption. Because dissolution of calcium citrate is not acid dependent, it is the preferred salt formulation over calcium carbonate.[104] The importance of adequate calcium and vitamin D intake to prevent osteoporosis with aging cannot be overstated. This is a particular concern in bariatric surgery patients who are eating less, often have pH abnormalities, and have a smaller absorptive surface available.[104,105] In some series, the average age of bariatric surgery in women is between the ages 40 and 50 years, which further compounds bone loss induced by menopause, especially in women not receiving hormone therapy. Monitoring of bone loss via dual-energy x-ray absorptiometry should be performed for certain women considered at risk for osteoporosis.[106] The potential for decreased drug absorption should also be considered, and therapeutic effect of medications may require monitoring in patients who undergo bariatric surgery (Table 32-5).[104] Furthermore, it is important to consider the various dosage formulations available. For many patients who may not be able to tolerate large tablets, liquid or chewable dosage forms, nonoral route is usually the preferred method of administering medications.

Pregnancy After Bariatric Surgery

Eighty percent of patients having bariatric surgery are women of childbearing age.[97] Pregnancy after bariatric surgery has not been associated with adverse perinatal outcomes.[107] A small retrospective study did not find any differences in pregnancy or neonatal complications between women who conceived in the first year after surgery or 1 year after surgery.[108] Additionally, no differences in obstetric characteristics or pregnancy outcomes were noted with women who underwent either open or laparoscopic weight-loss surgical procedures, with the exception of a higher rate of cesarean delivery in women who had bariatric surgery.[109] Pregnancy outcomes after laparoscopic-adjustable gastric banding are consistent with general community outcomes, for both mothers and newborns, rather than outcomes of severely obese women.[110] Monitoring and, if necessary, band adjustments during pregnancy provided more favorable maternal weight outcomes. Furthermore, pregnant mothers should be monitored for increased risk of anemia, folate deficiency, vitamin B_{12} deficiency, calcium deficiency, and inadequate protein intake.[97] It is critical that nutritional counseling be individualized during pregnancy to assist women in maintaining adequate nutritional intake to prevent associated vitamin, iron, and protein deficiencies.[97] Because infants of obese women are at higher risk of **neural tube defects**, it is important to ensure adequate folic acid 400 mcg supplementation before and during pregnancy to prevent neonatal complications.[97]

Contraception

Women are generally advised to postpone conception 2 years after surgery until weight loss has been optimized and nutritional status is stabalized.[97] Some women may have higher risk for pregnancy as they become more sexually active or their fertility may increase because of correction of hormonal factors. It is possible that absorption of oral contraceptives could be decreased, but there have been no studies to date in women postbariatric surgery. Alternative hormonal contraception options are the contraceptive patch or vaginal ring. In addition to avoiding potential absorption problems, these dosage forms may facilitate adherence by bypassing the need to take an oral tablet on a regular schedule. If a barrier method is chosen, the condom is most effective for both pregnancy and sexually transmitted diseases prevention. For women who experience significant weight loss >6.8–9.1 kg (15–20 lb), a contraceptive diaphragm will need to be refitted. It is not known whether it is necessary to stop hormonal contraception before surgery because the potential increased risk of venous thromboembolism perioperatively with today's lower estrogen formulations has not been assessed. The American College of Obstetricians and Gynecologists (ACOG) recently issued recommendations about thromboprophylaxis in patients undergoing gynecologic surgery, and in the absence of data specific to female bariatric surgery patients, these might be taken into consideration. Their recommendations state that prothrombotic clotting factor changes appear to persist for 4–6 weeks after discontinuing oral contraceptive use. The risk of stopping oral contraception before surgery should be balanced against that of unintended pregnancy. In women continuing to take oral contraceptives, heparin prophylaxis is an option.[111] Because

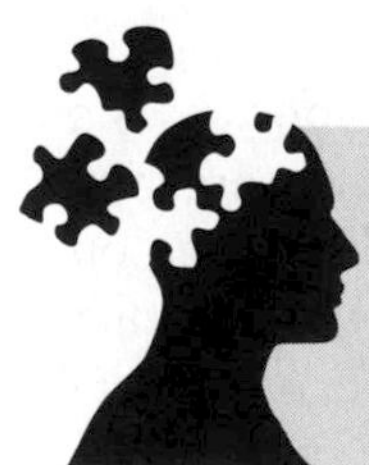

Therapeutic Challenge:

Which oral contraceptive is most appropriate for women with severe obesity before and after bariatric surgery?

Table 32-5. Selected Agents with Potential for Decreased Absorption in Patients Who Have Undergone Bariatric Surgery

Drug	Possible Site(s) of Absorption	Management
Enalapril	Hydrolyzed to active form, enalaprilat, in stomach; absorbed in small intestine[a]	May exhibit decreased activity; consider other angiotensin-converting-enzyme inhibitors
Ketoconazole	Likely absorbed in stomach because acidic medium required for absorption[b]	Absorption likely to be negligible; consider alternative agents[c]
Lamotrigine	Likely stomach and proximal small intestine due to rapid and complete absorption[c]	Monitor for and advise patients of decreased efficacy
Metformin	Slowly and incompletely absorbed in duodenum[d]	Increased monitoring of blood glucose; drug requirements can decrease as weight loss occurs
Metoprolol tartrate	Absorbed rapidly and completely, indicating stomach and duodenums[e]	Monitor blood pressure; medication requirements may decrease as weight loss occurs
Niacin	Primarily absorbed in duodenum[f]	Administer with low-fat snack to maximize absorption
Olanzapine	Stomach[g]	Monitor for decreased efficacy; switching to orally disintegrating tablet will not increase absorption (still absorbed in stomach)
Quetiapine fumarate	Exact location unknown, but likely stomach and duodenum due to rapid absorption[h]	Monitor for decreased efficacy
Ramipril	Unknown; decreased absorption documented in patients with steatorrhea and malabsorption[i]	Consider other agents; monitor blood pressure in the postoperative period; need for antihypertensives may decrease as weight loss occurs
Simvastatin	Absorption site unknown, but must be hydrolyzed to the active form in stomach[j]	Consider other agents; monitor serum lipids
Zlopidem	Absorbed rapidly and completely; absorption affected by food[k]	Absorption time may increase, resulting in delay to effect; take on an empty stomach

Source: Adapted from reference 104.
[a]Vasotec (enalapril) package insert. Morrisville, NC: Biovail Pharmaceuticals; August 2002.
[b]Data on file. Titusville, NJ: Janssen Pharmaceutica.
[c]Lamictal (lamotrigine) package insert. Research Triangle Park, NC: GlaxoSmithKline; August 2005.
[d]Vidon N, Chaussade S, Noel M, et al. Metformin in the digestive tract. *Diabetes Res Clin Pract.* 1988;4:223-229.
[e]Lopressor (metoprolol tartrate) package insert. Suffem, NY: Novartis; November 2004.
[f]Data on file. Cranbury, NJ: Kos Pharmaceuticals; August 2005.
[g]Data on file. Indianapolis, IN: Eli Lilly and Company; October 2005.
[h]Seroquel (quetiapine fumarate) package insert. Wilmington, DE: AstraZeneca; December 2005.
[i]Data on file. Bristol, TN: King Pharmaceuticals; February 2004.
[j]Vickers S, Duncan CA, Chen IW, et al. Metabolic disposition studies on simvastatin, a cholesterol lowering prodrug. *Drug Metab Dispos.* 1990;18:138-145.
[k]Ambien (zolpidem) package insert. New York, NY. Sanofi-Synthelabo; March 2004.

of lack of supporting evidence, ACOG does not recommend discontinuation of menopausal hormone therapy before gynecologic surgery.[112]

Patient Education

- The first 12–18 months after surgery are a "window of opportunity" for relatively fast, large weight loss.
- Although the stomach is smaller, its size will eventually stretch to some degree.
- Hunger is less due to less of the stomach hormone ghrelin, which drives appetite.
- It is critical to develop a new lifestyle.
- New eating habits must include smaller portions.
- Greatly decreased portion size and caloric intake are required long term.
- Protein intake must be adequate to meet daily minimum requirement.

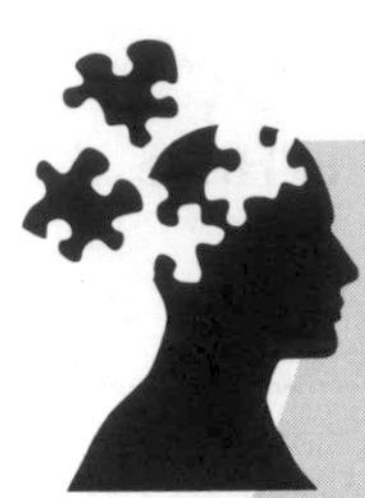

Therapeutic Challenge:

What risk factors would warrant initiation of thromboprophylaxis in patients undergoing bariatric surgery? Which anticoagulants would be the best choice, at what dose, and for what duration? Should anticoagulants be administered perioperatively in women without history of thromboembolic events?

- Protein should be consumed first because stomach space is limited.
- Ensure adequate fluid intake.
- Adequate vitamin and nutritional supplementations are lifelong requirements.
- Large amounts of carbonated beverages can significantly stretch the new stomach.

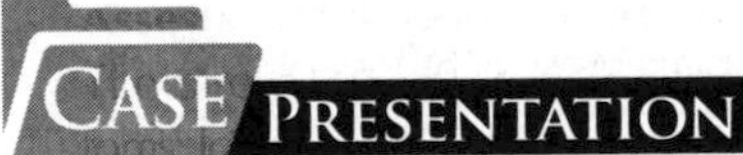

Patient Case: Part 2

Assessment:

J.C. is having a Roux-en-Y, which is a restrictive and malabsorptive procedure with the capacity to decrease stomach acid and affect availability of intrinsic factors. Therefore, she will require supplementation of vitamin B_{12} by sublingual, nasal, or injectable route.

She is presently taking estrogen therapy via a nonoral route and would like to continue (less likely to affect clotting factors without first-pass metabolism). Minimum elemental calcium requirement in women on estrogen therapy is 1,200 mg daily, in divided doses. J.C. should also be supplementing vitamin D_3 800–1,000 International Units/day. She will not require iron supplementation because of her postmenopausal status. Use of antidiabetic medications should be reevaluated postsurgically by daily glucose monitoring because dietary carbohydrate intake is expected to be very small.

Plan:

1. Metformin must be discontinued before surgery. Continuation of antidiabetic medications may not be necessary as patient will consume much less food and calories postsurgery.
2. Ibuprofen, aspirin, and any medication or supplement that could interfere with blood clotting must be discontinued 2 weeks before surgery. Patient may need to temporarily withhold nonsteroidal anti-inflammatory drugs because of tablet size and gastric irritation postsurgery.
3. Enoxaparin 40 mg will be given subcutaneously every 12 hours starting after surgery for 7 days.
4. Start daily chewable multivitamin, calcium citrate 200 mg 6 times daily, vitamin D_3 400 International Units, and vitamin B_{12} 1,000 mcg sublingually as soon as the supplements can be tolerated.

Rationale: Patients undergoing surgery for obesity are at significant risk for thromboembolic complications.[52] Low-molecular-weight heparin has been used postbariatric surgery, but large series of data are not available. Enoxaparin 40 mg every 12 hours has been shown to decrease the incidence of postoperative deep vein thrombosis (in one case series) when used along with other preventive measures (early ambulation and intermittent pneumatic compression devices).[111] Supplementation with calcium citrate is preferred over calcium carbonate because of decreased gastric acid secretion after surgery.

Monitoring: Weight loss, fasting blood glucose, folic acid deficiency, vitamin B_{12} deficiency, and dumping syndrome.

Patient education: Vitamins and minerals will need to be taken daily for the rest of her life. She is to use either chewable or liquid form. In addition to a multivitamin, she should take calcium citrate plus vitamin D, vitamin B_{12}, and folate. For the first 4 weeks postsurgery, diet will be primarily liquid or puréed. She will need to consume 60 g of protein daily. Skim milk is a good low-calorie protein source (with lactase enzyme supplementation if lactose intolerant). When eating a regular diet, fiber-containing cereal or fiber supplements are advisable. Eat slowly, allowing 30 minutes for each meal, taking frequent pauses.

In response to the exponential rise in numbers of bariatric surgeries performed, the American College of Chest Physicians recently included recommendations for periprocedural anticoagulation with bariatric surgery in the 8th edition of clinical practice guidelines on antithrombotic therapy.[113] The American College of Obstetricians and Gynecologist has for the first time issued a practice bulletin on bariatric surgery and pregnancy."[114]

Summary

Obesity is increasing worldwide, and with it comes attendant morbidity and mortality. Women are affected by this disease—some from childhood—throughout the lifespan. Extreme obesity is a chronic disorder that appears to be intractable and is associated with significant health concerns. Therapeutic programs to address this condition most likely require lifelong adherence.

References

Additional content available at
www.ashp.org/womenshealth

33 Gastrointestinal Disorders

Brian A. Hemstreet, Pharm.D., BCPS; Charmaine D. Rochester, Pharm.D., CDE, BCPS

Learning Objectives

1. Describe the clinical presentation and pathophysiology of irritable bowel syndrome (IBS).
2. Identify the desired therapeutic goals for women with IBS, and recommend appropriate nonpharmacologic and pharmacologic interventions.
3. Explain the unique features of and underlying causes for gastroesophageal reflux disease (GERD) in women.
4. Identify the desired therapeutic goals for women with GERD, and recommend appropriate nonpharmacologic and pharmacologic interventions.
5. Compare and contrast the underlying pathophysiologic and clinical features of Crohn's disease (CD) and ulcerative colitis (UC) in women.
6. Review the pharmacologic options for the treatment and maintenance of inflammatory bowel disease.
7. Educate women with gastrointestinal disorders on appropriate lifestyle modifications, importance of adherence, drug adverse effects, and drug interactions.

Gastrointestinal (GI) symptoms are among the most prevalent symptoms resulting in visits to outpatient clinics in the U.S.[1] Recent data demonstrate that disorders and symptoms such as gastroesophageal reflux disease (GERD), constipation, irritable bowel syndrome (IBS), rectal bleeding, and inflammatory bowel disease (IBD) were within the top 16 GI diagnoses made in outpatient clinics in 2002.[1] Given that millions of patients seek help each year for such varied GI-related conditions, a substantial burden is placed on the health-care system.[1,2] Based on the prevalence of both IBS and GERD not only in the U.S. but specifically within the female patient population, these disorders will be commonly encountered in clinical practice. Although less prevalent than IBS and GERD, IBD often requires intensive and prolonged drug therapy, with the potential for serious adverse effects relevant to the female population. For these reasons, this chapter will focus on the management of IBS, GERD, and IBD, with particular focus on treatment of female patients.

Irritable Bowel Syndrome

IBS, also called spastic colon, nervous colon, irritable colon, intestinal neurosis, or mucus colitis, is a functional bowel disorder.[3] Functional bowel disorders are GI disorders identified only by symptoms related to the middle or lower GI tract with no identified underlying pathophysiology.[4]

IBS is defined as a chronic, relapsing, but benign disorder characterized by recurrent abdominal pain, altered bowel habits, and features of disordered defecation in the absence of detectable organic disease.[4] There are various subtypes of IBS defined predominantly by stool patterns. Irritable bowel syndrome with constipation (IBS-C) describes a patient with hard or lumpy stools in ≥25% of bowel movements with loose (mushy) or watery stools occurring in <25% of bowel movements. Irritable bowel syndrome with diarrhea (IBS-D) describes loose (mushy) or watery stools in ≥25% of bowel movements with hard or lumpy stool in <25% of bowel movements. Mixed IBS (IBS-M) describes hard or lumpy stools in ≥25% and loose (mushy) or watery stools in ≥25% of bowel movements, and unsubtyped IBS (IBS-U) describes insufficient abnormality of stool consistency to meet criteria for IBS-C, D, or M.[4] Data suggest that IBS-D and IBS-M subtypes are more prevalent than IBS-C, and some patients switch between subtypes.[5]

The prevalence of IBS is about 10% to more than 20% in the U.S. and Europe.[4-6] Only 25% to 50% of patients with IBS seek medical care.[7] When compared with men with IBS, women with IBS have a much lower quality of life, and women are 2 times more likely to be diagnosed with IBS than men.[6,8] The age at which IBS presents

CASE PRESENTATION

Patient Case: Part 1

Chief symptom: I have had an "irritable colon" for more than 30 years.

History of present illness: T.L. is a 50-year-old woman who presents to the clinic with a symptom diary, which was given to her at the last visit to record her baseline symptoms. She states her bowel symptoms have worsened in the past 3 months. Weekly symptom diary shows the following:

Stool description: Hard, pelletlike stool more than 75% of the time (she documented one loose stool) in the past week.

Stool frequency: Four bowel movements per weekly record.

Symptoms: Straining, bloating.

Gas: Belching and flatus.

Pain: Abdominal cramping; rectal pain (describes a hard object in her rectum).

Emotional status: Sad, depressed, anxious, fatigued.

Stressors: She lost her husband in a motor vehicle accident 4 months ago.

Women (menstrual cycle, ovulation, menstruation): Menopause.

Food: Fruits, breads, rice, vegetables, dairy products, poultry.

Beverages: Caffeine, fruit juices.

Past medical history: IBS × 30 years, history of iron-deficient anemia (diagnosed 1 year ago).

Family history: Noncontributory.

Social history: No alcohol or tobacco use; drinks 5 cups of coffee daily.

Medications: Dicyclomine 20 mg orally twice daily, amitriptyline 25 mg orally daily, $FeSO_4$ 325 mg orally 3 times daily.

Allergies: NKDA.

Vitals: 110/70 mm Hg; Weight 140 lb; Height 5′5″; Pulse 80; RR 20.

Physical exam: Within normal limits.

Current labs: All normal.

ranges between late teens to mid-40s.[9] Women describe problems with social relationships, work, travel, domestic activities, leisure activities, and sexual intercourse, whereas men report difficulties with finances and work.[6] Management of IBS is thought to be different in women than men because of the higher prevalence in women, a possible effect of the menstrual cycle on symptom severity, and recent drug studies showing more effective drug therapy in women when compared with men.[8]

IBS has an estimated annual direct medical cost of $8 billion and indirect costs of $20 billion.[10,11] There is no cure for IBS.[12]

CLINICAL PRESENTATION

Patients with IBS present with abdominal discomforts associated with altered bowel habits. Patients typically report diarrhea with loose, mushy, or watery stool; constipation with hard or lumpy stool; straining during a bowel movement; alternation between diarrhea and constipation; urgency; feeling of incomplete evacuation; passing mucus during a bowel movement; abdominal discomfort, which is relieved with defecation; and abdominal pain, bloating, or fullness.[6,12,13] Many patients report extracolonic symptoms, such as low backache, constant lethargy, nausea, thigh pain, urinary frequency, urgency or urge incontinence, and dysmenorrhea or dyspareunia.[13] Women are more likely to report symptoms of constipation, distension, mucus, nausea, and psychological health problems, whereas men report diarrhea more commonly.[10] Healthcare providers should investigate further if a patient presents with "alarm" symptoms, as these are atypical of IBS and are indicative of organic disease. These include rectal bleeding or any visible or occult blood in the stool; anemia; weight loss >10 lb; late age of onset; acute onset; family history of colon cancer; family history of IBD; chronic severe diarrhea; signs of infection, pain, or diarrhea that awakens/interferes with sleep; or any abnormal physical findings on examination.[12-15]

PATHOPHYSIOLOGY

Although the symptoms of IBS are clearly established, its etiology remains unclear as patients demonstrate significant differences in symptom frequency, severity, and subtypes (e.g., IBS-C vs. IBS-D). The literature reports early physical and psychological abuse as an association with IBS development.[15] Other etiologic factors include genetics, environmental influences (e.g., stress), postinfection, abnormal bacterial flora overgrowth, and abnormal serotonin signaling.[6,16-20]

Several studies show that impairment or imbalance in serotonergic signaling can affect GI motility, secretion, and visceral sensitivity, possible as a result

Table 33-1. Rome III Diagnostic Criteria for Irritable Bowel Syndrome[4,23]

Recurrent abdominal pain or discomfort[a] need to have originated at least 6 mo before the diagnosis of IBS, and these symptoms should have occurred for at least 3 or more days/mo in the last 3 mo, which should be associated with two or more of the following:

- Improvement with defecation, and/or
- Onset associated with change in frequency of stool, and/or
- Onset associated with a change in form (appearance) of stool

[a]Discomfort means an uncomfortable sensation not described as pain. The diagnostic criteria is fulfilled for the last 3 months with symptoms onset at least 6 months before diagnosis.

of defects or deficiencies in serotonin production or its receptors. These changes can manifest in symptoms such as abdominal pain, altered bowel habits (constipation, diarrhea, or alternation between these two states), and bloating.[11]

There is evidence for differences in pathophysiology or response to treatment between men and women with IBS.[8] There is a greater efficacy of the agent 5-HT_3 antagonist alosetron in women with IBS-D when compared with men. In addition, there is a lower threshold for rectal distention postprandially in women with IBS compared with men.[8] Female sex is a risk factor for developing postinfectious IBS, which appears to be associated with a psychological profile, and the literature suggests a greater prevalence of depression, anxiety, and somatization in women compared with men.[8,21] In addition, women show differences in motility when compared with men. In pregnancy, there are changes in the **lower esophageal sphincter** (LES) pressure. Gastric emptying is slower in menstruating women than men of similar ages, and estrogens modulate the responsiveness of primary afferent neurons to substance P. Therefore, women with IBS experience greater pain sensation to most levels of pain stimuli compared with men, especially those women with a history of abuse.[8,22]

DIAGNOSIS

The Rome III criteria (Table 33-1) is used for diagnosing patients with IBS and is based solely on stool consistency.[23] The healthcare provider should carefully conduct a detailed family, medication, and medical history; physically examine the patient; rule out organic causes for the disorder; and evaluate for alarm symptoms before introducing therapy.[11]

A patient reporting a chief symptom of diarrhea and constipation may mislead healthcare providers. The patient may describe the stool as solid, leading the healthcare provider to classify the condition as IBS-C, but the patient's defecation may occur frequently throughout the day. To avoid misclassification, the Bristol Stool Form Scale or Bristol Stool Chart (Table 33-2) gives an accurate symptom description of the stool in the toilet.[4] Assuming no use of antidiarrheal agents or laxatives, the Bristol Stool Form Scale can be used to identify constipation as types 1 or 2 and diarrhea as types 6 or 7.[4]

GUIDELINES AND POSITION STATEMENTS

The American College of Gastroenterology (ACG) Functional Disorders Task Force on IBS updated the management of IBS guidelines in 2009 based on a systematic review of recent data.[5] In diagnosing patients with IBS, the healthcare provider should be assured that the diagnosis is correct and that the patient fulfills the symptoms of IBS (Table 33-1). Absence of alarm features—such as anemia; weight loss; and a family history of colorectal cancer, IBD, or celiac sprue—should be noted.[5] Colonoscopic imaging is recommended only in IBS patients who present with alarm symptoms to rule out organic diseases or for colorectal cancer screening of patients older than age 50 years.[5]

Table 33-2. The Bristol Stool Form Scale[4]

Type	Description
1	Separate hard lumps like nuts, hard to pass
2	Sausage shaped, but lumpy
3	Like a sausage, but with cracks on its surface
4	Like a sausage or snake, smooth and soft
5	Soft blobs with clear-cut edges (passed easily)
6	Fluffy pieces with ragged edges, a mushy stool
7	Watery, no solid pieces; entirely liquid

TREATMENT GOALS

The goals of therapy should be to improve global IBS symptoms (including abdominal discomfort, bloating, and altered bowel habits) and improve overall well-being, not just target a single symptom.[5,14] An effective healthcare provider–patient relationship is important for improved patient satisfaction, adherence to therapy, and symptom reduction.[24]

NONPHARMACOLOGIC THERAPY

The ACG Task Force does not encourage food testing or initiating or excluding specific diets for IBS patients despite the prevalent belief in the IBS population that certain foods worsen their IBS symptoms.[5] The ACG Task Force reviewed Chinese herbal mixture data, which appeared to show a benefit, but they suggested that there were too many confounders, including a lack of purity, publication bias, liver toxicity concerns, and other serious side effects.[5] Many studies have looked at evaluating the benefits of behavioral therapy, which include biofeedback, hypnotherapy, cognitive behavioral therapy, acupuncture, and relaxation therapy. Most of the behavioral therapy trials had significant flaws in their design and did not evaluate global assessment symptom improvement.[12] Trial results suggest that behavioral therapy may improve individual IBS symptoms, especially psychological symptoms among patients with comorbid psychological disorders.[14] The ACG Task Force recommended more work on acupuncture and herbal therapy studies before making any recommendations.[5]

PHARMACOLOGIC THERAPY

Therapy for IBS in a given patient is directed at the dominant symptom(s). Most of the currently available agents for IBS have not been subjected to randomized, controlled clinical trials, and some trials, although of good quality, had small numbers of patients.[5,13] Available agents include antispasmodics (dicyclomine, hyoscyamine), bulking agents (wheat bran, corn fiber, calcium polycarbophil, ispaghula husk, psyllium), peppermint oil, antidiarrheals (loperamide), antidepressants (selective serotonin reuptake inhibitors [SSRIs] and tricyclic antidepressants [TCAs]), serotonin agonists (tegaserod—restricted access), serotonin receptor antagonists (alosetron—emergency use only), prostones or type 2 chloride channel activators (lubiprostone).[5,11,13,14,19,25,26]

Abdominal Pain

Antispasmodic Agents

Antispasmodics, like dicyclomine and hyoscyamine, are anticholinergic agents that relax the smooth muscles of the gut, reducing motility, muscular spasms, and secretions by inhibiting acetylcholine. Antispasmodics are thought to reduce the visceral hypersensitivity and pain in IBS.[14] Most of the antispasmodics that were studied are unavailable in the U.S. Although hysocine has been studied, it differs from what is currently available in the U.S.[5] Peppermint oil, in a variety of preparations, also acts as an antispasmodic in IBS and has been used to provide short-term relief of abdominal pain and discomfort.[5] From many of the studies, the main side effects of antispasmodic agents—which include dry mouth, urinary retention, visual disturbances, and constipation—have not been clearly defined.[5] The ACG Task Force now suggests that there is some evidence for the short-term use of this drug class; however, many of the studies were unable to clearly distinguish the effects of the drugs on global and individual symptoms.[5]

Antidepressants

According to the literature, half of the patients with IBS have been described as either anxious, depressed, or hypochrondriacal.[21] TCAs and SSRIs have been evaluated in small studies for IBS. According to the literature, TCAs, such as amitriptyline, trimipramine, desipramine, and doxepin, may treat the chronic pain of IBS; however, most of the trials for TCAs were poorly designed.[14] The dosages for chronic pain include desipramine 150 mg orally at bedtime, amitriptyline 50 mg orally at bedtime, trimipramine 50 mg orally at bedtime, and doxepin 75 mg orally at bedtime.[27] Global improvements were not measured in most of the studies. Desipramine and doxepin showed improvement in abdominal pain, whereas amitriptyline was ineffective.[27-29] Desipramine may be useful in IBS-D patients because of its anticholinergic effect.[5] Constipation was significantly worse for desipramine-using patients compared with atropine-using patients.[28] TCAs cause constipation and should be used in caution in IBS-C patients.[14] Tiredness was significantly worse in trimipramine-using patients compared with control patients.[30] Evidence of the effectiveness of SSRI has been lacking. Results of a crossover trial of 23 nondepressed patients who were treated for IBS symptoms with citalopram 20 mg for 3 weeks followed by 40 mg for 3 weeks or placebo showed that after 3 and 6 weeks of citalopram therapy, patients had significant improvement in abdominal pain, bloating, impact of symptoms on daily life, and overall well-being compared with placebo. The authors noted only a modest effect on stool pattern, and they concluded that changes in depression or anxiety scores were unrelated to symptom improvement.[31]

Results of a two-part study showed that paroxetine (10 mg daily) in combination with a high-fiber diet was more effective than a high-fiber diet alone. The study was designed with a trial of a high-fiber diet alone (group 1; n = 98), which was followed by a trial of high-fiber diet in combination with paroxetine (n = 38) or placebo (n = 43) for the treatment of patients with nondepressed IBS.[32] Compared with placebo patients, the paroxetine-treated patients had overall improvement in well-being (63.3% vs. 26.3%; $p = 0.01$). However, abdominal pain, bloating, and social functioning did not improve with paroxetine. Although there was no improvement in abdominal pain, more paroxetine-treated patients wanted to continue their study medication for the improvement of overall well-being compared with placebo-treated patients (84% vs. 37%; $p < 0.001$).[32] Larger, prospective randomized trials will give more information on the effectiveness of SSRI therapy in patients with IBS. The presence of depression in patients is not a predictor of the response to TCA or SSRI therapy. According to the ACG Task Force, there is still a lack of evidence on the safety and tolerability of these agents in IBS patients.[5]

Constipation

Bulking Agents and Laxatives

Fiber and osmotic laxatives have been used to relieve constipation in patients with IBS-C or IBS-M.[33] In the general U.S. population, constipation is more often reported by women than men (estimated prevalence rate of 2.2:1) and by elderly patients older than 65 years of age.[34] Bulking agents, sometimes called fiber supplements, are frequently recommended. It has been traditionally recommended to treat constipation with a trial of fiber supplements. This recommendation is now controversial because some studies suggest that 40% to 70% of patients with IBS-C had improvement with placebo.[21] The British Society of Gastroenterology recommends patients with IBS-C should be given a trial of increased intake of dietary fiber, and those who fail to respond or are intolerant of the increased fiber should be tried with a fiber supplement.[21] The ACG Task Force and British Society of Gastroenterology now recommend the use of psyllium, a soluble fiber, which is moderately effective, but they reject the use of insoluble fiber such as wheat or corn bran.[5,21] Fiber is often discussed in terms of its solubility: soluble and insoluble.[14,35-37] Soluble fiber forms a gel when mixed with water (e.g., oats, psyllium husks, fruits such as apples and oranges, calcium polycarbophil). Insoluble fiber is insoluble in water (e.g., whole wheat products, corn bran, some seeds, nuts).

Psyllium (also known as Metamucil®, Fiberall®, Reguloid®, or Konsyl®) is often used as fiber supplementation. This agent can function as a laxative. It empties the bowels by absorbing water into the colon, increasing fecal bulk, which in turn induces peristalsis. Psyllium is usually started after the person has been unresponsive to dietary fiber. Psyllium is available over-the-counter (OTC) in dosages of 4 g taken orally 1–3 times a day. It should be avoided if there are any allergic reactions or any signs of obstruction, such as acute abdominal pain, nausea, or vomiting.

A systematic review of 17 randomized control trials found soluble fiber more effective than placebo for reducing constipation and global symptoms, but insoluble fiber was not better than placebo. Additionally, abdominal pain was not reduced with either fiber.[37] Some studies show that corn, wheat fiber, calcium polycarbophil, and psyllium were not effective in global IBS symptom improvement. However, the majority of psyllium (ispaghula husk) studies demonstrated global improvements, but this may have resulted from increasing frequency of bowel movement in IBS-C patients. Fiber products increase intestinal gas, bloating, flatulence, and abdominal discomfort. Only 10% of IBS-C patients will have improvement in pain with fiber.[21]

Data are lacking regarding magnesium salts and polyethylene glycol (PEG)–based laxatives for patients with IBS-C.[21] According to one study, low-dose oral PEG (13 g/sachet) was superior in efficacy and tolerability to oral lactulose (10 g/sachet), with less flatulence in patients with chronic constipation.[38] Stimulant laxatives are not recommended for regular use because of dependence and tachyphylaxis and should only be used occasionally.[21]

Tegaserod

Tegaserod is a 5HT-serotonin receptor agonist and was the first U.S. Food and Drug Administration (FDA)–approved agent for the treatment of IBS-C in women only. The main adverse effect is diarrhea. The recommended dosage is 6 mg orally twice daily.[14] Clinical trials demonstrated statistically significant improvement in global IBS symptoms for tegaserod-using women compared with placebo patients.[14] In subgroup analysis, tegaserod-using patients experienced less bloating, less abdominal discomfort, and improved satisfaction with their bowel habits compared with placebo-using patients. The trials demonstrated effectiveness for the treatment of IBS-C in women, but not in men or patients with IBS-M.[39-41]

Tegaserod was discontinued in March 2007 when the FDA issued a public health advisory because of an increased risk of heart attacks, strokes, and worsening chest pain. It was then made available under restricted access in July 2007 as a treatment investigational new drug (IND).[42] However, in April 2008, Novartis Pharmaceuticals voluntarily discontinued the availability of the drug under the treatment IND protocol and made it available only under an emergency IND.[43]An emergency was defined as a life-threatening situation or one serious enough to require hospitalization. For physicians to obtain tegaserod, they must seek approval from the FDA, or contact the FDA's Division for Drug Information about the emergency IND process at druginfo@fda.hhs.gov. Patients who have a prior history of heart attack, stroke, unstable angina, hypertension, dyslipidemia, diabetes, age >55 years, smoking, anxiety, obesity, depression, or suicidal ideation may have denial of authorization.[43]

Lubiprostone

Lubiprostone is now the only FDA-approved agent for IBS-C in the U.S. without restrictions. The drug was approved in April 2008 for adult women ages 18 years and older with IBS-C.[44] It is a locally acting type 2 chloride channel activator, which activates a specific chloride channel, CIC-2, lining the gut, causing increased intestinal fluid secretion; softened stool; improvement in gut motility; and reduction in abdominal pain, discomfort, and bloating. It is a member of a new class of compounds called prostones.[26,44-46]

Results of two randomized placebo-controlled trials demonstrated the safety and efficacy of lubiprostone in 1,154 patients diagnosed with IBS-C.[47] Most of the patients were women (92%), and all the patients enrolled in the studies were experiencing at least mild abdominal discomfort or pain that was associated with at least two of the following additional symptoms: 1) fewer than three spontaneous bowel movements per week that did not result from laxative use, 2) hard stools, or 3) moderate or severe straining with bowel movements. Results of the study showed that more patients treated with lubiprostone 8 mcg twice daily reported that their IBS symptoms were moderately or significantly relieved over a 12-week treatment period compared with patients who received placebo. The most common side effects included nausea, diarrhea, and abdominal pain. The efficacy of lubiprostone in men for IBS-C was not conclusively demonstrated, and lubiprostone is only approved for women who are not pregnant or nursing. The studies also assessed whether there was a rebound effect after withdrawal of lubiprostone, but withdrawal did not result in a rebound effect in patients.[26,44,47]

Lubiprostone is not to be administered to patients suffering from severe diarrhea or patients with known or suspected bowel obstruction. It is also approved for the treatment of chronic idiopathic constipation, but the dosage for that indication is 24 mcg orally twice daily.[26,44,45,48]

Diarrhea

Alosetron (Restricted Access Only)

The distribution of alosetron, a 5-HT_3 antagonist, was halted in 2000 because of concerns about ischemic colitis and serious complications of constipation. In 2002, it was FDA approved with restricted marketing for the treatment of women with severe IBS-D who failed to respond to conventional IBS therapy.[12,14,49]

In large, double-blind, placebo-controlled clinical trials, alosetron 1 mg orally twice daily was significantly more effective than placebo in improving bowel urgency, abdominal pain, and global symptom improvement in IBS-D.[11] The effectiveness of alosetron has not been demonstrated in men.

Physicians must enroll in a prescribing program and follow the program's requirements to obtain alosetron. Patients should receive the medication guide that discusses the benefits and risks of alosetron and instructions on how to take the medication. Both the physician and patient must sign the patient-physician agreement. Patients should have all their questions answered and receive a prescription with a sticker affixed to it to inform the pharmacist that the physician is enrolled in the prescribing program.[49] Pharmacists should ensure all patients have a medication guide, reinforce all the information with patients, and review the risks and benefits of alosetron. Pharmacists should also be aware that prescriptions should be written and not faxed or transmitted over the phone or computer. Physicians who enroll in the prescribing program must be able to diagnose and manage IBS, ischemic colitis, constipation and its complications, or refer to a specialist.[49] All serious events should be reported to the FDA.[50]

The dosage of alosetron is 0.5 mg orally twice daily, which can be increased to 1 mg orally twice daily with or without food. If a patient has no symptoms relief after 4 weeks, the drug should be discontinued. The main adverse effects are headache, nausea, stomach upset, and constipation. Serious reactions include obstruction, ileus, toxic megacolon, impaction, secondary bowel ischemia, perforation, and death. If the patient experiences symptoms of ischemic colitis (constipation, bloody stools, new or worsening abdominal pain), she should immediately stop taking alosetron and seek medical attention.[50] The risks increase in the elderly or debilitated and patients taking medications that decrease bowel motility. Alosetron should not be restarted in any patient who develops ischemic colitis.[50]

Loperamide

The ACG Task Force suggests that loperamide is not more effective than placebo and is ineffective for abdominal discomfort, pain relief, bloating, or improvement of global IBS symptoms.[5] Loperamide is the only antidiarrheal agent that has been evaluated for the treatment of IBS and is only effective for the symptom of diarrhea.[5,14] All of the trials were conducted before ROME classification, were shorter than 5 weeks, and had relatively small sample sizes. Loperamide showed no effectiveness in patients with IBS-M without pain, but it improved stool frequency and consistency in IBS-M patients with pain. Loperamide also improved stool frequency, consistency, and overall symptoms in patients with painless IBS-D. Patients with painless IBS-C had worse symptoms.[11] The dosage used in trials was 2–12 mg orally daily, and it is recommended to titrate loperamide until soft stool becomes firm.[14,51-53]

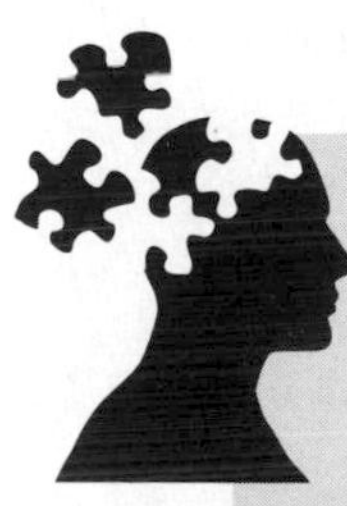

Therapeutic Challenge:

How do we manage patients given the fact that the agents with the best documented efficacy are only available on an emergency or restricted basis?

Bloating

Up to 96% of patients with a functional GI disorder such as IBS and 30% of the general population commonly report bloating, but bloating is more common in women.[54,55] Distension does not necessarily occur in these patients except in patients with IBS-C, but treatment options are not satisfactory.[55] Dietary changes may help, and patients should be advised to reduce wheat fiber, lactose or fructose, fat, carbonated drinks, and artificial sweeteners as necessary in their diet.[21,55] Treating constipation may be helpful, but laxatives like lactulose and fermentable fiber preparations worsen bloating. Hypnotherapy, antispasmodics, and antidepressants may have some benefit, but there is little evidence of efficacy.[55] Although tegaserod has shown consistent improvement in bloating, access is only for emergency use, and bloating would not be considered an emergency.[40,43,56,57]

Other Treatment Options

Dietary Supplements: Probiotics

Probiotics are dietary supplements containing viable bacteria and yeast, which are usually part of the body's normal microbial flora. The mechanism of action is unknown, but theoretically they are used to replenish normal flora and to provide relief for GI symptoms such as bloating, diarrhea, and constipation. Some examples of probiotics include *Bifidobacterium infantis*, *Lactobacillus acidophilus,* and mixed cultures.[19,58] According to the ACG Task Force, probiotics with lactobacilli is not effective for IBS, but bifidobacteria and certain probiotic combinations are efficacious.[5]

A multicenter, randomized, double-blind, placebo-controlled, dose-ranging clinical trial of 362 women with IBS ages 18–65 years was performed to confirm the efficacy of the probiotic bacteria, *B. infantis* 35624. The secondary objective was to determine the optimal dosage of the encapsulated formulation of the probiotic.[59] The study was conducted in adult women who met Rome II criteria for the diagnosis of IBS. Patients were randomized to four treatment arms of live bacterial cells of *B. infantis* 35624 (1×10^6, 1×10^8, 1×10^{10}, or placebo in a 1:1:1:1 ratio). Patients received identical capsules taken orally once daily for 4 weeks during the treatment phase of the study. A total of 330 patients completed the study. Of these, 55% were considered IBS-D, 20.7% were IBS-C, and 23.8% were IBS-M at baseline. At week 4, compared with placebo, *B. infantis* 35624 in a dose of 1×10^8 was associated with a significant improvement in abdominal pain and discomfort. Other dosages were not significantly different from placebo. In addition, symptoms of bloating/distension, sense of incomplete evacuation, passage of gas, straining, and bowel habit satisfaction were all significant with the 1×10^8 dosage compared with placebo.

To evaluate the probiotic based on IBS subtype, post hoc analyses were performed that showed significant bowel habit satisfaction improvement for both the IBS-D and IBS-C subtypes. There was only a trend toward efficacy in the IBS-M groups. The use of rescue medications was low in all treatment groups. When the investigators compared the improvement in global symptom assessment, it exceeded placebo by more than 20% ($p < 0.02$). This product is now sold as Align® as a supplement.

MONITORING AND FOLLOW-UP

Because of the heterogenous nature of IBS, symptoms change over time, and healthcare providers need to determine whether to treat patients "on demand," intermittently, or continuously.[60] One study reported patients' self-report in a symptom diary, which was evaluated every 4 weeks.[60] Results of the study show that two thirds of the patients remain with the same subtype after a 3-month follow-up, and only one half had the same symptom intensity. Patients with IBS-C and IBS-D tended to move toward IBS-M. Because of the variability in intensity and instability of symptoms manifestation, the authors suggested that an "on demand" medication be prescribed.[60]

The International Foundation for Functional Gastrointestinal Disorders has developed a symptom diary to help patients get a better understanding of their bowel disorder. They suggest the diary should be used for 2–4 weeks to record the patient's stool consistency (e.g., hard, pelletlike), stool symptoms (urge, straining, incomplete evacuation), stool frequency, continence, gas, pain, diet, medication, exercise, menstrual cycle (if a woman), and emotional status.[61,62] Healthcare providers can use the diary to determine the variability and intensity of the patients' symptoms and use their clinical judgment to schedule visits in such a manner to address the patient's concern while avoiding excessive physician visits.

PATIENT EDUCATION

Patients need education on all aspects of their medication and the etiology and pathophysiology of IBS. The pharmacist can play a significant role in developing a counseling program for patients with IBS. Some of the topics that pharmacists should address include the following:

1. Basic pathophysiology and etiology of IBS
2. Assurance that IBS is often a relatively benign disorder
3. Medication therapy, including benefits, risks, drug interactions, and adverse effects
4. The benefits of keeping a food diary and avoiding drug therapy or diet that could worsen the symptoms of IBS
5. The benefits of keeping a symptom diary and its benefits
6. When to call the physician or pharmacist
7. Health-promoting behaviors that can reduce anxiety

CASE PRESENTATION

Patient Case: Part 2

The patient has chronic IBS-C, which is currently unstable and uncontrolled on dicyclomine and amitriptyline. The symptoms may have worsened because of the psychological stress from the death of her husband. Several medications in her profile could also potentially worsen her constipation (amitriptyline and ferrous sulfate).

Plan:

1. Discontinue ferrous sulfate because labs are within normal limits.
2. Discontinue dicyclomine and amitriptyline, which are ineffective and can worsen constipation.
3. Consider initiating fiber (psyllium 6.4 g orally 3 times daily) with adequate water intake (at least six 8-oz glasses of water) in the diet.
4. If symptoms of constipation continue despite fiber use, consider adding lubiprostone 8 mcg orally twice daily.
5. Document IBS symptoms in a symptom diary for 2 weeks to re-evaluate stool consistency, frequency, and quality of life.
6. Re-evaluate patient in 2 weeks for symptom and global improvement.

SUMMARY

IBS is a chronic but benign disorder, and patients need a strong pharmacist– and physician–patient relationship for reassurance and education. Therapies for IBS are limited. Both tegaserod and alosetron agents with the best-documented efficacy studies now have emergency and restricted access, respectively. Lubiprostone is a new option for IBS-C, but experience with this agent is limited. Behavioral therapy has not been shown to be effective in IBS, but has been for patients with depression and anxiety. Probiotics have been gaining popularity, but more studies are needed. Future studies need to focus on evaluating newer agents for IBS to improve global symptoms and quality of life for patients with IBS.

Gastroesophageal Reflux Disease

(See Web Resources for Patient Case: Gastroesophageal Reflux Disease.)

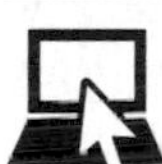

Additional content available at
www.ashp.org/womenshealth

A consensus of world experts developed a definition for GERD called the Montreal consensus or Montreal definition, which defined GERD as a "condition which develops when the reflux of stomach contents causes troublesome symptoms and/or complications."[63] According to this new definition, GERD can now be divided now into esophageal and extraesophageal syndromes.[64] Esophageal syndromes can be further subdivided into symptomatic syndromes (reflux chest pain syndrome, typical reflux syndrome) and syndromes with esophageal injury (reflux esophagitis, reflux **stricture,** Barrett's esophagus, and adenocarcinoma).[64] Extraesophageal syndromes can be further subdivided into established association (reflux cough, reflux laryngitis, reflux asthma, reflux dental erosions) and proposed association (sinusitis, pulmonary fibrosis, pharyngitis, and recurrent otitis media).[64] The underlying premise of this new definition shows that reflux is the cause of the troublesome symptoms and/or complications in GERD.[64] The consensus panel also distinguishes episodic heartburn from GERD in that they suggest that in a given patient without esophageal injury (benign nature), if the patient does not perceive their heartburn as "troublesome symptoms" because of less intensity or frequency of symptoms, then this heartburn will not be considered symptomatic esophageal GERD syndrome.[64]

The true prevalence of GERD is unknown because many patients do not seek medical treatment or their symptoms do not always correlate with disease severity.[65] One out of five persons in the U.S. (20%) suffers from heartburn or regurgitation on a weekly basis, and two out of five (40%) have heartburn or regurgitation at least once monthly.[66] In the U.S., it is estimated that the lifetime prevalence of GERD is 25% to 30%.[67] Pregnant women experience a high incidence of heartburn.[68,69] Whites have a higher incidence of esophageal adenocarcinoma than blacks or Native Americans.[70] The annual direct costs of managing GERD in the U.S. is $9 billion.[71] Lifestyle events—such as lying down or bending after meals, eating heavy meals, the presence of a hiatal hernia, exercising after meals, a history of esophageal surgery or esophageal strictures, cigarette smoking, alcohol intake, eating certain foods (chocolate, peppermint, tomato, citrus, high fat, spicy, onion, garlic, coffee), and/or psychological stress—can contribute to worsening GERD symptoms.[72]

CLINICAL PRESENTATION

Typical symptoms of GERD include a burning discomfort generally felt in the chest just behind the breastbone because of acid regurgitation of gastric contents rising up to the neck, which causes epigastric pain. Patients also report regurgitation, which is the effortless return of stomach contents into the esophagus.[73] Other symptoms include water brash or hypersalivation and belching.[74,75]

Gastroesophageal reflux disease is a chronic condition that affects both men and women. Studies suggest that the disease in women is no different from that in men. Women may have different symptoms and physical signs of the disease because of hormonal differences or varying levels of disease severity.[74] Women tend to have similar patterns of endoscopic severity of GERD compared with men, but they are less likely to develop Barrett's esophagus. In addition, the severity of the symptoms in women appear to be significantly more than in men and may contribute to earlier recognition of the disease.[74] According to the literature, heartburn has been reported to occur in about 22% of pregnancies during the first trimester, 39% during the second trimester, and 72% during the third trimester.[68] During pregnancy, women experience anatomic changes such as a decrease in LES tone mediated by progesterone, slowed gastric emptying, and increased intra-abdominal pressure from the expanded uterus.[69] A history of heartburn before pregnancy and multiparity predicts heartburn during pregnancy, but there is no association with weight gain during pregnancy.[68] In most cases, heartburn resolves after delivery and has not been identified as a risk factor for long-term GERD. It is unusual to have reflux complications during pregnancy, so upper endoscopy or other diagnostic tests are rarely needed for these women.[68]

Atypical Presentation

Atypical symptoms, now referred to as extraesophageal syndromes, include dysphagia, dental erosions, laryngitis, pharyngitis, bleeding, noncardiac or atypical chest pain, chronic hoarseness, chronic coughing, wheezing or asthma-like symptoms, and weight loss.[76] Alarm symptoms include chest pain accompanied by pain in the neck, jaw, arms, or legs; shortness of breath, weakness, irregular pulse, or sweating; continuous nausea, vomiting, or diarrhea; extreme discomfort in the stomach; vomiting of blood or black material; black or bloody bowel movements; difficulty swallowing (dysphagia) or pain with swallowing (odynophagia); weight loss; or anemia.[72] Patients should be immediately referred to a specialist with alarm symptoms, and the pharmacist should not initiate self-care in these circumstances.

PATHOPHYSIOLOGY

Many factors contribute to the pathogenesis of GERD, including gastric function bnormalities, transient LES relaxation, dysfunction of the antireflux barrier, autonomic nervous system disturbances, obesity and overweight, and abnormal esophageal transit and clearance.[77,78] Factors that contribute to GERD include the duration, magnitude of relaxation, and the pressure gradient across the LES.[77] The presence of a hiatus hernia is a strong predictor of prolonged esophageal acid exposure and abnormal acid clearance.[79] Food and beverages have also been demonstrated to affect the LES relaxation. Foods such as fats and chocolates can lower the LES tone, whereas food such as citrus juice, tomato juice, garlic, onion, and pepper can irritate the damaged esophageal lining. Cigarette smoking and alcohol can also affect the LES sphincter tone. Certain classes of medications, such as calcium channel blockers, anticholinergic drugs, iron supplements, nonsteroidal anti-inflammatory drugs, potassium, dopamine, sedatives, bisphosphonates, and beta-blockers, can lower the LES tone or irritate the esophagus.[72] Obese patients are more likely to have an increased intragastric pressure, as the higher the body mass index and waist circumference, the greater the intragastric pressure and gastroesophageal pressure gradient.[80] In summary, the patient is more likely to perceive a reflux episode as heartburn or regurgitation when the pH drop is large, the proximal extent of the refluxate is high, and the volume and acid clearance are prolonged.[77]

DETECTION, SCREENING, AND DIAGNOSIS

An initial trial of empiric acid–suppressing therapy is recommended for diagnosing patients with GERD if they have a typical presentation of GERD (see Table 33-3). The recommendations for diagnostic testing for esophageal GERD syndromes are to avoid misdiagnosis (patients with alarm features), identify complications of reflux disease (e.g., esophageal malignancy), and evaluate empirical treatment failures.[63] Occasionally it is a challenge to differentiate GERD-related symptoms from noncardiac chest pain. Patients should see a physician if they experience noncardiac chest pain as it may closely resemble cardiac pain. The chest pain usually occurs in the middle of the chest with a dull burning pressure sensation, but the pain does not radiate into the neck, shoulder, or arms. It can worsen after meals, when lying supine, or when exercising after meals. A short course of high-dose oral omeprazole has been demonstrated to be sensitive, specific for diagnosing GERD, and cost-effective in patients who present with noncardiac chest pain.[81,82]

Endoscopy, **ambulatory reflux monitoring**, and esophageal manometry are often used for further detection or diagnosis of GERD. Endoscopy allows direct visualization of the esophageal mucosa and is the only reliable method for the diagnosis of Barrett's esophagus, or strictures. Biopsy is added to confirm the presence of Barrett's epithelium and to evaluate for dysplasia.[72] If the endoscopy is normal, ambulatory reflux monitoring is recommended by the ACG.[63] The purpose of ambulatory reflux monitoring is to help confirm GERD in patients with persistent symptoms, whether typical or atypical, without evidence of mucosal damage when empiric therapy fails.[72] Esophageal manometry may be used to ensure accurate placement of ambulatory monitoring probes and may be helpful before antireflux surgery and to document the presence of effective esophageal peristalsis in patients in whom antireflux surgery is being considered.[72]

Table 33-3. H_2 Receptor Antagonists and Proton Pump Inhibitors[32]

Medications	Dosages
H_2RAs (prescription strength)	
Cimetidine	400–800 mg twice daily
Famotidine	20–40 mg twice daily
Nizatidine	150 mg twice daily
Ranitidine	150–300 mg twice daily
H_2RAs (over-the-counter strength)	
Cimetidine	200 mg twice daily as needed
Famotidine	10 mg twice daily as needed
Nizatidine	75 mg twice daily as needed
Ranitidine	75 mg twice daily as needed
Proton Pump Inhibitors (prescription strength)	
Omeprazole delayed release Omeprazole immediate release	20, 40 mg daily
Lansoprazole	30 mg daily
Pantoprazole	40 mg daily
Esomeprazole	20 mg daily
Rabeprazole	20 mg daily
Dexlansoprazole	30, 60 mg daily

TREATMENT GOALS

The therapeutic goals for GERD management include relieving GERD symptoms, healing the esophageal lesions and maintaining healing, improving the patients' quality of life, and preventing relapse of GERD symptoms and complications.[83]

NONPHARMACOLOGIC THERAPY

Nonpharmacologic therapies include lifestyle modifications, antireflux surgery, and endoscopic therapies. Healthcare providers usually recommend lifestyle modifications for GERD to decrease distal esophageal acid exposure, although there are no placebo-controlled randomized studies to demonstrate the true efficacy of these recommendations. Investigators note the 20% to 30% placebo response rate demonstrated in most clinical trials, which they usually relate to lifestyle modifications. These include elevating the head of the bed with 6- to 8-inch blocks; ceasing smoking; avoiding recumbency for 3 hours postprandially; reducing meal size and fat intake; avoiding spicy, acidic, and high-fat foods; and avoiding consumption of caffeine, chocolate, and carminatives (peppermint). Although recommended, few patients achieve satisfactory symptom control from lifestyle changes alone.[72,83-87] Recent studies show no improvement with smoking cessation, weight loss, or eating a low-fat diet in GERD patients.[63] The consensus is that there are no evidence-based data to suggest a benefit for all GERD patients, but in individual patients, if they benefit from an identified modification, they should make those changes (e.g., avoiding alcohol, coffee, or spicy foods) despite acid-adequate pharmacotherapy.[63]

Antireflux Surgery

Indications for antireflux surgery include failed medication therapy management, patient preference for surgery despite successful medication management, complications of GERD, the presence of a large hiatal hernia causing medical complications or atypical symptoms seen with 24-hour pH monitoring.[84] Studies show that 75% to 90% of patients show improvement for heartburn and regurgitation after surgery.[88] Despite complications from surgery—which include solid food dysphagia, bloating, diarrhea, nausea, and early satiety—patient satisfaction is usually high if they experience controlled GERD symptoms.[85] Within 3–5 years of surgery, 52% patients will return to antireflux medications.[89]

Endoscopic Therapies

Endoscopic therapy provides a minimally invasive therapeutic alternative to patients who want to avoid antireflux surgery or GERD medication therapy. There are several procedures that have been investigated, including radiofrequency, Stretta procedure, and the EndoCinch procedure. The goal of the procedure is to change the anatomy or physiology of the gastroesophageal junction, thereby decreasing reflux.[90] It has been reported that medication use for GERD has been eliminated or reduced in 50% to 75% of patients with these procedures.[91]

PHARMACOLOGIC THERAPY

Antacids

Antacids are an inexpensive option for patient-directed therapy for heartburn and regurgitation and are available without a prescription.[72] Antacids act primarily by neutralizing acid in the esophagus and stomach and inhibit the actions of the digesting enzyme pepsin. They provide a rapid onset of action of symptom relief (usually <5 minutes), but the buffering effects are only 20–30 minutes on an empty stomach and 60–90 minutes with food.[86,92] The presence of food in the stomach delays gastric emptying and prolongs the antacid effect. Because of the short duration of action, multiple doses of antacids are needed for symptom control throughout the day. Antacids are indicated for the temporary relief of patients with mild and occasional heartburn, but it is ineffective in patients with frequent and nocturnal heartburn.[92] The main ingredients in antacids are either sodium bicarbonate, magnesium hydroxide or magnesium gluconate, aluminum hydroxide, calcium carbonate, or combinations. Other additional ingredients may be added, such as alginic acid, which is designed to prevent esophageal injury by forming a foam barrier, and simethicone, which decreases gas discomfort. Bismuth subsalicylate relieves acid indigestion by acting topically in the stomach, but it is not considered an antacid (e.g., Maalox Total Stomach Relief® contains bismuth subsalicylate 525 mg/15 mL with no antacids). Patients should be educated that liquid antacids act faster than tablets and chewable antacid tablets.[86,92,93]

Magnesium-containing antacids can cause diarrhea, whereas calcium and aluminum cause constipation. Aluminum and magnesium are renally eliminated and should be avoided in patients with severe renal dysfunction. Bismuth subsalicylate darkens the tongue and stool, and healthcare providers should avoid this agent in salicylate-sensitive patients, those with renal dysfunction, children experiencing chicken pox or influenza because of the potential of Reye's syndrome, patients on warfarin therapy, or patients taking concomitant salicylate products. Drug-drug interaction could be avoided by separating the antacid dose from other oral medications by 1–2 hours. An acid-neutralizing capacity (ANC) of 40–80 mEq will provide adequate acid neutralization, and the goal is to choose the product with the highest ANC dosage in the smallest volume or number of tablets.[86,92,93]

H_2 Receptor Antagonists

The H_2 receptor antagonists (H_2RAs) are cimetidine, ranitidine, famotidine, and nizatidine, and they are all available OTC and in prescription strength (see Table 33-3). They reduce gastric acid by inhibiting the histamine receptors on the parietal cell. The onset of action is about 30–45 minutes, and the duration of action is about 6–10 hours. Because of tachyphylaxis, they should be taken only when necessary in patients with mild heartburn.[86,92] The efficacy of H_2RAs in regular or high dosages has been demonstrated. When used over 2–4 weeks, OTC H_2RAs were superior to placebo in providing adequate relief, complete relief, subjective improvement in breakthrough GERD symptoms as suggested by a decreased use of rescue antacids.[94] The H_2RAs can be used interchangeably. The OTC H_2RAs are useful before an activity that can potentiate a reflux symptom, such as exercise or a meal. The H_2RAs are not as effective as the PPIs in the treatment of esophagitis and more severe frequent heartburn symptoms.[73] Self-treatment should be limited to twice daily, and medical referral should be recommended if a patient fails to achieve the therapeutic goal after 2 weeks of therapy.

The adverse effects of H_2RAs include nausea, constipation, diarrhea, and headache, which disappear with continued use. Mental status changes, such as confusion and dizziness, have been described in elderly patients, especially those with renal and hepatic dysfunction. Famotidine and nizatidine are associated with fewer side effects in elderly patients when compared with ranitidine and cimetidine, but also must be dose adjusted for renal function.[95]

Cimetidine has the greatest potential of drug-drug interactions, as it inhibits several isoforms of the cytochrome P450 (CYP450) enzyme system and also alters the absorption of weak bases.[86,92]

Proton Pump Inhibitors

Proton pump inhibitors (PPIs) include omeprazole, pantoprazole, lansoprazole, rabeprazole, esomeprazole, and dexlansoprazole (see Table 33-3). Omeprazole is the only PPI that is available without a prescription. PPIs are weak bases that become protonated as they cross the parietal cell membrane, and they produce the activated form of the drug that binds covalently with the H^+/K^+ATPase enzyme, resulting in irreversible inhibition of acid secretion by the proton pump.[96]

The PPIs are well tolerated, and the most common adverse effects are headache, diarrhea, abdominal pain, and nausea. PPIs should be used with caution in patients with severe hepatic disease and are not recommended for use in breast-feeding mothers. Omeprazole is a pregnancy category C agent; the others are pregnancy category B medications.

Drug interactions with PPIs take place through two major mechanisms, which include an increase in intragastric pH and metabolism through the CYP450 enzyme system (CYP2C19 and to a lesser extent CYP450-3A4). PPIs interact with several weak acids and weak bases because of their action of increasing intragastric pH. The increased gastric pH can increase the absorption of weak acids by increasing their dissolution and of weak bases by decreasing their ionization. Drugs like nifedipine, digoxin, griseofulvin, and ketoconazole have the greatest potential for drug-drug interactions. The other PPIs also have drug-drug interactions to varying extents.[96]

PPIs have similar efficacy, and they have been shown to be more effective than H_2RAs and placebo in the healing of esophagitis and controlling GERD symptoms.[73,96] PPIs improve quality of life, reduce sleep disturbance, and increase work productivity compared with placebo.[97] They are more cost-effective than H_2RAs because of less frequent dosing requirements.[96] Patients on once-daily PPIs should take them before breakfast and those with nocturnal symptoms should take them before the evening meal. Patients require a trial of twice-daily oral dosing when once-daily dosing is ineffective, and it should be administered before the breakfast and the evening meal and not at bedtime.[72]

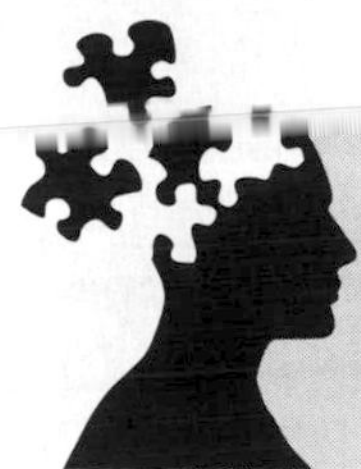

Therapeutic Challenge:

How should patients taking long-term PPI therapy be managed for the existing risk of hip fracture?

Long-term PPI therapy, particularly at high doses, has been associated with an increase in hip fractures in a study of 135,000 people 50 years and older. These patients were on high-dosage PPI therapy for more than 1 year and were found to be 2.6 times more likely to break a hip. However, those on smaller dosages for 1–4 years were 1.2 to 1.6 times more likely to break a hip.[98] Possible theories include the possibility of reduction of the amount of calcium dissolved in the stomach from hypochlorhydria or reduction of bone resorption through the interfering of acid production of osteoclasts.[98] In women ages 65 years and older, results of a trial showed that 1 week of omeprazole therapy showed a significant decrease in calcium absorption when compared with patients on placebo.[99] In a case-control study of more than 12,000 patients, it was concluded that the use of PPIs in patients without major risk factors for hip fractures did not increase the relative risk of hip fractures.[100] These results suggest that careful monitoring of patients with osteoporosis or high risk for osteoporosis or hip fractures (such as the elderly) should be recommended.

Promotility Agents

The currently available promotility agents include bethanechol, cisapride, and metoclopramide. Domperidone has been demonstrated to produce symptom relief of GERD, but is not commercially available in the U.S. Promotility agents can be used in selected patients as an adjunct to acid suppression, but they are not ideal monotherapy for most GERD patients.[72] Metoclopramide and bethanechol have significant central nervous system side effects, such as drowsiness, irritability, and extrapyramidal effects.[72] The FDA recently warned manufacturers to carry a black-box warning for metoclopramide as its chronic (long-term or high-dose) use, even after discontinuation, can cause tardive dyskinesia (involuntary body movements).[101]

Cisapride, which has also demonstrated relief from GERD symptoms, was withdrawn from the U.S. market because of reports of fatal cardiac arrhythmias and death. Cisapride continues to be available in the U.S. on a restricted basis through an investigational limited-access program to patients who meet clearly defined eligibility criteria. The program has three protocols available: adults, pediatrics, and neonates. These patients must demonstrate that they do not respond to all other standard treatment options or have severely debilitated conditions in which the benefits of cisapride might outweigh its risks. There are also strict guidelines for physicians.[102] Both metoclopramide and domperidone are dopamine receptor antagonists with equal efficacy, but unlike metoclopramide, domperidone has few central nervous system effects, and its main adverse effect is hyperprolactinemia in 10% to 15% of patients.[72]

MONITORING AND FOLLOW-UP

If drug therapy is discontinued, GERD symptoms return, and 80% of patients will have esophagitis relapse after 6–12 months.[103] After 2 weeks of therapy, patients should be monitored for efficacy of the treatment, adverse effects, and extraesophageal signs and symptoms. Maintenance therapy should keep the patient's symptoms under control and prevent complications. A full dose of H_2RAs given once daily is ineffective for GERD. Reduced doses of PPIs are ineffective for long-term therapy, such as alternate-day omeprazole or weekend therapy. Most patients will be controlled on GERD therapy, but if a patient is refractory to therapy, the healthcare provider should reconsider a GERD diagnosis.[63,72]

There are several rating scales used to monitor GERD symptoms over time. Patients can also be monitored by the GERD-specific quality-of-life questionnaires, such as the Patient Assessed Upper Gastrointestinal Quality of Life (PAGI-QOL) or the Quality of Life in Reflux and Dyspepsia (QOL-RAD).[104]

PATIENT EDUCATION

The pharmacist should educate the patient on the following topics:

1. The basic pathophysiology and causes of GERD
2. Modification of lifestyle (e.g., diet, weight loss, smoking cessation, alcohol reduction)
3. Drug therapy (e.g., side effects, administration with regard to meals, onset of action of the drug, drug-drug interactions, when to call the pharmacist or physician)
4. Alarm symptoms or red-flag signs and symptoms

SUMMARY

In the medical therapy of GERD, there has been no recent major breakthrough. PPIs have shown the greatest efficacy over H_2RAs for the treatment of GERD and erosive esophagitis. However, H_2RAs are effective for as needed use for breakthrough GERD symptoms or prevention of GERD symptoms if used 1 hour prior to heavy or spicy meals or exercise. More recently, interests in lifestyle and dietary recommendations have waned.

Inflammatory Bowel Disease

(See Web Resources for Patient Case: Inflammatory Bowel Disease.)

Additional content available at
www.ashp.org/womenshealth

IBD is a group of diseases that encompasses both Crohn's disease (CD) and ulcerative colitis (UC). Although each disease has some distinct characteristics, there may be overlap in clinical presentation and treatment. In general, CD may affect any area of the GI tract and may cause transmural inflammation of the intestinal wall. In contrast, UC is a inflammatory disease that is confined to the colon and rectum, and typically affects the mucosal layer of the intestinal tract.[105] The underlying pathophysiologic mechanisms of IBD are not entirely known, and this disease has been an intense focus of research. One major area of IBD that may significantly affect the female patient population is the surgical and pharmacologic management the disease and its complications. Likewise, management of patients who desire to become pregnant is also a challenging part of selecting drug therapy for the treatment of IBD.

In general, IBD is most common in urbanized developed countries, such as the U.S. and westernized countries in Europe.[105,106] In the U.S., the incidence of CD is reported as anywhere from five to 12 new cases per 100,000 population annually, whereas the prevalence is reported as approximately 50 per 100,000 population.[106-108] The incidence of UC in the U.S. has remained fairly constant over the last 50 years and is reported as two to 12 new cases per 100,000 population annually and affecting anywhere from 250,000 to 500,000 people.[108-109] Ulcerative proctitis, which affects only the rectum, accounts for up to 49% of UC cases and is variably included in epidemiologic studies of IBD, which may affect the true incidence and prevalence of UC.[110] Both types of IBD are described as having a bimodal distribution in initial diagnosis, with the initial peak occurring between 20 and 40 years of age, and the second between 60 and 80 years of age.[108] Both sexes are thought to be equally affected, although women may have a 20% to 30% higher incidence of developing CD and men may be at higher risk of developing UC.[110] Generally, IBD has been most prevalent in the white population, particularly in Ashkenzi Jews, although data suggest that in urbanized areas, the prevalence for black patients is approaching that of the white population.[110-113]

CLINICAL PRESENTATION

The hallmark of IBD is symptoms related to varying degrees of GI inflammation. Both forms of IBD can fluctuate between periods of activity and remission. Symptomatic patients may present with fever, abdominal pain, diarrhea, rectal bleeding, weight loss, or abdominal mass.[105,106,108] CD most commonly affects the terminal ileum and may be associated with transmural inflammation.[105] Because of these characteristics, patients may also present with malnutrition, pallor, cachexia, intestinal strictures, perineal fissures or abscesses, or intestinal **fistulae** or perforation.[105,107,112] Nutrient deficiencies may also develop secondary to malabsorption.[105,108] Patients with UC may have similar presentations, with fever, diarrhea, abdominal pain, passage of mucopurulent stools, and rectal bleeding being most common.[117] Patients may also experience weight loss, and proctitis is the predominating feature, with many reporting pruritus ani or tenesmus.[108] Because of the superficial nature of UC, perforation and fistulae formation are typically not present.[105] Patients with severe IBD, particular UC, may present with acute dilation of the colon, known as toxic megacolon, which can life threatening and often requires surgical intervention.[114] Both forms of IBD also increase the risk of developing colorectal adenocarcinoma.[105,114] Patients with IBD may also be at high risk for bone loss and fracture.[115,116] Female patients with IBD are reported to have higher rates of voluntary childlessness compared with the general population; however, rates of involuntary childlessness are reported as similar.[117] Fertility rates are reported as normal during times of disease inactivity and may be reduced proportionally to the disease activity in those with active IBD or in instances when the patient has undergone previous abdominal surgery for IBD.[117]

IBD is also associated with the development of extraintestinal manifestations that may affect the hepatobiliary system, skin, eyes, joints, and skeleton. Examples include primary sclerosing cholangitis, arthritis, ankylosing spondylitis, erythema nodosum, pyoderma gangrenosum, uveitis, iritis, or episcleritis.[107,118] The severity of IBD is generally defined as mild, moderate, severe, or fulminant. Classification takes into account the patient's symptoms, physical or laboratory signs of systemic toxicity, and frequency and characteristics of stools.[107,119,120] Patients with severe or fulminant disease are managed in the hospital setting, whereas patients with mild-moderate disease may be managed as outpatients.

PATHOPHYSIOLOGY

The true cause of IBD is unknown; however, many factors may influence the development and severity of the disease. Ultimately, the underlying disease process results in initiation of inappropriate inflammatory response within the GI tract, thought to be mainly directed against intestinal bacteria. Genetic predisposition to developing IBD has been supported by the discovery of several genes, such as *CARD15* and *DLG5*, that are involved with antigen recognition and regulation of the intestinal immune response.[120,121] Additionally, the incidence of IBD is reported to be 30–100 times greater in people with a first-degree relative who has IBD.[117] Higher concordance rates for CD have also been reported for monozygotic twins compared with dizygotic.[122]

CD is primarily a T helper type 1–mediated process, whereas UC is mediated by T-helper type 2 cells.[122-124] Abnormal regulation of the immune system and infiltration of the intestinal wall by various inflammatory cells have also brought forth the theory that IBD is an autoimmune disease.[122,125] Production of various proinflammatory cytokines is also an integral part of the disease progress that is regulated by the immune system. Overproduction of interferon-γ and tumor necrosis factor alpha (TNF-α) is well documented in CD, with TNF-α playing a major role in propagating the inflammatory cascade.[124,125] Additional evidence of autoimmunity is that up to 70% of patients with UC and 40% of patients with CD have a positive pANCA.[109,116] Transmembrane proteins, known as α4 integrins, are intimately involved with lymphocyte adhesion and migration, and represent a drug target for treatment in the inflammatory process.[123] Recent data also suggest that defects in the intestinal epithelial barrier may also contribute to development of IBD.[127]

Another major theory is that the inflammatory response seen in IBD is an inappropriate response directed against microorganisms. This may include commensal or acquired organisms and is supported by differences in fecal and mucosal organisms seen in patients with IBD compared with healthy patients.[128]

Candidate organisms include *Mycobacterium paratuberculosis*, *Listeria monocytogenes*, *Chlamydia trachomatis*, *Escherichia coli*, and *Cytomegalovirus*, amongst others.[121] Bacteria may translocate across the epithelial barrier, where they are presented to T cells as foreign antigens, thus triggering an immune response.[106] Evidence for a bacterial cause is supported by the fact that up to 60% of patients with CD may have antibodies to *Saccharomyces cerevisiae*.[122]

Other factors may also contribute to the development of IBD. It is still debated whether psychosocial factors, such as stress, play a role in the development and severity of the disease process.[129] Smoking is associated with an increased frequency of CD and can definitely worsen symptoms of CD, whereas smoking appears to have a protective effect on development and symptoms of UC.[105,110] Nonsteroidal anti-inflammatory drug use is associated with both development of IBD and worsening of symptoms.[130-132]

DIAGNOSIS

The pursuit of a diagnosis of IBD is largely driven by the presence of the clinical features described above. Supporting evidence for a diagnosis also includes laboratory-based tests, abdominal imaging, and endoscopy. Patients may have evidence of electrolyte derangements, blood loss, and leukocytosis secondary to IBD; therefore, serum chemistries, hemoglobin and hematocrit, platelets, and leukocytes should be assessed. Stool studies should be obtained to rule out infectious causes of diarrhea.[119] Serologic markers that evaluate inflammation, such as the **erythrocyte sedimentation rate** and C-reactive protein, may be obtained and can be used to monitor disease activity and response to therapy.[133] Additionally, pANCA and antibodies to *Saccharomyces cerevisiae* may also be evaluated. Radiographic studies, such as barium enema or computed tomography scan with contrast, can help to confirm disease location and identify potential complications.[107]

Endoscopic approaches are very useful to evaluate the extent and severity of the disease, obtain biopsy specimens, and to rule out other disease processes. CD may be present in the small and large intestine, as well as the rectum, whereas UC is confined to just the colon and rectum. Capsule endoscopy is preferred for evaluating small intestinal CD.[134] CD is associated with discontinuous inflammation, known as "cobblestoning" or "skip lesions," whereas UC is associated with superficial continuous inflammation.[105] UC that affects the rectal area is referred to as proctitis, whereas proctosigmoiditis affects both the rectum and sigmoid colon. Disease extending to the splenic flexure is referred to as "left-sided" disease, and **pancolitis** refers to involvement of the entire colon.[92,117] Biopsy specimens may reveal crypt abscess, which may be more common in UC, or caseating granulomas, which may be more indicative of CD and may also help to rule out carcinoma.[119,135] Future diagnostic options may include genetic profiling of the patient to evaluate course, outcome, and treatment.[120]

TREATMENT GOALS

The major treatment goals for patients with active IBD are to suppress the inflammatory response as quickly as possible and induce disease remission. Improvement in patient symptoms, prevention complications and adverse events, and improvement in quality of life are also other important goals of treatment. The choice of treatment will depend largely on the extent, location, and severity of the disease, as well on whether the patient is in the inpatient or outpatient setting. Several types of drugs are used for inducing as well as maintaining remission of both CD and UC. Surgical intervention may also be required in certain instances.

NONPHARMACOLOGIC MANAGEMENT

Most nonpharmacologic interventions deal with nutritional support of the IBD patient. Patients with long-standing disease may be at risk for serious malnutrition.[136] Enteral nutrition may be used to supplement caloric intake or as the primary means of intake if necessary.[137] Some evidence suggests that enteral nutrition may also have anti-inflammatory effects in patients with IBD.[138] Parenteral nutrition may also be required for those patients with prolonged severe disease or those who had had significant small bowel resection.[136] Probiotics may also help symptoms in patients with diarrhea, although this may be strain specific.[139,140] The most widely studied probiotic preparation in IBD is VSL #3, which contains eight bacterial species that are part of the human normal flora. These include strains of lactobacilli and bifidobacteria, as well as *Streptococcus salivarius*.[139] Studies in patients with UC demonstrate efficacy in patients unable to tolerate mesalamine, as combination therapy with balsalazide, and as preventative or maintenance therapy following antibacterial resolution of acute pouchitis.[139] Given that there are several probiotic preparations available on the market, patients may seek advice as to which agents may be effective for IBD. Lastly, patients with CD who have intestinal strictures should avoid excessive intake of high-residue foods, such as those high in fiber.[108]

Surgical intervention may be required in up to 40% of patients with UC and up to 80% of patients with CD.[141] This may be implemented to remove affected areas or malignancies, or surgically remove or repair complications, such as abscesses or fistulae. Whereas UC is curable with colectomy, CD is not and often recurs after surgical resection of affected areas.[142] Female infertility has been a major problem for those patients undergoing colectomy for UC who receive an ileal pouch–anal anastamosis.[143] This appears to be secondary to the development of adhesion formation in the pelvis. Better surgical techniques are being developed to focus on protecting the fallopian tubes during surgery. In vitro fertilization is effective for those patients who are infertile following surgery and wish to conceive.

DRUG THERAPY

Most drugs used in the treatment of IBD target the underlying inflammatory response. Agents that slow GI motility— such as loperamide, narcotics, or agents with significant anticholinergic properties— should be avoided in patients with untreated active IBD, as they may precipitate toxic megacolon.[114] Some drugs used to induced and maintain remission of IBD may be formulated to be given topically (rectally) as suppositories or enemas, whereas others are available as immediate- or delayed-release oral preparations, and some are available for intravenous administration. Extensive guidelines are available for the management of both CD and UC, and use of the following agents in IBD is summarized in Table 33-4.[107,119,144-147]

Aminosalicylates

The aminosalicylates are the most common drugs used in the management of IBD and can be used for both induction and maintenance of remission. The prototype drug is sulfasalazine, which consists of the active component mesalamine (5-ASA) linked to the carrier molecule sulfapyridine by a diazo bond.[148-150] When administered orally, the diazo bond is cleaved by intestinal bacteria, releasing the mesalamine component, which has a topical anti-inflammatory effect, and the sulfapyridine component is absorbed. Up to 80% of patients with mild to moderate extensive UC who receive 4–6 g/day of sulfasalazine can be expected to have a clinical response.[119] Newer agents use just the active mesalamine component and are formulated as delayed-release preparations. Some release in the small and large bowel (Pentasa) or the terminal ileum and colon (Asacol). Other, such as olsalazine (Dipentum), balsalazide (Colazal), and once-daily formulations of mesalamine (Lialda, Apriso) release in the colon.

Mesalamine

The mesalamine products are all generally considered to be as effective as sulfasalazine for treatment of active UC.[119] Use of higher daily dosages of mesalamine (4.8 g/day) results in better overall symptom improvement compared with lower dosages (2.4 g/day).[148] Oral sulfasalazine and mesalamine may be used to maintain remission in UC and are generally considered similar in effectiveness. Mesalamine is better tolerated than sulfasalazine and may be preferable for this indication.[119] Mesalamine suppositories (Canasa) treat the rectal area, up to 20 cm, whereas enemas (Rowasa) will reach to the splenic flexure and thus will treat left-sided disease.[147] In general, topical agents are more effective in treating distal UC compared with oral agents. Topical agents may also be combined with oral agents to treat both more extensive and distal symptoms.[147,148]

Sulfasalazine

In CD, sulfasalazine may be used, and it is most effective in patients with mild to moderate active colonic or ileocolonic disease.[107,150] Although mesalamine is often used for mild to moderate active CD because of its better tolerability compared with sulfasalazine, it is associated with variable efficacy.[107,148,150-153] Neither sulfasalazine nor mesalamine is very effective for maintenance of remission in CD. Mesalamine appears to lower the risk of relapse in patients with surgically induced remission but has reduced efficacy in medically induced remission.[150-153]

Sulfasalazine is less well tolerated than the mesalamine products and should not be used in patients allergic to sulfa-containing drugs. Adverse effects of sulfasalazine are thought to be due to the sulfapyridine component and include dose-related effects (such as nausea, anorexia, dyspepsia, folate malabsorption, and headache) and idiosyncratic effects (such as hypersensitivity reactions, hemolytic anemia, bone marrow suppression, pancreatitis, and pneumonitis).[149,154] Pregnant patients may receive sulfasalazine, but folate supplementation is required.[155-157] Olsalazine should be avoided in pregnancy, but the other mesalamine agents are generally considered safe.[156]

Corticosteroids

Corticosteroids are potent anti-inflammatory agents that inhibit production of proinflammatory

Table 33-4. Summary of Guideline Recommendations for Treatment of Inflammatory Bowel Disease[107,119,144-147]

Disease	Treatment Recommendations Based on Disease Severity and Location	
Ulcerative colitis	Mild-moderate	Distal: Topical (enema or suppository) or oral aminosalicylate (or combination of both) Extensive: Oral sulfasalazine 4–6 g/day or alternate aminosalicylate up to 4.8 g 5-ASA equivalent/day
	Moderate-severe	Oral or topical aminosalicylate as above PLUS Oral prednisone 40–60 mg daily for nonresponse to aminosalicylates OR Infliximab 5 mg/kg IV at 0, 2, 6 weeks
	Severe-fulminant	Hydrocortisone 100 mg IV 3 times daily, then Cyclosporine 4 mg/kg/day for nonresponse to IV corticosteroids after 7 days
	Maintenance	Topical or oral aminosalicylates; if no response use azathioprine or infliximab
Crohn's disease	Mild-moderate	Distal: Topical (enema or suppository) or oral aminosalicylate (or combination of both) Extensive: Oral sulfasalazine 4–6 g/day or alternate aminosalicylate up to 4.8 g 5-ASA equivalent/day Small Intestine/Ascending Colon Budesonide 9 mg/day
	Moderate-severe	Oral or topical aminosalicylate as above PLUS Oral prednisone 40–60 mg daily for nonresponse to aminosalicylates OR Infliximab 5 mg/kg IV at 0, 2, 6 weeks OR Adalimumab 160 mg SC week 0, then 80 mg SC week 2, then 40 mg SC every other week starting at week 4 OR Certolizumab 400 mg SC initially, then 400 mg SC at 2 and 4 weeks, days 1 and 2 OR Natalizumab 300 mg IV every 4 weeks if no response to prior therapies, including biologic agents
	Severe-fulminant	Hydrocortisone 100 mg IV 3 times daily, then Cyclosporine 4 mg/kg/day for nonresponse to IV corticosteroids after 7 days
	Maintenance	Topical or oral aminosalicylates, if no response use methotrexate, infliximab, adalimumab, certolizumab, or natalizumab (if no prior response to other therapies)

IV = intravenous; SC = subcutaneous.

molecules and are used for the acute management of active IBD. Corticosteroids are not, however, appropriate for use as maintenance therapy. Agents most commonly used in this class include prednisone, methylprednisolone, hydrocortisone, and budesonide.[145-150] Systemic absorption of these agents allows the treatment of inflammation regardless of the location in the GI tract, but also predisposes patients to serious adverse effects. Hydrocortisone suppositories and enemas (hydrocortisone) will treat distal disease. Budesonide has a substantial first-pass metabolism compared with the other steroids and is formulated as a delayed or release preparation that releases in the terminal ileum and ascending colon; thus, it is only effective for patients with CD affecting these areas.[148] Budesonide is considered more effective than mesalamine for induction of remission in patients with mild to moderately active CD.[150,151] Up to 69% of patients treated with budesonide 9 mg/day were in remission at 16 weeks compared with 36% of those treated with mesalamine 4 g/day.[152,153] Budesonide, at a dosage of 6 mg/day, is also effective in maintaining remission for 3–6 months in patients with mild to moderate CD. In severe UC, approximately 67% of patients can be expected to respond to intravenous corticosteroid therapy.[152] Corticosteroids have many significant adverse effects, such as adrenal suppression, glucose intolerance, edema, osteoporosis, and hypertension, among others, so exposure should be limited.[146,150] The incidence of these adverse effects may be reduced with the use of budesonide, given its lower extent of systemic absorption.[145,150,154]

Immunomodulators

The immunomodulators are immunosuppressant agents used in treatment of IBD and include 6-mercaptopurine (6-MP) and its prodrug azathioprine, as well as methotrexate, and cyclosporine. Azathioprine and 6-MP are immunosuppressant agents that are used primarily for maintenance of remission and for facilitating reduction of corticosteroid dosages in corticosteroid-dependent patients with UC and CD.[158] Their onset of action is slow, and effects may not be evident for at least 3 months; thus, these agents are not typically used for induction of remission.[146] These drugs tend to work best in CD, and evidence exists that azathioprine may be effective in maintaining remission for several years.[145,146,153,158] Toxicities may hinder long-term use and may include nausea, abdominal pain, leukopenia, thrombocytopenia, pancreatitis, and predisposition to infection. Toxicity may be enhanced in patients who lack the enzyme thiopurine-methyl transferase (TPMT), which is responsible for metabolism of these agents.[145] Patients should be tested for TPMT activity before initiating therapy with azathioprine.

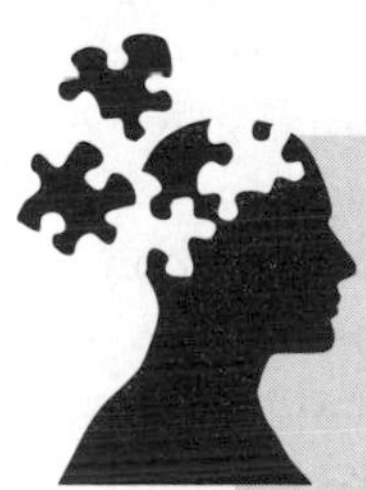

Therapeutic Challenge:

How long should potentially toxic agents, such as azathioprine and methotrexate, be continued when used for maintenance therapy of IBD?

Methotrexate

Methotrexate is an antimetabolite that inhibits dihydrofolate reductase and is used for induction and maintenance of remission in patients with CD and for facilitating reduction of corticosteroid dosages in corticosteroid-dependent patients.[145,159] It can be given weekly as oral tablets or as an intramuscular injection. Up to 65% of patients treated with methotrexate 15 mg weekly, given intramuscularly, may be maintained in remission after 40 weeks of treatment.[145] Methotrexate has several potential toxicities, including nausea, vomiting, leukopenia, hepatic fibrosis, and pneumonitis. Likewise, it is a known teratogen (category X) and is contraindicated for use in pregnancy.[145,148,155] Last, cyclosporine is a calcineurin inhibitor that is used primarily for patients who are refractory to traditional agents, including high-dose intravenous corticosteroids, as a means to induce remission and avoid colectomy.[145,160] It is typically given as an intravenous infusion for these indications. This agent has significant potential adverse effects, including hypertension, seizures, tremor, and nephrotoxicity. Azathioprine and 6-MP are both rated as pregnancy category D agents. Despite that fact they appear to be relatively safe in pregnant patients receiving the drug, initiation during pregnancy should be avoided if possible.[154-157] Breast-feeding should be avoided in patients receiving azathioprine, methotrexate, and cyclosporine.[156]

Biological Agents

Biological agents available for use in IBD include infliximab, adalimumab, and certolizumab. These agents are antibodies directed against TNF-α and are typically used for treatment of moderate to severe active disease, including fistulizing CD disease, in patients failing other therapies (such as immunosuppressants or steroids) and for maintenance therapy of remission thereafter.[145,161-163] Infliximab is a chimeric IgG1 antibody to TNF-α that contains human and murine sequences and can be used for both forms of IBD. Adalimumab is fully humanized and is only indicated for use in CD.[163] Certolizumab is a humanized PEGylated Fab' fragment containing sequences of amino acids in the complimentary determining regions derived from mouse anti-TNF-α antibody that are then inserted into a human variable region.[162] Unlike infliximab and adalimumab, certolizumab does not induce apoptosis of T cells or monocytes.[162] Certolizumab is indicated for use in CD. Infliximab is given intravenously, whereas adalimumab and certolizumab are given subcutaneously. The anti-TNF biological agents can cause infusion-related reactions, cause development and exacerbation of heart failure, and predispose patients to serious infections, including reactivation of latent infections such as tuberculosis or hepatitis B.[154,163] For this reason, they are not to be used without screening for latent infections, particularly tuberculosis, or in those with advanced heart failure. Antibodies may form to infliximab over time, which may be associated with reduction in effectiveness.[157] Because adalimumab is fully humanized, it has a role as an option for patients who have lost response to infliximab over time because of development of these antibodies to infliximab. All biological agents are extremely expensive. Infliximab, adalimumab, and certolizumab are rated as pregnancy category B, but it is not known whether these agents are excreted in breast milk; thus, they should be avoided during breast-feeding if possible.[126,155-157]

The anti-TNF-α biological agents are effective in both inducing remission in patients with moderate to severe active disease and maintaining remission. Infliximab has been the most widely used agent. Initial trials demonstrated that up to 65% of patients with moderate to severe active CD may clinically respond at 4 weeks following an initial dose of 5 mg/kg, with 41% response observed at 12 weeks.[145,146,161] In patients with CD who initially respond well to infliximab, maintenance therapy may lead to up to a 2 times greater chance of remaining in remission compared with placebo after 30 weeks of treatment.[145,152] Likewise, patients receiving infliximab are more likely to be able to discontinue chronic use of corticosteroids. Similar results are seen in patients with UC, including up to a 69% response rate at 8 weeks compared with placebo, as well as reductions in the need for colectomy.[164]

Several recent trials have evaluated the use of adalimumab for both treatment of active CD and maintenance of remission, including patients with loss of response to infliximab.[165-169] For induction of remission in patients with moderate to severe active CD, a dose of 160 mg subcutaneously, followed by 80 mg subcutaneously, resulted in 36% of patients in remission at 4 weeks.[168] In patients previously treated with infliximab, induction of remission at 4 weeks was observed in 21% of patients at 4 weeks.[165] For patients continued on adalimumab following induction of remission, a dose of 40 mg subcutaneously given every other week has been demonstrated to maintain remission in 36% to 79% of patients.[167,169]

Certolizumab has been demonstrated to be effective for both induction and maintenance of remission in patients with moderate to severe CD.[170,171] Clinical response was achieved in 37% of patients at 6 weeks who received 400 mg at 0, 2, and 4 weeks.[170] This is observed in patients with C-reactive protein concentrations >10 mg/L. In patients initially responding to certolizumab at 6 weeks, who were then given a dose of 400 mg every 4 weeks, remission was maintained in 62% of patients at 26 weeks.[171] Thus certolizumab provides another option for both treatment of active CD and maintenance of remission.

The newest biological agent to be approved for the treatment of CD is natalizumab. This agent was originally used for the treatment of multiple sclerosis and has also been studied in CD.[123,172,173] This agent interferes with leukocyte adhesion by targeting glycoproteins expressed on the cell surfaces called integrins. Natalizumab is a humanized monoclonal IgG antibody directed against the α_4 integrins.[123] This results in prevention of α_4 integrin–mediated leukocyte adhesion and prevention of leukocyte transmigration into areas of inflammation.[147] A recent trial of natalizumab in patients with moderate to severely active CD demonstrated that a dose of 300 mg intravenously every 4 weeks resulted in a significant clinical response rate of 48%.[165] In a similar trial of moderate to severely active CD, a dose of 300 mg intravenously every 4 weeks performed similarly to placebo.[166] However, a continuation of this trial demonstrated that 61% of patients who initially responded and were maintained on this dosage for 6 months maintained their initial clinical response over this time frame, with 44% observed to be in remission.[166] The role of natalizumab at this time is mostly in patients failing other therapies, including the anti-TNF-α biologic agents. Natalizumab should not be used in combination with anti-TNF-α biologic or immunosuppressant agents. One important aspect of treatment with natalizumab is that is has been associated with the development of progressive multifocal leukoencephalopathy. Because of this potential toxicity, this agent can only be prescribed through the manufacturer's registered prescribing program. Patients should be monitored closely for changes in mental status during therapy. Natalizumab is a pregnancy category C drug. Other biological agents targeting various cytokines are currently under development. These include agents targeting interleukin-12 and interleukin-23.[147]

Antibiotics

Antibiotics are the last class of agents that may be used in IBD. This is based on the fact that bacterial pathogens may play a role in the inflammatory response. Metronidazole and ciprofloxacin are the most studied agents. Data suggest that these drugs may be somewhat effective, particularly in patients with perianal or fistulizing CD; however, they are often used as adjunctive therapies.[107,148,174] The variable effects of antibiotic efficacy in treatment of active IBD are largely secondary to underpowered studies.[152] Antibiotics may need to be administered for long periods, and metronidazole in particular may be associated with significant adverse effects, such peripheral neuropathy.[154,174] Metronidazole is pregnancy category B agent; ciprofloxacin is rated category C.[157]

MONITORING AND FOLLOW-UP

Monitoring for response to therapy is largely based on improvement in patient symptoms, particularly stool frequency and characteristics, abdominal pain, and extraintestinal symptoms. Patients with active disease should be monitored within 4 weeks of initiating drug therapy to assess efficacy and toxicity. Once remission is achieved, patients may be seen 1–2 times per year. Given the propensity for many of the drugs used to treat IBD to cause adverse effects, appropriate symptom and laboratory monitoring should be implemented based on the chosen drug(s). Periodic endoscopy may also be indicated, based on the extent and severity of the disease, response to therapy, and presence of complications. Periodic assessment of quality of life and patient well-being should also be assessed.

PATIENT EDUCATION

There are several important aspects of both IBD and its treatment that female patients should be aware of. As IBD severity may affect fertility rates, patients should be aware that optimal times for conception are typically during periods of remission. Likewise, patients who become pregnant will need treatments that limit harm to the fetus. In addition, measures may need to be implemented to reduce toxicity of some treatments, as in the case of folate supplementation for patients receiving sulfasalazine or calcium supplementation for patients receiving corticosteroids. Given that some therapies, such as methotrexate, are teratogenic, education regarding appropriate contraceptive methods is essential. Proper education regarding which therapies are amenable to being used while a patient is breast-feeding is also an important aspect of IBD management. Advising patients regarding potential adverse effects and expected efficacy of drug therapies may also facilitate improved adherence to therapies.

SUMMARY

IBD is associated with severe inflammation in various parts of the GI tract. Both UC and CD are associated with significant symptoms and greatly affect patient's quality of life. Although the cause is unknown, most therapies focus on inducing and maintaining remission by targeting the underlying inflammatory response. Several drug classes can be used for these purposes, many of which are associated with significant toxicity. Surgical interventions for UC and use of some agents during pregnancy and breastfeeding appear to be the major areas in which female patients may be affected.

References

Additional content available at
www.ashp.org/womenshealth

34 Mental Health

Tracy L. Skaer, Pharm.D., FABFE, FASCP, FASHP; Carol M. Odell, MSN, FNP

Learning Objectives

1. Recognize the signs and symptoms (clinical presentation) of the mental illnesses discussed.
2. Formulate a treatment strategy based on an individual patient's needs.
3. Understand the guidelines as they relate to monitoring and follow-up and suicide prevention.
4. Know the sex-related issues facing mental illness diagnosis.

Mental illness has become a major health concern across the globe with women often having a higher predisposition than men. Some of the major mental illnesses affecting women today that are discussed in this chapter are depression, selected anxiety disorders, and body dysmorphic disorder (BDD). An estimated 19 million people in the U.S. experience depression each year, with twice as many women affected than men.[1] Anxiety disorders are among the most prevalent form of mental illness in the U.S. Some 30 million Americans (25%) will fulfill the diagnostic criteria for at least one anxiety disorder in their lifetime, with 15.7 million affected annually.[2] This amounts to a lifetime prevalence of nearly 15%. Women have a higher predisposition toward anxiety disorders, with >13% meeting the diagnostic criteria compared with 6% of men.[1,3] The impact of sex is profound, increasing the likelihood of developing an anxiety disorder by 85% in women compared with men.[3]

There is consistent documentation of high rates of psychiatric comorbidity among patients with mental illness, especially anxiety disorders.[3,4] Clinical studies have shown that ≥50% of patients with a primary anxiety disorder have at least one additional anxiety or mood disorder; 60% of patients with a principal anxiety or mood disorder have an additional **axis I disorder,** and 80% have a positive lifetime history.[5,6] Reported comorbidity rates for specific anxiety and mood disorders are even higher. For instance, 65% and 88% of general anxiety disorder (GAD) patients have a current or lifetime comorbid anxiety or mood disorder, respectively, with post-traumatic stress disorder (PTSD) patients at 92% and 100%.[5,6] It is therefore important to screen patients for other psychiatric comorbidities at the time of anxiety disorder diagnosis.

Etiology and Pathophysiology

The etiology of depressive disorders is complex, multifactorial, and has yet to be explained by a single social, developmental, or biological theory. Several factors appear to trigger or precipitate depressive episodes and changes in brain monoamine neurotransmitters; norepinephrine, serotonin, and dopamine have been related to patient symptomatology.[7] There are several theories and hypotheses on the pathophysiology of depression, including postsynaptic changes in receptor sensitivity, dysregulation, serotonin/norepinephrine link hypothesis, dopamine in depression, and biological markers; however, the true pathophysiology of this illness has yet to be fully discovered.

Anxiety symptoms are inherently present in the clinical presentation of several medical and psychiatric illnesses, often complicating the diagnosis at initial presentation. The modulation of normal and pathologic anxiety states is associated with multiple regions of the

CASE PRESENTATION

Patient Case: Part 1

S.T. is a 39-year-old woman who presents to the clinic reporting difficulty sleeping and loss of appetite. She says, "I can't sleep or think straight anymore. I feel like I'm going in slow motion; nothing seems to be any fun. Is this the way my life is going to be from now on? I'm beginning to wonder if it really is worth living."

HPI: S.T. is in the process of a divorce; she left her husband 6 months ago after 15 years of marriage. This was her first marriage, and the couple has had severe daily arguments for the last 4 years. She reports that she suffered from an acquaintance rape while in college and that she and her mother did not have a good relationship when she was younger and her mother was drinking. S.T. has become increasingly depressed since she left her husband. She has not been eating well, frequently does not eat at all, and has lost 15 lb. She cries frequently and has difficulty falling asleep. She lies awake at night crying and tossing and turning for hours before finally falling asleep. She is unable to concentrate as well as before and has become disinterested in reading novels, which she used to enjoy thoroughly.

PMH: S.T. suffers from hay fever but has no significant medical conditions; no previous history of psychiatric treatment but reports a lifelong history of occasional periods of intense sadness lasting several weeks. During these times, she would lose interest in her usual activities, sometimes taking time off from work to recover.

Family history: Mother is a recovering alcoholic (has not had a drink in 20 years) with bipolar disorder and chronic obstructive pulmonary disease. Father has diabetes, hypertension, and dyslipidemia. Her sister and brother are both in relatively good health.

Social history: Does not smoke, has an occasional drink with friends (~1/mo), and walks 20 minutes 4 times/wk.

Medications: Multivitamin daily; ibuprofen 200 mg (two tablets) as needed for pain or menstrual cramps; loratidine 10 mg daily as needed for allergies.

Allergies: NKDA.

Vitals: 5′5″, 110 lb (BMI 18.3), BP 116/76, HR 74, Temp 99°F, RR 14.

Physical exam: Within normal limits.

Laboratory values: Within normal limits.

brain, with abnormal function linked to norepinephrine, gamma-aminobutyric acid, and serotonin.[8,9] Ongoing research in the areas of neuroendocrinology, neurobiology, and neuroimaging has advanced a number of theories on the pathophysiology of anxiety disorders.[9] Data from these studies indicate that the modulation of normal and pathologic anxiety states is associated with multiple regions of the brain, including the amygdala, hippocampus, thalamus, and prefrontal cortex.[8,9]

Depression

CLINICAL PRESENTATION AND DIAGNOSIS

Women who experience some form of victimization (e.g., molestation, rape, physical abuse, sexual harassment) during their lifetime are more likely to develop clinical depression at some time as opposed to those who have not.[1] Other risk factors include a family history of the disorder (especially bipolar disorder), pregnancy, stressful life events (e.g., divorce, loss of loved one), chronic medical conditions (e.g., other mental illness, substance abuse, diabetes, chronic pain states, systemic lupus erythematosus, cancer, cardiovascular disease, stroke), medications (antihypertensives, oral contraceptives, steroids), personality (low self-esteem, overly dependent, self-critical, pessimistic), and gender (women are 2 times as likely as men to be diagnosed with depression).[7,10,11]

The two hallmark symptoms that are key to establishing a diagnosis of clinical depression include loss of interest in normal daily activities and/or depressed mood most of the day nearly all day.[10] The patient must have one of these hallmark symptoms plus at least three additional symptoms, including sleep disturbances, impaired thinking or concentration, changes in weight, agitation, fatigue or slowing of body movements, low self-esteem, less interest in sexual activities, and/or thoughts of death during the same 2-week period that represent a change from previously normal functioning. These symptoms cause clinically significant distress or impairment in occupational, social, or other areas of work/life and are not due to the direct physiologic effects of a substance or medication or a general medical condition such as hypothyroidism. The full criteria for diagnosis of a major depressive episode from the American Psychiatric Association's *Diagnostic and Statistical Manual of Mental Disorders, Fourth Edition, (DSM-IV)* can be found at the following website: www.behavenet.com/capsules/disorders/mjrdepep.htm.

The mean age of onset of major depression is 27 years.[7] Patients may appear saddened or depressed and are often quite pessimistic. A wide variety of physical symptoms, such as gastrointestinal problems (indigestion, constipation, or diarrhea), headache, and backache are often caused by depression.[10] Chronic fatigue is a common symptom, with decreased ability to perform normal daily tasks. Fatigue often appears worse in the morning and does not improve with rest. Of important note is that the elderly tend to report more somatic than affective symptoms and report loss of interest, pleasure, and emotion while denying change in mood.[7] Older adults may often experience cognitive impairment as part of the clinical syndrome, and symptoms of depression may stimulate pseudo/reversible dementia with concentration difficulties, memory loss, and distractibility.[7]

Left untreated, depression can lead to further disability, dependency and possible suicide (including both attempts and/or fatal).[10] Women attempt suicide more often than men, but men are more likely to succeed in killing themselves.[10] The rate of suicide is 4 times greater for men. Warning signs of a possible suicide are provided in Table 34-1. Factors that increase the risk of suicide for either sex include previous psychiatric admission; substance abuse; depression and/or feelings of hopelessness; family history of suicide or prior suicide attempts; anniversary of a loss; presence of a serious medical condition; lack of a social support system and/or refusal to seek help; and being widowed, unmarried, unemployed, or living alone.[12] It is important to take any threat of suicide seriously, even if the patient is already receiving treatment for depression.

Table 34-1. Suicide Warning Signs

- Pacing, agitated behavior, frequent mood changes, and sleeplessness for several nights
- Actions or threats of assault, physical harm, or violence
- Threats or talk of death or suicide, such as "I don't care anymore," or "You won't need to worry about me much longer."
- Withdrawal from activities and relationships
- Putting affairs in order, such as saying goodbye to friends, giving away prized possessions, or writing a will
- A sudden brightening of mood after a period of being depressed
- Unusually risky behavior, such as buying or handling a gun or driving recklessly

TREATMENT

Supportive psychiatric management techniques—including interpersonal psychotherapy, cognitive behavioral therapy (CBT), brief dynamic psychotherapy, marital and family therapy, stress-management programs, and lifestyle adjustments—are often used in the treatment of depression. The combination of psychotherapy and pharmacotherapy has been proven to be more effective than either invention alone.[7,10]

There are three treatment phases to consider in the treatment of depression: 1) the *acute* phase, lasting 6–10 weeks, in which the goal is remission of symptoms; 2) the *continuation* phase, lasting for 4–9 months after remission is achieved, in which the goal is to eliminate residual symptoms or prevent relapse; and 3) the *maintenance* phase, lasting at least 12–36 months, in which the goal is to prevent recurrence.[13] An alternative antidepressant should be considered for those patients not responding with appropriate dosing at the end of the acute treatment phase (at approximately 10–12 weeks).

There are now several antidepressant medications available on the market for the treatment of depression. The selective serotonin reuptake inhibitors (SSRIs—e.g., citalopram, escitalopram, fluoxetine, paroxetine, sertraline) and the serotonin-norepinephrine reuptake inhibitors (SNRIs—e.g., duloxetine, venlafaxine) are among the first chosen in therapy.[7,10] Bupropion, tricyclic antidepressants (TCAs—e.g., amitriptyline, desipramine, nortriptyline, protriptyline, imipramine), tetracyclics (e.g., maprotiline, mirtazapine), monoamine oxidase inhibitors (MAOIs—e.g., phenelzine and tranylcypromine), stimulants (e.g., methylphenidate, mixed amphetamine salts), lithium, and anticonvulsants (e.g., lamotrigine, carbamazepine) are also available if necessary.[1,7,8,10,13]

The selection of an antidepressant is largely dependent on presenting symptoms, the patient's history of response, pharmacogenetics (history of familial antidepressant response), patient's concurrent medical history, side-effect profile of the medication, potential for interaction with other medications, patient tolerance, and medication cost. Table 34-2 outlines some selected examples of medication interactions associated with the newer generation of antidepressants (SSRIs and SNRIs).[7,10,13] Of important note is their potential to cause **serotonin syndrome** when prescribed with antimigraine triptan class medications (commonly used in women) and increased risk of gastrointestinal bleeding when

Table 34-2. Selected Medication Interactions of Newer-Generation Antidepressants

Antidepressant	Potential Interaction	Effect
All SSRIs and SNRIs	Triptans, linezolid	Serotonin syndrome
All SSRIs and SNRIs	MAOIs	Hypertensive crisis, serotonin syndrome, delirium
SSRIs, SNRIs	NSAIDs, alcohol	Increased risk of gastrointestinal bleeding and/or ulceration
Fluoxetine, paroxetine, and fluvoxamine	Beta-blockers (e.g., metoprolol)	Bradycardia, possible heart block
Fluoxetine and fluvoxamine	Alprazolam	Increased plasma concentration and half-life of alprazolam; increased psychomotor impairment
Fluvoxamine	Warfarin	Increased hypothrombinemic response to warfarin
Fluvoxemine	Diltiazem	Bradycardia

NSAIDs = nonsteroidal anti-inflammatory drugs; MAOIs = monoamine oxidase inhibitors; SNRIs = serotonin norepinephrine reuptake inhibitors; SSRIs = selective serotonin reuptake inhibitors.

combined with nonsteroidal anti-inflammatory drugs (NSAIDs) and/or alcohol.

TCAs and MAOIs are generally not considered first line because of their negative side-effect profiles and additionally, in the case of MAOIs, dietary restrictions, the details of which have been well publicized in the literature.

Electroconvulsive therapy, consisting of 6 to 12 treatments administered either unilaterally or bilaterally 2–3 times weekly, is available as well for treatment-resistant patients and those who need a rapid response (i.e., are at high risk of suicide). Electroconvulsive therapy is considered generally safe and effective.[10,14] The most common side effect is confusion that lasts a few minutes to several hours post-therapy.[10,14]

Herbal and dietary supplements are becoming increasingly popular and present the healthcare provider with increasing challenges in finding appropriate therapy. Some of the popular supplements available include St. John's wort, s-adenosyl-methionine (SAM-e), 5-hydroxytryptophan (5-HT), and omega-3 fatty acids.[10] Although SAM-e and omega-3 fatty acids have very few side effects, interactive potential of St. John's wort with other medications can be problematic.[10]

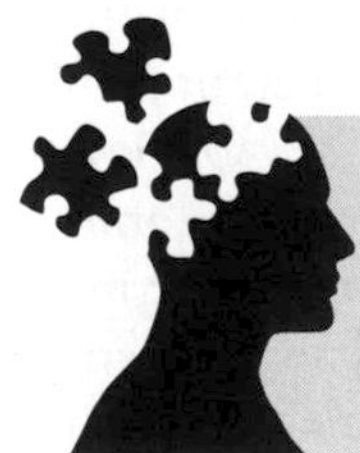

Therapeutic Challenge:

Which antidepressant should be used if a patient is pregnant or breast-feeding?

Interestingly, St John's wort has demonstrated efficacy in the treatment of mild to moderate depression.[15,16] However, if St John's wort is to be used, it should be administered under the guidance of a healthcare provider trained in the treatment of depression, and a single-source product should be used continuously from a reputable and trusted manufacturer.

Light therapy is available and very effective for those suffering from seasonal affective disorder (SAD). In this disorder, the patients suffer depressive episodes that recur at the same time each year, usually when daylight hours are shorter in the fall and winter months.[10]

A well-studied and publicly available treatment algorithm is the Texas Medication Algorithm Project (TMAP) for depression.[17] The TMAP has two different algorithms for the treatment of depression, depending on whether psychoses are present. The different stages of depression noted in the TMAP algorithms are a depiction of worsening illness and thus treatment-resistant cases. For future reference, the 2008 algorithms are publicly available on the following websites:

Nonpsychotic depression:
http://www.dshs.state.tx.us/mhprograms/pdf/TIMA_MDD_MDDAlgoOnly_080608.pdf;

Psychotic depression:
http://www.dshs.state.tx.us/mhprograms/pdf/TIMA_MDD_WPsychAlgoOnly_080608.pdf

MONITORING AND FOLLOW-UP

Adherence to therapy and close monitoring is vital to the successful treatment of depression. Patients

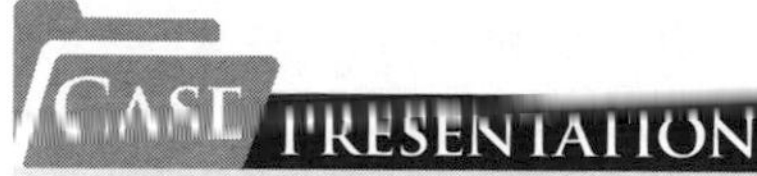

Patient Case: Part 2

S.T. meets the diagnostic criteria for depression with depressed mood, loss of interest in normal activities, sleep disturbance, weight loss, and impaired thinking. She is expressing some hopelessness as well and perhaps some slight suicidal ideation for her statement, "Is life worth living?". Her history of recent stress (impending divorce), victimization, occasional periods of sadness lasting for several weeks, and mother's diagnosis of bipolar disorder are all risk factors for depressive illness. S.T. is therefore in need of therapeutic intervention for her depression.

Plan: S.T. is enrolled in individual psychotherapy, with the rate of sessions per week and length of therapy to be determined by the counseling psychologist. Additionally, information and strong encouragement to enroll in one of the local 8-week stress-management programs is provided to S.T. Counseling on appropriate sleep hygiene is also provided for her insomnia difficulties (Table 34-3), and she is requested to keep a sleep diary. She is prescribed citalopram 20 mg/day and is scheduled to return to the clinic in 7–10 days for symptom re-evaluation. S.T. is given a prescription for eszopiclone 1 mg before bedtime if needed for sleep as a short-term remedy for her sleeping difficulties. Continued treatment for insomnia symptoms will be assessed at each sequential follow-up appointment.

must be carefully monitored for efficacy, suicidality, and how well they are tolerating the side effects of pharmacotherapy. Although many antidepressants provide some symptomatic relief within 7–10 days, their full antidepressant effect is usually not achieved until at least 30 days. Once depressive symptoms fully remit, pharmacotherapy should be continued for at least another 4–9 months for those newly diagnosed.[17,18] It may take from 9 months to a year or more to achieve the desired therapeutic outcome.

The risk of recurrence increases significantly with each sequential diagnosis of a depressive episode.[19,20] Data indicate that individuals who experience their fist episode of depression have a 28% likelihood of recurrence within 1 year; this risk increases to 90% in individuals who have had three previous depressive episodes.[17] Therefore, lifelong therapy may be required. Additionally, patients will benefit the most from pharmacotherapy if they are also enrolled in some form of psychotherapy and self-care program, such as stress management and/or lifestyle modifications. It is just as important for the patient to take the responsibility to address their illness as it is for the healthcare provider to prescribe appropriate therapy.

Anxiety Disorders

(See Web Resources for Patient Case: Generalized Anxiety Disorder.)

Additional content available at ***www.ashp.org/womenshealth***

The American Psychiatric Association's *Diagnostic and Statistical Manual of Mental Disorders, Fourth Edition, Text Revision (DSM-IV-TR)* classifies anxiety disorders into several categories: general anxiety disorder (GAD), panic disorder (with or without agoraphobia), agoraphobia, social phobia (also called social anxiety disorder), specific phobias, obsessive-compulsive disorder (OCD), post-traumatic stress disorder (PTSD), and acute stress disorder.[21] Women have a higher predisposition toward anxiety disorders, with >13% meeting the diagnostic criteria compared with 6% of men.[2-6] For the specific *DSM-IV-TR* criteria for any given anxiety disorder, please refer to the following website: www.behavenet.com/capsules/disorders/dsm4TRclassification.htm.

The most common characteristic features of these illnesses are anxiety and avoidance behavior.[22]

Table 34-3. Sleep Hygiene

- Follow a regular sleep pattern; go to bed and arise at about the same time each day
- Make the bedroom comfortable for sleeping; avoid temperature extremes, noise, and light
- Make sure the bed is comfortable
- Go to bed only when sleepy
- Engage in relaxing activities before bedtime
- Use the bed and bedroom for sleep and sexual activities only
- If tense, practice relaxation exercises
- If hungry, eat a light snack, but avoid eating meals or large snacks immediately before bedtime
- Eliminate daytime naps
- Avoid using caffeine after noon
- Avoid using alcohol or nicotine later in the evening
- If unable to fall asleep, do not become anxious; leave the bedroom, and participate in relaxing activities for 20–30 min

Moreover, there is an increased amount of evidence that hereditary factors play a significant role in the development of anxiety disorders.[23]

GENERAL ANXIETY DISORDER, PANIC DISORDER, AND SOCIAL PHOBIA

Clinical Presentation and Diagnosis

The clinical presentation of GAD includes some or all of the following symptoms:

- **Psychological and cognitive**—excessive anxiety, worries that are difficult to control, feeling keyed up or on edge, poor concentration, or mind going blank
- **Physical**—restlessness, fatigue, muscle tension, sleep disturbance, irritability
- **Impairment**—social, occupational, or other important functional areas, poor coping abilities

Of important note is that the diagnostic criteria for GAD requires persistence of these symptoms for at least 6 months with the essential feature of GAD being unrealistic or excessive anxiety and worry about a number of events or activities.[21,22] Those suffering from GAD have exaggerated worry and tension, even when there is little to nothing to provoke it.[23] They anticipate disaster and become overly concerned about finances, health, family problems, or difficulties at work.[23] The anxiety of apprehensive expectation is accompanied by at least three psychological or physiologic symptoms, and the persistent worry must cause significant distress and impairment in social, occupational, or other important areas of functioning.

Panic disorder affects about 6 million American adults and is twice as common in women as is men.[22,23] Panic attacks often begin in late adolescence or early adulthood, but not everyone who experiences panic attacks will develop panic disorder.[23] The clinical presentation of a panic attack includes some or all of the following symptoms:

- **Psychological**—depersonalization, derealization, fear of losing control, fear of going "crazy," fear of dying
- **Physical**—abdominal pain, diarrhea, chest pain or discomfort, chills, dizziness or light-headedness, feeling of choking, hot flashes, palpitations, nausea, paresthesias, shortness of breath, sweating, tachycardia, trembling, or shaking

It is characterized by sudden attacks of terror, usually accompanied by tachycardia, sweating, weakness, feeling faint, or dizziness. The patient may also feel flushed, chilled, experience paresthesias in their hands, nauseated, chest pain, or smothering sensations.[22] There is usually a fear of impending doom or fear of losing control. Panic attacks can occur at any time, even while sleeping.[22] These attacks usually peak within 10 minutes but can last longer. Obviously, those suffering from full-blown, repeated panic attacks can become disabled and should seek professional help before they start avoidance behaviors, which will create further restriction in their work/life.

The presentation of social phobia, also known as social anxiety disorder, involves the following possible symptoms:

- **Fears**—being scrutinized by others, being embarrassed, being humiliated
- **Some feared situations**—addressing a group of people, eating or writing in front of others, interacting with authority figures, speaking in public, talking with strangers, use of public facilities
- **Physical**—blushing (most common), "butterflies in the stomach," diarrhea, sweating, tachycardia, trembling

Social phobia is diagnosed when people become overwhelmingly anxious and excessively self-conscious in everyday social situations.[22,23] These patients have intense, persistent, and chronic fear of being watched and judged by others and of doing things that will embarrass themselves. They realize that the fear is excessive and unreasonable but can worry for days or weeks before a dreaded situation. This becomes so severe that it interferes with work/life and makes it difficult to maintain relationships, including friendships.[22,23]

Treatment

The treatment of anxiety disorder presents many challenges. Anxiety disorders often go untreated.[24] Careful diagnostic evaluation must be made, including full determination of all mental health issues present and whether there are other coexisting medical conditions. Substance abuse or depression are of particular importance and must be addressed in the treatment plan.

The British Association for Psychopharmacology (BAP) has published comprehensive, evidence-based guidelines for the pharmacologic treatment of anxiety disorders to aid healthcare providers in diagnosis and treatment.[25,26] (See www.bap.org.uk/consensus/anxiety_disorders_guidelines.pdf.) A brief overview of the BAP recommendations is presented in Tables 34-4, 34-5, and 34-6.

Table 34-4. Summary of British Association for Psychopharmacology Guidelines for Treating Generalized Anxiety Disorder

- Higher dosages of SSRIs or venlafaxine may be associated with greater response rates
- For longer-term pharmacotherapy, use an approach known to be efficacious in preventing relapse (best evidence is for escitalopram and paroxetine)
- Consider switching to another evidence-based treatment after nonresponse to initial treatment
- For nonresponders to acute treatment with an SSRI, switch to venlafaxine or imipramine
- Consider benzodiazepines after nonresponse to SSRI and SNRI treatment
- Consider combining pharmacotherapy treatment and CBT

CBT = cognitive behavioral therapy; SNRI = serotonin norepinephrine reuptake inhibitor; SSRI = selective serotonin reuptake inhibitor.

Table 34-5. Summary of British Association for Psychopharmacology Guidelines for Treating Panic Disorder

- Consider increasing the dosage if there is insufficient response
- Initial side effects can be minimized by slowly increasing the dosage
- Consider CBT with exposure, as this may reduce relapse rates
- For longer-term pharmacotherapy, use a clinical practice approach known to be efficacious in preventing relapse
- First-line pharmacotherapy is an SSRI; imipramine is a second-line choice
- When discontinuing pharmacotherapy, reduce the dosage gradually over a minimum of 3 months to avoid discontinuation and rebound symptoms
- Combinations to consider for poor responders:
  - Adding paroxetine or buspirone to psychological treatments after partial response
  - Adding paroxetine, while continuing with CBT, after initial nonresponse
  - Adding group CBT in nonresponders to pharmacotherapy approaches

CBT = cognitive behavioral therapy; SSRI = selective serotonin reuptake inhibitor.

Many patients with anxiety disorders also suffer from major depressive disorder (MDD). Thus, antidepressants, particularly the SSRIs and SNRIs, are now considered the first-line pharmacotherapy for those with both conditions.[25-35] An adequate trial of antidepressants in GAD, social phobia, and panic disorder is considered to be at least 8 weeks, with a maximal benefit possibly not demonstrated until 12 weeks.[25-35] Table 34-7 summarizes the medications of choice for GAD, panic disorder, and social phobia. Data also indicate the efficacy of the SNRI venlafaxine XR in the treatment of GAD, panic disorder, SAD, and PTSD, with less robust findings for OCD.[25,26,36,37]

Benzodiazepines (primarily clonazepam, lorazepam, and alprazolam) remain widely prescribed for the treatment of anxiety, although their side effects (i.e., sedation, poor coordination, cognitive impairment, potential for withdrawal symptoms) have serious implications.[23-28] They are more likely to be prescribed for women than men.[27,28] The BAP guidelines (Tables 34-4, 34-5, and 34-6) have them assigned as second or third line for maintenance therapy, depending on anxiety diagnosis, and buspirone has been reserved for primarily nonresponders.[25,26] Moreover, TCAs imipramine and clomipramine remain effective second-line agents for some anxiety disorders (Table 34-7).[25,26,33-35]

A critical review of the literature on the role of antiepileptic drugs (AEDs) in anxiety disorders was recently completed.[38] The authors stated that the strongest evidence has been demonstrated for

Table 34-6. Summary of British Association for Psychopharmacology Guidelines for Treating Social Phobia

- Routinely prescribed higher dosages of SSRIs is not recommended, but individual patients may benefit from higher dosages (evaluated case by case)
- Consider CBT with exposure, which may reduce relapse rates better than pharmacotherapy
- For longer-term pharmacotherapy, use a clinical practice approach known to be efficacious in preventing relapse
- Consider an SSRI or CBT first line; clonazepam is considered second line
- Consider CBT after initial pharmacotherapy response in patients with high risk of relapse
- After insufficient response, consider the following:
  - Adding buspirone after partial response to an SSRI
  - Benzodiazepines in patients who have not responded to other approaches
  - Combining pharmacotherapy with CBT

CBT = cognitive behavioral therapy; SSRI = selective serotonin reuptake inhibitor.

Table 34-7. Medications of Choice for Anxiety Disorders

Disorder	First-line Agent	Second-line Agent	Alternatives
GAD	Duloxetine, escitalopram, paroxetine, venlafaxine XR	BZDs, buspirone, imipramine, sertraline	Hydroxyzine, pregabalin
Panic	SSRIs, venlafaxine SR	Alprazolam, clonazepam, clomipramine	Phenelzine
SP	Escitalopram, fluvoxamine, paroxetine, sertraline, venlafaxine XR	Citalopram, clonazepam	Buspirone, gabapentin, mirtazapine, phenelzine, pregabalin

BZDs = benzodiazepines; GAD = generalized anxiety disorder; SP = social phobia/social anxiety disorder; SR = sustained release; SSRIs = selective serotonin reuptake inhibitors; XR = extended release.

pregabalin in social phobia and GAD, lamotrigine in PTSD, and gabapentin in social phobia. The available data for gabapentin in panic disorder are somewhat mixed. More study is needed to make a definitive recommendation. Thus, AEDs can be an alternative treatment possibility in some anxiety disorders.[38]

Monitoring and Follow-up

Despite the general efficacy of initial pharmacotherapy, no single antianxiety agent has been found to be effective for all patients. Treatment response rates (generally defined as 50% improvement in anxiety symptoms from baseline), although reaching 80% in many randomized, acute clinical trials, have been shown to be as low as 30% to 40% in some studies.[23-31] Treatment goals are now aimed at remission, which mandates resolution of clinical symptoms. Moreover, anxiety symptoms frequently persist over time, even when patients are appropriately diagnosed and treated. The key to successful intervention is that antianxiety therapy must be tailored to each individual patient's response.

OBSESSIVE-COMPULSIVE DISORDER AND POST-TRAUMATIC STRESS DISORDER

(See Web Resources for Patient Case: Obsessive Compulsive Disorder/Post-traumatic Stress Disorder.)

Additional content available at
www.ashp.org/womenshealth

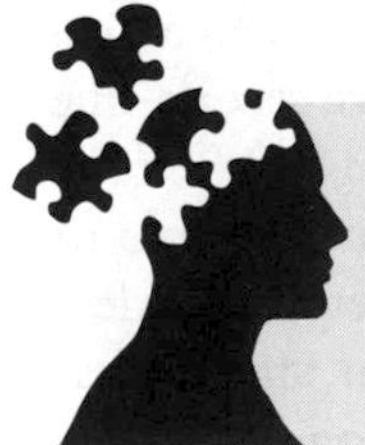

Therapeutic Challenge:

When should benzodiazepines be used in the treatment of anxiety disorders?

Clinical Presentation and Diagnosis

OCD patients have persistent, upsetting thoughts (obsession) and use rituals (compulsion) to control the anxiety caused by the obsessive thought patterns.[23,39] The clinical presentation of OCD includes the following:

- **Obsessions**—repetitive thoughts (e.g., feeling contaminated after touching an object, doubting whether the door was locked or appliances were shut off), images, or impulses (e.g., need for symmetry or putting things in specific order), sacrilegious thoughts
- **Compulsions**—repetitive activities (e.g., hand washing, checking, ordering, need to ask, need to confess), mental acts (e.g., counting, repeating words silently)

The most common obsession is the aversion to dirt or germs, which compels patients with OCD to wash their hands over and over again. If they are concerned about intruders, they may lock, unlock, and relock their doors many times before going to bed or leaving the home. Other common rituals include repeatedly checking things, touching things (especially in a particular sequence), or counting. Some other obsessions include frequent thoughts of violence and harming loved ones, persistently thinking about performing sexual acts the person dislikes, or having thoughts that are contrary to their religious beliefs. The OCD patient may be preoccupied with order and symmetry, have difficulty throwing things out, or hoard items needlessly.[23,39]

The majority of OCD sufferers have multiple obsessions and compulsions during the course of their illness, with a particular fear or concern dominating the clinical picture at any one time.[39] Most of these patients know that their behavior is excessive but some actually lack insight to assist them in recognizing that their compulsions and obsessions are unreasonable. The age of onset is late adolescence or young adulthood, although it can begin at any age; childhood onset is not uncommon and earlier for men than women.[39] The course is chronic and waxes and wanes in severity, often in response to work/life stress. Mood disorders (e.g., major depression), other anxiety disorders, eating disorders, substance abuse, and psychotic illness are often seen with OCD. Unlike other anxiety disorders already discussed, OCD affects men and women equally.[23]

In cases of PTSD, an individual must be exposed to a traumatic event that evoked an actual or perceived threat to the person's life or physical integrity and continues to elicit intense fear, helplessness, and/or horror.[40] Of important note is that PTSD was first brought to the attention of the public through its relationship to war veterans, but it can result from a variety of traumatic incidents.[23,40] Examples of traumatic events include combat, child or spousal/partner abuse/neglect, rape/sexual assault, terrorism, motor vehicle accidents, natural disasters, community or domestic violence, captivity, and torture. Patients with PTSD may have an exaggerated startle response or become emotionally numb (especially in relation to those whom they were previously close to), lose interest in things they used to enjoy, have trouble feeling affectionate, become more aggressive or violent, and be irritable. There is high avoidance behavior to placing themselves in situations that might remind them of the trauma. Anniversaries of the incident are quite difficult.

The common signs and symptoms of PTSD include the following:

- **Re-experiencing**—recurrent, intrusive distressing memories of the trauma, recurring, disturbing dreams of the event, feeling that the traumatic event is recurring (e.g., flashbacks), physiologic reaction to reminders of the trauma
- **Avoidance**—avoidance of conversations, thoughts, or feelings about the trauma; avoidance of activities that are reminders of the trauma and of people or places that arouse recollections; inability to recall an important aspect of the trauma, anhedonia, estrangement from others, restricted affect, sense of foreshortened future, praying
- **Hyperarousal**—decreased concentration, easily startled, hypervigilance, insomnia, irritability, or angry outbursts

Not every trauma victim will develop full-blown or even minor PTSD.[23,40] Symptoms usually begin within 3 months of the event but occasionally can emerge years later. Symptoms must last for more than a month to be considered PTSD, with a varying course of illness. Some PTSD patients recover within 6 months, whereas others have symptoms that last longer. Posttraumatic stress disorder can become chronic as well, requiring lifelong therapy. Women are more likely to develop PTSD than men, and there is some evidence of a genetic predisposition. As with other anxiety states, PTSD is often seen with other depression, substance abuse, or one or more of the other anxiety states.[23,40]

Treatment

The BAP evidence-based guidelines for the treatment of PTSD and OCD are provided in Tables 34-8 and 34-9, respectively.[25,26] SSRIs are considered first-line therapy for both disorders. Management of both of these anxiety disorders often requires psychotherapy and pharmacotherapy in combination as initial first-line therapy.[39-43] For those who do not respond to the first SSRI with increased dosages (for OCD), the best strategy is to try another SSRI or SNRI.[34,45] As with other anxiety disorders, an adequate trial of antidepressant pharmacotherapy for PTSD and/or OCD is 8–12 weeks.[46]

CBT is an established treatment for OCD and may be more effective than pharmacotherapy.[39] In CBT, the patient faces a feared object or activity without performing the compulsive ritual. CBT can be used instead of or in addition to SSRIs, depending on patient preference, compliance, or the presence of comorbid illness. CBT might prove valuable in cases of patients who opt out of pharmacotherapy to assist with prevention of relapse.[22,39,40,43]

The American Psychiatric Association and U.S. Departments of Defense and Veterans Affairs have all recommended **eye movement desensitization and reprocessing** (EMDR) as first-line therapy for all anxiety and/or stress trauma cases.[47] In addition, current guidelines from the International Society for Traumatic Stress Studies and the BAP guidelines designate EMDR as an effective treatment for PTSD, listing it among the primary treatments for trauma victims.[25,26,40,48-50]

Psychodynamic interventions (individual or group) may also prove useful for these patients, although their efficacy has not been fully evaluated. Psychodynamic interventions tend to focus on tasks of mourning losses, developing meaning to past and present experiences, facilitating acceptance of one's life, re-establishing self-coherence and awareness of self-continuity, and achieving increased self-confidence.[40] Mind-body interventions (e.g.,

Table 34-8. Summary of British Association for Psychopharmacology Guidelines for Symptom Prevention and Treatment of Post-traumatic Stress Disorder

PTSD Prevention

- Consider propranolol immediately and trauma-focused CBT in individuals with post-traumatic symptoms lasting >1 month
- Routine debriefing is not indicated

PTSD Treatment

- SSRIs are first-line pharmacotherapy
- EMDR is a psychological treatment alternative
- Antidepressants should be used in patients with coexisting severe depressive symptoms
- After initial insufficient response:
  - Consider combining pharmacotherapy and psychological treatment
  - Consider augmentation of antidepressants with atypical antipsychotic after initial non response

CBT = cognitive behavioral therapy; EMDR = eye movement desensitization reprocessing; PTSD = post-traumatic stress disorder; SSRIs = selective serotonin reuptake inhibitors.

Table 34-9. Summary of British Association for Psychopharmacology Guidelines for Treating for Obsessive Compulsive Disorder

- SSRIs are first-line pharmacotherapy
- Routinely combining pharmacotherapy and psychological approaches is not recommended for initial treatment, but consider adding an SSRI or clomipramine to psychological treatment when efficacy needs to be maximized
- After initial treatment failure:
  - Increase dosage of clomipramine or SSRI after initial nonresponse to standard dosing
  - Combine pharmacotherapy and exposure therapy or CBT
  - Augmentation of SSRIs with antipsychotics or pindolol

CBT = cognitive behavioral therapy; SSRIs = selective serotonin reuptake inhibitors.

mindfulness-based stress reduction, guided imagery, progressive muscle relaxation, meditation, yoga) may also be of great benefit to patients.[22,23,40]

Finally, augmentation pharmacotherapy with antipsychotic medications (haloperidol, risperidone, quetiapine, and olanzapine), clonazepam, or pindolol (OCD) might be the best choice for treatment-resistant cases.[44,51-57] Although the atypical antipsychotics (APs) (e.g., risperidone, quetiapine, olanzapine) are associated with reduced side effects compared with conventional antipsychotics, they are not without risk. All APs and first-generation agents (e.g., haloperidol, perphenazine) now carry a black-box warning of an increased risk of death in elderly patients with dementia-related psychosis.[58] The most significant potential adverse effects of APs include extrapyramidal symptoms (EPS), tardive dyskinesia, weight gain (a major cause of nonadherence), diabetes mellitus, dyslipidemia, and hyperprolactinemia.[59] Regarding the risk of EPS, clozapine is < quetiapine < olanzapine = ziprasidone < first generation antipsychotics (e.g., haloperidol, fluphenazine, perphenazine).[59] Risperidone has a higher EPS risk at higher dosages, but considerably less at lower dosages.[59]

Monitoring and Follow-up

OCD and PTSD patients require a significant amount of close monitoring and follow-up. OCD is often a chronic lifelong illness with a waxing and waning course.[40,44] Even those who improved over a period of years continue to have residual symptoms. Discontinuation of treatment for OCD is clearly associated with relapse, regardless of treatment duration.[59,60] Therefore, it is recommended that treatment be continued for OCD and PTSD patients for a minimum of 1–2 years in SSRI-responsive individuals.[26,44] Most importantly, these patients need routine psychotherapy and self-care techniques tailored to their individual needs.

BODY DYSMORPHIC DISORDER

(See Web Resources for Patient Case: Body Dysmorphic Disorder.)

Additional content available at
www.ashp.org/womenshealth

Clinical Presentation and Diagnosis

Body dysmorphic disorder (BDD) is a somatoform disorder that is characterized by a preoccupation with an imagined or exaggerated defect in physical appearance. The common feature of the somatoform disorders is the presence of physical symptoms that suggest a general medical condition and are not fully explained by a general medical condition, by the direct effects of a substance, or by another mental disorder.[61]

The diagnostic criteria for BDD are threefold: 1) preoccupation with an imagined defect in appearance; 2) this preoccupation causes clinically significant distress or impairment in social, occupational, or other important areas of functioning; and 3) the preoccupation is not better accounted for by another mental disorder.[61]

Treatment

Management of BDD includes medication, psychotherapy, CBT, and self-care. The literature suggests that SSRIs are successful in treating BDD, usually at higher dosages than needed for depression—fluoxetine at up to 80 mg/day or sertraline at up to 250 mg/day. The mean response to treatment time when SSRIs are used for BDD is 6–16 weeks.[62] CBT may also be helpful as treatment for BDD, often in addition to SSRIs.

Monitoring and Follow-up

BDD is considered a chronic condition and requires ongoing monitoring and follow-up. SSRI management every 2–3 months with a tailored, individual therapy schedule is reasonable.

Gender-Related Considerations for Mental Health

As mentioned earlier, women are twice as likely to develop major depression as compared with men.[1,2] Victimization and family history are also contributory factors. Women have a higher predisposition toward anxiety disorders, with >13% meeting the diagnostic criteria compared with 6% of men.[2-6] Women are approximately twofold more likely to meet lifetime criteria for panic disorder (5% vs. 2%), agoraphobia (7% vs. 3.5%), simple phobia (15.6% vs. 6.7%), PTSD (11.3% vs. 6%), GAD (6.6% vs. 3.6%), SAD (15.5% vs. 11.1%), and OCD (3.1% vs. 2%).[3-6] The impact of sex is profound, increasing the likelihood of developing an anxiety disorder by 85% in women compared with men.[3] There are no gender considerations for BDD, as it affects both men and women with equal frequency.

Mental Health Patient Education

Self-care, lifestyle adjustments, and overall wellness are key elements to successful treatment of patients with mental illness. Patients must be educated about their mental health, psychotherapy treatments, and medications such that they can come to recognize and cope with these illnesses, as well as be able to help themselves or seek professional help at the appropriate time. Patients need to understand the importance of maintaining compliance and continued therapy for several months or at least a year in many cases. Risk of relapse and the possible need for lifelong therapy must also be explained to the patient. Finally, it is important to keep in mind that mental health education must be individualized based on the specifics of each patient's care plan.

Summary

As evidenced by the case studies provided in this chapter, careful clinical screening, patient monitoring (e.g., treatment response, adverse events), and follow-up are absolutely essential in mental health. Anxiety and depression are usually prolonged and recurrent conditions that are rarely "cured" completely. Thus, mental health often requires a chronic disease management approach. The good news is that there are a number of treatment choices and combinations available. Current recommendations support the use of psychotherapy along with pharmacotherapy plus some form of stress-management intervention and self-care. Patients must be encouraged to take an active role in their treatment and make necessary lifestyle adjustments if needed. When treating mental illness, it takes a concerted effort by all parties involved to create a successful individualized care plan that may require significant adjustments over the life course of the illness.

References

Additional content available at
www.ashp.org/womenshealth

35 Sexual Disorders

Candace S. Brown, Pharm.D., MSN; Sandra R. Leiblum, Ph.D.

Learning Objectives

1. Differentiate between the female and male sexual response.
2. Compare and contrast criteria for the diagnosis of female sexual desire disorders, sexual arousal disorders, orgasmic disorders, and sexual pain disorders.
3. Describe how medical conditions, medications, and psychological factors contribute to female sexual dysfunction.
4. Apply consensus statements to appropriately classify female sexual disorders and female androgen deficiency.
5. Discuss psychological, hormonal, herbal, and educational treatments of female sexual disorder.

Normal Sexual Response: Sex Differences

Most healthcare providers are aware of the traditional human sexual response cycle of Masters and Johnson and Kaplan and Passalacqua.[1,2] This cycle depicts a linear sequence of discrete events, including desire, arousal, plateau of constant high arousal, peak intensity arousal, and release of **orgasm,** possible repeated orgasms, and then resolution. An alternative sexual response model for women has been suggested by Basson.[3] This model incorporates the importance of emotional intimacy, sexual stimuli, and relationship satisfaction. It acknowledges that compared with male sexual functioning, female sexual response is more circuitous and more affected by psychosocial issues. Women may enter the cycle at multiple points, and their goal is not necessarily orgasm, but personal satisfaction, which may include physical or emotional satisfaction or both.

Female Sexual Dysfunction

Recent population surveys highlight the fact that female sexual disorders are highly prevalent. Comparison between countries is problematic because different definitions and methodologies are used in different surveys. The National Health and Social Life Survey was conducted in 1992 and involved personal interviews with a probability sample of the U.S. population between the ages of 18 and 59 years.[4] The survey found that 43% of women reported significant sexual symptoms lasting several months in the preceding year. The most common concern was lack of sexual interest (reported by 33% of women), followed by difficulty reaching orgasm (24%) and problems with lubrication (19%). The survey did not include older women. Although there is a natural decline in sexual desire, intensity of orgasm, and reduced lubrication in postmenopausal women, a woman's sexuality in later years is often related to her function earlier in her life. As with women of any age, a significant change in sexual function suggests a need for further evaluation.

Clinical Presentation and Diagnosis

The Sexual Function Health Council of the American Foundation convened a consensus conference for urologic disease in 1998 to review and update the classification of female sexual disorders.[5] The consensus conference panel built on the existing framework of the World Health Organization International Classification of Disease-10 (ICD-10) and the *Diagnostic and Statistical Manual of Mental Disorders IV (DSM-IV)* of the American Psychiatric

Case Presentation

Patient Case: Part 1

A.L. is a 38-year-old white woman who reports low libido, which began 1 year earlier. She says she "never cares if I ever have sex again" and she goes to bed after her spouse is asleep to avoid sexual activity. She does not think about sexual activity and denies self-stimulation. She is distressed because she misses her desire and feels guilty because she feels she is disappointing her spouse. She has adequate lubrication, denies pain with intercourse, and is orgasmic.

Typical encounter: Intercourse once weekly on partner's initiation, when she feels he needs relief. Sexual activity on weekends when she is well rested and there is plenty of privacy and sufficient time.

HPI: Normal sexual desire before surgery. Also reports hot flashes and night sweats, as well as fatigue and decreased sense of well-being, which has improved since starting hormone therapy but remains somewhat troublesome.

PMH: Hypertension (controlled), hypothyroidism (controlled), mammogram and Pap test current and normal, status post **leiomyoma**, NKDA.

Surgeries: Total abdominal hysterectomy, bilateral salpingo-oophorectomy (TAH/BSO) because of fibroids 1 year ago; two vaginal deliveries.

Current medications: Lisinopril 10 mg daily × 2 years; levothyroxine 0.1 mg PO daily × 3 years; estradiol 0.5 mg PO daily × 1 year; estradiol cream 1 gPV 3x/wk × 1 year.

Past medications: Hydrochlorothiazide 25 mg BID × 1 year.

Social history: No tobacco, occasional alcohol, walks 20 minutes 3 times/week.

Psychiatric history: Nonsignificant for psychiatric disorder, individual or relationship counseling.

Family history: Mother—hypothyroidism; father—hypertension, diabetes.

Developmental/sexual history: Normal childhood with no sexual abuse, significant losses, or parental issues. Adequate sexual education about menses and sex. First sexual experience at 18 years with current partner and pleasurable.

Relationship history: Marriage of 19 years characterized by good communication, mutual respect, and commitment. Enjoy similar activities, have similar attitudes about child rearing, and finds spouse sexually attractive. Partner sexually functional. Has 10- and 12-year-old sons.

Stressors: Denies stressors such as finances, parenting, deaths, work, or illness.

Psychiatric exam/MSE: Normal speech, coherent thought process, average judgment/insight, and euthymic. MSE reveals a 38-year-old woman who appears her stated age, slightly overweight, oriented × 3, focused, of average intellect, and with intact memory.

Vital signs: 5′5″, 170 lb (BMI = 28), BP 124/80, HR 72, RR 16, Temp 98.6°F.

Pelvic examination: Mild vulvar atrophy with no evidence of episiotomy scars.

Laboratory values: Cholesterol, complete metabolic panel, TSH, CBC + differential WNL, estradiol 72 (35–500 pg/mL, premenopausal range), free testosterone 0.9 (1.1–6.3 pg/mL), SHBG 50 (40–120 nmol/L).

Association.[6,7] The former *DSM-IV* classifications were expanded to include psychogenic and organic cause of desire, arousal, orgasm, and sexual pain disorders. An essential element of this new classification system was the personal distress criterion, meaning that a condition was considered a disorder only if it created distress for the woman experiencing the condition.[5,8] Table 35-1 lists the most current classification system. With the upcoming release of the *DSM-V,* however, some revisions may occur.

Each sexual disorder is subtyped as lifelong vs. acquired type, generalized vs. situational type, and etiologic origin (organic, psychogenic, mixed, unknown). Subtyping is based ideally on evidence from the medical history, laboratory tests, and physical examination.

The Sexual Health Council of the American Foundation of Urologic Diseases convened a second consensus conference in 2003.[8-10] The recommendations from the second conference were based on using a circular model for female sexual disorders and in subtyping sexual arousal disorders. At present, the most widely accepted nomenclature for the diagnosis of women's sexual disorders continues to be the text revision of *DSM-IV*

Table 35-1. Classification of Sexual Dysfunction Disorders

- Sexual desire disorders
  - Hypoactive sexual desire disorder (sexual interest/desire disorder)
  - Sexual aversion disorder
- Female sexual arousal disorders
  - Subjective sexual arousal disorder
  - Genital sexual arousal disorder
  - Combined genital and subjective arousal disorder
  - Persistent sexual arousal disorder
- Female orgasmic disorder
- Sexual pain disorders
  - Dyspareunia
  - Vaginismus
  - Noncoital pain disorder
- Vulvodynia[a]
  - Generalized vulvodynia (essential dysesthetic vulvodynia)
  - Localized vulvodynia (vestibulodynia, vulvar vestibulitis syndrome)

Source: Adapted from references 5, 8, 9, and 12.

[a]Not classified as a sexual dysfunction disorder.

(DSM-IV-TR), published in 2000, and the first consensus conference.[5,7]

SEXUAL DESIRE DISORDERS

Hypoactive sexual desire disorder (HSDD), also known as sexual interest/desire disorder, is defined as the absence or diminished feelings of sexual interest or desire, absent sexual thoughts or fantasies, and a lack of responsive desire, which causes personal distress.[5,8-10] Motivations (e.g., reasons or incentives) for attempting to become sexually aroused are scarce or absent. The lack of interest is considered to be beyond a normative lessening with life cycle and relationship duration. What is considered crucial in the new definition is the persistent absence of receptive desire and motivation to be sexual along with personal distress about the condition.[10]

Sexual aversion disorder is defined as an extreme anxiety and/or disgust at the anticipation of/or attempt to have any sexual activity, which causes personal distress.

FEMALE SEXUAL AROUSAL DISORDERS

Female sexual arousal disorder (FSAD) is the persistent or recurrent inability to attain or maintain sufficient sexual excitement, causing personal distress, which may be expressed as subjective, genital, or combined genital and subjective arousal disorder.[5,8-10] Subjective sexual arousal disorder is the absence of or markedly diminished feelings of sexual arousal (sexual excitement and sexual pleasure) from any type of sexual stimulation. Genital sexual arousal disorder refers to symptoms of absent or impaired genital sexual arousal. Self-reports may include minimal vulvar swelling or vaginal lubrication from any type of sexual stimulation and reduced sexual sensations from caressing genitalia. Combined genital and subjective arousal disorder is absence of or markedly diminished feelings of sexual arousal from any type of sexual stimulation, as well as symptoms of absent or impaired genital sexual arousal.

Persistent sexual arousal disorder is defined as a spontaneous, intrusive, and unwanted genital arousal (e.g., tingling, throbbing, pulsating) in the absence of sexual interest and desire.[8-10] Any awareness of subjective arousal is typically unpleasant. The arousal is unrelieved by one or more orgasms, and the feelings of arousal persist for hours or days.

FEMALE ORGASMIC DISORDER

Female orgasmic disorder (FOD) is defined as the persistent or recurrent difficulty, delay in, or absence of attaining orgasm following sufficient sexual stimulation and arousal, which causes personal distress.[5,8-10]

This condition is usually further subdivided into either primary or secondary FOD. Primary orgasmic disorder refers to a woman's inability to achieve an orgasm under any circumstances. A secondary orgasmic disorder most often refers to an inability to reach climax only during intercourse, but otherwise can be achieved either with masturbation or during sexual foreplay. Inability to have orgasm via intercourse is common, occurring in approximately one third of women, and is only problematic if it distresses the woman.[11] Implicit in this definition is an acceptance that a woman does not have a release during her experience of arousal and this lack of release is distressing to her.

SEXUAL PAIN DISORDERS

Three types of sexual pain disorders have been classified. Dyspareunia is defined as persistent or recurrent genital pain associated with intercourse that causes interpersonal distress.[5,8-10] It may be related to the lack of elasticity and vaginal atrophy in the postmenopausal woman, but it is not caused exclusively by lack of lubrication.

Vaginismus is a recurrent or persistent involuntary spasm of the musculature of the outer third of the vagina that interferes with vaginal penetration and causes personal distress.[5,8-10] There is current debate about whether a vaginal spasm is responsible for the pain or whether it is a variable involuntary pelvic muscle contraction associated with phobic avoidance and anticipation or fear of the experience of pain.[8-10] Structural or other physical abnormalities must be ruled out.

Noncoital pain disorders are recurrent or persistent genital pain induced by noncoital sexual stimulation.[5,8-10] This category acknowledges that pain may be experienced by a woman during sexual activities other than intercourse.

VULVODYNIA

Vulvodynia is not listed as a sexual pain disorder by either *DSM-IV (DSM-IV-TR)* or the consensus conferences.[5,8-10] It is included in this chapter because this condition should be ruled out before making a diagnosis of a sexual pain disorder; vulvodynia is also discussed in Chapter 39: Genitourinary Disorders. Vulvodynia is defined as vulvar discomfort, most often described as burning pain, occurring in the absence of relevant visible findings or a specific clinically identifiable neurologic disorder.[12-14] It is not caused by commonly identified infection, inflammation, neoplasia, or a neurologic disorder.[14]

The classification of vulvodynia is based on the site of pain, whether it is generalized or localized, and whether it is provoked, unprovoked, or mixed. Two subtypes of vulvodynia have been described. Generalized vulvodynia ("essential dysesthetic vulvodynia") is associated with a constant diffuse pain affecting the **labia major, labia minora,** and/or **vestibule.** Localized vulvodynia ("vestibulodynia or vulvar vestibulitis") is characterized by focal pain aggravated by touch and pressure, intercourse, and speculum insertion.[12,13]

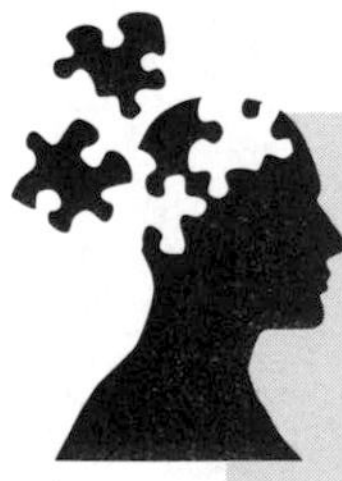

Therapeutic Challenge:

Can a woman be diagnosed with both HSDD and FSAD? If so, how would you decide which is the primary disorder and which is the secondary disorder?

Pathophysiology

Although there are still large gaps in our understanding of female sexual function, sex steroids and neurotransmitters in the central and peripheral nervous system appear to play a significant role.[15] In the central nervous system (CNS), the neurotransmitter dopamine appears to modulate sexual desire. In addition, dopamine, along with norepinephrine, increases the sense of sexual excitement and the desire to continue sexual activity.[16] Increasing levels of serotonin can diminish the effects of both dopamine and norepinephrine, whereas melanocortins, small protein hormones, may have a stimulatory effect on dopamine.[17] Estrogen and testosterone function may, at least in part, be modulated by the effects of serotonin activity in the hypothalamus and associated limbic structures.[16] Other hormones also are involved in CNS modulation of sexual behavior. These include oxytocin, which may enhance sexual receptivity and orgasmic response.[18] Conversely, the pituitary hormone prolactin negatively influences the sexual excitement phase and is inversely related to dopamine function (Figure 35-1).[17]

In the periphery, sex hormones are important mediators of genital structures and function.[15] Nitric oxide (NO) and vasoactive intestinal peptide

Figure 35-1. Central effect of neurotransmitters and hormones on sexual functioning. The symbols indicate a positive effect (+); negative effect (−); and unknown effect (?). (Adapted from reference 15; Munarriz R, Kim NN, Goldstein I, et al. Biology of female sexual function. *Urol Clin North Am.* 2002;29:685-693; and Clayton AH. Sexual function and dysfunction in women. *Psychiatr Clin North Am.* 2003;263:673-682.)

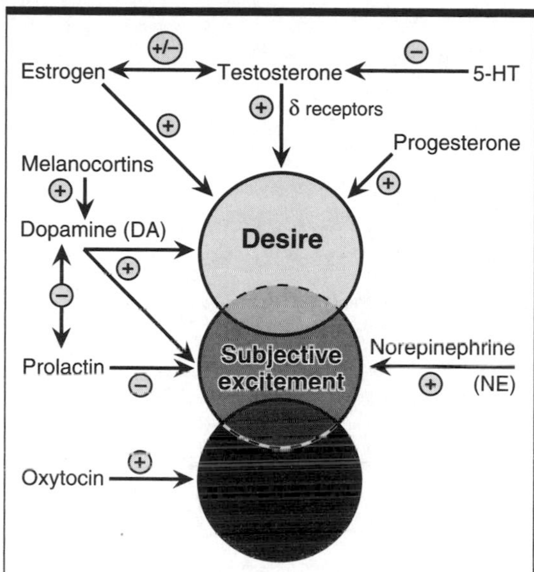

Figure 35-2. Peripheral effects of neurotransmitters and hormones on sexual functioning. The symbols indicate a positive effect (+); negative effect (−); and unknown effect (?). (Adapted from reference 15; Munarriz R, Kim NN, Goldstein I, et al. Biology of female sexual function. *Urol Clin North Am.* 2002;29:685-693; and Clayton AH. Sexual function and dysfunction in women. *Psychiatr Clin North Am.* 2003;263:673-682.)

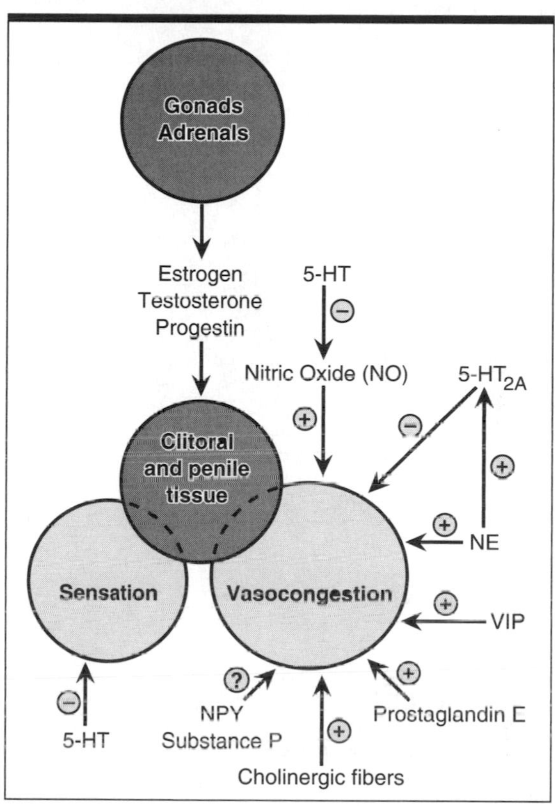

are implicated in engorgement of clitoral tissue following sexual stimulation; however, adequate levels of estrogen and free testosterone are needed for NO to stimulate **vasocongestion.** Peripheral serotonin has negative effects on vasocongestion, NO function, and sensation. Prostaglandin E and cholinergic fibers also induce vasocongestion (Figure 35-2).

MEDICAL CONDITIONS

Numerous medical conditions are associated with sexual dysfunction, including neurologic, cardiovascular, gynecologic, and endocrine disorders (Table 35-2).[19-22]

Neurologic disease frequently alters sexual response. Injuries to the spinal cord and peripheral nerves that link genitalia to limbic and cognitive centers can profoundly influence arousal and orgasmic function.[23] In epilepsy, expressions of hypersexuality and hyposexuality occur as a result of epileptogenic activity in the temporolimbic system. Multiple sclerosis affects all phases of sexual response, but Parkinson's disease is more likely to affect desire, whereas stroke most often produces inorgasmia.[22]

Female sexual dysfunction may result from cardiovascular and peripheral vascular disease because of insufficient blood flow to the genitalia, causing decreased genital congestion and swelling, with consequent vaginal dryness and dyspareunia.[19,20] Inorgasmia has also been reported in hypertension. Myocardial infarction is associated with low libido because of concerns over exacerbating heart problems.

Numerous gynecologic conditions can affect sexual functioning. Gynecologic malignancies, such as endometrial cancer, may cause abnormal bleeding and abdominal discomfort before the diagnosis, which may stop women from engaging in any type of sexual activity.[20] Additionally, radiation and chemotherapy used in gynecologic cancer treatment

Table 35-2. Medical Conditions Associated with Female Sexual Dysfunction

Medical Condition	Type of Sexual Dysfunction
Neurologic disorders	
Epilepsy	↓↑Desire
Head injury	↓Arousal,[a] dyspareunia
Multiple sclerosis	All types
Parkinson disease	↓Desire
Spinal cord and peripheral nerve injuries	↓Arousal, inorgasmia
Stroke	Inorgasmia
Cardiovascular disease	
Coronary artery disease	↓Arousal, dyspareunia
Hypercholesterolemia	↓Arousal, dyspareunia
Hypertension	↓Arousal, dyspareunia, inorgasmia
Myocardial infarction	↓Desire
Renal failure	↓Arousal, dyspareunia
Peripheral vascular disease	↓Arousal, dyspareunia
Gynecologic disorders/cancer	
Breast cancer	↓Desire
Endometrial cancer	↓Arousal, dyspareunia
Ovarian cancer	↓Desire, ↓arousal, dyspareunia
Primary ovarian insufficiency	↓Desire, ↓arousal, dyspareunia
Stress and urinary incontinence	↓Desire, dyspareunia
Uterine prolapse	Inorgasmia
Endocrine disorders	
Adrenal insufficiency	↓Desire, ↓arousal
Androgen deficiency	↓Desire, ↓arousal
Diabetes mellitus	↓Arousal, inorgasmia
Estrogen deficiency	↓Desire, ↓arousal, dyspareunia
Hyperprolactinemia	↓Desire, ↓arousal
Hypothyroidism/hyperthyroidism	↓Desire

Source: Adapted from references 19–22.

[a]Refers to genital arousal or genital lubrication, swelling, and tingling.

may have adverse effects on vaginal elasticity and thickness of the vaginal wall, causing dyspareunia and problems with sexual arousal.[24] Malignancies also are associated with psychological and social difficulties, and may impair self-image and decrease sexual desire. This issue is particularly important in conditions that may impair a woman's sense of sexuality, such as in breast or ovarian cancer.[25] Urogenital disorders, characterized by stress and urge incontinence or uterine prolapse, may also affect a women's comfort during sexual activity for fear of leakage or appearance of genitals, affecting all phases of sexual response.[21,22]

Hormonal changes associated with menopause and aging, such as estrogen or androgen depletion, often cause important physical and psychological adverse effects on female sexual response.[21] Estrogen depletion often leads to dyspareunia, sleep disturbances, mood swings, depression, and decreased desire. The thinning of the vaginal epithelium, atrophy of the vaginal wall smooth muscle, and elevated pH changes in the vagina may ultimately result in vaginal dryness and pain during intercourse. In androgen depletion, symptoms include muscle wasting, mood changes, and loss of sexual motivation, including a decrease in libido and a diminution in sexual fantasy.[21,26] Because diabetes leads to decreased peripheral perfusion and autonomic neuropathy, reduced arousal and inorgasmia occur. Other hormonal imbalances that may affect sexual desire and arousal are adrenal insufficiency, hyperprolactinemia, and thyroid dysfunction.[21,26]

MEDICATIONS

Neurotransmitters are involved in all three phases of the human sexual response, thus the pharmacology of the agent determines its sexual side effects (Figure 35-3).[27]

The sexual enhancing and sexual side effects in medications are related to whether they facilitate or inhibit these neurotransmitters. Table 35-3 lists medications that affect the three phases of the sexual response.

The most common medications associated with female sexual dysfunction are the selective serotonin reuptake inhibitors (SSRIs) (Table 35-2).[11,20,28,29] Delay or absence of orgasm with reduced sexual desire occurs in up to 70% of women taking SSRIs.[11,20,28] In general, any antidepressants that interfere with serotonergic pathways (nonselectively), such as SSRIs, or with acetylcholine pathways, such as tricyclic antidepressants, may inhibit all phases of the sexual response. In contrast, antidepressants that affect dopaminergic and (central) noradrenergic receptors, or selective hydroxytryptamine (5-HT_{1A} and 5-HT_2 receptors), are not likely to reduce sexual response.[11,20,28] Therefore, those antidepressants least likely to interfere with sexual response include non-SSRI antidepressants, such as nefazodone, mirtazapine, bupropion, venlafaxine (at doses of 150 mg or greater), duloxetine, and buspirone.[11,20,28]

Figure 35-3. Psychopharmacology of sex. In stage 1, desire, dopamine (DA), melanocortin, testosterone, and estrogen exert a positive influence, whereas prolactin and serotonin (5HT) have negative effects. In stage 2, arousal correlates with genital swelling and lubrication in women. Several neurotransmitters facilitate sexual arousal, including nitric oxide (NO), norepinephrine (NE), melanocortin, testosterone, estrogen, acetylcholine (ACh) and DA. As with desire, 5HT has a negative effect. Stage 3, orgasm, is inhibited by 5HT and facilitated by NE; DA and NO may have weak positive influences. (Reprinted with permission from reference 27.)

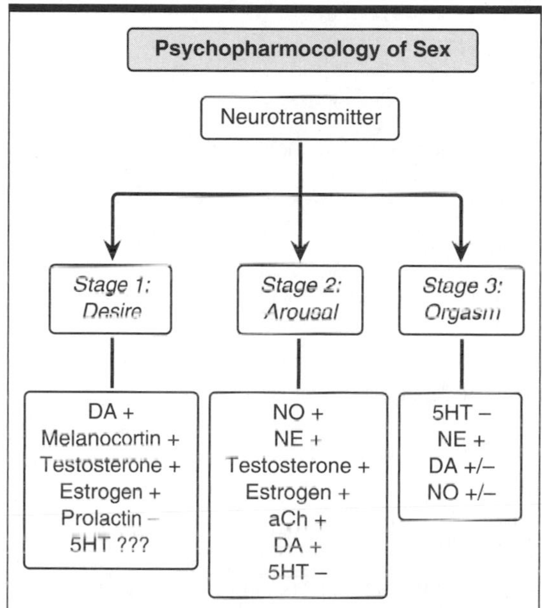

Other centrally acting medications—including psychoactive substances, such as antipsychotics, barbiturates, benzodiazepines, and codeine-containing opiates—may affect all stages of sexual function.[11,20,28,30,31] Anticonvulsants that induce P450 hepatic enzymes, such as carbamazepine and phenytoin, decrease desire by increasing sex hormone binding globulin (SHBG) and reducing free testosterone.[32] Anticholinergic agents, which interfere with acetylcholine function, such as antihistamines, impair genital arousal and lubrication.[11,20,28]

Antihypertensives that penetrate the blood-brain barrier, such as beta-blockers and centrally acting antihypertensives, as well as diuretics, may reduce sexual desire, arousal, and orgasmic function.[11,20,28,33]

Table 35-3. Medications Associated with Female Sexual Dysfunction

Pharmacologic Class	Type of Sexual Dysfunction
Anticholinergics	
Antihistamines	↓Arousal
Anticonvulsants	
P450 hepatic enzyme inducers	↓Desire
Antihypertensives	
Beta-blockers	All types
Centrally acting agents (clonidine, methyldopa)	All types
Diuretics	All types
Antilipemics	All types
Hormones	
Gonadotropin-releasing hormone agonists	↓Desire, ↓arousal
Progestins	↓↑Desire
Oral contraceptives	↓↑Desire
Estrogen agonists antagonists	↓Desire, ↓arousal
Opiates	All types
Psychoactive medications	
Antipsychotics	All types
Barbiturates	All types
Benzodiazepines	All types
Selective serotonergic reuptake inhibitors (SSRIs)	All types
Tricyclic antidepressants	All types

Source: Adapted from references 11, 20, and 28.

However, calcium channel blockers and angiotensin-converting enzyme (ACE) inhibitors are generally not considered to have sexual side effects.[11,20,28] Other cardiovascular agents, such as antilipemics, may induce sexual problems.[11,20,28]

Agents that interfere with the hypothalamic-pituitary-ovarian axis, such as gonadotropic-releasing hormone agonists, like leuprolide, are likely to inhibit desire and arousal.[11,20,28] Some estrogen agonists antagonists may have estrogen antagonistic activity in the vagina. Thus, raloxifene, tamoxifen, and phytoestrogens may reduce libido and exacerbate vaginal dryness and dyspareunia.[11,20,28]

The effect of oral contraceptives (OCs) on sexual desire is unclear. Reduced libido is biologically plausible, because OCs significantly decrease circulating androgens. However, OCs also provide positive effects on sexuality, such as decreased risk of pregnancy, decreased bleeding, decreased pain, or improved acne and hirsutism. One would anticipate that increased dosages of estrogen or progestin, mode of delivery (transdermal, vaginal ring), or the androgenic potency of progestins would affect sexual desire, but a review of the research does not show a consistent relationship with these factors.[34] Clearly, more research is warranted. Until then, healthcare providers must be cautious in attributing negative experiences to OCs and be willing to explore other explanations for the common experience of decreased libido.

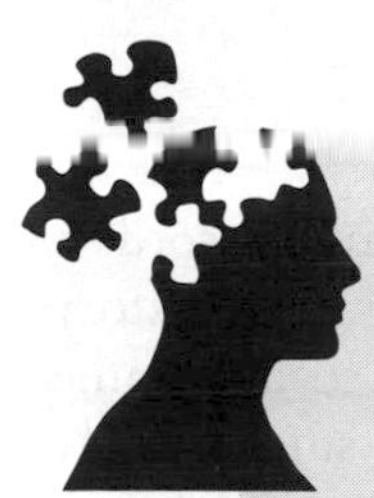

Therapeutic Challenge:

Some women report low sexual desire as a result of taking OCs. In what situation(s) may OCs have a positive effect on libido?

PSYCHOLOGICAL FACTORS

Individual Factors

Low libido frequently accompanies major depression. Women who report mood changes, sleep disturbance, fatigue, decreased concentration, low self-esteem, reduced interest in activities, decreased energy and motivation, and appetite or weight changes may report improvements in their sexual desire if their depression is effectively treated.

Women who are under stress often feel they do not have time to engage in sexual activity and may view it as just "another job." Those who work full time, take care of children, and carry major responsibility for domestic activities may feel resentful toward their partner. Other life stressors—such as financial, family or job problems, or family illness or death—may also affect sexual functioning.

Although alcohol and other recreational substances may temporarily produce a "disinhibiting" effect on women who are anxious about sexual activity, chronic substance abuse impairs sexual function.

Many researchers report a relationship between sexual or physical abuse and female sexual dysfunction.[35] Other psychological factors that commonly affect sexual response in women include body image concerns and concerns about pregnancy and sexually transmitted disease.

Relationship Factors

The most common cause of women's sexual dysfunction is partner dissatisfaction. A variety of factors may contribute to this, including poor communication, infidelity, control issues, partner substance abuse, and parental conflicts. Current sexual, verbal, or physical abuse may be a significant factor as well.

Lack of privacy because of the presence of children or relatives living with a couple may also affect a woman's comfort in engaging in sexual activity. Finally, partner dysfunction, such as **erectile dysfunction** or early or delayed ejaculation, may reduce a woman's motivation to be sexual.

Sociocultural Factors

Many women are raised to believe that premarital sexual activity is sinful. For these women, the transition to guilt-free sexual function may be difficult. Similarly, women receiving the message that sex is "dirty" may find it difficult to view sexual intimacy as an "act of love" in a committed relationship. A lack of positive sexual messages and education characterize the upbringing of women from diverse cultures and interferes with sexual spontaneity and pleasure for many women. With the increasing number of women immigrating from Africa and Asia to the U.S., female genital mutilation (or female circumcision) involving partial or total removal of the female genitalia is increasingly being seen.

Detection, Screening, and Diagnosis

SEXUAL HISTORY

A comprehensive sexual history is the essential first step in diagnosing female sexual disorders. Sexual inquiry should proceed from the general to specific and should provide adequate time to explore the patient's concerns.[36] The onset, duration, and precipitating factors for the patient's chief sexual symptom should be elicited, as well as the determination of whether the symptom is situational or generalized (present in all settings) and whether it is lifelong or acquired. It is important to ask why the patient is seeking treatment at this time, about the amount of distress, and about the woman's motivation for treatment, as these factors may affect compliance with therapy. It is useful to determine attempts to remedy the problem, including previous medical or psychological treatment.

A thorough medical history—particularly surgeries, neurologic, endocrinologic, cardiovascular, and genitourinary disorders—should be obtained to determine illness-induced contributory factors. A personal and family history of illnesses of hypertension, cardiovascular disease, cerebral vascular accidents, and cancer should be ascertained, as prescribing hormone therapy will depend on these factors. Current medications should be identified to determine any drug-induced sexual dysfunction. Past medications should be recorded to determine previous response and assess if a change in medications is required.

The psychiatric history should include previous treatments, hospitalizations, and suicide attempts as well any past or current history of substance abuse. Areas to be discussed during the family history include ethnicity, religion, and parental relationship, including cultural factors, such as beliefs about sexuality.

The development and sexual history should include childhood, adolescent, and adult categories. Childhood should include any losses, number of friends, family role, sexual knowledge, and sexual abuse. Response to pubertal changes, body image, masturbation, and onset of sexual activity should be elicited.

Relationship history should concentrate on the current relationship, including partner description, conflicts, loss of trust or infidelity, communication problems, control issues, conflicts over parenting, and intimacy. Current stressors and their relationship to the onset of sexual disturbance can be helpful to establish their association with the problem.

PHYSICAL EXAMINATION

Physical examination is crucial for diagnosing sexual pain disorders, including chronic pelvic pain, vaginal infections, vaginal atrophy, vulvodynia, and certain bladder conditions.[11,19] The role of a detailed physical examination for low sexual desire and orgasmic disorder is less obvious. Nevertheless, it can reassure the woman to know that the results of her physical examination are normal.

PSYCHOMETRIC TESTS

Sexual function is typically assessed via self-report (questionnaires or diaries) and healthcare provider interviews.[37] Both modes have their advantages and drawbacks: the accuracy of self-report depends on the willingness of the subject to provide truthful responses, whereas the interview can be subject to healthcare provider bias. A healthcare provider's perceived judgment or intimidation may significantly affects a woman's comfort level in discussing her sexual concerns.

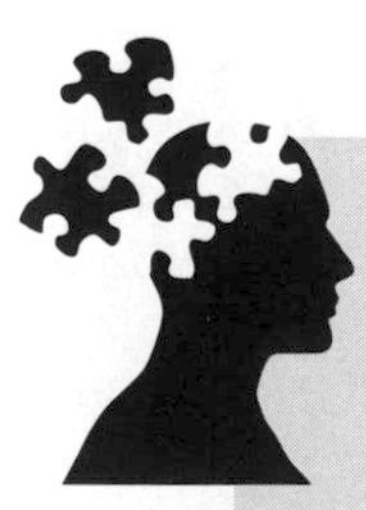

Therapeutic Challenge:

Which components of the sexual history would be appropriate for a pharmacist to elicit in a timely manner?

LABORATORY TESTING

Use of laboratory testing to detect sexual disorders is often unnecessary because the medical history and physical exam are often sufficient to determine diagnosis and treatment.[38,39] However, studies show that significantly more women with an estradiol level of <50 pg/mL report vaginal dryness, dyspareunia, and pain compared with women with an estradiol level of >50 pg/mL.[40] Prospective records of coital behavior and concomitant steroid analysis revealed that women with an estradiol level of <35 pg/mL reported reduced coital activity.[40] Follicle-stimulating hormone testing may be used to detect perimenopause, but it should not be used for monitoring hormone therapy because it is an inaccurate marker of estrogen status.

Plasma testosterone levels are insensitive and inaccurate unless the dialysis method is used. Consequently, most experts do not recommend obtaining levels for diagnosing low sexual desire in androgen-deficient women and suggest obtaining them only when adverse effects are noted with androgen therapy.[38,39]

If a healthcare provider decides to obtain testosterone levels, free rather than total testosterone is a better measure of bioavailable testosterone.[26] In women, only about 1% to 3% of testosterone is free in the blood, the remainder being bound to SHBG (about 65% to 75%) and albumin (about 25% to 35%).[41] Blood samples should be drawn in the morning, typically before 10 A.M., because a diurnal variation in testosterone secretion has been noted with peak levels found in the early morning.[38,39] Salivary testosterone assays are not recommended because of the imprecision of available assays and because they only represent a small fraction of the amount in circulation.[38,39]

When infertility or oligomenorrhea is present, prolactin levels are measured to account for low desire. When signs or symptoms are present (e.g., lethargy, feeling cold, weight gain), thyroid-stimulating hormone levels are measured.[38,39]

Guidelines and Position Statements

PRINCETON CONSENSUS STATEMENT ON FEMALE ANDROGEN INSUFFICIENCY

An international consensus conference on androgen deficiency in women was convened in Princeton, New Jersey, in 2001.[26] The objective was to evaluate the evidence for and against androgen insufficiency as a cause of sexual problems in women and to make recommendations regarding definition, diagnosis, and assessment of deficiency states through evaluating peer-reviewed literature. Three criteria were established for determining a diagnosis of androgen insufficiency:

1. Clinical symptoms of androgen insufficiency should be clearly present, such as a diminished sense of well-being or dysphoric mood; persistent, unexplained fatigue; and sexual function changes, including decreased libido, sexual receptivity, and pleasure.
2. Because estrogen effects are also strongly linked to mood, psychological well-being, and sexual function in women, a diagnosis of androgen insufficiency should be made only in women who are adequately estrogenized.
3. In the absence of a sufficiently sensitive assay or absolute threshold for androgen insufficiency in women, free testosterone values should be at or below the lowest quartile of the normal range for the reproductive age (20–40 years), in conjunction with the presence of clinical symptoms and adequate estrogen status. Selection of the lowest quartile criterion was based, in part, on the insensitivity of current assays at the lower ranges.

THE NORTH AMERICAN MENOPAUSE SOCIETY POSITION STATEMENT ON TESTOSTERONE THERAPY IN POSTMENOPAUSAL WOMEN

In 2005, The North American Menopause Society enlisted a panel of experts to review the medical literature and to establish recommendations on the use of androgens in women.[39] They concluded that postmenopausal women with decreased sexual desire along with personal distress and no other identifiable cause were possible candidates for testosterone therapy; however, testosterone treatment without concomitant estrogen therapy could not be recommended because of lack of evidence. The panel recommended that laboratory testing of testosterone levels should be used only to monitor for supraphysiologic levels before and during therapy, not to diagnose testosterone insufficiency. Although not U.S. Food and Drug Administration (FDA) approved, transdermal patches and topical gels or creams were preferred over oral products because of first-pass hepatic effects documented with oral formulations. Caution was advised for prescribing custom-compounded products and testosterone products formulated specifically for men because the dosing might be more inconsistent than it is with government-approved products. Suggested contraindications for testosterone therapy were women with breast or uterine cancer or those with cardiovascular or liver disease. The group recommended administering the lowest dose for the shortest time that met treatment goals and to counsel patients regarding the potential risk and benefits before initiating therapy.

ENDOCRINE SOCIETY CLINICAL PRACTICE GUIDELINE FOR ANDROGEN THERAPY IN WOMEN

In 2006, the Clinical Guidelines Subcommittee of the U.S. Endocrine Society convened to develop clinical practice guidelines for androgen therapy in women based on available evidence.[38] In contrast to the Princeton Consensus Statement on Female Androgen Insufficiency, the Endocrine Society subcommittee recommended against making a diagnosis of androgen deficiency in women because of the lack of a well-defined clinical syndrome and normative data on total or free testosterone levels across the lifespan that could be used to define the disorder. The subcommittee also disagreed with the Princeton Consensus and the North American Menopause Society recommendations for use of testosterone in postmenopausal women with sexual dysfunction because women initiating therapy may wish to remain sexually active indefinitely, and there was no current evidence of long-term safety.

Prevention

Being raised in a nurturing environment in which adult role models demonstrate affection, provide accurate sexual education, and consider sex to be both positive and healthy is an important prevention against sexual problems.

Goals and General Treatment Guidelines

Women should be educated on normal anatomy, sexual function, and normative sexual changes associated with aging, pregnancy, and menopause. To enhance stimulation and eliminate routine, the healthcare provider should encourage the use of erotic materials (videos and books); self-pleasuring; communication during sexual activity; the use of vibrators; discussion of varying positions, times of day, or places; and making a "date" for sexual activity.

The healthcare provider should encourage noncoital behaviors, such as sensual massage and other noncoital activities, to promote comfort and communication between partners with or without orgasm. For vaginal dyspareunia, recommendations include female astride (woman "on top") for control of penetration, 2% topical lidocaine, warm baths before intercourse, and biofeedback.[14] For deep dyspareunia, position changes are encouraged so that force is away from pain and deep thrusts are minimized; nonsteroidal anti-inflammatory drugs are suggested before intercourse.[11]

Psychological Treatment

Cognitive therapy may help challenge a woman's negative thoughts about herself and about her partner regarding sexual activity.[42] The essence of cognitive therapy consists of exploring unrealistic expectations, self-defeating attitudes, unjustified negative explanations, and illogical conclusions. Cognitive therapy helps correct these negative attitudes and misinterpretations. Examples of negative thoughts a woman may have about herself include "My body is not sexy enough" or "I won't satisfy my partner." Examples of negative thoughts a woman may have about her partner include "How long is this going to take?" or "This is all you're interested in."

Sensate focus, which involves structured exercises progressing from nongenital to genital touch, is often used as a mechanism to reduce anxiety and for a woman to learn more about her body. Relationship or marital therapy may also improve sexual difficulties by enhancing communication among partners.

Pharmacologic Therapy

ALTERING CURRENT THERAPY

Antidepressants

The most common approaches to treating sexual-induced side effects of antidepressants are to switch agents or use of antidotes.[43,44] Case reports indicate adjunctive medications, which treat SSRI-induced **anorgasmia**, include bupropion, yohimbine, amantadine, cyproheptadine, dextroamphetamine, sildenafil, and buspirone.[45-54] Of these drugs, bupropion has received the most research supporting its efficacy.

Antipsychotic

The newer atypical antipsychotics, such as clozapine, olanzapine, and quetiapine, appear to be associated with lower levels of sexual dysfunction than conventional antipsychotics, such as haloperidol, which cause prolactin elevation.[55] The atypical antipsychotic risperidone, which also increases prolactin levels, has higher rates of sexual dysfunction than do olanzapine and quetiapine.[44] Switching from a prolactin-elevating antipsychotic to olanzapine has been reported to restore normal sexual function.[56,57]

Antihypertensive Agents

Antihypertensives that penetrate the blood-brain barrier, such as beta-blockers and centrally acting antihypertensives, as well as diuretics may reduce sexual desire.[20,28,33,58,59] Patients receiving these agents may want to consider switching to calcium channel blockers and ACE inhibitors, which are generally not considered to have sexual side effects.[20,28,33,58,59]

HORMONAL SUPPLEMENTATION

Estrogen Therapy

Although estrogen has both central effects in improving libido and peripheral effects in stimulating genital arousal (Figures 35-1 and 35-2), studies have been inconclusive. Studies from the 1970s did not find any changes in satisfaction, orgasm, or frequency of sexual intercourse or masturbation.[60] More recent randomized controlled trials have reported beneficial effects of oral estrogen therapy (ET) on sexual enjoyment, orgasmic frequency, and vaginal lubrication, but no difference in coital frequency.[61] Another study evaluating transdermal estrogen noted improvement in satisfaction, increase in sexual activity and vaginal lubrication, decreased dyspareunia, but no change in arousal or orgasm frequency.[62]

Dyspareunia caused by atrophy is treated best by vaginal estrogen, either delivered as a cream, tablet, or ring. Many experts initiate systemic ET in the absence of contraindications in postmenopausal women with low libido. Because of the findings from the Women's Health Initiative data, current guidelines recommend that women considering ET should use the lowest effective dose of ET for the shortest duration consistent with the treatment goals of the individual.[63]

Androgen Therapy

The term *androgen* is generally applied to the class of C19 steroids, which are produced by the gonads and the adrenals in both sexes and include testosterone, dehydroepiandrosterone (DHEA), dehydroepiandrosterone sulfate, androstenedione, and 5 α-dihydrotestosterone (DHT).[64] Of the androgenic steroids, testosterone and DHT have the most potent biological activity. In women, approximately 25% of androgen biosynthesis takes place in the ovaries, 25% of androgen is produced by the adrenal gland, and the remainder is produced at tissues sites in the periphery.[64]

As stated previously in the guidelines and position statements section, there is controversy regarding androgen therapy in postmenopausal women.[26,38,39] However, postmenopausal women who present with symptoms of decreased sexual desire associated with personal distress and have no other identifiable cause for their sexual concerns may be considered for limited therapy.[39] Testosterone therapy without concomitant ET cannot be recommended, because there are no data on the safety and efficacy of testosterone therapy in women not using concomitant estrogen.[26,38,39]

No testosterone product is FDA approved in the U.S. for treating symptoms of sexual dysfunction in women. However, a few prescription testosterone-containing products are FDA approved for use by women and men, some of which are used off label to treat sexual desire disorders in postmenopausal women (Table 35-4).[21]

Oral Testosterone

When taken orally, micronized testosterone is generally not well absorbed and does not result in measurable blood levels.[39] Thus, a chemical process (e.g., methylation) is used to create testosterone derivatives that can provide better bioavailability when administered orally, as with methyltestosterone, which is infrequently used today.

The only testosterone-containing product with FDA approval to treat menopause-related symptoms is an oral tablet that combines esterified estrogens and methyltestosterone (Estratest, with 1.25 mg esterified estrogen plus 2.5 mg methyltestosterone; Estratest HS, with 0.625 mg esterified estrogens plus

Table 35-4. Androgen Therapy for Treatment of Postmenopausal Women with Hypoactive Sexual Desire Disorder

Formulation	Advantages	Disadvantages
Oral testosterone		
Esterified estrogen + methyltestosterone (Estratest®)	FDA approved for hot flashes Available orally	Liver dysfunction Decreases HDL
Compounded testosterone[a]		
Cream/ointment/gel	Increased sensation in genitalia	Variable absorption Local irritation to genitalia Formulation messy
Sublingual/buccal[b]	Well absorbed	Tachyphylaxis Gum-related adverse effects Unpleasant taste Limited experience
Pellets[b]	Well absorbed	Surgical incision for insertions Spontaneous extrusion
Transdermal testosterone[a,b,c]		
Gels (AndroGel®, Testim®)	Good skin tolerability Flexible dosing Convenient delivery system	Transferred by skin contact
Patches (Androderm®, Testoderm®)	Convenient delivery system	Skin irritation Visible
Injectable testosterone[a,b,c]		
Enanthate (Delatestryl®) Cypionate (Depo-Testosterone)	Inexpensive Allows flexible dosing	Requires IM injection Roller-coaster effect Tachyphylaxis

Source: Adapted from reference 21.
FDA = U.S. Food and Drug Administration; HDL = high-density lipoprotein.
[a]Supraphysiologic dosages (masculinizing effects).
[b]Not recommended.
[c]Not FDA approved in women.

1.25 mg methyltestosterone). This product is indicated for the treatment of moderate to severe vasomotor symptoms unresponsive to estrogen. However, it is often used off label to treat symptoms of sexual desire disorders in postmenopausal women, and data have shown some success.[65-67]

Oral estrogen and testosterone have been shown to be effective in improving sexual desire in three studies. In one study, 20 surgically or naturally menopausal women were randomized to receive either oral esterified estrogens (EE) (1.25) or EE plus oral methyltestosterone therapy (mT) over a 2-month period.[65] All women were using ET at baseline. At 8 weeks, methyltestosterone recipients had significantly improved sexual desire and satisfaction compared with baseline; the EE-alone group did not have a significant improvement from baseline.

Another study investigated the effect of adding oral mT (1.25 mg) to oral EE (0.625 mg) in 218 surgically and naturally postmenopausal women with HSDD in a 4-month trial.[66] Testosterone recipients had significantly increased levels and frequency of sexual interest compared with those receiving estrogen alone; however, other sexual function scores did not improve.

In a placebo-controlled, 6-month crossover trial, Floter and colleagues added oral testosterone undecanoate (40 mg/day) to oral estradiol valerate (2 mg /day) therapy for surgically induced postmenopausal women.[67] Compared with estrogen-alone recipients, testosterone-estrogen recipients had significantly improved overall sexual function, which included greater interest in and enjoyment of sexual activity. Testosterone levels obtained with testosterone undecanoate in this study were supraphysiologic.

All oral testosterone formulations undergo first-pass hepatic metabolism, increasing the risk of adverse effects on lipids and liver function.[39] Prolonged use of high doses of oral testosterone has been associated with liver dysfunction in women, including hepatomas and hepatocellular carcinomas.[39] Oral formulations also reduce high-density lipoprotein cholesterol levels and triglycerides in estrogen-treated women.[66]

Compounded Testosterone

Despite the lack of clinical trials and quality-control standards, custom-compounded testosterone creams, ointments, and gel forms are popular formulations for improving women's sexual desire.[68-70] For women, an appropriate dosage of compounded 1% testosterone gel, cream, or ointment is 0.5 g/day, which should deliver 5 mg of testosterone daily, one tenth the generally prescribed dosage for men.[39] The product can be applied directly to any skin surface (but commonly the clitoris, labia, thigh, arm, or abdomen) several times weekly. Genital application has the potential to increase sensitivity in the genital tissues but it is often associated with local irritation. In addition, some women find the formulation messy.

Whereas creams, gels, and ointments may result in unpredictable blood levels, sublingual/buccal tablets and pellets are well absorbed when properly compounded.[21,68,71-75] Sublingual and buccal testosterone formulations result in rapid absorption and turnover, requiring increased doses for an effect, and there is limited compounding experience with this formulation.[68] They may also cause gum-related adverse effects and produce an unpleasant taste. Risks of subcutaneous custom-compounded testosterone pellets include the surgical procedures required for insertion and removal, discomfort at the insertion site, and infection. All compounded dosage forms may result in supraphysiologic levels if large doses are applied.[68]

Transdermal Testosterone

Two testosterone transdermal gels (AndroGel® and Testim®) and two transdermal patches (Androderm® and Testoderm®) have been approved in the U.S. for use in men. These products deliver high doses of testosterone, which can cause masculinizing side effects in women. Patches, either whole or in part, should not be used by women. Some healthcare providers modify the gel dose for off-label use in women by reducing the amount applied, but it is difficult to accurate regulate the amount of testosterone delivered. When applied to the arm, abdomen, or thigh, gels may result in transfer to partner or child.[76]

Several testosterone-containing products appropriately dosed for women are being investigated for the treatment of sexual desire disorders in postmenopausal women. Transdermal patches delivering lower testosterone dosages (150–300 mcg/day) and transdermal gels (1%) are being investigated. Clinical trial reports indicate that a 300-mcg/day dosage for 3–6 months is generally safe and effective for the treatment of sexual desire disorder in surgically induced postmenopausal women receiving concomitant ET for up to 2 years.[77-81] However, there are insufficient long-term safety data regarding breast, endometrium, or heart safety to draw strong conclusions.

Injectable Testosterone

In the U.S., all testosterone products administered by intramuscular (IM) injection are approved for use only in men. Recommended dosages are inappropriate for women, although a smaller dosage may be used in women. Testosterone administered by IM injection often results in supraphysiologic levels immediately after administration, followed by low levels over time, creating a roller-coaster effec.[82] Peaks may result in both side effects and tachyphylaxis, leading to increased dosing requirements to obtain the same therapeutic effect. Resulting testosterone levels can be modified by adjusting the dosage and the injection frequency.

Sherwin and colleagues studied the efficacy of intramuscular testosterone and estrogen injections on sexual function in 53 surgically menopausal women. Women were randomized at the time of surgery to one of five groups: 150 mg testosterone enanthate plus estrogen, 10 mg estradiol valerate alone, 200 mg testosterone enanthate alone, placebo, or a control group.[82] The crossover design had 3-month active-treatment phases plus a 1-month placebo washout between the phases. In the treatment phases, adding testosterone significantly enhanced intensity of sexual desire, sexual arousal, and frequency of sexual fantasies compared with estrogen alone or placebo. The testosterone levels achieved with this formulation of intramuscular testosterone were often supraphysiologic for women.

Any recommendation for testosterone therapy should be accompanied by a full explanation of the potential benefits and risks of therapy. Commonly reported adverse effects are acne and excess facial hair.[39,83,84] With topical testosterone, hair growth or skin irritation may occur at the application site. Adverse changes in lipids and liver function tests have been observed with oral formulations.[39,83,84] High testosterone dosages causing supraphysiologic levels could result in lowering of the voice (which could be permanent), clitoral enlargement, excess body hair, edema, erythrocytosis, and liver dysfunction.[39,83,84] Psychological changes (e.g., increased anger or aggression) also are potential risks.[39,83,84] In general, adverse effects can be minimized if testosterone levels are maintained within appropriate physiologic ranges.[39,83,84] Testosterone therapy should not be initiated in postmenopausal women with breast or uterine cancer or with cardiovascular or liver disease.[38,83,84]

During testosterone therapy, monitoring should include a subjective assessment of sexual desire and satisfaction. Women also should be evaluated for potential adverse effects and blood levels obtained if these occur. Establishing baseline lipids and liver function tests should be obtained before initiating therapy, particularly with oral testosterone.[39] The tests may be performed 3 months after initiating therapy, and if levels are stable, once or twice yearly thereafter.[11] Testosterone treatment should be reduced or stopped if adverse events occur.[39] Pap tests and mammograms should be kept current.

Dehydroepiandrosterone

The passage of the 1994 FDA Dietary Supplement Health and Education Act allowed for the expanded availability of androgenic substances. Androgenic dietary supplements do not require regulatory review and have thus not undergone formal trials of efficacy and safety. Dehydroepiandrosterone and androstenedione are the two major androgen supplements currently available, although there are a growing number of "pro-androgen" supplements being introduced to the marketplace either through the internet or in stores without prescriptions. Although some efficacy data on DHEA in women with adrenal insufficiency are encouraging, data in healthy postmenopausal women are not adequate to establish the efficacy of this agent in this population.[39]

Tibolone

Tibolone is a synthetic steroid with estrogenic, progestogenic, and androgenic properties. Although it is not currently available in the U.S., it has been used in Europe for 20 years for treatment of symptoms of menopause.[85] In a recent randomized controlled trial, tibolone was shown to increase clitoral circulation and sexual function scores significantly as compared with conventional hormone therapy in postmenopausal women who had HSDD.[86]

VASOACTIVE AGENTS

PDE-5 Inhibitors

Small-vessel atherosclerotic disease of the vagina and clitoris may contribute to arousal disorders; thus, vasoactive medications have been explored for low arousal.[87] Selective inhibitors of phosphodiesterase (PDE-5 inhibitors) block PDE-5 activity, causing accumulation of 3', 5'-cyclic guanosine monophosphate in the corpora cavernosa, which leads to muscle relaxation.[88] Sildenafil has been prescribed to millions of men for treatment of erectile disorder and theoretically could be effective in women with inadequate genital blood flow.

However, current research on the use of sildenafil in women has shown inconsistent results. Three

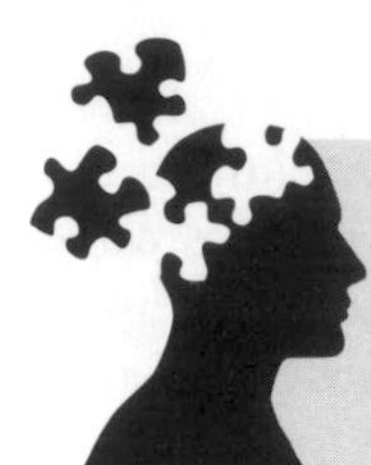

Therapeutic Challenge:

How would you counsel a woman presenting a prescription for sildenafil at the pharmacy?

studies have shown modest efficacy, one with premenopausal women with FSAD, one with postmenopausal women with sexual dysfunction, and one with women with spinal cord injuries.[89-91] However, two other studies in postmenopausal women with FSAD showed lack of efficacy.[92,93] Two studies have shown that sildenafil may improve sexual function in antidepressant-induced sexual dysfunction in both sexes.[94,95]

Nevertheless, sildenafil treatment is well tolerated, and no serious adverse effects have been reported in women. As with men, women who are using nitrates or have cardiovascular disease should not be prescribed PDE-5 inhibitors. Healthcare providers continue to intermittently report off-label uses of PDE-5 on a case-by-case basis. Such individualized treatment is likely to continue for some women until safer and more efficacious alternatives are available.

α-Adrenoceptor Antagonists

Phentolamine is a combined α_1- and α_2-adrenoceptor antagonist that was originally approved for the treatment of pheochromocytoma-induced hypertension and norepinephrine-related dermal necrosis.[88] The effects of oral phentolamine 40 mg were assessed in a placebo-controlled pilot study of six postmenopausal women with lack of lubrication or subjective arousal during sexual stimulation.[96] Mild improvements in subjective arousal and changes in vaginal blood flow were observed.

Prostaglandins

Prostaglandins improve arousal by relaxing the vaginal arterial smooth muscle and increasing vaginal secretions.[88] A placebo-controlled study of 79 postmenopausal women with sexual arousal disorder found that local application of the prostaglandin alprostadil 100 or 400 mcg resulted in a significant improvement over placebo in both subjective arousal and in somatic sensations following visual sexual stimulation.[97] The women receiving alprostadil 400 mcg reported significantly greater changes from baseline in genital warmth, tingling, level of sexual arousal, and sexual satisfaction.

CENTRAL NERVOUS SYSTEM–ACTING AGENTS

Apomorphine

The use of dopaminergic drugs, such as apomorphine, has been shown to have stimulatory effects on sexual behavior when given to patients with Parkinson disease. A sublingual formulation of apomorphine, a nonselective D1 and D2 dopamine receptor agonist, has been approved in Europe for the treatment of erectile dysfunction.[88] An intranasal formulation for the treatment of both male and female sexual dysfunction has been investigated in the U.S.

Flibanserin

Flibanserin is a postsynaptic 5-HT_{1A} agonist, a very weak partial agonist on dopamine and a 5-HT_{2A} antagonist.[85,98] It was initially investigated to treat depression but showed inconsistent effects in animal models. Because dopamine and these subtype receptors of serotonin are thought to be related to libido, a number of large clinical studies are ongoing in premenopausal women with HSDD.

α-Melanocyte-Stimulating Hormone

Recent findings indicate that effects on sexual dysfunction may be stimulated through melanocortin receptors in the brain. A nasally administered analogue of α-melanocyte–stimulating hormone, bremelanotide, was recently found to be effective in a small group of premenopausal women in improving both low sexual arousal and libido in an at-home setting.[99] Research suggests that melanocortin receptors are associated with complex pathways related to skin pigmentation, weight, and sexual response.[85]

LUBRICANTS AND MOISTURIZERS

Lubricants and newer vaginal moisturizes are available as over-the-counter products. Lubricants are generally considered temporary measures to relieve vaginal dryness during intercourse.[100] Short durations of action limit their usefulness as a long-term solution. Lubricants must be applied frequently for more continuous relief and require reapplication before sexual activity. Examples of lubricants include Astroglide®, KY® Jelly, Surgilube®.

Moisturizers are promoted for long-term relief of vaginal dryness rather than being just sexual aids. These products prolong contact with the vaginal surface, requiring only two to three applications a week and do not require reapplication before sexual intercourse. They also lower vaginal pH through their weak activity and buffering capacity. Examples of moisturizers include Replens and Liquibeads. Moisturizers provide an alternative to ET in high-risk groups, such as women with a history of breast cancer.

HERBAL PRODUCTS

Zestra™ is oil that contains natural botanical ingredients (borage seed oil, evening primrose oil, special extracts of angelica, coleus forskolin, antioxidants, and vitamin E) with natural fragrances.[88] (The recommended daily allowance for vitamin E is 15 mg; the upper limit of intake should not exceed 1,000 mg/day because it is a fat-soluble vitamin and supratherapeutic ranges may lead to flulike symptoms.) A small, randomized, double-blind, crossover study in 20 women (10 with FSAD) reported statistically significant improvements in Zestra™ relative to placebo in levels of arousal, desire, satisfaction, and sexual pleasure (irrespective of SSRI use for some study participants).[101] Zestra™ should be applied with general massage to the genitalia, clitoris, labia, and vaginal opening at least 3–5 minutes before vaginal intercourse for enhanced sexual experience.

ArginMax™ is a proprietary nutritional supplement consisting of extracts of ginseng, ginkgo, damiana, arginine, and vitamins and minerals. In a 4-week placebo-controlled study, women receiving ArginMax™ reported an improvement in sexual desire, clitoral sensation, and satisfaction with their overall sex life; a reduction of vaginal dryness; and an increase in frequency of sexual intercourse and orgasms without any significant adverse effects.[102] It should be noted that oral products that contain high doses of L-arginine should be used with caution in women with histories of oral or genital herpes because of a potentiating effect. In addition, ginseng should be used with caution in women with poorly controlled hypertension, and it may decrease the serum levels of warfarin.

Avlimil™ and Vigorelle™ are products that are advertised on the internet and magazines to enhance sexual desire. Avlimil™ is a tablet which contains multiple ingredients, including isoflavones; capsicum pepper; leaves from sage, red raspberry, and damiana; roots from ginger, licorice, valeriana, and black cohosh; and bayberry fruit. Vigorelle™ is a cream that contains damiana leaf, suma root, motherwort, wild yam, ginkgo biloba, and peppermint leaf. There are no studies using these products published in peer-reviewed journals.

MECHANICAL DEVICES

The Eros clitoral therapy device, a small handheld mechanical device increasing blood flow to the clitoris, labia, and vagina by creating a vacuum over the clitoris, is the only FDA-approved mechanical device for the treatment of female sexual dysfunction.[103] Clinical trials suggested that it improves genital sensation, lubrication, ability to experience orgasm, and sexual satisfaction.[103] This device requires a prescription, and its recommended use is 3–4 times a week, independent of sexual intercourse, for tissue-conditioning effects or before intercourse. Eros therapy may have a role as monotherapy or be used as adjunctive therapy, such a with estrogen and/or testosterone therapy.

Monitoring and Follow-up

Patients should be monitored for any changes in their medications, which may affect sexual function. Whenever androgen therapy is initiated, they should receive a baseline lipid profile and liver enzyme levels. Blood levels should be re-evaluated at 3 months, then once or twice yearly and whenever adverse effects are reported. Women should receive the lowest effective dose for the shortest time interval necessary. Women receiving PDE-5 inhibitors should be monitored for cardiovascular illnesses and any contraindicated medications.

Patient Education

Patients should be counseled and educated about

- The types of female sexual dysfunction and their prevalence
- Sexual side effects of medications
- The benefits and risks of testosterone therapy

Summary

Female sexual disorders are extremely prevalent, and new diagnoses are emerging that take into account both psychological and organic etiologies. A thorough sexual history is essential to determine psychological, interpersonal, and medical causes of disorders. Physical examination and laboratory

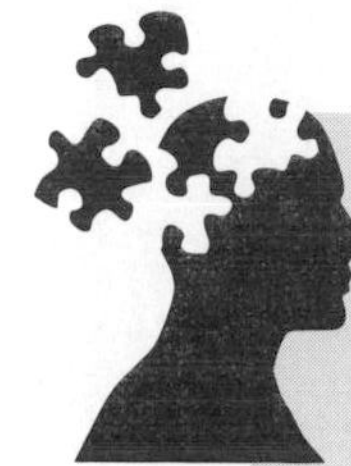

Therapeutic Challenge:

Why was Estratest® selected for this patient? What would be an alternative choice of androgen therapy?

Case Presentation

Patient Case: Part 2

Assessment: A.L.'s diagnosis is HSDD because she describes an absence of sexual interest, absent sexual thoughts, and a lack of responsive desire, which causes personal distress. Her HSDD is generalized because it applies to all situations (sexual activity with spouse and self-stimulation) and is acquired and of organic etiology because her desire decreased immediately following surgery. There is no evidence of disease-induced dysfunction (hypertension and hypothyroidism are controlled) or medication-induced dysfunction (ACE inhibitors unlikely to cause sexual dysfunction), and the onset of medical disorders and medication use are not consistent with the onset of HSDD. There is no evidence of interpersonal difficulties (e.g., depression/anxiety, stress, substance abuse, prior sexual or physical abuse), relationship concerns (e.g., relationship quality or conflict, lack of privacy, partner performance), or sociocultural factors (e.g., religious conflicts or inadequate education).

Plan: A.L. has symptoms consistent with HSDD and with female androgen insufficiency, including low libido, decreased energy, and decreased well-being, as described by the Princeton Consensus Statement.[26] There is no alternative explanation or cause for these symptoms (such as major depression or medical illness). She is adequately estrogenized on oral and topical ET, with estrogen levels of 72 pg/mL (35–500 pg/mL premenopausal). Her free testosterone is 0.9 (1.1–6.3 pg/mL) and SHBG is 50 (40–120 nmol/L), with free testosterone being in the lowest quartile of normal ranges for reproductive-age women, suggesting impaired testosterone production. She has no specific treatable cause of androgen insufficiency, such as medication-induced causes. Therefore, a trial of androgen replacement may be considered.

As her lipid profile and baseline liver enzymes were normal and mammogram and Pap test were done within the past year, she will be started on Estratest HS® daily. If she has significant vaginal atrophy, topical estrogen should be continued. Before initiating therapy, she will be counseled on the potential risks and benefits of androgen therapy. She will be re-evaluated in 3 months and have androgen levels, estradiol, lipid profile, and liver enzyme levels repeated at that time. Side effects, such as acne and hirsutism, will be monitored. If she responds to treatment and tolerates the medication, she will be tapered to the lowest effective dosage, with discontinuation of therapy recommended within 2 years, consistent with current recommendations.[83] Her lipid and liver enzyme levels will be obtained once or twice yearly, and she will be encouraged to obtain yearly Pap tests and mammograms.

testing can often rule out medical illness–related dysfunction. A pharmacist is in a key position to identify sexual-induced side effects to patients. Pharmacists should also be aware of the controversy regarding androgen therapy, off-label uses of medications for sexual dysfunctions, and herbal treatments.

References

Additional content available at ***www.ashp.org/womenshealth***

36 Substance-Use Disorders

Bethany A. DiPaula, Pharm.D., BCPP; Sneha Baxi, Pharm.D.

Learning Objectives

1. Identify prevalence and diagnostic issues of substance-use disorders that are relevant to women.
2. Compare and contrast the pharmacotherapy of substance-use disorders with an emphasis on sex-related issues.
3. Describe complications in treating substance abuse in pregnancy and lactation.
4. Discuss the complications of **dual diagnosis** (psychiatry and substance abuse) in women.

Epidemiology

The abuse of substances, including tobacco, alcohol, illicit drugs, and prescription drugs for nonmedical purposes, is prevalent across sexes, and the number of women with substance-use disorders has continued to increase. In 2006, it was estimated that illegal drugs were used by 9 million women in 1 year, and prescription drugs were abused by 3.7 million women without a medical purpose.[1] It is estimated that 9.9% of nonpregnant women and 3.9% of pregnant women report using illicit drugs. Although adult men are more likely to be current alcohol drinkers, female adolescents between the ages of 12 and 17 have a higher incidence of current drinking than male adolescents.[2] Women now make up one third of those with substance-use disorders (excluding nicotine dependence).[2,3] Adult men are twice as likely as women to be diagnosed with **substance dependence**; however, among adolescents, the rate of substance dependence is similar between the sexes. Unfortunately, substance experimentation and abuse is more common in teenage years through midlife, the same time that women are likely to become pregnant.[4]

Sex-Specific Issues

The demographics of men and women seeking treatment for **substance abuse** are relatively similar, although the latter are more likely to have custodial responsibilities for children.[5] Women face sex-specific barriers in obtaining adequate treatment because of psychosocial and financial problems, such as social stigma, history of trauma from physical and sexual abuse, lack of child care, and poor or no health insurance. Some substance-abuse treatment programs specifically exclude pregnant women because of increased liability with this patient population.[6] Among those in outpatient treatment (excluding methadone programs), women are more likely to be unemployed, have Medicaid as primary insurance source, and be admitted for drug abuse as opposed to alcohol.[5]

Developing treatment goals to meet the unique needs of women may improve treatment outcomes.[2,4] Some of the sex-specific programs that enhance treatment effects include childcare services, prenatal care, women-only programs, women's topics, and mental healthcare.[4,7] Implementing these services has resulted in improvements in pregnancy outcomes, substance use, psychiatric symptoms, employment, and medical benefits, including decreased risk for human immunodeficiency virus (HIV) transmission. Yet among available substance-abuse treatment centers, it is estimated that only about 13% provide child care, 12% offer prenatal care, 6% serve women only, 37% present sex-specific programming, and 19% supply pregnancy programming.[4]

Most of the trials assessing the benefits of pharmacotherapy for managing withdrawal or maintaining abstinence are in men or mixed sexes. Yet there are data to show that women have physiologic differences that directly affect medication pharmacokinetics, such as absorption, distribution, metabolism, and excretion. In addition, women's physical differences, such as greater adipose tissue, can significantly affect medication. Further, the biology of addiction may differ for women. The **National Institute on Drug Abuse (NIDA)** started to focus their efforts on supporting research on drug abuse in pregnant women in the 1970s and 1980s, and then the intersection of HIV/AIDS (acquired immunodeficiency syndrome) and drug abuse in pregnant and postpartum women. In the 1990s, National Institutes of Health (NIH) issued guidelines requiring sex analysis in phase 3 clinical trials in NIH-funded studies. This led to drug-abuse research that included women of all ages, regardless of pregnancy status, allowing sex differences to be studied.[8]

Substance-Use Disorders in Pregnant Women

There are little to no pharmacotherapy trials designed to focus solely on pregnant women. Pregnant women who have addictions should meet the criteria for substance dependence, have no specific contraindications, and provide informed consent after

Table 36-1. Pregnancy and Nursing Information for Medications Commonly Used to Manage Substance-Use Disorders[58]

Medication or Class of Medications	Treatment Option	FDA Pregnancy Category	Nursing Considerations
Benzodiazepines	Alcohol detoxification	D	Effect on nursing infant unknown and may be a concern.
Buprenorphine	Heroin detoxification Maintenance therapy	C	May reduce breast milk production in animals. Passes into human breast milk. Unclear whether compatible with breast-feeding; may want to avoid.
Bupropion SR	Smoking cessation	C	Excreted into breast milk. Should consider risks to infant before continuing breast-feeding.
Carbamazepine	Alcohol detoxification	D	Compatible with breast-feeding.
Clonidine	Alcohol detoxification Heroin detoxification	C	Passes into human breast milk. Unclear whether compatible with breast-feeding; may want to avoid.
Disulfiram	Alcohol—maintain abstinence	C	Unclear whether compatible with breast-feeding; may want to avoid.
Methadone	Heroin detoxification Maintenance therapy	C/D	Compatible with breast-feeding.
Naltrexone	Alcohol—maintain abstinence Heroin—maintain abstinence	C	Passes into human breast milk. Unclear whether compatible with breast-feeding; may want to avoid.
Nicotine replacement	Smoking cessation	D	Passes into human breast milk. Unclear whether compatible with breast-feeding. Must weigh risk of continued smoking while breast-feeding vs. risk of exposure to pharmacotherapy.
Valproic acid	Alcohol detoxification	D	Compatible with breast-feeding.
Varenicline	Smoking cessation	C	Unknown whether it is excreted in breast milk in humans but has been shown to pass into animal breast milk. Unclear what the effects will be on the infant; may want to avoid.

FDA = U.S. Food and Drug Administration; SR = sustained release.

fully being advised of the risks and benefits before being prescribed pharmacotherapy. In general, medication is dosed using the same guidelines for adults regardless of sex. Practitioners should be aware that some substances of abuse do not produce life-threatening withdrawal and may not have improved outcomes with pharmacotherapy. For instance, pregnant women who abuse stimulants (cocaine, amphetamines) or hallucinogens (marijuana, LSD) or disassociate anesthetics (PCP) in most cases should not receive pharmacotherapy.

Despite the fact that information is scant and issues complicated, the practitioner must strive to provide optimal care to the growing number of substance-dependent women. Therefore, this chapter reviews current practice with the understanding that further research is needed. The focus will be on sex-specific issues. The reader should refer to the summary tables (Table 36-1 and Table 36-2) and the referenced treatment guidelines for general assessment and treatment of substance-use disorders.

Tobacco Dependence in Women

EPIDEMIOLOGY

Tobacco products are designed to maximize the addictive potential of nicotine, a chemical that alters brain chemistry. It is a highly addictive substance that results in enormous health, societal, and economic burdens. In the U.S., approximately 45.1 million adults are current smokers; meaning about one out of every five adults is a smoker. The percentage difference among men (23.9%) and women (18.1%) is much narrower than in the past, making the importance of decreasing smoking-related diseases an important issue in women's health. The most common form of tobacco used by both men and women is the cigarette. In addition, there are many different types of tobacco, including spit tobacco, pipes, cigars, clove cigarettes, **bidis,** and water pipes; spit tobacco is more prevalent in men, accounting for about 0.2% use in women.

Table 36-2. General Nonpharmacologic Treatment Summary for Substance-Use Disorders[33]

Therapy	Description
Cognitive behavioral therapy	Attempt to manage dysfunctional thoughts, such as "my drug use is beyond control," and maladaptive behaviors, like continuing to accept offers from friends to use substances.
Motivational enhancement therapy	Motivates the individual to change by empathy and assessment of pros and cons of substance use.
Behavioral therapies	Comes from learning theory. Based on positive and negative reinforcement. The goal is to stop the pattern of substance use and exchange for behaviors that are unrelated or incompatible with substance use. Types of behavioral therapies include contingency management, community reinforcement, cue exposure and relaxation training, and aversion therapy.
Psychodynamic and interpersonal therapies	Associates detrimental symptoms and personality traits to trauma and deficits during development.
Group therapy	Uses many different types of therapy. Healthcare provider meets with more than one patient simultaneously, making efficient use of time. May be more beneficial for those with substance-use disorders than individual therapy.
Family therapies	Provides therapy to family members because dysfunctional families have been associated with poor outcomes for patients with substance-use disorders.
Self-help groups and 12-step–oriented approaches	Views substance dependence as an incurable, chronic illness. Uses physical, emotional, and spiritual components. AA (Alcoholics Anonymous) and NA (Narcotics Anonymous) are two examples.
Hypnosis	Mostly studied for smoking cessation but has not been clearly established as effective.

Smoking-related diseases are tremendously affecting the trends of morbidity and mortality. For example, until 1987, breast cancer was the leading cause of cancer deaths in women; now lung cancer is considered the leading cause of cancer deaths in both men and women. In addition to lung cancer death, cigarette smoking caused a total of 437,902 deaths in 2005, secondary to cardiovascular disease, respiratory disease, cancers of the lip, oral cavity, pharynx, esophagus, pancreas, larynx, cervix, uterus, bladder, and kidneys, as well as secondhand smoke, which killed 49,000 nonsmoking adults and 430 newborns because of sudden infant death syndrome.[9,10] An estimated 178,000 women die annually secondary to tobacco-related diseases. In addition, women who smoke have approximately a 30% higher chance of becoming infertile. Economically, annual loss of productivity costs secondary to smoking-related mortality for women are estimated to be $26,483 billion ($55,389 billion for men).[11]

One of the reasons for the higher use of tobacco among women is the marketing strategy employed toward women.[12] For example, ultralight cigarette advertisements are designed specifically to entice women to smoke cigarettes, implying that these cigarettes are not as harmful and using thin, beautiful women as role models. Additionally, popular magazines for woman are used to advertise cigarettes, appealing to the adolescent and older female population.

CASE PRESENTATION

Patient Case: Part 1

J.A. states: "I just found out I am pregnant and I can't stop smoking! I need to quit now!"

HPI: J.A. is a 33-year-old woman presenting to the pharmacy consult clinic for smoking cessation. J.A. has been smoking for one pack/day for 15 years without any quit attempts. J.A. found out 2 days prior that she is 6 weeks pregnant and is worried about the effects of smoking on the fetus.

PMH: Asthma, tobacco dependence.

Family history: Mother—diabetes type 2, hypertension; father—lung cancer secondary to tobacco use.

Social history: Tobacco—smokes one ppd × 15 years, no quit attempts; alcohol—one to two drinks/week, discontinue secondary to pregnancy; illicits—denies.

Medications: Prenatal vitamin daily.

CLINICAL PRESENTATION

Abrupt nicotine withdrawal is associated with various physiologic symptoms lasting 2–4 weeks after quitting. These symptoms include chest tightness, constipation, cough, depression, insomnia, irritability, frustration, anger, difficulty concentrating, fatigue, and hunger/weight gain. Many of these symptoms are alleviated in 1–2 weeks; weight gain occurs more gradually, mostly in the first 1–2 years after quitting. Women tend to gain more weight than men; studies show that typical weight gain is <10 lb, but about 10% of women may gain >30 lb. The risk factors associated with the most weight gain include being female, black race, age <55 years old, and smoking >25 cigarettes/day.[13] The mechanism behind this is that smoking increases metabolic rate and alters taste sensation. Quitting smoking in turn decreases metabolism, improves sense of taste, and food is often used as a substitution for hand-to-mouth habit. Therefore, it is important to address this issue with women who are quitting smoking. The pharmacologic agents assist with many of the withdrawal symptoms and could be incorporated with behavioral strategies, such as substituting cravings with a healthy snack or gum, distracting cravings by exercising, or by changing routine (i.e., showering directly after awakening instead of having coffee and a cigarette).

DETECTION, SCREENING, AND DIAGNOSIS

The clinical practice guideline clearly states that tobacco dependence is a chronic condition and relapses may be frequent. Therefore, every patient in every healthcare setting should be asked about tobacco use and this information documented. National surveys have shown that only about one third of adolescents who visit the doctor or dentist are counseled about the dangers of smoking, and pregnant women who smoke were identified at 81% of physician visits but received counseling at only 23% of those visits. Studies have shown that smokers who receive advice from a healthcare provider are 1.5–2.2 times more likely to successfully quit for more than 5 months.[14] Additionally, the importance of screening for tobacco use during adolescence and early adulthood is particularly important because of the likelihood of pregnancy. The importance of screening remains a priority in women older than age 35 as well because of the higher risk of cardiovascular events in women who smoke and are on estrogen-containing contraceptives.

The guidelines provide strategies for tobacco cessation intervention (also known as the five As) and strategies to promote motivation (the five Rs).

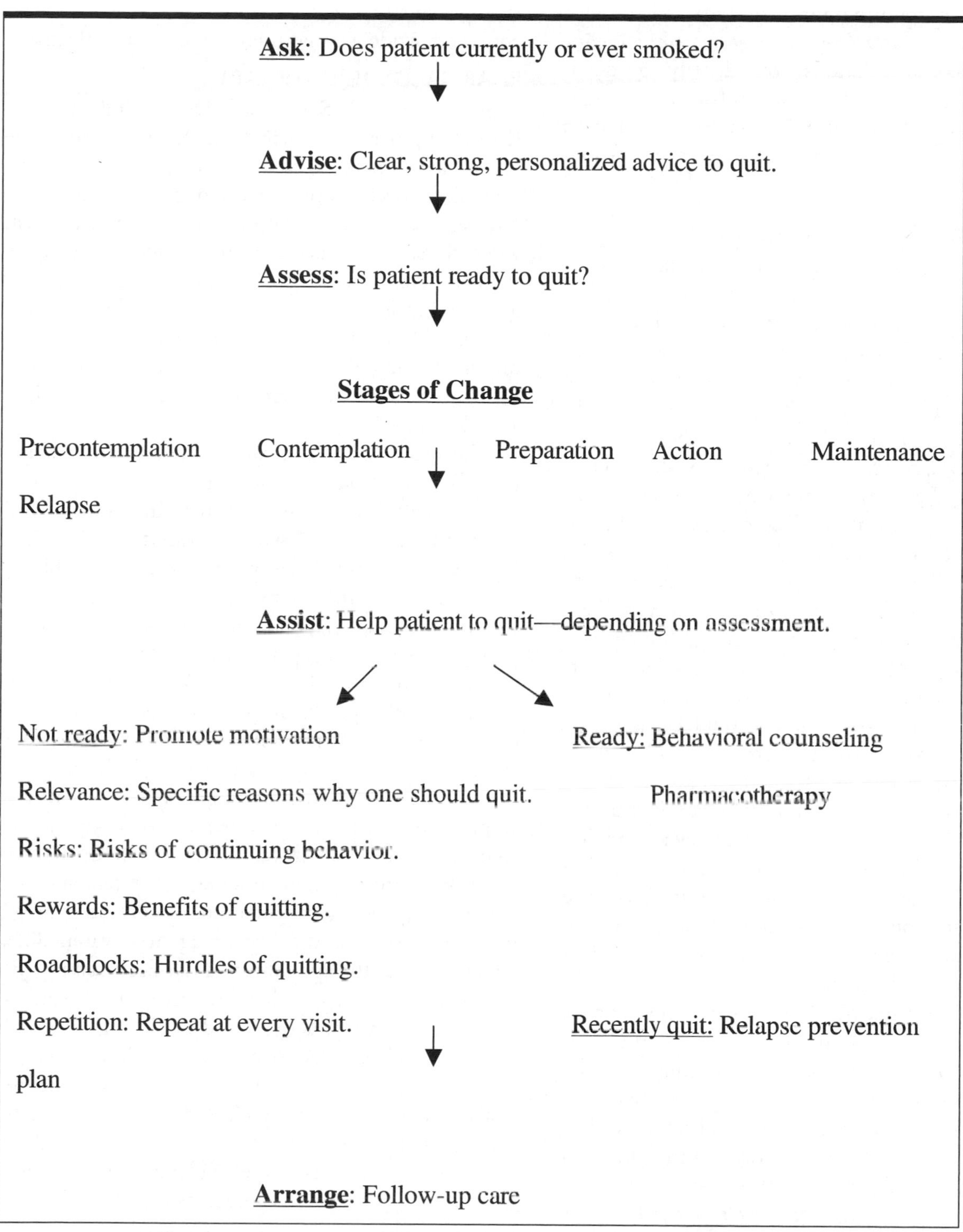

Figure 36-1 Five As, five Rs, and transtheoretical model of change.

The assessment component of tobacco cessation often incorporates the transtheoretical model of change. The five As, five Rs, and this model of change are summarized in Figure 36-1.[15,16] Screening and detection of tobacco use can be accomplished by using the first *A* at every visit: Ask.

GUIDELINES AND POSITION STATEMENTS

The clinical practice guideline sponsored by the Public Health Service, *Treating Tobacco Use and Dependence*, was recently updated in 2008.[14] The guidelines were originally developed in 1996 and updated in 2000. The updates reflect the ongoing research and publications about tobacco dependence and treatments, now accounting for 8,700 research articles. The *Treating Tobacco Use and Dependence* guideline provides recommendations for identifying, documenting, assessing, and treating tobacco use; highlights the importance of brief counseling for each patient at every encounter; and discusses various strategies for counseling.

NONPHARMACOLOGIC THERAPY

The approach to tobacco use and dependence treatment follows the aforementioned five As—Ask, Advise, Assess, Assist, and Arrange. Every tobacco user should be advised in a clear, strong, and personalized manner to quit. The next step is to assess the tobacco user's willingness to quit, which will determine the next intervention and *A*: Assist. If the patient is unwilling to quit, the healthcare provider's action should be to Assist the patient by using the five Rs for promoting motivation (Figure 36-1). If the patient expresses a desire to quit smoking, the STAR method can be used to Assist the patient. The STAR method consists of **S**etting a quit date, **T**elling friends and family about quitting, **A**nticipating challenges, and **R**emoving tobacco products from the environment. In addition, pharmacologic treatment and practical counseling should be used as a two-prong approach to the treatment of tobacco dependence. The guidelines state that patients should be offered the use of approved medication except in certain populations, including pregnancy and adolescence. Practical counseling should include modifications to behavior and discussion about abstinence, past quit attempts, triggers, and challenges to the attempt, which commonly include coffee, driving, meals, alcohol, and stress.

Although pharmacologic agents are recommended in almost all patients in the guidelines, there are nonpharmacologic methods for quitting as well. The most common nonpharmacologic method used is cold turkey, in which quitting is abrupt, and it is considered to be the least successful quitting method. There is also the tapering method, either by reducing the number of cigarettes by self-regulation or by smoking cigarettes with less nicotine. Although this method may lead to a gradual decrease in the number of cigarettes, oftentimes one starts to inhale more deeply to offset the lower amount of nicotine. Additionally, there are several self-help and group programs that provide counseling either in person, in groups, or on the Web. Other nonpharmacologic methods include acupuncture, hypnosis, aversion therapy, and massage therapy; however, there is no consistent evidence that these methods are effective.

PHARMACOLOGIC THERAPY

There are various U.S. Food and Drug Administration (FDA) approved pharmacologic agents to treat tobacco dependence, including nicotine replacement therapies, psychotropic agent, bupropion sustained release (SR), and a partial nicotinic receptor agonist, varenicline. The nicotine replacement therapies available over-the-counter include nicotine patch, gum, and lozenge. A nicotine inhaler and nasal spray are available with a prescription. The guidelines recommend using these agents for smoking cessation first line. Second-line therapies include nortriptyline and clonidine.[9]

The mechanism of nicotine replacement therapy (NRT) is to reduce withdrawal symptoms by delivering half the amount of nicotine, slowly and less variably, compared with a cigarette. By alleviating these withdrawal symptoms, patients are able to concentrate on incorporating behavioral strategies to stop the habit. A meta-analysis of studies comparing smokers using placebo vs. NRT showed that patients using any NRT were 1.77 times more likely to successfully quit.[17] In general, NRT is not recommended in patients with a recent cardiovascular event, and it is pregnancy category D (see Table 36-1 for summary of pregnancy and nursing information). Bupropion blocks neural dopamine or norepinephrine uptake in the central nervous system, thereby suppressing the dopaminergic reward system and decreasing the craving for nicotine. Bupropion is pregnancy category C. The newest agent is varenicline, which binds with high affinity and selectivity at $\alpha_4\beta_2$ neuronal nicotinic acetylcholine receptors, resulting in low-level agonist activity and inhibiting surges of dopamine release that decreases withdrawal symptoms and suppresses the reward center. Varenicline is also pregnancy category C. Although all the first-line agents for smoking cessation are similar in their effectiveness, there is some evidence that suggests women may not benefit as much as men from NRT.

ISSUES IN PREGNANCY AND LACTATION

Smoking while pregnant may result in perinatal death, low-birth-weight infants, preterm deliveries (about 30% more likely), preterm premature rupture of membranes, placenta previa, and risk of infertility.[18] Problems that arise from smoking while pregnant include impaired fetal oxygen delivery, carbon monoxide exposure from smoking, direct damage to fetal genetic material, direct toxicity from all the various chemicals found in a cigarette, sympathetic activation, increasing fetal heart rate, and decreasing fetal breathing movement. Nicotine acts as a neuroteratogen because it affects the brain, most likely causing deficits in learning, memory, and emotional and behavioral problems in childhood. Additionally, nicotine has been associated with higher incidence of attention deficit hyperactivity disorder, higher rates of depression in adolescents, and higher incidence of nicotine addiction later on in life. Nicotine levels are found to be 15% higher in the fetus than in the mother, and the delivery of nicotine continues through breast-feeding.[19]

Studies have shown that only 20% to 40% of women stop smoking during their pregnancy. It is most beneficial to quit before conception; however, quitting at any time will lead to health benefits. The clinical practice guidelines states that healthcare providers should offer psychosocial interventions and offer this throughout pregnancy, from preconception visits onward, including postpartum, because there is a high rate of relapse during this period. During the preconception phase, it is vital to educate women that smoking decreases fertility.

The first-line intervention for pregnant women should be cognitive behavioral therapy (CBT). Women with partners who smoke, have lower education, and are heavy smokers have a lower rate of success with CBT.[20] During this intervention, educational messages about the dangers of smoking on the health of the mother and fetus should be conveyed, as well as clear advice about quitting as soon as possible. Additionally, pregnancy-specific materials and social support should be used.

Pharmacotherapy should be considered as second line when a pregnant woman is unable to quit with behavioral counseling alone and the potential benefits outweigh risks of continued smoking. Nicotine replacement is classified as class D; however, some argue that NRT delivers a lower blood level of nicotine than cigarette smoking, and there are no other toxic chemicals. Generally, the shorter-acting NRT is preferred over the longer-acting dosage forms. The American College of Obstetricians and Gynecologists (ACOG) states that NRT may be considered in pregnant women for smoking cessation only after nonpharmacologic treatments have failed.[71] The clinical practice guidelines do not make a recommendation on the effectiveness of nicotine replacement therapy during pregnancy; however, they do comment that although nicotine is harmful to the fetus, there is increased exposure to other chemicals as well as the nicotine with smoking.[14] Bupropion is pregnancy category C because risk for congenital anomalies may be increased in the first trimester.

Case Presentation

Patient Case: Part 2

Assessment: J.A. is addicted to nicotine and has expressed an interest in quitting. She is not currently using any therapy for smoking cessation.

Plan: The five As should be applied to J.A.

Ask: J.A. reports smoking.

Advise: J.A. knows she must quit smoking because she is pregnant. Using motivational interviewing skills, J.A. should be recognized for realizing that she should quit and questioned as to why she thinks it is important to quit smoking generally and especially during her pregnancy. In addition to the effects of cigarette smoking to her unborn baby, the risk of uncontrolled asthma in her pregnancy should be discussed.

Assess: Is J.A. ready to quit? J.A. states she is ready to quit now, placing her in the preparation stage. It is also important to assess past and present tobacco use, and determine quit attempts. Motivation and confidence in quitting should be addressed, including specific reasons to want to quit smoking and barriers that may occur.

Assist: Work with J.A. to make a trigger plan, addressing patient-specific triggers and ways to modify behaviors. Additional issues should be addressed (i.e., weight gain). Pharmacotherapy should be addressed, and its appropriateness should be considered. Although pharmacotherapy should be offered to assist in smoking cessation to most patients, J.A. is not a candidate because she is pregnant. J.A. should be intensively counseled.

Arrange: Follow-up is key, and J.A. should be seen again within 2 weeks.

J.A. comes back for a follow-up visit with her husband, who is still smoking around her. She reports weight gain that she does not associate with her pregnancy and has continuous cravings for cigarettes.

First, J.A. should be commended on her smoking cessation. J.A. and her husband should be advised about the risks of secondhand smoke to her and the fetus. Her weight gain should be addressed;

(Continued on next page)

she should be advised that weight gain is normal in pregnancy and after quitting smoking, with an average of <10 lb. J.A. should be encouraged to make healthier food choices and to talk to a nutritionist to assure that the baby receives appropriate nutrition. Additionally, although J.A. reports cravings, behavior modifications should be continued. Considering that J.A. has quit for 2 weeks, the withdrawal symptoms and cravings should be decreasing. Pharmacotherapy is not recommended because of potential harmful risks to the fetus. Pharmacotherapy may be considered by some healthcare providers because cigarettes contain ingredients in addition to nicotine that may cause additional harm to the fetus.

Alcohol Dependence in Women

(See Web Resources for Patient Case: Alcohol Dependence.)

Additional content available at
www.ashp.org/womenshealth

EPIDEMIOLOGY

Few research studies focus solely on the management of female alcoholics. Many of the older trials are sex biased toward men, and women seem to be less likely to seek treatment, which may reduce their participation in studies.[21] As is the case with substance abuse in general, most pharmacotherapy trials for alcohol dependence exclude pregnant women. Although alcohol dependence appears to be more common in men, the difference in the ratio seems to be decreasing, suggesting a growing incidence in women. It is unclear if this increase is just an artifact of study design or a true shift in alcohol use.

The pattern of alcohol use does differ by sex. Of those who abuse alcohol, the rate appears to be highest in younger women.[3] Yet women develop substance-related disorders later in life, and they drink smaller amounts less frequently. The literature suggests that once a woman begins drinking excessively, she progresses more rapidly to alcohol-related social problems and medical illnesses and may experience greater alcohol-related drinking problems.[3,21,22] Women also seek treatment sooner than men.

CLINICAL PRESENTATION

Alcohol use results in sex-specific pharmacokinetic differences.[23] It takes less alcohol for women to become intoxicated.[5,23,24] There are several potential explanations, including metabolism, total body water, and hormonal fluctuations. The first-pass effect is reduced in women because of decreased alcohol dehydrogenase (ADH) activity, particularly in the gastric mucosa.[25] However, older men experience an age-related decrease in gastric ADH, resulting in less of a notable sex difference later in life.[22] In addition, women have proportionately lower muscle mass, body weight, and body water, resulting in sex-specific differences in volume of distribution.[22,23] Consequently, consuming the same amount of alcohol will produce higher blood alcohol concentrations in women.[22,23] Alcohol metabolism has also been linked to female hormonal fluctuations. The data are conflicting as to whether blood alcohol levels vary during the menstrual cycle.[26-29] It has been suggested that alcohol is eliminated most quickly during the midluteal phase of the cycle.[30,31] However, poorly designed trials with few subjects limit this conclusion, suggesting the need for further research. Higher estrogen phases have been linked with increased acetaldehyde levels.[32]

Female drinkers may progress to severe hepatic injury more rapidly and may be more susceptible to it.[5,23,27,33] The incidence and mortality rate is also increased in women who consume more than two standard unit drinks per day. Women who abuse alcohol are at greater risk for death than those women who do not have a history of abuse. Women with alcohol-use disorders have a higher incidence of sexual dysfunction and menstrual disorders, such as amenorrhea, anovulatory cycles, luteal phase dysfunction, and early menopause than those women without an alcohol-use disorder.[24]

DETECTION, SCREENING, AND DIAGNOSIS

Women are less likely than men to be identified as having an alcohol-use disorder.[34] The **CAGE**, the **Michigan Alcoholism Screening Test (MAST)**, **TWEAK**, and the **Alcohol Use Disorders Identification Test (AUDIT)** are used to screen for alcohol-use disorders. Other than TWEAK, these tools were not designed specifically for women. The CAGE (an acronym for **C**ut down, **A**nnoyance with criticisms about drinking, **G**uilt about drinking, **E**ye-opener) is a four-question screening tool that can be quickly self- or healthcare provider–administered. Two affirmative answers is generally considered a positive screen. The MAST is a 22-item, self-administered questionnaire. The length of the MAST may make it less convenient to use for screening. The TWEAK (an acronym for **T**olerance, **W**orried, **E**ye-opener, **A**mnesia, and **K**/Cut down) is a five-question modification of the CAGE and was designed specifically to screen pregnant women for drinking problems. The AUDIT is a 10-question, self-rated tool developed by the World Health Organization to screen for excessive drinking. The CAGE appears to be less sensitive in women.[34] The TWEAK and AUDIT may be more useful for screening women, especially when lower cutoffs are used.[35] All women, particularly in primary care and obstetric settings, should be routinely screened for alcohol-use disorders.[34]

GUIDELINES AND POSITION STATEMENTS

There are several published guidelines or position statements that directly or indirectly review the assessment and management of alcohol-use disorders.[3,36,37] However, there are no published guidelines that solely address sex-specific issues in alcohol dependence.

NONPHARMACOLOGIC THERAPY

Studies suggest that the benefits of pharmacotherapy are limited in patients with substance-use disorders unless adjunctive nonpharmacologic therapy is used.[3] Table 36-2 provides an overview of nonpharmacologic therapies used in the management of substance-use disorders. When comparing nonpharmacologic treatment effects on initiation, utilization, and outcomes, no sex-specific differences have been noted, except in employment outcomes.[38] The benefits of female-focused treatment have been hypothesized but not fully investigated.

PHARMACOLOGIC THERAPY

The goals of pharmacotherapy in alcohol dependence are to manage acute withdrawal and to maintain abstinence/prevent relapse. Benzodiazepines, carbamazepine, and, to a lesser extent, valproic acid are all considered treatment options in managing acute withdrawal (see Table 36-3 for review of pharmacotherapy). Benzodiazepines are generally regarded as the treatment of choice in preventing withdrawal, especially in those with moderate to severe symptoms. There are some data to suggest that women may require lower dosages of benzodiazepines because of a better response.[39] Older women metabolize benzodiazepines through oxidation faster than men.[39] However, there is no difference in the rate of glucuronidation. There may be hormonal effects as well. For instance, oral contraceptives may decrease the absorption and oxidation rate of benzodiazepines.[39]

Carbamazepine is a well-accepted alternative for managing withdrawal in those with milder symptoms. It is frequently the treatment of choice in an outpatient setting because of its low abuse potential. There are also limited data to support valproic acid for managing milder alcohol withdrawal.

Disulfiram, naltrexone, and acamprosate are pharmacologic alternatives for promoting continued abstinence. Disulfiram inhibits aldehyde dehydrogenase, causing a toxic reaction when an individual consumes alcohol. The agent has been used with minimal success, primarily in highly motivated alcoholic patients, for the prevention of relapse. Most of the trials that support the use of this medication have been conducted in men. Disulfiram should be avoided in women with nickel dermatitis because there appears to be an increased risk for hepatotoxicity.[39]

Naltrexone is an opioid antagonist. It is theorized that alcohol produces an endogenous opioid and resulting dopamine surge, which serves to reward and reinforce continued consumption.[3,40] Naltrexone may be beneficial because of its ability to block opioid receptors, lessening the reinforcing effects. Because naltrexone is a newer agent, many of the trials have included both men and women. Oral and long-acting injectable studies of naltrexone pharmacokinetics demonstrate no significant sex-specific difference.[41] Oral naltrexone appears to be equally effective for women.[42] However, one study found a greater rate of nausea in younger women treated with this agent.[43] Animal data suggest that micro-opioid receptor and endogenous beta-endorphin levels may change throughout the estrous cycle. The sensitivity of the endogenous opioid system may differ for women based on hormonal fluctuations.[43] Gastrointestinal upset has clearly been shown to increase nonadherence. Initiating naltrexone only after a sufficient period of abstinence, starting with a lower dosage such as 12.5 mg/day and increasing the dosage more gradually, may help to reduce nausea.

Acamprosate has been widely used in Europe and was recently approved in the U.S. for alcohol relapse prevention. Most of the studies include men and women, with no sex-specific efficacy differences noted.

ISSUES IN PREGNANCY/LACTATION

Pregnant women who drink >1 pint of liquor (8 oz of absolute alcohol) daily are at risk for tolerance and withdrawal. The latter can be life-threatening for mother and fetus.[6] Therefore, management of withdrawal should occur in an inpatient setting with appropriate medical care, including access to an obstetrician. It is unclear if benzodiazepines should be

Table 36-3. General Pharmacologic Treatment Summary for Substance-Use Disorders

Substance-Use Disorder	Pharmacotherapy of Choice	Alternative Pharmacotherapy
Nicotine dependence	• Nicotine replacement • Bupropion • Varenicline	• Nortriptyline • Clonidine • Combination
Alcohol withdrawal	• Detoxification using benzodiazepine taper • Diazepam or chlordiazepoxide if liver function tests are within normal limits and no history of hepatic disease • Lorazepam, temazepam, oxazepam (benzodiazepines that are conjugated, not oxidized) if history of alcoholic liver disease	• Carbamazepine, balproic acid—fewer data • Alternatives for outpatient detoxification in patients not at risk for severe withdrawal such as delirium tremens
Wernicke's encephalopathy	• Thiamine supplementation • Supportive therapy, if required	• None
Korsakoff's psychosis	• Antipsychotics • Long-term care, if required	• None
Alcohol dependence	• Naltrexone • Disulfiram • Acamprosate	• None
Heroin withdrawal	• Detoxification is one alternative for managing heroin withdrawal • Methadone taper • Buprenorphine taper • Clonidine taper—less efficacious in reducing withdrawal symptoms than methadone or buprenorphine but not controlled and lower abuse potential	
Heroin dependence	• Buprenorphine or methadone therapeutic substitution—involves substituting a legally prescribed opioid for opioid of abuse • Patient should not be detoxified if therapeutic substitution is to be used • Data suggest better outcomes with therapeutic substitution than detoxification	• Naltrexone—used to maintain abstinence once patient has been detoxified from all opioids

contraindicated in pregnancy. Diazepam is considered an FDA pregnancy category D drug. It crosses the placenta and enters the breast milk. Initially, there were reports of congenital malformations, such as cleft palate, when exposed during the first trimester. However, this association has since been challenged.[39] The data remain inconclusive. Babies born to diazepam-dependent mothers are at risk for neonatal abstinence syndrome. Periodic benzodiazepine administration during the third trimester has been associated with floppy infant syndrome.[4,39] However, repeated doses of 30–40 mg/day of oxazepam administered during the third trimester did not result in the birth of any infants with floppy infant syndrome.[4] Therefore, oxazepam may be a safer option. The agent has a shorter half-life, does not undergo oxidation, and has no active metabolites, which may make it a better tolerated alternative. In general, the risk of short-term benzodiazepine exposure, such as what is used for alcohol detoxification, may not be significant. On the other hand, delirium tremens can be life-threatening. The risk of benzodiazepine exposure vs. alcohol withdrawal for the fetus and mother must be closely weighed.

Carbamazepine is also considered an FDA pregnancy category D drug. There is an increased risk for serious congenital anomalies, such as neural tube, cardiovascular, and urinary defects, as well as cosmetic malformations, such as cleft palate. Studies in patients with epilepsy found a twofold increased risk for congenital malformations.[39] There are no studies looking at the risk of using this agent in pregnant women experiencing withdrawal. However, benzodiazepines appear to be a safer and more efficacious alternative, especially for severe withdrawal. If carbamazepine is indicated, folic acid should be coadministered because it reduces the risk for neural defects.

Valproic acid is an FDA pregnancy category D drug. It is also associated with neural tube defects. It is contraindicated during the first trimester of pregnancy. This agent should probably be avoided in pregnant women experiencing withdrawal given the availability of better investigated, safer alternatives.

Clonidine has been shown to relieve some of the alcohol withdrawal symptoms associated with autonomic hyperactivity. However, it does not prevent severe withdrawal or delirium tremens and can mask the early symptoms. Clonidine is an FDA pregnancy category C drug and does cross the placenta. It has not been associated with significant adverse events when administered to pregnant women during the second and third trimester for hypertension. It may be a good alternative for managing mild alcohol withdrawal symptoms on a short-term basis or as an adjunct to benzodiazepines in those with severe hypertension.[4] It should be avoided as monotherapy in women who are at risk for significant withdrawal.

Women with alcoholism are susceptible to developing Wernicke-Korsakoff syndrome. All pregnant women should receive a prophylactic regimen of thiamine, folic acid, prenatal iron, and vitamins.[6] Thiamine 100 mg/day is generally administered during detoxification as prophylaxis against this syndrome. There are no data to show that this dosage is considered teratogenic. Because Wernicke-Korsakoff syndrome is considered life-threatening, thiamine prophylaxis should probably be administered during alcohol detoxification of pregnant women.

Disulfiram is considered an FDA pregnancy category C drug. There may be congenital anomalies, especially during the first trimester of pregnancy. The data are limited and conflicting. The risk of continued alcohol use must be weighed against the teratogenic effects of disulfiram. However, guidelines suggest that this agent is contraindicated in pregnancy.[6] Given its limited proven efficacy, disulfiram should probably be avoided in pregnancy, unless clear benefit outweighs the risk of congenital anomalies.

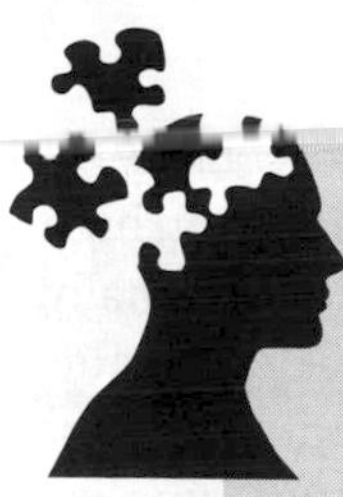

Therapeutic Challenge:

Under what circumstances would you recommend using benzodiazepines to detoxify a pregnant woman experiencing alcohol withdrawal?

Naltrexone and acamprosate are FDA pregnancy category C drugs. There are no controlled studies of either agent in pregnant women. However, a preliminary trial of naltrexone in pregnant women did not find any fetal abnormalities.[39]

Prescription Drugs

EPIDEMIOLOGY

An estimated 4.7 million American women used a prescription medication—including a pain reliever, tranquilizer, stimulant, or sedative—for nonmedical purposes in 2002; in 2004, about 2.4 million people aged 12 and older started taking an opioid without a prescription.[16,45] More than half of these abusers were women. Opioids, central nervous system depressants, and stimulants are the most commonly abused prescription medications. Studies suggest that women may be up to 55% more likely to be prescribed a medication with abuse potential, especially a narcotic or anxiolytic.[46] The rates among men and women are similar for abusing prescription drugs except in the adolescent age, when young women are more likely than men to use psychotropic medications. Data have also shown that there are higher rates of abuse and more emergency room visits and treatment admission in teenaged women. More than 50% of those being treated for sedative and tranquilizer dependence are women.[47]

Women may tend to abuse these medications more because of the higher likelihood of other vulnerabilities, including depression, anxiety, and trauma.[16] A study conducted at a large public university surveyed 4,580 full-time undergraduate students about the motives and source of acquiring prescription medications. No sex differences were found among the prevalence of nonmedical use of prescription opioids; however, men were doubly more likely to state their motive for opioid abuse was to get high and to experiment vs. relieve pain. Additionally, women reported that their leading source of obtaining prescription opioids was their parents, whereas men stated friends from other universities supplied the drugs.[48]

Treatment for prescription drug abuse is similar among women and men. There are two parts that need to be addressed: initiatives to control the increase of drug abuse and the treatment for withdrawal from the medication. The Drug Enforcement Agency (DEA) has implemented many methods to reduce the drug trafficking and increase education and resources for the public.[49] Medications to treat opioid withdrawal in nonpregnant women include methadone, buprenorphine, and buprenorphine/naloxone.

DETECTION, SCREENING, AND DIAGNOSIS

The physician and pharmacist can play a significant role in screening for prescription-medication abuse. The physician may choose to implement a medication or pain contract, which sets structured criteria for continuing pharmacotherapy. Pharmacotherapy is discontinued for patients who violate the contract. Pharmacists should educate patients about proper use of medication and side effects to increase the likelihood that the medication will be correctly used. In addition, the pharmacist should monitor for early refills and use of multiple prescribers and communicate any findings to the prescribing physicians.

GUIDELINES AND POSITION STATEMENTS

The U.S. Department of Health and Human Services/National Institute on Drug Abuse has published a *Research Report Series on Prescription Drugs: Abuse and Addiction*. Although there are some articles addressing withdrawal protocols, there is no specific guideline or position statement on prescription-drug abuse.

Illicit Drugs

EPIDEMIOLOGY

Based on findings from the National Survey on Drug Use and Health, the rate of illicit drug use in adults is higher (10.4%) in men than in women (5.8%).[50] Between 2006 and 2007, the incidence of heroin use in women dropped from 0.06% to 0.02%.[50]

Unlike with cocaine or hallucinogens, heroin dependence is one of the few addictions involving illicit drugs, which is routinely treated with pharmacotherapy. Pregnancy complicates treatment, resulting in sex-specific policies and recommendations. Consequently, the following section will focus solely on heroin dependence.

CLINICAL PRESENTATION

Based on findings from a single study, women who are alcohol or substance dependent report more comorbid medical conditions (e.g., cardiovascular, mood, nose/throat, central nervous system, skin, and gastrointestinal) than men.[51] In addition, women frequently begin using cocaine or opioids with substance-using partners and often start using at a younger age.[3] Women may prostitute themselves as a means of supporting their illicit drug use, which increases risk for transmission of sexually transmitted diseases, HIV, and hepatitis.

GUIDELINES AND POSITION STATEMENTS

There are published guidelines that directly or indirectly review the assessment and management of opioid dependence.[3,52] However, there are no published guidelines that solely address sex-specific issues in heroin dependence.

DETECTION, SCREENING, AND DIAGNOSIS

An objective measure, such as a toxicology screen, can be used to help detect opioid dependence. The CAGE-AID (CAGE Adapted to Include Drugs) and the Drug Abuse Screening Test (DAST) are screening tools for substance dependence.[35] The CAGE-AID is similar to the CAGE, which is used for alcohol dependence. However, the screening questions are asked about alcohol or drug use. Because the screening does not differentiate between alcohol or drug use, it is impossible to determine if a positive response is for alcohol, drugs, or both. The DAST is a 28-item tool that does not specifically differentiate between substances of abuse. Women who screen positive should receive a more complete psychosocial assessment.[35]

PHARMACOTHERAPY

The goals of pharmacotherapy are to reduce withdrawal symptoms, to maintain abstinence, or to provide substitution therapy. Studies suggest that the benefits of pharmacotherapy are limited in patients with substance-use disorders unless adjunctive nonpharmacologic therapy is used (Table 36-2).[3] Within 6–12 hours of the last heroin use, anxiety, rhinorrhea, lacrimation, sweating, and yawning can develop. Additional symptoms include mydriasis, restlessness, irritability, anorexia, shaking, chills, profuse sweating, pilomotor activity, nausea, vomiting, myalgias, and diarrhea. Symptoms generally peak in 48–72 hours and resolve within 7–10 days. Heroin detoxification is extremely uncomfortable but, for the most part, not considered life-threatening.

Some patients choose to withdraw without pharmacotherapy. The goal of medical detoxification is to use medication to reduce or ameliorate withdrawal symptoms. Clonidine, buprenorphine, and methadone are the most commonly used pharmacotherapy (Table 36-3). Clonidine is effective in reducing the autonomic withdrawal symptoms. However, both buprenorphine and methadone have been shown to be more effective than clonidine in reducing autonomic and subjective withdrawal. Naltrexone is an opioid-antagonist that has been used in combination for rapid and ultrarapid detoxification as well as to maintain abstinence. In theory, the reinforcing effects of heroin should be reduced as a result of the opioid receptor blockade. In reality, the long-term success rate of abstinence-based programs is extremely low.

The literature suggests that patients are more successful in remaining heroin-free when they receive opioid substitution therapy, such as methadone or buprenorphine. Methadone maintenance has been shown to reduce not only illicit drug use but improve social and health factors, such as decreasing criminal behavior and disease transmission, such as sexually transmitted diseases, HIV, and hepatitis. Women account for about one third of methadone-maintained patients. There are a limited number of sex-specific trials, but those that do exist suggest that women benefit from treatment.[39]

Buprenorphine is a relatively new treatment for heroin dependence. Consequently, many of the trials include women. Women maintained on buprenorphine had higher rates of abstinence from illicit opioids and treatment retention and lower number of positive urines than their male counterparts.[53]

ISSUES IN PREGNANCY/LACTATION

Because of the lack of significant surveys or studies, the prevalence rates for specific addictions during pregnancy are largely unknown. Although there are very few controlled trials, estimates of opiate use during pregnancy range from 1% to 21%.[54] Opioids pass through the placenta and can affect fetal metabolism and development.[3,54] There is a sixfold increased incidence of obstetric complications associated with opioid dependence. The largest drug transmission to the fetus occurs during the third trimester, when blood flow and transport are greatest. The fetal blood concentration of these substances average 50% to 100% of maternal levels but can exceed those of the mother. Exposure to illicit substances increases the risk for birth defects, cardiovascular disorders, decreased growth, prematurity, low birth weight, and still birth. As many as 60% to 90% of babies born to methadone-dependent mothers may develop neonatal abstinence syndrome.[55] Symptoms are similar to adult withdrawal syndrome, but the fetus may be more susceptible and also may experience poorly coordinated sucking, seizures, and death.

Pharmacotherapy can be used to detoxify or maintain pregnant patients (see Table 36-1 for a summary of pregnancy and nursing issues). There is at least one study that suggests that naltrexone is safe for detoxifying or maintaining abstinence in pregnant women.[39] However, treatment guidelines warn against administering narcotic antagonists except under overdose circumstances secondary to increased risk for abortion, preterm labor, or stillbirth.[6] One case report suggests that clonidine may be safe for inpatient detoxification of pregnant women.[39] Rapid detoxification can induce preterm labor and should probably be avoided.

Methadone is categorized as an FDA pregnancy category C/D drug and as maintenance therapy is generally considered the treatment of choice for heroin-dependent pregnant women. Methadone passes into the amniotic fluid, cord plasma, and newborn urine. However, the mother's varying opioid blood levels during illicit drug use can induce repeated withdrawal symptoms for the fetus. There have been case reports of spontaneous abortion and stillbirth after opioid detoxification. The risk seems to be the greatest during the first and possibly third trimester. One small study of detoxification of pregnant women suggested that third-trimester detoxification may not increase the risk for preterm birth.[56] This opens the door for debate as to whether detoxification might avoid neonatal abstinence syndrome and be a safer alternative for the baby. However, treatment guidelines recommend against medical withdrawal during pregnancy because of increased risk of fetal death.[6]

Most healthcare providers recommend methadone maintenance during pregnancy as the treatment of choice. Some of the cited advantages include reduction in illicit drug use and criminal behavior, provision of consistent blood levels preventing abstinence syndrome during pregnancy, improved maternal nutrition, increased participation in prenatal care, and decreased obstetric complications.[6] There are no recommended methadone dosages specific for pregnant women. Regardless of pregnancy status, women should be administered the lowest efficacious dosage, usually between 50 and 150 mg daily. However, NIDA suggests that dosages below 60 mg daily are not effective. Arbitrary low-dose policies for pregnant women may be associated with reduced program retention and should be avoided.[6] Methadone metabolism is increased during pregnancy. Consequently, pregnant women may require higher or more frequent doses (dosed twice a day), especially during the third trimester.[6,39,56,57] Methadone trough levels can offer some indication of whether the dosage is likely to provide withdrawal relief. Women with trough levels <0.24 mg/L and symptoms of withdrawal may require higher methadone dosages.[57]

Larger methadone dosages have been associated with greater neonatal withdrawal.[39] Lower maternal dosages of methadone generally produce more manageable neonatal symptoms. Symptoms can occur for up to 2–4 weeks after delivery. Methadone exposure while in utero may lead to lower birth weights and head circumference.[39] In addition, although these children may fall within the normal range of cognitive function at 1- and 2-year evaluations, they may still present with some developmental deficiencies compared with peers.[39] Medical, psychiatric, and socioeconomic factors confound the data, making it less clear whether there is a true association between methadone exposure and development.

The American Academy of Pediatrics Committee on Drugs lists methadone as one of the drugs compatible with breast-feeding, citing no signs or symptoms in infants and no effects on lactation.[58] Interestingly, heroin has been associated with significant adverse effects in breast-feeding infants, which further supports providing optimal treatment to prevent use or relapse.

Buprenorphine is considered an FDA pregnancy category C drug. Preliminary data suggest that it is relatively safe for mother and child during delivery or after birth.[39,59,60] Buprenorphine may offer a benefit over methadone because placental transfer appears to be reduced.[55] This medication is available for maintenance patients in two commercial formulations as monotherapy and in combination with naloxone to prevent diversion. Although naloxone is not generally orally absorbed, treatment guidelines suggest buprenorphine be administered as monotherapy for pregnant women receiving maintenance treatment to prevent fetal exposure to naloxone.[61]

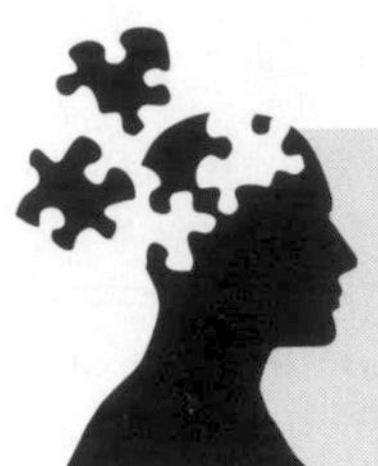

Therapeutic Challenge:

Should a pregnant woman who is currently dependent on heroin be detoxified or maintained?

Although infants are still susceptible to neonatal abstinence syndrome at birth, symptoms may be less severe with buprenorphine.[60,62] Onset of symptoms can range from 1–8 days after delivery, with greatest risk earliest in life. Transitioning pregnant women from short-acting opioids, such as heroin, to buprenorphine maintenance can be difficult. Buprenorphine is a partial opioid antagonist that can induce withdrawal if administered too soon after last heroin administration. One study concluded that opioid-dependent women in their second trimester of pregnancy can safely be transitioned to buprenorphine.[63] Buprenorphine has not been routinely investigated during the first or third trimester. The amount of buprenorphine and norbuprenorphine that passes into breast milk is relatively low and may have little effect on the infant. In addition, buprenorphine has a limited oral absorption and low bioavailability, which makes it less likely that infants would have significant oral absorption from breast milk. Further investigation is warranted, but buprenorphine during breast-feeding is not contraindicated and may be a safer alternative than methadone for breast-feeding mothers.[60,62]

Sex Differences: Co-occurring Disorders (Psychiatric and Substance-Use Disorders)

Patients with comorbid psychiatric and substance-use disorders are often known as dually diagnosed or co-occurring. Those with substance-related disorders have co-occurring axis I psychiatric disorders at a higher rate than the general population. The 2002 National Survey on Drug Use and Health found 2 million women with co-occurring substance-use disorders and a serious mental illness, which equates to about 2% of all adult women.[64] Women with co-occurring disorders are less likely to be employed than those women with only substance use.[65] Women with co-occurring disorders are more likely to have health insurance and have received psychiatric or substance-abuse treatment in the last year than their male counterparts.

Substance-abusing women seem to have a greater incidence of mood and anxiety disorders than men.[3] Alcohol-use disorders and depression frequently co-occur, particularly in women. Women may be more likely to report a history of depression that predates the alcoholism.[24] About 20% of substance abusers have comorbid post-traumatic stress disorder (PTSD), with women being more likely than men to be dually diagnosed.[3,65] Women are more likely to have a history of PTSD symptoms and victimization.[66] Women who have experienced trauma may use substances of abuse to self-medicate.[67]

The literature suggests that women with co-occurring disorders present differently from men. Women report psychosocial stress but are more likely to downplay their substance-use disorders.[66] At least one study suggests that methadone-maintained pregnant women with mood disorders have poorer substance-abuse treatment outcomes than those without mood disorders.[66] All women with substance-use disorders should be screened for psychiatric disorders such as depression and anxiety disorders, particularly PTSD.

It may be difficult to differentiate between primary and secondary depressive or anxiety symptoms while an individual is experiencing an abstinence syndrome. The decision to treat psychiatric symptoms in women who are withdrawing or are recently clean from substances of abuse should be made based on the severity of psychiatric symptoms, the certainty of the psychiatric diagnosis, and the projected benefits of treatment weighed against the risk of toxicity.[3] Potential indicators of a primary psychiatric disorder include persistence of psychiatric symptoms despite abstinence, history of psychiatric symptoms before substance abuse started or during intermittent periods of abstinence, family history of psychiatric disorders, and history of self-medication.[68]

Treatment strategies should include therapy for psychiatric and substance-abuse disorders concurrently. One trial of 107 women with PTSD and substance-use disorders found that those managed in an integrated program had better treatment outcomes for both the PTSD and the substance-use disorders.[67] When a primary diagnosis is less certain, pharmacotherapy to manage depression or anxiety should be withheld for 1–4 weeks. Once the psychiatric diagnosis is confirmed, the prevailing recommendation is to treat psychiatric and substance-related disorders concurrently. Medication selection is based on practice standards, safety, and abuse potential. Nonpsychoactive medications are psychotropics, such as lithium or antipsychotics, which regulate mood and thought over days to weeks and generally do not have much abuse potential.[69] Psychoactive medications, such as benzodiazepines, may have therapeutic benefit but produce rapid psychomotor effects and alteration in mood or thought with a high risk for abuse.[70] All substances of abuse are considered psychoactive. For mild to moderate psychiatric disorders, a stepwise approach is recommended: step 1, nonpharmacologic therapy; step 2, add nonpsychoactive medications if step 1 is unsuccessful; and step 3, add psychoactive medications if steps 1 and 2 are unsuccessful.[70] However, the guidelines recommend pharmacotherapy as a first-line treatment strategy for patients with acute or severe schizophrenia and mood disorders.

The length of therapy should be consistent with the recommended standard of care for those without a substance-use disorder. Antidepressants are the treatment of choice for generalized anxiety disorder, panic disorder, PTSD, social anxiety disorder, and depression, regardless of sex. However, anxiolytics, such as benzodiazepines, are frequently used as alternative or adjunctive therapy in most anxiety disorders (generalized anxiety, panic, social anxiety). Because of their abuse potential, benzodiazepines may not be a good alternative for women with co-occurring substance-use disorders. If they are prescribed, the pharmacist should counsel the patient about the risk of interactions, abuse, and abstinence syndrome.

Alcohol can significantly increase the risk of benzodiazepine toxicity, resulting in respiratory depression. Psychotropics with significant risk for overdose, such as tricyclic antidepressants, should be avoided in patients with co-occurring disorders. However, psychotropic medication should not be withheld from women who relapse, as long as there is no significant risk of toxicity from overdose or interaction. Nonadherence is a common medication problem in patients with co-occurring disorders.

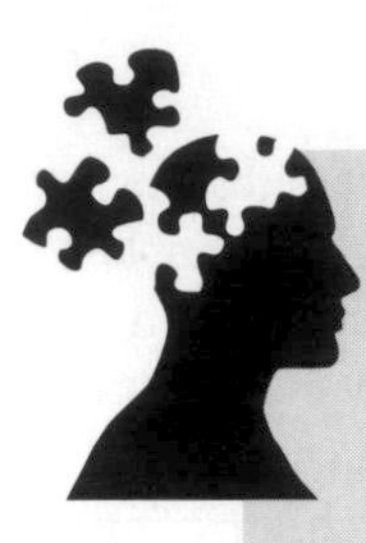

Therapeutic Challenge:

How do you differentiate between a primary and secondary depressive symptom in a woman with co-occurring disorders who is currently abusing substance(s) or alcohol?

Summary

Substance abuse among women is rising and becoming more comparable to the number of men with substance-use disorders. Many women with substance-abuse problems are of reproductive age and therefore may become pregnant. Special considerations must be measured in treating these women, including the pharmacologic and nonpharmacologic therapies used. In addition, mothers with substance-use disorders often require assistance in parenting skills and social services to reduce the likelihood of child abuse and neglect. Women with co-occurring disorders seem to be at greatest risk. The optimal treatment strategy should be nonpunitive. Women should be educated so that they can make an informed decision about whether to continue the pregnancy as well as available treatment resources.

References

Additional content available at ***www.ashp.org/womenshealth***

37 Immunity and Autoimmune Diseases

Gail Goodman Snitkoff, Ph.D.; Andrea K. Hubbard, Ph.D.; Jennie Broders, Pharm.D.; Arthur A. Schuna, MS, FASHP

Learning Objectives

1. Understand the epidemiology of autoimmune diseases in women.
2. Identify factors that predispose to autoimmune diseases.
3. Understand the different mechanisms of immune damage to host tissue.
4. Compare and contrast the medications used to treat these diseases.
5. Evaluate approaches to therapy.
6. Promote patient education.

Autoimmune diseases are defined by the American Autoimmune Disease Association as a varied group of chronic illnesses that involve almost every human organ system. This definition, however, continues to evolve as a reflection of ongoing research. These autoimmune diseases include more than 80 disorders and are the third most common category of disease after cancer and heart disease. They affect 5% to 8% of the population and are the fourth leading cause of disability among women.[1,2] It is estimated that 78.8% of individuals with autoimmune disease are women and that women are 2.7 times more likely than men to acquire autoimmune diseases. In fact, some specific autoimmune diseases pose an even greater risk for women (Table 37-1).[1] The most striking difference in sex is seen in Sjögren's syndrome (SS), systemic lupus erythematosus (SLE), autoimmune hepatobiliary disease, autoimmune thyroid diseases, and **scleroderma.** The middle tier of relatively common diseases includes rheumatoid arthritis (RA), multiple sclerosis (MS; see Chapter 41: Neurological Disorders), and myasthenia gravis. A final group includes sarcoidosis, ulcerative colitis, and insulin-dependent diabetes mellitus (IDDM).[1] Female prevalence in autoimmune diseases has been recognized for more than 100 years. More recently, autoimmune diseases were found to be the eighth leading cause of death for women between the ages of 15 and 64.

Although the cause of autoimmune diseases is unknown, there are numerous associations that can be made. Most important among these are **human leukocyte antigen (HLA)** alleles (Table 37-2). This association with specific HLA haplotypes is plausible because HLA class II molecules are required for antigen presentation to T cells. The autoantigen binds within the MHC molecule and is presented to specific T cells. Because HLA molecules bind to a restricted repertoire of antigens, if there is not an HLA molecule to interact with the antigen, the antigen will not be presented to the T cells.[3] In the absence of antigen presentation, an autoimmune response can not occur. The role of HLA and genetics in autoimmune disease is also demonstrated by the fact that children of women with autoimmune diseases may be at increased risk of autoimmune diseases but only rarely evidence the same autoimmune disease as their mothers.[4,5] Other major triggers may include antigenic mimicry between viral or bacterial antigens with host antigens, altered self-proteins, failure to regulate immune responses, and the production of natural antibodies. In addition, exposure to other environmental factors (sunlight, diet, allergens, environmental toxins) can also trigger autoimmune responses (Figure 37-1). It is also hypothesized that microchimerism may play a role in autoimmune diseases such as systemic sclerosis and autoimmune thyroiditis.[5]

As noted above, molecular or antigenic mimicry can be a trigger for autoimmune diseases. Immune responses to bacterial proteins have been

Table 37-1. Mechanism of Pathogenesis of Autoimmune Diseases More Common in Women

Syndrome	Pathogenic Mechanism	Consequence	Female: Male Ratio	Disease Prevalence Per 100,000
Antibody against Cell-Surface or Matrix Proteins				
Hashimoto's thyroiditis	Antibody to thyroid peroxidase/thyroglobulin; also T cell infiltrate	Hypothyroidism	50:1	21.8
Antiphospholipid syndrome	Antibodies to lipid membranes	Hypercoagulability syndrome	9:1	--
Primary biliary cirrhosis	Antibodies to mitochondria	Cirrhosis	9:1	0.9
Chronic active hepatitis	Antibodies to liver-kidney microsomal type 1 and liver cytosol proteins	Hepatitis	8:1	0.7
Graves' disease/ hyperthyroidism	Antibody to thyroid-stimulating hormone receptor	Hyperthyroidism	7:1	13.9
Myasthenia gravis	Antibody to acetylcholine receptor	Progressive muscle weakness	2:1	0.4
Chronic idiopathic thrombocytopenic purpura	Antibody to platelet integrin	Abnormal bleeding	2:1	--
Antibody to Soluble Antigens				
Systemic lupus erythematosus	Antibody to DNA, histones, ribosomes. and RNA	Glomerulonephritis, vasculitis, skin rashes	9:1	7.3
Sjögren's syndrome			9:1	4
Mixed connective tissue disease	Antinuclear antibodies, antibodies to ribonuclear protein	Symptoms overlapping those of systemic lupus erythematosus, rheumatoid arthritis, and Sjögren's syndrome	8:1	--
Rheumatoid arthritis	Antibodies to filaggrin; rheumatoid factor (anti-IgG antibodies)	Arthritis, vasculitis, rheumatoid nodules	4:1	23.7
T Cell–Mediated Disease				
Hashimoto's thyroiditis	T-cell infiltrate, also antibody to thyroid peroxidase; thyroglobulin	Hypothyroidism	50:1	--
Rheumatoid arthritis	Unknown synovial antigens	Arthritis	4:1	--
Scleroderma	T-cell infiltration of the skin with the production of TGF-β	Hardening of the skin	3:1	0.8
Multiple sclerosis	Myelin basic protein, proteolipid protein, myelin oligodendrocyte glycoprotein	Progressive muscle weakness, invasion of the brain by CD4 + T cells	2:1	3.2

Source: Adapted in part from reference 11.

Table 37-2. Association of Host Susceptibility Factors with Autoimmune Diseases[1]

Disease	Environmental Factors	Human Leukocyte Antigen (HLA) Association
Multiple sclerosis	Epstein Barr virus (EBV), measles virus	HLA-DRB1, HLA-DR2 HLA-DQ6
Lyme arthritis	*Borrelia burgdorferi*	
Type I diabetes	Coxsackie virus B4, rubella virus, cytomegalovirus (CMV), mumps virus	HLA-DR3 HLA-DR4
Rheumatoid arthritis	*E. coli,* mycobacteria, EBV, hepatitis C virus	HLA-DRB1 HLA-DR4
Systemic lupus erythematosus	EBV	HLA-DR2, HLA-DR3
Myocarditis	CMV, chlamydia	
Rheumatic fever/myocarditis	Streptococci	
Chagas' disease/myocarditis	*Trypanosome cruzi*	
Myasthenia gravis	Herpes simplex virus, hepatitis C virus	HLA-DR3
Guillain-Barré syndrome	CMV, EBV, *Campylobacter spp.*	
Graves' disease	*Yersinia enterocolitica*	HLA-DR3
Hashimoto's thyroiditis	*Yersinia enterocolitica*	HLA-DQB1, HLA-DQA1
Sjögren's syndrome		HLA-DR3
Addison's disease		HLA-DR3

investigated, and it has been shown that infection can activate autoimmune T cells as well as elicit antibodies, which cross-react with normal host proteins. For some diseases, such as myasthenia gravis, it has been demonstrated that there are a large number of cross-reactive epitopes from a variety of different microbial pathogens, suggesting that myasthenia gravis may be triggered by different pathogens in different patients.[3] Table 37-2 shows the currently identified correlations between infectious diseases and autoimmune diseases.

Altered protein or protein expression and post-translational or covalent modification of proteins have also been shown to play a role in autoimmunity. As examples, both glycosylation of human collagen type II and citrullination of the guanidinium side chains of arginine have been implicated in RA. This modification of normal tissue can occur for other large molecules with autoimmune consequences (SLE, SS, RA, Hashimoto's thyroiditis, type I diabetes, and Addison's disease, among others).[3] For example, methylation of DNA GG pairs as a mechanism for suppressing gene expression is a process influenced by a variety of factors. Patients with SLE have very low total T cell DNA methylation, which suggests more activated genes.[6]

Additionally, autoimmunity may arise because of mutations in the genes responsible for control of cellular and immune functions. The autoimmune regulator gene (AIRE) is responsible for the ectopic display of normal antigens in the thymus. This display of antigens is important for negative selection of the T cells and maintenance of self-tolerance. Mutations in this gene may lead to autoimmune diseases, such as autoimmune polyendocrinopathy candidiasis ectodermal dystrophy. Mutations in other regulatory proteins, such as CTLA-4, lymphoid protein tyrosine phosphate nonreceptor type 22, and TNF-α have been associated with SLE, Graves' disease, and RA. Changes in the transcription factor FoxP3, which is expressed in T regulatory cells (CD4+, CD25+), can cause systemic autoimmunity and polyendocrinopathy when mutated.[3]

Figure 37-1. Interrelationship between triggers for autoimmune diseases.

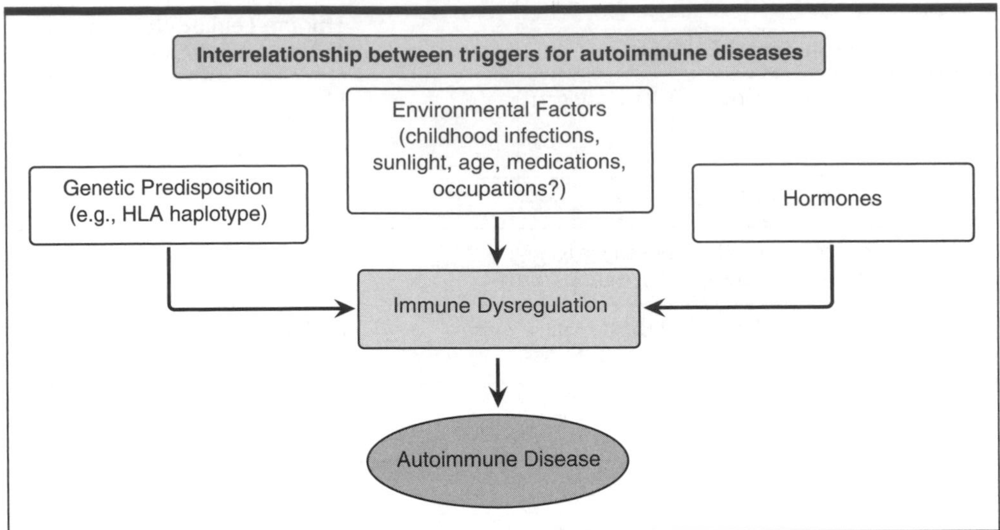

Release of sequestered antigens through trauma (in particular ophthalmic injury) and defects in **apoptosis** or protein degradation by proteosomes may also lead to the release of normally sequestered antigens, resulting in the development of autoimmunity. It has been demonstrated that exposure of an individual to nucleosomes, which are normally sequestered, leads to the development of anti-DNA antibodies, which are characteristic of SLE.[3]

B-1 B cells (CD5+ B cells) are able to synthesize and secrete natural antibodies, which can bind to a broad range of antigens, including autoantigens. These antibodies may be cross-reactive with self-antigens (the epitopes are similar to the nonself epitope) or may bind to self-antigens identical to the antigen that stimulated them (molecular mimicry). These antigens may also be truly polyreactive, binding to antigens of diverse structures, including proteins, nucleic acids, phospholipids, and polysaccharides. Whatever the case, these natural antibodies are found in SLE, SS, and RA.[3]

Microchimerism is defined as the bidirectional trafficking of maternal and fetal cells during pregnancy that may persist in individuals for decades after childbirth. These small populations of cells or DNA from the fetus that persist in the woman have been implicated in the pathogenesis of autoimmune disease. This hypothesis arises from the fact that systemic rheumatic diseases share clinical similarities with chronic graft-vs.-host disease. Although the mechanisms of pathogenesis that is due to microchimerism are unknown, microchimeric cells could function as effector cells or targets of an immune response.[4]

Although differences in sex hormone levels between women and men do not explain the broad predilection of autoimmune diseases for women, there does appear to be a relationship between fluctuations in hormone levels, pregnancy, and status of autoimmune disease. Indeed, it has been suggested that immune events occurring during pregnancy to maintain maternal peripheral tolerance to the semi-allogeneic fetus may explain the improvement in symptoms of RA in pregnant women. Depending on the specific autoimmune disease, symptoms may improve, worsen, or remain unchanged when a woman becomes pregnant. For example, the attenuation of symptoms associated with RA and MS is reported to occur during pregnancy. Among women with RA, 70% of pregnancies result in lessening of signs and symptoms of this disease, with peak improvement observed in the second or third trimester. Disease does return postpartum, usually within 3 months of delivery.[7] Pregnancy in women with SLE may provide no benefit or worsening of disease symptoms.[8] Moreover, some studies suggest that SLE occurs more frequently in women who have taken oral contraceptives and in postmenopausal women taking hormone therapy. Women with SLE are at increased risk for several obstetric complications, including preterm labor and fetal death. The fetus may also be affected by autoantibodies that cross the placenta to elicit neonatal lupus syndrome and neonatal thyrotoxicosis. Autoimmune thyroiditis is often increased in incidence postpartum. In 1% of infants born to mothers with Graves' disease, the effects can be especially harmful because of the transplacental transfer of maternal antibodies directed against the thyroid stimulating hormone (TSH) receptor.[7] Most autoimmune diseases other than RA and SLE do not peak in occurrence in women during their reproductive years but rather later in life. The impact of estrogens on the immune response has long been recognized and suggests that women produce a more vigorous immune response with increased antibody production.[9] This observation is supported by the fact that the hormonal environment during pregnancy appears to favor a T_H2 (humoral) response.[9] Indeed, estrogens and androgens have been found to directly influence whether a T_H1 or T_H2 immune response develops by interacting with hormone receptors on immune cells.[10] In addition, estrogen receptors are highly expressed in SS salivary glands.[8] Sex hormones can also modulate the hypothalamic pituitary adrenal (HPA) axis and thus affect the stress response.[9]

Prevention of these autoimmune diseases under discussion is not an option because an exact cause of these diseases is unknown.

Immune Mechanisms Underlying Autoimmune Diseases

Autoimmune diseases are mediated by the same mechanisms as normal immune responses and typically involve activation of both B and T cells. The difference is not in the type of response, but in the specificity toward self-antigens rather than pathogenic or nonself-antigens. Often pathogenesis is associated with a single effector mechanism, such as antibody (Ab) or T-cell responses, although some autoimmune diseases, such as RA and Hashimoto's thyroiditis, may have multiple pathogenic mechanisms.

Pathogenesis in diseases mediated by antibodies may have numerous mechanisms, depending on the type of antigen (cell associated or soluble) and the effect of Ab on the antigen or cell. In diseases in which Ab binds to self-surface or matrix proteins, Ab can either modulate the effects of the protein to which it binds (antagonist or agonist) or initiate inflammatory responses. Receptors to which Ab binding has been demonstrated include the receptor for TSH, the acetylcholine receptor, and insulin receptors. Ab binding to receptors for TSH in the thyroid gland can act as an agonist, stimulating overproduction of thyroid hormone as seen in Graves' disease. In contrast, Ab to the acetylcholine receptor can cause muscle cells to internalize and degrade the receptors, leading to the progressive muscle weakness seen in myasthenia gravis. In addition, both hypo- and hyperglycemia have been associated with Abs directed to the insulin receptor.

Abs directed to cell-surface and basement membrane proteins that are not receptors may activate macrophages and complement, leading to inflammation and cell lysis. When Abs are directed toward basement membranes, as in Goodpasture's syndrome and *Pemphigus vulgaris,* there is inflammation and tissue damage, whereas Abs directed to antigens on the surface of red blood cells and platelets lead to hemolytic anemia and thrombocytopenia, respectively. In all of these cases, inflammation and cell loss are the result of activation of complement or Fc-mediated phagocytosis. Activation of complement on nucleated cells does not induce lysis but rather complement components, such as C3a and C5a, which act as chemoattractants for macrophages and neutrophils. Activation of complement through the Fc portion of Ab may further activate these cells to release cytokines and oxygen radicals, as well as to initiate the synthesis of prostaglandins and leukotrienes.

Abs can also be directed toward soluble antigens, such as proteins (including immunoglobulin G [IgG]), DNA, histones, ribosomes, and RNA. These diseases are generally classified as systemic in nature because multiple organ systems are involved. Pathogenicity in these diseases is due to inflammatory responses resulting from the formation of immune complexes by soluble antigen-Ab interactions and activation of complement and macrophages by these complexes. When immune complexes form, they are usually cleared by macrophages. It is when these complexes are not cleared that disease results. Failure to clear the complexes can occur when 1) there is a large amount of antigen, leading to the formation of a large quantity of immune complexes; 2) there is chronic infection and persistence of antigen; and 3) immune complexes form because of ubiquitous self-antigen, resulting in tissue damage (as occurs in SLE). The presence of the immune complexes leads to Ab-mediated inflammation and tissue damage by macrophages. In addition, autoreactive T cells develop. These cells are important because they are not only able to activate self-reactive B cells but also may act as effector cells and directly damage host tissue.

Effector T cells specific for self-antigens can also be harmful to the host. These cells can act in three ways. First, as mentioned above, activated T cells may stimulate self-reactive B cells to produce and secrete antibody, thus maintaining Ab production to autoantigens and sustaining disease pathogenesis. Other

T cells, such as inflammatory T cells, may activate macrophages, stimulating an inflammatory response, whereas cytotoxic T cells can directly damage host cells by inducing cell death through apoptosis. Autoreactive T cells are directly involved in the pathogenesis of diseases such as MS, RA, and Hashimoto's thyroiditis. A summary of the mechanisms of autoimmune diseases for which women are at increased risk is presented in Table 37-1.

The diseases included in this review were chosen based on their prevalence in women, the variety of organs targeted, and the underlying pathogenic immune mechanisms (i.e., humoral and cell mediated).[11]

Rheumatoid Arthritis

CLINICAL PRESENTATION

Initial presentation of RA in patients is insidious with vague, often nonspecific symptoms, including weakness, fatigue, anorexia, and musculoskeletal symptoms. This prodrome may last for weeks before arthritis pain, **synovitis,** and joint stiffness develop. Early symptoms include morning joint stiffness of more than 1 hour daily and joint pain or swelling of three or more joints for a duration of 6 weeks or more. Joints especially affected include the interphalangeal and metacarpophalangeal joints of the hands, the wrists, the elbows, the knees, and the feet. The patient may present with an asymmetric involvement initially and usually evolves to a symmetric disease over time. In about 10% of the population, there is rapid onset of arthritis accompanied by lymphadenopathy and splenomegaly. Patients with RA are subject to acute and chronic pain, which may lead to disability, depression, and impaired social functioning.[12-17] The disease course is variable in each patient, with a persistent but fluctuating disease activity. Patients also have a decreased life expectancy and an increased risk of cardiovascular disease. Effective treatment of RA, particularly with methotrexate, appears to reduce this risk.[18]

In addition to joint symptoms, RA is a systemic disease that may affect other organ systems. **Rheumatoid nodules** are frequently seen later in the course of the disease and are often found on extensor tendons. They may also be present in the lung. Pulmonary fibrosis and pleural effusion may also be seen. Patients may develop chronic obstructive pulmonary disease. Vasculitis may occur in patients late in the course of the disease. Invasion of the blood vessel wall by inflammatory cells may reduce blood flow to organs and tissues fed by those vessels, leading to infarction of tissue. Small vessel vasculitis at distal fingers and toes, particularly around nail beds, may occur. Clinically relevant complications from this small vessel disease is rare, although skin ulcers may occur, requiring treatment. Ocular findings include scleritis and episcleritis. Nodules may develop on the sclera. Pericarditis may be seen, which can lead to effusion and tamponade in severe cases. Cardiac conduction abnormalities and aortic valve problems may also occur. Felty's syndrome is RA associated with splenomegaly and neutropenia. Lymphadenopathy may be seen in patients with very active disease. Rarely, amyloidosis can be seen but usually late in the disease course.

CASE PRESENTATION

Patient Case: Part 1

M.V.S. is a 34-year-old woman who was previously in good health. Over the past 2 months, she reported symmetric stiffness and pain in her hands, knees, and hips every morning. Stiffness lasted about an hour until she had showered and dressed. After her wrists and fingers began to swell, she sought advice from her primary care physician, who suspected RA. Before visiting her physician, she attempted to control the pain and impairment with ibuprofen 400 mg 4 times daily.

A blood sample revealed that she was positive for RF (titer of 1:160). Her white blood cell count was 4,720 and her ESR was 87. CRP (6.4 mg/dL) and anti-CCP (320 units/mL) were also elevated. Blood pressure, pulse, and rate of respiration were all normal. She also presented with lymphadenopathy and reported that she was losing weight and experiencing unusual fatigue. Urinalysis was normal.

PATHOPHYSIOLOGY

RA causes chronic inflammation of the joints as well as inflammation in tissue around the joints (e.g., tendons, bursae). It is a relapsing and remitting disease. Inflammation causes damage to both articular and periarticular bone.[19] It is believed that the initiating event in the pathophysiology of RA is nonspecific damage to the synovium that is due either to infection or trauma. The resulting inflammation causes the activation of T cells, especially CD4+ T_H cells. It is believed that these effector T cells migrate back to the joint, where they recruit and activate macrophages, neutrophils, B cells, and additional T cells. There is considerable evidence supporting this view, including the large numbers of CD4+ T_H cells found in the synovium, the association of RA with specific MHC class II alleles (important for activating CD4+ T_H cells), and the finding that the disease can be ameliorated by suppression of T cell responses.[15]

The activated CD4+ T_H cells differentiate primarily into T_H1 effector cells, which secrete interferon (IFN)-γ a proinflammatory cytokine, and express CD40 ligand. The combination of IFN-γ and CD40 ligand activates macrophages in the synovium to produce additional proinflammatory cytokines, including interleukin (IL)-1 and tumor necrosis factor (TNF)-α. The release of these cytokines increases inflammation in the joints and contributes both to the local inflammation and systemic manifestations of the disease. The role of TNF-α in the pathogenesis of RA is demonstrated by the ameliorating effect of blocking this cytokine in the signs and symptoms of RA.[15] The presence of these cytokines leads to activation of the endothelial cells of the local blood vessels, and recruitment and activation of additional macrophages and neutrophils. These activated phagocytic cells produce oxygen radicals, matrix metalloproteinases, prostaglandins, and leukotrienes, which further damage tissue and increase inflammation within the joint.

Within the synovium there is also an accumulation of B cells. These cells are stimulated in the joint by activated T cells and produce Abs and **rheumatoid factor (RF)** (anti-IgG Ab). The local production of Abs and RF leads to the formation of immune complexes that activate complement. Complement activation results in the production of the anaphylatoxins C3a and C5a, which also serve to increase inflammation within the joint.

The inflammation seen in RA results from the interaction of T_H1 cells, phagocytic cells, and B cells, leading to the production of inflammatory mediators such as cytokines, immune complexes, and activation of complement. Additional signs of the disease, such as joint remodeling, may be due in part to the presence of prostaglandins and activation of osteoclasts.

Many of the auto-Abs produced in RA are similar to those seen in SLE and SS and therefore are not diagnostic for RA. For example, RF is also found in patients with SS and SLE, whereas antinuclear Abs seen in SLE and SS can be detected in individuals with RA. Anticyclic citrullinated protein (anti-CCP) antibodies have similar sensitivity to RF (50% to 85%) but greater specificity (90% to 95%). Anti-CCP antibodies are usually present earlier in the disease than RF. The presence of positive antibodies for both RF and anti-CCP is highly diagnostic for RA.

As a result of chronic inflammation, a variety of characteristic changes occur in the joints, including pannus formation; damage to ligaments, tendons, and the joint capsule; and cartilage degradation. Tendon contractures, joint deformity, and bony ankylosis (fusion) may result from chronic inflammation.

RA is associated with excess mortality, which is estimated at approximately 25%.[18] RA itself is seldom the cause of death, and most deaths in RA are caused by comorbidities.[20] Cardiovascular disease is the most important comorbid cause of death, with an incidence of 42% in RA patients.[21] Other comorbidities include infections (9%), renal disease (8%), pulmonary disease (7%), and gastrointestinal disease (4%).

DIAGNOSIS

Diagnosis is made using both clinical signs and symptoms combined with laboratory findings. Joint pain and swelling, morning stiffness >1 hour in duration, rheumatoid nodules, and radiographic changes including periarticular osteopenia and erosions are signs and symptoms of RA. Nodules and radiographic changes are usually late manifestations of the disease.

Laboratory tests helpful in diagnosing RA include RF, anti-CCP antibody, C-reactive protein (CRP), and erythrocyte sedimentation rate (ESR). CRP and ESR may be increased in any disease associated with inflammation or infection. RF is not specific and often may be normal early in the disease. Anti-CCP antibody is highly specific, with 90% to 95% of patients with a positive antibody test having RA. If both tests are positive, the predictive value of the tests is even higher. In all cases, these blood test results must be considered together with the patient presentation. Although RF is not diagnostic for RA, it is found in more than two thirds of the patients with RA, as well as in 5% of healthy patients and in 10% to 63% of patients with SLE. In addition, >20% of healthy individuals 65 or older are RF positive.[15,22]

In a study that compared anti-CCP Abs to RF for diagnostic performance, RF was more sensitive but less specific than anti-CCP antibodies. By combining RF assay with anti-CCP assay, the predictive performance increased; this was also true when one of the serologic assays was combined with the presence of swollen joints.[23] Although citrullinated peptides have been found in synovial tissues from RA patients (and some non-RA controls), the role of anti-CCP antibodies in disease pathogenesis of RA is unknown. It is not clear if these autoantibodies are involved in ongoing immune stimulation or are a consequence of synovial inflammation.[24]

TREATMENT GOALS

Therapy for RA should strive for remission or near remission of symptoms and return to full function in ability to do activities of daily living. Effective treatment should slow or halt radiographic progression. No treatment can reverse damage that has already been done, and this must be recognized in patient evaluation.

Therapeutic Drugs

Current pharmacologic therapies for RA include nonsteroidal anti-inflammatory drugs (NSAIDs), glucocorticoids, disease-modifying antirheumatic drugs (DMARDs), and biologic agents. NSAIDs include aspirin, naproxen, ibuprofen, and etodolac. The efficacy of NSAIDs partially depends on the inhibition of the enzyme cyclo-oxygenase, critical in the metabolism of arachidonic acid in the cell membrane to proinflammatory prostaglandins. Glucocorticoids may diminish pain and swelling in most patents. Their administration must be balanced with potential side effects, such as osteoporosis, increased blood sugar, increased blood pressure, cataracts, and others. It is important to note that although NSAIDs and corticosteroids may provide symptomatic relief, they are not considered effective in preventing joint damage in RA. For this reason, nearly all patients with RA need DMARDs or biologic therapy. It has been shown that early initiation of DMARDs results in better outcomes. It is recommended all patients begin this therapy within 3–6 months of onset of symptoms.

DMARDs can include methotrexate (7.5–25 mg/wk), leflunomide (10–20 mg daily), hydroxychloroquine (200 twice daily), and sulfasalazine (0.5–1.5 g twice daily). Of these compounds, methotrexate has been the anchor drug of therapy for RA for decades and is often used in combination with sulfasalazine, hydroxychloroquine, and biologics.

Biologic response modifiers, the newest class of medications to treat RA, include TNF-α inhibitors (etanercept [50 mg subcutaneously weekly], infliximab [3 mg/kg intravenously at 0, 2, 6, and then every 8 weeks], adalimumab [40 mg subcutaneously every 2 weeks]), an IL-1 receptor antagonist (anakinra [100 mg subcutaneously daily]), an inhibitor of T-cell activation (abatacept [500–1,000 mg, dose dependent on weight, given 0, 2, and then every 4 weeks intravenously]), a monoclonal antibody against B cell CD20 (rituximab [1 g intravenously given twice over 2 weeks and repeated when disease flares]), and an antibody against the IL-6 receptor (tocilizumab [4–8 mg/kg intravenously every 4 weeks]). Tocilizumab is the newest in biologic response modifiers.[13]

Although DMARD therapy is effective in promoting/maintaining disease remission, DMARDs may take several months for onset of action. Thus, glucocorticoids are often used as bridge therapy. Combining methotrexate with TNF-α inhibitors, sulfasalazine, or hydroxychloroquine has been shown to have a good efficacy-to-toxicity ratio in patients who do not respond well to a single DMARD agent.[12-14]

Dosing Strategies

Combinations of these drugs have proven to be more effective than single treatments (Figure 37-2).[25-27] Combination therapy using methotrexate as the "anchor drug" and combined with any of the TNF blocking agents, sulfasalazine, or hydroxychloroquine has demonstrated better efficacy than single-agent therapy. In one trial, a combination of methotrexate, sulfasalazine, hydroxychloroquine, and prednisone for initial therapy was superior to sequential monotherapy or stepwise additions of DMARDs and equivalent to infliximab + methotrexate for initial therapy.[27] Combinations of methotrexate + biologics have also been found to be superior to biologic monotherapy in terms of RA outcomes. Adding methotrexate to infliximab has been shown to reduce the development of antibodies to this chimeric anti-TNF-α agent.[25] Anakinra as monotherapy has a modest effect in controlling RA inflammation for most patients. Usage of this drug is so minimal that it is not discussed in the American College of Rheumatology recommendations for the use of nonbiologic and biologic DMARDs in RA, although there are clinical situations in which it may be considered.[13] The combination of anakinra and TNF antagonists is not advised as it may increase infections, local reactions, and neutropenia.[25]

Figure 37-2. Treatment paradigm for patients with RA. Predictors for bad prognosis include functional limitation, extra-articular disease, erosions on radiograph, elevate RF, and/or anti-CCP antibody.[13] MTX = methotrexate; DMARD = disease modifying antirheumatic drug; anti-TNF = tumor necrosis factor inhibitor; NSAID = nonsteroidal anti-inflammatory drug; HCQ = hydroxychloroquine.

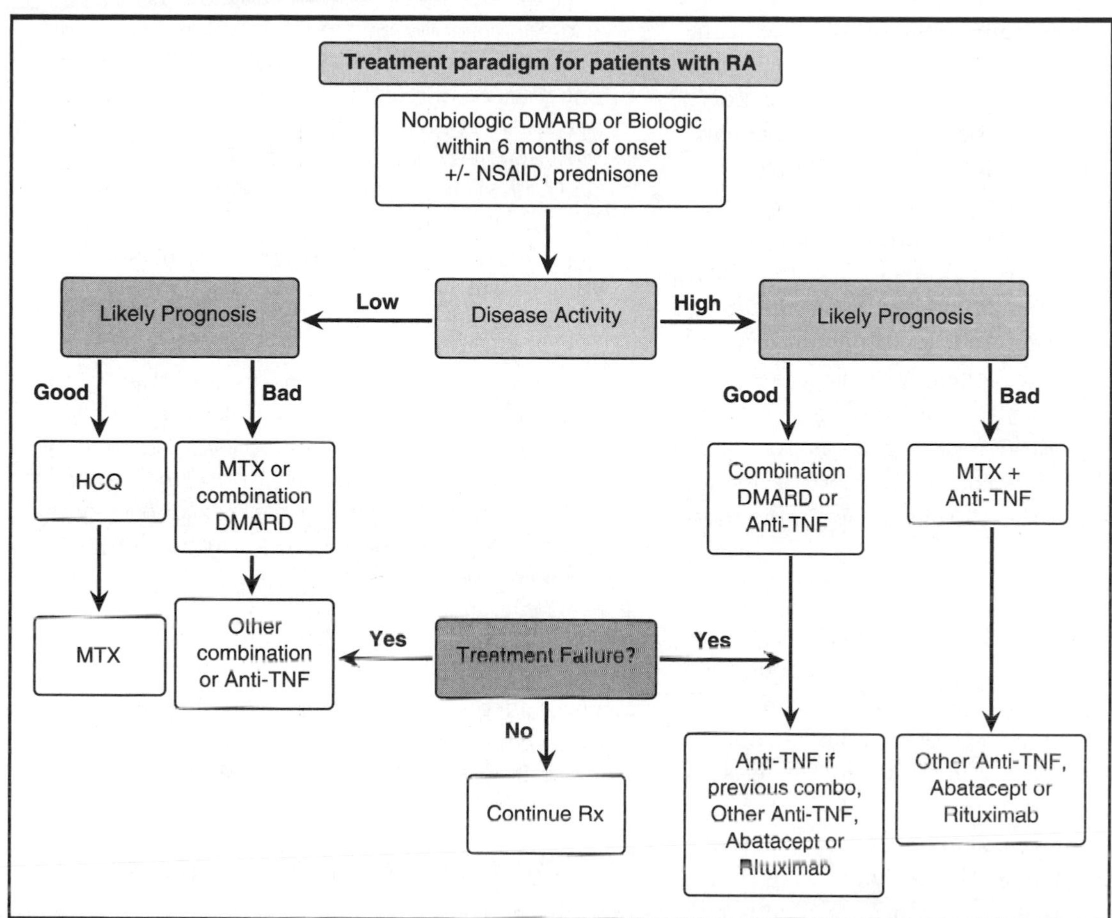

Adjunct Therapy

Patients requiring chronic corticosteroids should be given supplemental calcium and vitamin D to minimize bone loss. Annual bone density studies should be done, and patients who develop osteopenia or osteoporosis should also be given a bisphosphonate. Some clinicians would begin a bisphosphonate as a preventive measure before osteopenia develops. As immunosuppression may reduce ability to produce an antibody response, immunization should be done before starting therapy when possible. Live vaccines are contraindicated with rituximab therapy and should be administered before beginning therapy or just before the next course of therapy in a patient who has already received treatment. Folic acid may be administered with methotrexate to reduce the risk of toxicity. Patients should have tuberculin skin tests before starting biologic therapy as tuberculosis has been reported in patients started on these therapies. Skin-test–positive patients should receive adequate treatment with isoniazid before starting a biologic agent. Because of the increased risk of coronary artery disease in RA, coronary risk factors should be treated aggressively.

Therapeutic Monitoring

Monitoring of therapeutic outcomes includes assessment for improvement in clinical signs and symptoms of RA. This includes reduction of pain and swelling in affected joints, reduced stiffness, decreased fatigue, and other nonspecific symptoms. Assessment of patient ability to perform daily activity is also useful. Laboratory monitoring is of little benefit in assessing patient response to therapy. Laboratory monitoring for drug toxicity is necessary for many of the drugs used. Also, patients should be asked about symptoms that may suggest adverse effects to treatment. Radiographs of affected joints should show little or no progression over time with effective treatment.

Treatment of Rheumatoid Arthritis in Pregnancy

RA disease activity tends to decrease during pregnancy, especially during the third trimester, making it possible to reduce or eliminate anti-inflammatory therapy. Methotrexate and leflunomide are contraindicated during pregnancy and should be discontinued before conception. Leflunomide has a long elimination half-life because of enterohepatic circulation. It is recommended that cholestyramine be used to eliminate the drug before a planned pregnancy. NSAIDs should be discontinued during the last trimester because of premature closure of the ductus, changes in fetal renal function, and pulmonary hypertension. Hydroxychloroquine, sulfasalazine, and low-dose prednisone are generally considered to be safe. Limited data are available for biologic agents in pregnancy. To date, case reports suggest no increased risk to the fetus, but the lack of substantial evidence should preclude use of these drugs except in the most severe RA.[28-30]

Patient Education

Patients should be advised to scale back on physical activities when the disease flares and counseled to rest when fatigued or when a joint is inflamed. Gentle range-of-motion exercises should keep the joints flexible. During remission, low-impact aerobics may increase muscle strength and improve overall health. Drug therapy is usually a lifetime necessity, with treatment aimed at significantly reducing symptoms to allow patients to maintain normal activities. Patients need regular monitoring to assess for disease progression and drug toxicities. Women taking leflunomide or methotrexate need to avoid pregnancy because of teratogenicity and embryotoxicity. As immunosuppression increases patient risk for infection, patients should be instructed to contact their healthcare provider at the first sign of infection for treatment recommendations.

SUMMARY

RA is a relapsing, remitting autoimmune disease that affects a disproportionate number of women. The goal of therapy is to slow progression of the disease and to maintain remission. DMARDs, either as single agents or in combination, should be initiated early in diagnosis. NSAIDs and glucocorticoids can be used as bridge therapy during the slow onset of action of DMARDs. Biologic response modifiers are often combined with DMARDs such as methotrexate and may be effective when DMARDs fail to achieve adequate responses. Ongoing surveillance must be conducted for increased susceptibility to infectious diseases and other comorbidities.

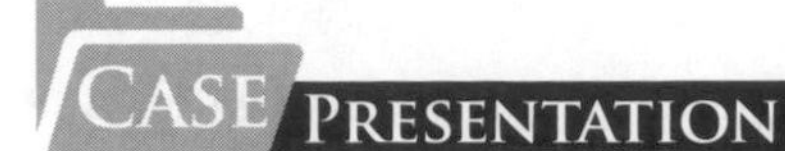

PRESENTATION

Patient Case: Part 2

The symptoms and laboratory findings for this patient were consistent with the diagnosis of RA. She had symmetric swelling and pain with morning stiffness of 1 hour. Her positive RF, anti-CCP antibody, and elevated CRP and ESR supported the clinical diagnosis. The patient sought care from a rheumatologist who prescribed prednisone (10 mg twice daily) and hydroxychloroquine (200 mg twice daily). Symptoms did not abate, and after 4 months, methotrexate (15 mg/wk) was added to her regimen, as well as folic acid (1 mg/day) to reduce risk of toxicity. Liver enzymes, other serology, and a differential leukocyte count were evaluated every 8 weeks. With the disease in remission, prednisone was tapered and discontinued. M.V.S. got married. However, she was unable to remain on methotrexate during her two pregnancies. Shortly after the birth of her second child, she added infliximab (3 mg/kg intravenously at 0, 2, 4, and then every 8 weeks) to her treatment of methotrexate and hydroxychloroquine.

Systemic Lupus Erythematosus

(See Web Resources for Patient Case: Systemic Lupus Erythematosus.)

Additional content available at
www.ashp.org/womenshealth

CLINICAL PRESENTATION

SLE is a multisystem autoimmune connective tissue disorder with a peak age at onset in young women between late teens and early 40s. Women of African or Asian ancestry are at greatest risk for developing this disorder. Other risk factors include early age at menarche (<10 years), any use of oral contraceptives, and irregular menses at ages 18–22.[31]

Initial presentation of SLE involves one or more organ systems and systemic manifestations, including muscle aches and arthritis, fatigue, low-grade fever, malaise, loss of appetite, and weight loss, which are seen in approximately 95% of SLE patients. Although arthritis is common, erosive joint damage

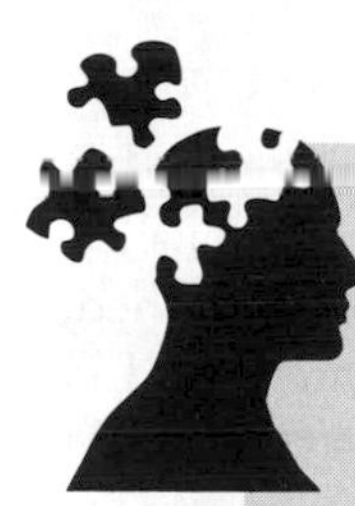

Therapeutic Challenge:

The choice between conventional DMARD therapy and biologic agents in early active RA is not all that clear-cut. What factors need to be considered in choosing between these classes in patients not previously treated?

is rarely seen. Virtually all organ systems may be involved in SLE, and cutaneous manifestations, including photosensitivity, malar (butterfly) rash, and mouth/nasal ulcers are present in 70%, 50%, and 40% of patients, respectively. Cardiopulmonary manifestations occur in 60% of SLE patients, with the most common being pleuritis and pericarditis. **Raynaud's phenomenon** and **alopecia** occur in 40% to 50% of patients. Involvement of multiple organ systems is common (e.g., pleuritis, pneumonitis, nephritis, cerebritis), with nephritis as one of the leading causes of death in the first 10 years after diagnosis.[32] Central nervous system involvement may have a broad range of manifestations, including cognitive dysfunction, headache, seizures, stroke, visual disturbances, and psychiatric illness. Lupus nephritis often is asymptomatic, and frequent monitoring for changes in renal function or proteinuria may serve as markers for renal disease. Acute loss of kidney function may occur as a result of thrombosis of the renal artery or vein. Hematuria may result from cystitis, interstitial cystitis in the bladder, or as a complication from cyclophosphamide therapy to treat SLE. SLE patients are also at increased risk of heart attack, stroke, and transient ischemic attacks, as well as infections, secondary lymphoproliferative disorders (leukemia, lymphoma), and breast cancer.[32] It is not known if these increased risks are due to immunosuppressive drug treatment or the autoimmune disease itself.[33,34]

Cutaneous manifestations of SLE include malar and discoid rashes, oral ulcers, alopecia, and inflammation of the subcutaneous fatty tissue (panniculitis). Discoid lupus is a localized form of the disease, with most patients just having involvement of the skin. Erythema with inflammation occurs in well-marginated patches and is followed by subcutaneous atrophy in the affected regions of the skin. Alopecia of scalp lesions is usually seen. Only about 5% go on to develop SLE, even though more than one half of them are positive for antinuclear antibody (ANA), whereas up to 20% of patients with SLE also exhibit discoid lesions. Photosensitivity is common in SLE, and sun exposure may induce flares of the disease.

Drug-induced lupus usually just has skin and musculoskeletal symptoms and usually is reversible within several months of stopping the offending agent. Hydralazine, procainamide, and quinidine, as well as TNF inhibitors, are associated with this variant of SLE. It has also been suggested that viral illness may induce lupus or induce a flare in patients with SLE in that patients often report symptoms before onset of SLE or disease flare. Epstein-Barr virus (EBV) has been implicated, as 100% of children and young adults with SLE have EBV DNA.[35]

Patients may have antiphospholipid antibody syndrome in association with SLE. Patients with this syndrome have one or more antibodies to phospholipids that may be detected on testing. Clinically, these patients present with venous or arterial thrombotic disorders or recurrent early fetal loss. Thrombocytopenia may also be noted.

Anemia associated with chronic disease is common. Patients may develop immune-mediated hemolytic anemia that is due to development of antibodies to red blood cells, resulting in early red cell lysis. Antibody-mediated leukopenia and thrombocytopenia may also occur.

PATHOPHYSIOLOGY

Pathogenesis of SLE is the result of sustained production of autoantibodies and formation of immune complexes. The mechanisms by which these antibodies are stimulated and produced are numerous and include dysfunction in apoptosis, T-cell signaling, and cytokines. The antibodies to nuclear components may be due to defective removal of apoptotic debris by macrophages. This leads to the presentation of normally sequestered self-antigens and activation of self-reactive B and T cells, resulting in the production of autoantibodies, in particular ANAs, which are present in 98% of individuals with SLE. In addition, patients with SLE have high levels of interferon-α Defects in receptors for type I interferons leading to decreased signal transduction have been demonstrated. These defects in signal transduction can lead to abnormal cytokine production. There is also a decrease in function of T regulatory cells, which may lead to proliferation of T helper cells and increased activation of B cells.

The pathogenic autoantibodies in SLE include anti-dsDNA and anti-SM Abs, which are specific for SLE. Other autoantibodies (e.g., anti-SS-A, anti-SS-B) often found in patients with SLE are not specific for the disease. Nephritis is the most important and serious manifestation of SLE and is usually asymptomatic. Proteinuria and active urine sediment with red blood cell casts may be found in urinalysis. Kidney biopsy is important for diagnosing the amount of renal involvement and determining the treatment options.[31] Nephritis in SLE patients is generally ongoing, requiring retreatment when the disease flares. In addition, nephritis predisposes to accelerated atherosclerosis, hypertension, and dislipidemia.[32] SS is often associated with SLE.

Mortality remains a major concern among patients with SLE at a rate 3 times higher than among the general population. Arteriosclerotic disease is also a major health concern, as are side effects of certain therapies (e.g., glucocorticoids).

LABORATORY FINDINGS

The presence of antibodies in patients with symptoms consistent with SLE makes the diagnosis highly likely. ANAs are present in 76% of patients at onset and in 94% at any time. There is also an increased frequency of other ANAs, such as anti-SS-A(Ro), anti-SS-B(La), anti-Sm, anti-RNP, and antiphospholipid antibodies.[36] Other serologic indicators can include elevated ESR and CRP. However, the absence of ANA, anti-dsDNA Abs, or anti-SS-A(Ro) Abs, even in symptomatic individuals, makes the diagnosis of SLE less likely.[32]

TREATMENT GOALS

The goal of pharmacologic and nonpharmacologic therapy is to preserve organ function, improve patient quality of life, and reduce patient symptoms.

Drug Therapy

Patients with SLE are initiated on NSAIDs and corticosteroids. Other agents may be administered to patients singly or in combination. These would include hydroxychloroquine, azathioprine, methotrexate, cyclophosphamide regimens, mycophenolate mofetil, and/or rituximab. Common clinical practice recommends placing most if not all patients initially on hydroxychloroquine.[37] Other therapies would be considered in patients with more severe disease or if hydroxychloroquine is ineffective. Cyclophosphamide is reserved for patients with life-threatening complications from SLE, such as lupus cerebritis, severe nephritis, or other organ-threatening vasculitic complications.

Rituximab has been found to be effective for SLE in a large number of uncontrolled trials and published case series. However, two recent, as yet unpublished, controlled trials in patients with nonrenal SLE (EXPLORER) and renal lupus nephritis (LUNAR) failed to detect statistical differences in treatment comparing rituximab to conventional therapies. Some reasons for this lack of response may have been due to variation in trial methodology. Both studies enrolled participants with relatively mild disease, and treatment with corticosteroids and immunosuppressives in the two treatment arms may have further decreased the likelihood of detecting differences between rituximab and placebo.[38-41] Literature to support use of other biologics for the treatment of SLE is lacking at this time.

Adjunct Therapies

Screening for osteoporosis and intervention (bisphosphonates, calcium, vitamin D) in patients requiring chronic steroid use is important adjunct therapy. In addition, patients should be advised to apply high sun protection factor (SPF), broad-spectrum sunscreen (≥30) and to wear protective clothing. Comorbidities—including infections (especially urinary tract), atherosclerosis, hypertension, dyslipidemias, diabetes, avascular necrosis, and malignancies (especially non-Hodgkin's lymphoma)—require treatment. Patients with positive antiphospholipid antibodies and history of clotting disorders, and women with a history of recurrent fetal loss need long-term anticoagulation. If Raynaud's symptoms are a problem, dihydropyridine calcium channel blockers and losartan may be of some value to reduce symptoms. Heat-conservation measures—including wearing coats, gloves, and hats during cold weather and avoiding sudden temperature changes in summer or winter—is also of benefit.

Therapeutic Monitoring

Measures useful in monitoring lupus activity and flare-ups include the appearance of new clinical signs and manifestations of the disease. Laboratory tests, including creatinine or blood urea nitrogen to monitor changes in renal function, and urine tests for protein or active urinary sediment that may suggest nephritis, are needed. Periodic complete blood counts should be done. Assessment of patient global disease activity should be periodically done.

Drug Therapy in Pregnancy and Lactation

Methotrexate, leflunomide, mycophenolate mofetil, and cyclophosphamide are all contraindicated in pregnancy and lactation because of teratogenicity.

Cyclophosphamide use may result in ovarian failure. Hydroxychloroquine may be safely used during pregnancy. Azathioprine is not converted to an active metabolite in the fetal liver and may be continued during pregnancy. Prednisone may also be used throughout pregnancy safely. High-dose corticosteroids increase risk for drug-related complications to fetus and mother. Disease flares during pregnancy increases fetal risk and may result in spontaneous abortion and preterm delivery. There are little data on the use of biologic agents in pregnancy or lactation. In patients with antiphospholipid antibody syndrome, warfarin is contraindicated in pregnancy because of teratogenicity and risk for fetal bleeding. It does not appear to impose risk for breast-fed infants. Careful planning should take place in childbearing decisions in patients with SLE to optimize treatment to those drugs that will be safe yet effective in controlling the disease.

Patient Education

Patients should be counseled to have realistic expectations of the disease and its treatments, to identify symptoms and signs of flares, and to comply with the medication plan, including keeping medical appointments. Patients should also balance adequate rest with exercise, cease smoking, avoid extensive ultraviolet light exposure, avoid physical exhaustion, and use hormone therapy/oral contraceptives with caution. Pregnant women with SLE may experience an increased risk of miscarriages, pre-eclampsia, intrauterine growth restriction, fetal death, and preterm delivery.[31]

SUMMARY

SLE is a relapsing, remitting autoimmune disease that affects a disproportionate number of women. Both DMARDs and NSAIDs have been shown to be effective in these patients. Hydroxychloroquine is an anchor therapy for patients with SLE. In patients with more severe disease or life-threatening complications, high-dose corticosteroids, cyclophosphamide, or rituximab may be needed. Adjunctive therapy for SLE-related comorbidities may be needed.

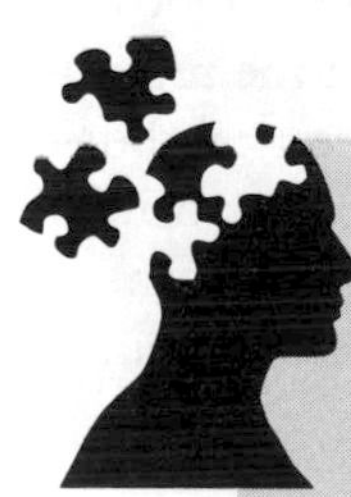

Therapeutic Challenge:

Perhaps one of the biggest challenges is managing the patient with active disease who wishes to become pregnant. Develop a therapeutic and monitoring plan to address drug therapy concerns and safety of the fetus.

Sjögren's Syndrome

(See Web Resources for Patient Case: Sjögren's Syndrome.)

Additional content available at
www.ashp.org/womenshealth

CLINICAL PRESENTATION

Patients with SS present with symptoms consistent with decreased exocrine gland function, including decreased tear production, leading to dryness and irritation of the eyes; slit-lamp examination may reveal punctuate corneal ulcers. Oral symptoms of SS include dry mouth and difficulty swallowing dry food. Patients are susceptible to increased dental decay and oral candidiasis. Salivary gland enlargement may be seen in half of patients. This may be episodic and usually is not associated with tenderness. Nasal and throat symptoms may also occur, with chronic dry cough being the most common. Interstitial lung disease and dyspnea may also occur and may be associated with abnormal pulmonary function tests. Vaginal dryness has been reported in half the women with SS and may lead to painful intercourse as well as increased bacterial and candidal infection. Dry skin (xerosis) is seen in more than half of patients, and 10% may develop cutaneous vasculitis. Raynaud's phenomenon is reported in 37% of patients. Half of patients develop joint or muscle pain. A fibromyalgia-like presentation may be seen. Both central and peripheral nervous complications may occur, including neuropathy, neuralgia, and central neurologic deficit. Renal complications include nephritis and cystitis. Dysphagia is frequently seen because of reduced saliva formation, resulting in difficulty moving the food bolus past the throat. Lymphoma is 16–44 times more likely in patients with SS, which may be classified as primary or secondary when it is associated with another systemic immunologic disease. Ninety percent of all patients with SS are women.

PATHOPHYSIOLOGY

SS is a chronic autoimmune disease that is slowly progressive and may take 8–10 years to develop into full-blown disease. SS elicits inflammation of the lacrimal glands, leading to decreased production of tears and eye dryness. There is also inflammation of the salivary glands and parotid glands, leading to dry mouth. The disease is characterized by autoantibodies and cellular infiltration of exocrine glands by activated B and T cells. Extraglandular features include fatigue, musculoskeletal symptoms, Raynaud's phenomenon, gastrointestinal manifestations, parenchymal involvement, neurologic involvement, gynecologic problems, and vasculitis. Dysregulation of exocrine gland epithelial cells causes them to produce and secrete proinflammatory cytokines and chemokines as well as display HLA class II molecule and costimulatory molecules (B7). SS is associated with specific HLA class I (e.g., B8) and class II (-DR3, -DRw52, and -DQA1) molecule. SS that is not associated with other connective tissue autoimmune disease is known as primary SS. However, when SS is associated with other diseases, such as RA, SLE, scleroderma, Hashimoto's thyroiditis, gastroesophageal reflux disease, lymphoma (rarely), and primary biliary cirrhosis, it is referred to as secondary SS.

DIAGNOSIS GUIDELINES

Diagnosis of SS is established based on the presence of eye or mouth dryness and on the occurrence of autoantibodies against the ribonucleoprotein complexes Ro/SS-A and La/SS-B. Detecting dryness of the eye can be tested by measuring the eye's ability to wet a small testing paper strip under the eyelid (Schirmer's test). **Rose Bengal stain** is used to measure ocular integrity and will stain surface cells of the cornea and conjunctiva that are devitalized. Detecting dryness of the mouth is measured by a salivary flow test, sialometry. Biopsy of minor salivary gland may show characteristic lymphocytic invasion of the gland and glandular atrophy. Serologic markers can include detection of ANA, anti-SSA(Ro), anti-SSB(La) autoantibodies, RF, and increased ESR.[42,43] The presence of anti-SSA(Ro) and anti-SSB(La) antibodies are part of the diagnostic criteria for this disease.

TREATMENT GOALS

Goals of treatment are to reduce local and systemic manifestations of SS. Treatment to alleviate symptoms includes topical therapy for dry eyes and dry mouth, therapy for the wide variety of systemic symptoms and arthritis, and pain management. Replacement therapy for ocular dryness can include tear substitutes, lubricating ointments, and methylcellulose inserts (the latter two for night-time use). Topical cyclosporine eye drops may result in improved tear formation for some patients. Plugging of lacrimal punctal ducts, which drain tears from the eye, may be beneficial. Replacement therapy for dry mouth includes salivary substitutes and lubricating agents. Use of sugar-free lozenges or gum may help stimulate natural saliva. Systemic stimulation of salivary gland function includes cholinergic agonists, such as pilocarpine and cevimeline. Systemic anti-inflammatory therapy including—corticosteroids, NSAIDs, and hydroxychloroquine—may also be of benefit for arthritis symptoms. Management of extraglandular manifestations is reviewed in Mavragani et al.[43]

Therapeutic Drugs

Current pharmacologic therapies for SS include the following as replacement therapy (artificial tears, eye lubricants, vaginal lubricants), local stimulators of tear production (cyclosporin ophthalmic emulsion 0.05%, one eye drop twice daily), systemic stimulants of glandular function (pilocarpine 5 mg 4 times a day; or cevimeline 30–60 mg 3 times a day), systemic anti-inflammatory agents (hydroxychloroquine 200–400 mg/day), and prednisone (varying dosages). Neither infliximab nor etanercept showed any evidence of efficacy in patients with primary SS. A promising new treatment for patients with primary SS is rituximab, a monoclonal antibody directed against the B-cell surface marker CD20. This drug depletes B cell, reducing antibody formation.[44]

Therapeutic Monitoring

The effectiveness of therapy is evaluated by subjective improvements in dry eyes, dry mouth, and other symptoms.

Patient Education

Patients should be counseled to increase fluid intake, avoid medications (e.g., anticholinergics) that exacerbate dryness, and monitor oral care through frequent visits to the dentist (use of sugar-free lozenges, gum, chlorhexidine mouthwash, fluoride gels). Good oral hygiene with regular brushing and flossing of teeth is necessary. Use of eye lubricants, artificial tears, and saline nasal sprays may help relieve dry mucous membranes. Avoiding low humidity will reduce mucous membrane as well as skin dryness. Pain in the mouth is not a symptom of xerosis and may suggest candidiasis. Painful or irritated eyes not relieved by ocular replacement therapy may suggest blepharitis. Both of these conditions warrant health provider evaluation.

SUMMARY

SS is a chronic autoimmune disease that is slowly progressive and may take 8–10 years to develop into full-blown disease. If diagnosed as the sole autoimmune disease, it is primary SS, and when associated with other autoimmune diseases, it is secondary SS. Diagnosis is fairly specific, and there are multiple drugs available for treating the symptoms.

Graves' Disease

(See Web Resources for Patient Case: Graves' Disease.)

Additional content available at
www.ashp.org/womenshealth

CLINICAL PRESENTATION

The clinical signs and symptoms of Graves' disease are the same as those for any hyperthyroid disorder, including nervousness, heat intolerance with excessive perspiration, agitation, palpitations, tachycardia, weight loss with increased appetite, tremor, irregular menstrual flow, and goiter.[43] Also associated with Graves' disease is ophthalmopathy, which typically presents in 25% of patients. Graves' ophthalmopathy (exophthalmos) is characterized by enlarged extraocular muscles and eye discomfort but may extend to proptosis and double vision in severe cases. These patients may be at risk for corneal abrasions. Approximately 3% of patients develop Graves' dermopathy, characterized by reddening and swelling of the skin, especially on the shins and tops of feet.[45,46]

PATHOPHYSIOLOGY

Autoimmune thyroid diseases are the most common autoimmune diseases and affect about 1.5% of the population. Of affected individuals, >90% are women. Graves' disease is an autoimmune disease that is influenced by genetic factors (HLA-DR, HLA-A DQ, and CTLA-4), environmental factors (including stress, smoking, and increases in iodine consumption), and, in women, the postpartum period.[45,47] The etiology of the disease stems from the presence of antithyroid antibodies acting as receptor agonists, also know as thyroid-stimulating immunoglobulins (TSI), and anti-TSH receptor antibodies (TRAb).[45-48] The development of these antibodies is linked to the loss of suppressor activity by CD4 T regulatory cells preceding the development of clinical hyperthyroidism.[47] By inhibiting the mechanism regulating thyroid hormone production, TSH is suppressed, and thyroid hormones thyroxine (T4) and tri-iodothyronine (T3) are overproduced. As these thyroid hormones regulate metabolism, patients may present with metabolic symptoms, including weight loss and heat intolerance. Goiter is also caused by this overabundant yield. Rarely, patients with Graves' disease develop autoimmune cytotoxic T cells, which may result in spontaneous hypothyroidism.[45]

DIAGNOSIS

Diagnosis of Graves' disease is based on a thyroid scan, measurement of serum TSH levels, presence of antithyroglobulin antibodies (TSI and TSH-R Ab), and levels of free T4. Because of negative feedback inhibition of the pituitary by elevated thyroid hormones, blood levels of TSH are low or at undetectable levels (<0.1 units/mL). Therefore, the finding of low TSH and high T4 in the presence of Graves' ophthalmopathy can be diagnostic. Antithyroglobulin antibodies are elevated, and TSI/TRAb are found in about 65% of patients with Graves' disease.[45,46] Confirmation of Graves' disease can also be made through a 24-hour radioiodine uptake, in which diffuse uptake is noted.[48]

TREATMENT GOALS

Treatment Options

There are three treatment options for patients with Graves' disease: antithyroid drugs, radioactive iodine, and surgery. Methimazole and propylthiouracil (PTU) are antithyroid drugs that decrease the production of T4. Normal levels are achieved with methimazole in 5–6 weeks, whereas PTU is effective in lowering T4 level in about 8 weeks. Oral radioactive iodine is given one time to ablate the hyperactive gland. The gland becomes normal in 8–12 weeks. All oral treatment options are contraindicated in pregnancy and lactation because of fetal risk. In these cases, surgical thyroidectomy, whether partial or full, may be a useful alternative to radioactive iodine. Radioactive iodine therapy is the treatment of choice in Graves' hyperthyroidism because of remission and side effects associated with antithyroid medications and complications that can arise with surgical removal.[48]

Dosing Strategies

Antithyroid medication dosages range depending on the severity of hyperthyroidism and symptoms the patient is experiencing. Methimazole is given in dosages of 10–60 mg/day, typically divided in three doses to minimize side effects, but can be administered once daily because of its long half-life. Propylthiouracil is dosed 300 mg/day for mild disease and upward of 900 mg/day in severe disease, administered in three to four divided doses. Patients should be monitored closely every 2–4 weeks while on either drug, with a goal to reduce total T4 levels to normal. The medication dosage should be gradually tapered over time as patients reach euthyroid levels, typically in 8–12 weeks after therapy initiation. Many patients require only 50–150 mg of PTU or 5–15 mg of methimazole daily of maintenance therapy once reaching euthyroid levels.

Radioactive iodine therapy is the treatment of choice to eradicate or reduce thyroid- and antibody-producing cells. This therapy is safe and effective to treat Graves' disease. Typically, this ablative therapy will cause patients to become hypothyroid and require thyroid replacement for the rest of their lives. Radioactive iodine therapy is contraindicated in pregnancy, and women should wait at least 6 months after treatment to become pregnant; however, there is no evidence that radioactive iodine therapy has any adverse effects if used properly.[47] Evidence does suggest a link of ophthalmopathy symptoms initially worsening after radioactive iodine therapy because of an initial increase in TRAbs from cell ablation. This therapy should be used with caution in patients who have known Graves' ophthalmopathy. Pretreatment with antithyroid medication should be considered to reduce risk these side effects.

Adjunct Therapy

For Graves' ophthalmopathy, symptomatic relief is generally sufficient. Patients can administer cool compresses to the eyes, wear sunglasses, use lubricating eye drops, and elevate the head of the bed to reduce pressure. If symptoms persist, oral corticosteroid therapy can be administered. Both PTU and methimazole require at least 2–4 weeks to suppress elevated T4 and T3 levels, during which time β-adrenergic antagonist therapy remains the cornerstone of symptom control. Atenolol is the drug of choice because of its long half-life; however, any beta-blocker may be adequate.

Therapeutic Monitoring

Monitoring TSH levels as well as levels of T3 and T4 are important with any type of therapy. Initially, these levels should be monitored frequently (every 2–4 weeks); then, as a patient stabilizes, every 6–12 months. As hypothyroidism may develop long after treatment with radioactive iodine treatment, TSH needs to be monitored periodically, probably for life, in patients treated.

Patient Education

Patients should be advised to monitor for signs of hypothyroidism or hyperthyroidism. Measures of thyroid function should be conducted annually.

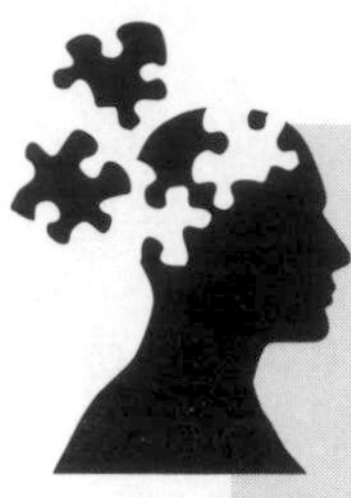

Therapeutic Challenge:

A 26-year-old woman with Graves' disease was treated with I^{131}. Two months later, she became pregnant in spite of measures taken to prevent pregnancy. What patient counseling measures and recommendations could be made?

SUMMARY

Graves' disease is an autoimmune disease of the thyroid occurring more frequently in women. Early detection and management is important in this disease. It can be treated with antithyroid drugs, radioactive iodine, or surgery. Adjunctive ophthalmopathy can also be treated with artificial tears and nondrug approaches.

Hashimoto's Thyroiditis

(See Web Resources for Patient Case: Hashimoto's Thyroiditis.)

Additional content available at
www.ashp.org/womenshealth

CLINICAL PRESENTATION

Hashimoto's thyroiditis mimics the classic symptoms of hypothyroidism, including fatigue, weakness, depression, cold intolerance, dry hair, dry skin, weight gain (10–20 lb), and menorrhagia, but is associated with elevated serum autoantibodies to thyroid peroxidase and thyroglobulin. Late in the disease, the symptoms may evolve to include hoarseness, swelling, thickening of the skin, constipation, decreased concentration, pericardial effusion, bradycardia, and heart failure. Heart failure is rare in patients without pre-existing heart disease but may worsen in patients with concomitant disease. Rare complications are myxedema, coma, and death. Physical examination often shows a firm, irregular, nontender goiter.

PATHOPHYSIOLOGY

Hashimoto's thyroiditis is the most common cause of goiter in the U.S. and is characterized by a lymphocytic infiltrate of the thyroid gland. It is familially linked, similar to Graves' disease, which can progress to Hashimoto's thyroiditis in about 15% of patients.[45] The association with HLA-DR2 and DR5 suggests a genetic predisposition also shown through the disease stratification among families. It is more common in women than men and often presents in adulthood. Hashimoto's thyroiditis is characterized by an infiltration of activated $CD4^+$ and $CD8^+$ T cells, as well as antibody-producing B cells in the thyroid. The destruction of the thyroid tissue is likely due to CD^+ T cell–induced apoptosis, either because of granzymes or perforin, as well as the effects of inflammatory cytokines, such as TNF-α.[49] The marked infiltrate and accompanying inflammation lead to destruction of the thyroid gland. Hashimoto's thyroiditis has been shown to often coexist with other autoimmune diseases, such as type 1 diabetes mellitus, celiac disease, RA, MS, and vitiligo.[49]

DIAGNOSIS

Hashimoto's thyroiditis is objectively diagnosed by an increase in serum antibodies to thyroglobulin and thyroid peroxidase protein. Autoantibodies are detectable in 95% of patients with Hashimoto's thyroiditis.[48] These serologic measures are typically accompanied with increased levels of TSH and low levels of free T4 thyroid hormone, in addition to an abnormal thyroid scan and ultrasound. With the influx of lytic cytotoxic T lymphocytes and antibody to thyroglobulin and thyroid peroxidase protein, the thyroid gland is destroyed, in turn causing the pituitary gland to produce higher-than-normal levels of TSH.[50]

TREATMENT GOALS

Treatment Options

This disease is treated with thyroid hormone therapy with the synthetic thyroid hormone levothyroxine at an average dosage of 1.6 mcg/kg or 100–125 mcg orally every day.[48]

Dosing Strategies

Thyroid hormone replacement dosages must be carefully adjusted according to individual requirements and response. Typically, patients begin on levothyroxine 75 mcg daily, and doses are titrated to normalize TSH. However, levothyroxine requirements decrease with age because of diminished thyroid hormone metabolism. Therefore, patients older than 50 years of age may require levothyroxine replacement ≤1 mcg/kg/day, with a starting dosage of 50 mcg daily and titrated to normalize TSH.[51] Many medications will interact with levothyroxine. Cationic medications (including iron, calcium, and aluminum hydroxide) and medications that bind as their mechanism of action (e.g., cholestyramine) can decrease the absorption of levothyroxine. These medications that reduce the absorption of levothyroxine should be administered 4 hours apart from levothyroxine. Protein binding by anticonvulsants and metabolism increases by rifampin are other ways medication can interact with levothyroxine.[48] Thyroid-stimulating hormone levels should be monitored more frequently if any interacting agents are added to therapy.

Therapeutic Monitoring

Levothyroxine is recognized by the U.S. Food and Drug Administration as a compound with a narrow therapeutic range and should be carefully monitored for clinical symptoms and laboratory changes. Substitution between brands/manufacturers may result in the need for dosage changes. Thyroid-stimulating hormone levels should be monitored at least 6 weeks after any dosage adjustment or brand change. Monitoring free T4 levels can be helpful in patients who continue to have some functionality of their thyroid gland.[48] Hypothyroid symptoms can resolve with TSH levels of 3–4 micro-International Units/mL; however, the goal is to normalize TSH (1–2 micro-International Units/mL), which will resolve symptoms.

In women, long-term supertherapeutic levothyroxine sodium therapy has been associated with decreased bone mineral density because of increased bone resorption. This is noted in postmenopausal women on greater-than-replacement dosages or in women who are receiving suppressive dosages of levothyroxine sodium. The increased bone resorption may be associated with increased serum levels and urinary excretion of calcium and phosphorous, elevations in bone alkaline phosphatase, and suppressed serum parathyroid hormone levels. Therefore, it is recommended that patients receiving levothyroxine sodium be given the minimum dosage necessary to achieve biochemical response (i.e., TSH = 1–2 micro-International Units/mL).

Therapy in Pregnancy

In pregnancy, hypothyroidism can cause significant complications, including an increased risk of fetal death and pre-eclampsia, as well as placing the mother at further risk for postpartum hemorrhage. Levothyroxine is safe to use during pregnancy; however, some women have changes in their levothyroxine requirements during pregnancy.[48] Laboratory TSH levels should be monitored throughout pregnancy for proper dosage adjustments.

Patient Education

As with Graves' disease, self-monitoring is important for proper treatment of Hashimoto's thyroiditis. Patients should be aware of all the symptoms and vigilant to any changes, including, but not limited to, moderate weight gain, fatigue, depression, or cold intolerance. Levothyroxine sodium should be administered on an empty stomach, preferably ½–1 hour before breakfast or the first meal of the day. If the patient cannot tolerate the medication on an empty stomach, levothyroxine may be dosed with food as long as the patient is consistent with this administration for absorption purposes and titrations may be made appropriately. Levothyroxine may be crushed and placed in a small amount of water for patients with difficulty swallowing tablets.

SUMMARY

Hashimoto's thyroiditis is an autoimmune disease that results in destruction of the thyroid tissue. It is diagnosed in patients who have autoantibody serologic measures and elevated TSH. Ultrasound may be useful in identifying goiters. Treatment of Hashimoto's thyroiditis requires levothyroxine to replace the hormone that the thyroid gland is no longer able to produce in adequate amounts.

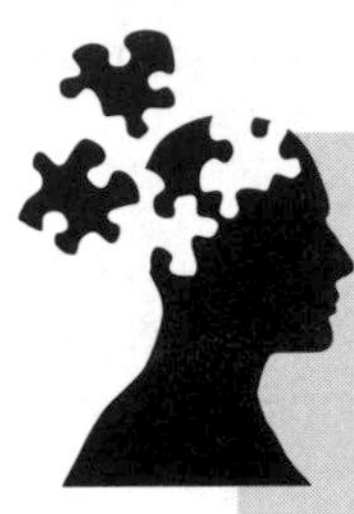

Therapeutic Challenge:

A 43-year-old woman with positive antithyroid antibodies has a TSH of 3.53, normal T4, and no symptoms of hypothyroidism. Should she be supplemented with levothyroxine?

Chapter Summary

Autoimmune diseases, many of which predominantly affect women, present with a variety of signs and symptoms and varying severity. These diseases do not share common underlying immune mechanisms of damage, nor is there a common environmental factor or HLA haplotype. Early patient education by healthcare professionals is critical in ensuring enhanced quality of life. For many, prescribed drugs can also dramatically slow disease progression. Finally, adjunct and nonpharmacologic intervention strategies should be a common element in disease management. The one course of treatment that is not available to patients with autoimmune diseases is prophylaxis. Because the causes and triggers of these chronic diseases are multiple and speculative, prevention is not possible.

References

Additional content available at ***www.ashp.org/womenshealth***

38 Sexually Transmitted and Infectious Diseases

Lisa D. Inge, Pharm.D., BCPS, AAHIVE; Kimberley C. Brown, Pharm.D., AAHIVE; Raymond Cha, Pharm.D.

Learning Objectives

1. Identify cultural, ethnic, and racial differences in rates of sexually transmitted diseases in women.
2. Recognize the symptoms associated with common sexually transmitted diseases, along with human immunodeficiency virus/acquired immunodeficiency virus and pelvic inflammatory disease in women.
3. Recommend an appropriate first-line treatment option for the identified sexually transmitted diseases in women.
4. Describe any potential interventions that should be taken to care for HIV-positive women and treatment management of pregnancy in HIV-positive women.

The Centers for Disease Control and Prevention (CDC) estimates that there are 19 million new sexually transmitted infections each year in the U.S.[1] These conditions are common, costly, and yet preventable.[1] Women remain disproportionately represented in identified sexually transmitted disease (STD) cases, subsequently accounting for more serious complications when compared with men.[2] A recent study identified that one in four adolescent girls in the U.S. has had or is infected with an STD.[3] A number of factors contribute a woman's increased risk. These include the asymptomatic nature of many of these diseases in women; greater susceptibility, especially in younger women between the ages of 15 and 24 years (as a result of both physiological and emotional maturity); lower socioeconomic status; and the potential for sexual coercion.[2] Additionally, the secrecy of sexuality, especially among women in a variety of cultures, tends to limit the potential for educational initiatives that assist in decreasing risks.[2]

Compared with men, women have a greater risk of contracting nearly all STDs when exposed.[4] This is particularly true in the case of human immunodeficiency virus (HIV) transmission from men to women.[5] Moreover, the presence of almost any STD increases a woman's risk of contracting HIV.[6] Identification of women who may be classified as high risk, as well as all of those already infected, is essential. High-risk populations include those who have a history of a prior STD, have new or multiple sex partners, use condoms inconsistently, are commercial sex workers, or have a history of drug use, as well as those with partners who possess such high-risk characteristics.[7]

Screening and Prevention

Women with symptomatic infections frequently seek medical treatment, but those who are asymptomatic usually go undetected and thus remain untreated. All high-risk patients, as well as those who are treated for a prior STD, should receive education and counseling on STD prevention, asymptomatic or symptomatic screening as per recommended treatment guidelines, and subsequent treatment of any diagnosed STD. This process diminishes the risk for reinfection and potential complications. Furthermore, all partners should also be screened and treated when possible.[7] (See Web Resources for STD Guidelines Resources.)

Additional content available at
www.ashp.org/womenshealth

Methods of primary STD prevention may also include vaccination along with distribution and use of certain barrier methods, particularly

Case Presentation

Patient Case: Part 1

T.B. is a 23-year-old woman who presents to your inner-city clinic with the chief symptom of pain upon intercourse and vaginal discharge. She explains that she supports herself with employment at a phone sex organization. She often finds herself involved in "relationships" with some of her "special" connections. When discussing the risks involved in these relationships, she admits that many of these men do not want to wear condoms. She denies the use of female condoms as she likes the feel of skin. Her last sexual encounter was about 8 days ago. She denies any fevers or chills but reports pain with sexual intercourse.

PMH: Two prior episodes of gonorrhea and a reactive rapid plasma regain (RPR) of 1:32 from her last clinic visit about 3 months ago. Her treatment history for the two cases of gonorrhea is documented along with a prior RPR titer result from 3 years ago that was 1:2 after treatment of a prior syphilis infection.

Social history: Doesn't smoke, drinks socially (four to six drinks a week).

Medications: None.

Allergies: NKDA.

Vitals: Height: 5′, 6″; Weight: 134 lb; BP: 124/83; Pulse: 67.

Physical exam: Pain upon vaginal exam.

Laboratory tests: Pregnancy test negative. A vaginal swab of the cervix produced bloody discharge that tested positive for both chlamydia and gonorrhea by nucleic acid amplification tests (NAATs). Herpes simplex virus (HSV) culture results pending.

condoms. Secondary prevention methods involve screening, diagnosis, and treatment of particular segments of sexually active populations to reduce disease transmission. Education, however, remains the cornerstone for prevention in both patient populations. Community outreach programs and primary care visits for yearly preventive service offer excellent opportunities for multiple prevention activities, including education.

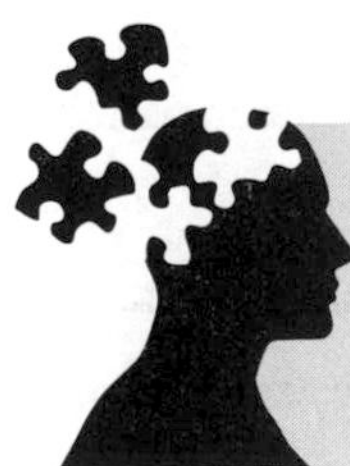

Therapeutic Challenge:

What must be considered when attempting to develop recommendations or plans for STD prevention?

To assist healthcare providers in identifying methods for STD prevention, a number of national organizations have developed their own risk-assessment and counseling recommendations. (See Web Resources for National Sexually Transmitted Infection Recommendations.) One of the key preventive approaches supported by the CDC includes the promotion of abstinence, monogamous relationships, pre-exposure vaccination when available, and consistent and correct use of condoms.[7]

Additional content available at ***www.ashp.org/womenshealth***

A starting point for all preventative recommendations is to obtain a routine sexual history from every patient. This will assist with identifying potential risk factors while also offering opportunities for screening and prevention counseling. Key components of these discussions may be found in *Contraceptive Technology* (18th edition) or in the curriculum offered by the CDC's STD/HIV Prevention Training Centers at www.std.hivpreventiontraining.org. The CDC's Sexually Transmitted Diseases Treatment Guidelines support questions that focus on the "five Ps" as a means of starting a patient discussion. These include a patient's history and number of past and current partners, the methods used for pregnancy and STD prevention, types of sexual practices, and questions pertaining to past STDs. Patient responses to these questions will assist in guiding the types of educational discussions necessary while also offering the healthcare provider a means of risk-factor assessment for STD screening. Each of the STDs, including HIV, has specific recommendations for screening and treatment, which may be assessed on the previously mentioned websites.

Finally, providers and laboratories are required to report all confirmed cases of chlamydia, gonorrhea, syphilis, and HIV to the local health department. These epidemiologic programs are responsible for investigation of local contacts as well as identifying prevalence, surveying behavior, and monitoring antimicrobial resistance patterns of currently recommended agents and clinical outcomes. The data collected also assist in formulating future treatment guidelines, particularly empiric recommendations for future therapeutic interventions.

Treatment Goals

There are specific treatment options for each STD, yet the goals of such interventions are similar. These include a biological cure or eradication when possible, elimination of clinical symptoms or manifestations, prevention of subsequent complications or outbreaks, and prevention of transmission.[7] Treatment of one particular disease also reduces the risk of acquisition of other STDs, including HIV.[4,7]

Assessment and recommendations pertaining to screening and management of STDs should consider the general symptomatic groupings as a starting point. However, it is important to remember that some infected women are asymptomatic, especially with infections exhibiting a longer latency period. The patient's sexual and travel history may correlate with incubation periods or symptomatic onset of particular diseases. The CDC STD treatment guidelines attempt to group the common diseases by symptomatology (ulcers, urethritis or cervicitis, and vaginal discharge). The identification and treatment of HIV in women has become a growing problem that continues to challenge those infected and affected, and the medical community as a whole. HIV's risk of coinfection with any STD cannot be overstated.

Genital Ulcers

SYPHILIS

Epidemiology

Syphilis is caused by *Treponema pallidum*, a spirochete, which produces a systemic infection that presents with periods of clinical disease and latency in infected individuals. From 2006 to 2007, the number of primary and secondary syphilis cases increased 10% in women (continuing a trend that started in 2005).[8,9] Although men who have sex with men remain at greatest risk of infection, both black and Hispanic women are disproportionately represented in comparison with white women.[1]

Clinical Presentation

Acquisition of syphilis occurs by mucocutaneous transmission. Exposure may occur from an infectious lesion during sexual contact, although congenital transmission is also possible. An incubation period of 9–90 days is expected before a painless, nonpurulent, and indurated ulcer appears at the site of inoculation. In women, this ulcer or chancre is often located on the labia minora but can occur vaginally or on the cervix, lasting for a variable number of weeks before resolving on its own without treatment.[10] Only 30% to 40% of primary syphilis cases are diagnosed during this early stage, especially in women if the chancre is a vaginal or cervical ulcer.[10] The disease may then transgress into secondary syphilis in 25% of patients.[11] This can occur anywhere from just before the time the lesion heals to within 6 months.[12] During this stage, hematogenous dissemination occurs in 75% of patients, resulting in a maculopapular or papular rash that is evident on the palms, soles, trunk, face, and extremities.[12,13] This offers a second period for diagnosis. Other generalized symptoms may include fatigue, malaise, sore throat, fever, and lymphadenopathy, along with the potential for additional organ involvement.[10] Should a diagnosis at this stage be missed or inappropriate treatment be prescribed, the patient can progress to an asymptomatic period of latent syphilis. This may be further designated as early latency or late latency. The CDC defines early latency as the period within 1 year, whereas the World Health Organization (WHO) classifies it as 2 years from time of exposure.[7] Any period after either of these is considered late latency. Progression within this stage may result in additional organ involvement, including cardiovascular complications, gummatous lesions on any organ, and, more commonly, neurosyphilis, which affects both the brain and spinal cord.[7,10,13] However, women are about half as likely to develop the cardiovascular and neurosyphilis complications when compared with men.[14] Last, HIV-positive patients do not present with fewer stages but have a tendency for the stages to overlap, as ulcers are often larger, deeper, and more numerous, taking longer to heal in this population.[7,13,15]

Pathophysiology

The mechanism of attachment of *Treponema pallidum* remains under investigation. This organism has the ability to transverse intact mucous membranes or uses microscopic tears to enter its host, disseminating systemically within hours. The diagnostic symptoms are a result of the host's immune response to the organism and can present as the chancre, rash (vessel vasculitis), and potential **gummas** of tertiary syphilis. The greater the *T. pallidum* load, the greater the immune response. Research has identified interferon gamma as one of the primary inflammatory mediators that triggers the macrophage involvement and stimulates the antibodies produced. Yet this immune response may only serve to assist in opsonization by macrophages and not offer protection from reinfection.[16]

Diagnosis

Diagnosis during the primary stage may occur by examining a section of the lesion or exudates by direct fluorescent antibody or dark-field microscope for *T. pallidum* as a definite diagnosis.[7,17] Nontreponemal tests include RPR and venereal disease research laboratory (VDRL) serology to determine an immune response to the cardiolipin (regain). These tests are used for screening and disease monitoring only.[7] The results are reported as dilutions, with a greater dilution indicating greater *T. pallidum* counts. False negatives may occur, as these tests may be negative for up to 6 weeks after primary infection. False positives are rare but may occur in other medical conditions, particularly autoimmune disorders but also in other infectious conditions. Thus, conformational testing methods rely on the detection of treponemal antibodies for a definitive diagnosis of infection. These treponemal tests include both the fluorescent treponemal antibody and *T. pallidum* particle agglutination and are reported as positive or negative. All patients with suspected neurosyphilis, active tertiary syphilis, or HIV infection with late latent syphilis should have a lumbar puncture performed, as well for cerebral spinal fluid biochemical tests, blood counts, and VDRL tests for diagnostic purposes.[7,15,17]

Once treponemal tests are positive, they will remain positive for the patient's lifetime. However, treatment effectiveness may be monitored by the fold change in either of the nontreponemal tests (RPR or VDRL). This effectiveness is defined by a fourfold reduction in titers when repeating the RPR in 6–12 months. Anything less should be considered a treatment failure.[7,18,19] Although early treatment often results in a nonreactive result within 1–2 years after treatment, latent or late syphilis patients may have lifelong, low-level detectible titers. Monitoring for late syphilis includes using VDRL titers at 3 and 6 months and biannually after that for a total duration of 2 years.[7]

Automated enzyme immunoassay tests for the detection of treponemal antibodies have increased in popularity as a screening test likely because of convenience and perhaps cost. However, this testing method cannot differentiate between past and current infections in patients who have had a prior infection, as it remains positive for life. Although this test is not recommended as a first-line screening test by the CDC, when used it should be followed by a confirmation nontreponemal test to differentiate between past and current infections. Any fourfold or greater increase in titer from a past infection is considered a new infection.[20]

Treatment

Treatment of syphilis includes intravenous (IV) penicillin G, which may be used during any stage. In cases of early syphilis, a single intramuscular (IM) injection of 2.4 million units of benzathine penicillin G is sufficient treatment.[7,18,] For cases where in which the infectious time period is >1 year or there is no prior documentation of a negative RPR test within 1 year identified, late syphilis treatment should be recommended. Late syphilis requires a series of three weekly injections of 2.4 million units of benzathine penicillin.[7,18] An exception to the use of IM injections is neurosyphilis, in which 3–4 million units of penicillin is given intravenously every 4 hours or 24 million units continuous IV infusion is given over 10–14 days; this remains the preferred regimen to achieve cidal levels in the central nervous system (CNS).[7,19] All patients who receive treatment for syphilis are at risk for the Jarisch-Herxheimer reaction.

The Jarisch-Herxheimer reaction is more prevalent with secondary syphilis, occurring with rates of 70% to 90%, and occurs to a lesser extent in other stages.[21] This reaction is an immune response generated by the release of the infectious organisms. Typically, this reaction occurs within 2 hours of administration of therapy and can potentially last for up to 12–24 hours after treatment completion.[22] Symptoms may include fevers as high as 103°F, chills, myalgias, headaches, and tachycardia. Prophylactic treatment can include anti-inflammatory medications. Sixty milligrams of prednisone administered to patients with symptomatic neurosyphilis or to pregnant women reduces this reaction.[23] Treatment alternatives for penicillin-allergic patients include doxycycline 100 mg twice daily for 14 days for early syphilis or 4 weeks for late syphilis, tetracycline 500 mg 4 times daily for 14 days, and ceftriaxone 1–2 g IM or IV for 8–10 days. Those patients who are HIV-positive, suspected of having neurosyphilis, or are pregnant should be desensitized to penicillin for its treatment use.[7,19]

GENITAL HERPES

Epidemiology

The herpes simplex virus (HSV) may be further designated as type 1 (HSV-1) or type 2 (HSV-2). HSV-1 is most often associated with oral ulcers acquired at a younger age. The seroconversion after oral infection with HSV-1, a rate of up to 70% in some developed countries, can offer some protection against HSV-1 genital infections.[24] It can also reduce the severity of the genital HSV-2 infection, which is typically sexually acquired at an older age.[25] For those infected with HSV-2 first, protection against HSV-1 is conferred.[26] Surveillance data from 2000 estimated that 20% of the U.S. population was infected with HSV-2, a cause of infectious lesions of the genital tract as well as the oropharyngeal and anal area.[27] This equates to at least 50 million people being infected with the HSV-2, accounting for an incidence of 1 million to 2 million infections and 600,000–800,000 clinical cases yearly.[7,28] Women in particular remain at greater risk of acquisition of HSV-2 when compared with men, with a population infection rate of 23% vs. 11%.[25]

Clinical Presentation

HSV infection may be associated with periods of painful blisters and cervicitis, commonly referred to as "outbreaks," alternating with asymptomatic periods. Outbreaks can begin with prodromal symptoms that include local pain, tingling, and burning before outbreaks. The frequency and severity of these outbreaks, as well as the risk for subclinical shedding, vary depending on the genital HSV subtype. HSV-1 tends to produce fewer and less severe outbreaks when compared with HSV-2 infections.[29] Although either HSV subtype can cause cervicitis, HSV-2 has been identified as the cause of cervicitis in 15% to 20% of women and is more severe in HSV-2 infection. However, primary infection with either HSV-1 or HSV-2 can also result in severe symptoms.[28,30]

Up to 70% of all new infections are a result of transmission from individuals who are asymptomatic with subclinical levels of viral shedding.[31] Viral secretions may be found primarily on the lips, the genital and anal areas, and, less commonly, other exposed mucosal surfaces. In women, these lesions can occur on the cervix as well as the exterior genitalia. During primary HSV-2 exposure, the number of outbreaks averages at least five per year in most infected persons without prophylactic medication (depending on the infected individual's immune status).[32] Additionally, 80% of primary HSV genital infections in women involve the cervix along with an additional dysuria.[33] Symptoms of HSV urethritis and/or cystitis include severe pain, itching, dysuria, and vaginal and urethral discharge, along with lymphadenopathy. Most primary lesions heal within 2 weeks without treatment.[34] Although the lesions may heal, an additional means of transmission remains because of subclinical shedding. There is less shedding for genital infections with HSV-1 vs. HSV-2.[7] Women may also have fewer reoccurrences than men.[35] Recurrence in women tends to be less common and presents with the same prodromal symptoms of tingling, pruritus, pain, and vaginal discharge and dysuria.[7,36] A complication of HSV is aseptic meningitis, which occurs more frequently in women than men.[33]

Pathophysiology

Transmission of both HSV subtypes occurs as a result of close contact with viral secretions from infected individuals to recipient mucosal membranes. This viral shedding may be a result of active, subclinical, or asymptomatic infection. Although HSV-1 has previously been associated with oral lesions, the incidence of genital lesions is increasing, perhaps as a result of lack of immunologic protection offered by HSV-1 acquisition at an earlier age.[25,37,38] Once the virus enters the mucosal surface cells, it begins to replicate near the site of entry. The virions then cause cell fusion, and the formation of a multinucleated giant cell results. This replication and fusion process causes damage to the endothelial cells, resulting in detachment of this skin layer and the symptomatic "blistering."[39] The inflammatory response results in viral transmission through the dermis to the peripheral sensory neurons. Virions can then ascend the peripheral nerves and enter the local nerve root ganglia, where they remain latent for a variable amount of time. Later, these virions may descend down the same neural axon to any mucosal areas that the axon peripheral infiltrates. Thus, symptoms are not linked to a particular area but depend on the area of infiltration of the infected neuron. HSV may also replicate in the ganglia and be transported to the local lymph nodes, where it is held in check in immunocompetent patients.[40]

Diagnosis

General screening for HSV infection is not recommended.[7] However, diagnosis of HSV and viral typing is possible during outbreaks by using viral cultures, HSV antigen detection, or polymerase chain reaction (PCR) testing. The use of direct fluorescent antigen tests or older enzyme-linked immunoassays is specific but lacks sensitivity and viral typing ability. Newer HSV type-specific laboratory-based tests are available but may need to be requested when testing is ordered. The Tzanck smear (a cytologic detection of cell change) is no longer a recommended diagnostic test.[7] Additionally, the use of serologic testing allows healthcare providers to identify HSV infection in cases in which clinical diagnosis should be confirmed or ulcers are atypical, or in those patients who lack the typical external lesions (i.e., partner testing). Limitations of some serologic testing methods include the lack of specific viral typing, along with the risk of false negatives in patients exposed within the prior 12 weeks.[28] Recent STD guidelines acknowledge the recommended tests that are commercially available.[7]

Treatment

The recommended antiviral symptomatic or preventative treatment options include acyclovir, famciclovir, and valacyclovir. All have been proven effective

Table 38-1. STDs Treatment Options

Herpes Simplex Virus

Non-HIV Infected Individuals

	Acyclovir	Famciclovir	Valacyclovir	
Initial Therapy				
	400 mg orally TID[a]	250 mg orally TID[a]	1 g orally BID[a]	
	200 mg orally 5 times a day[a]			
Suppressive Therapy				
	400 mg orally BID daily	250 mg BID daily	500 mg or 1 g orally daily	
Episodic Recurrent Therapy				
	400 mg orally TID × 5 days	125 mg orally BID × 5 days	500 mg orally BID × 3 days	
	800 mg orally BID × 5 days	1000 mg orally BID × 1 day	1 g orally daily × 5 days	
	800 mg orally TID × 2 days			

HIV Positive Individuals

Suppressive Therapy				
	400–800 mg orally BID to TID	500 mg orally BID	500 mg orally BID	
Episodic Treatment Options				
	400 mg orally TID[b]	500 mg orally BID[b]	1 g orally BID[b]	

Chlamydial Infections

Recommended	**Azithromycin 1 g orally once**	**Alternative**	Erythromycin base 500 mg orally QID[c]	Ofloxacin 300 mg orally BID[c]
	Doxycycline 100 mg orally BID[c]		Erythromycin ethylsuccinate 800 mg orally QID[c]	Levofloxacin 500 mg orally daily[c]

Gonococcal Infections[e]

Recommended Agents	**Ceftriaxone 125 mg IM**	**Alternative Nonoral Agents**	**Cefotaxime 500 mg IM**
	Cefixime 400 mg (oral tablet/suspension)		**Cefoxitin 2 g IM**
Alternative Oral Agents	**Cefpodoxime 400 mg**		**Spectinomycin 2 g IM with probenecid 1 g orally[d]**
	Cefuroxime axetil 1 g		

Source: Adapted from reference 7.
[a] 7–10 days for episodic treatment.
[b] Prescribed for 5–10 days.
[c] All noted therapy should be prescribed for 7 days.
[d] In cases of severe penicillin allergy.
[e] Also treat for chlamydia unless infection is ruled out.

for episodic treatment, thus reducing pain, symptoms, and viral shedding during the first treatment regimen of 7–10 days.[7,41] The recommended treatment durations and prophylactic dosing for both HIV-negative and HIV-positive patients may be found in Table 38-1. The decision of which agent to use should be based on the cost and convenience of dosing because both influence the likelihood of patient adherence. It is important to note that HIV-positive patients require higher dosages and longer treatment durations. Treatment of severe infections in both immunocompetent and immunosuppressed patients, such as those requiring hospitalization or CNS infections, require intravascular acyclovir be used until clinical improvement is observed. After that point, use of oral formulations may commence. Treatment durations will vary, but a minimum of 10 days is recommended.[7] Additionally, a small number of immunosuppressed patients (<1%) may develop resistant virus, prompting the use of an agent that does not use thymidine kinase. Options include topical cidofovir gel 1% applied daily to the lesions for 5 consecutive days or intravenous foscarnet 40 mg/kg dosed every 8 hours until clinical resolution.[7,41]

The use of continuous suppressive therapy should be discussed with patients who are experiencing multiple episodic outbreaks yearly or those who wish to diminish the risk of HSV-2 transmission to seronegative partners.[7] The use of 500 mg of valacyclovir daily has resulted in more than a 50% reduction in both clinical and subclinical viral shedding. Additionally, the use of suppressive therapy with 500 mg twice daily or 1 g daily of valacyclovir has shown promise in potentially reducing the risk of HIV transmission by reducing the viral shedding of both HSV and HIV viral load in women with CD4+ lymphocyte counts >450 cells/mm.[4,41-44]

Cervicitis

CHLAMYDIA

Epidemiology

Chlamydia trachomatis, a gram-negative obligate intracellular bacterium, remains the most common infectious disease in the U.S. with a rate 3 times higher for women than men.[1] Data collected from family-planning clinics within the U.S. estimated an infection rate of 6% for women between the ages of 15 and 24 years old.[1] However, these infection rates are 7 times higher for black women compared with white women, with an overall infection rate of among U.S. women being 13%.[45] Other high-risk populations include those of Hispanic and American Indian/Alaska native origin.[1]

Clinical Presentation

Chlamydia has an incubation period that extends 7–21 days.[46] Although chlamydia infections are asymptomatic in 70% to 75% of women with endocervical infection, symptoms may include cervicitis, urethritis, endometritis, salpingitis, and a perihepatitis (**Fitz-Hugh-Curtis syndrome**).[47] In cases in which symptoms are present, an odorless, mucoid vaginal discharge may be noted. Other localized symptoms of cervicitis include pain or minor bleeding with sexual intercourse or vaginal examination. Urethritis is also possible, presenting with dysuria and whitish, clear, or mucopurulent urethral discharge and negative urine cultures. Fifty percent of women with cervicitis can also have endometritis.[46] Without treatment, the infection progresses up the genital track, resulting in pelvic inflammatory disease (PID). PID complications include an infertility rate of 20%, chronic pelvic pain, tubal scarring, and ectopic pregnancy as a result of the inflammatory and scarring process.[1] Infection during pregnancy places the baby at risk for conjunctivitis and pneumonia.[7] Infrequently, untreated women develop **Reiter syndrome,** a triad of conjunctivitis, urethritis/cervicitis, and asymmetric reactive arthritis, which may be more prevalent in certain HLA-type individuals and is 5 times greater in men than women.[48] This arthritis occurs in conjunction with urethritis or cervicitis, conjunctivitis, and painless mucocutaneous lesions commonly seen on the palms and soles. The duration of this syndrome typically lasts anywhere from 3–4 months, but some synovitis may extend to a year. Treatment with antichlamydial therapy reduces relapse and complications, including perihepatitis (Fitz-Hugh-Curtis syndrome).[48,49]

Pathophysiology

The cell membrane of chlamydia includes important major outer-membrane proteins (MOMPs) that may play a role in attachment (a recombinant *Chlamydia trachomatis* MOMP binds to heparan sulfate receptors on epithelial cells), as well as cell wall lipopolysaccharides (LPS) and several heat shock proteins found in other gram-negative bacteria.[50] The MOMPs may serve as method of adherence to the epithelial cells along with other currently unidentified proteins. After attachment of the bacteria or the elementary body to the host cell, these organisms are ingested by phagocytosis. Within the cell, these bacteria replicate and grow. Once maturation is complete, the infected cell bursts, releasing the infectious agent. The LPS found on these organisms assists in triggering a cytokine response, subsequently resulting in an extensive inflammatory response.[51] Symptoms are a likely manifestation of this inflammatory response and parasite replication, which ultimately destroys the infected cells. The result of this process includes cervical discharge that contains large numbers of lymphocytes and mononuclear cells lacking any parasite.

Screening and Diagnosis

Routine screening is recommended for all sexually active women <25 years of age as well as high-risk individuals.[7] A first-void urine or vaginal/endocervical swab is the specimen of choice to send for a nucleic acid amplification test (NAAT). This testing method allows specimen collection to be done by the patient or the healthcare provider with minimal concern for technique or transit time. Additionally, the presence of >10 white blood cells (WBCs) in vaginal fluid without trichomonas should offer a suspicion of chlamydial or gonococcal infection with the inflammatory response.[7]

Treatment

First-line agents include a one-time dose of azithromycin or oral doxycycline for 7 days, both of which are extremely effective in nonpregnant women, but cost-effectiveness and treatment adherence should be taken into consideration.[7] Treatment alternatives include erythromycin base or ethylsuccinate, ofloxacin, or levofloxacin.[7] Pregnant women should not receive doxycycline, ofloxacin, or levofloxacin but may use azithromycin, amoxicillin or erythromycin (not estolate) as treatment options. Dosing may be found in Table 38-1. All individuals with confirmed chlamydia should be prescribed one of the recommended treatment options for *Neisseria gonorrhoeae* listed in Table 38-1 unless this diagnosis is otherwise ruled out.[7] Patients should also be asked to abstain from sexual intercourse for 7 days. Sex partners within the last 60 days should also be treated to avoid reinfection after treatment completion.

GONOCOCCAL INFECTIONS

Epidemiology

Neisseria gonorrhoeae is a gram-negative coccobacilli bacterium responsible for gonorrhea. It is the second most common STD in the U.S., with approximately 600,000 new infections reported per year.[1,7] The number of identified cases peaked in 1975, subsequently declining by 74% in 1995.[1] Since that time, the number of cases has remained fairly stable. Regional disparities exist within the U.S., particularly with the southeast being overly represented, although infectious cases have increased in the western U.S. as well. CDC surveillance data from 2001 to 2005 also points out that black woman between the ages 15 and 19 are the population most affected.[1]

Clinical Presentation

Gonococcal infections in women are responsible for urethritis, cervicitis, pharyngitis, and PID. Cervicitis remains the most common site of infection in women and may present as an odorless vaginal discharge, vaginal bleeding, or pain, particularly during intercourse. Symptoms usually appear within 10 days of infection.[52] Some women remain asymptomatic despite local cervical inflammation, but discharge and bleeding can occur upon vaginal exam. This organism can also colonize the urethra in 70% to 90% with cervical infections, which also becomes the primary infectious location in women posthysterectomy.[52,53] Infection can also involve the **Bartholin gland ducts.** Ten to twenty percent of women with untreated infections will develop PID, the result of ascending infection.[52] The complications of PID can be chronic pelvic pain, ectopic pregnancy, and infertility.[1] In addition to PID, perihepatitis (Fitz-Hugh-Curtis syndrome) is also possible, as this organism moves up the fallopian tubes to the liver, resulting in right upper quadrant pain and tenderness. Gonococcal infections can involve the pharynx and rectal areas. However, some cases of rectal involvement are a result of the perineal contamination by vaginal secretions.

Healthcare providers should have a low threshold for screening and empiric treatment in high-risk populations. Untreated gynecologic infections can progress to disseminated gonococcal infections of bacteremia, arthritis, and meningitis in some patients. These disseminated gonococcal infections are 4 times more common in women then men, perhaps a result of the frequency of asymptomatic infection, although other factors—such as recent menstruation, pregnancy or immediate postpartum state, congenital or acquired complement deficiencies, and systemic lupus erythematosus—may play a role as well.[54,55] Dissemination with arthritis presents in two forms. The first is a triad of tenosynovitis (inflammation of wrist, fingers, ankle, and toes), dermatitis (commonly transient pustular or vesicular), and migratory polyarthralgias. The second is purulent arthritis without rash.[56,57]

Pathophysiology

Infection with *N. gonorrhoeae* occurs in four stages: attachment, local invasion, proliferation, and local inflammation or dissemination. Attachment is assisted by the bacterial pili and Opa (opacity related proteins or protein II), which attach to the epithelial receptor. Once attached, the bacteria are engulfed by parasite-directed endocytosis. However, the polymorphonuclear leukocyte response and phagolysosomal fusion are blunted. This allows bacterial replication in both the endothelial cell as well as the phagosome as **facultative parasites.** These bacteria also produce extracellular enzymes that damage host cells. Other bacterial components involved in the inflammatory process include the lipo-oligosaccharide of the outer membrane and peptidoglycan fragments. This inflammatory response may play a role in the arthritis associated with this bacterium. Dissemination can occur as a result of bacterial alterations, which is presumed to make it resistant to the normal activation of the complement cascade, resulting in bacterial cell death.[58]

Screening and Diagnosis

As is recommended with chlamydia, routine gonococcal screening is recommended for all high-risk, sexually active women <25 years of age in addition to those older possessing similar risk factors.[7] Diagnosis can be made by gram stain from a cervical swab in only 50% at best, making the culture and NAAT the preferred diagnostic methods.[30] The NAAT may be performed on urine or vaginal swabs as well as cervical swabs. As a result of the potential for cross-reactivity with other normal bacterial colonization, use of NAAT is not recommended for rectal or pharyngeal diagnosis.[7] However, bacterial cultures offer the ability to determine antimicrobial resistance. Patients diagnosed should undergo multiple other STD screening, which should include chlamydia, syphilis, and HIV.[7]

Treatment

Fluoroquinolones are no longer recommended as first-line therapy because of increasing drug resistance, which is estimated to be 38.3% in the U.S.[59] A one-time dose of either ceftriaxone 125 mg IM or cefixime 400 mg (suspension or tablet) orally is the preferred treatment for infections of the cervix, urethra, and rectum.[59] Alternative treatment regimens include cefotaxime 500 mg IM, cefoxitin 2 g IM, or spectinomycin 2 g IM with probenecid 1 g orally for patients allergic to cephalosporins. Oral alternatives may include cefpodoxime 400 mg and cefuroxime axetil 1 g.[7] A one-time dose of intramuscular ceftriaxone 125 mg is the treatment of choice for both anogenital and pharyngeal gonorrhea.[59] Additionally, unless chlamydial infection has been ruled out, presumptive empiric therapy with doxycycline or azithromycin should be added to the prescribed regimen.[59] In cases of bacteremia, arthritis, or meningitis, intravenous ceftriaxone 1 g IM or IV every 24 hours is the recommended regimen. IV treatment should be continued for 24–48 hours after determination of clinical improvement followed by either cefixime 400 mg or cefpodoxime 400 mg orally. Follow-up may be recommended in patients who remain symptomatic because of reinfection or treatment failure, those with a history of treatment nonadherence, and pregnant women.[60]

Vaginal Discharge

BACTERIAL VAGINOSIS

Epidemiology

Vaginitis is a common medical problem in women that is responsible for approximately 5 million to 10 million office visits per year.[61] The prevalence of this disease is underestimated, as 50% of cases are asymptomatic.[62,63] Despite recent advancements, the diagnosis and treatment of patients with vaginitis remains problematic for practitioners.[63-66] The most common infectious causes of vaginitis includes yeast infection, bacterial vaginosis, and trichomonas infection. Because of the associated risk with sexual transmission, the focus will be on bacterial vaginosis.

Pathophysiology

Bacterial vaginosis has a complex and poorly understood pathophysiology. Overall, symptomatic bacterial vaginosis results from overgrowth of certain bacterial species, concurrent with a decrease in normal flora and lactobacilli.[7,66,67] Furthermore, lactobacilli that produce hydrogen peroxide are replaced with nonproducing species. Hydrogen peroxide from lactobacilli combines with chlorine, a halide present in cervical mucus, to produce a nonspecific antimicrobial host defense.

Pathogens associated with this infection include *G. vaginalis, Mycoplasma hominis, Mobiluncus* species, *Bacteroides* species other than *B. fragilis,* and other anaerobic gram-positive cocci, such as Prevotella and Peptostreptococcus.[7,66] Also, organisms can be present in asymptomatic cases. For example, *G. vaginalis* carrier rates can be as high as 10% to 40% of normal women.[68]

STD clinics report a varied but high range of bacterial vaginosos.[69,70] However, the role of sexual transmission of bacterial vaginosis is obscure. Male sexual contacts of women with bacterial vaginosis have been shown to carry similar organisms, but treatment of sex partners does not reduce the risk of recurrence.[7,71] Furthermore, bacterial vaginosis has also been diagnosed in virginal adolescents.[72]

The prevalence of bacterial vaginosis also varies with the method of contraception. The use of an intrauterine device has been associated with higher rates of bacterial vaginosis compared with other means of contraception, although higher rates of bacterial vaginosis have also been reported among women who do not use any form of contraception.[73,74]

Bacterial vaginosis has been associated with a number of complications, including an increased rate of abnormal Pap tests, preterm delivery, postpartum endometritis, and PID.[69,75-80] The association of bacterial vaginosis with PID is controversial. Premature rupture of membranes and preterm delivery of low-birth-weight infants has also been reported with bacterial vaginosis in several case controls and cohort studies.[77,79] Treatment of bacterial vaginosis with antimicrobials has been shown to reduce prematurity and premature rupture of membranes, and increase newborn weights. Postpartum endometritis following cesarean delivery occurs at a 5 times greater rate in women with bacterial vaginosis than in women without this diagnosis.[77]

Clinical Presentation

Women with bacterial vaginosis have an extremely variable clinical presentation. A vaginal discharge is frequently the most noticeable symptom, accompanied by irritation, pruritus, odor, or urinary symptoms, such as dysuria or frequency.[7,66,69] The discharge can be thick to watery, and white to yellow or gray. The clinical examination is marked by the lack of vulvar and groin involvement and normal-appearing vaginal rugations.

Diagnosis

Inter-healthcare provider variability in making the diagnosis of bacterial vaginosis and the association with upper reproductive tract complications emphasizes the importance of accurate methods.[66,80,81] The gold standard for diagnosing bacterial vaginosis is the Nugent system, which involves a gram-stain scoring system.[68,82] This scoring system, from 0 to 10, grades the severity of bacterial vaginosis using the most reliable bacterial morphotypes to create a summary score of the alteration in vaginal flora. A score of 0–3 represents normal flora, 4–6 is indeterminate, and 7–10 is diagnostic of bacterial vaginosis. The presence of small gram-negative rods or gram-variable rods and the absence of longer lactobacilli on a Gram stain of the vaginal discharge is also highly predictive of bacterial vaginosis. However, this method of diagnosis is impractical, and *G. vaginalis* is commonly found in asymptomatic women.

Treatment

According to guidelines from the CDC, treatment of bacterial vaginosis is indicated to reduce symptoms and prevent infectious complications associated with pregnancy termination and hysterectomy. Treatment also may reduce the risk of HIV transmission.[7] Thus, it is reasonable to treat asymptomatic patients who are scheduled for hysterectomy or pregnancy termination or who are at increased risk for HIV infection. Other asymptomatic patients need not be treated. Until recently, the standard treatment of symptomatic disease was metronidazole, 500 mg orally twice a day or 250 mg orally 3 times a day for 7 days, resulting in a cure rate of up to 90%.[66,69] Alternatively, a single oral 2-g dose of metronidazole can be given, but this therapy has a higher recurrence rate. For adherent patients, one of the longer treatment courses is preferable and has greater efficacy than the single-dose regimen. All patients should receive education on avoiding alcohol consumption during treatment and for at least 24 hours and ideally 72 hours after completing treatment.

The availability of topical preparations has precluded the administration of systemic therapy in many patients because of their high efficacy.[7] The topical preparations are only minimally absorbed, reaching 2% to 5% of the mean peak serum concentration of systemic therapy, resulting in much lower toxicity. Metronidazole 0.75% vaginal gel twice a day for 5 days has the advantage of fewer systemic reactions. Other regimens include clindamycin 2% cream vaginally for 7 nights.[7] The topical sulfonamide creams have been used for many years in the therapy of bacterial vaginosis, but there are no data to support their use.[66,69]

The preferred treatment of bacterial vaginosis during pregnancy is metronidazole, 250 mg orally 3 times a day for 7 days, or 2 g orally in a single dose.[7] The use of clindamycin 300 mg orally twice a day for 7 days is a less desirable alternative in most women, as it can result in a higher incidence of diarrhea and adverse events, but it can also be used in pregnancy. However, clindamycin vaginal cream is not recommended because of the finding of an increase in preterm birth. Topical treatments for bacterial vaginosis in pregnancy may not be adequately effective to reduce preterm delivery, and systemic therapy may be required.[69]

TRICHOMONIASIS

Epidemiology

Trichomoniasis is the most common nonviral STD in the world. Approximately 180 million women are affected worldwide, with varying prevalence rates of 5% to 74% across different populations.[83,84] The annual incidence in the U.S. has been estimated to be 3–5 million cases, with an overall prevalence of up to 2.8% in young women.[85,86] Risk factors for trichomoniasis is multifactorial and may include race, older age, previous STDs, prostitution, pregnancy, and other socioeconomic factors.[84,87] Concomitant STD infection is common, with rates of 10% to 28% for chlamydial and gonorrheal coinfection.[84] Trichomoniasis is also a substantial cofactor for HIV infection.

Clinical Presentation

Significant complications associated with trichomoniasis include vaginitis, cervicitis, urethritis, PID, and adverse birth outcomes, such as low birth weight, stillbirth, and neonatal death. Some pregnant women with trichomoniasis may present with premature rupture of membranes or preterm labor.[84,88]

However, symptomatic trichomoniasis occurs in less than half of infected patients but manifests most commonly with vaginal discharge that may be malodorous or discolored.[89,90] Cervical pathology, such as mucopurulence, erythema, and friability, can be commonly seen with trichomoniasis. Colpitis macularis, or "strawberry cervix," is particularly associated with *T. vaginalis* infection. *T. vaginalis* has been isolated from all genitourinary structures and has been associated with urinary tract infection and colonization.[84,87,89,90]

Pathophysiology

The exact pathophysiology of trichomoniasis has not been not completely identified to date. However, what is known is that *T. vaginalis* possesses proteolytic enzymes that assist in breaking down the protective mucous barrier at pHs in the range of 4.5–7.0. Once the parasite penetrates the mucous layer, it may either adhere to epithelial cells by use of surface adherin proteins or use identified phospholipase A to lyse nucleated mammalian cells and red blood cells. This process results in the observed tissue damage and inflammation.[91] This inflammatory response assists in increasing the risk of HIV transmission by recruitment of lymphocytes and macrophages with CD4+ receptors, direct damage to the mucosal barrier including potential microhemorrhages, and increased rates of HIV viral replication in those already HIV positive, which increases the risk of HIV transmission.[92]

Diagnosis

For diagnosis, specimens can be obtained by either the patients themselves or by healthcare providers from the lateral walls and fornices. A wet mount should be prepared as quickly as possible from vaginal specimens and microscopically assessed for *T. vaginalis*'s characteristic tumbling motility. Although inexpensive and rapidly performed, wet mounts prove to exhibit low sensitivity (60% to 70%) for the detection of *T. vaginalis* isolates.[93] Although delayed (3–7 days) and more costly, culture remains the gold standard for its sensitivity of detecting *T. vaginalis*. Papanicolaou tests perform with low sensitivity at 61%, with a positive predictive value that correlates directly with trichomoniasis prevalence in the given population.[94-96] In general, it is not recommended as a screening test, and its specificity is highly operator dependent. PCR methods have exhibited high sensitivity and specificity, but their expense and availability has hindered their widespread use. Two U.S. Food and Drug Administration (FDA)-approved, point-of-care tests are now available and include OSOM Trichomonas Rapid Test and the Affirm VP III. These tests produce results within 10 and 45 minutes, with sensitivities and specificities >83 and 97%, respectively.[96-98]

Treatment

Nitroimidazoles (metronidazole or tinidazole as a single 2-g oral dose) represent definitive therapy for trichomoniasis, with cure rates of up to 97% to 100%.[84,96] The CDC has estimated that 5% of clinical *T. vaginalis* isolates exhibited some degree of metronidazole resistance. For resistant strains, the CDC has proposed an escalation-based metronidazole therapeutic algorithm for the management of infections with resistant strains.[96] Oral tinidazole, intravaginal furazolidone, intravaginal nitroimidazoles, or topical paromomycin may be potential alternatives for such resistant isolates.[99] Treatment relapse usually represents reinfection by an untreated partner in 36% of instances.[84,96,100] Previously unrecognized chronic or drug-resistant infections are also possible. In pregnancy, the risks and benefit of nitroimidazoles use is controversial and requires considerable assessment because of their mutagenic and carcinogenic potential.[84]

Pelvic Inflammatory Disease

PID, the infection and inflammation of a woman's upper genital tract, is frequently associated with infertility, ectopic pregnancy, and chronic pelvic pain among women of childbearing age. PID is diagnosed in approximately 8% of American women in their lifetime, and more than 1 million women in the U.S. are treated annually for this disorder.[1]

PID occurs when microorganisms ascend from the lower genital tract and infect the uterus, fallopian tubes, and ovaries. Generally, PID has a polymicrobial etiology that can include *Chlamydia trachomatis, Neisseria gonorrhoeae,* anaerobic gram-negative rods, *Mycoplasma genitalium,* and pathogens associated with bacterial vaginosis.

Because of its polymicrobial nature, PID is often treated empirically with broad-spectrum antibiotics. Guidelines of the CDC recommend outpatient treatment of PID with ofloxacin, levofloxacin, ceftriaxone plus doxycycline, or cefoxitin and probenecid plus doxycycline, all with optional metronidazole for full coverage against anaerobes and bacterial vaginosis.[7] In a meta-analysis of 34 treatment trials published primarily between 1985 and 1992, four inpatient regimens and one outpatient regimen were found to have pooled clinical cure rates ranging from 92% to 95% and microbiological cure rates ranging from 91% to 100%.[101] These inpatient regimens included the following drugs: clindamycin and aminoglycoside, cefoxitin and, cefotetan and doxycycline, and ciprofloxacin. A fifth inpatient regimen, which included metronidazole and doxycycline, was found to have much lower rates of clinical and microbiological cure.[101] One outpatient regimen (cefoxitin, probenecid, and doxycycline) was included in this meta-analysis and was found to have a pooled clinical cure rate of 95% and a microbiological cure rate of 91%. Among the recent trials of treatment for PID, regimens including ofloxacin, moxifloxacin, azithromycin, and clindamycin-ciprofloxacin all yielded high rates of clinical cure and eradication of *N. gonorrhoeae* and *C. trachomatis,* although microbiological cure data among women with PID that is due to anaerobes are limited.[102]

Because anaerobic gram-negative rods and anaerobic gram-positive cocci are frequently isolated among women with bacterial vaginosis, there may be consideration for the use of antimicrobials with an-

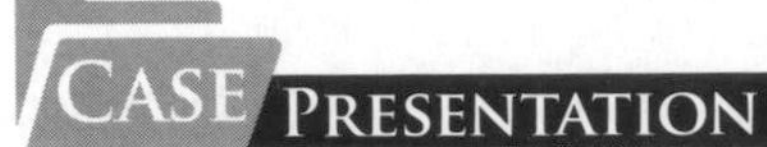

CASE PRESENTATION

Patient Case: Part 2

T.B. has multiple risk factors for acquisition of an STD. These include her prior history of multiple STDs, the potential involvement with multiple sexual partners, and her refusal to use condoms. Although she has no symptoms of painful lesions, which would be consistent with HSV infection, it is important to remember that not all women present with exterior lesions. T.B.'s diagnosis should prompt the healthcare provider to recommend an HIV test, as most STDs increase the risk of HIV acquisition. T.B. is also at risk for bacterial vaginosis based on her age and sexual activity, including the lack of barrier contraceptives.

Recommendation: A series of three weekly injections with 2.4 million units of benzathine penicillin G is sufficient to treat her syphilis. She may be offered ibuprofen and 60 mg of prednisone for a current or prior Jarisch-Herxheimer reaction during her prior syphilis treatment. The treatment of choice for T.B.'s coinfection is ceftriaxone l25 mg IM as a single dose for her gonorrhea and 1 g azithromycin (chlamydia). T.B. should also receive an HIV test as she is a high-risk patient.

Rationale: With a confirmed reactive RPR, T.B. should receive treatment for syphilis. Medical documentation of a prior negative RPR within the past year is not available and thus she should be treated for late latent syphilis unless she is HIV positive or is expressing symptoms of tertiary syphilis.

T.B.'s vaginal secretions sent for NAAT are positive for both gonorrhea and chlamydia, which is not surprising because coinfection is common in 40% of patients diagnosed with either infectious agent. If diagnostic testing is unable to be completed, empiric treatment for both may be prescribed based on symptoms and risk of coinfection. Although treatment for chlamydia with doxycycline may be cheaper, this patient's potential for poor treatment adherence to a 7-day regimen is a concern. The cost-effectiveness analysis must take into account the likelihood of treatment completion.

Monitoring: T.B. has at high risk of reinfection unless she uses some of the counseling points of STD prevention. It is recommended that she be retested for gonorrhea and chlamydia in 3 months. Repeat RPR testing should be done within 6–12 months to confirm the effectiveness of this treatment by a fourfold drop in titers.

Patient education: T.B. should receive extensive prevention counseling in addition to the multiple STD diagnostic tests. Should her HSV culture come back positive, patient counseling may include a discussion on the risk of transmission even when there are no symptoms (subclinical viral shedding). Should T.B. experience multiple outbreaks per year or if she was HIV positive, suppressive therapy would be recommended to reduce transmission of both the HSV and HIV to her partners as well as prevent future HSV outbreaks.

T.B. should also be followed up shortly for pharmacotherapeutic assessment of her current treatment of cervicitis, as both gonorrhea and chlamydia species play a significant role in PID. She should be screened regularly for abnormal Pap tests and counseled on the use of barrier contraceptives and the risks of preterm delivery, postpartum endometritis, and PID.

aerobic coverage. Trials of metronidazole showed it to have limited efficacy, perhaps because poor tolerability limits adherence. Regimens with shorter duration and monotherapy regimens are promising and may increase compliance and decrease sequelae. However, there is currently limited evidence for the recommendation of alternative therapies for the treatment of anaerobic PID. Although azithromycin provides coverage against a range of anaerobic and aerobic pathogens, fluoroquinolones, including ofloxacin, have generally been found to have limited activity against anaerobes. Neither azithromycin nor fluoroquinolones are optimal for the treatment of gonococcal PID, because increasing drug resistance is being reported.[45]

Whether currently prescribed antibiotic regimens for PID are effective in the prevention of subsequent reproductive morbidity is unknown. Ultimately, microbe-directed and -optimized treatment is important to preserve fertility following PID and to prevent recurrent and persistent infection, ectopic pregnancy, and chronic pain, improving the long-term prognosis for women who have PID.

Human Immunodeficiency Virus/Acquired Immunodeficiency Syndrome

EPIDEMIOLOGY

Recent statistics from the Joint United Nations Program on HIV/AIDS (human immunodeficiency virus/acquired immunodeficiency syndrome) have estimated that approximately 17.7 million people

CASE PRESENTATION

Patient Case: Part 3

T.B. returns to clinic 1 month later reporting persistent malaise, nausea, and vomiting for 1 month. She initially thought she had the flu, but when her symptoms continued for more than a week, she sought medical attention from the local emergency room. She reported that several labs were obtained at her emergency room visit (she is unaware of the what tests were obtained or the results), but her symptoms have not yet subsided. Today, she denied the company of sick contacts, foreign travel, or new medications or foods.

Vitals: Stable.

Physical exam: Well dressed and nourished, alert and oriented × 3. Evaluation of review of systems revealed a maculopapular rash on her trunk and abdominal guarding.

Laboratory values: Recent labs indicate that she is HIV positive. Her other labs are listed below:

VL CD4/%

Feb: 10,200 copies/mL 299 cells/mm^3 (15%)

Genotype: Wild type virus

CBC with diff, CMP

Lipids: Within normal limits

hCG + (first trimester per ultrasound)

Questions that should be considered for this patient include whether she should be treated, her options for therapy, and what steps should be taken to prevent perinatal transmission to the fetus.

or 48% of the total population living with HIV are women.[103] Rates of HIV infection in the U.S. have increased among adult women and account for more than one fourth of all new HIV/AIDS diagnoses.[104] Since 2000, the number of AIDS cases have increased exponentially, with rates for women and men increased by more than 10% and 7%, respectively. Recent statistics have also documented that HIV disproportionately affects black and Hispanic women between the ages of 15 and 39. These two ethnic groups represent <25% of all U.S. women, yet they account for more than 79% of AIDS cases in women.[105]

POSITIVE PREVENTION

The most effective way to prevent transmission of HIV is to prevent exposure. Education regarding protective behaviors (abstinence or consistent use of male or female condoms, avoidance of shared injection equipment) is of paramount importance. Healthcare providers and supportive staff should assess the patient's previous prevention methods and sexual practices. This assessment should include frank, nonjudgmental questions about sexual behaviors, alcohol use, and illicit drug use. After potential risks are identified, ongoing education, counseling, and risk reduction counseling should be offered.

Providers should review special points of interest, such as appropriate contraceptive methods to reduce unintended pregnancy and safer sexual practices to protect against STDs and HIV superinfection. A report by Wortley and colleagues found that in seven states, 20% of HIV-infected women were not diagnosed before delivery. They also found that 36% of the study population had no prenatal care and were substance abusers.[106] Both infected and noninfected women should be counseled appropriately on the risks of transmission and HIV in pregnancy. Transmission from an infected man to an uninfected woman is 8 times more likely to occur than in the reverse situation.[107] The risk of transmission between discordant couples who were counseled on the proper use of condoms showed lower rates of transmission than those who did not use condoms at all. Furthermore, investigators from a Ugandan study reported that transmission between discordant couples with low viral load was also rare (VL <1,500 copies/mL).[108] Methods such as artificial insemination and methods of semen processing can also be considered for those partners who are trying to become pregnant.[109]

Postexposure prophylaxis in nonoccupational exposures may afford protection from HIV after sexual contact or IV drug use. Persons who have been involved in unanticipated sexual contact or IV drug use exposure within 72 hours may be candidates for nonoccupational exposure prophylaxis (nPEP). The Department of Health and Human Services (DHHS) guidelines on Non-Occupational Exposure Prophylaxis suggest that an exposed person should receive at least 28 days of highly active antiretroviral therapy (HAART). Healthcare providers must assess each individual case for initiation of nPEP in persons whose exposure is >72 hours. Healthcare providers must balance the decision to initiate nPEP on the potential toxicities of the regimens, the cost-effectiveness, and the patient's willingness to adhere, as few patients remain on nPEP for the full 28 days.[110]

MODES AND FACTORS INFLUENCING TRANSMISSION

The two principle ways in which adult women ages 15–39 acquire HIV are through injection drug use and heterosexual contact with an HIV-infected partner.[111] In 2004, the CDC estimated that 70% of U.S. cases were attributed to heterosexual contact and 28% to injection drug use.

Transmission of HIV is affected by several different factors: host, recipient, and viral characteristics. The most fundamental host characteristics that may affect transmission are genital viral burden, stage of infection, and the presence of resistance, which may be inherited or acquired. A study of heterosexual individuals found that the likelihood of infection increases exponentially with an increase of 1 $\log_{10}$ of the viral load. Viral shedding in sanctuary sites is also increased during the acute stage of infection, as antibodies and cytotoxic T lymphocytes start to occur after the acute phase.[112] Aspects that increase the risk of the recipient are exposure to blood, such as genital ulcer disease (may facilitate transfer of HIV by impairing natural barriers to infection), trauma during intercourse, and menstruation (because of hormonal changes and irritation to the genital mucosa) of during intercourse. In this country, studies have shown that during unprotected heterosexual intercourse with an HIV-infected partner, women have a greater risk of becoming infected than uninfected men who have heterosexual intercourse with an HIV-infected woman. In other parts of the world, however, this is not necessarily true. In Uganda, for example, one study demonstrated that the risk of HIV transmission from woman to man was the same as from man to woman. This difference may be due to the lack of circumcision in Ugandan men.[113] However, female-to-female transmission from oral-anal, oral-vaginal, sex-toy related, and digital intercourse have also been reported, but is significantly less than heterosexual contact.[114,115]

Uninfected individuals may also have characteristics that may make them more likely to become infected with HIV. In addition to the aforementioned information (that STDs increase the risk of HIV transmission), the susceptibility of the host can be increased as a result of irritation in the genital or rectal mucosa, sex during menstruation, and bleeding during intercourse. In addition, contraceptive methods have been evaluated to investigate if there is a direct correlation between hormonal contraceptives and risk of acquiring HIV. This has been attributed to the hormones potentially causing thinning of the vaginal lining, interaction of hormones on the immune system, and increased cervical shedding.

CLINICAL PRESENTATION AND PATHOPHYSIOLOGY

HIV presents in different stages during the course of infection: primary infection or acute antiretroviral syndrome, asymptomatic infection, symptomatic infection, AIDS, and death. After seroconversion and without treatment, a person with HIV may advance from asymptomatic infection to AIDS within 8–10 years.[116] During acute infection, both men and women may experience a flulike illness, rash, rapid weight loss, fatigue, night sweats, lymphadenopathy, and oral candidiasis. Early in the epidemic, women appeared to have more a rapid progression of illness than men and also presented with a different constellation of opportunistic conditions. Sex-specific manifestations include recurrent or persistent vaginal candidiasis, menstrual changes, PID, human papillomavirus infections, cervical abnormalities, and cervical cancer.[117] Other symptoms may be the appearance of genital lesions, such as warts, ulcers, or herpetic blisters. The presence and recurrence of gynecologic infections are sometimes the first clinical manifestations of HIV and can occur early in infection.

Recent data suggest that opportunistic infections and rates of progression of disease are similar between sexes.[118,119] Women may be less likely to present for care early in the disease because of the burden of being the primary caregiver in a family affected by HIV. This often creates a barrier to accessing healthcare and interferes with their ability to adhere to treatment. Thus, they tend to have more sequelae related to HIV infection. Although women tend to have HIV RNA levels that are 30% to 50% lower than men who had comparable CD4 counts, the lower level of viremia is not associated with a better prognosis in terms of disease progression and survival.[118,119]

LABORATORY INDICATORS AS PREDICTORS OF TREATMENT INITIATION AND MONITORING

After initial diagnosis, a complete history, a physical, and extensive labs should be obtained. Together, these will provide clues as to the severity of immunodeficiency, activity of HIV, and other comorbid conditions that may affect the progression of HIV or cause various complexities with treatment. The following list of labs may be crucial in identifying comorbid illnesses, which may affect disease progression and influence antiretroviral choices.

- HIV 1/2 antibody testing (if confirmation is not available)
- Baseline complete blood count (CBC) with differential
- Urinalysis
- Syphilis, hepatitis, toxoplasmosis, cytomegalovirus serologies (Pap test in women)
- Tuberculin skin test (PPD)
- Chemistries, including BUN/SCr, LFTs, and albumin
- CD4 (absolute number and percentage), CD4/CD8 ratio, CD8
- HIV viral load (via PCR or bDNA)
- Glucose-6-phosphate dehydrogenase (G6PD) if indicated
- Fasting lipids
- HIV genotype (if the VL is >500–1,000 copies/mL)

The effects of antiretroviral therapy should be monitored both clinically and through laboratory markers. The main goals of therapy are suppression of the patient's viral load to <50 copies/mL and restoration of immunologic function. Ideally, the CD4 count should be monitored every 3–6 months to determine when to start antiretrovirals and opportunistic infection prophylaxis, and to assess the response to therapy (generally a 100–150 cell/mm^3 increase should be seen per year until the threshold is reached). The viral load should be checked at baseline, 2–4 weeks after starting therapy, and then every 3–4 months after the patient's viral load is suppressed to <50 copies/mL.[116]

If taken properly and consistently, antiretrovirals should completely suppress the viral load. Uncontrolled viremia in the face of drug exposure can promote resistance. Resistance occurs because of mutations or changes in the proteins of the enzymes that the virus needs for replication (i.e., reverse transcriptase, integrase, protease), thus changing the active or binding site for antiretrovirals. Often suboptimal drug levels—either because of nonadherence, problems with absorption or penetration into sanctuary sites, pre-existing or acquisition of resistant virus transmitted from another HIV-infected individual, and drug interactions—can cause loss of virologic

Table 38-2. When to Start Antiretroviral Therapy

Clinical Category or CD4+ Count	Recommendation
• History of AIDS defining illness • CD4 count <350 cells/mm^3 • Pregnant women • Persons with HIV associated nephropathy, co-infected with Hepatitis B (when treatment is indicated) Treatment with fully suppressive antiviral drugs active against both HIV and HBV is recommended	Antiretroviral therapy should be initiated
Patients with CD4 count between 350 and 500 cells/mm^3 who do not meet any specific conditions listed above, treatment should be recommended In certain cases the clinician may consider treatment when the CD4 count is >500 cells/mm^3	The optimal time to initiate therapy in asymptomatic patients with CD4 count >350 cells/mm^3 is not well defined; patient scenarios and comorbidities should be taken into consideration

Source: http://aidsinfo.nih.gov/contentfiles/AdultandAdolescentGL.pdf. Accessed December 2, 2009.

control. There are three resistance tests that are used in current practice: the genotype, phenotype, and virtual phenotype. It is important to note that interpretation of resistance testing should be done by an experienced HIV provider.[120]

Pharmacists can play an important role in guiding patients to properly adhere to therapy and can provide techniques to aid in adherence. Other ways a pharmacist can contribute to the care of these patients are by monitoring for proper dosing, laboratory abnormalities, drug interactions, and overlapping toxicities, which will provide better outcomes for patients and thereby prevent the emergence of resistant HIV. This will lower the economic burden on the healthcare system and will provide the best outcomes for patients.

POSITION STATEMENTS AND TREATMENT GOALS

Table 38-2 notes when to begin antiretroviral therapy. The goal of therapy in an HIV patient is to reduce morbidity and mortality by suppressing the viral load and increasing immunologic function. Providers often refer to the expert opinion of national and international treatment guidelines to direct the management of their patients. The DHHS has issued a position statement regarding treatment in adults, adolescents, children, and pregnant women, which is updated frequently (www.aidsinfo.nih.gov). The International AIDS Society has developed guiding principles for the management and treatment of HIV infection (http://www.iasusa.org/). Both of the guidelines suggest implementation of treatment based on immunologic suppression, symptoms, and virologic status.

For example, the following should initiate HAART, as soon as the patient and provider are comfortable with treatment and long-term adherence:

- Patients with an AIDS-defining illness
- Those who are symptomatic (regardless of their immunologic status)
- Pregnant women
- Patients with HIV-associated nephropathy
- Patients coinfected with HBV when treatment is indicated, or
- Asymptomatic patients with CD4 counts <350 cells/mm^3

Treatment can also be offered to asymptomatic patients with CD4 counts >350 cells/mm^3, however, a healthcare provider must weigh the benefits vs. the risks of therapy. (Please see each reference for detailed information regarding initiation and

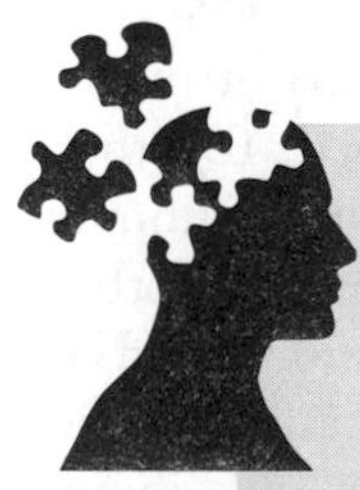

Therapeutic Challenge:

For what opportunistic infections should a practitioner consider initiating prophylaxis in patient with a CD4 count of <200 cells/mm^3?

changing antiretrovirals in HIV-infected persons.) Further, the recommendation of when to start antiretroviral therapy is the same for HIV-infected men and women.

Providers must take several aspects into account before designing a regimen for patients who are treatment naïve or experienced. Comorbid conditions, ability to adhere to a complex regimen, other medications, previous resistance, intolerances, and lifestyle are just a few factors that should be considered. It is important in both cases that expert advice from an HIV provider be sought.

ADHERENCE

Studies have found that >95% adherence is necessary to maintain viral suppression below the level of detection. Adherence to antiretroviral medications can be challenging, given the pill burden, potential toxicities, and complex dosing schemes. If adherence is not achieved, patients may be at risk for incompletely suppressed HIV and drug resistance. Regimens with once-daily dosing and fewer pills per dose, as well as patient education about the importance of adherence, will likely improve outcomes. Furthermore, counseling about potential side effects, offering ancillary medications for side effects (e.g., antiemetics) if they occur, and providing access to ongoing encouragement and consultation by phone or office visit are also beneficial.

PHARMACOLOGIC TREATMENT

Highly active antiretroviral therapy has significantly reduced the number of cases as well as the number of deaths attributed to AIDS. The retrovirus can only replicate in living cells and uses the host cell's replication enzymes to reproduce. However, HIV uses some of its own enzymes to facilitate transfer from a single-stranded RNA genome to a double-stranded DNA (before the cell can begin viral replication). Currently there are six classes of antiretroviral agents that target the viral enzymes and membrane proteins necessary for replication: nucleos(t)ide reverse transcriptase inhibitors (NRTIs), non-nucleoside reverse transcriptase inhibitors (NNRTIs), protease inhibitors (PIs), fusion inhibitors, chemokine coreceptor antagonists (CCR5 antagonists), and integrase inhibitors, which each have a distinct mechanism of action and related adverse effects (Table 38-3).

Given the various mechanisms of action, the most activity is seen when agents of different classes are used in combination. The current DHHS guidelines recommend the use of two nucleosides (tenofovir/emtricitabine) plus either a non-nucleoside (efavirenz) or a protease inhibitor (atazanavir, darunavir, fosamprenavir, or lopinavir/ritonavir) for treatment-naïve individuals. Similarly, the International AIDS Society recommends the above as initial therapy and also suggests the use of saquinavir. Guidance on treating treatment-experienced patients must be driven by resistance data, comorbid conditions, lifestyle restraints, drug interactions, active opportunistic infections, or intolerances.

Antiretroviral Toxicities

Despite the fact that HAART improves overall survival and immune status, many patients find it difficult to manage complications related to HAART. Initially, patients are plagued with side effects, such as gastrointestinal effects, CNS effects, and malaise, which can impede normal daily activities.

Note that antiretrovirals are being used as part of combination drug regimens. It is important to recognize that the antiretroviral-associated toxicities and side effects do not exist in a vacuum. Many long-term survivors are now noticing the toxic effects of long-term use and are developing diabetes mellitus, coronary artery disease, lipid abnormalities, renal failure, fat redistribution, and peripheral neuropathy. When using the antiretrovirals, consideration must be given to 1) how the toxicities and side effects may affect or be affected by the other components of the HIV regimen, and 2) toxicities and side effects of the non–HIV-related medications prescribed by the physician for the patient.

The NRTIs are associated with mitochondrial toxicity via inhibition of DNA polymerase gamma (the enzyme responsible for mitochondrial synthesis). This translates to potential lactic acidosis, peripheral neuropathy, myopathy, pancreatitis, and hepatic steatosis. Lipodystrophy is another syndrome that may occur after NRTI use, and it too is attributed to mitochondrial toxicity. Each nucleoside inhibits the production of mitochondrial DNA in differing amounts; ddC > ddI > d4T > ZDV > 3TC

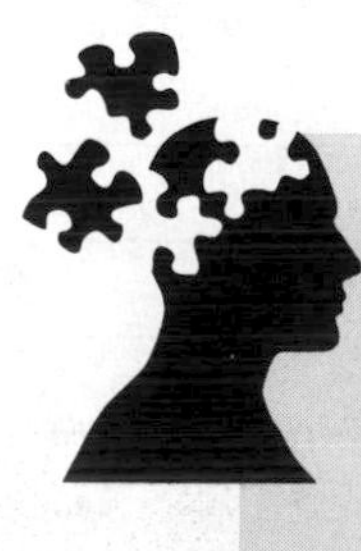

Therapeutic Challenge:

When identifying methods for increasing STD/HIV treatment adherence, what factors need to be taken into account before the development of the program?

Table 38-3. Advantages and Disadvantages of Antiretroviral Regimens

	Advantages	Disadvantages
NNRTIs	Extensive experience	Low genetic barrier to resistance with first generation NNRTIs Drug interactions High rate of rash reactions
ETR (2nd generation NNRTI)	May still be susceptible when NNRTI resistance is present; well tolerated	Pill burden, multiple drug interactions
EFV	Potent Low pill burden daily Once daily dosing	CNS toxicity Teratogenic in first trimester
NVP	Extensive experience in pregnancy No food effect	ADR: Hepatotoxicity + rash Contraindicated in women with baseline CD4 count >250, men >400
PI	Class—extensive experience Saves the NNRTI class as a future treatment option	ADR—lipodystrophy Multiple drug interactions GI intolerance
ATV	Once daily dosing Low pill burden No hyperlipidemia	ADR: Jaundice + PR interval prolongation Drug interaction with TDF and EFV
LPV/r	Potency Coformulated with RTV	ADR: GI intolerance Reduced levels in pregnancy
FPV/r	Low pill burden No food effect Once daily dosing	ADR: Skin rash
IDV/r	No food requirement BID dosing with RTV boosting	ADR: Nephrolithiasis Requirement for PO fluid
NFV	Substantial experience in pregnancy	ADR: Diarrhea High rate virologic failure Food requirement
DRV	Well tolerated, high barrier to resistance	ADR: Rash, food requirement
SQV/r	Improved GI tolerance with newer formulation	ADR: GI intolerance
Integrase Inhibitors		
RAL	Well tolerated, low pill burden	Low barrier to resistance
CCR5 Inhibitors		
MVC	Well tolerated, low pill burden	Low barrier to resistance, expensive resistance testing

(*Continued on next page*)

	Advantages	Disadvantages
Entry Inhibitors		
T20	Well tolerated, no food requirement	Low barrier to resistance, injection site reactions
NRTIs		
AZT/3TC/ ABC	Coformulated No food effect Preserves PI and NNRTI options	Higher rate of virologic failure if used alone ADR: ABC hypersensitivity
AZT/3TC[a]	Extensive experience Coformulated No food effect	ADR: GI intolerance + narrow suppression (AZT) HBV flare when 3TC stopped
d4T/3TC[a]	No food effect Once daily	ADR of d4T[b] HBV flare when 3TC stopped
TDF/3TC[a] or FTC	Well tolerated Once daily TDF + FTC coformulated	HBV flare when TDF, 3TC or FTC stopped
ddI/3TC[a]	Once daily	ADR: ddI[b] Food effect HBV flare when 3TC stopped
ABC/3TC[a]	Once daily No food effect Coformulated	ADR: ABC hypersensitivity HBV flare when 3TC stopped

[a]FTC is similar to 3TC; has longer intracellular half life and has less extensive experience.
[b]ADRs—d4T lipoatrophy, lactic acidosis, peripheral neuropathy; ddI—peripheral neuropathy, pancreatitis, and lactic acidosis.

= FTC = ABC = TDF.[121] Of note, all nucleosides carry the following black box warning: "Lactic acidosis and severe hepatomegaly with steatosis, including fatal cases, have been reported with the use of antiretroviral nucleoside analogues alone or in combination." Risk factors for developing metabolic acidosis are female sex, obesity, and prolonged exposure. In addition, some studies indicate that an acute infection, pregnancy, and other factors may lead to the development of the syndrome as well. Finally, the risk of lactic acidosis appears to be increased with the concomitant use of stavudine (d4T) and didanosine (ddI) (especially in pregnant women), and this combination is no longer recommended.[122]

Non-nucleosides are often chosen as a part of a regimen because of their potency, clinical outcome data, advantageous pharmacokinetics, low pill burden, and favorable short- and long-term side-effect and toxicity profiles (relative to the PIs). As a class, patients may be at risk for developing rash (which may require close monitoring and even discontinuation because of risk of Stevens-Johnson syndrome) or hepatotoxicity (nevirapine > efavirenz > etravirine). It is important to note that nevirapine has the potential for sex-related toxicity. Women with CD4 counts >250 cells/mm^3 have been documented as having a threefold higher risk of developing symptomatic hepatic events within the first 6 weeks of treatment vs. in men with CD4 counts >400 cells/mm^3.[123] The most commonly used NNRTI, efavirenz, is noted for causing psychiatric and CNS side effects, including depression, anxiety, hallucinations, dizziness, drowsiness, insomnia, vivid dreams, and nightmares. Black women have been noted to have increased levels of efavirenz that are due to the CYP2B6 polymorphism. Furthermore, cases of neural tube defects in human newborns have been associated with efavirenz therapy (pregnancy category D). This agent should be avoided during the first trimester of pregnancy and should only be used if no other alternatives are available.[124] Currently etravirine is only indicated in the presence of NNRTI resistance. In clinical studies, this agent appeared to have a higher incidence of rash in women than in men (28% vs. 16%), but there were no differences as far as the severity of the rash or discontinuations because of rash.[125]

As a class, the PIs are associated with a risk of lipodystrophy (fat and metabolic changes), hepatotoxicity (liver injury), hyperglycemia, hyperlipidemia, increased bleeding in patients with hemophilia, osteopenia or osteoporosis, and gastrointestinal disturbances (most notably nausea, vomiting, and diarrhea). Other PI specific adverse events include nephrolithiasis, hyperbilirubinemia, and jaundice.[116]

Studies have shown that raltegravir is generally safe and well tolerated. In Phase II studies in treatment-experienced patients (BENCHMRK 1 and 2), the most commonly reported treatment-related adverse effects were diarrhea, nausea, fatigue, headache, and itching. Other reported adverse effects included constipation, flatulence, and sweating. Overall, the adverse effects of raltegravir were comparable with those in the placebo arm.[116]

Injection site reactions are frequently seen with enfuvirtide. Injection site reactions (itching, swelling, redness, hard or painful nodules) are usually mild to moderate in nature but occasionally may be severe. The subcutaneous injections should never be given in the same location twice. Other effects that may be seen with enfuvirtide therapy are bacterial pneumonia and hypersensitivity reactions.[116]

Maraviroc, a CCR5 antagonist, was approved in 2007 via phase III studies (protocols 1027 and 1028). Adverse events that occurred more often than placebo were cough, pyrexia, upper respiratory tract infections, rash, musculoskeletal symptoms, abdominal pain, and dizziness. Additional adverse events that occurred with once-daily dosing at a higher rate than both placebo and twice-daily dosing were diarrhea, edema, influenza, esophageal candidiasis, sleep disorders, rhinitis, parasomnias, and urinary abnormalities.[116] The usage of this drug may be limited in advanced disease because of the number of CXCR4 proteins on the CD4 cell in advanced disease.

Overall, nausea, vomiting, lactic acidosis, hepatotoxicity, fat redistribution, and rash have all been reported as having an increased frequency and severity in women.[126] Unfortunately, the major focus of clinical trials evaluating the efficacy and safety of antiretrovirals have included limited numbers of women, so we may not understand the full extent of differences in side-effect profiles between sexes. The mechanism behind this increase in side effects is unknown but could be attributed to hormonal differences or unique pharmacokinetic profiles.[127] Another possible etiology may be that higher concentrations and decreased clearance may be linked to changes in metabolism for NNRTIs and PIs, and thus to an increase in adverse effects (cytochrome P450 enzyme system).

Pharmacokinetics and Drug Interactions

Limited information is known about the pharmacokinetic and pharmacodynamic differences between women and men. Further studies are needed to investigate the differences, but distinctions occur in drug disposition, effectiveness, and rates of metabolism. Contributing factors that may account for differences in drug disposition are lower body weight and organ size, more body fat, lower gastric acid secretion, and a lower glomerular filtration rate. These variations may explain why drug penetration into the female genital tract differs because of each drug's different physicochemical characteristics, and why differences in resistance patterns have been isolated in blood and the genital tract.[128,129] Further investigation in each of these areas is needed, and without confounding variables such as age, ethnicity, menstrual cycle, and concomitant medications.

Various drug-drug interactions affecting the metabolism of antiretrovirals have been well described in the literature. Sex may modestly affect the metabolism and effectiveness of some antiretroviral agents (women have been shown to have higher concentrations and decreased clearance relative to men of some NNRTIs and PIs, and have an increase in volume of distribution during pregnancy). This is mainly due to slight variations in hepatic enzyme expression, endogenous and exogenous hormones, and changes in expression of p-glycoprotein and other transporters.[130] NNRTIs and PIs are inhibitors, inducers, and substrates of the cytochrome P450 enzyme system and p-glycoprotein, and may have drug interactions with other antiretrovirals as well as non–HIV-related medications. Furthermore, these agents are highly protein bound and have varying abilities to cross the blood–brain barrier. An example of a specific drug interaction that would affect women would be oral contraceptives. Oral contraceptives, which contain ethinyl estradiol, have reduced concentrations when used in conjunction with NNRTIs. Protease inhibitors have been shown to decrease concentrations of these oral contraceptives as well.[131] Patients should be reminded to use a second form of birth control to prevent unwanted pregnancies. See Table 38-4 for further drug-drug interactions.

The NRTIs are primarily renally eliminated (except abacavir), but some have been shown to have interactions with other antiretrovirals (i.e., tenofovir and atazanavir) or even other concomitant medications. Differences in NRTIs are more difficult to predict, as NRTI must be triphosphorylated into the active anabolite. These anabolites are difficult to measure; thus, there is limited information of differences in men and women.[131]

PREGNANCY AND HUMAN IMMUNODEFICIENCY VIRUS

Many studies have reviewed the effects of pregnancy on the progression of HIV infection and the effects of HIV on pregnancy. To date, data about disease progression during pregnancy has been inconclusive. Earlier studies found that pregnancy and HIV increased the chances of progression of the disease, whereas studies during the HAART era have shown no effect. Recently, an article by investigators at Vanderbilt University found that pregnancy in HIV infection was found to have a protective effect. Patient characteristics that may have led to these results were that patients were younger, had higher CD4 counts, had immune activation, and were more likely to adhere to clinic visits and HAART. Further investigation is needed, but these results confirm that HIV-infected women who are pregnant may not be putting themselves at increased risk.[132]

Approximately one half of all pregnancies that occur in the U.S. are unplanned.[133] On average, 25% to 30% of births to HIV-infected mothers are transmitted via pregnancy, labor, delivery, or breastfeeding. The rates of mother-to-child transmission (MTCT) are increased if the mother has advanced disease, the p24 antigen has occurred in acute infection, there are high viral loads, and there are low CD4 counts. Other factors that can preclude MTCT are IV or intranasal drug use, severe inflammation of fetal membranes, and a prolonged rupture of membranes before delivery. Given the proven efficacy of the use of HAART during pregnancy (transmission rates as low as 1% to 2%), many HIV-infected persons elect to have children (with either infected or uninfected partners). If prenatal care is not sought early and antiretrovirals are taken during the last 6 months of the pregnancy, the rate increases to 4%.[134] Conversely, rates of MTCT are decreased significantly when HAART is used before conception and during the pregnancy. When prescribing antiretroviral agents to women of childbearing age, it is important to consider the risks and benefits of each potential agent (efficacy in reducing transmission and teratogenicity risk) (Table 38-4). The DHHS Guidelines on Reducing Perinatal HIV Transmission advises that antiretrovirals that cross the placenta and result in adequate systemic drug levels should be used during the antepartum period. Combination therapy with zidovudine should be strongly considered if there are no contraindications to its use. This agent should also be given during labor, and to the child for 6 weeks or until there have been multiple negative-antigen confirmation tests.[134] The first landmark trial to report the decrease in MTCT using zidovudine was the Pediatric AIDS Clinical Trials Group (PACTG) 076 trial in 1994.[135] In this study, zidovudine was shown to decrease MTCT by more than two thirds. Zidovudine was given in three stages. First, zidovudine was given to the mother orally after 14 weeks of gestation and continued throughout the pregnancy. Second, zidovudine was given intravenously during delivery (intrapartum treatment). Finally, the newborn was given zidovudine orally for 6 weeks following birth (postpartum treatment).

Nevirapine can also be considered as initial therapy if the woman's CD4 count is <250 cells/mm^3 and should only be used in higher CD4 counts if the benefit outweighs the risk of hepatotoxicity. It may also be given during labor to the mother and as a "one-dose prophylaxis" to the newborn for 2–3 days after birth. A Ugandan study (HIVNET 012) showed that a single dose of oral nevirapine given during labor and another dose to the child within 3 days of birth prevented MTCT in about 50% of the study population.[136,137] However, because resistance

Table 38-4. Antiretroviral Agents: Pharmacokinetic and Toxicity Data

Agent	FDA Cat.	Experience in Pregnancy
Nucleoside/nucleotide reverse transcriptase inhibitors		
ABC	C	No studies; concern for hypersensitivity
ddI	B	Well tolerated; usual pharmacokinetics; concern for lactic acidosis; avoid ddI + d4T
FTC	B	No studies
3TC	C	Well tolerated; usual pharmacokinetics
d4T	C	Well tolerated; usual pharmacokinetics; concern for lactic acidosis; avoid ddI + d4T
TDF	B	No studies; animal studies show bone abnormalities
ddC	C	No studies; teratogenic in animals
ZDV	C	Well tolerated; preferred agent
Non-nucleoside reverse transcriptase inhibitor		
DLV	C	No studies
ETR	B	No studies
EFV	D	Teratogenic; 4/142 birth defects; avoid in 1st trimester
NVP	B	Well tolerated; contraindicated as initial Rx with CD4 >250; single dose with labor causes high rates of resistance
Protease inhibitors		
APV	C	No studies; oral solution is contraindicated
ATV	B	Limited data; concern for elevated indirect bilirubin; studies underway
FPV	C	No studies available
IDV	C	Low levels and theoretical concern for elevated indirect bilirubin
LPV/r	C	Large amounts of data; extensive experience; need to increase dose
NFV	B	Well tolerated; extensive experience; use 1250 mg BID
RTV	B	No studies available
SQV	B	Levels are low; use SQV: RTV 1000/100 mg BID
TPV	C	No studies available
DRV	B	Limited data; studies underway
Integrase Inhibitors		
RAL	C	Limited data; studies underway
Entry Inhibitors		
T20	B	Limited data available
MVC	B	No studies available

Source: Reference 134.

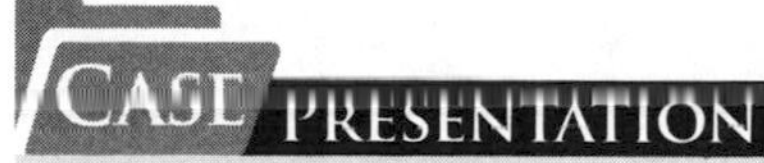

Patient Case: Part 4

Assessment: T.B.'s most recent HIV test was positive, and she is pregnant. The goals of therapy, treatment, and monitoring are the same for pregnant HIV-infected women as nonpregnant HIV-infected women (suppress the viral load and increase the immune response). Based on recommendations from the DHHS guidelines, treatment is indicated because she is pregnant (regardless of her viral load or CD4 count). She has no other comorbid conditions, and her CBC, CMP, and lipids are within normal limits. Because she is treatment naïve and has no transmitted resistance per her most recent genotype, she has several available options for therapy.

Key points that should be considered are treatment of the mother's HIV infection, potential adverse effects to the mother and fetus, and prevention of transmission. A direct correlation exists between elevated viral load values and increased risk for transmission. Transmission has been observed across a wide range of HIV RNA levels (including those with nondetectable viral load values). However, there are limited data of the use of certain agents in pregnancy. Ideally, a provider should choose agents that will have adequate levels given the change in the volume of distribution during pregnancy and counsel each patient on the importance of starting antiretroviral therapy. Furthermore, longer duration of therapy (i.e., starting therapy at or before 28 weeks) offers additional protection. When selecting a new regimen, the healthcare provider must assess the potential to prevent MTCT. There are limited data about the safety, efficacy, pharmacokinetics, and long-term effects of antiretrovirals used during pregnancy.

Appropriate laboratory monitoring, evaluation of comorbid illnesses and symptomatology, and pharmacokinetics profiles of agents should be considered before making a definitive decision.

Zidovudine and nevirapine monotherapy were the first agents documented to decrease transmission rates. However, recent data suggest that combination therapy is more effective than single-drug regimens for reducing perinatal transmission.

Recommendation: Lopinavir/ritonavir 600 mg/100 mg orally and zidovudine/lamivudine 300 mg/150 mg orally twice daily.

Rationale: A PI-based regimen is preferred given that the NNRTI options would not be recommended in this case (efavirenz—related to neural tube defects in the first trimester of pregnancy [pregnancy category D]; nevirapine—T.B's CD4 count >250 cells/mm³, which may increase her risk of hepatotoxicity). Two options for protease inhibitors include nelfinavir and lopinavir/ritonavir. Previously, nelfinavir was not recommended in pregnancy given the process-related impurity (EMS) was found to be a potential human carcinogen (class 2B). Now both nelfinavir and lopinavir/ritonavir are options for use of a protease inhibitor in pregnant women. Lopinavir/ritonavir would be preferred given that the results from efficacy data that showed that nelfinavir was inferior to lopinavir/ritonavir in several head-to-head studies. Twice-daily dosing of lopinavir/ritonavir is necessary to maintain adequate levels given the change in pharmacokinetics in pregnancy. Furthermore, zidovudine has been shown to drastically reduce the risk of MTCT when included as a part of HAART and should be included in all regimens unless there is severe toxicity or resistance is present. Oral zidovudine should be used as a part of combination therapy during the antepartum period and should be initiated at 14–34 weeks of gestation. Other nucleoside options include lamivudine or emtricitabine. Lamivudine and zidovudine are components of the fixed dose combination Combivir, which would lower pill burden, increase adherence, and reduce cost. Providers should pay special attention to monitoring for bone marrow suppression and gastrointestinal symptoms with zidovudine.

Monitoring: TB's viral load and CD4 count should be obtained at baseline and 2–8 weeks after initiating therapy. At least a 1 $\log_{10}$ drop in her viral load should be seen with the subsequent readings. A goal viral load of undetectable (VL <50 copies/mL) should be obtained at least by 16–24 weeks. For patients on a stable regimen, the VL should be obtained every 3–4 months after reaching an undetectable status (goal of <50 copies/mL). If she does not reach a VL <50 copies/mL after 16–24 weeks, resistance or nonadherence should be considered. Resistance testing is not advised for persons with a viral load <1,000 copies/mL. Immune reconstitution does not occur as rapidly, thus the goal is 100 cells/mm³ after the first year of viral suppression. Other labs to assess for potential toxicities should be obtained at regular intervals, or sooner if symptoms develop (e.g., lactic acid, CBC, LFTs).

can develop quickly in women who take single-dose nevirapine, this may reduce the number of therapeutic options for the mother and may also be transmitted to newborns during breast-feeding. Thus, it is not recommended as first-line therapy in developing countries.

CASE PRESENTATION

Patient Case: Part 5

T.B. is nonadherent during most of her pregnancy while on lamivudine/zidovudine and lopinavir/ritonavir. A week before delivery, her viral load was 15,000 and her CD4 count was 436. What further steps should be taken to prevent perinatal transmission?

Vaginal delivery should not be considered given that T.B.'s viral load was not undetectable (VL <50 copies/mL). A C-section should be performed and antiretrovirals continued during delivery. According to the PACTG 076 trial, oral zidovudine should be switched to IV zidovudine, and the infusion should start at least 3 hours before surgery. Lamivudine and lopinavir/ritonavir should be continued orally. Nevirapine should be avoided given its low barrier to resistance (only one point mutation needed to confer resistance across the class). Furthermore, because of the long half-life of the agent, drug levels may be detectable for many days after single-dose therapy.

To prevent transmission after delivery, T.B. must be educated not to breast-feed the infant at any time. Furthermore, oral zidovudine should be given to the infant for at least 6 weeks or until a confirmatory negative result has been obtained. Based on labs a week before delivery, T.B. does not need antiretrovirals for her own health. Thus, these medications can be discontinued to prevent resistance given her previous nonadherence. She should continue to be monitored every 3–4 months as stated previously.

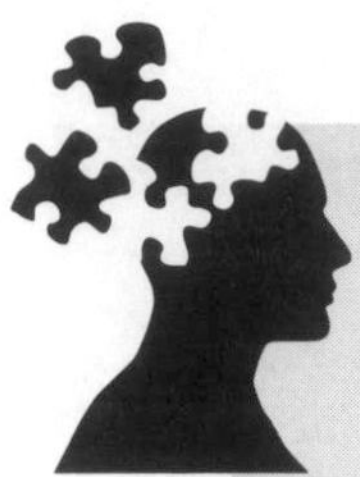

Therapeutic Challenge:

Compare and contrast HIV testing for a newborn, child, and adult.

Perinatal guidelines drugs that are not recommended in pregnancy include didanosine, stavudine, tenofovir, and efavirenz (pregnancy category D). As previously mentioned, the risk of lactic acidosis in pregnancy is increased when using the nucleoside combination of stavudine and didanosine. Tenofovir has limited data in this population and has been linked to possible bone disorders. Women should also avoid efavirenz-containing regimens during the first trimester because of the risk of teratogenicity based on animal studies and case reports.[138] Other studies that have evaluated other antiretrovirals have determined that adverse pregnancy outcomes have been reported (low birth weight, preterm birth, and intrauterine growth retardation).[139]

Manufacturers of nelfinavir released a "Dear Doctor" letter in regards to potential concerns related to the presence of ethyl methane sulfonate (EMS) and provided guidance on the use of nelfinavir in pregnant women and pediatric patients. EMS, a process related impurity, was found to be a potential human carcinogen (class 2B), and data from animal studies indicate EMS is teratogenic, mutagenic, and carcinogenic (however, there are no data from humans). At that time, Pfizer and the DHHS recommended that pregnant women who needed to begin antiretroviral therapy should not be offered regimens containing nelfinavir until further notice. Those who were taking nelfinavir were advised to switch to an alternative medication unless the benefits of continuation outweigh the risks.[135] As of March 31, 2008, all nelfinavir manufactured and released by Pfizer now meets the new final EMS limits established by the FDA for prescribing to all patient populations, including pregnant women and pediatric patients. Nelfinavir may now be prescribed for pregnant women and for new pediatric patients.

Data regarding the safety and efficacy of antiretrovirals as they relate to pharmacokinetics are limited. As stated previously, the volume of distribution is increased in pregnancy, which can cause variations in drug levels. Suboptimal drug levels have been documented with nelfinavir, saquinavir, indinavir, and lopinavir/ritonavir. This may be due to induction of the cytochrome P450 system, changes in gastrointestinal transit time, and an increase in drug transporters.[131] Because of the fact that there are limited data on antiretroviral use in pregnancy, more investigation is indicated. For the most up-to-date research and guidelines, visit www.aidsinfo.nih.gov.

Cesarean sections (C-sections) have also been shown to decrease MTCT transmission. A study published in the *Lancet* suggested that transmission rates for C-sections were 1.8% and 10.5% in those that had planned vaginal delivery.[140] Although C-sections appear to reduce the rates of transmission on the whole, it is unknown whether the rates of transmission are reduced even further for those women who have viral loads <1,000 copies/mL. Therefore, the risks vs. benefits must be weighed when considering the potential risks of invasive surgery. Furthermore, mothers need to be counseled that breast-feeding should be avoided in developed countries.

PATIENT EDUCATION

It is important to take every medication as prescribed. Missing some medication doses can increase the risk of developing drug-resistant virus, which places the mother and the baby at risk. If the patient is unable to tolerate the medication because of nausea, vomiting, or any other side effects, she should contact her doctor so that a solution to the problem may be developed. Most women who receive this treatment will not have an infected baby. After the patient delivers her baby, she may or may not continue taking antiretroviral therapy. More information will be discussed with the patient at that time.

Summary

Diagnosis and management of STDs in women offer a good challenge for the healthcare provider. These infections are often asymptomatic and underdiagnosed. Additionally, the transmission risk for many of these organisms is often disproportionate between men and women, placing women at greater risk of contracting multiple STDs. However, with the proper prevention and treatment interventions, the risk the complications or risk for MTCT can be diminished and in most cases potentially eliminated.

References

Additional content available at
www.ashp.org/womenshealth

39 Genitourinary Disorders

Susan K. Bowles, B.Sc.Pharm., Pharm.D., M.Sc.

Learning Objectives

1. Describe the physical, psychosocial, and economic consequences of urinary incontinence.
2. Compare and contrast medications used in the treatment of urinary incontinence, including alpha-agonists, serotonin-norepinephrine reuptake inhibitors, and anticholinergics.
3. Formulate a comprehensive clinical plan including nonpharmacologic and pharmacologic therapy for a patient with urinary incontinence.
4. Describe the physical and psychosocial consequences of interstitial cystitis.
5. Compare and contrast medications used in the treatment of interstitial cystitis.
6. Formulate a comprehensive clinical plan, including nonpharmacologic and pharmacologic therapy for a patient with interstitial cystitis.
7. Formulate a comprehensive clinical plan, including nonpharmacologic and pharmacologic therapy for a patient with vulvodynia.

The term *genitourinary disorders* refer to numerous diseases of the genital and/or urinary tract. For the purpose of this chapter, the discussion of genitourinary disorders in women will be limited to **urinary incontinence (UI),** interstitial cystitis, and vulvodynia.

Urinary Incontinence

EPIDEMIOLOGY

The overall incidence and prevalence of UI is difficult to determine accurately because of the reluctance of patients to discuss their symptoms, the unwillingness of healthcare professionals to approach the subject with patients, inconsistencies in the definition of UI across various studies, and the specific population studied. Nevertheless, there is considerable evidence that UI is a common problem for women. Although the true prevalence of UI is not known, it appears to increase with age.[1] Data from the **EPICONT** study suggest a prevalence of <10% in women between ages 20 and 24, increasing to between 25% to 40% in women older than age 65 years.[2] These data are consistent with those of other studies, which estimate a prevalence of 10% to 40% in younger women, increasing to 17% to 55% among older women.[3]

CLINICAL PRESENTATION

Several classifications of UI have been described, but there are five basic types that are generally agreed on. These are stress incontinence, urge incontinence (also referred to as overactive bladder or detrusor instability), overflow incontinence, functional incontinence, and mixed incontinence. As the underlying pathophysiology of each of these different types of UI differs, their clinical presentation also differs. Among the different classifications of UI, stress, urge, mixed, and functional incontinence are most common in women.[1,3,4]

Typically, stress incontinence occurs with increased intra-abdominal pressure, such as is related to coughing, laughing, sneezing, or lifting moderately heavy objects, resulting in a small to moderate amount of urine loss.[1] Urge incontinence is characterized by the loss of moderate to large amount of urine, usually accompanied by the inability to delay voiding upon perceiving the sense of bladder fullness.[1] Overflow incontinence is associated with dribbling of small amounts of urine, hesitancy in initiating urination, and a sense of incomplete bladder emptying after voiding.[3] Functional incontinence occurs in people who would otherwise be continent, but for various reasons are unable to sense the need to void or reach toileting facilities.[3] Mixed incontinence occurs when patients have two or more underlying pathologies causing their bladder control problems. It is not unusual for patients to have a mixed picture, with stress and urge incontinence commonly occurring together in women.[1,4]

CASE PRESENTATION

Patient Case: Part I

R.A. is a mildly obese, 62-year-old woman who presents to the urology clinic for a joint consult with the continence care nurse and clinical pharmacist for an assessment of urinary incontinence and multiple urinary tract infections.

HPI: R.A. has experienced UI for about 10 years, beginning approximately 1 year after menopause. Initially, R.A. would experience "leaking" urine only when she coughed or laughed, but her symptoms have gradually worsened over the years such that she now loses urine when she picks up heavy grocery bags, her cats, or small grandchildren. She also reports a feeling of incomplete bladder emptying after voiding, which she recalls as having started about 3 months ago. Since that time, she finds that there are days when she "dribbles" constantly, even when sitting in a chair. She has been treated for three urinary tract infections in the past 6 months. R.A. currently uses incontinence absorbent products (guards) to manage her symptoms, which she finds prevents urine from staining her clothing and furniture, but she worries about odor and has curtailed many of her social and volunteer activities because of this. She even considered missing her granddaughter's fourth birthday party because of her symptoms.

PMH: Three normal pregnancies, all delivered vaginally, without complications, while in her early to mid-20s. Type II diabetes mellitus was diagnosed 3 years ago, hypertension 8 years ago. She is also experiencing postherpetic neuralgia resulting from an episode of herpes zoster 3 months ago.

Current medications: Metformin 850 mg 3 times daily, glyburide 10 mg twice daily, ramipril 7.5 mg daily, amitriptyline 25 mg in the morning and 50 mg at bedtime. She has received three courses of ciprofloxacin for culture-positive *E. coli* urinary tract infections in the past 6 months.

Fluid and caffeine intake: Over the past 3 months, R.A. has restricted her fluid intake to 3 cups of caffeinated coffee/day. On those days when she has a social activity planned, she will not have anything to drink.

Allergies: No known drug allergies.

O/E:

Vitals: Height 5′5″, weight 176 lb, BP 132/76, HR 66 regular, RR 16, Temp 37.0°C.

Neuro: Reports burning pain on trunk following dermatome of herpes zoster infection.

Ab: Bladder palpable, otherwise unremarkable.

GU: Urine spurt noted with Valsalva maneuver. Pelvic exam is within normal limits.

All other systems unremarkable.

Labs: FBS 111 mg/dL, HbA1C 6.8%.

Urinalysis—no bacteria or pyuria.

All other labs within normal limits.

Abdominal ultrasound reveals postvoid residual of approximately 230 mL.

In addition to the five types of UI described above, some healthcare providers would include a sixth type, that of neurogenic bladder. This refers to bladder dysfunction arising from neurologic injury or disease.[5] However, symptoms and pathophysiology can be classified broadly into either detrusor over- or underactivity as outlined in the section on pathophysiology.[5]

PATHOPHYSIOLOGY

Normal Bladder Physiology

To understand the pathophysiology of UI, it is important to first understand the basic physiology of the bladder. The basic innervation of the bladder is outlined in Figure 39-1. Normal bladder function is a result of interactions between the sympathetic, parasympathetic, and somatic systems. Filling of the bladder occurs with sympathetic stimulation of β-adrenergic receptors located in the bladder wall.[6] At the same time, stimulation of α-receptors in the bladder neck and internal urethral sphincter cause contraction of these structures, preventing urine from leaking into the urethra.[6] Stretch receptors, located in the bladder wall, are then activated when urine volume reaches approximately 200–400 mL.[7] These stretch receptors send a signal to the micturition center of the central nervous system, causing the sensation of needing to void. Activation of the parasympathetic system stimulates muscarinic receptors in the bladder, causing bladder contractions. At the same time, parasympathetic stimulation relaxes the internal and external sphincters, decreasing outflow resistance pressure, allowing the bladder to empty, which occurs when the intravesical pressure of the bladder exceeds outflow pressure in the urethra.[7] Voluntary contraction of the external sphincter and relaxation of

Figure 39-1. Basic anatomy and innervation of the bladder.

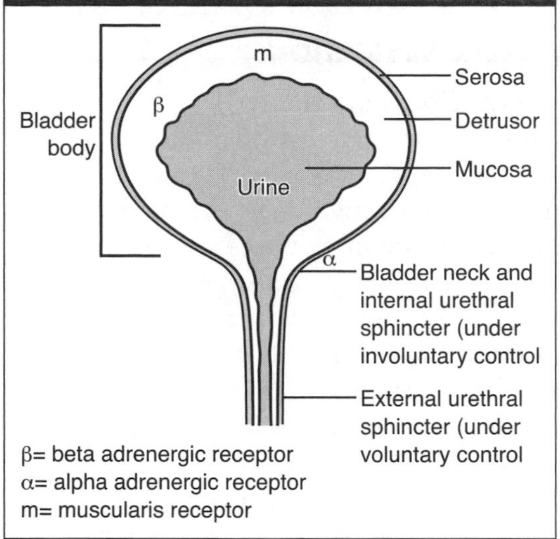

the bladder allow the individual to delay voiding, mediated through somatic control of the external sphincter and suppression of the parasympathetic nervous system in higher cortical brain centres.[6,7] Urinary incontinence occurs when one or more of these functions are disrupted.[7]

There are several potential mechanisms by which UI can occur, each of which will require a different therapeutic approach. Therefore, it is important that pharmacists understand these differences to outline an appropriate therapeutic plan for individual patients. Broadly, the pathophysiology of UI can be classified as either under- or overactivity of the bladder or urethra.[8,9]

Stress Incontinence

The primary mechanism of stress incontinence is that of urethral underactivity, related to either decreased tone of the internal urethral sphincter or hypermobility of the bladder neck, with most women exhibiting components of both.[1] As outlined in the section on clinical presentation, stress UI occurs during episodes of elevated intra-abdominal pressure, which then increases the intravesical pressure of the bladder. Normally, sudden changes in bladder pressure are counteracted by closure of the internal urethral sphincter. Stress UI occurs when the intravesical pressure of the bladder exceeds that of the urethra.[1,8] Hypermobility refers to displacement of the bladder neck and urethra occurring with increases in intra-abdominal pressure. Typically, elevations in intra-abdominal pressure result in the urethra being compressed against the muscles of the anterior vaginal wall, providing support for the bladder neck and urethra.[1,7] When these muscles are weakened, the bladder neck and urethra are not properly supported, causing them to slip out of place, resulting in incomplete closure of the urethral sphincter and leakage of small amounts of urine.

Urge Incontinence

The basic mechanism of urge UI is that of bladder overactivity, characterized by uninhibited contractions of the bladder during the filling and storage phase.[8,9] Although there are several neurologic disorders (e.g., dementia, multiple sclerosis, Parkinson disease) associated with urge UI, most women experiencing this disorder have no identifiable pathology.[1,10,11]

Older women diagnosed with urge UI may present with a particular problem in that they experience uninhibited contractions of the bladder, but at the same time bladder contractility is impaired.[12] This has previously been referred to as bladder hyperactivity with impaired contractility. It is now considered to be primarily a function of detrusor underactivity, although symptoms may initially present as those of urge UI.[12]

Overflow Incontinence

Overflow UI is related to bladder underactivity or outflow obstruction. When the bladder fills to capacity, it cannot empty completely because of poor contractility of the bladder muscle and/or obstruction around the urethral sphincter.[7,8] Incontinence occurs when the intravesical pressure exceeds resistance outflow pressure and urine leaks into the urethra.[7] Overflow UI is much more common in men than women, most often associated with benign prostatic hyperplasia. However, women can experience overflow UI as a result of urogenital malignancies, in the presence of prolapsed genitourinary organs, or if they develop an atonic or neurogenic bladder because of peripheral neuropathy, such as diabetic neuropathy.[7,13]

Functional Incontinence

As outlined in the section on clinical presentation, functional incontinence occurs in people who would normally be continent but cannot sense the need to void or are unable to reach toileting facilities. Numerous factors have been associated with functional incontinence, with the most common including dementia, delirium, dexterity problems, impaired mobility, and environmental barriers (e.g., stairs).[8,9]

Transient Incontinence

Some forms of UI are transient, arising from a variety of reversible causes as outlined below, using the mnemonic DIAPPERS[14]:

- D Delirium—Impaired cognition decreases awareness of need to void and ability to get to toilet.
- I Infection—Inflammation and irritation of the bladder increase frequency and urgency.
- A Atrophic vaginitis/urethritis—Estrogen deficiency can lead to increased frequency and urgency.
- P Pharmaceuticals—See Table 39-1.
- P Psychological—Related to impaired self-care abilities in severe depression or psychosis.
- E Excess urine output—Polyuria increases frequency and urgency. Hyperglycemia and medications are common causes.
- R Restricted mobility—Decreased ability to reach toileting facilities.
- S Stool impaction and constipation—Distention of the sigmoid colon and rectum can interfere with neural control of bladder contractions.

Of interest to pharmacists is the potential for medications to precipitate or exacerbate incontinence. Problematic medications for female UI and the mechanisms by which they precipitate or exacerbate UI are outlined in Table 39-1.

LONG-TERM COMPLICATIONS

Psychosocial Consequences

Urinary incontinence can have a profound impact on psychosocial and emotional well-being. Individuals may restrict their activities, especially in settings where they are unsure of restroom availability.[15] Interpersonal relationships can also suffer, with particular impact on intimacy, as persons avoid sexual activity because of concern about odor and urine leakage.[16-18] These factors contribute to increasing social isolation, poor self-esteem, and depression, all of which negatively affect quality of life.

One of the most important psychosocial consequences of UI is the apparent relationship between institutionalization and UI in older adults. Qualitative data indicate that UI is a major contributor to caregiver burden.[19] This qualitative evidence is supported by quantitative data indicating that UI is an independent risk factor for institutionalization.[20,21]

Consequences to Physical Health

Just as UI can affect psychosocial and emotional well-being, it is also associated with serious health

Table 39-1. Medication Effects on Urinary Incontinence in Women

Medication	Effect on Urinary Tract
ACEI	Causes cough ⇒ ⇑ intra-abdominal pressure ⇒ stress UI in susceptible individuals
α-Adrenoreceptor antagonists (e.g., prazosin, terazosin)	⇓ Urethral sphincter tone Used to treat overflow UI in men with BPH but can worsen stress UI
Antipsychotics	Hyperglycemia related to atypical agents ⇒ polyuria, frequency, urgency ⇓ Mobility if parkinsonism ⇓ Awareness of need to void if sedation
Caffeine	Polyuria, frequency, urgency
Diuretics	Polyuria, frequency, urgency
Ethanol	⇓ Awareness of need to void due to CNS effects Polyuria, frequency, urgency
Sedative-hypnotics	⇓ Awareness of need to void if sedation or drug-related delirium Impair mobility
Tricyclic antidepressants	Anticholinergic activity ⇓ bladder contractions ⇒ worsen overflow UI, especially if **atonic bladder** Noradrenergic activity ⇑ urethral sphincter tone ⇒ worsen overflow incontinence

ACEI = ACE inhibitor; BPH = benign prostatic hyperplasia; CNS = central nervous system; UI = urinary incontinence.

consequences. Skin breakdown or worsening of existing pressure sores, increased frequency of urinary tract infections, and increased risk of renal failure are among the most common problems. There are also other, less obvious, health-related consequences, such as an increased risk of falls and fractures, particularly with urge UI.[22] Frail older women may also be at particular risk of dehydration if they, or their caregivers, restrict fluids in an attempt to reduce UI.

DIAGNOSIS

Goals of Diagnosis

When approaching the diagnosis of UI, it should be kept in mind that this disorder is not a disease, but a symptom resulting from disruption of normal bladder function. As such, the goals of the diagnostic process are threefold:

1. To identify potentially reversible causes of incontinence
2. When reversible causes of incontinence have not been identified, to determine the underlying etiology of persistent incontinence to outline an appropriate therapeutic plan
3. To identify conditions requiring specialized care

Basic Assessment

Pharmacists can assist the assessment process by reviewing a symptom checklist (Figure 39-2a) with patients, explaining the use of and providing a bladder diary (Figure 39-2b) for quantification of symptoms, and completing a medication history to identify any drugs precipitating or exacerbating UI.

In addition to identifying specific symptoms and quantifying their frequency, the diagnostic evaluation consists of the following:

- Physical examination that is focused on identifying the cause of UI. Includes assessment of the abdomen, perineum, and pelvic structures/organs. A stress test involves observation of the urethral opening when the patient coughs/strains with a full bladder.[23] A tissue can be held to the urethral opening, with a wet test positive for stress UI. Alternatively, healthcare providers will observe the urethral opening for a urine spurt, which is also indicates stress UI.[9]
- Postvoid residual by ultrasound or catheterization, especially in women with symptoms of incomplete bladder emptying. A postvoid residual of >200 mL is considered abnormal and suggestive of either poor contractility of the bladder muscle or outflow obstruction.[1]
- Gynecologic history—prior gynecologic surgeries, malignancy, radiation, childbirth (number of vaginal and cesarean deliveries).
- Other urogynecologic surgeries or procedures (i.e., bladder suspensions or placements of cystoceles).
- History of comorbid conditions, with particular emphasis on diabetes, neurologic disorders associated with UI, and genitourinary malignancy.
- Laboratory tests, including urinalysis, fasting glucose, serum creatinine, blood urea nitrogen, electrolytes.
- Determination of how UI is affecting the person's life.
- Functional assessment to identify functional causes of UI, such as poor manual dexterity to unfasten clothing when toileting, poor mobility, physical accessibility of toileting facilities.

Specialized Testing

Cystometry can be performed to measure bladder pressure during filling, which is helpful in the diagnosis of urge incontinence. The bladder is filled with water or saline, with the first sensation of bladder filling, bladder fullness, and bladder capacity recorded.[1] Abnormalities identified during this process provide information about individual bladder capacity and the ability to inhibit bladder contractions.[1] Other specialized testing is usually reserved for those with an uncertain diagnosis, for those with sterile hematuria or pyuria, upon failure of the therapeutic plan after a reasonable trial, when surgery is being considered as a treatment option, and in the presence of comorbid conditions complicating UI treatment (e.g., spinal cord injury, other neurologic disorders, genitourinary malignancy).[23]

GUIDELINES

Numerous guidelines exist regarding the diagnosis and management of UI. Many have not been updated in recent years and do not reflect the most recent evidence regarding treatment options. Furthermore, few guidelines specifically address UI in women. To address this gap, the American College of Obstetricians and Gynecologists (ACOG) published a Practice Bulletin for the Clinical Management of Urinary Incontinence in Women in 2005.[4] This Practice Bulletin offers healthcare providers recommendations on specialized testing, nonpharmacologic treatment options (behavior modifications, pelvic muscle exercise), pharmacologic treatment, and surgical interventions. However, recommendations for pharmacologic treatment do not address the newer anticholinergic agents or duloxetine.

Figure 39-2a. Symptom checklist. (Reproduced with permission from the Canadian Continence Foundation.)
Fill this out and bring it along to discuss with your healthcare professional. Knowing the symptoms will help him or her decide on your best course of treatment. Sometimes incontinence is a symptom of another condition. Describe your symptoms and how they affect your life. Talk openly about your options.

1. Do you lose urine when you don't want to?
   Yes ☐ No ☐ Not sure ☐
2. When you need to urinate, is there an urgency about doing it right away?
   Yes ☐ No ☐ Not sure ☐
3. Does leakage happen when you laugh, cough or sneeze, or lift something heavy?
   Yes ☐ No ☐ Not sure ☐
4. How long have you been losing urine?
   Weeks ☐ Months ☐ Years ☐ Not sure ☐
5. Have you ever been diagnosed with a urinary tract infection or enlarged prostate?
   Yes ☐ No ☐ Not sure ☐
6. Do you experience burning when you urinate?
   Yes ☐ No ☐ Not sure ☐
7. Do you leak urine on the way to the bathroom or toilet?
   Yes ☐ No ☐ Not sure ☐
8. Do you lose urine in your bed at night?
   Yes ☐ No ☐ Not sure ☐
9. Do you go to the bathroom frequently to avoid losing urine?
   Yes ☐ No ☐ Not sure ☐
10. Do you use disposable pads, adult diapers, or anything else to absorb urine?
    Yes ☐ No ☐ Not sure ☐
11. Do you dribble after urinating?
    Yes ☐ No ☐ Not sure ☐
12. Do you have difficulty starting to urinate?
    Yes ☐ No ☐ Not sure ☐
13. How many times at night do you awaken to go to the bathroom?
    0–2 times ☐ More than 2 times ☐ Not sure ☐
14. Is your bowel function normal (i.e., no constipation, diarrhea, or pain)?
    Yes ☐ No ☐ Not sure ☐
15. Are you taking pills? (Make a list of all your medications or bring your pills to your healthcare professional)
    Yes ☐ No ☐ Not sure ☐
16. Do you avoid going to activities because of your incontinence (such as shopping, golfing, or gardening)?
    Yes ☐ No ☐ Not sure ☐
17. Does your incontinence affect your ability to exercise?
    Yes ☐ No ☐ Not sure ☐
18. Does urine loss interfere with getting a good night's sleep?
    Yes ☐ No ☐ Not sure ☐
19. Has incontinence affected your personal relationships?
    Yes ☐ No ☐ Not sure ☐

Try to think of any other information that might help your healthcare professional properly diagnose and treat your urinary incontinence. Complete and accurate information is very helpful!

Figure 34-2b. Sample voiding diary. (Reproduced with permission from the Canadian Continence Foundation.)

BLADDER DIARY
Supplied by the Canadian Continence Foundation

Complete this 2-day diary, and bring it to your healthcare professional to discuss.

Name: ______________________________

Date: ______________________________

Medications: ______________________________

____

____

____

____

Bladder Diary DAY 1

	Amount Voided		Did you feel a strong urge to go?		Leakage		Drinks	
Time	How many times?	How much?	Yes	No	How many times?	How much?	Which drink?	How much?
SAMPLE	3	A lot	X		1	A little	Water	One glass
6–8 a.m.								
8–10 a.m.								
10–12 p.m.								
12–2 p.m.								
2–4 p.m.								
4–6 p.m.								
6–8 p.m.								
8–10 p.m.								
10–12 p.m.								
12–2 a.m.								
2–4 a.m.								
4–6 a.m.								

Number of pads used today ______________

PREVENTION: PELVIC FLOOR MUSCLE TRAINING

Pelvic floor muscle training (PFMT; also known as Kegel exercises) is frequently used in the prevention of UI in the postnatal period. Postpregnancy PFMT can be effective in reducing the occurrence of UI if patients undergo specific training, have follow-up to ensure that the exercises are performed correctly, and if patients adhere to the exercise program such that six to eight contractions are done 3 times daily on a regular basis.[24,25] Pharmacists can assist new mothers by referring them to appropriate healthcare professionals for PFMT and providing follow-up for adherence to the exercise regimen.

TREATMENT GOALS

Most women consider complete restoration of continence to be the ideal treatment goal. This is achievable for some patients, but it is not a realistic expectation for all. As such, the desired outcome for these individuals is relief of the most bothersome aspects of UI. For treatment goals to be achieved, patients and healthcare professionals both must participate in the decision-making process, with an understanding that achieving the agreed treatment goals is a long-term, stepwise process involving commitment on the part of both parties.

NONPHARMACOLOGIC INTERVENTIONS

Absorbent Products

Absorbent products are used to protect clothing, bedding, and furniture, which can provide patients with a greater sense of confidence. Unfortunately, many patients consider these products as their only option for the management of UI and do not disclose their symptoms to healthcare professionals. As these products should be considered as a supportive therapy only, patients presenting with queries about absorbent products should be referred to their primary care provider for a basic assessment of their UI. In addition, many women do not use appropriate absorbent products for their UI, relying solely on menstrual pads. This often occurs because of cost concerns, as absorbent products are more expensive. However, menstrual products do not provide adequate protection; they can worsen skin irritation as they do not wick moisture away from the surface adequately and are subject to greater leakage than incontinence products.[26] Patients with UI incontinence should receive counseling about the availability of products designed specifically for UI and be referred to appropriate healthcare providers. It is important to reassure patients that UI can always be improved with appropriate assessment and treatment.

The selection of a particular absorbent product is dependent on the type and severity of UI, sex, functional status, convenience, cost, and patient preference.[27] Guards or shields are appropriate for stress UI with only small amounts of urine leakage.[27] Undergarment briefs are best for urge UI, in which larger volumes of urine are lost.[27] Some products are sex specific and should be selected accordingly.

The importance of skin care needs to be stressed to patients and caregivers when absorbent products are being used, because their use may increase the risk of skin irritation and breakdown. It is recommended that absorbents be checked every 2 hours and changed every 2–4 hours. Skin should be thoroughly cleaned with a gentle, moisture-containing cleanser, using a clean soft or disposable washcloth.[28] Scrubbing should be avoided so as to not abrade the skin. After drying, a barrier cream or ointment should be applied to protect against the development of **incontinence-related dermatitis.** Appropriate barrier products can contain petrolatum, zinc oxide, and dimethicone, individually or in combination. Alternatively, a skin sealant (copolymer film product) can be used for persons at increased risk of skin breakdown because of frequent or high-volume episodes of UI, but the most effective skin protectant has not been determined.[28] In the presence of mild-to-moderate incontinence-related dermatitis, the use of a skin sealant and products containing ingredients shown to promote wound healing (Balsam of Peru, castor oil, trypsin) are recommended.[28] When dermatitis is complicated by candidiasis, cutaneous antifungal agents should also be used, applied before the use of the barrier cream or sealant.[28] Patients and caregivers should be counseled on the signs of early skin breakdown and instructed to report them to their primary care provider immediately.

Lifestyle Modification

Lifestyle modifications are an important adjunct in the treatment of UI, and counseling women regarding these interventions is important to the management of UI. Specific interventions that have been shown to be effective include weight loss in obese women, reduction of caffeine consumption, and monitoring fluid intake.

Obesity is a risk factor of stress UI, as increased weight is associated with elevated intra-abdominal pressure.[29] For obese women, a weight loss of 5% to 10% total body weight can reduce the number of incontinent episodes.[29,30]

Caffeine use and fluid intake are linked, and each must be considered in the context of the other. Caffeine acts as a diuretic, increasing urine production, potentially exacerbating stress and urge UI. Many women significantly reduce their fluid intake in an effort to reduce their UI. However, what fluid intake they have over a 24-hour period may consist primarily of caffeinated beverages. Reducing fluid intake to below 750 mL/day can increase urine concentration, serving to increase the sense of frequency and urgency. This reduction in fluid intake works in combination with the diuretic effect of caffeine, resulting in worsening UI. Minimizing caffeine intake and increasing fluid intake to at least 750 mL/day reduces symptoms of frequency and urgency, and volume of urine lost during incontinence episodes.[31-33] More importantly, women report an increased quality of life and greater sense of control over their symptoms.[32,33]

Pelvic Floor Muscle Training

The ACOG Practice Bulletin on Urinary Incontinence in Women recommends PFMT as an effective treatment for adult women with stress and mixed UI.[4] A formal training program of at least 3 months in duration with follow-up by a trained healthcare professional (continence care nurse or specialized physiotherapist) is important to ensure proper technique.[34] As proper technique and adherence to the treatment regimen are important, PFMT may not be an option for some women, such as those with cognitive impairment.

Behavioral Therapy

Behavioral therapy includes bladder training and prompted voiding, which involve teaching the individual to prolong the interval between voiding according to a timetable tailored to meet the person's ability to cooperate. Prompted voiding is used more often in older persons who may not possess the cognition necessary to recognize the need to void, requiring assistance from caregivers. Compliance with behavioral therapy, either by the patient themselves or caregivers providing assistance, is essential to its success.

Behavioral therapies are frequently used in conjunction with other interventions, including medications. Both have been recommended by the AGOG Practice Bulletin for treatment of urge and mixed UI as a noninvasive treatment strategy and are effective in reducing the number of incontinence episodes.[4,35,36]

Surgery

A comprehensive discussion of surgical treatment options is beyond the scope of this chapter. However, surgery is considered necessary for some women experiencing stress UI.[4] Surgical interventions involve stabilizing the urethra and bladder neck or enhancing urethral resistance with bulking agents.[9]

PHARMACOLOGIC INTERVENTIONS

Drug therapy is specific for the type of UI that a person is experiencing, with the mechanism of action aimed at the underlying pathophysiology, as discussed above. Therefore, it is essential that the type of UI be accurately identified for women to achieve the maximum benefit from their UI medications. It is also important to understand that drug therapy does not necessarily restore continence but reduces the overall number of incontinence episodes. Table 39-2 briefly outlines key points about medications commonly used to manage UI.

Stress Incontinence

Three classes of drugs are used in the management of stress UI: the alpha-adrenergic agonists, vaginally administered estrogen products, and the **serotonin-norepinephrine reuptake inhibitor (SNRI)** duloxetine (Table 39-2.)

The alpha-adrenergic agonists act directly on alpha-receptors in the bladder neck, thereby increasing sphincter tone. This pharmacologic property has led to interest in the use of these agents for the management of stress UI. Before its withdrawal in 2000, phenylpropanolamine (PPA) was often used in combination with estrogen, with some benefit suggested for women with mild to moderate stress incontinence.[37-39] With PPA no longer available, pseudoephedrine became the only remaining option. However, there are limited data on efficacy, and use is largely based on extrapolation of information supporting the use of PPA, which has recently been questioned.[40] Furthermore, there is concern that pseudoephedrine may also increase the risk of stroke in addition to its potential adverse cardiac effects.[41] Therefore, the use of alpha-adrenergic agonists are not recommended for routine use.

The use of systemic estrogen therapy in postmenopausal women does not appear to reduce UI and may even be associated with worsening UI.[40,42,43] Systemic estrogen therapy is also accompanied by significant adverse effects, such as increased risk of breast and endometrial cancers. Furthermore, women taking estrogen replacement may be at increased risk

Table 39-2. Treatment Options for Urinary Incontinence

Type of Incontinence	Drug	Dosage	Mechanism of Action	Place in Therapy
Stress	Pseudoephedrine	15–60 mg 3 times daily	⇑ Tone of bladder sphincter	Limited evidence; avoid in patients with hypertension, diabetes, pre-existing cardiac arrhythmias, and those taking MAOIs
	Estrogen	Estradiol 25 mcg vaginal tablet daily × 14 days then once weekly Estradiol vaginal cream 2–4 g daily for 1–2 wk followed by 1 g administered 1–3 times/wk CEE vaginal cream 0.5–2 g daily, 3 wk on and 1 wk off	⇓ Symptoms associated with atrophic vaginitis (dysuria and frequency most often reported)[44]	No role for systemic therapy; avoid if previous history of breast cancer, active thromboembolic disease, or history of thromboembolism with previous estrogen use
		Estradiol 2 mg vaginal ring every 3 mo		Vaginal ring useful for women with cognitive impairment or physically unable to use vaginal tablets or cream
	Duloxetine	40–80 mg once daily or divided twice daily Available as DR capsules		Off-label indication; can ⇑ blood pressure; avoid if poorly controlled hypertension Do not use if CrCl <30 mL/min, pre-existing hepatic disease, or history of alcohol abuse May ⇑ risk of suicide even if no pre-existing mental illness Taper therapy rather than abruptly stopping to avoid discontinuation syndrome Be aware of potential drug interactions with CYP450 2D6 and 1A2 substrates/inhibitors
Urge			All anticholinergic agents act on muscarinic receptors in the bladder wall to decrease bladder contractility	Choice of agent dependent on patient-specific factors All agents have potential to cause confusion among older women, especially those with pre-existing cognitive impairment[48] Older persons with detrusor underactivity, who may present with some symptoms of urge UI, are at ⇑ risk of retention with anticholinergic agents[12]
	Oxybutynin	Immediate-release tablets 2.5–5 mg twice to 4 times daily Sustained-release tablets 5–30 mg once daily Transdermal patch 3.9 mg/day applied twice a wk		Be aware of potential for CYP3A4 inhibitors to decrease oxybutynin metabolism ⇒ ⇑ anticholinergic effects Sustained-release products demonstrate ⇓ dry mouth but caution should be used with these agents in those with cognitive impairment, regardless of formulation

(*Continued on next page*)

Type of Incontinence	Drug	Dosage	Mechanism of Action	Place in Therapy
	Tolterodine	Immediate-release tablets 1–2 mg twice daily Sustained-release tablets 2–4 mg once daily		Maximum dose 1 mg twice daily if CrCl <30 mL/min, in hepatic cirrhosis, or if concomitant use of known CYP450 3A3 inhibitors; monitor closely for anticholinergic adverse effects Sustained-release formulation subject to dose dumping if administered concomitantly with antacids; effect not observed with PPIs or H2 antagonists
	Trospium chloride	20 mg twice daily		Predominately renal elimination ⇒ maximum dosage 20 mg/day if CrCl <30 mL/min, and monitor closely for adverse effects Best administered on an empty stomach Hydrophilic agent but no apparent difference in CNS effects[48]
	Solifenacin	5–10 mg once daily	Selective for the M_3 muscarinic receptor	Maximum dosage 5 mg daily if CrCl <30 mL/min, moderate hepatic disease, or concomitant use of known CYP3A4 inhibitors, and monitor closely for adverse effects Avoid in severe hepatic disease
	Darifenacin	7.5–5 mg once daily	Selective for the M_3 muscarinic receptor	Maximum dosage 7.5 mg daily if concomitant use of known CYP 3A4 inhibitors, and monitor closely for adverse effects
Overflow	Tamsulosin	Controlled release tablet 0.4 mg daily	Act on α-receptors at internal sphincter to ⇓ outflow obstruction	Tamsulosin and terazosin are the only α-adrenoreceptor antagonists studied to date in women with outflow obstruction
	Terazosin	1 mg at bedtime for 1 week then titrate by 1 mg increments every wk to maximum of 5 mg daily		Symptomatic postural hypotension can be dose limiting; initiate at lowest possible dosage to minimize "first-dose" effect; maximum dosage studied in women is 5 mg daily

CEE = conjugated equine estrogens; CNS = central nervous system; CrCl = creatinine clearance; DR = delayed release; MAOIs = monoamine oxidase inhibitors; PPIs = proton-pump inhibitors; UI = urinary incontinence.

of stroke and myocardial infarction. Therefore, only vaginally administered estrogen products are recommended in the management of stress UI, especially for postmenopausal women whose symptoms are exacerbated by atrophic urethritis or vaginitis. Although vaginally administered estrogen may be recommended, it is important to understand that its use does not cure or even reduce the frequency of incontinent episodes.[40] Rather, it decreases specific symptoms that are important to some women, particularly dysuria and frequency, over the course of 1–3 months.[44]

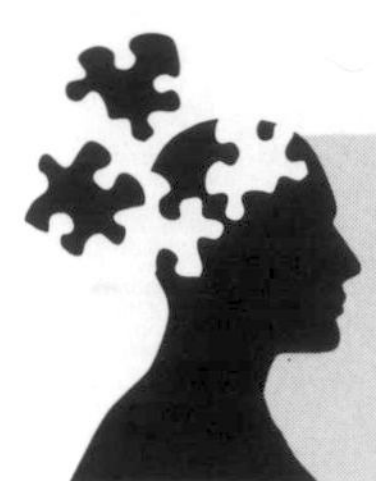

Therapeutic Challenge:

What is the benefit of combining PFMT with duloxetine in the treatment of stress incontinence?

Although not approved for use in stress UI, duloxetine, originally developed as an antidepressant, is sometimes used in the management of stress UI. It exhibits dual serotonin and noradrenergic reuptake activity, acting centrally on the micturition center and may also act directly on the urethra via peripheral adrenergic activation.[45] Duloxetine has been shown to exhibit a modest effect on stress UI. Dosages of 40–80 mg daily, administered over 3–12 weeks, resulted in a 50% reduction of incontinent episodes but did not resolve UI.[40,46] Nausea is the most commonly reported adverse effect, potentially reducing persistence to therapy.[46] Patients should be counseled not to discontinue therapy abruptly, as a discontinuation syndrome has been described.[45] Pharmacists should also be aware of potential clinically important drug interactions resulting from concomitant use of potent cytochrome P450 1A2 and 2D6 inhibitors and contraindications to duloxetine as outlined in Table 39-2.[45]

Urge Incontinence

The anticholinergic agents are considered as first-line drug therapy in the management of urge UI. As the primary problem in urge UI is bladder overactivity, anticholinergic medications act on muscarinic receptors in the bladder to reduce bladder contractility. As outlined in Table 39-2, five agents are approved for use in urge UI: oxybutynin, tolterodine, trospium, darifenacin, and solifenacin. Use of oxybutynin and tolterodine in the treatment of urge UI demonstrates modest efficacy in comparison with placebo, with an approximate reduction of 0.5–1 incontinence episodes per day, although some women did experience complete resolution of their symptoms.[40,47] Comparative studies between the newer agents (darifenacin, trospium, and solifenacin) and older anticholinergics (oxybutynin and tolterodine) are limited, but what data are available suggest similar efficacy across the class.[48] Additionally, there is little evidence to suggest that the specific characteristics of the newer agents (Table 39-2) reduce adverse effects and improve tolerability.[48] Therefore, the choice of agent and formulation is largely dependent on patient-specific characteristics, such as comorbid disease states, concomitant drug therapy, and adherence considerations.[9] Patient preference is also important, including not only the side-effect profile, but also cost considerations, as many insurance plans do not cover extended-release products. Another important consideration is that of underlying dementia, as these medications can worsen cognition without providing much benefit, especially in the late stages of disease when patients are completely dependent on caregivers for their basic activities of daily living.[48]

Adverse effects represent an extension of the anticholinergic activity of these drugs, with dry mouth, blurred vision, constipation, confusion, memory problems, and tachycardia being the most common side effects.[9,48]

Anticholinergic-related adverse effects can reduce persistence of therapy, with the sustained-release formulation of tolterodine demonstrating the least number of early withdrawals because of side effects in a meta-analysis of clinical trials.[49] However, the duration of most of these studies was only 12 weeks. Longer-term, population-based studies are needed to determine if there are truly any differences in persistence of therapy between agents.

When therapy is initiated, the lowest possible dosage should be used, with dosing increases based on tolerance and efficacy. Once the maximum tolerated dosage is reached, it should be maintained for a minimum of 4 weeks to provide an adequate therapeutic trial.[9] If one drug is not well tolerated, or if therapy fails, then switching to another agent may be beneficial for some women.[9]

Overflow Incontinence

Overflow UI is not common in women, but it can occur, most frequently from obstruction secondary to pelvic organ prolapse. The use of α-receptor antagonists has been studied in a small number of women with functional bladder neck obstruction for whom surgery was not an option. The use of both terazosin and tamsulosin was observed to reduce obstructive

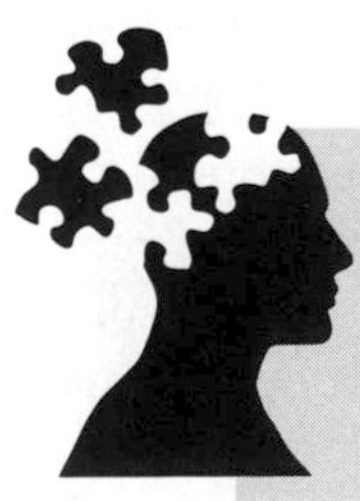

Therapeutic Challenge:

What is the benefit of combining bladder training with anticholinergic medications in the treatment of urge incontinence?

symptoms and postvoid residual volumes.[50,51] However, the impact on the number of incontinent episodes has not been determined.

Adverse effects of the α-receptor antagonists are largely an extension of their pharmacologic activity, with symptomatic orthostatic hypotension being the most bothersome. Importantly, terazosin can exhibit a "first-dose" effect and should therefore be initiated at the lowest possible dosage, titrated slowly upward as tolerated.[52,53] Throughout the dosage titration period, women should be counseled to get out of bed slowly, dangling their feet over the bed for a few minutes before standing. They should also exercise caution when standing from a sitting position.

Rhinitis is another common adverse effect related to the pharmacologic activity of the α-antagonists, which many patients find problematic. It is important to counsel them not to treat symptoms with over-the-counter decongestants with α-agonist activity, which can counteract the effect of terazosin and tamsulosin.

MONITORING AND FOLLOW-UP

Monitoring and follow-up are important to evaluate the effectiveness of treatment, improve adherence, and assess potential adverse effects of drug therapy. Monitoring for effectiveness of treatment strategies is similar, regardless of the specific treatment or type of UI experienced. The symptom checklist and the voiding diary are key components to ongoing monitoring of therapy. The symptom checklist can provide an objective assessment for both patient and healthcare professional in determining if the most bothersome symptoms have improved over time, whereas the voiding diary can be used to determine if the number of incontinent episodes have declined with treatment. In addition to monitoring symptoms and the number of incontinent episodes, it is important to determine if therapy has resulted in resumption of normal activities that may have been curtailed as a coping mechanism.

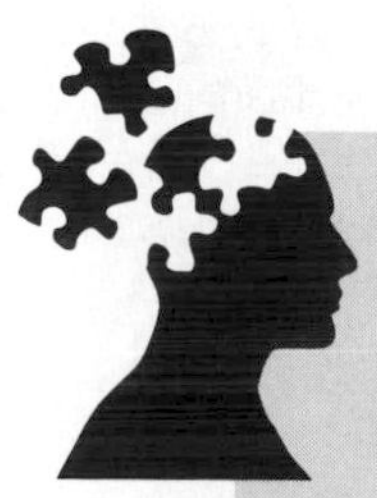

Therapeutic Challenge:

What is the efficacy of alpha-antagonists in comparison with surgery in women with overflow UI caused by prolapsed pelvic organs?

Adherence to both nonpharmacologic and drug treatment strategies is important. Pharmacists can promote adherence to nondrug treatment, such as PFMT, by referring women to continence care nurses or physiotherapists when appropriate.

Clinical trials suggest that persistence to pharmacologic therapy for UI is influenced by adverse effects. Therefore, it is important to identify side effects early to ensure time for an adequate therapeutic trial. Pharmacists should also be aware of clinically important drug interactions and dosing considerations (Table 39-2) that increase the risk of adverse events occurring. Women taking duloxetine for stress UI should have their blood pressure monitored regularly, especially after dosing increases. Because of the potential increased risk of suicide associated with drugs exhibiting **selective serotonin reuptake inhibitor (SSRI)** activity, including duloxetine, pharmacists have a responsibility to discuss this with women when therapy is initiated, with periodic follow-up to assess for suicidal ideation. Side effects of the anticholinergic agents used to treat urge UI are related to their pharmacologic effect. In particular, older persons who may be vulnerable to the cognitive effects of anticholinergic agents should be monitored for changes in memory. If cognitive changes are suspected, a cognitive assessment should be completed, including collateral history from a reliable caregiver. Constipation can also be problematic for those taking anticholinergic agents, with potential to worsen UI in some patients. Women should be counseled about appropriate preventative measures, which take into account their daily fluid and dietary fibre intake. For some patients, laxatives may be necessary.

PATIENT EDUCATION

Patient education is important to dispel the myths around UI, particularly that it is an untreatable disorder. There are several organizations that have developed written educational material that can be provided to patients (Table 39-3). As UI is a complex condition and there is a large amount of information available to patients, education is probably best delivered over several sessions in conjunction with follow-up visits. Patient education is also important for adherence to both nonpharmacologic and pharmacologic therapies. Because adherence to treatment regimens is essential to improving symptoms, patients need to be full partners in the decision-making process. This can be accomplished by carefully explaining each treatment option in detail and reviewing the specifics of what is involved, including potential benefits and risks in realistic terms.

Table 39-3. Organizations Providing Educational Material

Organization	Web Address
National Association for Continence	www.nafc.org
Simon Foundation for Continence	www.simonfoundation.org
National Institute of Diabetes and Digestive and Kidney Diseases	www.niddk.nih.gov Follow A to Z index for links on urinary incontinence in women and interstitial cystitis/painful bladder syndrome
Interstitial Cystitis Association	www.ichelp.org
National Vulvodynia Association	www.nva.org
Office of Research on Women's Health—Vulvodynia	http://orwh.od.nih.gov/health/vulvodynia.html
Women's Health Matters	www.womenshealthmatters.ca Follow A to Z index for links to urinary tract and kidney disorders. Follow A to Z index for links to pelvic health and disease

CASE PRESENTATION

Patient Case: Part 2

Assessment: R.A. has mixed stress and overflow UI. The stress component is evidenced by her symptoms: loss of small amounts of urine with increases in intra-abdominal pressure (laughing, coughing, picking up her grandchildren) and the urine spurt observed with the Valsalva maneuver (which increases intra-abdominal pressure) on physical examination. The overflow component is evidenced by symptoms of sensation of incomplete bladder emptying, dribbling urine without increased intra-abdominal pressure, and a high postvoid residual of >200 mL as measured by ultrasound. The stress component is likely to be persistent but treatment responsive, whereas the overflow component is probably transient, related to R.A.'s use of amitriptyline for treatment of postherpetic neuralgia.

Plan:

1. Discontinue amitriptyline, and consider use of another treatment option for postherpetic neuralgia, such as gabapentin or pregabalin. Other tricyclic antidepressants, such as desipramine, should be avoided.
2. Initiate a course of PFMT for 6–8 weeks with follow-up by continence care nurse to ensure proper technique and adherence.
3. Reduction of caffeine intake over the next 3–6 weeks, replacing her 3 cups of caffeinated coffee/day with water or noncaffeinated beverages, up to 750–1,000 mL of noncaffeinated fluid/day.

Rationale: Amitriptyline is a tricyclic antidepressant agent. Although effective in the management of postherpetic neuralgia, it exhibits significant anticholinergic activity. Anticholinergic agents act on the muscarinic receptors of the bladder, inhibiting normal contractions, resulting in high postvoid residual volumes, and precipitating symptoms of overflow UI. Pelvic floor muscle training, when performed with proper technique and when the patient is adherent to the exercise regimen, can improve symptoms of stress UI. Reduction of caffeine intake and adequate fluid intake will also improve symptoms of stress UI by decreasing bladder irritation.

Monitoring: Pain associated with postherpetic neuralgia, reduction in postvoid residual volume to <150 mL, symptom checklist to identify improvement in symptoms of sensation of incomplete bladder emptying, resolution of dribbling not associated with increased intra-abdominal pressure, fewer episodes of urine loss with laughing, coughing, or lifting grandchildren.

Patient education: Provide reassurance that UI can be treated and improved. Review proper technique for PFMT exercises. Gradually eliminate caffeinated beverages over next few weeks and replace with water or noncaffeinated fluids, up to 3–4 glasses/day. Advise regarding appropriate absorbent products with discussion regarding good skin care to prevent skin irritation.

Interstitial Cystitis

EPIDEMIOLOGY

Similar to UI, the epidemiology of interstitial cystitis is poorly understood. However, it is estimated that approximately 1 million Americans suffer from interstitial cystitis (also known as painful bladder syndrome) (**IC/PBS**), with women accounting for 90% of those affected.[54] Current evidence suggests a genetic component, as the prevalence of IC/PBS is higher in those with family members affected in comparison with the general population.[55] There also seems to be a higher prevalence associated with certain comorbid conditions, including endometriosis, inflammatory bowel disease, irritable bowel syndrome, vulvodynia, and anxiety/panic disorders.[54,56]

IC/PBS can be very disabling for many women, negatively affecting occupational and social functioning as well as intimate relationships.[57] All of this can have a significant impact on mental health and quality of life.[58]

CLINICAL PRESENTATION

IC/PBS is characterized by chronic suprapubic pain, which is often relieved by voiding.[54,57] Other common symptoms include frequency, urgency, **nocturia,** and **dyspareunia.**[54,59] Many of these symptoms, such as frequency, urgency, and dyspareunia, are related to **high-tone pelvic floor muscle dysfunction.**

Before diagnosis of IC/PBS, patients are often treated for recurrent urinary tract infections, as urinalysis demonstrates pyuria and/or hematuria, but the urine culture is negative.[54]

Typically, patients present with a subacute onset, followed by a period of symptom exacerbation and spontaneous remission.[60] Certain factors have been associated with worsening symptoms, including stress, cigarette smoking, and specific foods/beverages.[54,56] Symptoms also seem to exacerbate just before menses in some women.[60]

PATHOPHYSIOLOGY

Numerous theories exist regarding the pathophysiology of IC/PBS, none of which have been definitively proven. Of these theories, three are considered to be the most reasonable. The first is that the bladder lining has been damaged secondary to some insult, resulting in an inflammatory response, involving mast cells and neuropathic changes.[60] Alternatively, it is thought that a deficient bladder epithelium results in the bladder lining being more permeable to irritants.[60] Finally, IC/PBS has been considered as an autoimmune condition.[60] In general, most experts consider IC/PBS to result from a combination of each of these pathologies.[60]

DIAGNOSIS

The diagnosis of IC/PBS is largely a diagnosis of exclusion, in which other conditions—urinary tract infection, bladder cancer, urinary tract stones, sexually transmitted infections, and endometriosis—are ruled out as the cause of suprapubic pain. Physical examination (including pelvic exam) and history of symptoms is important to differentiate IC/PBS from these disorders. The clinical criteria for diagnosis include the following[56]:

- At least 6 months of suprapubic pain/discomfort
- Pain is worsened with bladder filling and relieved by voiding
- Urinary frequency, urgency, and nocturia in the absence of urinary tract pathology

A symptom questionnaire, such as the O'Leary-Sant Symptom Index and Problem Index or the Pelvic Pain and Urgency/Frequency Patient Symptom Scale, can be useful for patients to describe and quantify their symptomatology.[61]

Specific laboratory tests include a urinalysis and urine culture to rule out urinary tract infections.[61] When indicated by history, vaginal cultures to rule out sexually transmitted infections should be done.[60] Specific diagnostic tests, such as bladder biopsy, cystoscopy, and urodynamics, may aid in the diagnosis of some individuals but are not considered necessary for most patients.[61] In recent years, the **potassium sensitivity test (PST)** and **anesthetic challenge** have been added to the diagnostic workup. However, their sensitivity and specificity in identifying IC/PBS have been questioned.[54]

TREATMENT GOALS

At present, there is no cure for IC/PBS. As such, the primary goal of treatment for IC/PBS is that of symptom relief, allowing patients to resume their normal activities. Treatment is most effective when patients and healthcare providers function as equal partners in the care process.

NONPHARMACOLOGIC INTERVENTIONS

Nonpharmacologic interventions are important to the management of IC/PBS. In particular, dietary changes can improve symptoms for many women. A number of foods (Table 39-4) have been associated

Table 39-4. Foods Associated with Symptom Exacerbation in Interstitial Cystitis/Painful Bladder Syndrome

- Acidic beverages/foods, such as apples, cranberries, pineapple, and tomato
- Aged cheese
- Alcohol
- Artificial sweeteners
- Chili, hot peppers, horseradish, and other spicy foods
- Citrus fruits and juices
- Coffee, tea, cola, and other caffeinated beverages
- Soda and other carbonated beverages
- Vitamin C

Source: Adapted from reference 62.

with symptom exacerbation in IC/PBS.[62] Because foods can affect each patient differently, it is suggested that all high-risk foods be eliminated from the diet for 1–2 weeks, then gradually reintroduce them one by one, allowing for identification of a specific offending food.[54]

Behavioral interventions, such as timed voiding and bladder training, are useful to reduce symptoms of frequency and urgency but do not result in any appreciable reduction in pain.[63,64] Physical therapy for those experiencing symptoms related to increased tone of the pelvic floor musculature is helpful to reduce pain.[65] Stress results from IC/PBS for some women and is an important precipitant symptom exacerbation for others. Although the effect of stress management on symptoms has not been studied, reducing stress may improve symptoms and improve the overall sense of well-being for some women. In particular, women report that participation in an IC/PBS support group as a beneficial coping strategy.[58]

PHARMACOLOGIC INTERVENTIONS

A number of different agents have been used to manage the symptoms of IC/PBS. These include oral amitriptyline for pain management, used alone or in combination with other therapies; oral therapy aimed at specific pathologies (hydroxyzine, pentosan polysulfate); and intravesical administration of compounds thought to act directly on the bladder lining **(dimethyl sulfoxide [DMSO])**. Medications commonly used in the management of IC/PBS are outlined in Table 39-5. A recent systematic review suggests that amitriptyline, pentosan polysulfate, and DMSO are effective treatments for IC/PBS but questions the role of hydroxyzine.[66] At present, only pentosan polysulfate and DMSO are approved therapies in the management of IC/PBS.

MONITORING AND FOLLOW-UP

The purpose of monitoring and follow-up is to determine if a given therapy is effective in managing symptoms and identify any adverse effects related to medications. As there is a lag time for effect of some treatments, this needs to be taken into consideration. The effectiveness of therapy can be followed using symptom scales specific to IC/PBS.

PATIENT EDUCATION

Perhaps the most important aspect of patient education is the diagnosis itself. Women with IC/PBS often remain undiagnosed for several years, and recognition of their symptoms as a real disease can be very reassuring.[67] It is important to explain that although there is no cure for IC/PBS, there are a number of effective therapies available. Education of

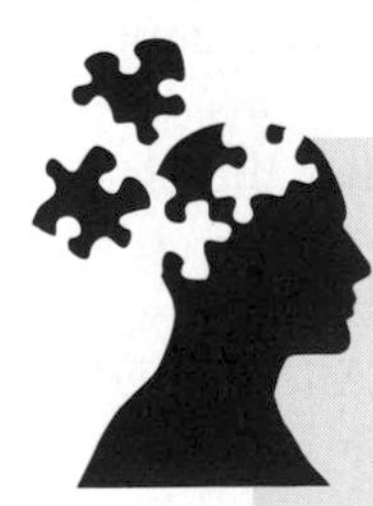

Therapeutic Challenge:

Is there a role for combining pentosan and amitriptyline in the treatment of IC/PBS?

Table 39-5 Treatment Options for Interstitial Cystitis/Painful Bladder Syndrome

Drug	Dosage	Mechanism	Comments
Amitriptyline	25 mg QHS titrated to target dosage of 75 mg	Treats neuropathic pain of IC/PBS; anticholinergic properties ↓ frequency/urgency; antihistaminic properties may suppress mast cell degranulation resulting from inflammatory response of bladder	Cognitive and cardiac effects may limit treatment in some women; dry mouth and sedation can ⇓ persistence to therapy
Hydroxyzine	25 mg QHS titrated to 25 mg QAM and 50 mg QHS	Antihistaminic properties may suppress mast cell degranulation	Sedation can be dose limiting and ⇓ persistence to therapy; requires 3–4 mo treatment before therapeutic benefit observed
Pentosan polysulfate	100 mg TID or 150 mg BID	Replenishes bladder mucosa; antihistaminic properties may suppress mast cell degranulation	GI upset most common adverse effect; best taken on an empty stomach; hair loss can be bothersome for some women
DMSO	50 mL of 25% to 50% solution instilled directly into bladder (sodium bicarbonate, a steroid, and heparin are often added)		Weekly treatments for 6–8 wk followed by treatments every 2 wk for 3–6 mo; may cause ⇑ symptoms (pain, frequency/urgency) transiently for initial two to three treatments; recent data suggest that concentrations <50% DMSO are beneficial[56,67]

BID = 2 times a day; DMSO = dimethyl sulfoxide; GI = gastrointestinal; IC/PBS = interstitial cystitis/painful bladder syndrome; QAM = every morning; QHS = every night; TID = 3 times a day.

spouses and other family members is essential, pointing out that although the patient might appear well, there are times in the course of the disease when she will be quite debilitated because of her symptoms.[67] Contact information for reputable organizations providing patient information regarding IC/PBS can be found in Table 39-3.

Vulvodynia

EPIDEMIOLOGY

Chronic vulvar pain is increasingly recognized as a common disorder, estimated to affect from 3% to 15% of women.[68-71] One of the difficulties in determining the prevalence of this disorder has been multiple terminology for vulvar pain syndromes. Recently, the International Society for the Study of Vulvovaginal Disease (ISSVD) defined vulvodynia as "vulvar discomfort, most often described as burning pain, occurring in the absence of relevant visible findings or a specific, clinically identifiable, neurologic disorder."[72]

CLINICAL PRESENTATION

As implied by its definition, vulvodynia presents as discomfort or pain in vulvar area, frequently described as burning, but it can also be described as sharp, prickly, and occasionally as pruritic.[73] The level of pain can range from mild to severe. Factors reported to worsen pain include sexual intercourse, wearing tight clothes, riding a bicycle, use of tampons, and prolonged sitting.[73] Women typically report that pain occurs suddenly, often taking hours to days to resolve.[73]

PATHOPHYSIOLOGY

A number of different etiologies for vulvodynia have been proposed.[74,75] These include the following:

- Embryologic abnormalities
- Genetic, hormonal, or immune factors
- Infection
- Neuropathic changes
- Urinary oxalates

With no specific etiology identified, it is believed that vulvodynia occurs as a response to several different factors.[74,75]

DIAGNOSIS

Vulvodynia is a clinical diagnosis of exclusion when no other cause of symptoms can be identified. A thorough history should be taken, with specific questions regarding the nature and duration of symptoms, and any previous treatments. Although some women will find discussion of their sexual history uncomfortable, it is an important to identify how symptoms are affecting their sexual activity. Past medical and surgical history should also be taken.[74,75]

Physical exam of the vulva should not reveal any mucosal or skin irritation, but erythema can be present.[73] The cotton swab test, with gentle pressure applied to several areas, usually elicits some degree of discomfort, with the location and severity of this discomfort helpful in monitoring treatment over time.[73-75] Vaginal secretions should be tested to rule out fungal and other infectious causes of symptoms.[73-75]

NONPHARMACOLOGIC INTERVENTIONS

Vulvar care measures are important to minimize local irritation and include the following[74]:

- Wearing 100% cotton underwear, avoiding underwear while sleeping
- Using mild soaps for bathing and cleaning the vulva with water only
- Avoiding the use of other potential vulvar irritants (perfumes, dyes, shampoos, and detergents)
- Avoiding hair dryers on the vulvar area, patting the area dry after bathing
- Applying preservative-free emollients to the vulvar area after bathing
- Rinsing and drying the vulvar area after voiding
- Using adequate lubrication during intercourse
- Applying cool gel packs to the vulvar area to relieve pain

Other nonpharmacologic treatment strategies include physical therapy, biofeedback, and therapeutic ultrasonography.[74]

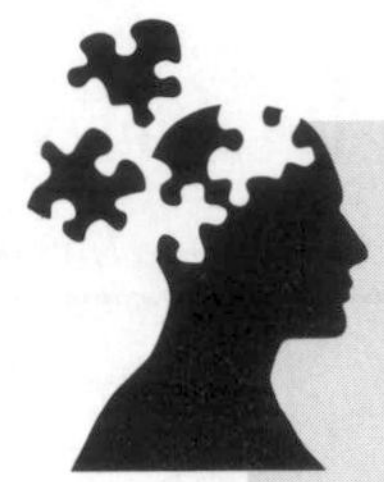

Therapeutic Challenge:

What is the effect of combination therapy of biofeedback and gabapentin in the treatment of vulvodynia?

PHARMACOLOGIC INTERVENTIONS

Oral medications used to manage the symptoms of vulvodynia are directed at its neuropathic pain component. Amitriptyline is considered as the first-line agent and is effective in relieving pain.[76] Alternative treatments include gabapentin and pregabalin.[77,78] Regardless of which therapy is used, patients should be counseled that it may take 2–3 weeks before pain control is achieved.

A variety of topical therapies, applied directly to the vulva, have been used to manage symptoms. Of these, local anesthetics seem to provide some benefit. In particular, overnight application of 5% lidocaine ointment significantly reduced symptoms.[79] Patients should be instructed to use a cotton ball to apply the ointment to the vulvar area (pictures can be helpful when counseling to describe the specific area) at bedtime and leave it on overnight.[75] As lidocaine can be absorbed systemically, application of large amounts of ointment should be avoided to reduce the potential of lidocaine toxicity. The local anesthetic benzocaine should be avoided because of high rates of contact dermatitis.[75]

Summary

Genitourinary disorders are common among women, often having a profound impact in psychosocial and emotional well-being. Although no cure exists for UI, IC/PBS, or vulvodynia, effective therapies exist for each.

References

Additional content available at ***www.ashp.org/womenshealth***

40 Bone and Joint Disorders

Mary Beth O'Connell, Pharm.D., BCPS; Nima M. Patel, Pharm.D., BCPS;
Sharon L. Hame, MD

Learning Objectives

1. Explain sex differences in pathophysiology, risk factors, epidemiology, and treatment for sports injuries, osteoporosis, and osteoarthritis.
2. Educate girls and women on prevention of sports injuries, osteoporosis, and osteoarthritis.
3. Use screening and diagnostic tools to identify osteoporosis and modifiable risk factors.
4. Individualize drug therapy for girls and women with sports injuries, female athlete triad, osteoporosis, and osteoarthritis.
5. Monitor medication therapy for these musculoskeletal disorders and resolve any medication related problems identified.

Sex differences exist for musculoskeletal disorders, the extent and impact of which are still being unraveled. As a result, specialties such as orthopedics and sports medicine are generating sex-specific data and therapies. Although historically women have competed in some sports, only recently have the numbers of women athletes and female athletic support greatly increased. This is partially related to Title IX, federal legislation passed in 1972.[1,2] Title IX was approved to overcome sex inequity within federally funded education programs, including sports, and has increased female participation in both high school and college sports.[2] Despite these changes, women's overall participation in all sports still continues to be less than that of men.[3] Sports injury rates for women and men are difficult to compare because women and men participate in different sports. Where comparisons have been made, sex differences have been reported in anterior cruciate ligament (ACL) injuries, female athlete triad, and stress fractures. (See Web Resources for Patient Case: ACL Tear, Female Athlete Triad, and Stress Fractures.)

Additional content available at
www.ashp.org/womenshealth

Osteoporosis and osteoarthritis also have sex differences. Women experience more bone loss related to hormone deficiency starting in midlife. Although women have more osteoporosis than men, the mortality rate after a fragility fracture is greater for men than women.[4] Osteoarthritis (OA) also affects more women than men.[5] Sex differences in treatment include timing and types of orthopedic devices and surgery.[6,7] Healthcare providers must be aware of sex differences for all musculoskeletal disorders so that they can provide appropriate care from diagnosis to treatment.

Anterior Cruciate Ligament Tears

EPIDEMIOLOGY

Sex differences related to the ACL and its injury are one of the predominant topics in sports medicine today. The incidence of noncontact ACL injury in sports with pivoting or cutting maneuvers is 2–8 times greater in women than in men.[8,9] About one out of every 100 high school female athletes will injure her ACL during her 4-year career. As she advances to college, her risk is one in 10.[10] Between 100,000 and 150,000 ACL reconstructions are performed in the U.S. each year.[11-13] Functional outcomes have been reported to be equal among women and men.[14,15] The long-term effects of this injury, such as post-traumatic OA, have a dramatic impact on the health of women throughout life.

CASE PRESENTATION

Patient Case: Part 1

R.T. is a 70-year-old woman in clinic today reporting bilateral knee pain that is limiting her activities.

HPI: R.T. reports morning stiffness and worsening of pain with activity. Several days ago, she nearly fell when her knees gave away walking down the stairs. She uses acetaminophen, but it provides minimal pain relief.

PMH: Coronary artery disease, hypertension, dyslipidemia, knee osteoarthritis, and osteoporosis; frequent knee injuries while playing sports in high school and college. She used ice and bandages without medical attention—the standard of care when she was young. She has never had any type of radiology examination of her knees.

Family history: Noncontributory.

Social history: No alcohol or tobacco.

Medications: Lisinopril/HCTZ 20/25 mg daily; aspirin 81 mg daily; atorvastatin 40 mg daily at bedtime; acetaminophen 500 mg two tablets 4 times a day.

Allergies: NKDA.

Vitals: 5′2″, 210 lb (BMI 38.4), BP 118/84, HR 70, Temp 98.6°F, RR 18.

Physical exam: Significant for crepitus on motion and height loss of 2″. R.T. does not report any stomach ulcerations, bleeding, or fractures.

Laboratory values: All within normal limits.

Procedures: DXA T-scores from 3 years ago were spine −2.3 and hip −2.7.

CLINICAL PRESENTATION

A patient with an ACL injury typically describes a "pop" in the knee following a twisting activity and presents with a painful, swollen knee and limited mobility. Chronic ACL tears might not have knee swelling but can have mobility limitations.

RISK FACTORS

Risk factors for ACL injury can be divided into environmental, anatomic, hormonal, and neuromuscular. Environmental risk factors include type and availability of equipment and braces, the type of shoe, playing surface, and the interaction between footwear and playing surfaces. Anatomic, hormonal, and neuromuscular differences exist between men and women and might account for the increase in ACL tears in women. **Knee valgus** and foot pronation, which are more common in women, and the geometry of a woman's ACL within the notch have been implicated. Estrogen and progesterone receptors have been identified on the ACL, and although hypothesized to play a role, no definitive association has been proven.[16] However, ACL injuries tend to cluster around the perimenstrual and preovulatory stages of the menstrual cycle.[17-19] More recently, neuromuscular influences are being investigated. For example, women and girls land from a jump with the knee straight vs. the knee bent for men.[12]

DETECTION, SCREENING, AND DIAGNOSIS

After an acute injury, knee effusion and limited range of motion are observed on physical examination. Ligamentous injury can be difficult to assess initially, sometimes requiring multiple examinations. A positive **Lachman test** and **anterior drawer test** are indicative of a tear. Chronic ACL tears are easier to diagnose as the patient might have full range of motion and no effusion and therefore more able to tolerate testing maneuvers. Radiographs should be obtained and in an acute injury might show an effusion. Magnetic resonance imaging should also be obtained to confirm the diagnosis and identify any associated injuries, such as medial and lateral collateral ligament and meniscal injuries, that are often associated with ACL injury.

PREVENTION

Prevention of ACL injury has focused on improvements in equipment (e.g., shoes, braces) and on neuromuscular training. Based on limited data, successful prevention programs include **plyometrics** with attention to proper landing technique; increased stretching and strengthening exercises; aerobic conditioning; improved balance, agility, and proprioception; and awareness of how ACL injury occurs.[20]

TREATMENT

Treatment of an ACL tear varies with patient age and activity level. The treatment goal is to establish a functional, stable knee.

Nonpharmacologic Treatment

The early stages of treatment should include cold therapy, bracing, and physical therapy to improve range of motion and regain muscular control. For long-term treatment in those who do not undergo surgery, bracing and activity modification can be beneficial.[21]

Pharmacologic Treatment

Short-term pain medication, including nonsteroidal anti-inflammatory drugs (NSAIDs) and opioids (Table 40-1) might be required for 2–3 days following an injury. The NSAIDs should be discontinued before any surgical procedure because of their platelet inhibition. Long-term pain medication is usually not required for this injury unless post-traumatic arthritis develops.

Surgical Treatment

Reconstruction of the ACL is recommended in most young active patients after the knee has stabilized, which occurs 2–6 weeks postinjury. Grafts for reconstruction can be **autografts** (bone patella, quadriceps, or hamstring tendons) or **allografts** (those above and Achilles, anterior tibialis, or posterior tibialis tendons).

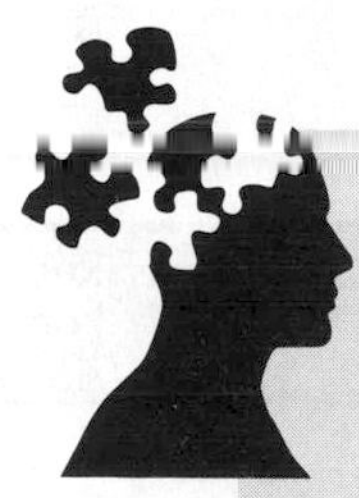

Therapeutic Challenge:

How do NSAIDs inhibit platelet action? What effect do cyclooxygenase-2 (COX-2) inhibitors have on platelet action?

Femoral nerve blocks before surgery can reduce the amount of anesthesia used during surgery and postoperative pain medication. Postoperative pain medication includes opioids (Table 40-1) for typically 2–7 days. Cold therapy can also be used to decrease swelling and pain. Traditional NSAIDs are not recommended in the early postoperative period because of their increased risk for bleeding.

Table 40-1. Pharmacotherapy for Bone and Joint Pain Management

Drug	Dosage	Advantages	Limitations
Acetaminophen	500–1,000 mg 1–4 times daily	Can be used safety in patients with GI disorders, bleeding, and renal disease; sustained release products exist	Lack of long-term efficacy in OA patients; use caution and usually lower dosages (≤ 2 g/day) in patients with liver disease and regular ethanol use; use of ≥2 g daily with warfarin can alter INR; lacks anti-inflammatory effects
NSAIDs:			
Diclofenac[a]	25–50 mg BID–TID	Reduces pain related to inflammatory process more effectively than acetaminophen	Should be taken with food and sufficient fluids; might take 1–2 wk to see anti-inflammatory effects; high incidence of GI-related bleeding and renal failure when used long term; cardiovascular safety concerns
Diclofenac XR	100–200 mg daily		
Etodolac	300–400 mg BID–TID		
Etodolac XL	400–1,000 mg daily		
Ibuprofen	200–800 mg TID or QID		
Meloxicam	7.5–15 mg daily		
Naproxen	200–500 mg BID		
Nabumetone	500–750 mg daily BID		
COX-2:			
Celecoxib	100 mg daily or BID 200 mg daily	Reduces pain as effectively as NSAIDs and might have lower risk of GI-related bleeding	Contraindication following CABG surgery and history of sulfonamide allergies; increased risk of myocardial infarction and stroke at high dosages; can also cause renal insufficiency; greater cost than NSAIDs
Nonacetylated salicylates:			
Choline magnesium trisalicylate	500–1,500 mg BID–TID, <4.5 g daily	Reduces pain and inflammation	Tinnitus and CNS toxicity; can monitor salicylate concentration (except for diflunisal); some products have high cost
Salsalate	500–1,500 mg BID–TID, <3 g daily		
Diflunisal	250–1,000 mg BID, <1.5 g daily		

(*Continued on next page*)

Drug	Dosage	Advantages	Limitations
Topical capsaicin	Apply 0.025% to 0.075% to affected area TID or QID	Reduces pain for hand and knee OA; usually no systemic side effects	Need to continue therapy for 2–4 wk for efficacy; local pain, stinging, and erythema can occur with first doses and poor adherence
Glucosamine Glucosamine with chondroitin	1,500 mg/day in divided doses 1,200 mg/day in divided doses	Pain relief with combination therapy in patients with moderate to severe symptoms; minimal side effects; lack of drug interactions; may also be disease modifying	Conflicting efficacy data; need to continue therapy for 2–3 mo for efficacy; some data suggest chondroitin affects bleeding time
Adenosylmethionine (SAMe)	200 mg TID	Can decrease depression; however, higher dosages required (400–1,600 mg daily)	Butanedisulfonate salt has best absorption (5%); adverse effects at higher dosage including GI symptoms, headache, anorexia, dry mouth, sweating, nervousness, tiredness; can cause serotonin syndrome when given concomitantly with other medications known to increase serotonin; drug interactions with levodopa, and medications increasing serotonin
Methylsulfonylmethane (MSM)	500 mg tid–3 g BID	No known drug or disease interactions	GI symptoms, headache, fatigue, insomnia, difficulty concentrating, pruritus
Opioids Codeine Hydrocodone Morphine Morphine SR Oxycodone Oxycodone CR	Various 15–30 mg q 4–6 hr prn 2.5–5 mg q 4–6 hr prn 10 mg q 3–4 hr prn 15–30 mg q 12 hr 2.5–5 mg q 6 hr prn 10–20 mg q 12 hr	Reduction of pain without GI or renal toxicities; combination products with acetaminophen and ibuprofen; some long-acting products	Nausea, constipation, sedation, dizziness, pruritus, respiratory depression, and tolerance; oxycodone sustained release has significant abuse potential; codeine—nausea and GI upset are common; codeine has a ceiling effect and for some patients with 2D6 polymorphism it is ineffective
Tramadol	50–100 mg 1–4 times daily	Reduction in pain without GI or renal toxicities; lower addiction potential than opioids	Contraindications—CrCl <30 mL/min and severe hepatic dysfunction; flushing, headache, dizziness, insomnia, muscle weakness, and constipation; seizures, especially with concomitant use of tricyclic or SSRI antidepressants and opioid analgesics; can cause serotonin syndrome when given concomitantly with other medications know to increase serotonin; immediate release products—reduce dosage by 50% in patients with renal insufficiency; do not use the extended-release product

BID = twice daily; CABG = coronary artery bypass graft; CNS = central nervous system; COX = cyclo-oxygenase; CR = controlled release; CrCl = creatinine clearance; GI = gastrointestinal; INR = international normalized ratio; NSAIDs = nonsteroidal anti-inflammatory drugs; OA = osteoarthritis; prn = as needed; QID = 4 times daily; SR = sustained release; SSRI = selective serotonin reuptake inhibitor; TID = 3 times daily; XR = extended release.

[a]Also available as a combination product with misoprostol.

MONITORING AND FOLLOW-UP

Initially, close follow-up is required after surgery to ensure proper wound healing and adequate knee range of motion. Physical therapy is generally prescribed for 6–12 months. Patients treated nonsurgically also require close follow-up for any signs of frank knee instability and injury to additional structures. All patients need to be monitored for post-traumatic arthritis.

PATIENT EDUCATION

Patient education is vital to successful injury treatment. Patients should be given ACL recovery and prevention information from pamphlets, videos, and or websites. (See Web Resources for Good Bone and Joint Disorders Websites.)

Additional content available at
www.ashp.org/womenshealth

The Female Athlete Triad

EPIDEMIOLOGY

The female athlete triad was first described in 1992, with prevalence now as high as 62% in female athletes.[22,23] Disordered eating, amenorrhea, and osteoporosis compose the triad, and all can occur on a spectrum.[22,24]

PATHOPHYSIOLOGY

The pathogenesis is not fully understood, but the concept of a negative energy balance—in which calories expended outweigh calories consumed—is the most supported theory at this time. Inadequate caloric intake appears to be the primary mechanism that predisposes female athletes to menstrual dysfunction and resulting detrimental bone effects, including osteoporosis.[25,26]

A wide range of eating behaviors has been seen in the female athlete triad. Diet pills, diuretic and laxative abuse, excessive exercise, food preoccupation, anorexia nervosa bulimia, unrealistic fears of weight gain, and a distorted body image might accompany the eating issue (see Chapter 31: Nutrition and Eating Disorders). The second component of the triad is primary (delayed onset) or secondary (absence of menses for more than three consecutive months after menarche) amenorrhea. Any factor that could influence the hypothalamus–pituitary–ovarian axis can affect menses (see Chapter 11: Menstruation Disorders). Such factors include energy deficit, low leptin concentration (a hormone involved in metabolism and reproductive function) during caloric restriction, and the physical and psychological stress of training and competing.[27,28] Low leptin concentrations have been shown to suppress the hypothalamic release of gonadotrophin-releasing hormone and markedly diminish the release of ovarian estrogen.[28] Eating disorders and estrogen deficiency predispose women to the third component of the triad, osteoporosis.

DETECTION, SCREENING, AND DIAGNOSIS

The female athlete triad can be difficult to diagnose, occurring in girls and women participating in any sport or strenuous activity. Screening should be done at preparticipation physicals or annual health screening exams.[25] Physical signs can be rare but include low weight, bradycardia, orthostatic hypotension, dry hair and skin, hirsutism, parotid gland enlargement, the **Russell's sign,** and erosion of dental enamel.[29] An electrocardiogram might show prolonged QT intervals in patients with severe eating disorders. If the triad is suspected, laboratory testing should include thyroid-stimulating hormone, complete blood count, chemistry panels, follicle-stimulating hormone, luteinizing hormone, estradiol, testosterone, urine pregnancy test, and dexamethasone suppression testing.[25] Sometimes dual energy x-ray absorptiometry (DXA) of the hip and spine will be ordered to evaluate bone mineral density (BMD). Radiographs of any suspected stress fractures should also be obtained.

TREATMENT

Treatment goals include establishing a positive energy balance, re-establishing normal menstrual function, and preventing osteoporosis. A team approach including family members is frequently used.[25] Pharmacists could assist with nutrient and caloric supplements and identifying and resolving medication-related problems secondary to hormone therapies. Individualized treatment of the athlete will depend on how each

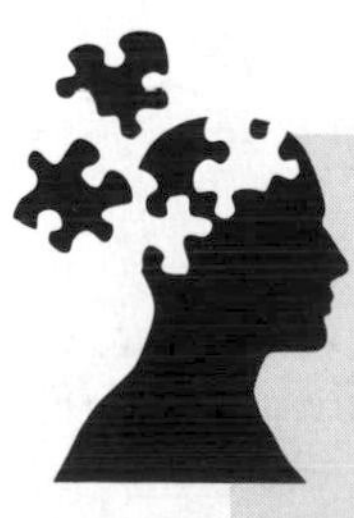

Therapeutic Challenge:

What effect do the various antidepressants have on patient weight? How long does it take for an antidepressant medication to work for a patient with anorexia nervosa or bulimia nervosa?

component of the triad has been affected. Correcting the energy balance in the athlete combined with setting weight goals and frequent visits to a healthcare provider is a solid basic approach (see more specific nutrition information in Chapter 31: Nutrition and Eating Disorders). Appropriate psychological counseling for athletes with eating disorders is recommended.

Pharmacologic treatment for this disorder has had limited effects on the outcome of the triad. Antidepressants have been used in cases of anorexia nervosa and bulimia nervosa, but these have not been shown to improve BMD.[25] Regulating the menstrual cycle has been difficult, as hormone therapy (HT), including oral contraceptive pills (OCPs), have produced inconsistent results. No prospective study on women with anorexia nervosa treated with HT or OCPs has shown an increase in BMD.[30-33] However, the American College of Sports Medicine's most recent position on the female athlete triad states that OCPs (see Chapter 19: Hormonal Contraception) can be considered in an athlete with functional hypothalamic amenorrhea older than age 16 years if BMD is decreasing, despite adequate nutrition and body weight.[25] General use of OCPs is not recommended for improving bone health. Although bisphosphonates are successful in older adults, they should not be used in the young athlete as they have unproven efficacy in women of childbearing age, they might have harmful effects on a developing fetus, and long-term effects are unknown.[34,35] Daily nutritional supplements, including calcium (1,000–1,300 mg) and vitamin D (400–1,000 units), are also important in the prevention and treatment of osteoporosis in the premenopausal athlete.

STRESS FRACTURES

(See Web Resources for Stress Fractures.)

Additional content available at
www.ashp.org/womenshealth

Osteoporosis

EPIDEMIOLOGY

Although osteoporosis affects both sexes, women are 4 times more likely than men to develop the disease (8 million women vs. 2 million men) and experience a fracture (1.42 million fractures for women, 0.68 million for men).[36,37] Because menopause is associated with accelerated bone loss, women experience more bone problems that begin earlier in life than men. Aging increases bone loss in both sexes (e.g., osteoporosis: 4% of women 50–59 years increasing to 44% to 52% of women 80 years or older).[38,39] Because women live longer than men, the impact of age-induced osteoporosis and fractures are greater in women. However, women have longer survival after a hip fracture than men.[4]

CLINICAL PRESENTATION

Osteoporosis is a silent disease until height decreases or fractures occur. Height can decrease secondary to asymptomatic or painful vertebral fractures, which sometimes cause spine curvature. Wrist fractures occur throughout adult life, whereas vertebral fractures generally occur after menopause and hip fractures occur mostly in older age. Depression, low self-esteem, and fear of falling can result with advanced disease. Fractures result in pain and immobility and can lead to loss of independence, nursing home placement, and death.

PHYSIOLOGY AND PATHOPHYSIOLOGY

Bone physiology and pathophysiology are still being unraveled. Basically, the osteoblasts receive a signal to produce RANKL (receptor for activator of nuclear factor kB ligand) that adheres to the RANK receptors on osteoclasts, causing their differentiation, maturation, and bone resorption actions.[40,41] Various hormones (e.g., estrogen, vitamin D, parathyroid hormone, calcitonin) and cytokines (e.g., growth factors, prostaglandins) stop bone resorption by causing osteoprotegerin to be created by osteoblasts. Osteoprotegerin binds RANKL and inhibits bone resorption. Osteoblasts create osteoid, which is mineralized over the next 3–4 months, creating new bone. When this system is balanced, no bone loss occurs. Women have smaller bone size and lower peak bone mass than men, which gives women greater likelihood of developing osteoporosis and experiencing fractures.[42]

Certain conditions cause an imbalance in bone physiology. Bone loss occurs during pregnancy, but most mothers correct bone loss after delivery without long-term consequences. During pregnancy, calcium absorption increases to help meet needs of mother and fetus, but during lactation, calcium is obtained from bone resorption.[43] Prudent care involves increased calcium intake during pregnancy and breastfeeding. Estrogen deprivation during menopause triggers increased bone resorption, with bone formation incapable of meeting demands, thus a bone loss.[44] With aging, bone formation is incapable of meeting demands and also creates bone loss.

RISK FACTORS

A major risk factor for osteoporosis is female sex. Other major risk factors included in the World Health Organization (WHO) fracture risk algorithm (FRAX) are age, low femoral neck BMD, previous minimal trauma fracture, low body mass index (BMI), current or history of glucocorticoid use, alcohol use (3 or more drinks/day), current smoking, rheumatoid arthritis, parental history of hip fracture, and certain secondary causes.[45,46] Ethnicity and race influence osteoporosis prevalence, with Native American women having the highest prevalence (12%), followed by Asian (10%), Hispanic (10%), white (7%), and black (4%) women.[47]

Medications can also cause osteoporosis, with glucocorticoids being the most problematic.[48,49] Other medications causing bone loss are excessive thyroxine, certain anticonvulsants, depot medroxyprogesterone acetate (can be reversible effect), some chemotherapy, cyclosporine, gonadotropin-releasing hormone agonists or analogs, long-term unfractionated heparin, aromatase inhibitors, and some highly active antiretroviral therapy for HIV (human immunodeficiency virus). Recent medications associated with increased fracture risk include long-term proton pump inhibitor (PPI) therapy and selective serotonin reuptake inhibitors.

DETECTION, SCREENING, AND DIAGNOSIS

Screening for osteoporosis includes height measurements, peripheral BMD testing, FRAX, and questionnaire assessments. Height loss >1.5 inches suggests spine bone loss; however, the measurement needs to be done accurately. (See Web Resources for Measuring Height Accurately At Home.)

Additional content available at
www.ashp.org/womenshealth

In community pharmacies, peripheral ultrasound or DXA measurements can be used for osteoporosis screening in postmenopausal women, perimenopausal women with at least one major risk factor, and men aged 65 years and older. Peripheral T-scores <−1 warrant a central DXA test.[50] Peripheral testing should not be used for diagnosis and monitoring. The FRAX assessment tool calculates a person's likelihood of developing a major osteoporotic or hip fracture within the next 10 years.[51] Central DXA (hip and spine) is the gold standard test for diagnosis and monitoring.[45,52] This test uses a minimal amount of radiation. The test yields a T-score that compares patient's bone mass with the young, average sex-specific reference standard. Based on WHO recommendations, normal bone mass is a T-score between −1 and 1, low bone mass (osteopenia) is a T-score between −1 and −2.5, and osteoporosis is a T-score at or below −2.5. A Z-score is also provided to compare bone mass with the average same age and sex group and can suggest secondary causes. Central DXA testing is indicated for all women 65 years and older, perimenopausal and postmenopausal women with risk factors, patients with or suspected of a low trauma fracture after 50 years of age, patients with secondary causes from medications or diseases, consideration for prescription osteoporosis medications, and monitoring response to therapy.

GUIDELINES AND POSITION STATEMENTS

The most recent guideline is from the National Osteoporosis Foundation (NOF) with important statements from the North American Menopause Society.[45,53,54] The NOF guidelines recommend osteoporosis treatment when the T-score is <−2.5, after a hip or vertebral fracture, or when the T-score is between −1.0 and −2.5 with a FRAX score of ≥20% for a major osteoporotic fracture or ≥3% for hip fracture within the next 10 years.

GOALS

For infants, girls, adolescents, and women in their 20s and early 30s, the primary goal is to obtain maximal bone mass. After achievement of peak bone mass, the goal is to maintain bone mass. During menopause, the goal is to eliminate/minimize accelerated bone loss secondary to estrogen deprivation. Throughout the rest of life, the goal is to minimize bone loss and prevent fractures, which includes fall prevention.

NONPHARMACOLOGIC PREVENTION AND TREATMENT

A positive bone healthy lifestyle—defined as adequate calcium and vitamin D intake from food or supplements (Table 40-2), exercise (weight-bearing or isometric), no smoking, minimal to no alcohol use, and limited caffeine intake—is required throughout life.[45,55,56] Both sexes have diets insufficient in calcium and vitamin D, partially related to decreased milk and increased carbonated beverage ingestion. Patients with lactose intolerance can have low calcium intake that is due to decreased dairy product intake. At least 15 minutes of daily sunlight with the correct ultraviolet radiation on extremities and face (without sunscreen) can increase vitamin D conversion in skin. Adequate vitamin D ingestion should result in a 25(OH) vitamin D concentration >30 ng/mL (75 nmol/L).[57,58] Patients

Table 40-2. Calcium and Vitamin D Requirements

Age	Sex	Calcium Requirements[a]	Vitamin D Requirements
Birth–6 mo	Both	210 mg	400 units[b]
6 mo–1 yr	Both	270 mg	400 units[b]
1–3 yr	Both	500 mg	400 units[b]
4–8 yr	Both	800 mg	400 units[b]
9–18 yr	Both	1,300 mg	400 units[b]
19–50 yr	Both	1,000 mg	200 units[a,c]
Pregnant or nursing	Female	1,000 mg	200 units[a,c]
≥51 yr	Both	1,200 mg	800–1,000 units[d]

[a]Institute of Medicine 1997 adequate intakes.[55]
[b]American Academy of Pediatrics 2008 recommendations.[56]
[c]Most experts consider these doses too low; new recommendations coming from National Institutes of Health mid-2010.
[d]National Osteoporosis Foundation 2008 recommendations.[45]

might require dosages as high as 2,000–4,000 units/day to achieve therapeutic vitamin D concentrations.[57,59]

Because falls can lead to fractures, fall prevention is important.[38,60,61] Vitamin D is also required for muscle function and can help with fall prevention. Medications known to increase fall risk need to be identified and replaced if possible. Home improvements can also decrease falls. (See Web Resources for Fall Prevention Material, Calcium Content of Selected Food and Beverages, and Vitamin D Content of Selected Foods and Beverages.)

Additional content available at ***www.ashp.org/womenshealth***

PHARMACOLOGIC TREATMENT

Because most diets are insufficient in calcium and vitamin D, almost everyone will require supplementation to achieve required amounts (Table 40-2). Vitamin D insufficiency (25[OH] vitamin D 13–29 ng/mL) and deficiency (25[OH] vitamin D <13 ng/mL) need to be corrected, sometimes requiring high vitamin D doses.[45,58,62] Assessment of adequate supplementation is probably prudent as well. Usually adequate calcium intake and calcium supplementation result in higher BMDs than placebo or inadequate intake, but no fracture risk reduction has been documented with calcium therapy alone.[63] Calcium combined with adequate amounts of vitamin D (i.e., ≥800 units daily) has been associated with decreased fracture risk.[59,64,65] Low adherence with supplementation decreases fracture risk reduction.

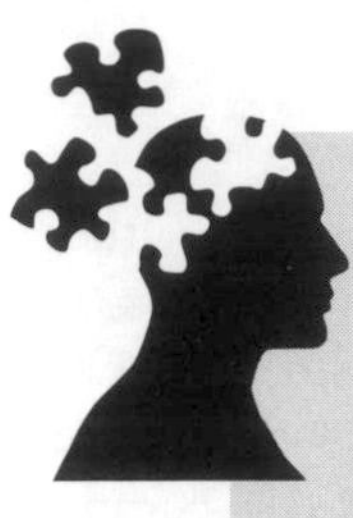

Therapeutic Challenge:

What vitamin D dosing strategies are used to treat vitamin D insufficiency or deficiency? How would you correct vitamin D deficiencies if the patient had liver or renal impairment?

Bisphosphonates are considered the drug of choice for osteoporosis treatment and are supported with pharmacoeconomic analyses.[45,66,67] They all increase spine and hip BMD and reduce vertebral and hip fracture risk.[38,68,69] Zoledronic acid decreased subsequent vertebral and nonvertebral fractures and decreased mortality in patients with a previous hip fracture.[70]

Adherence with bisphosphonates is suboptimal, leading to decreased fracture risk and increased healthcare costs.[71-73] To improve adherence, weekly and monthly oral bisphosphonates, quarterly intravenous ibandronate, and yearly intravenous zoledronic acid were developed. Duration of bisphosphonate therapy is still unknown. Bisphosphonate drug holidays (i.e., stopping therapy until bone markers document increased bone resorption again, which might be in 1–2 years) are being explored.

Overall bisphosphonates are safe if used correctly. Based on limited long-term safety data, treatment is generally considered safe for up to 10 years. Healthcare providers need to frequently re-educate patients about correct product ingestion and assess adherence.

For patients who can not use or tolerate bisphosphonates, raloxifene, calcitonin, and teriparatide are alternatives.[38,68,74] Raloxifene has a breast cancer prevention indication that most likely will influence its use for osteoporosis prevention and treatment in women at high risk for breast cancer.[75] Both raloxifene and calcitonin only have vertebral—not hip—fracture prevention data. Teriparatide is the only medication that can increase bone mass and improve bone strength and architecture.[74,76] Because the product is a daily injection and is expensive, its use is reserved for patients with severe (sometimes defined as BMD T-score <–3 or –3.5) or unresponsive osteoporosis. Bisphosphonates are usually used before or after teriparatide administration, since concomitant use with most bisphosphonates results in less BMD gains.

Some data exist for phytoestrogens to increase BMD, but the quantities required are greater than average American intakes and no fracture data exist. Women can use these products but should try for soy protein intake of 20–60 g or isoflavone intake of 35–120 mg daily. Phytoestrogen safety in women with current or past breast cancer has not been confirmed.

Estrogens, with and without a progestogen (HT), decrease hip, vertebral, and nonvertebral fractures.[53] Estrogens are U.S. Food and Drug Administration indicated for osteoporosis prevention; however, this approval came before the Women's Health Initiative trials. Because HT in older postmenopausal women can increase risk for cardiovascular disease, breast cancer, thromboembolic events, and stroke, the risk is greater than the fracture prevention benefit. Estrogen therapy is thus not recommended primarily for osteoporosis therapy but only for short-term therapy for menopausal symptoms using the lowest possible dosage.

MONITORING AND FOLLOW-UP

Repeat central DXA can be used after about 1–2 years of therapy to assess response. Current research is exploring bone biomarkers to assess medication effectiveness within 1–3 months after therapy initiation. Medication profiles should be monitored for adherence, with barriers to nonadherence identified and resolved. Adequate intakes of calcium and vitamin D should be ensured at each patient encounter as the efficacy of osteoporosis prescription medications was determined with concomitant supplement ingestion.

PATIENT EDUCATION

Bisphosphonate therapy is complex, requiring oral and written patient information and frequent reassessment of correct administration. Many good websites exist for patient and provider information. (See Web Resources for Good Bone and Joint Disorders Websites.)

Additional content available at
www.ashp.org/womenshealth

Osteoarthritis

EPIDEMIOLOGY

Joint disorders are more common in women and decrease quality of life with pain and disability. Approximately 7.2 million adults reported disability from arthritis and rheumatism with rates of this disability 2 times higher in women than men.[77] In women, the rates of arthritis vary by ethnicity and race.[78] The highest rates were reported in non-Hispanic white women followed by non-Hispanic black women. The lowest rates were reported among Asian women.

Osteoarthritis is the most common chronic joint condition in the U.S. and the leading cause of joint pain and disability. After age 55 years, women are affected more than men, with more joints involved and greater severity. Women have more hand, foot, and knee OA involvement, whereas men have more hip OA.[5] Severe knee OA greatly increases in women after menopause.[79] Osteoarthritis prevalence is estimated to double by 2020 as the U.S. population ages and the obesity epidemic grows.[80]

RISK FACTORS

Generally accepted OA risk factors include advancing age, obesity, postmenopausal status, higher BMD, occupations with repetitious tasks, sports activity, previous injury, and genetic factors.[5] Sudden major injury or stereotyped repetitive activity that exceeds the ability of periarticular muscle and tendon to withstand such use can damage the cartilage causing OA. Evidence supports that jobs in which workers have to do tasks repeatedly (e.g., crouching, squatting, pincer grips) and in sports, especially endurance sports with repeated joint use, have higher prevalence of hand, knee, and hip OA.[81] Young female athletes with ACL tears are subsequently at increased risk for knee OA.[82] Increased risk for knee OA is stronger in overweight women than men. Women had twice the risk of radiographic knee OA than did men with risk increasing for every 5-unit increase of BMI and every 10-lb increase in weight. Many studies have noted an inverse relationship between osteoporosis and OA.[83] The mechanism behind this association is unknown. Elevated BMD in OA patients does not protect from fracture, possibly because risk of falling is still increased.

CLINICAL PRESENTATION

Osteoarthritis presentation is similar between sexes. Typically, patients report joint pain that worsens with weight-bearing activity and improves with rest. Morning stiffness and **gelling** is often experienced with periods of inactivity. Women with arthritis report greater prevalence of activity and work limitations, psychological distress, severe joint pain, and decreased function on quality-of-life instruments before surgery than their male counterparts.[84,85]

PATHOPHYSIOLOGY

Causes of OA are not completely understood, although biomechanical stresses affecting cartilage and subchondral bone and biochemical changes in the cartilage and synovial membrane play an important role. Larger knee cartilage volume in men compared with women after adjustments of age, height, weight, and bone volume suggests that men are naturally more protected from knee OA than women.[86]

DETECTION, SCREENING, AND DIAGNOSIS

Diagnosis uses the clinical, radiologic, and synovial fluid analysis criteria developed by the American College of Rheumatology.[87-89] On examination, patients exhibit tenderness on palpation, bony enlargement, crepitus on motion, and limitation of joint motion. Healthcare providers will commonly ask the patient to rate the improvement or worsening of activity and mechanical pain on visual analog scales and have them describe duration of stiffness after inactivity and ability to carry out activities of daily living (i.e., opening jars). Laboratory testing is not routinely done unless needed to rule out other etiologies, such as inflammatory arthritis, gout, or pseudogout. Patients with OA do not exhibit an active inflammatory process such as seen with rheumatoid arthritis. Radiography is used in clinical practice to confirm diagnosis, although it is less sensitive and specific than physical examination. In advanced disease, narrowing of joint space, **osteophytes,** and sometimes changes in subchondral bone is visible on plain radiographs. Synovial fluid examination is indicated to rule out other inflammatory joint conditions. A white cell count below 2,000/mm^2, clear and viscous fluid, and low erythrocyte sedimentation rate (indicating lack of inflammatory process) is consistent with OA diagnosis.

GUIDELINES AND POSITION STATEMENTS

The American evidence-based guidelines for hip and knee OA medical management were last published in 2000.[89] Since then, more research exists on treatment options, including nutraceuticals, and new safety concerns exist for COX-2 inhibitors and NSAIDs. The most current guidance is the 2008 Osteoarthritis Research Society International evidence-based, expert consensus recommendations for hip and knee OA management.[90]

PREVENTION

Obesity is the most modifiable risk factor for knee OA. Weight loss of approximately 5.1 kg over a decade decreased the risk of developing OA by >50% in women of medium height, especially in women with baseline BMI above 25.[91]

Avoiding major joint injuries might also prevent disease. Ending jobs that require bending and carrying is an unrealistic prevention goal, but identifying particular job tasks that lead to later OA and altering the way these tasks are performed could help reduce OA incidence. Training errors are major cause of knee injury during sports participation, along with failure to do stretching and lack of graduated training. Athletes should be educated to use of proper equipment and protective gear, to cross-train, and to vary activities.

GOALS AND TREATMENT

Medications currently do not prevent progression to advanced disease. Thus, goals of OA therapy are to avoid further joint injury, control pain and swelling if present, minimize disability, improve quality of life, and educate the patient about her role in the management team. Overall treatment of OA does not differ between sexes, but some data suggest that older women were more likely to be prescribed NSAIDs and selective COX-2 inhibitors than older men.[92]

Nonpharmacologic Treatment

Nonpharmacologic therapy encompasses patient education, weight loss, exercise, physical and occupational therapy, assistive devices, and thermal modalities. Regularly scheduled rest will prevent pain from overexertion. At least a 5% weight reduction, improved diet and exercise, and quadriceps strengthening have resulted in decreased joint pain and increased function.[89,90,93,94] Although effective, these modalities are underutilized. A referral for physical or occupational therapy improves functional limitation in OA patients. A cane can unload an affected knee or hip and diminish the pain with walking.

Thermal modalities can alleviate pain. Heat applied in a number of ways can increase blood flow and ease pain and stiffness. Cold can reduce inflammation if present, numb the area, decrease muscle spasms, and provide pain relief.

PHARMACOLOGIC TREATMENT

Acetaminophen is the drug of choice for OA pain (Table 40-1). Although comparative trials have demonstrated better pain control with NSAIDs and COX-2 inhibitors compared with acetaminophen, they are reserved as second-line therapy because of gastrointestinal (GI), renal, and cardiovascular (CV) toxicities that limit their long-term use, especially in seniors.[89,90] Acetaminophen also does not affect

Table 40-3. Pharmacotherapy for Osteoporosis Prevention and Treatment

Drug	Dosage	Advantages	Limitations
Calcium (most common salts used are carbonate [40% elemental calcium] and citrate [21% elemental calcium])	300–500 mg elemental calcium 2–3 times/day to achieve adequate intakes	Sometimes easier than ingesting foods, especially for those who are lactose intolerant or have dyslipidemia Chewable or dissolving tablet, liquid	Citrate tablets are more expensive, and more tablets needed to achieve adequate intakes; constipation, gas, bloating, kidney stones (rare); proton pump inhibitors can decrease calcium absorption from carbonate salts; iron, tetracycline, quinolones, bisphosphonates, phenytoin, and fluoride have decreased absorption with concomitant therapy; oxalates, phytates, sulfates, and fiber (variable) can decrease calcium absorption
Vitamin D	400–1,000 units 1–2 times/day to achieve therapeutic 25 (OH) vitamin D concentrations (≥30 ng/mL) 50,000 units 1–2 times weekly until replete for deficiency	More accessible than vitamin D fortified foods	Hypercalcemia (uncommon); inactive compound that must be metabolized in liver to 25(OH) vitamin D and then in kidneys to 1,25(OH) vitamin D, the active moiety; if severe renal or hepatic failure, different vitamin D analogs are required for therapy; phenytoin, barbiturates, carbamazepine, and rifampin increase vitamin D metabolism with some metabolites inactive; cholestyramine, colestipol, orlistat, and mineral oil decrease vitamin D absorption
Bisphosphonates			
Alendronate	5 mg daily, 35 mg weekly (prevention) 10 mg daily; 70-mg tablet, 70-mg tablet with vitamin D 2,800 or 5,600 units, or 70 mg in 75-mL liquid weekly (treatment)	Reasonably safe, some 7- to 10-year safety data for risedronate and alendronate, respectively Much bone mineral density data and hip and spine fracture prevention data Weekly, monthly, quarterly, and yearly administration to improve adherence Ibandronate has a company-sponsored phone, e-mail, and postal service reminder system free to patients	All foods and beverages except water decrease its absorption; therefore, take with a full glass of water, not juice, coffee, tea, on an empty stomach; remain upright for at least 30–60 min; do not take with any other medications; calcium and minerals decrease its absorption; contraindications are renal function <30–35 mL/min (controversial), and esophageal disorders or severe gastrointestinal problems (oral); nausea, heartburn, pain, irritation, ulceration, perforation, and bleeding with oral therapy; muscle aches and pains (uncommon) but discontinue if severe; transient, flulike symptoms with intravenous administration; osteonecrosis of the jaw (rare)
Ibandronate	150 mg monthly, 3-mg intravenous infusion quarterly		
Risedronate	5 mg daily, 35 mg weekly, 75 mg on two consecutive days once monthly, 150 mg monthly		
Zoledronic acid	5-mg 15-min intravenous infusion yearly		
Raloxifene	60 mg daily	Indication for estrogen-positive breast cancer prevention Small lipid-lowering effect	Black box warning for fatal stroke; only vertebral fracture prevention; hot flushes, leg cramps, venous thromboembolism, and peripheral edema; cataracts and gallbladder disease rare
Calcitonin	200 units intranasal daily, alternating nares every other day	Some analgesic effect after a fracture and for metastatic bone pain	Only vertebral fracture prevention; rhinitis, epistaxis; refrigerate until used
Teriparatide	20 mcg subcutaneously daily for up to 2 yr	Only product that builds new bone Pen device for administration	Expensive; limited use for only 24 mo; daily injection; discard pen 28 days after being opened; refrigeration required; pain at injection site, nausea, dizziness, leg cramps, increase in uric acid (rare) and calcium; contraindications are bone cancer, Paget disease, open epiphyses, pregnancy or breast-feeding, hypercalciuria or unexplained increased alkaline phosphatase, and prior skeletal radiation

platelets and has decreased risk of drug interactions (e.g., ACEIs/ARBSs). When this therapy fails, NSAIDs or COX-2 inhibitors can be used.

Two recent guidelines make recommendations on long-term use of NSAIDs in light of GI and CV risk.[95,96] For patients with low GI and CV risk, a traditional NSAID alone may be acceptable. For patients with low GI and high CV risk, full-dose naproxen (500 mg twice daily) may have a lower potential for CV risk than other NSAIDs. In patients with high GI and low CV risk, a COX-2 inhibitor plus PPI may offer the best GI safety profile, although it is more expensive than NSAID-plus-PPI therapy. Finally, when both GI and CV risk are high and NSAID therapy is absolutely necessary, naproxen plus a PPI would be preferred. The American Heart Association recommends a stepped-care approach, with COX-2 inhibitors being the last alternative in patients with known CV disease or risk factors for ischemic heart disease.[97]

Risk factors that increase NSAID-induced GI bleeding include age >65 years, comorbid medical conditions, oral glucocorticoid or anticoagulant therapy, and history of peptic ulcer disease or upper GI bleeding.[89] To reduce NSAID-induced GI toxicity, PPI or misoprostol therapy can be concomitantly used, or the patient can be switched to a selective COX-2 inhibitor.[98-101] In patients at very high risk for adverse events—defined as a previous GI bleed—an NSAID plus a PPI produced similar GI adverse event prevention to a COX-2 inhibitor.[102] A COX-2 inhibitor plus PPI showed greater effectiveness in preventing recurrent ulcer bleeding in very-high-risk patients than celecoxib alone.[103] Of note, use of low-dose aspirin abolishes the GI-sparing benefits of COX-2 inhibitor.[100]

Cardiovascular safety concerns exist with COX-2 inhibitors and some NSAIDs. The COX-2 inhibitors should be used with caution in patients with underlying CV disease.[90,104,105] Naproxen might be safer than diclofenac and ibuprofen for patients with CV disease.[106-109] Patients with underlying CV disease who require NSAID therapy should also be offered low-dose aspirin for CV protection.[110]

The effects of immediate-release and enteric-coated aspirin might be attenuated by NSAIDs, particularly ibuprofen, based on an in vitro study. The proposed mechanism is NSAIDs competing with aspirin for a common binding site on COX-1. Timing of administration might be important. The interaction was not measured if the NSAID is taken

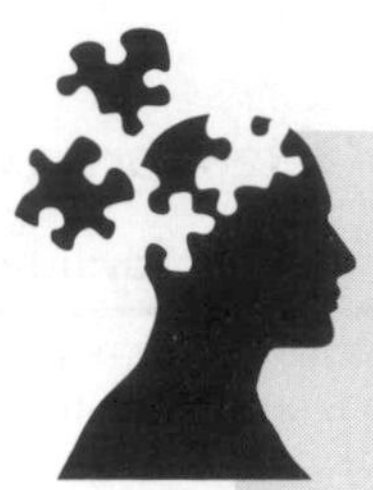

Therapeutic Challenge:

Should patients be put on non-naproxen NSAIDs at the expense of increased CV risk?

8 hours before or at least 30 minutes after the immediate-release aspirin; however, separated dosing by up to 12 hours did not correct the drug-drug interaction with enteric coated aspirin.[97,111,112] Further research is required to know the true clinical concern and options for resolution.

Nonacetylated salicylates inhibit prostaglandin synthesis to a lesser degree than NSAIDs and therefore can be considered for patients with mild renal insufficiency.[89] These agents do not affect platelet aggregation.

Topical capsaicin therapy can be considered for patients with mild to moderate pain who do not respond to acetaminophen and do not want systemic therapy.[89,90] The 0.025% concentration is better tolerated than 0.075% concentration. Because penetration is low in the hip area, this product might not be effective for hip OA.

Osteoarthritis is the leading medical condition for which persons use alternative therapies. Glucosamine and chondroitin sulfate are the most widely used supplements for OA.[113] Systematic reviews have showed both effectiveness and no effect, with large heterogeneity for studies included.[114,115] Glucosamine with or without chondroitin was less effective than celecoxib 200 mg daily. A large meta-analysis concluded chondroitin alone has minimal to no effect.[116] Clinical data suggested no increase in blood glucose in patients with diabetes.[117] If at 6 months no benefit is seen, the product should be discontinued.

Adenosylmethionine (SAMe) has shown effectiveness greater than placebo and comparable to NSAIDs and COX-2 inhibitors for OA.[118-120] This nutraceutical is endogenous to the body but can decrease with aging or as a result of nutritional deficits. Proposed mechanisms for OA are increase cartilage growth and repair, increase proteoglycans, and antagonize tumor necrosis factor. Celecoxib produced better OA knee pain relief in the first month, but similar pain relief with SAMe was documented after 2 months of therapy.[119]

Methylsulfonylmethane (MSM) is a compound found naturally in small amounts in green plants, fruits, and vegetables and is promoted as having anti-inflammatory and analgesic effects.[121] The nutraceutical is usually sold in combination supplements containing glucosamine with or without chondroitin. Some data support modestly reduced pain and swelling but no joint stiffness reduction.[122,123] A recent review concluded MSM trials provided positive but not definitive evidence that MSM is superior to placebo for mild to moderate knee OA.[124]

For patients who have failed therapy or are not candidates for NSAIDs, COX-2, and over-the-counter products, therapy with opioids or tramadol can be considered.[6,90] Opioids have many side effects and addiction concerns. No long-term trials have used opiates for OA pain. These agents are often combined with either acetaminophen or NSAIDs to achieve synergistic analgesic activity. Tramadol is a synthetic opioid agonist that also inhibits reuptake of norepinephrine and serotonin, and despite its opioid pharmacology, surveillance programs have failed to demonstrate significant abuse. Because tramadol is a weak opioid agonist, the degree of opioid-related adverse effects is reported to be lower.

Intra-articular (IA) corticosteroids can be considered for patients who present with acute exacerbations of pain unresponsive to oral agents or with effusions and physical signs of inflammation.[90,125,126] Data support use primarily for knee OA because little data exist for hip OA. The onset of efficacy of IA corticosteroids is rapid (24–48 hours), with maximal efficacy realized in <1 week and lasting up to 4 weeks.[127] Adverse reactions include postinjection flare that can be decreased with ice and analgesics, steroid articular cartilage atrophy, joint sepsis (rare), tendon rupture, and some systemic side effects like hypertension and hyperglycemia. Most experts recommend not using corticosteroid injections more than 4 times annually.

Hyaluronic acid (HA) is a high-molecular-weight glycosaminoglycan, a major component of synovial fluid and cartilage. Viscosupplementation with IA injections of HA can help restore the viscoelasticity of the synovial fluid and promote functional hyaluronan, improving mobility and function, and reducing pain.[127] The data evaluating efficacy of HA are inconsistent.[128-130] These injections are characterized by delayed onset but prolonged duration of symptomatic benefit when compared with IA corticosteroid injections.[90,130] Side effects include mild to moderate pain at the injection site, effusions, and iatrogenic joint infection (rare).

Because postmenopausal women have more OA, HT was considered to be protective, but most evidence questions this hypothesis.[131,132] Based on the Women's Health Initiative trials, the authors concluded that HT might influence joint health, but the effect is limited to unopposed estrogen.[133] The American College of Obstetricians and Gynecologists states that HT does not have a role in OA prevention or treatment.[134]

SURGERY

Surgery is reserved for patients in whom symptoms cannot be managed with nonpharmacologic or pharmacologic therapies. Joint replacement is underused by both sexes, but for women, the degree of underuse is three times greater. Sex differences have been reported in offering and performing hip and knee arthroplasty. Canadian physicians were 2 times more likely to recommend total knee arthroplasty to a male patient than to a female patient.[7] The possible reasons proposed included conscious attitudes or overt discrimination based on sex (taking women's symptoms less seriously), unconscious bias (women don't receive the same benefit as men from total knee arthroplasty), and different presentation style (women tend to speak more openly and personally, and men are more factual and businesslike). Although arthroplasty in the U.S. is greater in women than men, this is partially due to higher incidence of OA in women. However, when accounting for prevalence, more men had arthroplasty than women, even though the women had worse symptoms and greater disability.[135] Possible reasons for this difference is later-stage OA presentation by women, lack of social support, different patient willingness to undergo surgery, and communication differences with physicians and surgeons.[136]

MONITORING AND FOLLOW-UP

Follow-up visits for OA should address response to treatment. Patients should be asked to rate their average pain level over the last month on a scale of 0–10. If little improvement in symptoms or function is reported, a different treatment approach should be considered. Patients on anti-inflammatory therapy should be vigilantly monitored for GI bleeding, CV events, and renal dysfunction.

PATIENT EDUCATION

Patient education is a vital component of OA management. Good websites provide detailed information regarding OA and treatment options. Education pamphlets are widely available from government and health organizations, pharmaceutical companies, and patient advocacy groups (e.g., the Arthritis Foundation). Self-management programs have demonstrated

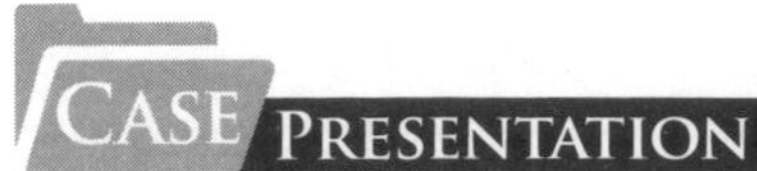

Patient Case: Part 2

Disease assessment:
Osteoarthritis—Knee pain related to activity, as described in this woman, is typical of OA. As a young athlete, she might have had serious knee injuries that were never diagnosed, like an ACL tear, which is a risk factor for OA. Other causes of knee pain should be ruled out by medical exam. A visual analog scale can be used to quantify pain. Assessment of limitations with activities of daily living might be helpful to explore OA-induced physical disabilities. Radiographs are not routinely ordered but might be useful to confirm diagnosis.

Osteoporosis—This patient should have another spine and hip DXA exam to evaluate not only BMD but rate of bone loss.

Drug therapy assessment:
Osteoarthritis—Adherence to acetaminophen should be ascertained as well as use of any over-the-counter and nutraceutical pain products.

Osteoporosis—The amount of calcium and vitamin D in her diet and use of such supplements should also be ascertained. A 25(OH) vitamin D level might be helpful to assess vitamin D status and need for therapy.

Nondrug therapy:
Osteoarthritis—Patient should be encouraged to lose at least 5 kg to have an impact on OA knee pain. Walking about a mile a day should decrease knee pain, improve physical function, minimize further bone mass loss, and potentially decrease falls. The patient can be referred to physical therapy for an evaluation of function and for exercises to strengthen the quadriceps.

Osteoporosis—Weight-bearing, resistance, and balance exercises are also warranted. Because she has dyslipidemia, dairy products would not be a good calcium source unless they were low in fat. She could drink calcium- and vitamin D–fortified juices and eat low-sugar, high-fiber calcium- and vitamin D–fortified cereals.

Drug therapy and rationale:
Osteoarthritis—The patient has failed first-line OA therapy with acetaminophen. Because of her age, CV history, and concomitant aspirin therapy, R.T. can try first glucosamine 750 mg twice a day. After an adequate trial of about 6–8 weeks, therapy should be reevaluated. If no relief is apparent after 6 months, the glucosamine should be stopped. If there is no or partial relief, a low-dose naproxen with a PPI can be tried because she doesn't have renal failure or past GI disorders. Although naproxen is preferred in high-risk CV patients, if ibuprofen is used, it should be taken ½–1 hour after or at least 8–11 hours before the immediate-release aspirin.[138] Because of her CV history, a COX-2 inhibitor would not be a good first choice. The patient could also try topical therapy with capsaicin if she does not wish to undertake risk of NSAID therapy.

Osteoporosis—Using bisphosphonate therapy in senior women with BMD-documented osteoporosis is cost-effective. Seniors need higher intakes of vitamin D to help prevent bone loss, fractures, and falls. Because R.T. has no contraindications for bisphosphonates, she can use a weekly or monthly product, with final choice dependent on prescription medication coverage. Her combined diet and supplement use should result in 1,200–1,500 mg of calcium and minimally 800–1,000 units of vitamin D daily.

Monitoring:
Osteoarthritis—Monitoring parameters for knee OA include pain and physical activity. NSAID monitoring also includes renal function, liver function tests, CV events, and GI ulcer bleeding.

Osteoporosis—If a 25(OH) vitamin D level was ordered, this test can be repeated after 3–4 months of vitamin D supplementation. If still low, more aggressive high-dose vitamin D replacement might be warranted. Height loss and fracture occurrence can be evaluated at each clinic visit. Assessment of bisphosphonate administration and adverse effects such as muscle pains and GI problems should be assessed with each medication refill. A repeat DXA in 2 years can be performed to assess for efficacy and need for teriparatide therapy.

a 20% to 30% benefit, which is as great as NSAID therapy.[137] (See Web Resources for Good Bone and Joint Disorders Websites.)

Additional content available at
www.ashp.org/womenshealth

Summary

Girls and women are at significant risk for bone and joint disorders. Girls and athletes should be queried for eating disorders, amenorrhea, and appropriate stretching and equipment use to identify and or prevent ACL injuries, female athlete triad, and stress fractures. Learning correct ways to stretch, strengthen, and exercise can decrease sports injury risks and future OA. Throughout life, a bone-healthy lifestyle can decrease the risk of osteoporosis. Prevention and treatment medications do exist for bone and joint diseases, some of which need to be individualized for the patient based on age, comorbidities, and polypharmacy. Healthcare providers can play an important role in preventing bone and joint disorders, identifying and resolving medication-related problems when they develop, and providing patients with disease and medication information.

References

Additional content available at
www.ashp.org/womenshealth

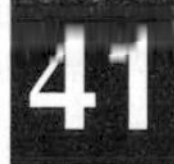

41 Neurological Disorders

Sarah L. Johnson, Pharm.D.; Jacquelyn L. Bainbridge, B.S.Pharm., Pharm.D.; Melody Ryan, Pharm.D., MPH; Edna Elise Moore, MSN, ARNP, WHNP-C; Dennis Parker Jr., Pharm.D.; Baochau Nguyen, Pharm.D.; Debbie Rodriquez, RN, Pharm.D.

Learning Objectives

1. Compare and contrast the disease-modifying therapies in regard to multiple sclerosis and pregnancy.
2. Describe which antiepileptic drug therapies can be used concurrently in women on oral contraceptives.
3. List the common differential diagnoses for chronic fatigue syndrome.
4. Define the types of headaches discussed, and recommend a pharmacologic treatment for each.
5. Explain common strategies used to prevent ischemic stroke in women.
6. Discuss the role of pharmacologic therapy in the treatment of fibromyalgia.

Common neurologic conditions such as multiple sclerosis, epilepsy, stroke, fibromyalgia, chronic fatigue syndrome, and headache disorders appear in this chapter. These conditions often have unique characteristics seen in the female population that distinguish them from other neurologic conditions. These differences affect treatment, the condition itself, or both.

Multiple Sclerosis

Multiple sclerosis (MS) is a chronic, progressive, unpredictable, neurologic disease that affects the **central nervous system (CNS).** There are four clinical subtypes of MS: **relapsing-remitting multiple sclerosis (RRMS), secondary progressive multiple sclerosis (SPMS), primary progressive multiple sclerosis (PPMS),** and **progressive relapsing multiple sclerosis (PRMS).** RRMS accounts for 85% of MS cases and is characterized by clearly defined acute attacks (also called exacerbations, relapses, or flares) with full or partial recovery. Periods between disease relapses are characterized by clinically silent disease progression. A relapsing-remitting course that later becomes steadily progressive is called SPMS; attacks and partial recoveries may continue to occur. SPMS is characterized by less recovery following attacks, persistently worsening functioning during and between attacks, and a decrease in the number of attacks (or none at all) accompanied by progressive disability. Approximately 50% of patients with RRMS will develop SPMS within 10 years, and 90% will develop SPMS within 25 years.[1] PPMS is characterized by progression of disability from onset, without plateaus or remissions or with occasional plateaus and temporary minor improvements. Patients with PPMS usually have onset of disease starting in their late 30s or early 40s and a less favorable prognosis. There does not appear to be a sex preference for this type of MS. PRMS occurs in <5% of MS patients and shows progression of disability from onset but with clear acute relapses, with or without full recovery. The discussion in this chapter will primarily focus on the most prevalent type of MS, which is RRMS.

EPIDEMIOLOGY

There are approximately 400,000 people living with MS in the U.S., 2.5 million worldwide; 70% to 75% of the MS population is female.[1,2] The majority of patients with MS will be diagnosed between the ages of 20 and 50 years.[1,2] Patients diagnosed younger than the age of 16 years account for approximately 5% of all cases, and diagnosis older than the age of 50 years accounts for approximately 9.4% of all cases.[1,2] The risk of developing RRMS begins at puberty and decreases with perimenopause. Whites have a higher rate of MS than other ethnic groups.[1] MS occurs more frequently in higher latitudes (above 40°F) compared

Case Presentation

Patient Case: Part 1

M.J. is a 32-year-old white woman who presents with a chief symptom of right-sided weakness and numbness; she has urinary urgency and occasional incontinence.

HPI: For the last few years, M.J. has noticed significant changes in her neurologic function, particularly heat intolerance precipitating a stumbling gait and a tendency to fall. She reports visual changes that occur periodically and sometimes are associated with pain. Two months ago, while under a lot of stress, she became sick with the flu, and her symptoms worsened. At that time, she could not hold objects in her hands and had significant tremors and severe exhaustion. She developed a right hemisensory deficit after several days of work. She now wears incontinence protection during the day. She also has persistent balance problems with dizziness and is extremely fatigued.

PMH: Noncontributory.

Family history: Mother has MS.

Social history: Single, no children, drinks one glass of wine 2–3× per week, denies tobacco or illicit substance use.

Medications: Multivitamin daily, intrauterine contraceptive device.

Allergies: No known drug allergies.

Vitals: Height: 68″; weight: 135 lb; BP: 120/74; HR: 68; Temp: 98.2° F;RR: 16.

Physical exam: Moderately distressed woman, moderately anxious.

Review of systems

Genitourinary: Urinary urgency with occasional incontinence × 2 weeks.

Neuro exam: Patient is alert, cooperative and oriented. Cranial nerves II-XII: intact PERRLAs; visual acuity 20/20 both eyes, fundoscopic examination normal, optic disc normal, EOMs: mild nystagmus on horizontal gaze.

Motor tone and strength: 5/5 left upper and lower extremities. 3/5 upper and lower extremities. deep tendon reflex (DTR): brisk 3+.

Sensory examination: Mild decrease in pinprick sensation on right upper and lower extremity. Positive Babinski bilaterally.

Coordination: Severe unsteadiness on tandem gait, moderate unsteadiness on casual gait, Romberg maneuver positive.

Laboratory values: Oligoclonal bands present in CSF; negative urinalysis; basic metabolic panel/hematology within normal limits.

Imaging results: Multifocal white matter disease.

with lower latitudes.[1] Men typically present with MS later in life and have a less favorable prognosis. MS is 2–4 times more common in women than men.[1,3] This strong sex preference is likely multifactorial and involves immune, hormonal, and genetic factors.

Sex issues in MS encompass basic pathogenesis and clinical, therapeutic, and psychosocial aspects of the disease. The prototypical patient with RRMS is a young, white woman of childbearing age. This makes pregnancy, breast-feeding, contraception, and menstrual-associated disease features important issues that should be taken into consideration.

CLINICAL PRESENTATION

MS is often characterized by episodes of neurologic dysfunction followed by periods of stabilization or partial to complete remission of clinical symptoms. These symptoms (relapses or exacerbations) can appear over a few hours or days, can be gradually worsening over a period of a few weeks, or can present acutely. Symptoms will persist, slowly resolve over weeks to months, or may resolve completely.

Common clinical features of MS are double or blurred vision, ocular pain, numbness, weakness in one or two extremities, instability in walking, tremors, bladder dysfunction, and heat intolerance (Table 41-1). Sensory alterations, such as numbness in the feet, hands, or affecting one side of the body, and generalized heat intolerance are suspicious of MS. Clinical features can vary greatly between patients and can change in severity and frequency throughout the course of the disease.

PATHOPHYSIOLOGY

MS is an autoimmune disease that attacks the myelin sheath in the CNS, which consists of the brain and spinal cord. Over time, the attacks damage the myelin sheath and lead to the formation of scar tissue (lesions). These lesions can slow down nerve impulses, block them all together or destroy the nerve. It is unknown what triggers the immune system reaction, but some experts believe it is the result of an abnormal immunologic response to an infectious agent or unknown environmental factors in people who have a genetic predisposition to MS. The differences in

Table 41-1 Clinical Features Associated with Multiple Sclerosis

Type of Dysfunction	Examples
Motor	Weakness
	Spasticity
Cerebellar	Incoordination
	Ataxic gait
	Scanning speech
	Loss of balance
Sensory	Dysesthetic pain
	Paresthesia (typically in the hands and feet)
	Numbness
	Trigeminal neuralgia
Urinary	Urgency/incontinence
	Incomplete emptying
	Increased frequency of urination
	Frequent urinary tract infections
Ophthalmic	Optic disc pallor
	Atrophy
	Blurred vision
	Diplopia
	Nystagmus
	Other visual field defects
Cognitive emotional	Emotional lability
	Depression
	Anxiety
Fatigue	Heat intolerance
Sexual	Erectile dysfunction
	Ejaculatory dysfunction
	Vaginal dryness
	Changes in sensations
	Inability to achieve orgasm

MS between sexes may be at least partly explained by the biological differences between men and women. There are intrinsic differences in density of neurons; size of regional brain areas and cell clusters; cell receptor expression; neurotransmitter systems; cerebral blood flow patterns; response to stress, hunger, and satiety; and cortical activation patterns between men and women.[2,4] Women have higher global brain white matter content, larger gray matter volumes, and smaller white matter volume than men.[3,4] As men age, they develop greater increases in white matter content and losses of gray matter volume than women. According to a recent study, men have larger upper cervical cord volumes than women.[5]

Women show stronger immune responses and have higher baseline immunoglobulin levels, higher CD4+ T-cell numbers, greater production of Th1 cytokines, and more sustained responses to antigenic challenge.[6,7] This heightened immune response cannot be explained completely by sex hormones. Females of all species, vertebrates and invertebrates, show this effect despite the fact that invertebrates lack sex hormones. Women have higher serum levels of prolactin and growth hormone, which stimulates autoimmunity.[8-12] Liver-derived insulin growth factor 1 is also higher in women, although this growth factor promotes recovery and repair of injured neural tissue.[8-12] Sex hormones have a direct function on lymphocytes and macrophages, which may influence immune response.[13,14] Estrogen enhances B cell function, whereas testosterone is inhibitory. Plasma immunoglobulin M levels are significantly greater in women than men.[13,14]

There are three major classes of sex hormones, and they all share the same precursor: cholesterol. All three classes are present in both sexes and play important roles in the development and functioning of the nervous and immune systems through complex processes. For example, sex hormones affect axon growth and myelination, neurotransmission, neural remodeling, motor coordination, and regulation of brain apoptosis.[2] Sex hormones modulate immune responses and the hypothalamic–pituitary–adrenal gland axis. Estrogen receptors are distributed widely in the CNS compared with progestin and androgen receptors. At low concentrations, estrogen facilitates immune responses, but at high concentrations, it suppresses immune responses.

Several genes have been linked to MS that are influenced by sex. For example, the major histocompatibility class II human leukocyte antigen DR2 haplotype, which is a susceptibility gene, is more common in female patients with MS.[11,12] There may be a relationship between MS and polymorphisms in the estrogen receptors.[8,9,14] There may be genes that are protective against MS as well.[15]

DIAGNOSIS

There is no single test that can be used to identify and diagnose MS. There are two features that are necessary for a diagnosis of MS: signs of disease in different parts of the nervous system and signs of at least two separate disease relapses. This is accomplished through a complete review of the patient's medical history, clinical examination of the nervous system, and diagnostic tests. Diagnostic tests that are useful in the diagnosis of MS include **magnetic resonance imaging (MRI),** evoked potentials (EPs), and evaluation of the **cerebrospinal fluid (CSF).** MRI is useful for identifying lesions in the CNS, EPs can identify problems with nerve conduction, and evaluation of the CSF can detect oligoclonal bands and elevated levels of immunoglobulin G (IgG).[16-19]

Table 41-2. FDA Approved Drug Therapies Used in the Treatment of Multiple Sclerosis

Drug Class	Drug	Dosage	FDA Pregnancy Category	Comments
Disease-modifying therapies	Interferon-beta-1a Avonex Rebif	 30 mcg intramuscular (IM) injection once weekly 44 mcg subcutaneous (SC) injection 3 times/wk	C Abortifacient in some animal models; no negative fetal effects have been documented; unknown if excreted in breast milk	Common side effects: Flulike reactions (> in young women with small body mass); injection site reactions (redness, induration, fibrosis, and lipoatrophy)
	Interferon-beta-1b Betaseron Extavia	250 mcg SC injection every other day		
	Glatiramer acetate	20 mg SC injection daily	B Based on database of 245 pregnancies[252]; no negative fetal effects have been documented, but risk cannot be ruled out	Injection site reactions (redness, induration, fibrosis, and lipoatrophy)
	Mitoxantrone	IV infusion	D Known to cause birth defects if either parent is receiving treatment at time of conception; excreted in breast milk	Changes in menstrual pattern Amenorrhea: maximum lifetime dose is 140 mg/m^2 Contraception should be used during and for 6 mo after treatment by men and women
	Natalizumab	300 mg IV infusion every 4 wk	C	Only available through the TOUCH™ prescribing program Risk of progressive multifocal leukoencephalopathy
Glucocorticoids (for the treatment of acute relapses)	Methylprednisolone		C	Implications of use in pregnancy and breast-feeding Side effects: striae, acne, fat redistribution, bone disturbances, and cataracts
Symptomatic therapies	See Table 41-3	Beyond the scope of this text		Implications of use in pregnancy and breast-feeding Drug interaction side effects: cosmetic, sexual

FDA = U.S. Food and Drug Administration; TOUCH = Tysabri outreach (unified commitment to health and is a restricted distribution program focused on safety).

PHARMACOLOGIC TREATMENT

The treatment of MS is complex, and numerous factors must be considered before initiation. This decision is best analyzed by the individual patient's neurologist. There are no established guidelines for the treatment and management of MS available. The **American Academy of Neurology (AAN)** and **National Multiple Sclerosis Society (NMSS)** have issued consensus statements and expert opinion papers to guide healthcare providers in the treatment decision process. Disease management consists of **disease-modifying therapies (DMTs)** and symptomatic treatments. For a review of these treatments, refer to *Pharmacotherapy: A Pathophysiologic Approach*, 7th edition.[20] For the purposes of this discussion, we will focus on the sex-based treatment issues (Table 41-2 and Table 41-3).

For women who wish to become pregnant and are currently using DMT, there is no clearly defined policy for how long they should be off DMT before trying to conceive. The general recommendation has been 1 month. It is unknown when DMT therapy should be restarted after giving birth. If a woman is not breast-feeding, then therapy can be started immediately. There is no documented differential response to DMT based on sex; however, several studies suggest that more research is needed in this area.[21,22] A study of interferon (IFN)-β1a in SPMS showed that women responded better than men.[21] In the post hoc analysis of primary progressive MS PROMISE trial, men showed significantly less progression on glatiramer acetate therapy, but this effect was not seen in women.[22]

Glucocorticoids are typically used for the treatment of acute relapses. Methylprednisolone is the agent most commonly used. Glucocorticoids should not be used during the first trimester of pregnancy because of a negative effect on organogenesis. They may be used during the second and third trimester of pregnancy, but they should be reserved for the treatment of serious exacerbations. Glucocorticoids cross the placenta and may cause transient neonatal leukocytosis or immunosuppression. Excessive use may slow postnatal growth and has been shown to cause birth defects in some animal models. Glucocorticoids are contraindicated in breast-feeding as they are excreted in breast milk. Common adverse effects of glucocorticoids, especially when used long term at high dosages, include hypertension, atrophic condition of the skin, impaired wound healing, fluid retention, muscle weakness, cataracts, and depression. Serious consequences include hyperglycemia, osteoporosis, seizures, and glaucoma. These effects only add to the physical and psychological burden of living with MS. Supplementation of calcium and vitamin D, regular physical activity, bone density monitoring, and treatment for osteoporosis when appropriate are recommended.

Symptoms of MS vary greatly between patients, depending on the pathology. Symptoms—such as

Table 41-3. Treatment Options for Specific Multiple Sclerosis Symptoms

Spasticity	Bladder Symptoms	Sensory Symptoms	Fatigue	Tremor
Baclofen	Oxybutynin	Carbamazepine	Amantadine	Propranolol
Dantrolene	Dicyclomine	Phenytoin	Modafinil	Primidone
Diazepam	Desmopressin acetate	Amitriptyline	Armodafinil	Isoniazid
Tizanidine	Self-catheterization	Gabapentin	Antidepressants	
Gabapentin	Imipramine	Lamotrigine	Methylphenidate	
Pregabalin	Amitriptyline	Pregabalin	Dextroamphetamine	
Botulinum toxin type A	Prazosin		4-Aminopyridine	
	Botulinum toxin type A			
	Solifenacin			
	Darifenacin			
	Trospium			
	Hycoscyamine			
	Tolterodine			

spasticity, bladder dysfunction, fatigue, and sexual dysfunction—also vary in the frequency and severity in which they occur. These symptoms may be a result of drug therapy or a symptom of the disease. Drug therapy is commonly prescribed for MS symptom management. Women who are pregnant, trying to become pregnant, or breast-feeding may not be the best candidates for drug therapy. A well-accepted rule is that drug therapy be avoided or minimized during pregnancy and breast-feeding.

The two most common symptoms that benefit from sex-based treatment are bladder dysfunction and sexual dysfunction. Up to 90% of men and 72% of women experience sexual problems, and up to 75% of both experience bladder dysfunction.[2] These symptoms can be treated with pharmacologic and nonpharmacologic treatment. If left untreated, these symptoms may result in a significant decrease in quality of life for the patient and her partner. Bladder dysfunction that leads to a high postvoid residual may cause urinary tract infections (UTIs). If left untreated, UTIs can lead to urosepsis and death.

MS is a chronic, progressive disease that can result in significant disability to the patient. Quality of life is an important factor in the management of MS. In addition to the physiological problems, there are a multitude of issues related to health maintenance and preventative healthcare, as well as psychosocial issues that vary between sexes and may be overlooked. MS has an impact on the families and caregivers of these patients, similar to other chronic diseases. Patients with MS have a suicide rate 7.5 times that of the general population. Patients with MS may have difficulty performing regular tasks that are important for health maintenance. For example, female patients with MS may have difficulty performing self breast examinations because of sensory deficits in their fingers. Patients may have difficulty losing or maintaining their weight because of mobility limitations. Daily activities can be difficult and frustrating, leading to depression, social isolation, and dependency on others. Employment may be difficult to find and maintain. The healthcare provider can help in the prevention, identification, and management of these issues.

SEX DIFFERENCES

Up to 80% of patients who have MS report disease fluctuations during their menstrual cycle.[23,24] The most common report is an increase in symptoms the week before or during the week of menstruation. There have been rare reports of relapses associated with specific phases of the menstrual cycle.[25]

There are limited data available on contraceptive use in MS. Oral contraceptive use is associated with fewer symptoms, less disability, and lower risk for developing MS. There is a concern that patients with limited mobility may be at higher risk for a deep vein thrombosis, especially if they are older than 35 years of age and smoke. Barrier methods such as diaphragms or sponges may be difficult for patients with paresthesias and spasticity. Intrauterine devices (IUDs) are not recommended because sensory changes may make it difficult to determine if the IUD has migrated. Condoms appear to be safe and effective for female patients. Male patients may have difficulty with the usage of condoms because of decreased manual dexterity or decreased sensation.[26]

Pregnancy is one of the most important sex issues in MS and is the focus of many studies and reports. Until the 1950s, women were advised against pregnancy because of presumed negative effects on the disease. MS has no effect on pregnancy (i.e., no risk to the fetus). However, pregnancy does have an effect on MS. The major effect of pregnancy on MS is a decrease in disease activity. The Pregnancy in MS (PRIMS) trial was the first prospective study of 254 women (269 pregnancies) who were followed for up to 2 years after delivery.[27] The study looked at the relapse rate during pregnancy and for the first 2 years postpartum.[28] The annual relapse rate prepregnancy was 0.7 and decreased to 0.2 during the third trimester. During the first 3 months postpartum, the relapse rate increased to 1.2. Despite the increase in risk, 72% of women did not experience a relapse during that period. The annualized relapse rate did not differ significantly from the prepregnancy rate for the other 21 months.[27-29] Three clinical predictors have been identified that correlate with occurrence of a postpartum relapse: increased relapse rate in the year before pregnancy, increased relapse rate during pregnancy, and a higher Expanded Disability Status Scale score at the onset of pregnancy.[30] Other studies have confirmed these findings.[31] The postpartum period is recognized as carrying a high risk for relapse. Prophylactic treatment may be beneficial in preventing a postpartum relapse. Several studies suggest that treatment with **intravenous (IV)** immunoglobulin or IV methylprednisolone may decrease the risk of postpartum relapse.[32-34] Initiating interferon therapy is expected

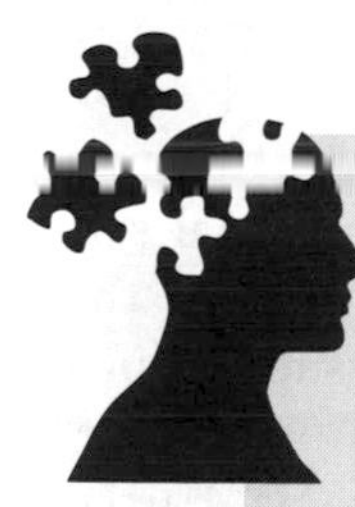

Therapeutic Challenge:

Your patient, who has MS and is currently on Avonex®, informs you that she would like to become pregnant and is planning to breast-feed. How would you manage the patient's drug regimen with regard to her pregnancy status?

to have the same effect; however, if the woman is breast-feeding, then interferon therapy is contraindicated, although this has not been formally studied.

There is no recommendation on breast-feeding because of limited data regarding the effect of breast-feeding on MS. The data that exist for breast-feeding are conflicting and have found no effect or a decrease in relapses.[35,36]

There are very little data regarding menopause and MS. Perimenopause is generally the time when patients will transition from relapsing to progressive MS; it can also increase the risk of osteoporosis because of increased bone loss. This is especially important for patients who have limited mobility. Hormone therapy is an option for patients; however, there is limited evidence to support their use as a treatment for MS.

SUMMARY

MS is a complex, chronic, and progressive disease. The typical patient with MS is a young woman of reproductive age. Issues regarding contraception, pregnancy, and breast-feeding are very important and will have a significant impact on the disease state itself and options for treatment. The subtype and disease progression may be affected by sex. Although the reasons for the sex differences remain unknown, it is clear that more research is needed to improve treatment and solve the enigma surrounding this disease.

CASE PRESENTATION

Patient Case: Part 2

M.J. is exhibiting signs consistent with RRMS. It is important to note that the diagnosis of MS is often a diagnosis of exclusion. Diagnosis can be a long complex process, depending on the how the patient initially presents. Decisions regarding treatment can be complex and should be thoroughly discussed with the patient as there are multiple factors that can affect treatment options. In general, patients should be referred to a neurologist with specialized training in the management of MS whenever possible. A complete discussion of the treatment options is beyond the scope of this text. Therefore, a simplified version of treatment recommendations is provided with a focus on the sex-related issues.

Recommendations:

1. Educate the patient on disease pathophysiology, prognosis, and management.
2. Treat patient with IV corticosteroids for the acute relapse (exacerbation).
3. Recommend starting a DMT (interferon beta or glatiramer acetate) for long-term management, provided that she is not currently pregnant.
4. Counsel patient regarding pregnancy while using a DMT. Evaluate current contraceptive method, and consider switching to another method.
5. Discuss treatment options for urinary dysfunction.
6. Evaluate and monitor patient for depression, and treat as necessary.
7. A social worker can assist the patient with family, psychosocial, and financial issues.
8. The patient may benefit from physical therapy.
9. Educate the patient on other resources, such as websites, local support groups, and local and national organizations.
10. Encourage patient to take control of her disease and promote self-care.

Epilepsy

(See Web Resources for Patient Case: Epilepsy.)

Additional content available at
www.ashp.org/womenshealth

Epilepsy is a common neurologic disorder that affects approximately 1% to 3% of the population during the lifespan. The risk of epilepsy from birth to age 20 is 1% and afflicts 3% of the population by age 75.[37] Patients with epilepsy may live in constant fear of the unexpected nature and unpredictability of when their next seizure may occur, as well as of numerous side effects that are associated with current **antiepileptic drugs (AEDs).** Epilepsy is a highly stigmatized disorder and often is accompanied by financial and social hardships. Women with epilepsy carry an even larger burden because neuroactive ovarian steroid hormones may alter the patient's epilepsy. Epilepsy affects sexual development, menstrual cycle, contraception, fertility, and reproduction. Bone loss related to AEDs may also lead to osteoporosis.

EPIDEMIOLOGY

The incidence and prevalence of epilepsy is similar in men and women. Men may appear to have a significantly higher incidence (by about 15%) than women.[38] The higher prevalence of epilepsy in men may be due to a higher rate of neurologic disorders, such as head trauma, cerebrovascular disease, traumatic brain injury, and alcohol-related epilepsy.[39]

CLINICAL PRESENTATION

In most cases, a healthcare provider will not be able to witness the actual seizure. In this situation, a family member, significant other, or friend is the best resource for information and is essential for a thorough history of the seizures. Often the patient is amnesiac to the actual seizure because awareness is impaired more than 50% of the time.[40] For this reason, a thorough history of the seizure and the events before (preictal) and after (postictal) the seizure should be ascertained.

There are several types of seizures. Most seizure types can be classified as generalized or partial seizures. Generalized seizures affect both sides of the brain and produce a loss of consciousness. Subtypes of generalized seizures include tonic, clonic, tonic-clonic, myoclonic, absence, and atonic. Partial seizures affect a focal area of the brain. They are the most common type of seizure and can include movement, sensory, or emotional symptoms. Visual and auditory hallucinations can be a part of the seizure. Partial seizures can be divided into simple partial and complex partial subtypes. Patients with simple partial seizures retain awareness, whereas patients with complex partial seizures experience impaired or loss of consciousness. Partial seizures can spread and cause a generalized seizure, and are classified as partial seizures that secondarily generalize. Table 41-4 lists the seizure types and associated symptoms.

Table 41-4. Types of Seizures and Associated Symptoms

Generalized Seizures	Symptoms
Generalized tonic-clonic	Unconsciousness, convulsions, muscle rigidity
Absence	Brief loss of consciousness (a few seconds), blank stare, rapid blinking, repetitive eye and extremity movements
Myoclonic	Sporadic (isolated) jerking movements, usually on both sides of the body
Clonic	Repetitive, rhythmic jerking movements on both sides of the body
Tonic	Muscle stiffness, rigidity
Atonic	Sudden and general loss of muscle tone, particularly of the arms and legs Brief loss of consciousness
Partial Seizures	
Simple	Awareness is retained
a. Simple motor b. Simple sensory c. Simple psychological	a. Jerking, muscle rigidity, spasms, head-turning b. Unusual sensations affecting the vision, hearing, smell, taste, or touch c. Memory or emotional disturbances
Complex	Awareness is impaired; automatisms such as lip smacking, chewing, fidgeting, walking, and other repetitive, involuntary but coordinated movements
Partial seizure with secondary generalization	Symptoms that are initially associated with a preservation of consciousness that then evolves into a loss of consciousness and convulsions

Several epilepsy syndromes are more common in women, including childhood absence epilepsy, photosensitive epilepsy, and juvenile myoclonic epilepsy.[39] Seizures may be precipitated by the menstrual cycle (catamenial pattern) and hormonal fluctuations from puberty through menopause.

PATHOPHYSIOLOGY

The pathophysiology of epilepsy in men and women is the same; however, hormonal differences can exacerbate the frequency of seizures. Estrogen increases neuronal excitation and decreases inhibition in the short term through its membrane effects and in the long term at a genomic level.[41] Estrogen binds to the A receptor for gamma aminobutyric acid (GABA-A), causing an alteration in chloride conductance so that the GABA-mediated neuronal inhibition is less effective. Estrogen also alters messenger RNA for GABA amino decarboxylase, which is an enzyme that is responsible for controlling the rate of GABA synthesis and decreasing the number of GABA-A receptor units. In addition to affecting GABA, estrogen also binds to the N-methyl-D-aspartate receptor to increase excitation in the medial temporal lobe.

When progesterone binds to the GABA-A receptor, unlike estrogen, it results in an increased inhibitory effect and a decreased excitatory effect in the temporal lobe. At the genomic level, progesterone increases GABA production and the number of GABA subunits to cause an overall increase in neuronal inhibition.

There are often abnormalities in the basal concentrations of pituitary gonadotropins and ovarian steroids found in epileptic women compared with nonepileptic women. Hypothalamic dysfunction and pituitary release of luteinizing hormone is altered in response to gonadotropin-releasing hormone. These alterations are seen in epileptic women without regard to drug therapy.

DIAGNOSIS

The diagnosis of epilepsy is not different for women than for men. Diagnosis is made by a detailed clinical neurologic examination, electroencephalogram (EEG), and, in some cases, an MRI or 24-hour video EEG. There are currently no laboratory tests that are utilized in the diagnosis although they have utility in ruling out other conditions that are treatable causes of seizures. For example, infections, hypoglycemia, and altered electrolytes may cause seizures.

GUIDELINES

Guidelines from the AAN for the recommendation of treatment for women of childbearing age and those who are pregnant or attempting to conceive have been developed because of the potential teratogenic effects of AEDs.[42-45] They are as follows:

- Women should supplement with folic acid 0.4 mg or greater per day before conception and during pregnancy.[44]
- Women should be educated on reliable methods of contraception, including a discussion regarding drug interactions between AEDs and oral contraceptives.
- Current drug therapy should be evaluated if a woman is planning to become pregnant.
- During pregnancy, monotherapy at the lowest effective dosage should be used to reduce the risk of major congenital malformations and poor cognitive outcomes in the child.
- Changing drug therapy during pregnancy increases the risk of allergic reactions and other serious adverse events and increases the risk of a polytherapy exposure.
- Obtaining serum levels of lamotrigine, carbamazepine, and phenytoin should be considered, and obtaining serum levels of levetiracetam and oxcarbazepine (as the monohydroxy derivative) may be considered, using the level of the AED as a guideline in addition to the clinical presentation of the patient.[44] This is due to changes in volume of distribution, alterations in protein binding, and clearance of the AED that occur during pregnancy.
- With any AED, monitoring serum levels during pregnancy should not be discouraged and can be done on a monthly basis.
- In clinical practice, supplemental vitamin K_1 at 10 mg/day during the last month of pregnancy is given to women on enzyme-inducing AEDs, or the neonate can be given 1 mg of vitamin K_1 intramuscularly at birth. There is limited evidence to support or disprove this practice.[44]
- Valproic acid and its derivatives (valproate, divalproex) should be avoided because of the increased risk of birth defects and poor cognitive outcomes in the child.[43]
- Breast-feeding is recommended, as the benefit outweighs the risk associated with complications of AED exposure in the infant. The exception would be if the infant is lethargic, has failure to thrive, or if changes in weight are noted.

PHARMACOLOGIC TREATMENT

When selecting pharmacologic therapy, there are many factors that need to be taken into consideration, such as seizure type, epilepsy syndrome, concomitant medications, comorbid diseases, lifestyle, and individual preferences. Goals of therapy include eliminating or decreasing the frequency of seizures, minimizing side effects, making rationale cost-effective decisions, optimizing a patient's quality of life, matching seizure disorder with appropriate AED, and using monotherapy when possible. Table 41-5 lists AEDs commonly used in clinical practice and the corresponding seizures they treat.[46,47] Tables 41-6 and 41-7 list the evidence-based recommendations for the treatment of epilepsy and refractory epilepsy using the newer AEDs.[48,49] At the time the articles for Tables 41-6 and 41-7 were written, lacosamide, rufinamide, and vigabatrin had not been approved by the U.S. Food and Drug Administration (FDA). Side effects of the medications may include cognitive impairment, alterations in weight, nystagmus, sedation, osteopenia, blood dyscrasias, tremor, and rash. Many of the newer AEDs have fewer adverse effects and drug interactions than the older AEDs. For complete treatment recommendations, see evidence-based guidelines from the AAN 2004 for the treatment of new-onset epilepsy and refractory epilepsy.[48,49]

In addition to drug therapy, there are some alternative treatments available. The vagal nerve stimulator has been offered as nonpharmacologic therapy to

Table 41-5. Commonly Used Antiepileptic Drugs by Seizure Type[46,47]

Antiepileptic Drug	GTC	Partial: Simple	Partial: Complex	Absence	FDA Pregnancy Risk Category
Phenytoin (Dilantin®)	X	X	X		D
Carbamazepine (Tegretol®, Carbatrol®)	X	X	X		D
Phenobarbital	X	X	X		D
Ethosuximide (Zarontin®)				X	Not categorized
Gabapentin (Neurontin®)	X	X	X		C
Pregabalin (Lyrica®)	X	X	X		C
Felbamate (Felbatol®)	X	X	X	X	C
Oxcarbazepine (Trileptal®)	X	X	X		C
Valproic acid, divalproex (Depacon®, Depakote®, Depakene®)	X	X	X	X	D
Lamotrigine (Lamictal®)	X	X	X	X	C
Topiramate (Topamax®)	X	X	X	X	C
Tiagabine (Gabitril®)		X	X		C
Levetiracetam (Keppra®, Keppra XR®)	X	X	X	X	C
Zonisamide (Zonegran®)	X	X	X	X	C
Primidone	X	X	X		D
Lacosamide (Vimpat®)		X	X		C
Rufinamide (Banzel®)[a]					C
Vigabatrin (Sabril®)[b]			X		C

GTC = generalized tonic-clonic; FDA = U.S. Food and Drug Administration; XR = extended release.

[a]FDA approved for the treatment of Lennox-Gastaut syndrome.
[b]FDA approved for the treatment of infantile spasms.

Table 41-6. Evidence-Based Recommendations for the Treatment of New Onset Epilepsy Using Newer Antiepileptic Drugs[48]

Antiepileptic Drug	Partial		Absence
	Simple	Complex	
Gabapentin (Neurontin®)	X	X	
Lamotrigine (Lamictal®)	X	X	X
Levetiracetam (Keppra®)			
Oxcarbazepine (Trileptal®)	X	X	
Tiagabine (Gabitril®)			
Topiramate (Topamax®)	X	X	
Zonisamide (Zonegran®)			

patients with pharmacoresistant epilepsy, with goals of decreasing seizure frequency, seizure duration, and drug-drug interactions and eliminating adverse effects. In the U.S., it is indicated as adjunctive therapy in patients at least 12 years of age with refractory partial onset seizures. This treatment option should only be considered if the patient has persistent seizures despite treatment with several AEDs. The best surgical outcome is in patients with mesial temporal lobe epilepsy. The ketogenic diet or a modified version has been studied primarily in children with intractable epilepsy and is a valid treatment; however, adherence to this diet is difficult. It consists of a diet high in fat, low in carbohydrate and low or normal in protein. The ketogenic diet is not commonly used among adult patients, and its efficacy is unknown.[50]

MONITORING AND FOLLOW-UP

Patients on any treatment for epilepsy need to be monitored carefully. Baseline measurements should be taken before initiation of drug therapy and should include liver function tests and complete blood count (CBC) with differential and platelet count. Monitoring requirements will differ depending on which AEDs are prescribed; therefore, a credible drug reference should be consulted to determine appropriate monitoring schedules. Once drug therapy is initiated, some AEDs will require monitoring of the serum level. AED serum levels should be monitored if the patient is not responding to drug therapy, if the patient reports signs or symptoms associated with toxicity, if there is a suspected drug interaction or when switching from brand to generic or between generic manufacturers. A serum level should also be drawn when the patient is on stable dosage and is having good seizure control (relevant to the patient) to be used as a reference point related to dosage and specific medications. A neurologic exam to assess toxicity should be performed at each follow-up visit.

Table 41-7. Evidence-based Recommendations for the Treatment of Newly Diagnosed and Refractory Epilepsy Using Newer Antiepileptic Drugs[48,49]

Antiepileptic Drug	Partial		Primary Generalized
	Adjunctive	Monotherapy	
Gabapentin (Neurontin®)	X		
Lamotrigine (Lamictal®)	X	X[a]	
Levetiracetam (Keppra®)	X		
Oxcarbazepine (Trileptal®)	X	X	
Lacosamide (Vimpat®))	X		
Tiagabine (Gabitril®)	X		
Topiramate (Topamax®)	X	X	Only GTC
Zonisamide (Zonegran®)	X		

GTC = generalized tonic-clonic.

[a]Conversion monotherapy.

Patients should be counseled on the importance of pharmacoadherence and nonpharmacologic methods for seizure management. Sleep deprivation, nonadherence to AEDs, and stress (physical or emotional) can affect seizure control in patients with epilepsy.

PATIENT EDUCATION

If a patient has epilepsy, she may want to educate her family, friends, and coworkers on how to respond if they witness a seizure. The following general guidelines should be used:

- Stay calm.
- Do not restrain the person. Don't try to keep the person from moving.
- Take away items that could cause injury if the person falls or bumps into them.
- Don't move the person to another place.
- Gently turn the person on his or her side so any fluid in the mouth can safely come out. Never try to force the person's mouth open or put anything in it.
- Call a doctor or ambulance if the person is not known to have a history of epilepsy or if the seizure lasts longer than 10–15 minutes, as most seizures are not life-threatening.
- When the seizure is over, observe the person for signs of confusion. Allow the person to rest or sleep if he or she wishes.

SEX DIFFERENCES

When selecting an AED for women, care must be taken to consider concomitant disease states and medications, pregnancy, and lactation. Women taking **cytochrome P450 (CYP450)** enzyme-inducing AEDs (carbamazepine, phenobarbital, phenytoin, primidone, felbamate, rufinamide, oxcarbazepine at dosages >1,200 mg/day, and topiramate at dosages >200 mg/day) have a fivefold increased rate of oral contraceptive failure.[51,52] This higher failure rate is due to increased steroid hormone metabolism and binding. Women on enzyme-inducing AEDs who wish to remain on oral contraceptives should use a product containing at least 50 mcg of estrogen to overcome the increased metabolism of the sex hormone.[53] Other options include switching to another AED with negligible effects on sex hormone metabolism (topiramate in dosages <200 mg/day, levetiracetam, gabapentin, zonisamide, or lacosamide), using a local hormone-releasing device, such as Mirena® (levonorgestrel-releasing intrauterine system) or nonhormonal methods of contraception. Mirena® may be a good option because progesterone acts locally by releasing in the uterus.[54-56] Lamotrigine can slightly affect the serum concentration of levonorgestrel levels in some patients, and oral contraceptives can decrease the effect of lamotrigine. This becomes clinically significant if the patient experiences lamotrigine side effects during the placebo week of the oral contraceptives. One way to minimize this effect is to use a nonhormonal method of birth control or an extended cycle oral contraceptive, such as Seasonale® (levonorgestrel/ethinyl estradiol), so that the menstrual cycle occurs only 4 times per year. Another option is to adjust the dosage of lamotrigine during the placebo week.

Epilepsy is different in women than in men because of differences in sex steroid hormones and other physiologic differences. In animal models, estrogen increases overall neuronal excitation, whereas progesterone enhances overall inhibition. It is presumed that this is the case in humans and can explain catamenial seizures and the change in seizure pattern at puberty and menopause. Fluctuations in the ovarian sex hormones affect seizure frequency.[57]

Puberty may bring on its own set of unique problems to women who have epilepsy. There are conflicting data on whether a relationship between seizure frequency and puberty exists. Puberty has been reported to increase or decrease seizure frequency.[58-60]

Catamenial seizures are seizures that are associated with the menstrual cycle. These seizures may occur just before or during the first few days of menstruation. Higher estrogen-to-progesterone ratios may be the reason for the increase in seizure frequency. In addition, water retention, electrolyte imbalances, and poor sleep may be contributing factors. Catamenial epilepsy occurs in about 12% of women with epilepsy.[61] There are three patterns of catamenial epilepsy: seizures around the start of menses (days 0–3 of the menstrual cycle), seizures occurring at the end of the follicular phase (days 10–14), and seizures occurring at the end of the luteal phase (days 24–28).[62]

If a woman with a seizure disorder becomes pregnant, there is a 30% chance that her seizures will worsen because of the pregnancy. Children with a family history of epilepsy have a twofold to threefold increased risk of developing epilepsy than those without a family history.[39] Women taking AEDs are at a slightly greater risk for a spontaneous abortion, miscarriage, or preterm delivery (see Table 41-5 for pregnancy categories for common medications used in epilepsy).[40] The physiologic changes during pregnancy may alter the AED concentrations in the blood via decreased gastric tone and motility, nausea, vomiting, increase in plasma volume, and increase in renal clearance. A greater reduction in phenytoin is seen during pregnancy compared with carbamazepine and valproate because of the effects of pregnancy on liver enzymes. It is important to monitor the patient's seizure activity and serum drug concentration and adjust the dosage as needed during pregnancy. As a general rule of thumb, the serum concentration of any AED can decrease as the gestation period reaches the third trimester. The serum concentrations of AEDs quickly return to prepregnancy levels after delivery. Dosage adjustments should be done before toxicity, including sedation, occurs.

In one of the largest class I studies, the absolute risk of major congenital malformations (cleft lip and palate, neural tube and cardiac defects) in infants born to epileptic mothers treated was reported as 2.2% for carbamazepine, 3.7% for phenytoin, 3.2% for lamotrigine, and 6.2% for valproate.[43,63] The frequency of major malformations in women who did not take AEDs was 1.62%. Prospective registries have been established to learn more about pregnancy and the outcome of the fetus in women taking AEDs. The North American registry reported a 7.8% (n = 65) incidence of major congenital malformations in women who were on phenobarbital monotherapy during the first trimester.[64] In 123 pregnancies, major birth defects were seen in 8.9% of valproate exposures.[65]

In 414 pregnancies, lamotrigine given during the first trimester as monotherapy was associated with 2.9% of major birth defects, which is similar to the risk in the general population. The risk increased to 12.5% for women who were taking lamotrigine and valproate during the first trimester.[66] Another study using the North American registry reported that 16 of 149 (10.7%) infants exposed to valproate monotherapy during the first trimester had a major birth defect. There is a threefold risk of a major birth defect in women who take valproate as monotherapy during the first trimester compared with women who use lamotrigine, and the risk is 7 times greater than the general population.[67] In a British study, researchers reported that 41 of 249 (16.5%) children, 6–16 years of age, from 163 mothers who were exposed to valproate during the first trimester had lower verbal IQ scores compared with children who had been exposed to phenytoin or another AED. In this study, 22% of those exposed to valproate had IQ scores in the extremely low or mentally impaired range, which is significantly higher compared with the general population, which is only 2% to 3%.[68] Valproate is not recommended during pregnancy unless absolutely necessary and should be used at the lowest possible dosage. Monotherapy with any AED is preferred over polytherapy, if possible. Additionally, an AED with a low peak serum concentration is preferred over an AED with a high peak.

Women with epilepsy are more likely to experience infertility, hormonal contraceptive failure, and adverse pregnancy outcomes. Hypo- and hypergonadotropic hypogonadism and polycystic ovarian syndrome (PCOS) may be key factors affecting fertility. Women taking CYP450 enzyme-inducing AEDs have decreased serum concentrations of estradiol, testosterone, and dihydroepiandrostenedione. Menstrual cycle irregularity can decrease fertility. Women with epilepsy may be at an increased risk for developing PCOS, but this has not been adequately studied.[39] Diagnosis requirements for this disease are serologic evidence for hyperandrogenism and anovulatory cycles. Hirsutism, cystic acne, male pattern baldness, and axial obesity are associated with this disease.

Sexual dysfunction can occur in women with epilepsy. A short standard sexual history should be part of the assessment of women with epilepsy. Social development and self-esteem may be decreased as a result of the social stigma regarding epilepsy. This can be a significant factor in quality of life, especially among adolescent women. Enzyme-inducing AEDs increase hepatic synthesis of estradiol, sex hormone–binding globulin, and testosterone, which can contribute to sexual dysfunction.

Patients with high seizure activity experience menopause significantly earlier in life. During menopause, about 40% of epileptic women report a worsening of their seizure disorder, 27% report improvement, and others report no effect.[60,69,70] Women with frequent partial or tonic-clonic seizures were more likely to be effected adversely from menopause. Natural progesterone may be beneficial in this population.[61] Currently, menopausal-related seizures and catamenial epilepsy are treated with conventional AEDs and acetazolamide.

In one study examining more than 8,000 community-dwelling women ≥65 years, those using AEDs were 75% more likely to experience a fall than women who did not use AEDs.[71] This is especially problematic because women with epilepsy taking an enzyme-inducing AED (carbamazepine, phenobarbital, phenytoin, oxcarbazepine >1,200 mg/day, and topiramate >200 mg/day) are at increased risk for fractures, osteopenia, osteoporosis, and osteomalacia. Valproate causes osteoporosis because it is a CYP450 enzyme inhibitor and has been associated with findings that reflect increased bone resorption.[72] Enzyme-inducing AEDs greatly increase the metabolism of vitamin D, which is vital to bone health. Analysis of blood from people with epilepsy show abnormalities including hypocalcemia, hypophosphatemia, elevated serum alkaline phosphatase, elevated parathyroid hormone, and reduced levels of vitamin D.[73] Bone turnover is accelerated. Women with a small bone frame are at an increased risk of bone fractures. Bone density and vitamin D level monitoring should be considered for all patients, particularly women on long-term (>5 years) AEDs. There are no consensus guidelines and little research has been conducted regarding the management of bone health in epilepsy and during AED therapy.[74] Other mechanisms besides vitamin D deficiency have been shown to contribute to bone loss; therefore, the patient's overall bone health must be evaluated, including calcium and vitamin D intake and weight-bearing exercise. Treatment with bisphosphonates, hormone supplementation, selective estrogen receptor modulators, calcium and vitamin D supplementation, and calcitonin may be recommended for women with bone loss.

SUMMARY

Epilepsy and AEDs can affect every aspect of a woman's sexual and reproductive life: the menstrual cycle, contraception, fertility, pregnancy, menopause, sexual function, and bone health. If practitioners are vigilant in treating their patients with epilepsy according to the guidelines and stay current with the latest research, many women with epilepsy will have a greater quality of life.

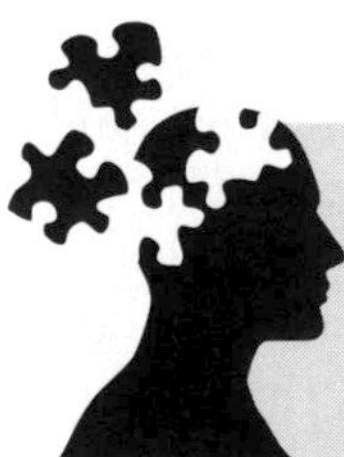

Therapeutic Challenge:

Your patient comes to see you in epilepsy clinic; she has been stable and seizure free, on a regimen of valproate and carbamazepine, and tells you that she is pregnant. Would you modify her drug regimen? Why or why not? If you choose to modify the regimen, how would you change it?

Stroke

(See Web Resources for Patient Case: Stroke.)

Additional content available at
www.ashp.org/womenshealth

Although stroke is the third leading cause of death for men and women in the U.S., women do not generally perceive themselves to be at risk for stroke. In a survey, 34% of women said that breast cancer was the greatest health problem facing women today.[75] In reality, stroke accounted for 91,487 female deaths in 2004 compared with 40,539 women dying from breast cancer.[76] A clear understanding of the similarities and differences between men and women with regard to stroke will enable healthcare providers to improve the stroke awareness of women.

EPIDEMIOLOGY

In the U.S., 46,000 more women than men have strokes each year, with 373,000 women sustaining stroke in 2004.[76] Men are at a greater risk for stroke at younger ages, but women have a longer life expectancy and thus account for a greater absolute number of strokes and 61% of stroke deaths. The male-to-female incidence rate increases from 1.25 at ages 55–64 to 0.76 when ≥85.[76] Race also affects stroke risk, with black women having a stroke incidence of 4.9 per 1,000 population compared with white women with an incidence of 2.3 per 1,000 population.[76]

RISK FACTORS

Many epidemiologic studies have focused on those factors that predispose individuals to stroke, some of which affect men and women differently. Women are generally 10 years older when they present with stroke.[77-80] Women are less likely than men to have a history of myocardial infarction, arterial peripheral disease, or sleep apnea and are less likely to smoke and abuse alcohol.[76,77,80]

Atrial fibrillation is a strong risk factor for stroke.[76] In some studies of atrial fibrillation, women have a greater risk for subsequent stroke.[77-83] Other studies have not shown sex to be a risk factor.[84,85] Hypertension approximately doubles the risk of stroke.[76] More men have hypertension until age 45; after age 54, women are more likely to have hypertension.[76] Elevated cholesterol is a stroke risk factor, but the evidence has come from male-dominated studies. Recent data demonstrate a relationship between lipid levels and stroke risk for women.[86] This trend was only detectable in women who were not using hormone therapy. Diabetes mellitus is also a risk factor for stroke. Migraines that present with visual auras increase stroke risk 1.5 times over women without migraine. Smoking and the use of oral contraceptives dramatically add to this risk.[87,88]

Understanding of the role of estrogen in stroke risk is evolving. Premenopausal women have a lower stroke risk than men. However, during pregnancy and the first 6 postpartum weeks, stroke risk is 2.4 times greater than for nonpregnant women.[76] Oral contraceptives containing <50 mcg of estrogen double the risk of stroke, whereas those with >50 mcg estrogen increase the risk of stroke 4.5 times that of a woman not taking oral contraceptives.[89] The risk increases with age, with greatest risk occurring in those older than 30 years. Smoking, hypertension, and obesity each further increase the risk of stroke compared with women who do not use oral contraceptives.[90] Hormone therapy appears to have no stroke-prevention benefit and may actually double the risk of stroke.[91-95]

CLINICAL PRESENTATION

Ischemic strokes usually have a sudden onset. The most common symptoms of stroke are numbness or weakness of the face, arm, or leg, usually on one side of the body; confusion; difficulty speaking or understanding; trouble seeing in one or both eyes; trouble walking; dizziness; loss of balance or coordination; and severe headache with no known cause.[96] Presenting signs and symptoms for ischemic stroke can be different between women and men. Women were more likely to report nontraditional stroke symptoms, such as pain and altered mental status, or to present with headache.[97,98] These less common presenting symptoms may lead to delay in diagnosis and differences in treatment of acute stroke.

PATHOPHYSIOLOGY

Given the differences between men and women in ischemic stroke epidemiology, one might expect significant differences in pathophysiology as well. Other than differences in risk factors between the sexes, few pathophysiological differences have been found. Cell cultures of neurons show male neurons are more susceptible to glutamate or peroxynitrite injury, even without sex steroids present.[99] The addition of estrogen in animal models of both sexes decreases tissue damage from ischemia.[99] However, the Women's Health Initiative study did not show a benefit of postmenopausal estrogen treatment on ischemic stroke; therefore, direct application of the basic science data to clinical care is unclear.[100]

DIAGNOSIS AND WORKUP

The diagnosis and workup of stroke is not different for women than for men. A practice guideline has been promulgated by the American Stroke Association to assist with diagnosis and workup.[101] If airway, breathing, and circulation are stable, a good history should be obtained, including a precise time of onset, if possible. A general physical examination should include vital signs, oxygen saturation, examination for carotid bruits, and cardiac examination. The neurologic examination is usually quite detailed and helps to localize the lesion as well as describe any deficits caused by the event. As part of this exam, the National Institutes of Health Stroke Scale is often administered.[102] All patients should have blood work for glucose, electrolytes, CBC, prothrombin time, activated partial thromboplastin time, and cardiac enzymes. An EEG and a brain computed tomography (CT) scan or MRI should also be performed. Additional imaging may include magnetic resonance angiography, transcranial Doppler ultrasonography, and carotid duplex sonography; and catheter angiography may be performed to detect vascular abnormalities or in preparation for intra-arterial procedures such as **carotid endarterectomy**.

Data regarding differences in the diagnostic workup between men and women is conflicting. In one European study comprising 4,499 patients, women had fewer investigations (imaging, Doppler, echocardiogram, angiography) than men.[77] A study of diagnostic evaluations for stroke in rural Texas demonstrated that women were less likely to have echocardiography (OR = 0.64, 95% CI 0.24–0.98) or any carotid imaging (OR = 0.57, 95% CI 0.36–0.91) than men after adjustment for other factors.[103] In contrast, a study in Sweden found that both sexes had equal rates of CT scanning and admission to designated stroke units.[78]

PREVENTION OF STROKE

Both primary and secondary stroke prevention is a cornerstone of treatment. The American Stroke Association has issued guidelines for the primary and secondary prevention of ischemic stroke.[104-106] In both primary and secondary prevention, a review of patient-specific risk factors to reduce all modifiable risks is paramount. Prevention of a first stroke also requires use of either warfarin or aspirin to avoid clot formation in atrial fibrillation. Therapy is chosen based on stroke risk factors, estimated bleeding risk, patient preferences, and access to high-quality anticoagulation monitoring.[105] As detailed above, the prevalence of atrial fibrillation may be different in men and women, but treatment recommendations are the same for both sexes. In men, aspirin is not recommended for primary stroke prevention in the absence of atrial fibrillation because of data demonstrating a lack of benefit and a nonsignificant increased risk of hemorrhagic stroke.[107,108] The Women's Health Study found women receiving aspirin 100 mg every other day had a reduced risk of stroke compared with women receiving placebo.[109]

After an initial ischemic event, attention shifts to secondary stroke prevention. Patients should be prescribed a platelet-active medication such as aspirin, clopidogrel, ticlopidine, or aspirin combined with sustained-release dipyridamole to prevent future strokes. Of these medications, only ticlopidine has been examined for benefit by sex, with women having a greater benefit.[110] However, ticlopidine is still not considered a first-line antiplatelet therapy in women.[106] Additional reduction of risk factors is important in secondary stroke prevention. No sex differences are seen in secondary prevention between men and women. Detailed guidance has been prepared by the American Stroke Association for secondary prevention.[106]

NONPHARMACOLOGIC THERAPY

Nonpharmacologic therapies for ischemic strokes include carotid endarterectomy, Mechanical Embolus Removal in Cerebral Ischemia™ (MERCI) clot retrieval system, and carotid artery angioplasty and stenting. Carotid endarterectomies are surgical procedures that remove stenosing plaques from the carotid arteries, thereby reducing stroke risk. The MERCI™ clot retrieval system is a mechanical device inserted into the cerebral artery to physically extract the clot obstructing blood flow. Sex differences have only been detected with carotid endarterectomies.

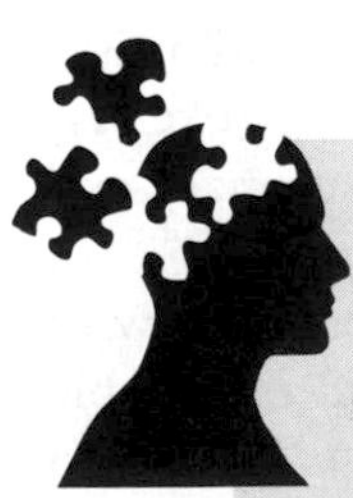

Therapeutic Challenge:

Based on the stroke studies discussed above, low-dose aspirin has been shown to reduce the risk of stroke in women but not men. Why would this be the case?

Two studies have revealed sex differences in surgical outcomes. Women with symptomatic carotid stenosis (i.e., those sustaining a transient ischemic attack, nondisabling stroke, or retinal infarction) only showed a benefit from carotid endarterectomy if their arteries were ≥70% occluded.[111] Asymptomatic men with >60% carotid stenosis appear to benefit more from surgery than women.[112]

PHARMACOLOGIC TREATMENT OF ACUTE EVENTS

The goal of acute treatment of stroke is to restore normal blood flow in the ischemic area. IV recombinant tissue plasminogen activator (tPA) can significantly alter the morbidity and mortality of stroke; however, it must be given within 3 hours of stroke onset and has numerous other exclusion criteria to minimize the likelihood of hemorrhagic events.[101] A 2008 study by the European Cooperative Acute Stroke Study investigators recently showed benefit from tPA administered up to 4.5 hours after onset of stroke symptoms.[113] Additional exclusion criteria are imposed on patients receiving tPA within the 3- to 4.5-hour time window.[114] Women appear to receive greater benefit from tPA; reopening of cerebral arteries after tPA administration occurred in 94% of women and only 59% of men in one study.[115] There may be sex-related differences in access to tPA treatment. In one study, only 40% of women arrived to the emergency department within 3 hours compared with 47% of men, and the time elapsed before seeing a physician was longer for women.[116] Male patients are treated with tPA more often; however, women may be more likely to refuse treatment with this agent. In a study that presented subjects with hypothetical situations regarding use of tPA, women were less likely to accept treatment with tPA (79% vs. 86%).[117]

PATIENT EDUCATION

Patient education for stroke prevention revolves around understanding and responding to stroke warning signs and reduction of stroke risk factors. Some potential counseling points follow:

- Know the warning signs of stroke, as discussed above.
- If you experience any of these warning signs, call 911 without delay.
- Eat a healthy diet, including nutritious foods from all the food groups.
- Exercise every day.

- Control your weight.
- Know your goal blood pressure and have your blood pressure checked regularly.
- Stop smoking.
- Control your cholesterol through diet, exercise, and/or medications.
- Limit alcohol intake to no more than two drinks per day.
- Do not discontinue medications without discussion with your healthcare provider; even though aspirin is available without a prescription, it is an important medication to prevent future strokes.
- Report any unusual bruising or bleeding to your healthcare provider.

OUTCOMES

Stroke is the most common cause of adult disability in the U.S.[76] Women have a longer length of hospitalization and are more likely to be discharged to a rehabilitation hospital or long-term care facility.[77,80] Approximately twice the number of women have poststroke depression.[118] Finally, women have frequently been shown to have a higher rate of mortality following ischemic stroke.[76,77]

SUMMARY

Stroke is a devastating event in the lives of women. There are differences between sexes in risk factors such as hypertension, atrial fibrillation, and migraine with visual aura. Estrogen use has emerged as a strong risk factor for stroke in women. Women present more frequently with nontraditional signs and symptoms of stroke. Women may benefit more than men from treatment with tPA; however, they receive treatment less frequently. Additionally, there appear to be differences in response to the antiplatelet therapies of aspirin and ticlopidine between men and women, the cause of which has not been elucidated. Much research regarding sex differences in the field of ischemic stroke remains to be done, but it is clear that considering men and women to be the same for risk factors, presentation, and treatment is an unacceptable stance.

Chronic Fatigue Syndrome

(See Web Resources for Patient Case: Chronic Fatigue Syndrome.)

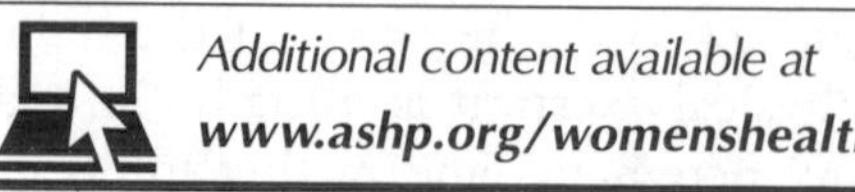

Additional content available at
www.ashp.org/womenshealth

Chronic fatigue syndrome (CFS), also known as myalgic encephalopathy, is challenging to diagnose and manage, for patients and healthcare providers. There is limited evidence-based research and a lack of education among healthcare providers regarding the diagnosis and treatment of CFS. Patients often present with a variety of symptoms that wax and wane over time. The symptoms are vague and mimic numerous other conditions. Recognition is challenging, which often delays a definitive diagnosis. Patients diagnosed earlier have a greater chance for recovery than those diagnosed more than 5 years after the onset.[119] Therefore, it is imperative that healthcare providers be able to recognize, diagnose, and manage this complex condition.

Epidemiologic data estimate that up to 4 million people in the U.S. meet the diagnostic criteria for CFS.[120] Women are affected 2–5 times more often than men, and the incidence peaks between the ages of 40 and 59 years.[119-122]

CLINICAL PRESENTATION

The severity of symptoms experienced by individuals with CFS varies, but symptoms can lead to impairment of functionality. The hallmark symptom of CFS is chronic fatigue lasting more than 6 months. Other symptoms used for the diagnosis of CFS include postexertional malaise lasting >24 hours, unrefreshing sleep, impaired memory or concentration, muscle pain, joint pain without redness or swelling, headache, tender cervical or axillary lymph nodes, and sore throat.[123] Other symptoms include irritable bowel syndrome (IBS), chills, night sweats, cognitive impairment, chest pain, shortness of breath, chronic cough, blurry vision, photosensitivity, ocular pain, dry eyes, orthostatic instability, arrhythmias , vertigo, coordination problems, fainting, depression, irritability, mood swings, anxiety, panic attacks, jaw pain, vertigo, tinnitus, changes in hearing, recurrent infections (i.e., Candida, sinusitis, otitis), weight loss or gain, and allergies/sensitivities to foods, alcohol, odors, chemicals, medications, or noise.[121,123,124]

PATHOPHYSIOLOGY

The pathophysiology of CFS is unknown at this time. Research efforts are focused on finding the cause(s) and treatments as well as defining the physiologic mechanism of the syndrome. One study reported that patients with CFS had significantly higher production of nuclear factor-kappa beta (NF-κβ), which is the major intracellular mechanism in white blood cells that regulates inflammation and oxidative stress.[125] Another study reported finding abnormalities of the ribonuclease L pathway in patients with CFS.[126] This pathway is an enzyme-mediated mechanism that helps the body fight infection. Recent and ongoing studies have identified a number of possibilities, such as dysfunction of the hypothalamic–pituitary–adrenal (HPA) axis, sympathetic nervous system, and immune system.[127-134]

The etiology of CFS is unknown, but several theories have been proposed. The theory that is gaining the most acceptance by experts is that genetically susceptible individuals are exposed to a triggering event. A triggering event can be an infection, traumatic injury, emotional trauma, hormonal changes, environmental conditions, and/or chemical exposure. The event results in a dysregulation of the usual HPA axis and sympathetic response. This dysregulation, combined with the cumulative wear and tear on the body, results in a high allostatic load, which then manifests as the multisystem effects of CFS. Other factors that may play a role in CFS are immune dysfunction, mitochondrial dysfunction, anaerobic energy conversion, and oxidative stress.[121,123,124] Several viruses have been identified as causal agents in patients with onset of CFS postinfection: herpes viruses, enteroviruses, Ross River virus, and Q fever.[135-137] The Centers for Disease Control and Prevention has published findings of specific gene mutations in individuals with CFS revealing potential genetic factors that may increase susceptibility to this condition.[138]

DIAGNOSIS

Diagnosing CFS can be challenging for many reasons. There is no diagnostic laboratory test or serum biomarker to confirm the syndrome. The symptoms of CFS can vary greatly between patients, and the symptoms are also common in many other conditions. Therefore, CFS is a diagnosis of exclusion.

The first definition for CFS, the Holmes Criteria (1988), was designed specifically for research and required idiopathic chronic fatigue, eight of eleven symptoms, or two physical findings and four symptoms.[139] The Fukuda Criteria (1994 International criteria) required unexplained chronic fatigue lasting more than 6 months and the exemption of other causes, specifically psychiatric disorders. Further, four of the following eight symptoms must be present: arthralgias, cognitive dysfunction, lymphadenopathy, myalgias, new onset headache, nonexudative pharyngitis, postexertional malaise, and unrefreshed sleep.[140] The Revised International Criteria (2003) allows for a history, but no current finding, of psychiatric disorders. Other criteria include Oxford (1992), Australia (1990), and Canadian (2004).[141]

Laboratory testing is used primarily to exclude other possible causes. Tests that should be considered include CBC with leukocyte differential, comprehensive metabolic panel, phosphorus, erythrocyte sedimentation rate (ESR), C reactive protein (CRP), thyroid-stimulating hormone (TSH), free T4, antinuclear antibody (ANA), rheumatoid factor (RF), and urinalysis.[121,123,124,142] General practitioners without keen knowledge of CFS should consider referring the patient to a CFS specialist or rheumatologist for initial diagnosis and treatment.

Some patients with CFS have orthostatic intolerance; therefore, cardiology testing with the tilt-table test can be useful.[143] In addition to orthostatic intolerance, there are several comorbid conditions with CFS that if identified can assist in the treatment of CFS. These conditions include metabolic syndrome, hormone imbalances/dysregulation, vitamin D and B12 deficiencies, IBS, gastroesophageal reflux disease, and celiac disease.[144]

LONG-TERM COMPLICATIONS

There are limited data available regarding CFS; so the long-term complications are unclear. The clinical course of CFS appears to be different in areas of outbreaks or epidemics and appears to have an increased rate of full recovery.[145,146] CFS does not appear to be associated with an increased mortality rate.[147,148] However, without treatment (pharmacologic or psychological), a full recovery is unlikely.

TREATMENT GOALS

In 2007, the National Institute for Clinical Excellence (NICE) published guidelines on the diagnosis and management of CFS. These guidelines can be obtained through NICE (http://www.nice.org.uk). Currently, there is no known cure for CFS. The primary goal is to focus on the management of bothersome symptoms. This can be accomplished using pharmacologic and nonpharmacologic methods.

NONPHARMACOLOGIC TREATMENT

Cognitive behavioral therapy (CBT) and graduated exercise therapy have been shown to be beneficial in the management of CFS. Graduated exercise therapy is a structured exercise program that is designed and adjusted to fit the needs of the individual patient. Physical exertion is initially limited to 2- to 5-minute increments and resting intervals of 5 minutes, which should be gradually increased over time. Efforts exceeding this may evoke a severe exacerbation.[149,150] Cognitive behavioral therapy may include modifications of the work schedule to allow a slower pace with frequent periods of reclined rest, education about and implementation of good sleep hygiene, and dietary modifications to eliminate food sensitivities, such as wheat, caffeine, milk products, soy, citrus, fruit, peanuts, and artificial sweeteners. In addition, patients with depression respond well to counseling but may still require treatment with antidepressants. Patients are encouraged to maintain social connectivity to prevent social isolation.

Many CFS specialists instruct patients to use supplements, vitamins, and minerals (i.e., high-dose B12 injections, coenzyme Q10, nicotinamide adenine dinucleotide [NADH], lipid replacements, magnesium, zinc, calcium, multivitamins, omega-3, dehydroepiandrosterone [DHEA], vitamin D); however, this practice has not been formally studied. Complementary therapies include massage, acupuncture, yoga, and meditation.[123,124,135,150]

Pharmacologic Treatment

No medications are currently approved for the treatment of CFS. Several agents have been investigated or are currently being investigated. Antivirals may be considered if chronic viral syndromes are suspected; however, not all patients respond to antiviral therapy because of the heterogeneous nature of CFS. The investigational agent Ampligen® (Poly I: Poly C12U) has shown promise, especially if given before 2 years of illness.[151] Ampligen is a double-stranded RNA with broad antiviral and immunomodulatory properties that is under investigation for conditions such as CFS, HIV (human immunodeficiency virus), and certain types of cancer.[152] Table 41-8 lists commonly used medications that are used for symptom

Table 41-8. Medications Commonly Used for Chronic Fatigue Syndrome and Fibromyalgia[a]

Depression	Fatigue	Neuropathic Pain	Pain	Insomnia	Muscle Relaxants	Postural Orthostatic Hypotension
Bupropion	Amantadine	<u>Duloxetine</u>	*Nonopiate*	<u>Amitriptyline</u>	<u>Cyclobenzaprine</u>	Fludrocortisone
Citalopram	Methylphenidate	<u>Gabapentin</u>	Acetominophen	Eszopiclone	Metaxalone	Midodrine
Duloxetine	Mixed amphetamine salts	Lamotrigine	Naproxen	Mirtazapine	Methocarbamol	
Escitalopram	Modafinil	<u>Pregabalin</u>	Ibuprofen	Tizanidine	Orphenadrine	
<u>Fluoxetine</u>		<u>Tramadol</u>	Meloxicam	Trazodone	Tizanidine	
<u>Paroxetine</u>		<u>Milnacipran</u>	Celecoxib	Zaleplon		
Sertraline			*Opiate Derivative*	Zolpidem		
Venlafaxine			Tramadol			
			Opiate			
			Codeine			
			Fentanyl			
			Hydrocodone			
			Oxycodone			
			Propoxyphene			
			Morphine sulfate			
			Local Anesthetics			
			Lidocaine			

<u>Underlined</u> = evidence-based recommendation.

[a]Patients with chronic fatigue syndrome and/or fibromyalgia may need to start at half of the typical recommended dose, as these patients may have increased sensitivity to medications.

management in clinical practice. Symptoms of CFS are numerous and widely variable between patients; therefore, multiple drugs may be needed to adequately control symptoms. Symptoms should be prioritized and addressed accordingly. Sleep problems, if present, should be addressed first.

Patients with CFS have variable response rates to medications and may be more sensitive to side effects. A thorough medical and drug history should be helpful in identifying patients with very low drug thresholds. It may be prudent to initiate drug therapy using the lowest recommended dose or half-dose and gradually escalate based on the patient's response and tolerability. If symptoms worsen significantly during a trial of drug therapy and improve once it is discontinued, consider this a patient intolerance and switch to a different product (perhaps a different manufacturer). Fillers may differ in generic preparations or contain added colors or dyes that may elicit a sensitivity or allergic response.

Monitoring and Follow-up

Patients should be seen every 4–6 weeks until symptoms stabilize or improve. Laboratory tests are based on symptoms and drug use. Providers may find managing CFS time-consuming or frustrating, as many patients suffer rejection by family and friends. Compassion and understanding enhance patients' cooperation and provide them with hope for improvement.

PATIENT EDUCATION

Patient education is a vital component and should be emphasized at each visit. Patients should be educated about the disease state, treatment goals, and treatment options. Patients should be informed of the proper use of their medications, common side effects, management of side effects, drug interactions, food interactions, signs/symptoms of allergic reaction, serious side effects, and when they should start to notice a benefit from the medication. If side effects become intolerable or symptoms significantly worsen, the patient should be instructed to notify their healthcare provider for instructions on proper discontinuation of the medication. It will be important to try to differentiate between an unpredicted flare or relapse of CFS vs. a true sensitivity reaction to the medication.

Decreased cognitive function can be a symptom of the disease or a side effect from drug therapy. Patients should be counseled on how to manage cognitive problems; for example, they may find it useful to take notes during their appointments and write down questions in between visits to aid with memory and progress. A pillbox may be utilized to help patients keep track of and manage their medication usage. A pillbox should be placed in a convenient and visible location to serve as a reminder for the patient.

SEX DIFFERENCES

Very little research has been published on sex issues. Women have higher occurrences of enlarged lymph nodes (60% vs. 30%), fibromyalgia symptoms (36% vs. 12%), disability (22% vs. 0%), and unemployment (35% vs. 0%).[153,154] Men have more pharyngeal inflammation (42% vs. 22%) and prevalence of lifetime alcoholism (90% vs. 9%).[153,154]

Information regarding reproductive issues in women with CFS is limited and remains unexplored. Recommendations are based primarily on opinions and observations of the experts. A 2004 retrospective study using a self-reported questionnaire found that 41% of women experienced no change in their CFS symptoms, 30% reported improvements, and 29% reported worsening of symptoms during pregnancy.[155] Anecdotally, pregnancy has been reported to be beneficial for CFS symptoms.[156] Polycystic ovary syndrome and anovulatory cycles are reported more often in women with CFS.[157] Dysmenorrhea appears to correlate highly with CFS. There is preliminary evidence that indicates women with CFS may have higher rates of endometriosis, which can affect fertility.[157] Women with CFS may be at higher risk for first-trimester spontaneous abortion.[155,157] There may be a higher risk of developmental delay in offspring of women with CFS, which may be due to low cortisol levels.[153,155,157,158] Theoretically, the labor process could precipitate a relapse due to stress and exhaustion. Maintaining vascular volume with IV fluids, pain management, and stress reduction may prevent or moderate this potential.[156] Epidural anesthesia may be a good option to conserve energy and prevent a relapse, especially in cases of prolonged labor.[156]

Although not formally studied, women may be at an increased risk of a severe relapse 3–6 months postpartum. The relapse may be related to physiologic changes and/or the cumulative effects of sleep deprivation and stress. It is unknown whether CFS affects breast-feeding or what the effects of breast-feeding are on CFS. The primary concern during pregnancy and lactation is the effect that the drugs may have on the infant. A complete review of drugs should be done before conception, if possible, to determine if any should be discontinued and, if necessary, to make a plan to taper off of them. Exacerbations or reoccurrences have been reported in women during menopause.[159] Preliminary research suggests that children born to women with CFS are at a higher risk of developing CFS (5.5%) or chronic fatigue (11.4%).[160]

SUMMARY

Chronic fatigue syndrome is a complex disease and is not well understood. Treatment is aimed at managing symptoms. Information regarding sex differences and women's health issues is scarce. Diagnosis and management of this disease can be quite challenging for the healthcare provider.

Fibromyalgia

(See Web Resources for Patient Case: Fibromyalgia.)

Additional content available at
www.ashp.org/womenshealth

Fibromyalgia (FM) is a central pain disorder characterized by chronic widespread pain. Initially, this condition was called myofascitis, muscular rheumatism, and fibrositis. It was classified by the Arthritis Foundation as soft-tissue rheumatism. The name was subsequently changed to fibromyalgia because of the absence of inflammation. Approximately 2% to 6% of the U.S. population is affected by FM, and the majority of sufferers are women.[161,162] Women (3.4% to 10.5%) are more often diagnosed with FM than men (0.5%).[161,162] Onset is primarily between 30 and 55 years of age. In women 60–70 years of age, the prevalence of FM is more than 7.0%.[162]

CLINICAL PRESENTATION

The hallmark symptom of FM is bilateral widespread muscle and joint pain and a heightened painful response to gentle stimuli. Unexplained fatigue, sleep disturbances, and activity intolerance are common symptoms. Several features of FM overlap with other chronic conditions, such as CFS, IBS, and temporomandibular joint pain, depression, anxiety, chronic pelvic pain, irritable bladder, hypothyroidism, restless legs syndrome, Raynaud's disease, and vertigo.[161,163]

PATHOPHYSIOLOGY

The pathophysiology of FM is not well understood. There are two major theories that attempt to explain the symptoms of fatigue and pain in fibromyalgia. The pathophysiology related to fatigue is the same as for CFS. This theory does not fully explain the hypersensitivity to pain that is common to fibromyalgia. Patients with FM have central hyperexcitability of the nociceptive system, causing a lowered pain threshold such that even light touch can produce pain with an increased duration.[164] Several physiological mechanisms have been identified, including increased levels of substance P, excitatory amino acids, and neurotrophins in the CSF.[165-167] As new information is uncovered, it is becoming clear that the pathophysiology of FM is extremely complex. To be able to prevent or treat this syndrome, we first need to determine the underlying mechanisms.

The etiology of FM is unknown. There are several theories that are similar to the theories discussed for CFS. Dysfunction in the autonomic nervous system and HPA axis results in chemical/hormonal imbalances, altered nerve input, and weakened responses in tissues and cells. It is speculated that the dysfunction could be related to chronically high levels of stress or emotional strain (e.g., abuse). Other factors that may play a role in the etiology of FM include genetic predisposition, sleep disturbances, central dopamine dysfunction, abnormal serotonin metabolism, deficient human growth hormone secretion, and environmental and psychological factors.[162,168-180] Additional theories include postviral syndrome, trauma reaction, autoimmune reaction, and chemical or environmental reaction.[181]

DIAGNOSIS

The 1990 American College of Rheumatology criteria for the diagnosis of FM requires a history of chronic widespread pain (>3 months) affecting all four quadrants of the body (left, right, upper, lower) and pain at 11 of 18 designated tender points using 4 kg/cm of force (enough to blanch the thumb of the provider).[182,183] Clauw argues that because this criteria was designed for research as opposed to clinical use, strict adherence regarding tender points is not necessary to diagnose FM.[184]

Similar to CFS, FM is a diagnosis of exclusion. There is no specific test that can be used to diagnosis FM. Laboratory testing is recommended to rule out other conditions that could be causing the patient's symptoms. Laboratory testing may include CBC with differential, ESR, creatine kinase, TSH, free T4, RF, and ANA. Practitioners may also choose to test for muscular enzymes and Lyme disease or order nerve conduction studies to rule out peripheral neuropathies or nerve entrapment.

LONG-TERM COMPLICATIONS

Limited research exists on long-term consequences and mortality in FM patients. Quality of life for patients with FM is significantly lower compared with those with rheumatoid arthritis.[185] Studies also reveal accelerated aging of the brain with significant increased loss of gray matter volume correlating to the length of illness.[186] Studies on increased occurrence of cancer in patients with widespread pain have returned conflicting results. Decreased hip bone mass has been found in patients, possibly because of limitations in weight bearing.[187] If premature mortality does exist, it is possibly related to a sedentary lifestyle.[188]

TREATMENT GOALS

In 2007, the European League against Rheumatism published evidence-based recommendations for the management of fibromyalgia syndrome.[189] In 2005, the American Pain Society published guidelines for the management of FM in adults and children, which are only available through the APS (http://www.ampainsoc.org). Both sets of guidelines were developed to aid healthcare providers in the diagnosis and treatment of FM. There is no cure for FM, and treatment goals are aimed at controlling symptoms through pharmacologic and nonpharmacologic therapies.

NONPHARMACOLOGIC TREATMENT

Pharmacologic therapy primarily addresses the pain associated with fibromyalgia. Nonpharmacologic therapy helps the patient to maintain a healthy lifestyle through education, CBT, and exercise, which can help minimize many symptoms associated with fibromyalgia, such as poor sleep and decreased physical and social activity. Education, aerobic exercise, and CBT have been shown to be effective treatments.[190] There is limited evidence supporting the use of strength training and hypnotherapy.[191,192] Cognitive behavioral therapy is used to help patients manage stress, improve sleep, and identify maladaptive illness behaviors. Cognitive behavioral therapy can also be beneficial for the treatment of depression and social isolation. The use of vitamins, supplements, and other complementary therapies is often recommended in clinical practice and may be beneficial in some patients; however, this has not been formally studied.

PHARMACOLOGIC TREATMENT

Many patients will require the use of pharmacologic treatments to help manage the pain associated with fibromyalgia. Many of the agents used for pain can also be beneficial on fatigue and sleep disturbances. Many drugs have been investigated, but few have proven to be efficacious. There are three commercial products that have FDA approval for the treatment of fibromyalgia: pregabalin, duloxetine, and milnacipran. Gabapentin, which is related to pregabalin, also has evidence to support its use in fibromyalgia.[193] Tricyclic antidepressants, specifically amitriptyline and cyclobenzaprine, appear to be effective for the treatment of fibromyalgia.[194,195] Duloxetine and milnacipran are serotonin-norepinephrine reuptake inhibitors (SNRIs). These agents provide the additional benefit of treating depression. The selective serotonin reuptake inhibitors (SSRIs) fluoxetine and paroxetine have some evidence of efficacy.[196-199] It is important to note that SSRIs are not interchangeable with SNRIs. When switching agents, patients should be titrated down off one medication while titrating up on the other. Other agents that have been studied with less compelling evidence include tramadol and pramipexole.[200-202]

Nonsteroidal anti-inflammatory drugs (NSAIDs), opioids, benzodiazepines, hypnotics, and sedatives are commonly used in clinical practice; however, there is no evidence to support their use.[197,203,204] In addition, there is potential for abuse of these agents, as many of them are controlled substances.[205]

Monitoring and Follow-up

Monitoring and follow-up are similar to that for CFS and are based on symptoms and medications.

PATIENT EDUCATION

Patients should be educated about their disease and realistic treatment goals should be set. Emphasis should be placed on nonpharmacologic therapies to help patients cope with their illness. If possible, a patient's spouse, family, and friends should be involved in the educational process. A thorough discussion of the effectiveness of pharmacologic therapies should be reviewed. In addition, patients should be educated about the proper use of these medications, including side effects (common and serious), duration of treatment, and drug interactions (including vitamins, supplements, and herbals).

SEX DIFFERENCES

There is limited information available on sex differences in FM. Women are more likely to be affected

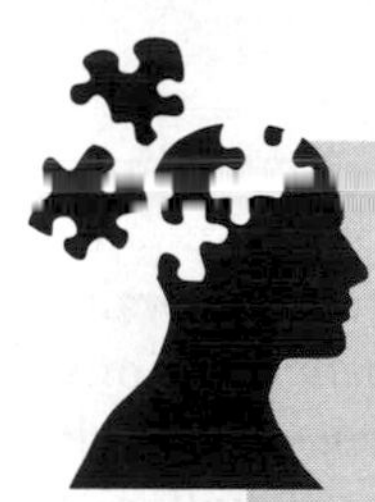

Therapeutic Challenge:

What strategies could be implemented to increase patient and practitioner awareness in the diagnosis and treatment of CFS and FM?

by fibromyalgia compared with men (ratio 9:1).[161,162] Rape increases the risk of FM in women, with victims 3.1 times more likely to develop this condition.[206] Individuals exposed to continuous high levels of stress—such as negative life events or sexual, physical, or emotional abuse—may be predisposed to FM.[207]

There is limited information regarding reproductive issues and FM. Women with FM report more reproductive health issues, such as breast cysts, dysmenorrhea, premenstrual syndrome, and bladder infections.[208] Sexual dysfunction is a common problem and may be related to fatigue and depression.[208] Sexual intercourse may be painful because of the decreased tolerance to pain.[208] In addition, many of the medications used to manage pain and depression can cause sexual dysfunction. The effect of pregnancy on FM is largely unexplored. One study reported that symptoms of FM worsened during pregnancy and within 6 months of delivery.[208] One study reported that 72% of patients experienced a worsening of symptoms premenstrually.[209] Symptoms may worsen during menopause as well.[210,211]

SUMMARY

For every patient with CFS or FM, there are many other patients who have not been diagnosed. Thus, it is very likely that these conditions are more prevalent than currently reported in the literature. FM can coexist with CFS and many other conditions. FM and CFS are manageable conditions that, when treated and managed, can significantly improve the quality of life for these patients. There is little understanding about the etiology and pathophysiology of these conditions, and there are few effective treatments. Education of patients and providers along with future research will be important in managing patients with FM or CFS.

Headache

(See Web Resources for Patient Case: Headache.)

Additional content available at
www.ashp.org/womenshealth

Headache disorders are one of the most ubiquitous and painful disease states. Headache disorders encompass a variety of clinical syndromes that vary in terms of severity, duration, frequency, location, and symptoms. Guidelines for the diagnosis and subclassification of specific headache types have been established by the International Headache Society (IHS)[212]; however, investigators have employed various definitions of headache, which makes epidemiologic data difficult to interpret. A higher prevalence of migraine has been reported in women (18.2%) compared with men (6.5%) older than 12 years.[213] For the purposes of this discussion, we will focus on the common headaches of women, with an emphasis on migraine.

Migraine headache is a chronic syndrome that disproportionately affects adult women, and clearly ovarian hormones play a role in the pathogenesis.[214-217] Headache patterns appear to correlate with changes in the hormonal milieu throughout the lifespan in women.[217] Before puberty, the incidence of migraine is similar for boys and girls.[218] In women, migraine develops most commonly in the second decade, and the majority report some relationship between headache attacks and their menstrual cycle.[217,219] Migraine frequency also is affected by pregnancy, oral contraceptive use, and menopause.[217,219]

Tension-type headaches (TTHs) are common among men and women and occur at a slightly higher rate in women (1.2:1).[220] TTHs can be present concomitantly with migraine or other types of headaches.

CLINICAL PRESENTATION

In clinical practice, many of the symptoms associated with migraine and TTH can overlap, making it difficult to distinguish between the two. Additionally, both headache types can be triggered by similar factors. For example, stress, alcohol, and menstruation can trigger a migraine or TTH. Other common factors that trigger migraine or TTH include fatigue, sleep deprivation, increased sleep (i.e., sleeping in on weekends), odors, certain foods, and skipping meals. Some patients may suffer from both types of headache disorders.

PATHOPHYSIOLOGY

The pathophysiology of headaches is poorly understood. There is an ongoing debate regarding whether migraine and TTH are separate entities or if they are on opposite ends of the same continuum. Migraine headaches are believed to occur as a result of primary neuronal dysfunction.[221] Experimental models suggest that substance P, calcitonin gene-related peptide, other vasoactive polypeptides, and serotonin play an important role in the pain and vasodilation that occurs during a migraine.[222,223] There is evidence that central sensitization and cutaneous allodynia are common in migraine patients. Genetic and environmental factors may also play a role in the pathogenesis.[224] TTH is believed to be a result of heightened sensitivity of pain pathways in the central and possibly peripheral nervous system.[225-227] Muscular factors and nitric oxide may be key players in the pathogenesis of TTH.[228-230] Genetic factors may play a role in the development of chronic TTH but appear to have a minimal role in episodic TTH.

A common trigger of migraines in women is menstruation. This has led to the term **menstrual migraine (MM),** which is not recognized by the IHS as a specific headache type. The term refers to the association of migrainous attacks that occur around the time of the menstrual cycle and are further categorized into pure MM and menstrually-related migraines. Pure MMs are attacks that occur *only* around the time of menstruation. Menstrually related migraines are attacks that occur at time of menstruation as well as at other times.[219]

Although the exact mechanism of MM has not been fully elucidated, the decline in estrogen levels during the late luteal phase is thought to be the primary culprit in its occurrence. Most women report a decline in migraine attacks during pregnancy and after menopause when estrogen levels are more stable.[231] Somerville found that an intramuscular injection of estradiol given just before the onset of menses (when levels of estrogen fall) delayed the onset of MM.[232,233] Another investigation has shown that perimenstrual administration of estrogen effectively treats MM.[234] Although the mechanism is unclear, estrogen is involved in opioid regulation and prostaglandin synthesis, and has effects to modulate serotonergic tone, all of which may play a role in the pathogenesis of MM.[215,235]

Chronic daily headaches (CDHs) are headaches that occur more than 15 days per month. They are often associated with medication overuse. There is a debate regarding whether the overuse of medications is the cause or result of CDH.[236-238] The two primary theories for the pathophysiology of **medication overuse headache (MOH)** are that continuous exposure to analgesics causes antinociceptive tolerance, which leads to diminishing effectiveness, and that medication tolerance and dependence results in repeated "mini-withdrawals" that result in a rebound headache with fluctuations in serum drug levels. Medication overuse is a risk factor for developing CDH but by itself will not induce CDH. Common medications associated with MOH include opioids, triptans, ergots, aspirin, acetaminophen, caffeine, and barbiturates. Patients with MOH often have headache pain that is refractory to treatment, and improvement of symptoms occurs on gradual removal of the offending agent.[239]

DIAGNOSIS

TTHs typically last from 30 minutes to 7 days and are characterized as bilateral, nonpulsating, and mild to moderate pain. Tension-type headache is usually not aggravated by physical activity and is not associated with nausea or vomiting. Phonophobia or photophobia are rarely present, but not both. Migraines can last from a few hours to several days and are characterized by unilateral (can be bilateral), pulsating, and moderate to severe pain. Migraines are aggravated by physical activity and are associated with nausea/vomiting, phonophobia, and photophobia. Before the headache attack, migraineurs may experience a premonitory phase characterized by food cravings, depressive symptoms, and fatigue. Similar symptoms may occur just after headache pain has subsided (recovery phase). Some patients have an aura, which is often described as a visual disturbance (flickering, partial loss of vision) or temporary focal neurologic symptoms (numbness, tingling), that occurs at initiation of the headache pain. Approximately 18% of migraine sufferers experience migraine with aura.[240] For a complete discussion of headache subtypes and diagnostic criteria, please refer to the International Classification of Headache Disorders published by the IHS.[212]

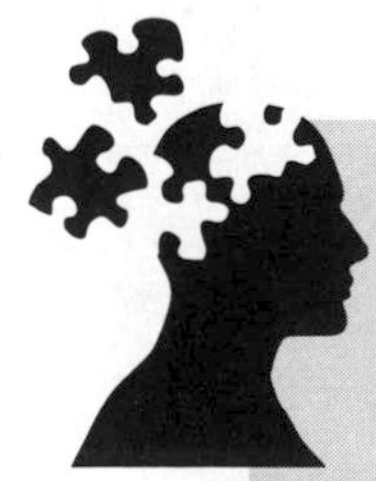

Therapeutic Challenge:

Should oral contraceptives be used in a patient experiencing migraine headaches with aura? Why or why not?

LONG-TERM COMPLICATIONS

There appears to be an association between migraine headache and the risk of cardiovascular complications. Large cohort studies have found an association between migraine headache and the risk of cardiovascular complications, such as stroke and myocardial infarction.[87,241] In an evaluation of patients with migraine headache in the Women's Health Study, women who reported a history of migraine with aura were found to be at a twofold increased risk of death from cardiovascular disease. No such association was found in women with migraine without aura.[242] Several plausible mechanisms for these associations have been noted. Patients with migraine with aura have been found to have an unfavorable ischemic cardiovascular risk profile (hypertension, dyslipidemia). Furthermore, an increase in prothrombotic factors and genetic polymorphisms may also play a role in the higher risk of ischemic events associated with migraine headaches.[218,243]

TREATMENT GOALS

The main goal of treatment for headache disorders is prevention. Other goals include reducing the frequency, severity and duration of the headache. This can be accomplished using pharmacologic and nonpharmacologic therapies.

NONPHARMACOLOGIC TREATMENT

Nonpharmacologic therapy should be emphasized to all patients, especially those who are pregnant, breastfeeding, or have contraindications to drug therapy. Patients should be encouraged to identify and avoid migraine triggers. A headache diary can be useful in helping patients identify their specific triggers. Lifestyle modifications can be taken to avoid those triggers, such as smoking cessation, eating meals on a regular basis, getting appropriate amounts of sleep, avoiding caffeine, and using stress-management techniques. These techniques include biofeedback, meditation, acupuncture, massage therapy, and application of hot and cold packs.[244]

Pharmacologic Treatment

Pharmacologic treatments are useful in reducing the intensity and frequency of headache pain, which can have a significant impact on the patient's quality of life. Pharmacologic therapy can be divided into two categories: acute and prophylactic therapy. Acute therapy is used to treat attacks as they occur and should be offered to all patients. Prophylactic therapy is aimed at preventing the attacks. Prophylactic therapy should be considered for patients with headaches that are frequent (two or more per month), severe, or debilitating or those with uncommon migraine conditions, such as hemiplegic migraine, basilar migraine, migraine with prolonged aura, or migrainous infarction. Prophylactic therapy should also be considered for patients who have contraindications to or have failed other treatments. Additionally, if MOH is suspected, if the patient experiences intolerable side effects, or if it is requested by the patient, prophylactic therapy could be considered. Medications with supporting evidence for their use for the prevention of migraines are listed in Table 41-9. Medications that have conflicting evidence or no evidence to support their use are listed in Table 41-10. For a general review of pharmacological treatments for migraine, refer to *Pharmacotherapy: A Pathophysiologic Approach*, 7th edition.[245]

SEX/SEX DIFFERENCES

In general, the treatment strategies for women with headache disorders are the same as men. The AAN has published guidelines for the management of migraine headaches (available at http://www.aan.com/practice/guideline). There are special considerations that should be given when selecting appropriate treatments for women because headaches are affected by menstruation, pregnancy, menopause, and the use of oral contraceptives. Each of these considerations will be discussed as they relate to the treatment of headaches, with an emphasis on migraine.

Menstrual Migraine

Many women with MM have migraines that occur in a predictable nature in reference to the onset of menses. Therefore, the most common practice to manage these headaches is through "miniprophylaxis," which involves the use of drugs given prophylactically a few days before the onset of the expected headache. The most studied approach has been with the use of triptans, and the available evidence demonstrates that these drugs are effective in the treatment of MM.[246] For women who have predictable menstrual cycles, treatment with a long-acting triptan (frovatriptan, naratriptan) should start 2–3 days before the anticipated headache and continue for a total of 5–6 consecutive days. Other common strategies include the use of NSAIDs, ergot alkaloids, and estradiol perimenstrually. In some patients it may be necessary for daily preventative therapy. In severe cases of MM, it may be necessary to use a miniprophylaxis method in addition to daily preventative therapy.

Table 41-9. Evidence-Based Recommendations for the Prevention of Headache[253]

Class 1 Evidence[a]	Class 2 Evidence[b]	Class 3 Evidence[c]
Beta-blockers	*Beta-blockers*	*Anticonvulsants*
Propranolol	Atenolol	Carbamazepine
Timolol maleate	Nadolol	*Calcium channel blockers*
Metoprolol	*SSRI*	Diltiazem
Tricyclic antidepressants	Fluoxetine	Nicardipine
Amitriptyline	*SNRI*	Nifedipine
Antiepileptic Drugs	Venlafaxine	Verapamil
Divalproex sodium	*Anticonvulsants*	Nimodipine
Valproic acid	Gabapentin	*α-adrenoreceptor antagonists*
Topiramate	*5-Hydroxytryptamine agonists (MM)*	Clonidine
5-Hydroxytryptamine agonists	Naratriptan	
Frovatriptan[d]	Zolmitriptan	
5-Hydroxytryptamine antagonists	*Miscellaneous*	
Methysergide	Coenzyme Q10	
Miscellaneous	Feverfew	
Petasites hybridus root (butterbur)	Riboflavin (Vitamin B_2)	
	Angiotensin-converting enzyme inhibitor	
	Lisinopril	
	Angiotensin-receptor blocker	
	Candasartan	
	Antihistamines/leukotriene antagonists	
	Cyproheptadine	
	Histamine	
	NSAIDs	
	Aspirin	
	Flurbiprofen	
	Fenoprofen	
	Ibuprofen	
	Ketoprofen	
	Mefenamic acid	
	Naproxen	

SSRI = selective serotonin reuptake inhibitor; SNRI = serotonin-norepinephrine reuptake inhibitor; MM = menstrual migraine; NSAIDs = nonsteroidal anti-inflammatory drugs.

[a]Class I: prospective, randomized, controlled clinical trials with masked outcome assessment in a representative population.
[b]Class II: prospective matched group cohort studies with masked outcome assessment in a representative population.
[c]Class III: controlled trials in a representative population where outcome is independently assessed.
[d]For short-term prophylaxis of MM.

Combined Oral Contraceptives

There are limited data available with regard to combined oral contraceptives (COCs) and headaches. Few studies have looked at the impact of COC use on headaches. COCs can induce, alter, or alleviate migraines, and the response is unpredictable. Common strategies used in clinical practice include the use of low-dose monophasic continuous COC or the addition of estrogen therapy around the time of menstruation. Low-dose monophasic continuous COCs are well tolerated but can cause irregular bleeding. The recommendation for dosing is to use three to

Table 41-10. Medications Not Recommended for Use for the Prevention of Migraine[253]

Class IV[a]	Medication
Anticoagulants	Acenocoumarol, coumadin, picotamide
Anticonvulsants	Lamotrigine, tiagabine, clonazepam, oxcarbezapine
Antidepressants	Doxepin, imipramine, nortriptyline, protriptyline, fluvoxamine, paroxetine, sertraline, mirtazepine, phenylzine
Beta-blockers	Acebutolol, bisoprolol, pindolol
5-Hydroxytryptamine antagonists	Methylergonovine
Other	Acetazolamide, lanepitant, montelukast, omega-3 fatty acids, vitamin E

[a]Evidence from uncontrolled studies, case series, case reports expert opinion or no evidence.

four cycles of COC, skipping the placebo days, followed by one pill-free interval. There is a commercial product available that extends the cycle to 91 days (Seasonale®). There are several commercial products that provide low-dose estrogen during the placebo week (e.g., Mircette®, Kariva®, Apri®, Desogen®, and Cyclessa®). Women who are not using oral contraceptives may benefit from the use of estrogen patches. The patch should be started 4 days before menses and used for a total of 4 days.[247] The use of COCs may not be appropriate for all women. Women who are ≥35 years, morbidly obese, have limited mobility, smoke, or have certain medical conditions (such as inherited blood-clotting disorders, diabetes, hypertension, dyslipidemia, or coronary artery disease) may not be candidates for COCs because of the increased risk of stroke. Medications that induce the CYP450 enzymes may increase the metabolism of the COC, thereby decreasing its effectiveness.

Pregnancy

Women who are taking prophylactic therapy and contemplating pregnancy should discuss how to safely taper off their medication with their physician to avoid unnecessary medication exposure to the fetus. Most women with migraines will experience a reduction in the frequency of attacks during pregnancy, especially after the first trimester.[248] Some women will have no change or an increase of attacks that may require treatment. During pregnancy, nonpharmacologic therapies should be used to prevent and treat headache attacks. Acetaminophen may be used safely in pregnancy. Nonsteroidal anti-inflammatory drugs should be limited to use in the first trimester. The antiemetics granisetron, metoclopramide, and ondansetron can be used to treat nausea. Triptans can be considered as a treatment option, but patients should be counseled that although there have not been any reports documenting risk to the fetus, risk cannot be ruled out. Triptans are vasoconstrictive, which may increase the risk of abortion in some individuals. Therefore, the risks and benefits must be considered. Prophylactic therapy during pregnancy is not recommended and should only be used for those patients with severely disabling or frequent attacks. Several of the medications used as prophylactic therapy are known to cause harm to the fetus. Valproic acid and its derivatives (valproate and divalproex) are known to be teratogenic and are listed as an FDA pregnancy category D. Beta-blockers and amitriptyline have been associated with fetal and neonatal abnormalities.[249] Ergot derivatives are category X and contraindicated in pregnancy. Table 41-11 lists medications commonly used in the prevention and treatment of headache and the corresponding FDA pregnancy categories.

Breast-Feeding

There are very little data available regarding treatment of headaches and breast-feeding. Therefore, drug therapy should be avoided during breast-feeding. Drugs should only be used if the benefit outweighs the risk. If drug therapy cannot be avoided while breast-feeding, then it is important to discuss ways to minimize drug exposure to the infant.

Menopause

Migraines may worsen during perimenopause because of fluctuating hormones. After natural menopause, two thirds of women will have an improvement in their migraines.[250] Surgical menopause worsens migraines in two thirds of women. Hormone therapy can alleviate or worsen migraines.[251]

Table 41-11. Pregnancy Risk Factors for Common Medications Used in Headache Treatment[254]

Medication	Risk Factor Category[a]	Comments
Analgesics		
Acetaminophen	B	
Aspirin	C/D	Aspirin risk factor D in full dose in third trimester
Caffeine	B	
NSAIDs		Risk factor D if used in third trimester or near delivery
Ibuprofen	B/D	
Naproxen	B/D	
Opioid Analgesics		Risk factor D if used in high dosages or for prolonged periods near delivery
Butorphanol	C/D	
Codeine	C/D	Potential for abuse
Hydrocodone	C/D	
Meperidine	B/D	
Morphine	C/D	
Oxycodone	B/D	
Serotonin Agonists		All ergot derivatives are contraindicated
Ergot alkaloids	X	
Triptans	C	
Antiemetics		
Metoclopramide	B	
Granisetron	B	
Ondansetron	B	
Promethazine	C	
Prochlorperazine	C	
Isometheptene	C	
Barbiturates		Butalbital is risk factor D if used in high dosages or for prolonged periods near delivery
Butalbital	C/D	
Beta-Blockers		Category D if used in second or third trimester
Atenolol	D	
Metopropolol	C/D	
Nadolol	C/D	
Propranolol	C/D	
Calcium Channel Blockers		
Verapamil	C	
Tricyclic Antidepressants		
Amitriptyline	D	
SSRIs		
Fluoxetine	C	
Paroxetine	D	

(*Continued on next page*)

Medication	Risk Factor Category[a]	Comments
Anticonvulsants		
Divalproex sodium	D	
Gabapentin	C	
Levetiracetam	C/D	
Topiramate	C	
Other		
Dichloralphenazone	B	
Magnesium sulfate	B	
Feverfew		May cause uterine contractions and abortion; avoid use[255]
Butterbur		Likely unsafe when used orally; butterbur preparations containing hepatotoxic pyrrolizidine alkaloid (PA) constituents may be teratogenic and hepatotoxic; information available is insufficient or unreliable about the safety of using butterbur products that do not contain hepatotoxic PAs during pregnancy[256,257]

NSAIDs = nonsteroidal anti-inflammatory drugs; SSRIs = selective serotonin reuptake inhibitors.

[a]Based on definition used by the Food and Drug Administration.

SUMMARY

Headache disorders are common in the general population. Migraine and TTH occur more frequently in women than men. They can occur throughout the lifespan but are most apparent during the reproductive years. Special considerations should be given to women presenting with headache disorders to identify appropriate therapies for their stage of life.

Chapter Summary

Many neurological disorders, such as multiple sclerosis, epilepsy, stroke, chronic fatigue syndrome, fibromyalgia, and headache disorders, have unique characteristics seen in the female population. This implies that there may be a benefit to gender based treatment. When recommending drug therapy it is important to consider the influence of hormones and reproductive goals of the patient. To date, attempted strategies to identify disease and treatment differences between genders has been less than ideal. Although research in this area has increased there is still much work that needs to be done.

References

Additional content available at ***www.ashp.org/womenshealth***

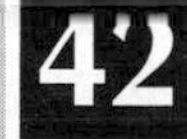

42 Dermatologic Conditions

Neha Shah, MD; Lee E. West, B.S.Pharm.; Kyle Anderson, MD; Bethanee J. Schlosser, MD, Ph.D.; Ginat W. Mirowski, DMD, MD; Dennis P. West, Ph.D., FCCP, CIP

Learning Objectives

1. List the warning signs of melanoma using the ABCDE mnemonic.
2. Describe the basic differences in female skin physiology.
3. Differentiate between the three major types of skin cancer.
4. Compare and contrast the unique types of acne in women and treatment options.

Primary **cutaneous** structural and anatomic differences between men and women include biochemical composition, mechanical properties, functional differences, difference in response to exogenous triggers, cutaneous microvasculature, sensory function, and skin color. Moreover, societal issues forge differences between men and women in relation to skin care. Exemplary of these differences is the fact that women receive more than 90% of cosmetic dermatology procedures in the U.S., although recently the number of men receiving these procedures has increased. Dermatology procedures are often used to improve skin appearance in those with sun damage, chronological aging, and cosmetically disfiguring skin disorders. Besides wrinkles and skin discoloration, signs of skin aging also may include development of varicose veins and actinic keratoses. Open communication between physician and patient is necessary to ensure the patient has realistic expectations of myriad dermatology procedures. Moreover, a combination of different treatment modalities is often used to achieve the most favorable outcomes.

Clinical Presentation

ACNE

Acne is a common condition that affects a majority of adolescents and young adult women that usually occurs on the skin of the face and trunk. Acne is related to four main factors: inflammation, follicular hyperkeratinization, increased secretion of **sebum,** and the *Propionibacterium acnes* colonization of the pilosebaceous unit. Other contributors to the formation of acne include genetic and hormonal factors. Acne can have various clinical presentations including pustules, **nodules,** inflammatory **papules,** and noninflammatory **comedones.**[1] Acne severity may be described from mild to moderate to severe. Mild acne includes closed and open comedones with few inflammatory lesions. Moderate acne exhibits more papules and pustules. Severe acne includes numerous lesions, **cysts,** nodules, and scarring.

Although most adolescents are affected by acne at some point, women are affected by acne into adulthood more commonly than men. There are various etiologies that have been suggested for the presentation of acne in adults. These include, but are not limited to, drug reactions, abnormalities of the endocrine system, and the usage of certain cosmetics. There may be subtle differences between persistent acne (acne that persists from adolescence into adulthood) and late-onset acne.

Lesions of persistent acne typically involve the lower third of the face and neck and are usually deep and tender, and are inflammatory

CASE PRESENTATION

Patient Case: Part 1

A 26-year-old woman presents reporting adult onset **acne** that has persisted for nearly 2 years.

HPI: She indicated that she has tried numerous over-the-counter (OTC) medications and remedies to no avail and has had minimal results with the medication prescribed by her primary care physician: topical clindamycin/benzoyl peroxide about 6 months ago. She used this regimen for nearly 2 months and gave up when she felt that she was not improving and that her facial flushing and persistent malar-distributed erythema was more pronounced than before. She states that her facial redness is definitely more pronounced after hot water to her face and after drinking hot liquids. She reports that she had no significant acne in high school or college and that her parents and siblings do not have a history of any significant acne.

PMH: Noncontributory.

Family history: Noncontributory.

Social history: No tobacco; one or two glasses of wine about 3 times each week. She is an attorney who works an average of 65 hr/wk and travels by air about 3 times/mo.

Medications: Oral contraceptive (generic norethindrone and ethinyl estradiol) for about 2½ years.

Allergies: NKDA.

Vitals: Height, weight, BMI, BP, HR, temp, and RR were within normal range.

Physical exam: Numerous scattered inflammatory lesions on the forehead, central face, and chin. Face is not excessively oily, and lesions are mostly erythematous and papulopustular with a few nodular lesions.

Laboratory values: None.

nodules and papules.[2] Late-onset acne initially presents for the first time at about 25 years of age or later. Late-onset acne may manifest cyclically at premenstruation and concentrates in the chin and perioral region, whereas noncyclical late-onset acne does not follow any pattern.

ROSACEA

Rosacea is a noncontagious, common chronic skin disorder that usually affects the central facial area and sometimes the eye. Vascular changes in facial skin result in intermittent or persistent erythema. Acneform eruptions may be present, including papules, pustules, cysts, and sebaceous hyperplasia. Rosacea varies from mild to severe, consists of several subtypes, and may exhibit exacerbations as a result of external factors, stress, or unknown reasons.[3]

It is estimated that more than 14 million people in the U.S. are affected by rosacea, typically developing after age 30. The reported incidence of rosacea has increased significantly in recent years, possibly because of the maturing of "baby boomers" or more people seeking treatment because of increased awareness. Rosacea affects women more commonly than men, but men tend to develop more severe disease.[4] Erythematotelangiectatic (redness with telangiectasias) rosacea (subtype I) is more prevalent than papulopustular rosacea (subtype II).

The primary symptoms of rosacea, usually in the central facial area, include transient erythema (flushing), nontransient erythema, papules and pustules, and telangiectasia.[5] Primarily located on the cheeks, nose, chin, and forehead, it is less commonly found behind the ears, on the chest, neck, back, and the extremities. The clinical features of rosacea vary with type, duration, age, and periods of flare. **Pruritus** is not usually associated with rosacea.

Pathophysiology

ACNE

Pathophysiology of acne in women includes increased sebum production, comedo formation, *Propionibacterium acnes* colonization, and inflammation (Figure 42-1 for the mechanism of formation of acne lesions). Knowledge of pathophysiology should influence treatment. Primary pathophysiologic factors in acne are sebaceous hyperplasia with seborrhea, ductal hypercornification, *Propionibacterium acnes* colonization of the duct, and inflammation and immune response.

Acne therapy is directed at one or more of the four mechanisms for lesion formation:

1. Reducing sebum production
2. Preventing clumping of keratinocytes
3. Decreasing *P. acnes*
4. Decreasing inflammation

The development of acne includes an innate phase initiated by interleukin-1α. The next phase of acne development results in comedo formation, and the final phase includes observable inflammation.[6] Acne scarring is caused by the loss of collagen, such

Figure 42-1. Mechanism of formation of acne lesions. Treatment involves interrupting one or more of these pathways, e.g., reducing sebum production with isotretinoin or reducing *P. acnes* levels with antibiotic use.

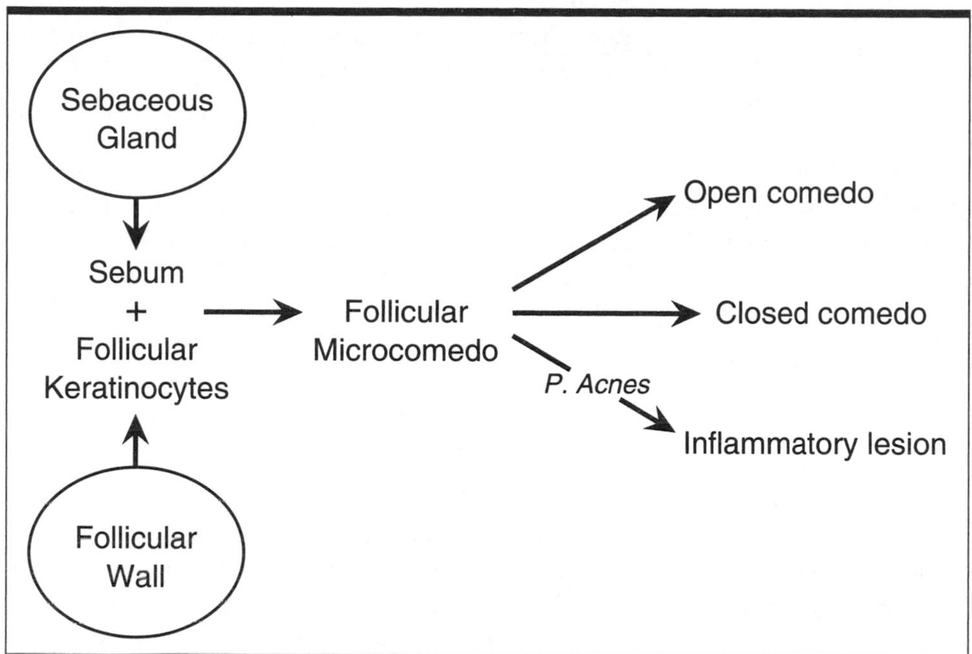

as ice pick scars, or excess of collagen, resulting in keloids or hypertrophic scars. Acne can also occur around menopause, which includes inflammatory papules and nodules that are deep. Adult acne in women is usually very difficult to treat because of its persistence. Thus, it is important for patients to adhere strictly to treatment and management of acne.[2]

ROSACEA

Although there is much speculation about inflammatory mechanisms in rosacea, there are several well-known factors that may aggravate the condition. Inflammatory mediators such as substance P, histamine, serotonin, bradykinin, and prostaglandin have been considered possible factors in rosacea. One theory postulates that rosacea symptoms represent an inflammatory process, a neutrophilic dermatosis, in which inflammatory mediators, especially neutrophils, and immune cells mediate the vascular, inflammatory, and hyperplasia of rosacea.[7]

It is also postulated that the facial flushing in rosacea may be caused by direct action of vascular smooth muscle or mediated indirectly through local innervation and vasomotor activity.[8] The incidence of migraines is up to 3 times more common in rosacea patients than in nonrosacea patients, indicating a possible microcirculatory disturbance.[4]

Phymas occur more frequently in men than women.[9] A higher incidence in men is possibly due to androgenic influence.[9]

Hair follicle mites, *Demodex folliculorum* and *Demodex brevis,* are normally occurring human parasites that feed on sebum in the hair follicle and are found in increased numbers in rosacea. Although it is not clear what role *Demodex* plays in rosacea, some theories include aggravation of rosacea by inducing inflammatory or allergic reactions, blockage of hair follicles, and introduction of bacteria carried by mites.[10]

Guidelines and Position Statements

Current published guidelines exist for acne from the American Academy of Dermatology and from the Global Alliance to Improve Outcomes in Acne, and for rosacea from the American Acne and Rosacea Society.[11-14]

Prevention

ACNE

Most treatments work primarily to prevent the formation of new acne lesions and have minimal impact on existing lesions.

Stress

Studies confirm what many patients suspect: Stress tends to aggravate acne.[15] In response to stress, immunoreactive nerve fibers may stimulate sebaceous gland activity and provoke inflammatory reactions via mast cells.[16]

Diet

There is no evidence that diet, with the exception of ingestion of iodine, has any influence on the development of acne. However, it is important to minimize contact of acne-prone skin areas with oils that may enhance the likelihood of follicular plugging. Patients need to be advised to keep greasy fingers away from the facial area.

ROSACEA

Although some known triggers for rosacea—such as ultraviolet (UV) radiation from the sun and spicy foods that trigger cutaneous vasodilation—may be avoided, flares often still occur. Several external triggers have been identified that may exacerbate rosacea. The trigger factors vary in individual patients. It may be helpful for a patient to determine which factor or factors affect her by keeping a diary of flushing occurrences and the factors present on that occasion. Avoidance of trigger factors can prevent some rosacea symptoms and benefit quality of life.

Several external triggers have been identified that may exacerbate rosacea, including weather (sun exposure, heat, cold, humidity, and wind), food (spicy foods, fruits, dairy products, and vegetables), alcohol, hot beverages, exercise, hot baths, stress, and cosmetics (soaps, shampoo, moisturizers, perfume, aftershave, and sunscreens).

Cosmetics

Facial skin in rosacea patients is very sensitive to many ingredients in ordinary cosmetics. Products for sensitive skin should have minimal amount of ingredients, avoiding the more irritating chemicals and potential allergens.[17] Identifying some typical irritants may be helpful. Ideally, products for use on the face should be noncomedogenic, nonacnegenic, nonirritating, hypoallergenic, and cosmetically acceptable.[18]

Sunscreens

Sun exposure is the most prevalent aggravating factor for rosacea; therefore, use of sunscreens to areas of rosacea involvement is emphasized. Careful selection is necessary because sunscreen ingredients may cause irritation in a particularly sensitive skin area. The least irritating products are those containing zinc oxide or titanium dioxide. Protective agents, such as dimethicone and cyclomethicone, may mitigate sunscreen irritation in some patients.[19]

Treatment

ACNE

Acne therapy is directed at one or more of four mechanisms for lesion formation: reducing sebum production, preventing clumping of keratinocytes, decreasing *P. acnes*, and decreasing inflammation. The treatment options in Table 42-1 represent general recommendations for acne management. Many acne treatments are avoided during pregnancy because of risk-to-benefit issues. Female patients should be advised which medications pose risks if pregnancy is a possibility. Systemic antiacne treatments are not commonly used during pregnancy. If acne treatment is needed during pregnancy or in women trying to become pregnant, oral and topical erythromycin are acceptable options.

Topical Treatment

A majority of acne patients are treated with topical therapy. Most commonly prescribed in mild acne, topical therapies include benzoyl peroxide, topical antibiotics, and topical retinoids. Inflamed lesions are treated best by benzoyl peroxide or topical antibiotics. Benzoyl peroxide or topical retinoids work most effectively on noninflamed lesions. Combination topical preparations are commercially available and may be best suited for patients with both inflammatory and noninflammatory lesions.[6]

During pregnancy, topical therapy is the preferred method for acne treatment. Not all topicals, including some OTC products, are safe in pregnancy. According to the U.S. Food and Drug Administration (FDA) Pregnancy Category Rating, erythromycin, clindamycin, metronidazole, and azelaic acid are Class B (no evidence of increased risk in humans), whereas benzoyl peroxide, tretinoin, and adapalene are classified as Class C (animal studies show increased fetal risk, and human studies are lacking but potential benefits may warrant use of the drug in pregnant women despite potential risks). Tazarotene is a Class X drug (studies in animals or humans have demonstrated fetal abnormalities and/or there is positive evidence of human fetal risk based on adverse reaction data from investigational or marketing experience, and the risks involved in use of the drug in pregnant women clearly outweigh potential benefits).

Systemic Treatment

Antibiotics

Oral antibiotics are prescribed for moderate to severe inflammatory acne and often in combination with topical agents that reduce follicular plugging.

Table 42-1. Acne Therapy by Lesion Type and Severity[13,14]

Severity	Lesion Type	First choice	Alternatives	Alternatives for Women	Maintenance
Mild	Comedonal	**TR**	Alternative TR or AA or SA	TR	**TR**
Mild	Papular/pustular	**TR + TA**	Alternate TA agent + alternative TR or AA	TR + TA	**TR**
Moderate	Papular/pustular	**OA + TR ± BPO**	Alternate OA + alternate TR ± BPO	Oral antiandrogens + TR/azelaic acid ± TA	**TR ± BPO**
Moderate	Nodular	**OA + TR + BPO**	Oral isotretinoin or alternate OA + alternate TR ± BPO/AA	AN + TR ± OA ± alternative TA	**TR ± BPO**
Severe	Nodular/conglobate	**Oral isotretinoin**	High-dose OA + TR + BPO	High-dose AN + TR ± alternative TA	**TR ± BPO**

AA = azelaic acid; AN = oral antiandrogen; BPO = benzoyl peroxide; OA= oral antibiotic; SA = salicylic acid; TA = topical antimicrobial; TR = topical retinoid.

The mechanism of action reduces the inflammatory mediators and reduces *P. acnes* colonization. Antibiotic resistance has become a significant problem in recent years, which has lead to combination benzoyl peroxide and topical antibiotics. Several studies have shown decreased antibiotic resistance with combination therapy using benzoyl peroxide resulting in increased efficacy of topical antibiotics. Recommendations to help prevent the development of resistance include the following[20]:

Avoid monotherapy; use with topical retinoids and/or benzoyl peroxide.

- Use oral antibiotics for moderate to severe acne.
- Recommend an average minimum oral antibiotic treatment of 6–8 weeks to determine efficacy and maximum treatment up to 18 weeks.
- Retreat with the same antibiotic; treat with benzoyl peroxide topically for 1 week between treatments to reduce resistant organisms.
- Do not use concurrent topical and systemic antibacterial treatment with chemically dissimilar antibiotics.
- Use with hormonal therapy in women if appropriate.
- Counsel patients on the importance of compliance.

Isotretinoin

Because isotretinoin is embryotoxic and teratogenic, it is known to cause major fetal malformations. Consequently, iPledge™, a computer-based registry, was developed to help prevention pregnancies during therapy. Patients, healthcare providers, and pharmacies must all be registered with the program before the drug is dispensed, and certain conditions must be met every month, especially by women of childbearing age, including a pregnancy test and monitoring of liver function.

Severe nodulocystic acne that is unresponsive to conventional therapy is best treated with oral isotretinoin. Studies have shown a 90% decrease in nodular lesions as well as a decrease in facial scarring. Isotretinoin works by decreasing the activity and size of sebaceous glands. The most common adverse effect is excessive drying of the face and mucous membranes. Hepatotoxicity and hypertriglyceridemia have been reported, leading to requirements of periodic monitoring of liver function tests and lipid levels. Isotretinoin is highly teratogenic; therefore, strict documentation of two different forms of birth control is required for women of childbearing capability.

Hormonal Therapy

Hormonal therapy (see Chapter 19: Hormonal Contraception is an excellent choice for women who need oral contraceptives for gynecologic reasons, for female patients with moderate to severe acne or with seborrhea/acne/hirsutism/alopecia symptoms, useful as part of combination therapy in women with or without endocrine abnormalities, and sometimes used in women with late-onset acne.

Hormonal therapy is designed to decrease sebum production by decreasing androgenic stimulation of the sebaceous gland and acts to normalize follicular desquamation. This therapy, useful in treating acne in women with elevated or normal serum androgens, consists of agents that block androgen production as well as antiandrogens.[21] Other hormonal therapies include enzyme inhibitors and oral isotretinoin.

Estrogen therapy is of limited use in female patients because of the high dosage of estrogen required for suppression of sebum production as well as increased side effects. Nevertheless, oral contraceptives are used as an alternate treatment for moderate acne in women. The dosage required is greater than that required to suppress ovulation. Acne responds to as low as 0.035 mg of ethinyl estradiol, but higher dosages may be required for enhanced efficacy. Norgestimate and ethinyl estradiol in combination have been shown to decrease androgen production by increasing sex hormone–binding globulin. Moreover, the oral contraceptive that contains drospirenone has also been reported to be an effective approach in selected women.

Antiandrogens

Antiandrogens are androgen receptor blockers. Pregnancy should be avoided during antiandrogen therapy. Examples of antiandrogens are spironolactone and flutamide. Spironolactone, an antiandrogen and inhibitor of 5α-reductase, reduces sebum production. Dosage for acne therapy for women with therapy-resistant acne is up to 100 mg twice daily. Side effects are dose dependent and can be lessened by initiating therapy with dosages as low as 25 mg/day. Side effects include hyperkalemia, irregular menses, breast tenderness, headache, and fatigue. Flutamide, an androgen receptor blocker, is used in combination with oral contraceptives in acne therapy for women. The use of this drug is limited because of reports of fatal hepatitis requiring monitoring of liver function during therapy.

ROSACEA

Early treatment often inhibits progression from mild to severe forms, but because early symptoms are usually mild, rosacea diagnosis and treatment is often delayed until some progression of severity has occurred. In some cases, patients mistake rosacea symptoms for acne and may self-treat with acne therapy products. Although rosacea and acne therapy do have some common treatment approaches, some nonprescription products, especially alcohol-based topicals, may aggravate rosacea and induce undue irritation in an already easily irritated skin.

Rosacea severity may fluctuate with stress and age, and even if signs and symptoms are calmed, it may be necessary to continue treatment. Chronic indefinite therapy with topical or oral medications is not uncommon in the management of rosacea. Treatment goals are to reduce rosacea signs and symptoms, such as inflammatory lesions, erythema, flares, burning, and stinging.

Telangiectasias do not respond to topical or oral treatment, and some laser procedural approaches may be indicated. Pharmacologic agents used successfully for the treatment of erythema, papules, and pustules of rosacea typically have anti-inflammatory activity, and some also act as antioxidants.[22] Antibiotic therapy may be beneficial in early stages of rhinophyma, but surgery may be the best option for advanced rhinophyma. See Table 42-2 for treatment options for rosacea signs and symptoms.

Sex Differences

STRUCTURAL AND ANATOMIC DIFFERENCES

Skin thickness in men is consistently greater than that in women. Although male skin gradually thins with age, women maintain constant skin thickness until onset of menopause, at which point skin begins to thin.[23] Women have a lower baseline skin collagen density than men, and even though both sexes lose collagen at the same rate with aging, women have the visual appearance of aging faster than men because of this disproportionate decrease in collagen.[24]

There are no significant sex differences in subcutaneous fat during adolescence, but after puberty, subcutaneous fat in women begins to increase in comparison with relative body mass. Women's distribution of fat is quite different from that of men. Men tend to accumulate fat in the upper body and the abdomen, whereas women tend to accumulate fat in gluteal and lower-body areas more readily.[25] These differences in fat distribution between men and women are related to lipoprotein lipase, which catalyzes lipids into lipoproteins. Lipoprotein lipase activity and mRNA levels in women are greater in the gluteal regions compared

Table 12-2. Treatment Options for Rosacea Signs and Symptoms

Symptom/Sign	Systemic Treatment	Topical Treatment	Other
Flushing	Clonidine β-blockers (atenolol, nadolol propranolol)	—	—
Erythema	Metronidazole Tetracycline Azathioprine	Metronidazole Azelaic acid Tacrolimus	Cosmetics (cover or camouflage)
Papules/pustules	Tetracycline Isotretinoin	Metronidazole Sodium sulfacetamide with or without sulfur Azelaic acid	—
D. folliculorum	Ivermectin	Crotamiton cream Permethrin cream Ivermectin	—
Ocular	Tetracycline	Antibacterials	—
Rhinophyma	Isotretinoin	—	Surgery Laser
Telangiectasias	—	—	Surgery Laser

with men, in whom lipoprotein lipase activity is increased in the abdominal regions.[26]

The stratum corneum is the outermost layer of the skin, which is composed of dead cells that lack a nucleus. It contains high levels of sphingolipids, including lipid ceramides. Men have been shown to have little to no change in sphingolipid concentration throughout life, whereas women have been shown to have significant increases in ceramides 1 and 2 and a decrease in ceramides 3 and 6 from puberty to adulthood. After menopause, changes occur that result in an increase in ceramide 3 and a decrease in ceramide 2.[27] Moreover, lipid changes in stratum corneum are correlated with changes in female hormone patterns. These changes in ceramide levels in women can affect important barrier functions of the stratum corneum, which include protection against transepidermal water loss (TEWL) and solutes as well as prevention of entry of harmful substances. Although altered skin ceramides are also implicated as a possible aggravating factor in several skin disorders, including psoriasis and atopic dermatitis, this relationship to sex differences is unclear. Some commercially available topical formulations contain lipids similar to endogenous intracellular ceramides and are used in the treatment of such skin disorders.[28]

MECHANICAL PROPERTIES

In general, mechanical properties of the skin, including the stratum corneum, are consistent between men and women.[29] Skin friction properties—known as skin smoothness, an important cosmetic indicator—have shown no overall sex differences. Skin elasticity and torsion extensibility have also not shown significant differences between the sexes.[30,31] Of note, as one measure to assess skin integrity, separation of dermal and epidermal layers of skin through controlled suctioning proved that women have longer onset to blistering times then men. This feature may be both age dependent and hormone related.[32]

FUNCTIONAL DIFFERENCES

With hydration, extensibility of female skin increases, whereas male skin does not. This may be due to differences in dermal thickness, female skin being thinner on average.[33] Some sex differences are seen with sebum secretion, men having been found to have increased sebum secretion.[34] For example, the hormone-dependant pilosebaceous unit in the skin shows a male-predominant increase in activity during puberty. Several hormones, including thyroid-stimulating hormone, corticotropin, follicle-stimulating hormone, and luteinizing hormone, are indirect activators of sebaceous glands. Sebum secretion is generally higher over the entire lifespan of men vs. women. After the age of 50 years, male sebum secretion remains nearly constant, whereas sebum secretion of women measurably decreases. The most probable cause of this decrease may be related to ovarian hormones. Likewise, testosterone activity is not shown to correlate with sebum secretion.[35]

DIFFERENCES IN RESPONSE TO EXOGENOUS TRIGGERS

Reported cases of irritant dermatitis in women may be increased over that of men. A probable cause may relate to differences in exposure to agents that may be responsible for occupational irritant dermatitis. When testing skin irritability using a primary irritant such as sodium lauryl sulfate, no sex differences are found. Also, there are no sex differences evident in studies that have compared normal subjects with those with hand dermatitis. Moreover, there is no increase in susceptibility between male and female subjects to develop cumulative irritant dermatitis.[36-38] However, significant differences are found in women when correlating irritant dermatitis with hormonal changes. Increased levels of TEWL are one indicator of skin barrier disruption. Of note, lower TEWL occurs on days when estrogen and progesterone secretion are high. During lower secretion of estrogen and progesterone, higher levels of TEWL are demonstrated. These findings indicate that skin barrier function is diminished in the days before menses in comparison with the days before ovulation.[39]

CUTANEOUS MICROVASCULATURE

Differences are found in the cutaneous microvasculature between men and women, and these changes may be related to hormone differences, as evidenced throughout the aging process as well as during pregnancy and the menstrual cycle. In addition, vascular disorders, such as Raynaud's phenomenon, are more prevalent in women during reproductive years.[40] Skin blood flow also varies with the menstrual cycle. Blood flow is highest in the preovulatory phase and lowest during the luteal phase. Another indicator is a woman's response to cold temperatures. The greatest vasoconstriction response from the cold and the longest recovery time is during the luteal phase. Estrogen may also affect circulation by stimulation of the sympathetic nervous system because a lower resting blood flow is noted in women younger than age 50.[41,42] An underlying cause of this change in blood flow may be due to estrogen-associated increased sympathetic tone because of activation of $\alpha 2$-adrenoreceptors rather than a structural or functional difference. When skin is tested by an endothelium-dependent vasodilator, a higher response is seen premenopause rather than postmenopause, implying that changes in skin vasculature correlate with aging in women.[43]

Vasodilatation of the skin occurs more rapidly in women than men. However, the degree of vasodilatation is not seen to be different in men and women.[44] Another measurement of skin vasculature is transcutaneous oxygen pressure. This measurement determines changes of blood flow in the skin based on oxygen pressure changes. Higher levels of transcutaneous oxygen pressure are found in postpubescent females compared to postpubescent males, but no changes are found between prepubescent girls and boys.[45,46]

SENSORY FUNCTION

Sensory functions of the skin include changes, such as heat, cold, pain, and pressure, resulting in external responses. Women are able to distinguish between smaller changes in temperature and to be more sensitive to changes in pain than men. Cutaneous receptors mediate thermal and pain responses. Another sensation is pain through skin pricking, with women having a lower threshold of pain in adulthood; however, both sexes increase pain sensation thresholds as aging continues.[47] Possible explanations include sex differences in the function and structure of the nervous system and differences of the skin vasculature.[24]

SKIN COLOR

Interestingly, skin color has been found to be lighter in women than men worldwide. The skin color of both men and women darkens during aging. Factors that may account for these differences are carotene, hemoglobin, differences in **melanin,** and hormonal factors. Other external factors that may contribute include exposure to sun and type of clothing. This progression includes a change from infancy, when where both boys and girls darken. After puberty, women begin to lighten; men lighten as well, but not to the same degree. Throughout late adulthood, both sexes begin to progressively darken. Effects of testosterone and estrogen cause the skin to darken.[24] Skin color is often referenced by phototype—i.e., self-described reaction to sun exposure (Table 42-3).

HAIR GROWTH

There are also differences in hair distribution and density between men and women. Factors that affect hair density include the environment and hormones. Androgen-sensitive hair growth in the body includes areas such face, scalp, axilla, and pubic regions. This is evident in hormone-related conditions such as hirsutism, a female condition of excess hair

Table 42-3 Skin Phototypes Based on Reaction to Sun Exposure

Skin Type	Description	Generalized Characteristics
1	Always burns easily, never tans	Light skin color, often blue eyes, very light skin
2	Usually burns easily, tans minimally	Light skin color, often blue eyes, fair skin
3	Burns moderately, tans gradually	Light brown skin
4	Burns minimally, tans readily	Moderate brown skin, olive skin
5	Rarely burns, tans profusely	Deeply pigmented, dark olive skin
6	Never burns	Darkly pigmented, brown/black skin

Source: Adapted from Fitzpatrick TB. The validity and practicality of sun-reactive skin types I through VI. *Arch Dermatol.* 1988;124:869-871.

growth that is due to increased levels of testosterone, which can be triggered by obesity and age.[48]

There are multiple causes of hirsutism, ranging from excess androgens, nonandrogenic causes, medication side effects, and idiopathic causes, with excess androgens accounting for 75% to 85% of cases. Examples of disease states giving an increase in androgens are polycystic ovary disease, which accounts for 80% of patients with excess androgens; 21-hydroxylase deficiency; insulin-resistant hyperandrogenic syndrome; Cushing's syndrome; hyperprolactinemia; and androgen-secreting tumors of the ovaries or adrenal glands. Medications associated with hirsutism are cyclosporine, phenytoin, oral contraceptives containing progesterone, penicillamine, danazol, metoclopramide, methyldopa, reserpine, and phenothiazines.

Androgenetic Alopecia: Female Pattern Hair Loss

Female pattern hair loss is a condition that affects women throughout the aging process. The range of severity can include the frontal scalp and crown, but in more severe cases can also affect parietal and occipital regions. Hair loss develops gradually and can develop as early as teenage years throughout late middle age. Hair thinning usually occurs at the outset of the scalp. In addition, there is a reduction in the density of the hair along with a widening of the central part.

Causes of female pattern hair loss include genetic factors, suggesting that hair loss is inherited in a polygenic fashion. This may explain the wide range of symptomatology, although studies suggest that there may be some relationship as women diagnosed with hyperandrogenism more commonly experience balding. Balding can also occur as a symptom of an androgen-secreting tumor. Women with female pattern hair loss may be socially stigmatized and can experience low self-confidence and negative body image. Medical treatment available includes oral antiandrogen therapy and topical minoxidil. These treatments cannot fully reverse hair loss but in optimal situations stimulate modest hair growth.[49]

Skin Cancer

In general, skin cancer broadly includes malignant melanoma and nonmelanoma skins cancers (squamous cell carcinoma and basal cell carcinoma). Risks, prevention, and treatment of skin cancers demonstrate some differences between men and women. Basal cell carcinoma is the most common type of skin cancer, followed by squamous cell carcinoma. These skin cancers result in a very low mortality in comparison with other cancers. A key distinction in this relationship is what stage the cancer is when diagnosed and what type of treatment is used. Common risk factors include lighter complexion, origination in Northern hemisphere, and sun exposure.[50] Risk increases with the amount of UV exposure from unprotected time in the sun, as well as from tanning beds, and includes frequent airplane travel. An increased incidence of squamous cell carcinoma is noted after extensive x-ray exposure, such as seen with radiation therapy, or after traumatic burns. Basal cell carcinoma and squamous cell carcinoma both originate in epithelial cells.

MALIGNANT MELANOMA

Although malignant melanoma is one of the less common types of skin cancer, it is unfortunately one of the more serious. The major risk factor for malignant melanoma is exposure to sun, particularly exposure to UV rays.[51] Sun exposure affects DNA of cells, including melanocytes, the pigment-producing cells of the body. Once the DNA of these cells is mutated, the cells begin to grow abnormally and invade surrounding tissues. Diagnoses of melanoma would include skin biopsy and pathologic determination of cancer cells. Early-stage melanoma can be diagnosed and treated with high success rates. Treatment of early-stage, nonmetastasized melanoma is surgical excision. Melanoma, like other cancers, metastasize and spread to other regions of the body, specifically internal organs, lymph nodes, blood, and bones. Once this occurs, the success rate of treatment is much lower and usually includes interferon therapy, along with other treatments that are currently being studied.[51,52]

Genetic risk factors for melanoma include a family history of the disease. The presence of moles, specifically atypical moles that do not present usual signs of skin cancer, may prove to be malignant. A change in birthmarks or moles may be significant. For pigmented lesions of the skin, warning signs of melanoma include asymmetry (one half unlike the other half); border irregular, scalloped, or poorly defined; color varied from one area to another (shades of tan and brown, black; sometimes white, red, or blue); diameter (melanomas are usually >6 mm, the size of a pencil eraser, when diagnosed, but they can be smaller); and evolving (a mole or skin lesion that looks different from the rest or is changing in size, shape, or color). A useful mnemonic to remember the warning signs of melanoma is ABCDE (Asymmetry, Border, Color, Diameter, and Evolving). In general, melanoma lesions have the following characteristics:

- A **A**symmetric in outline
- B Have an irregular, scalloped, or poorly defined **B**order
- C Nonuniform **C**olor (may be tan, brown, black; or, less commonly, may be white, red, or blue)
- D **D**iameter >6 mm
- E A history of **E**volving in size, becoming itchy or painful

Of these screening guidelines, size is the least predictive factor because skin cancers may initially be very small in size.[51,52]

Although melanomas may commonly originate from birthmarks or moles, they can occur at any anatomic site, such as subungual (under the nails), palmar-plantar surfaces, and mucous membranes, including vulvar tissue. Skin cancers of the vulva and other mucous membrane tissue have a worsened prognosis and thus deserve careful screening. Because men and women differ in clothing styles and skin area exposed to radiation from the sun, the more common anatomic sites for cutaneous melanoma in women are the upper back and legs.[51,52]

The risks and prevention for malignant melanoma are the same during pregnancy as for nonpregnant women. Studies have not shown an increased risk of melanoma or any decrease in survival rate for patients with melanoma during pregnancy. Pregnant must be as vigilant women as nonpregnant women in skin self-exams for abnormal moles. Although diagnosis is often initiated by dermatology, early- and late-stage melanoma care and treatment are managed by oncology.

Sex-differentiated melanoma is well described through the example of vulvar melanoma, which represents <1% of all melanomas even though it is disproportionately more common as a vulvar disorder. Vulvar melanoma is commonly diagnosed around age 60 and usually includes a family history of melanoma. Vulvar melanoma may be located on the labia minora, labia majora, clitoris, or periclitoris region. Most commonly, vulvar melanomas are located on the labia majora and minora. Symptoms of vulvar melanoma may include bleeding, mass, lump, swelling, abscess, discharge, pruritus, pain, dysuria, nonhealing sore, spotting, alteration of urine stream, and foul odor. Risk factors for vulvar melanoma usually do not include exposure to sun, but other risk factors are being investigated along with genetic associations. Vulvar melanoma may occur concurrently with cutaneous melanoma.[53] Treatment of all stages of vulvar melanoma usually is managed by oncology/gynecology and not by dermatology, even though initial diagnosis may occur in dermatology.[54]

SQUAMOUS CELL CARCINOMA

Actinic keratoses, precursor cells for squamous cell carcinoma, are more commonly found on men than women, are usually found on sun-exposed areas of the body, and are manifested as erythematous, scaly, and patchy. Because approximately 5% of actinic keratoses progress to squamous cell carcinomas, it is recommended to remove actinic keratoses when feasible.[55] Although squamous cell carcinomas usually develop on sun-exposed areas, it is possible to develop squamous cell carcinomas on non–sun-exposed areas. When this occurs, there is a higher risk for metastasis and thus a graver prognosis. Other sites that have a higher risk of squamous cell carcinoma include skin ulcers, radiation therapy sites, and prior burn sites.[55]

BASAL CELL CARCINOMA

Because basal cell carcinoma also tends to occur on sun-exposed areas, sex differentiation mostly relates to clothing styles and area of repeatedly exposed skin. Consequently, basal cell carcinoma commonly occurs on the nose and other facial sun-exposed areas, but a bit less commonly in women because of increased use of cosmetics and sunscreens. Basal cell carcinoma manifestations include papulonodular and ulcerative lesions. Although basal cell carcinoma may be locally invasive and destructive to surrounding tissue, it is rarely judged to be metastatic. Common anatomic sites for basal cell carcinoma include nasolabial fold, eyelids and periorbital region, pinna, forehead, scalp, and postauricular region.[56]

Hormone-related Skin Changes

AGING SKIN

Degenerative Changes

Aging skin and sex differentiation is a real phenomenon. Degenerative changes that occur naturally with aging are inhibited by the ability of estrogen and sex steroids to help the regeneration of dermal fibroblasts and proper blood supply to tissues. Especially for women, the presence of estrogen receptors in the skin confirms some element of estrogen-dependent skin activity. For instance, once the influence of the estrogen is removed at menopause, there is an acceleration of skin-related aging changes. Clinical signs include loss of elasticity, reduction of epidermal thickness, reduction in collagen content, elastic fiber degeneration, increased wrinkling, and dryness. Other changes that occur with aging include decreased growth of body hair and decreased sebum production. Aging of the skin may be viewed as related to photoaging and chronological aging. Photoaging refers to changes of the skin associated with sun exposure, whereas chronological aging is based on natural degenerative changes of the skin.

Skin aging on a molecular level involves changes in the skin that take place after UV damage. Skin healing after UV damage is very similar to healing that takes place after wound damage. These changes affect components of the microinflammatory model of skin aging. Once skin damage occurs, normal cellular immune responses begin the migration of immune cells, proliferation and differentiation of cells, and enhanced immune-response activities in cells. Most of these cellular responses are directed at the healing of the extracellular matrix. Once dead cells of the extracellular matrix are removed, new extracellular matrix components are made but may not fit the original cell matrix, resulting in an imperfect structure that is seen in many UV-damaged cells.[57] On a more microscopic level, when infectious agents penetrate the skin's barrier, the immune system responds by removing these agents. This removal includes the killing of cells through the release of collagenases and reactive oxygen species. Release of toxic free radicals into surrounding cells affects fibroblast and keratinocyte function.[57] Continual progression of this cycle following UV damage over time accelerates skin aging.

Collagen Content and Wrinkling

Collagen content of skin is an important consideration because it decreases with both chronologic aging and photoaging.[57] Sex differentiation is quite important to collagen content in skin because in the initial 5 years after menopause, approximately 30% of collagen is lost. During the next 20 years, an additional 2% is lost every year.[58]

Women's skin is more vulnerable to manifestations of reduced collagen content, as made evident by wrinkling. Skin thickness is decreased as elastic fibers and collagen production are decreased. The prevalence of dry skin in older persons can also be attributed to a decrease in ceramide levels.[59] When aging epidermis begins to fail to maturate fully, its structure becomes looser, and as **corneocyte** cohesion lessens, there is more epidermal water loss and drier skin. Application of moisturizers or emollients is an important part of skin maintenance as a person ages.[60]

Exfoliants

Exfoliant ingredients include salicylic acid, also called beta hydroxy acid, and the alpha hydroxy acids,

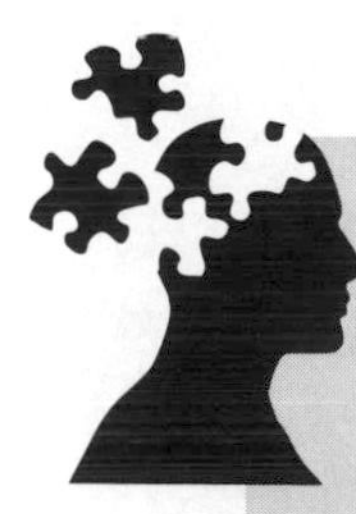

Therapeutic Challenge:

What benefit or risk exists for the use of hormone therapy in women going through menopause and age-related skin changes?

which include glycolic, lactic citric, malic, mandelic, and tartaric acids. The purpose of exfoliants is to increase sloughing of corneocytes from the stratum corneum by decreasing cell cohesion between.[61] By removing some of these drier outer cells, there may be some improvement in surface wrinkles, melasma, and dryness.

Antioxidants

Antioxidants are used for anti-aging and not for moisturizing properties. Oxygen radicals, such as hydrogen peroxide, are formed in skin and are damaging to surrounding tissue that contains natural antioxidants, such as catalase and ascorbic acid, to prevent oxidative damage. It is unknown whether these naturally occurring antioxidants are effective in topical application.

Dryness

Skin dryness also relates to sex differences. Women's skin is more vulnerable because many changes related to dry skin are dependent on circulating levels of estrogen. Changes that occur because of photoaging include wrinkles and furrows, **solar lentigines,** telangiectasias, change in pigmentation, purpura, actinic keratoses, nonmelanoma skin cancers, and melanomas. Changes that can be attributed to chronological aging include dryness, increased fragility, decreased epidermal and dermal thickness, fragmentation of elastic fibers, decreased sebum production, decreased number and function of apocrine sweat glands, and decreased growth of body hair.[62] Loss of estrogen affects the pilosebaceous unit, resulting in hair loss. This process occurs through estrogen's regulation of the telogen-anagen transition of the hair follicle.[57]

In premenopausal skin, there is a high content of glycosaminoglycans located in the extracellular matrix. Because of the hydrophilic nature of these glycosaminoglycans, water is attracted to dermis. This supports skin hydration and maintains suppleness. Thus, the loss of glycosaminoglycans because of postmenopausal decreased circulating estrogen increases the potential for dryness, wrinkling, and suppleness.[58]

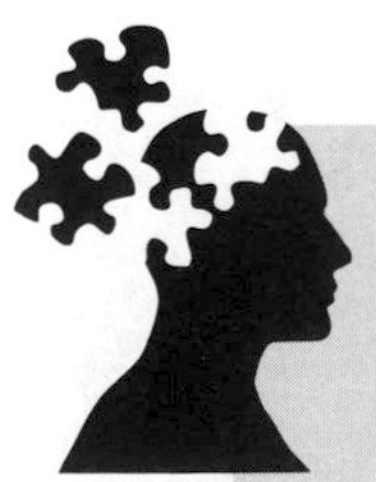

Therapeutic Challenge:

What benefit or risk exists for the use of alpha hydroxy acids for the treatment of surface wrinkling?

Moisturizers

Types of moisturizers include occlusives, humectants, hydrophilic matrices, and sunscreens. The additives found in moisturizers include exfoliants, antioxidants, humectants, emollients, and bioactive ingredients.

Vulvodynia

Vulvodynia is a general term that can imply many different underlying conditions (see Chapter 39: Genitourinary Disorders). Determining the type and cause of vulvodynia is the most essential step in deciding treatment options.[63] Symptoms include a wide range of discomfort, including burning, itching, pain, irritation, rawness, and soreness. Vulvodynia can occur with or without an underlying cause. Primary vulvodynia usually occurs without an underlying cause, whereas secondary vulvodynia can present as a symptom of another condition.[64] Secondary vulvodynia is associated with an observable lesion in the vulvar or vaginal area. There are three dermatologic conditions that can present as vulvodynia: dermatitis, psoriasis, and lichen sclerosis.[63] Vulvar pain can also be experienced acutely by small vulvar fissures and is the most common cause of vulvodynia.

Other conditions that can result in vulvar pain include desquamative inflammatory vulvovaginitis, chronic vulvovaginal candidiasis, vulvar aphthae, drug eruptions, bullous and autoimmune disease, atrophic vulvovaginitis, group B streptococcal vaginitis, allergy to seminal fluid, genital herpes, Crohn's disease, and vulvar varices. Primary vulvodynia can be caused by conditions such as neuropathy, referred pain syndrome, pelvic floor dysfunction, and sometimes psychiatric considerations with a normal vulva. Primary vulvodynia usually is a more chronic condition. Many of the women experience dyspareunia, which can result in lack of interest in sex. Primary vulvodynia is divided into two categories based on whether the symptom of dyspareunia is present.

Pregnancy

There are recognizable skin changes that occur in relation to pregnancy-related hormonal changes in women. Some conditions commonly occur during pregnancy. These conditions include melasma (chloasma), pruritic urticarial papules and plaques (PUPP) of pregnancy, and *Herpes gestationis*. As an example, one of the most common skin disorders in pregnancy that may involve pharmacotherapeutic approaches (often after pregnancy and nursing are completed) is melasma.

Melasma

Melasma presents in three clinical patterns—malar, mandibular, and centrofacial—and is common in women of skin phototypes 4–6 (Table 42-3) in areas of prevalent UV exposure.[65] Typical cases of melasma include a gradual and symmetric progression of pigmentation to adjacent areas. Symptoms typically improve in winter and can worsen during summer.[66] Possible causes of melasma include genetic predisposition, use of oral contraceptives, pregnancy (because of the fluctuations of female hormones), endocrine dysfunction, and exposure to UV light.[65]

A form of melasma, called chloasma or the "mask of pregnancy," is specific to the pigment disorder seen during pregnancy. Women that experience chloasma during pregnancy may have symptoms disappear within a few months after giving birth. There are cases in which chloasma persists. Theories suggest that pregnancy-induced melasma is due to increase in hormones of the ovary, placenta, and pituitary.[67] Moreover, increases in estrogen, progesterone, and melanocyte-stimulating hormone result in increased melanin synthesis.[68]

Keratinocytes are cells that make up the outer layer of the skin: the epidermis. Melanocytes synthesize melanin, which is stored in melanosomes. These melanosomes are contained within keratinocytes. Melanosomes function in melanin synthesis by containing the enzyme tyrosine, which converts the reaction of L-dopa to L-dopa-quinone.[69] Thus, the concentration of melanin-containing keratinocytes along with the amount of melanin contained in each cell result in pigmentation of the skin. When this system dysfunctions, it results in the hypermelanin typical of melasma.

Diagnosis of melasma includes viewing the skin under a Wood's lamp to help determine if the melasma is mixed, epidermal, or dermal, but it is an inexact determination. Determination of the type of melasma is an important aspect when deciding treatment options. There are many types of treatment options available, from creams to lasers to peels; all have different mechanisms of action. Common to many treatment options is the importance of general management, including the possible cessation of birth control pills, use of phototoxic drugs, scented cosmetics, the use of a broad-spectrum sunscreen, and avoidance of UV exposure when possible.

Many treatment options are available for the treatment of melasma with various mechanisms of action. The first category of drugs includes tyrosinase inhibitors, which affect the pathway for melanin synthesis. These include hydroquinone, tretinoin, azelaic acid, and kojic acid. Potential side effects are allergic or contact dermatitis, skin scaling, pruritus, and nail bleaching. Corticosteroids have also been shown to be briefly effective against melasma, although the exact mechanism is unknown. In addition, corticosteroids are known to have a short-term effect on melasma, usually with re-emergence of symptoms after discontinuation of the drug.

Chemical peels work on a different aspect of the problem. Rather then affecting melanocytes or **melanogenesis**, chemical peels work by nonspecific removal of melanin and top layers of the stratum cornea. Intense pulsed light therapy has been shown to be effective toward superficial melasma. Laser treatment works through thermal damage by selective heating of melanin-producing cells.[65] Photodynamic therapy has been found to be beneficial as well.

CASE PRESENTATION

Patient Case: Part 2

Assessment:

- Moderate inflammatory late-onset acne with underlying rosacea.
- Potential for mild postinflammatory acne scarring.
- Topical clindamycin/benzoyl peroxide appropriate but inadequate; generic oral contraceptive not indicated for acne.

Plan:

- Nondrug therapy includes avoidance of trigger factors and preventive measures as may be applicable for acne and rosacea:
    - Although highly variable and controversial, destressing and well-balanced dietary measures are viewed by some as perhaps stabilizing approaches but are not necessarily well-founded preventive measures.
    - Some trigger factors identified for some rosacea patients include weather (sun exposure, heat, cold, humidity, and wind), food (spicy foods, fruits, dairy products, and vegetables), alcohol, hot beverages, exercise, hot baths, stress, cosmetics (soaps, shampoo, moisturizers, perfume, aftershave, and sunscreens).
- Drug therapy includes continuation of clindamycin/benzoyl peroxide with a change in

(Continued on next page)

oral contraceptive regimen consisting of 3 mg drospirenone and 0.02 mg ethinyl estradiol (Yaz®), one tablet daily as directed for contraception and acne; in addition, subantimicrobial doxycycline, 40 mg orally once a day (an encapsulated beaded formulation that provides continuous subantimicrobial serum levels while producing anti-inflammatory activity) is efficacious orally once daily for rosacea.

- Rationale for drug regimen includes the need for achievement of better control of inflammatory acne to minimize the potential for acne scarring; subantimicrobial doxycycline selected to control underlying rosacea.
- Monitoring includes routine ob/gyn visits and labs relative to oral contraceptive use, and periodic dermatology physical exams and labs such as a serum metabolic panel and complete blood count as appropriate for indefinite use of oral low-dose doxycycline.

Patient education: It is important that patients be counseled concerning the importance of treatment to prevent worsening of symptoms. Rosacea is more than a "flush and blush" cosmetic problem. It can be a physically and emotionally devastating condition. Although there is no cure for rosacea, most cases are successfully managed with topical or systemic therapy along with avoidance of trigger factors. Also, understanding which trigger factors affect a patient and ways to avoid or mitigate these factors may improve quality of life. Recommendations for appropriates sunscreen and cosmetic use are quite useful in the therapeutic approach to the treatment of rosacea. Another important aspect of therapy that addresses self-esteem may include the use of corrective cover cosmetic products.

Although many patients may be self-conscious or even physically uncomfortable with flushing and redness, they may be reluctant to discuss what they feel others may perceive to be a minor problem. A healthcare practitioner can significantly contribute to patient education by discrete questioning and sympathetic listening.

Summary

Women more commonly seek dermatologic medical care than do men. Although age-related deterioration of skin in both men and women relates to environmental and genetic etiologies, signs and symptoms of skin changes in women across their lifespan include skin atrophy, wrinkling, laxity, and dryness. The cutaneous physiologic differences between men and women point to important considerations in choosing appropriate pharmacotherapeutic approaches in sex-related skin disorders.

References

Additional content available at ***www.ashp.org/womenshealth***

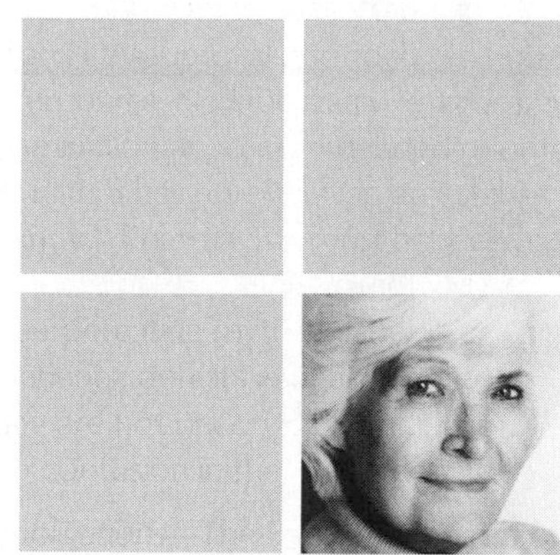

SECTION SEVEN

Cancer in Women

43 Breast Cancer

Chad Barnett, Pharm.D., BCOP; Janet L. Espirito, Pharm.D., BCOP

Learning Objectives

1. Discuss the presentation, pathophysiology, screening, and diagnosis of breast cancer.
2. Identify high-risk patients, and discuss options for appropriate breast cancer prevention therapy.
3. Compare and contrast therapeutic approaches for treatment of early-stage, locally advanced, and metastatic breast cancer, with a focus on pharmacologic interventions.
4. Develop an appropriate treatment plan in patients receiving adjuvant therapy for breast cancer.
5. Recommend an appropriate follow-up for long-term survivors of breast cancer.

Although great strides have been made in the prevention, screening, and treatment of breast cancer in the past two decades, it is a significant women's health issue in the U.S. and throughout the world. Research in the breast cancer arena has improved techniques for earlier diagnosis. Innovative treatments have improved outcomes in patients with early-stage disease and overall survival of those diagnosed with metastatic breast cancer, as well as helping them to maintain a good quality of life.

Epidemiology

Breast cancer is the most commonly diagnosed malignancy in American women and is the second leading cause of cancer death in the U.S. In 2009, it is estimated that 194,280 women will be diagnosed with and 40,610 women will die of the disease.[1] Breast cancer is a significant women's health issue, as one in eight women will be diagnosed with the disease during her lifetime.[2] Although breast cancer incidence rates steadily increased over the past few decades, the incidence has started to plateau. Mortality rates are declining as a result of screening mammography and effective adjuvant therapy.[3]

Etiology and Risk Factors

The etiology for breast cancer is largely unknown, although several risk factors have been identified. The two most common risk factors are female sex and increasing age. The median age of diagnosis of breast cancer is 61 years.[2] The association between breast cancer and estrogen has been recognized for more than a century, although the exact mechanism is not known. Experimental and human data strongly suggest that estrogen plays a role in the pathogenesis of breast cancer.[4] Exogenous hormone replacement also increases risk, particularly estrogen plus progestin, as demonstrated by the results of the Women's Health Initiative (WHI) Hormone Trials.[5,6] Thus, an increased risk of breast cancer is associated with factors that increase cumulative exposure of breast tissue to estrogen, such as early menarche, late menopause, older age at first live childbirth, and prolonged hormone therapy. Other risk factors include family history of breast cancer at a young age, exposure to therapeutic chest wall irradiation, benign proliferative breast disease, and genetic mutations in the breast/ovarian cancer susceptibility genes *BRCA1* and *BRCA2*.[7]

Approximately 5% to 10% of breast cancers are due to hereditary gene mutations, with the majority of these due to germline mutations

CASE PRESENTATION

Patient Case: Part 1

K.B. is a 61-year-old woman presenting for evaluation of a new mass in her left breast.

HPI: K.B. first noticed a palpable breast mass on self-examination approximately 12 months ago but was unable to have this further investigated because of loss of health insurance. The patient describes the mass as intermittently painful. A mammogram was performed before her current visit that was suspicious for malignancy.

PMH: Hypertension.

Family history: No history of malignancy in immediate family members.

Social history: Denies alcohol use and is a nonsmoker.

Endocrine history: Menarche age 11; menopause age 58; first child age 36; $G_1P_1A_0$. Last Pap test at age 40. No prior history of hormone therapy.

Medications: Hydrochlorothiazide 25 mg daily, multivitamin daily.

Allergies: NKDA.

Vitals: BP 128/73, P 91, RR 17, T 36.9°C; Ht 5′4″, Wt 165 lb.

Laboratory values: WNL.

Physical exam: Normal, with the exception of a 2.5-cm mass at the two o'clock position, approximately 3 cm from the nipple margin, not fixated to skin; no nipple retraction or discharge is visualized; the mass is exquisitely tender to palpation; 1.5 cm, nontender, palpable mass in the axilla noted.

Imaging:

Diagnostic bilateral mammogram—There is a mass measuring 2.6 cm in longest dimension located at the two o'clock position in the left breast suspicious for malignancy, American College of Radiology Category V. In the right breast, no dominant mass, distortion, or suspicious calcifications are identified.

Unilateral ultrasound left breast and left axilla with biopsy— Suspicious lesion in the left breast is 2.5 cm in diameter. Suspicious lymph nodes are noted in the axilla. A fine needle aspiration of the largest lymph node was performed. In the infraclavicular region, a few hypoechoic lymph nodes were also seen, and a biopsy was performed.

Core needle biopsy of left breast mass—Left breast, two o'clock: infiltrating ductal carcinoma, modified Black's nuclear grade 2 (moderately differentiated), ER 90%, PR 91%, Her2 overexpression 1+, Her2 FISH negative (no amplification), Ki67 30% (moderate).

Fine needle aspiration (FNA) of left axillary and infraclavicular lymph nodes—Adenocarcinoma consistent with breast primary.

Bone scan—No definite evidence of osseous metastases.

Ultrasound liver—No lesions suggestive of metastases.

Chest CT— No evidence of pulmonary metastases.

Patient assessment—K.B. is 61-year-old women presenting with unilateral breast mass with local invasion to lymph nodes.

in the *BRCA1* or *BRCA2* genes. In women with a known deleterious *BRCA* mutation, this may confer a 35% to 84% risk of breast cancer by age 70.[8] This is significantly greater than the 12% risk of breast cancer in the general population.

Several risk assessment models exist to help estimate a woman's risk of developing breast cancer. The Breast Cancer Risk Assessment Tool from the National Cancer Institute (www.cancer.gov/bcrisktool/Default.aspx) is an example of one tool that calculates a woman's 5-year and lifetime risk for invasive breast cancer. This is based on a statistical model known as the Gail Model, which takes into account a woman's personal medical history, reproductive history, and family history of breast cancer among first-degree relatives.[9] This model had only been validated for white women, but has now been updated for black women.[10] It may not, however, provide accurate information for other racial groups or those with known gene mutations. Other risk-assessment models have been developed to estimate the likelihood of a clinically significant *BRCA* mutation. Genetic testing for *BRCA* mutations is clinically available, and recommendations for who should receive referral for genetic counseling and *BRCA* testing have been published.[8,11] Genetic testing is limited, as not all causes of hereditary breast cancer can be detected by current methods, and there is limited information about the clinical significance of particular mutations.

Clinical Presentation

A breast lump is the most common clinical presentation and reason for which women seek medical attention. The mass is usually solid, firm, and painless. Some patients may have palpable regional lymph nodes. Less common symptoms include breast pain, nipple discharge, retraction or ulceration, change in breast shape or size, skin warmth, erythema, or edema. With increased use of screening mammography, many asymptomatic women will be diagnosed as a result of an abnormal **mammogram.**

The majority of breast cancers present as early stage, when the cancer is confined to the breast or local-regional lymph nodes. Some patients may present with locally advanced breast cancer (LABC), with extensive tumor volume or lymph node involvement. A small number of patients, <10%, will have metastatic disease at diagnosis, when there is evidence of cancer at sites distant from the breast. Common sites of breast cancer metastases include the bone, lung, liver, and brain.

Figure 43-1. The normal breast

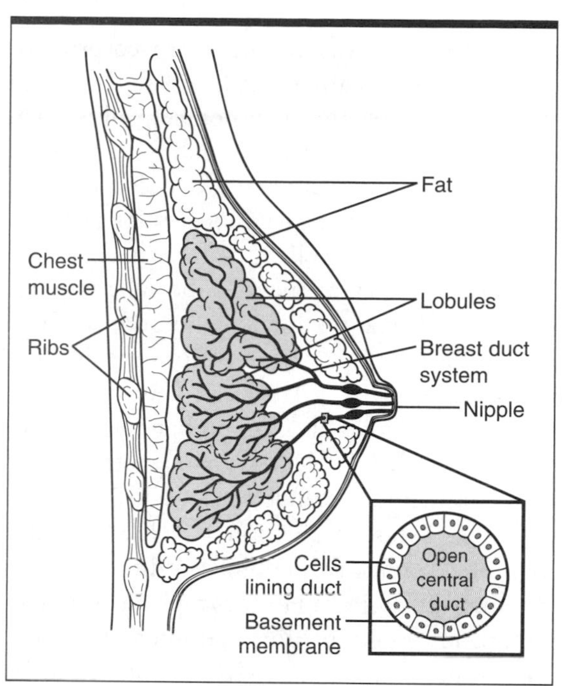

Pathophysiology

The breast is mainly composed of lobules and ducts (Figure 43-1). Carcinomas of the breast are broadly divided into two major groups: invasive and noninvasive carcinomas. The development of malignancy is believed to be a multistep process in which normal cells undergo gradual changes resulting in malignant transformation. When tumor cells remain confined within the basement membrane and show no evidence of invasion, these are referred to as noninvasive (or in situ) carcinomas. The majority of in situ carcinomas are either ductal (also known as intraductal carcinoma, or ductal carcinoma in situ, or DCIS), or lobular (lobular carcinoma in situ, or LCIS).

Invasive—or infiltrating—carcinomas occur when tumor cells have penetrated through the basement membrane to invade the breast stroma and have the ability to metastasize. The invasive carcinomas consist of many histiologic subtypes. Invasive (or infiltrating) ductal carcinomas are the most common type, accounting for about 75% of all breast tumors, whereas invasive (or infiltrating) lobular carcinomas account for 5% to 10%. Subtypes that account for the remaining cases include mucinous, tubular, medullary, papillary, and other rare histologies.[12]

Inflammatory breast cancer (IBC) is a not a histologic subtype, but a clinical diagnosis distinguished by rapidly progressing changes of the breast and skin that typically develop over weeks to months. The characteristic presentation includes breast warmth, erythema and edema, and thickened skin with a *peau d'orange* (skin of an orange) appearance that is due to dermal lymphatic invasion of tumor cells. There may or may not be a palpable underlying mass. It can be mistaken for cellulitis, an abscess, or infection, but may be distinguished from an infection by the lack of fever. Women who have persistent symptoms following antibiotic therapy for infection should seek further medical attention.[13] It is often aggressive and difficult to treat. Fortunately, IBC is a relatively rare presentation, accounting for 1% to 5% of all breast cancers.

Paget's disease of the breast is another clinically unique presentation, which involves eczematous changes of the nipple and areola, such as crusting and scaling. This is usually associated with an underlying carcinoma that may be invasive or in situ.

Breast Cancer Screening

The underlying premise for breast cancer screening is to discover malignant lesions before they become symptomatic or spread outside the breast, when there is the greatest chance of improved survival. Smaller tumors are more likely to be in an early stage of disease and may have an improved prognosis with appropriate treatment.[14] It should be noted that breast cancer screening will not help all women who participate; therefore, the evaluation of possible risks vs. benefits is a crucial part of decision making. Risks may include unnecessary biopsies for noncancerous abnormalities, as well as treatment of noninvasive cancers that may or may not become invasive if left untreated.[14] Many guidelines to address these issues have been developed from various medical organizations, including the American Cancer Society (ACS) and the National Comprehensive Cancer Network (NCCN).[14-16] Well-known methods for breast cancer screening include breast self-evaluation (BSE), clinical breast evaluation (CBE), and film mammography. Innovative methods of breast cancer screening such as digital mammography, computer-aided detection programs for mammography, and magnetic resonance imaging (MRI), continue to be evaluated.

BSE is a noninvasive procedure that allows women to actively participate in the screening process for breast cancer. Data from large, randomized trials have shown that BSE performed by trained women did not reduce breast cancer-specific or all-cause mortality.[17] Despite these data, routine BSE may still detect new breast lesions between other breast cancer detection methods. Therefore, the ACS recommends that beginning in their 20s, women should be informed about the benefits and limitations of BSE.[14] Women who choose to participate in BSE should receive instruction on proper technique, and their technique should be reviewed periodically.[14] Also, it is acceptable for women not to perform BSE or to perform it irregularly.[14] Women should be instructed to promptly report any new breast symptoms to a healthcare professional.

Although the practice of CBE is recommended by several national organizations, little data regarding the efficacy of clinical breast examinations exist from randomized clinical trials.[18] The ACS recommends that for average-risk asymptomatic women in their 20s and 30s, CBE should be included as part of a periodic health examination, preferably at least once every 3 years.[14] Also, information should be provided about benefits and limitations of BSE and CBE and the importance of reporting any new breast symptoms to a healthcare professional.[14] Women at increased risk of breast cancer may benefit from CBE earlier in life or with greater frequency.[16]

Meta-analyses that have evaluated the value of screening mammograms in randomized trials have shown statistically significant reductions in breast cancer–related mortality of 20% to 35% for women 50 to 69 years of age.[19] It is thought that this decrease in mortality results from the ability of mammographic screening to detect smaller tumors with more favorable histologic features than lesions found outside of screening.[18] Mammographic screening also reduces breast cancer–related mortality in women 40 to 49 years of age, but to a lesser extent.[18] The ACS and NCCN recommend that women with average risk of breast cancer begin annual screening with mammography at the age of 40.[14,16] In high-risk women, ACS recommends consideration of mammographic screening beginning at age 30 (or rarely, younger ages) or with shorter mammography intervals (i.e., every 6 months).[14]

Because of its high sensitivity for detecting breast cancer in high-risk, asymptomatic, and symptomatic women, MRI has been investigated for breast cancer screening. For patients designated as high risk of developing breast cancer, screening with MRI of the breast has recently been recommended by the ACS.[15] MRI has been shown to be highly sensitive in diagnosis compared with mammography. However, MRI has also been associated with significantly lower specificity compared with mammography, which has resulted in more recalls and biopsies.[15] Other disadvantages of MRI include increased cost and limited access to high-quality MRI breast screening in the community.[15]

Diagnosis

If a suspicious abnormality is visualized on a screening mammogram or if a patient is found to have symptoms—such as a palpable abnormality, skin changes, or nipple discharge—a bilateral diagnostic mammogram should be performed.[20] To create a uniform system of reporting mammography results, the Breast Imaging Reporting and Data System (BI-RADS) was developed by the American College of Radiology.[19] Based on mammographic findings, additional testing may be recommended. A focused ultrasound or breast MRI is often used as an adjunct to mammography to further characterize an abnormal lesion.[16,20] For BI-RADS categories suspicious of malignancy, tissue diagnosis is required. Core needle biopsy (biopsy obtained through a hollow needle) or excisional biopsy (removal of the entire lump or suspicious area) with ultrasound, stereotactic, or MRI guidance is typically performed for definitive diagnosis of the breast lesion.[16] Fine-needle aspiration (removal of fluid through a thin needle) can be used to identify the presence of cancer cells but cannot be used to distinguish between noninvasive and invasive breast cancers.[21] The patient is then treated (or observed) according to results of pathologic analysis. Determination of tumor grade, hormone-receptor status (estrogen receptor [ER] and/or progesterone receptor [PR] positivity), and human epidermal growth factor 2 (HER2) receptor expression from biopsied tissue is critical for selection of appropriate patients for hormonal and targeted treatments.[7]

Additional workup for diagnosis and staging includes a thorough history and physical, complete blood count, platelet count, and liver function tests.[7] If the patient has signs or symptoms related to the bone, lung, or abdomen, or an elevated alkaline phosphatase level, the patient should undergo bone scanning, chest imaging, or abdominal scanning with computed tomography (CT), MRI, or ultrasound to rule out the possibility of distant metastases.[7] Patients with LABC should routinely receive the above-mentioned imaging tests because of a higher risk of systemic metastases.[7]

Prevention

Estimating the risk of breast cancer for an individual woman is a difficult task. Specific characteristics that can be considered as high risk for development of breast cancer include known genetic mutations (such as *BRCA1* or *BRCA2*, p53, or PTEN mutations), more than two first-degree relatives with breast or ovarian cancers, history of LCIS, or a history of thoracic radiation.[22] The management of LCIS is controversial because it is not generally considered a preinvasive cancer, but rather a risk factor for the development of breast cancer. Also, patients with a 1.7% or greater 5-year actuarial risk of breast cancer calculated by the modified Gail model are considered to be a high-risk population.[22] Available strategies to reduce the risk of breast cancer in certain high-risk patients can be broadly classified as either surgical or medical methods of risk reduction.

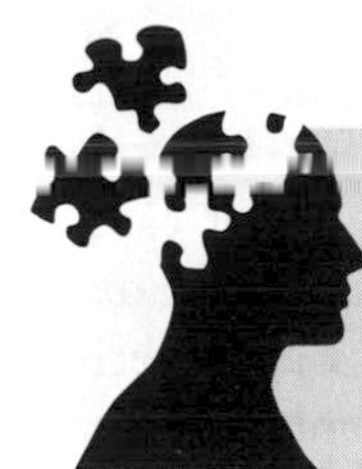

Therapeutic Challenge:

F.G. is a 36-year-old woman with a family history of breast cancer. Her grandmother died of ovarian cancer at the age of 54. Her sister was diagnosed with early-stage breast cancer. She tests positive for BRCA2 and presents to the clinic to learn about her options to "guarantee" prevention of breast cancer in her lifetime. What is her best option to prevent breast cancer?

Surgical methods for breast cancer risk reduction include bilateral total mastectomy and bilateral salpingo-oophorectomy (BSO). **Mastectomy** can reduce the risk of developing breast cancer by at least 90% in patients with genetic risk factors.[23] BSO has shown a reduction in *BRCA* mutation–associated gynecologic cancer of 85% to 95% and a reduction of breast cancer risk by 50% to 68% in retrospective and prospective cohort studies.[24] It should be noted that neither of these procedures entirely eliminate the risk of breast or ovarian cancers.

The selective estrogen receptor modulators (SERMs) tamoxifen and raloxifene have been studied for chemoprevention of breast cancer. The NSABP Breast Cancer Prevention (P-1) Trial was a prospective, randomized clinical trial that evaluated the efficacy of tamoxifen compared with placebo for breast cancer prevention in 13,175 high-risk women. After 48 months of follow-up, treatment with tamoxifen resulted in a 49% relative risk reduction and 21% absolute risk reduction of invasive breast cancer compared with placebo.[22] However, adverse events related to tamoxifen must be considered. A meta-analysis of tamoxifen prevention studies in women at high risk for the development of breast cancer found a 2.4-fold increase in endometrial cancers, 1.9-fold increase in deep vein thromboses, and 1.5-fold increase in cerebrovascular accidents for patients that received tamoxifen.[25]

Raloxifene has also been studied for the prevention of breast cancer in women at high risk. The NSABP Study of Tamoxifen and Raloxifene (STAR) trial randomized 19,747 high-risk, postmenopausal women to receive either tamoxifen or raloxifene therapy for 5 years. The reduction in incidence of invasive breast cancers was similar with tamoxifen and raloxifene; however, there were numerically fewer cases of noninvasive cancer (DCIS, LCIS) in the tamoxifen group.[26] Patients in the raloxifene group experienced significantly fewer episodes of thromboembolic events, uterine hyperplasia, hysterectomies, cataracts, and cataract surgeries compared with patients that received tamoxifen.[26] The incidence of uterine cancer was numerically decreased in the raloxifene group, but did not reach statistical significance.[26]

It has been estimated that only 5% to 30% of eligible high-risk women agree to take tamoxifen following the recommendation by a primary healthcare provider.[25] Benefits from therapy must be weighed with potential risks from surgery or medication, as this patient population is at high risk of, but does not have, breast cancer.

Staging/Prognosis

Staging of breast cancer provides a critical guide not only to prognosis, but also to treatment based on a patient's individual risk factors. The most recent revision to the American Joint Committee on Cancer (AJCC) Staging System for Breast Cancer occurred in 2002 and incorporated developments in imaging, surgical procedures, and biochemical assays.[27] Breast cancer is staged based on the tumor-node-metastasis (TNM) system and is separated into clinical and pathologic staging. Clinical staging includes physical examination and imaging data to make treatment recommendations (Table 43-1).[27] Pathologic staging occurs after surgery. This includes the elements of clinical staging, but also adds data from pathologic examination of the primary tumor and regional lymph nodes.[27]

Table 43-1. TNM Staging

Tumor

TX	Primary tumor cannot be assessed	
T0	No evidence of primary tumor	
Tis	Carcinoma in situ	
	Tis (DCIS)	Ductal carcinoma in situ
	Tis (LCIS)	Lobular carcinoma in situ
	Tis (Paget's)	Paget's disease of the nipple with no tumor
T1	Tumor 2 cm or less in greatest dimension	
	T1mic	Microinvasion 0.1 cm or less in greatest dimension
	T1a	Tumor more than 0.1 cm but not more than 0.5 cm in greatest dimension
	T1b	Tumor more than 0.5 cm but not more than 1 cm in greatest dimension
	T1c	Tumor more than 1 cm but not more than 2 cm in greatest dimension
T2	Tumor more than 2 cm but not more than 5 cm in greatest dimension	
T3	Tumor more than 5 cm in greatest dimension	
T4	Tumor of any size with direct extension to (a) chest wall or (b) skin, only as described below	
	T4a	Extension to chest wall, not including pectoralis muscle
	T4b	Edema (including *peau d'orange*) or ulceration of the skin of the breast, or satellite skin nodules confined to the same breast
	T4c	Both T4a and T4b
	T4d	Inflammatory carcinoma

(*Continued on next page*)

Tumor			
Node			
NX	Regional lymph nodes cannot be assessed (e.g., previously removed)		
N0	No regional lymph node metastasis		
N1	Metastasis to movable ipsilateral axillary lymph node(s)		
N2	Metastases in ipsilateral axillary lymph nodes fixed or matted, or in clinically apparent ipsilateral internal mammary nodes in the *absence* of clinically evident axillary lymph node metastasis		
	N2a	Metastasis in ipsilateral axillary lymph nodes fixed to one another (matted) or to other structures	
	N2b	Metastasis only in clinically apparent ipsilateral internal mammary nodes and in the *absence* of clinically evident axillary lymph node metastasis	
N3	Metastasis in ipsilateral infraclavicular lymph node(s) with or without axillary lymph node involvement, or in clinically apparent ipsilateral internal mammary lymph node(s) and in the *presence* of clinically evident axillary lymph node metastasis; or metastasis in ipsilateral supraclavicular lymph node(s) with or without axillary or internal mammary lymph node involvement		
	N3a	Metastasis in ipsilateral infraclavicular lymph node(s)	
	N3b	Metastasis in ipsilateral internal mammary lymph node(s) and axillary lymph node(s)	
	N3c	Metastasis in ipsilateral supraclavicular lymph node(s)	
Metastasis			
MX	Distant metastasis cannot be assessed		
M0	No distant metastasis		
M1	Distant metastasis		
Stage Groupings			
Stage 0	Tis	N0	M0
Stage I	T1	N0	M0
Stage IIA	T0	N1	M0
	T1	N1	M0
	T2	N0	M0
Stage IIB	T2	N1	M0
	T3	N0	M0
Stage IIIA	T0	N2	M0
	T1	N2	M0
	T2	N2	M0
	T3	N1	M0
	T3	N2	M0
Stage IIIB	T4	N0	M0
	T4	N1	M0
	T4	N2	M0
Stage IIIC	Any T	N3	M0
Stage IV	Any T	Any N	M1

Treatment

DUCTAL CARCINOMA IN SITU

Treatment Goals

The goals for treatment of DCIS are the prevention of invasive breast cancer or the treatment of an invasive component while still localized in the breast. Because of improvements in breast cancer screening, the incidence of DCIS has increased dramatically and now accounts for approximately 20% of breast cancers diagnosed by mammography.[28] Management of DCIS is somewhat controversial. It is estimated that fewer than half of DCIS cases will develop into invasive disease.[29] Even when appropriately treated, approximately half of all local recurrences after resection of DCIS are invasive.[21,28] Therefore, treatment of DCIS can be regarded as preventive for invasive breast cancer.

Surgery

Long-term, cause-specific survival with mastectomy appears to be equivalent to that of local excision and whole breast irradiation.[7] Local excision is also referred to as **lumpectomy,** segmental mastectomy, or breast-conserving therapy (BCT).

Mastectomy is now reserved for patients with large tumors, multifocal disease, or diffuse microcalcifications on preoperative mammograms.[21] Mastectomy should also be considered if the patient cannot undergo radiation therapy or if surgical margins are persistently positive (residual cancer cells remain close to the edge of the resected surgical specimen) with BCT.[21] Axillary lymph node dissection (ALND, surgical removal of lymph nodes in the axilla) is not recommended in patients with pure DCIS because the incidence of lymph node involvement is low.[7] Sentinel node biopsy (SNB), the technique of sampling the first draining lymph node(s) from the tumor, is controversial in this patient population, and more clinical data are needed to describe its role in patients with DCIS.[30]

Radiation Therapy

The need for radiation therapy (RT) for DCIS is dependent on the type of surgical procedure. Patients who undergo mastectomy generally do not require subsequent RT. The addition of RT following breast-conserving therapy has shown a benefit in reduction of ipsilateral (same side) recurrence in patients with DCIS in several large, randomized clinical trials.[21] The NCCN recommends the use of radiation after BCT in patients with DCIS 0.5 cm or greater in diameter.[7]

Hormonal Therapy

Tamoxifen also has shown benefit in prevention of ipsilateral and contralateral (opposite side) breast cancer recurrence in patients with DCIS. The NSABP B-24 trial compared 5 years of tamoxifen to placebo in 1,804 patients with DCIS treated with wide local resection followed by radiation.[31] After 7 years of follow-up, use of tamoxifen resulted in a 48% reduction in invasive breast cancer–related events compared with placebo.[21,29] A subsequent analysis of this trial suggests a benefit of tamoxifen in patients with hormone receptor–positive DCIS. The NCCN recommends consideration of tamoxifen use in patients with DCIS treated with BCT or mastectomy.[7] Results from clinical trials evaluating additional hormonal therapies for treatment of hormone receptor-positive DCIS are eagerly awaited.

EARLY STAGE BREAST CANCER (STAGE I, IIA, IIB, AND T3N1M0)

Treatment Goals

The ultimate goal for the treatment of early-stage breast cancer (ESBC) is eradication of the disease (cure). Local therapies, such as surgery and radiation, are used to eliminate disease from the breast. Systemic chemotherapy and/or hormonal therapies are used in the postoperative setting (adjuvant therapy) or preoperatively (neoadjuvant therapy) to eradicate any potential micrometastatic disease and prevent recurrences.

Surgery

For ESBC, surgery represents the primary modality for cure. Modified radical mastectomy (MRM, mastectomy with axillary lymph node dissection) and BCT with axillary lymph node mapping are medically equivalent treatment options for patients with ESBC, with similar disease-free survival (DFS) and overall survival (OS) with 18 years of follow-up in clinical trials.[7,30] It should be noted that the outcomes of BCT are only equivalent to MRM if the patient also receives postsurgical breast irradiation.[30] Absolute contraindications to BCT include previous moderate to high doses of RT to the chest wall or breast, pregnancy with the need to use RT during pregnancy, diffuse suspicious or malignant-appearing microcalcifications on mammogram, persistent positive margins, and multicentric cancer (tumor in more than one breast quadrant).[7] Relative contraindications to BCT include active connective tissue disease involving the skin, tumors >5 cm (due to poor cosmesis following resection or need for neoadjuvant chemotherapy), and focally positive margins.[7] Patient preference is a critical component of decision making as well. In selected patients, neoadjuvant chemotherapy may allow for BCT in patients who were not previously candidates for the procedure.[32]

Assessment of lymph node status is a critical component of staging and is the most important factor for prognosis. Patients with stage I or II breast cancer must undergo a lymph node mapping procedure, either ALND or SNB.[7] An SNB involves only excising the sentinel node(s), defined as the first node or nodes in the lymph node basin into which the primary tumor drains.[30] Comorbidities, including lymphedema and nerve injury, can result from ALND.[30] The NCCN recommends SNB as the preferred procedure for pathologic assessment of the lymph nodes in patients with stage I or II breast cancer.[7] Several requirements exist for SNB procedures, including the availability of an experienced SNB surgical team and clinically negative lymph nodes.[30] If a patient is found to have a positive lymph node or the sentinel lymph node cannot be identified, an ALND should be performed or axillary radiation should be administered.[7]

Radiation Therapy

Postsurgical breast irradiation following BCT is the standard of care in patients with ESBC.[30] The NCCN recommends postmastectomy RT in patients with four or more metastatic axillary lymph nodes, tumors >5 cm, and positive margins after mastectomy.[7] Although controversy exists, NCCN recommends consideration of radiation to the chest wall and supraclavicular area after mastectomy in women with one to three positive axillary lymph nodes.[7] In patients who receive adjuvant chemotherapy, radiation is typically administered after chemotherapy is completed.[33]

Hormonal Therapy

Patients whose tumors express ER and/or PR receptors may derive significant benefit from the use of various hormonal therapies. Tamoxifen has long been the gold standard for the adjuvant treatment of ESBC in premenopausal and postmenopausal women.[33] However, the advent of aromatase inhibitors (AIs) has dramatically changed the practice of adjuvant hormonal treatment in postmenopausal women. Hormonal therapy is largely appropriate for patients with hormone receptor–positive invasive tumors regardless of patient age, lymph nodes status, or whether chemotherapy will be administered.[7] However, it may be omitted in patients with tumors <0.5 cm or in well-differentiated tumors 0.6–1 cm without unfavorable prognostic features, such as lymphovascular invasion, high nuclear grade, and high histologic grade.[7] Hormonal therapy is typically administered after surgery, chemotherapy, and radiation, if indicated.

Tamoxifen therapy with or without ovarian suppression is the standard of care in premenopausal patients with ESBC.[7] AIs are considered to be ineffective in the presence of functioning ovaries and therefore are not indicated in premenopausal patients.[34] Tamoxifen is typically taken once daily for 5 years because of decreased efficacy and increased toxicity with longer therapy.[33] A large overview analysis conducted by the Early Breast Cancer Trialists' Collaborative Group (EBCTCG), which included approximately 145,000 patients in 194 clinical trials, revealed that approximately 5 years of tamoxifen therapy resulted in a 39% reduction in disease recurrence and 31% reduction in death after 15 years of follow-up (ER-positive disease only).[35] Ovarian suppression in premenopausal patients may be achieved by surgical removal of the ovaries (oophorectomy), ovarian radiation, or administration of luteinizing hormone–releasing hormone (LHRH) agonists.[34] An overview analysis of four clinical trials with a median follow-up of 6.8 years comparing tamoxifen with an LHRH agonist (i.e., goserelin) to an LHRH agonist alone demonstrated a significant improvement in progression-free survival (PFS) and OS with combination therapy in patients with advanced breast cancer.[34] However, whether combination therapy is superior to tamoxifen alone is uncertain, and studies are ongoing.

Several large, randomized clinical trials have demonstrated superiority of AIs over tamoxifen in the adjuvant treatment of postmenopausal women with ESBC.[36] Options for treatment include the nonsteroidal AIs (anastrozole and letrozole) and steroidal AI (exemestane). Anastrozole and letrozole currently have data supporting the initial use of these agents in the adjuvant treatment of ESBC, resulting in significant improvements in DFS. When compared with tamoxifen, AIs are associated with an increased number of fractures, osteoporosis, and musculoskeletal symptoms.[37] Tamoxifen is associated with increased hot flashes, vaginal symptoms, endometrial cancers, ischemic cerebrovascular events, and venous thrombosis compared with AIs.[37]

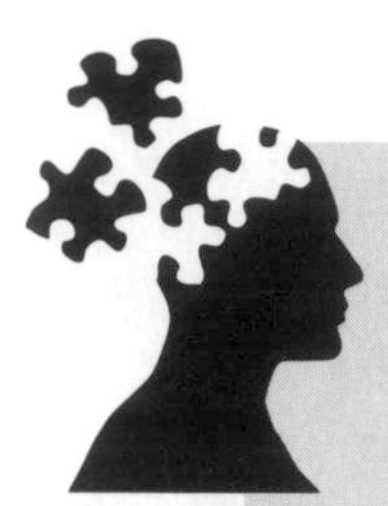

Therapeutic Challenge:

What is the optimal duration of treatment with AIs in the adjuvant setting? What are the benefits and risks?

Several trials have also evaluated the use of AIs after tamoxifen therapy for postmenopausal women in the adjuvant setting. Both anastrozole and exemestane have significantly improved DFS when switched following 2–3 years of tamoxifen.[37] Extended therapy with an AI after 5 years of tamoxifen has also been evaluated. Letrozole has resulted in significantly improved DFS in all patients and improved OS in patients with lymph node–positive breast cancer when compared with placebo after 5 years of tamoxifen therapy.[37]

All of these trials illustrate the importance of AIs in the adjuvant treatment of postmenopausal patients with hormone receptor–positive ESBC. However, many questions, such as the optimal sequencing strategy or preferred AI, still remain. The results of clinical trials addressing these issues are eagerly awaited.

Chemotherapy

The administration of adjuvant or neoadjuvant chemotherapy depends not only on the patients' risk factors for breast cancer recurrence, but also should include the expected risks and benefits of therapy for the patient. Clinical and pathologic staging incorporates the two most important independent risk factors for disease recurrence: tumor size and nodal status.[27] Further prognostic information can be gained through pathologic analysis, including tumor grade, hormone receptor status, and HER2 receptor status.[20] The decision-making process should include patient-related factors as well, such as age, performance status, comorbid conditions, and organ function (renal, hepatic, and cardiac function).[33] According to the NCCN guidelines, patients with tumors >1 cm or positive lymph nodes are appropriate candidates for systemic chemotherapy, with the addition of hormonal therapy in patients whose tumors are hormone receptor-positive and biologic therapy for patients whose tumors overexpress HER2.[7] Validated risk-calculation tools are available, such as the Adjuvant! (www.adjuvantonline.com) web-based program.[38] This program allows incorporation of patient- and tumor-specific information to estimate 10-year relapse and mortality benefits for various treatment regimens.[38] In selected patients, treatment decisions are also made based on newer gene-based assays, such as Oncotype DX and Mammoprint, that assist in determination of patient benefit from chemotherapy.[38] Oncotype DX is a 21-gene assay used in patients with hormone receptor–positive, lymph node–negative breast cancer to predict the risk of breast cancer relapse and to identify patients who may benefit from adjuvant chemotherapy followed by hormonal therapy. The assay produces a recurrence score, which places patients into low-, intermediate-, or high-risk categories. Based on the risk of recurrence, patients in the low-risk category may have minimal benefit from chemotherapy in addition to hormonal therapy and may be spared from chemotherapy administration.[39]

Chemotherapy has been a critical treatment modality for patients with ESBC since clinical trials conferred significant benefits in the 1970s.[38] Since that time, the combination of chemotherapeutic agents (polychemotherapy) has become the cornerstone of ESBC. In general, these regimens are typically administered for a period of 4–6 months.[33] Duration of therapy and the specific agents administered are based on the anticipated risk of breast cancer recurrence and potential harm to the patient. Chemotherapeutic agents commonly used in the adjuvant setting include anthracyclines, taxanes, alkylating agents, and antimetabolites.[33] Common chemotherapy regimens used in the adjuvant or neoadjuvant treatment of breast cancer are listed in Table 43-2.

The incorporation of anthracycline compounds in polychemotherapy has become the standard of care in the adjuvant and neoadjuvant treatment of ESBC. The overview analysis by the EBCTCG showed that approximately 6 months of anthracycline-based chemotherapy reduced the annual risk of breast cancer death by 38% for women younger than 50 years of age and by approximately 20% in women 50–69 years of age.[35] Also, compared with cyclophosphamide, methotrexate, and fluorouracil (CMF) chemotherapy, anthracycline-based regimens significantly reduced recurrence and breast cancer-related mortality to a greater extent.[35] Doxorubicin and epirubicin are anthracyclines commonly used in the treatment of breast cancer. There has been considerable debate among experts regarding which anthracycline is

Table 43-2. Selected Chemotherapy Regimens for Early-Stage and Locally Advanced Breast Cancer

Regimen	Drugs	Doses	Frequency	Cycles
Node negative				
CMF	Cyclophosphamide	600 mg/m² IV	Every 21 days	4–6
	Methotrexate	40 mg/m² IV		
	Fluorouracil	600 mg/m² IV		
AC	Doxorubicin	60 mg/m² IV	Every 21 days	4–6
	Cyclophosphamide	600 mg/m² IV		
FAC	Fluorouracil	500 mg/m² IV	Every 21 days	6
	Doxorubicin	50 mg/m² IV		
	Cyclophosphamide	500 mg/m² IV		
FEC	Fluorouracil	500 mg/m² IV	Every 21 days	6
	Epirubicin	100 mg/m² IV		
	Cyclophosphamide	500 mg/m² IV		
Node positive				
AC/FAC/FEC	As above			
AC→Pac	Doxorubicin	60 mg/m² IV	Every 21 days	4
	Cyclophosphamide	600 mg/m² IV		
	Paclitaxel	175–225 mg/m² IV 80 mg/m² IV	Every 21 days Every 7 days	4 12
FEC→Doc	Fluorouracil	500 mg/m² IV	Every 21 days	4
	Epirubicin	100 mg/m² IV		
	Cyclophosphamide	500 mg/m² IV		
	Docetaxel	100 mg/m² IV	Every 21 days	4
TAC	Docetaxel	75 mg/m² IV	Every 21 days	6
	Doxorubicin	50 mg/m² IV		
	Cyclophosphamide	500 mg/m² IV		
Dose-dense AC→Pac	Doxorubicin	60 mg/m² IV	Every 14 days	4
	Cyclophosphamide	600 mg/m² IV		
	Paclitaxel	175 mg/m² IV	Every 14 days	4

Source: Adapted from references 7 and 48.

IV = intravenous.

superior in the treatment of ESBC. However, these agents have not been compared in randomized controlled trials, and therefore superiority cannot be assessed.[38] As with any cytotoxic chemotherapy agent, the benefits of anthracycline therapy must also be compared with the risks of short- and long-term toxicities.

Taxanes are among the most effective chemotherapy agents for breast cancer in the metastatic setting, and their use in the adjuvant setting has become standard of care in patients with lymph node–positive breast cancer. Paclitaxel and docetaxel have both produced significant improvements in DFS when added sequentially to anthracycline-containing regimens in several large, randomized clinical trials.[40] Additionally, concomitant use of docetaxel with anthracycline-based regimens has shown significant improvements in DFS.[40] There is much debate over not only which taxane is superior, but also what dosage and schedule is optimal. Clinical trials are under way to address these questions.

Neoadjuvant chemotherapy may allow for surgical resection in patients with inoperable breast cancers.[32] The success of neoadjuvant chemotherapy in locally advanced and inflammatory breast cancers has led to research in patients with ESBC.[32] Neoadjuvant administration of chemotherapy in patients with operable breast cancer can result in downstaging of tumors before surgery, which may allow more patients to be eligible for BCT.[32] Other potential advantages of neoadjuvant chemotherapy include the ability to eradicate micrometastases and to assess response to treatment.[32] Chemotherapy regimens administered in the neoadjuvant setting are similar to those utilized in the adjuvant setting (Table 43-2).

Dose intensity is a concept that has been studied in patients with breast cancer to improve outcomes after chemotherapy.[41] Dose intensity can be achieved by either increasing the dose of a drug at a fixed schedule or by decreasing the frequency of administration at a fixed dose. The later method is referred to as dose-dense chemotherapy and has been evaluated in the adjuvant setting. Dose-dense regimens are given every 2 weeks in place of a conventional every-3-week schedule and require support with myeloid growth factors. Studies have shown significant improvements in DFS and OS with dose-dense chemotherapy compared with conventional chemotherapy, at the expense, however, of increased toxicities.[41] It is unclear whether the benefit of dose-dense chemotherapy seen in clinical trials is from the anthracycline or taxane portion. Paclitaxel given on a weekly schedule has produced superior results compared with conventional (every 3 weeks) paclitaxel in adjuvant, neoadjuvant, and metastatic settings.[41] Ongoing clinical trials will help to address the place of dose-dense chemotherapy for the treatment of breast cancer.

Targeted Therapy

Trastuzumab is a humanized monoclonal antibody targeted against the HER2 receptor.[42] The use of trastuzumab, either as a single agent or in combination with chemotherapy, has been shown to increase OS in patients with HER2-positive metastatic disease.[42] Since its approval in the metastatic setting, the results of four large, randomized clinical trials have shown dramatic benefits of adjuvant trastuzumab use in ESBC. These studies included treatment of patients with node-positive disease as well as patients with node-negative breast cancer at high risk for recurrence and demonstrated statistically superior DFS and OS with trastuzumab when compared with nontrastuzumab containing regimens.[42] In the U.S., approval of trastuzumab in patients with ESBC by the U.S. Food and Drug Administration (FDA) resulted from a combined analysis of the North Central Cancer Treatment Group (NCCTG) N9831 and NSABP B-31 trials. Patients in these trials received anthracycline- and taxane-based chemotherapy with or without trastuzumab. Trastuzumab was administered concomitantly with paclitaxel and then continued as monotherapy for a total of 52 weeks of treatment.[42] The addition of trastuzumab resulted in significant improvements in DFS and OS at 2 years of median follow-up compared with patients who did not receive trastuzumab.[42] Similarly to other adjuvant trials with trastuzumab, there were higher rates of cardiac events, which were predominately manifested as heart failure.[43]

LOCALLY ADVANCED BREAST CANCER

Goals

The ultimate goal for the treatment of patients with LABC remains cure, but this may be more difficult to achieve than in patients with ESBC.

Surgery

LABC can be defined as patients with bulky tumors with or without extensive lymph node involvement. These patients may be divided into patients with operable and inoperable disease. The advanced state of disease in these patients makes treatment a challenge, as these patients are at a substantially higher risk of treatment failure, breast cancer relapse, and mortality.[44] Traditional surgical treatment of patients with LABC is MRM. However, BCT may be possible in carefully selected patients with LABC with the use of neoadjuvant chemotherapy.[30]

Radiation

Several randomized clinical trials have shown that RT after mastectomy reduces the risk of locoregional failure by approximately two thirds.[45] The criteria for RT in patients with LABC is the same as for patients with ESBC. Given that patients with LABC are at increased risk for recurrence, RT is commonly administered.

Hormonal Therapy

Appropriate adjuvant hormonal treatments, as previously described, should be administered in patients with hormone receptor–positive LABC.

Chemotherapy

Because of the extent of disease in this patient population, neoadjuvant chemotherapy is indicated to allow for resection of inoperable tumors or more complete surgical resection of operable tumors in the breast and lymph nodes.[46] In patients with lymph node involvement, chemotherapy should include both an anthracycline and taxane.[46] Common chemotherapy regimens used in treatment of LABC are listed in Table 43-2. Regimens given in the neoadjuvant setting are similar to those given in the adjuvant setting.

Targeted Therapy

Adjuvant trastuzumab has shown benefits in patients with LABC similarly to ESBC.[42]

METASTATIC BREAST CANCER

Goals

Because metastatic breast cancer (MBC) is largely considered incurable, the goals of treatment are primarily palliative. Treatment goals in patients with MBC are to prolong survival, delay disease progression, relieve symptoms, and improve or maintain quality of life.[47]

Surgery

In patients with MBC, surgery is primarily palliative.[48] In select cases, surgery may be appropriate for patients with brain metastases, spinal cord compression, fractures, or isolated metastases.[48]

Radiation

RT is highly effective in the management of pain from bone metastases in patients with MBC.[48] Additional indications for palliative RT are local control of metastases to the brain, spine (cord compression), and viscera.[48]

Hormonal Therapy

Given the palliative nature of treatment, initial use of hormonal therapy is indicated in patients with hormone receptor–positive MBC because of improved tolerability over chemotherapy.[33] Endocrine therapies are typically administered sequentially until the patient has resistance to endocrine agents or clinical factors that necessitate the use of chemotherapy. In addition to the AIs and tamoxifen, fulvestrant, progestins (megestrol or medroxyprogesterone), androgens (fluoxymesterone), and estrogens (diethylstilbestrol, conjugated estrogens) are available therapies for postmenopausal patients with MBC.[33] Therapies for premenopausal women include tamoxifen with or without an LHRH agonist, followed by ovarian suppression in combination with agents indicated for postmenopausal patients.[7,33]

With the variety of endocrine agents available for treatment of MBC, the sequencing of agents has become more complex. In patients who have not had previous exposure to an AI, anastrozole and letrozole both have data showing superior outcomes as first-line therapy when compared with tamoxifen and are considered the treatment of choice in newly diagnosed postmenopausal patients with hormone receptor-positive MBC.[33] AIs have also proven to be beneficial following tamoxifen in the second-line treatment of MBC. For patients who have experienced disease progression on a nonsteroidal AI, exemestane or fulvestrant are appropriate options based on published data.[33] Fulvestrant, an estrogen receptor down-regulator, has shown to have equivalent efficacy to anastrozole in tamoxifen-resistant patients with MBC.[49] After second-line therapy, there are little data to support specific sequencing of hormonal agents, and selection is generally based on previous exposure and tolerability.

Chemotherapy

The management of MBC with chemotherapy remains a significant challenge. An increasing number of patients have been previously exposed to anthracyclines and taxanes, two of the most active chemotherapeutic classes for treatment of breast cancer. Still, other classes of cytotoxic agents are available for symptom palliation and prolongation of survival (Table 43-3). Chemotherapy is the initial treatment of choice in patients with hormone receptor–negative MBC. Indications for chemotherapy in patients with hormone-positive MBC include rapid disease progression, visceral crisis resulting in symptoms, or endocrine refractory disease.[7,33] There are little data to suggest that combination chemotherapy is superior to sequential single-agent therapy in the metastatic setting, and combination treatment often results in increased toxicity.[7] However, combination chemotherapy may be beneficial in patients requiring a rapid response, including those with extensive visceral involvement with hepatic or pulmonary metastases.[41]

Anthracyclines possess significant activity in the first-line treatment of MBC, with single-agent response rates (RRs) of 30% to 40%.[50] These may be used as monotherapy or in combination with other agents. The taxanes also possess significant activity for treatment of patients with MBC, with objective RRs of 50% or greater.[50] Taxane therapy after anthracycline failure is considered standard of care in patients with MBC.[50] Capecitabine is an oral prodrug of fluorouracil with single-agent activity in patients with MBC who have had previous exposure to an anthracycline and taxane. Ixabepilone is a member of the epothilone class of compounds. Ixabepilone in combination with capecitabine improved PFS compared with capecitabine alone in patients with anthracycline- and taxane-resistant breast cancer. It has also demonstrated efficacy as a single agent in patients with breast cancer resistant to anthracyclines, taxanes, and capecitabine.[51] Other agents with activity in MBC include gemcitabine, vinorelbine, liposomal doxorubicin, and albumin-bound paclitaxel (Table 43-3). Chemotherapy is generally continued until disease progression or intolerable toxicities.

Targeted Therapy

Trastuzumab was approved by the FDA in combination with paclitaxel for first-line treatment of MBC based on the results of a large phase III trial. This multinational, randomized phase III clinical trial compared weekly trastuzumab administration with anthracycline- or taxane-based chemotherapy to chemotherapy alone as first-line therapy in patients with HER2-positive MBC.[52] Trastuzumab therapy significantly improved time to progression, duration of response, and median survival. However, trastuzumab increased the risk of heart failure, particularly in patients who received concomitant anthracyclines. Since that time, many chemotherapeutic agents have been studied in combination with trastuzumab for MBC, including docetaxel, vinorelbine, and gemcitabine.

Lapatinib is an oral, small molecule dual tyrosine kinase inhibitor that blocks downstream signaling pathways of both HER2 and epidermal growth factor receptor (EGFR).[53] Lapatinib is indicated for patients with HER2-positive advanced or metastatic breast cancer who have received prior therapy including an anthracycline, a taxane, and trastuzumab. A phase III, randomized, open-label clinical trial that included 324 patients showed a significant improvement in DFS with lapatinib plus capecitabine compared with capecitabine alone.[54] The most commonly occurring adverse events with lapatinib are diarrhea, rash, nausea, and fatigue.[55] The potential for adverse events with drug interactions also exist with lapatinib. Lapatinib undergoes first-pass metabolism catalyzed by CYP3A4/5 and has the potential to interact with many other medications, including certain antibiotics, anticonvulsants, and antihypertensives.[53]

Bevacizumab is a humanized monoclonal antibody that targets the vascular endothelial growth factor (VEGF) receptor.[56] Vascular endothelial growth factor is a potent angiogenic growth factor that induces proliferation and inhibits apoptosis of endothelial cells.[56] The ECOG 2100 trial evaluated bevacizumab with paclitaxel compared with paclitaxel alone as first-line treatment of in 680 patients with MBC. The addition of bevacizumab to paclitaxel resulted in an increased RR and PFS compared with paclitaxel alone. OS was not significantly different. Significant adverse events reported with the use of bevacizumab include hypertension, proteinuria, thrombosis, bleeding, impaired wound healing, and gastrointestinal perforation.[57]

Bisphosphonate Therapy

Bone metastases can occur in 70% of patients with MBC and are associated with severe skeletal complications.[58] Bisphosphonates inhibit normal and pathologic osteoclast-mediated bone resorption, reducing bone destruction. Potent bisphosphonates, such as pamidronate and zoledronic acid, have shown to be beneficial in reducing skeletal related events (SREs) in patients with MBC with bone involvement.[58] These SREs were defined as pathologic fracture, spinal cord compression, bone surgery, radiation to treat bone pain, and hypercalcemia of malignancy.[58] Adverse events associated with bisphosphonate therapy include mild to moderate flulike symptoms with initial infusions, renal toxicity, and, rarely, osteonecrosis of the jaw.[59]

Table 43-3. Selected Chemotherapy Agents and Regimens for Treatment of Metastatic Breast Cancer

Regimen	Drugs	Doses	Schedule	Frequency
FAC/FEC	See Table 43-2			
Paclitaxel		175 mg/m² IV	Day 1	Every 21 days
		80–100 mg/m² IV	Day 1	Every 7 days
Paclitaxel + bevacizumab	Paclitaxel	90 mg/m² IV	Days 1, 8, 15	Every 28 days
	Bevacizumab	10 mg/kg IV	Days 1 and 15	
Docetaxel		60–100 mg/m² IV	Day 1	Every 21 days
		40 mg/m² IV	Day 1	Every 7 days
Abraxane (albumin-bound paclitaxel)		260 mg/m² IV	Day 1	Every 21 days
Capecitabine		1,000–1,250 mg/m² PO	Twice daily for 14 days, then off for 7 days	Every 21 days
Doxil (liposomal doxorubicin)		30–50 mg/m² IV	Day 1	Every 21–28 days
Capecitabine + Docetaxel	Capecitabine	1,000–1,250 mg/m² PO	Twice daily for 14 days, then off for 7 days	Every 21 days
	Docetaxel	75–100 mg/m² IV	Day 1	Every 21 days
Ixabepilone		40 mg/m² IV	Day 1	Every 21 days
Ixabepilone + Capecitabine	Ixabepilone	40 mg/m² IV	Day 1	Every 21 days
	Capecitabine	1,000 mg/m² PO	Twice daily for 14 days, then off for 7 days	Every 21 days
Gemcitabine		800–1,200 mg/m² IV	Days 1, 8, and 15	Every 28 days
Vinorelbine		25 mg/m² IV	Day 1	Every 7 days
Trastuzumab		8-mg/kg loading dose, then 6 mg/kg IV	Day 1	Every 21 days
		4-mg/kg loading dose, then 2 mg/kg IV	Day 1	Every 7 days

Source: Adapted from references 7 and 48.

IV = intravenous; PO = by mouth.

Monitoring and Follow-up

ROUTINE MONITORING FOR SURVIVORS

The goals for monitoring and surveillance of patients following treatment of their breast cancer are to detect potentially curable locoregional recurrences or new primaries, to monitor for symptoms of metastatic disease, and to assess treatment-related side effects. For women without an inherited genetic predisposition, the risk of developing a new, second primary breast cancer is about 0.5% to 1% per year. The risk of recurrence is related to tumor stage and grade. Recommendations for appropriate follow-up and management of patients following treatment of breast cancer have been published.[60,61] A careful history and physical examination performed by a clinician experienced in the surveillance of cancer patients and in breast examination should be performed every 3–6 months for the first 3 years, every 6–12 months for the next 2 years, and annually thereafter. For patients who have had breast-conserving surgery, continuation of yearly mammograms is recommended unless otherwise indicated. A referral for genetic counseling is recommended for patients at high risk for familial breast cancer. Patients should perform monthly breast self-examination to check for any new lumps and be educated regarding symptoms of distant disease. As breast cancer metastasis is most common in the bone, lung, liver and brain, symptoms of metastasis may include bone pain, chest pain, abdominal pain, dyspnea, jaundice, or neurologic symptoms. Regular gynecologic care is recommended for all women, and patients receiving tamoxifen should report any unusual vaginal bleeding, pelvic pain, or pressure. Routine use of blood tests, tumor markers, and radiographic imaging studies are not recommended in asymptomatic patients, as these tests have not been shown to improve disease-free or overall survival or quality of life.

More than 2 million women in the U.S. are alive with a history of breast cancer, including those with active disease and those who are cured. As more women are surviving breast cancer, many will be faced with survivorship issues related to the treatment of their malignancy, including cardiovascular health, bone health, vasomotor symptoms, and fertility.[61]

CARDIOVASCULAR

Congestive heart failure or dilated cardiomyopathy can occur as a result of exposure to anthracycline-based chemotherapy regimens.[62] The use of trastuzumab also increases the risk of cardiotoxicity. When given either sequentially or in combination with chemotherapy, trastuzumab contributes to about a 1% to 4% increase in the risk for cardiotoxicity in women with HER2-positive breast cancer treated for early-stage disease.[62] Tamoxifen decreases serum lipids and is reported to decrease the risk of myocardial infarction, but increases the risk of thromboembolic and cerebrovascular events. Before major surgeries, consideration should be given for temporary discontinuation of tamoxifen to reduce the risk of postoperative thrombosis. AIs are not associated with an increased risk of thromboembolic events, but some studies report a greater incidence of hypercholesterolemia or cardiovascular adverse events.[63] Longer follow-up data and results from additional trials will provide further information on the impact of AIs on cardiovascular health.

Both cardiovascular disease and breast cancer are significant causes of death in American women, particularly for those with shared risk factors or who have received cardiotoxic therapies for their malignancy. Continual assessment of cardiovascular risks with appropriate monitoring and treatment is important for all women, including those with or without a history of breast cancer.

BONE HEALTH

Many women are at risk for osteoporosis and fractures either because of their age or as a result of their breast cancer treatments.[64] The risk of osteoporosis is increased in premenopausal women who undergo premature menopause and in postmenopausal women who receive treatment with AIs. Options for management will be discussed in detail in Chapter 47: Management of Treatment Complications.

VASOMOTOR

Breast cancer survivors are faced with a number of issues related to estrogen deficiency and menopause, including hot flashes, vaginal dryness, genitourinary atrophy, dyspareunia, and osteoporosis.[61] Adjuvant endocrine therapies can exacerbate these symptoms. Hormone therapy is generally contraindicated in women with a history of breast cancer, and treatments for menopausal symptoms are limited.[65,66] Options for management will be discussed in detail in Chapter 45: Ovarian Cancer.

FERTILITY

Approximately 25% of breast cancers are expected to occur in women <50 years of age.[67] For women diagnosed in their childbearing years who wish to conceive, the possibility of treatment-related infertility should be discussed before beginning treatment. Options for fertility preservation exist.[68]

Premenopausal patients should use precautions against pregnancy while receiving treatment. In women receiving tamoxifen, nonhormonal methods of contraception are necessary because tamoxifen is teratogenic. It should be discontinued several weeks to months before trying to conceive. Similarly, precautions against pregnancy should be taken in women receiving adjuvant trastuzumab because of limited safety data.[69] Immunoglobulins do cross the placenta, and there are known HER2 receptors on the heart.

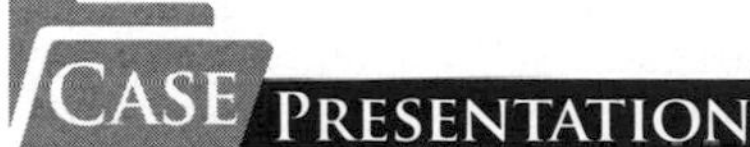

Patient Case: Part 2

Diagnosis: KB has stage IIIC (T2, N3, M0) breast cancer. Her risk factors for the development of breast cancer include early age of menarche, late age of natural menopause, and late age of first birth.

Treatment plan:

1. Because this patient has node-positive breast cancer, she should receive treatment with an anthracycline- and taxane-based neoadjuvant chemotherapy regimen. Reasons for use of specific chemotherapy regimens are complex, and many regimens are appropriate (Table 43-2).
2. Patient should have surgery with either modified radical mastectomy or BCT, with axillary lymph node dissection.
3. Patient should have radiation therapy to the chest wall, axillary lymph nodes, and infraclavicular nodal regions.
4. Because this patient is postmenopausal and has hormone receptor–positive breast cancer, adjuvant hormonal therapy with an AI is indicated. AIs approved for initial therapy include anastrozole 1 mg orally daily and letrozole 2.5 mg orally daily for 5 years.

Patient monitoring: A careful history and physical examination performed by a clinician experienced in the surveillance of cancer patients and in breast examination should be performed every 3–6 months for the first 3 years, every 6–12 months for the next 2 years, and annually thereafter. For patients who have had breast-conserving surgery, continuation of yearly mammograms is recommended unless otherwise indicated. Patients should perform monthly breast self-examination to check for any new lumps and be educated regarding symptoms of distant disease.

Patient education: Patient education for patients with breast cancer varies greatly and is dependent on the types of therapies indicated for treatment. Patients should be thoroughly counseled regarding potential adverse events and management of side effects from surgery, radiation therapy, chemotherapy, targeted therapy, or hormonal therapy, as indicated.

Summary

Breast cancer is a significant women's health issue in the U.S. and throughout the world. New approaches to breast cancer diagnosis, prevention, and treatment have enhanced clinical outcomes and care of patients with this malignancy. Screening for breast cancer with mammogram in women older than 40 years of age and MRI of the breast in women at high risk for development of breast cancer has allowed for the identification of tumors that are more likely to be in an early stage of disease, when they are potentially more curable. Advances in breast cancer treatments—including chemotherapy, surgery, radiation therapy, hormonal therapy, and targeted therapy—have improved outcomes in patients with early-stage disease and have helped those with metastatic disease live longer and with a more favorable quality of life.

References

Additional content available at ***www.ashp.org/womenshealth***

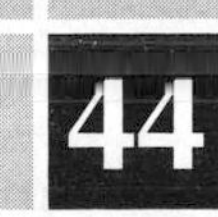

44 Endometrial Cancer

Claire M. Mach, Pharm.D.; Lynn Cloutier, RN, MSN, ACNP, AOCN

Learning Objectives

1. Evaluate the risk factors for endometrial cancer.
2. Explain when an evaluation for endometrial cancer would be necessary based on signs and symptoms.
3. Define the role of surgery, radiation, and chemotherapy in the treatment of endometrial cancer based on current guidelines and stage of disease.
4. Compare and contrast chemotherapy options for women with advanced or recurrent endometrial cancer.
5. Describe the long-term complications associated with the treatment of endometrial cancer.

Endometrial cancer is the most common genital tract malignancy in women, and the likelihood of the development of endometrial cancer for a woman during her lifetime is 1 in 37.[1] It is estimated 42,160 new uterine cancer cases will be diagnosed in 2009, with 7,780 women dying of the disease. The incidence of endometrial cancer remains constant; however, more women are dying of the disease. The death rate from endometrial cancer has increased significantly since 1987.[2,3] This may be due to both the aging of the American female population and obesity. More than 90% of worldwide cases present in women age 50 or older. The highest incidences are in North America and Europe. Rates are low in southern and eastern Asia and most of Africa.[4] In as many as 80% of women, the disease is diagnosed when the cancer is confined to the uterus. If endometrial cancer is caught early, when disease is limited to the uterus, the overall 5-year survival is nearly 90%, but for women presenting with advanced-stage disease, the prognosis is very poor, with a 5-year overall survival of only 27%.[5]

Peak incidence of this disease occurs in the sixth and seventh decades of life. However, 20% of the time the disease occurs in women who are premenopausal, with approximately 5% younger than the age of 40.[6] Young women are more likely to present with early-stage, lower-grade tumors and less likely to have serous histology when compared with older patients.[7,8]

Epidemiology

Chronic exposure to unopposed estrogen through either endogenous sources or exogenous administration is hypothesized to be the most common pathway leading to endometrial cancer. Endogenous estrogens rise in postmenopausal women because of increased production of androstenedione or a greater peripheral conversion of androstenedione to estrone. In absence of progesterone, estrogen effect on endometrial cells promotes increased mitotic activity and subsequent replication errors that ultimately produce **endometrial hyperplasia,** somatic mutations, and potentially endometrial cancer.[9] Endometrial hyperplasia leads to some degree of cellular atypia. Depending on the degree of atypia, invasion of the basement membrane may occur, resulting in endometrial cancer. Type I endometrial cancers are preceded by the premalignant change called *complex atypical hyperplasia*.[6,10-13] This change is a spectrum ranging from endometrial hyperplasia without atypia, to endometrial hyperplasia with atypia, to well-differentiated endometrial cancer.[14] Type I endometrial cancer is estrogen dependent and appears most often in pre- and perimenopausal women. It is well differentiated and therefore has a better prognosis. It is associated with conditions that elevate estrogen levels, such as **hyperestrinism,** diabetes, liver disease, hypertension, obesity,

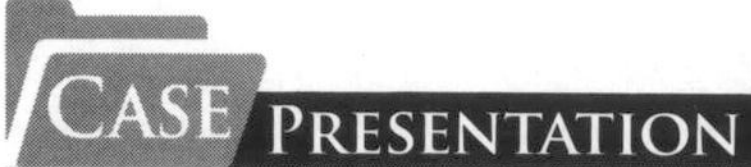

CASE PRESENTATION

Patient Case: Part 1

H.G. is 60-year-old Hispanic woman who presents with uterine bleeding lasting several days per month.

HPI: The patient believed this bleeding to be a menstrual cycle, though she had not had a cycle for 5 years. The bleeding progressed to continuous flow with passage of clots. The patient sought care from her primary physician. An endometrial biopsy (EMB) was taken, and the patient was referred to a gynecologic oncologist.

PMH: Menarche at age 11; gravida 2, para 1; menopause at age 55.

Family history: Unremarkable.

Social history: Married, one child, denies tobacco use, some alcohol use.

Medications: Once-daily aspirin, calcium with vitamin D, multivitamin.

Allergies: Codeine.

Vitals: 5′1″, 143 kg, BP 116/69, temp 37°C, RR 23.

Physical exam: Some discomfort and bleeding with exam. Uterus enlarged. No palpable ovarian masses. Otherwise, rest of exam within normal limits.

Lab values: CBC and chemistries within normal limits.

Pathology: The EMB performed by the patient's primary physician showed well-differentiated adenocarcinoma of the endometrioid type. Estrogen receptor (ER) and progesterone receptor (PR) demonstrated approximately 70% of tumor cell nuclei staining moderately to strongly for ER, and approximately 20% of tumor cell nuclei staining moderately to strongly for PR.

Preliminary assessment: H.G. has confirmed endometrial cancer and additional diagnostic testing—including computed tomography (CT) of chest, abdomen, and pelvis, and chest x-ray (CXR)—were ordered to assist in treatment planning.

infertility, and other menstrual cycle disorders.[15] Type II endometrial cancer is not estrogen dependent and is most often diagnosed in postmenopausal women, thin and fertile women, or in women with normal menstrual cycles. Those endometrial cancers not associated with endometrial hyperplasia tend to be unusually aggressive and less responsive to treatment. Often this type of endometrial cancer is of either serous or clear cell histology.[6]

Etiology

The etiology of endometrial cancer is multifactorial and not fully understood. Obesity is a major risk factor for endometrial cancer. Women who are 30 lb overweight have a risk 3 times that of the general population, and women who are 50 lb or more overweight are 5 times more likely to develop endometrial cancer than the general population.[10] Obesity causes a profound change in the hormonal environment of a woman's body through conversion of androgens to estrogens through several pathways, such as extraglandular aromatization of androstenedione to estrone, of which the net result is increased unopposed estrogen effect.[16] A higher body mass index (BMI) at baseline and adult weight gain are associated with increased endometrial cancer risk.[17] The effect of adiposity on endometrial carcinogenesis is a continuous and cumulative process throughout the entire life, with women who are consistently overweight through adulthood having a greater risk than women who become overweight in late adulthood (after the age of 60).[18] There are conflicting reports associated with the effect of hypertension increasing the risk of endometrial cancer. Most often, the hypertension is an effect of increased BMI, and when adjusted for, is not a consistent association.

Women who have not delivered a child are twice as likely to develop endometrial cancer as those who have.[19] It appears that the high levels of progesterone during pregnancy may offer the protection not observed in nulliparous women. Early age at menarche, late age of natural menopause, and longer span of ovulation are associated with increased risk for endometrial cancer.[20] Chronic anovulation in conjunction with a hyperandrogenic state results in constant stimulation of endometrium from peripheral conversion of androgens to estrogen, which increases risk for endometrial cancer. Without ovulation and progesterone secretion of the corpus luteum, women are at risk for the development of estrogen-driven endometrial cancers.[21]

Noninsulin-dependent diabetes is associated with a state of insulinemia, which is associated with a hyperestrogenic state. Women with diabetes have an approximate twofold higher risk for developing endometrial cancer. The risk is increased more than sixfold among obese diabetic women when compared with normal-weight women without diabetes. The most unfavorable combination is women with diabetes, obesity, and low physical activity having approximately a 10 fold higher risk in comparison with women without diabetes, normal weight, and a high level of physical activity.[22]

There is increased risk in those whose family has a history of endometrial cancer, especially those members diagnosed at an early age. Hereditary nonpolyposis colorectal cancer (HNPCC) or Lynch syndrome is caused by mutations in DNA mismatch repair genes in MSH2, MLH1, PMS1, PNS2, and MSH6. Those women with this syndrome are at a 40% to 60% risk of developing endometrial cancer, and women are at an equal or higher risk of developing endometrial cancer than colon cancer.[23-26] Women who undergo risk-reducing surgery have a 33% lower risk compared with women who undergo increased surveillance. Risk-reducing surgery is an effective strategy for preventing endometrial cancer in those women with HPNCC.[25]

The National Surgical Adjuvant Breast and Bowel Project (NSABP-27) warrants early screening for those women taking tamoxifen. The primary therapeutic effect of tamoxifen is derived from its antiestrogenic properties, but this medication also has estrogenic activity. The increased relative risk of developing endometrial cancer for women taking tamoxifen for breast cancer is 2–3 times higher than a matched population in women older than the age of 50 years.[27] There is currently conflicting evidence for the role of the *BRCA1* gene in the development of endometrial cancer; however, there is a possible association of an increased risk for endometrial cancer in women with a *BRCA1* mutation taking tamoxifen.[28]

Race has also been identified as a risk factor for endometrial cancer. A higher percentage of black women is initially diagnosed with advanced endometrial cancer as well as the more aggressive subtype.[19]

Clinical Presentation

The most common symptom women will present with to their gynecologist is abnormal vaginal bleeding. Younger pre- or perimenopausal women have **menorrhagia,** and postmenopausal women have resumption of vaginal bleeding after some time in menopause. As these are symptoms most individuals will not ignore for a long period, endometrial cancer is detected early in the majority of women. The presence of other symptoms—such as abdominal fullness and pressure, as well as organ dysfunction—are usually indicators of more advanced stage disease.

Patterns of Metastasis

Metastasis of endometrial cancer occurs in one of three routes. Metastasis occurs by direct extension to adjacent structures, including the rectum and bladder. It can occur via the lymphatic system to the pelvic lymph nodes, aortic lymph nodes, and ovaries, and it can occur hematogenously to distant sites, including the lungs and liver.[23] The most frequently observed sites of relapse are lymph nodes, vagina, peritoneum, and lung.[29] Most recurrences are detected through symptoms alone and are most often at distant sites.[30] Recurrent disease may be more difficult to treat than primary disease and usually recurs within the first 3 years after initial treatment.[10,30,31] Significant predictors of poor outcome in recurrent disease are multiple sites of disease and liver and splenic metastases. Increasing age and higher tumor grade at primary surgery, as well as rapid relapse, also predict a less favorable outcome in recurrent disease.[29] Healthcare providers should evaluate hormone receptor status of recurrent disease, location of the recurrence (including proximity to rectum and bladder), and emphasize quality of life in treatment decisions with the patient. Recurrent disease is potentially salvageable with radiotherapy alone or in combination with surgery or chemotherapy.[29] Most often, the management of advanced or recurrent disease is palliative and prognosis poor despite surgical treatment and irradiation.[32,33] The median survival of women enrolled in trials for recurrent or metastatic endometrial cancer is only approximately 12 months.[33]

Pathophysiology and Carcinogenesis

Endometrial carcinoma forms in the inner lining of the uterus and usually takes years to develop. It may originate in a small area (e.g., within an endometrial polyp) or in a diffuse multifocal pattern. Early tumor growth is characterized by an exophytic and spreading pattern. Growth is characterized by friability and spontaneous bleeding, even at early stages. Later tumor growth is characterized by myometrial invasion and growth toward the cervix (Figure 44-1).

Screening

The American Cancer Society (ACS) and the National Cancer Institute (NCI) do not recommend routine screening for endometrial cancer in most

Figure 44-1. Endometrial cancer myometrial invasion.

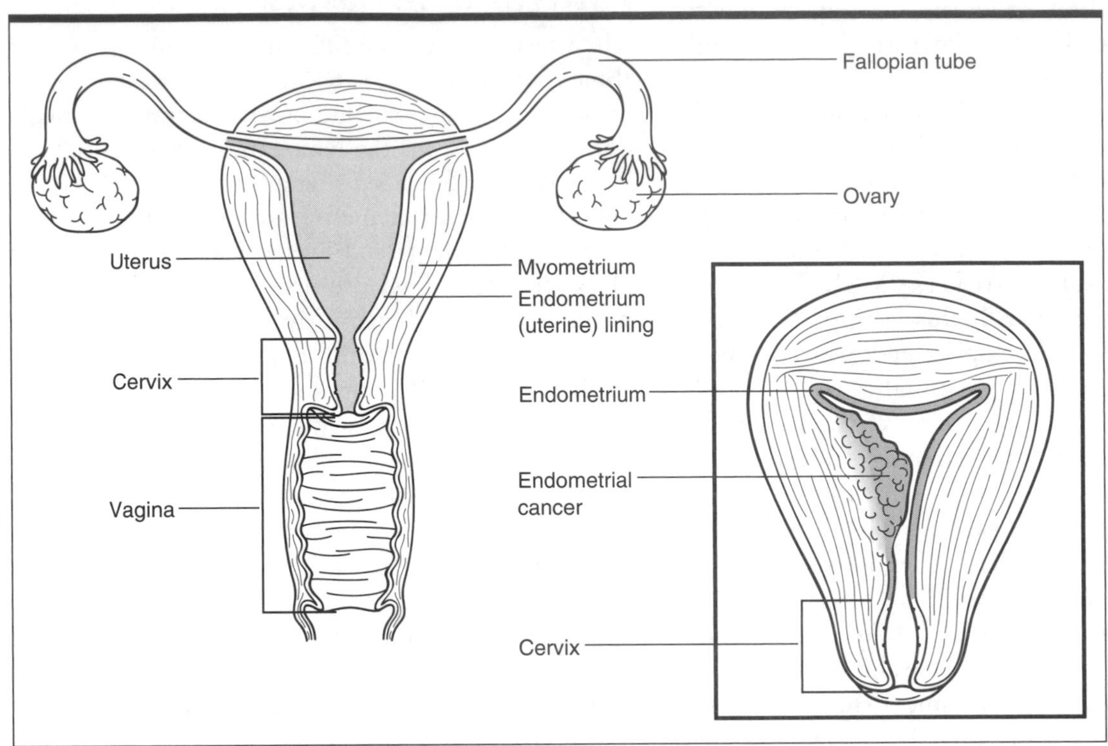

women. The ACS recommends that at the time of menopause, women at average risk should be informed about risks and symptoms of endometrial cancer and strongly encouraged to report any unexpected bleeding or spotting to their physicians.

The ACS recommends screening for women at very high risk for endometrial cancer because of three risk factors: known HPNCC genetic mutation carrier status, substantial likelihood of being a mutation carrier or mutation is known to be present in the family, or absence of genetic testing results in families with suspected autosomal dominant predisposition to colon cancer.[34] Women at high risk for endometrial cancer who carry a genetic predisposition to the disease should be offered annual screening and extensive counseling about risks, benefits, and limitations of screening beginning at age 35. Unfortunately, there is no standardized algorithm for screening in high-risk women.[35,36]

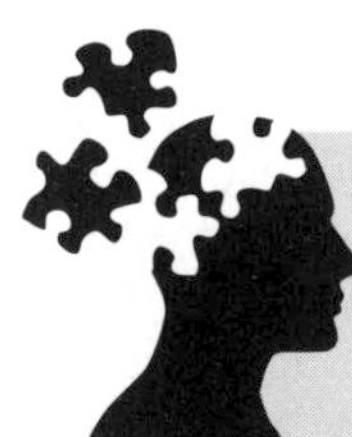

Therapeutic Challenge:

R.G. is a 34-year-old woman who recently married and presents to your clinic for family planning options. Both she and her spouse would like to wait another year before having children. R.G. has a father who died of colon cancer at age 56 and a mother with history of endometrial cancer diagnosed at age 47, but she was cured. R.G. tests positive for HPNCC. What are her fertility options?

Diagnosis of Endometrial Cancer

Workup for dysfunctional bleeding includes transvaginal ultrasound (TVUS), endometrial biopsy (EMB), and **dilatation and curettage (D&C);** it may also include hysteroscopy. A TVUS can be used in the initial diagnosis of endometrial cancer in postmenopausal women who may have difficulty tolerating in-office EMB and can assist in determining if a women should undergo biopsy. TVUS is used to determine endometrial thickness, in that an endometrial lining of >4–5 mm requires further evaluation; however, persistent bleeding and an endometrial lining of <4–5 mm does not reliably exclude endometrial cancer.[37] TVUS does offer reasonable accuracy of predicting cervical and myometrial invasion from endometrial cancer.[13] It often does not provide useful diagnostic information for premenopausal women as they normally have a thick endometrium. An EMB is the preferred diagnostic exam in both pre- and postmenopausal women because of high sensitivity, low complication rate, and low cost. EMB should be performed whenever abnormal bleeding is encountered in a postmenopausal woman or in a premenopausal woman with uncontrollable menorrhagia. If cervical involvement is suspected, a cervical biopsy should be performed. A D&C must be performed in those patients with high suspicion of endometrial cancer whose EMB is negative. Hysteroscopy is the inspection of the uterine cavity by endoscopy and is often used in conjunction with D&C. This is useful in evaluating the endometrium for polyps or for visualization of the endometrium if bleeding persists. The use of this diagnostic tool when endometrial cancer is suspected is controversial in that extrauterine spread to the abdominal cavity through the fallopian tubes may possibly occur during the procedure.[38,39] Once diagnosis is reached, further evaluation of extent of disease can be achieved through TVUS, cystoscopy, proctoscopy, CT, and magnetic resonance imaging (MRI) as dictated by suspicion of disease. These imaging modalities can determine if invasion of rectum, bladder, or cervix has occurred.

The preoperative assessment of the majority of women scheduled to undergo surgery for treatment of endometrial cancer may consist only of an extensive history and physical exam; laboratory studies, which include CBC, electrolytes, BUN, creatinine, glucose, and renal and liver function tests; and a chest x-ray.[3] However, patients with endometrial cancer often have comorbidities, such as obesity, hypertension, diabetes, and cardiopulmonary disease, placing them at high risk for undergoing surgical procedures. The workup of women deemed to be high-risk surgical candidates should include testing to evaluate for medical issues in addition to any testing required to assess the extent of disease.

Histology and Pathology

Seventy-one percent of endometrial cancers are type I or endometrioid adenocarcinoma. Mutations of DNA-mismatch repair genes (MLH 1, MSH2, MSH6), PTEN, k-ras, and ß-catenin genes are found in 20% of these types of tumors.[40] Type II endometrial cancer is more aggressive, with high-grade features and p53 mutations. These tumors have a worse prognosis, are nonendometrioid and more lethal, and account for 10% to 20% of patients with endometrial cancer.[41] The pathway of activation is through the ERBB2 (Her-2/neu) oncogene and mutation of the p53 tumor suppressor gene.[6,12] Endometrial intraepithelial carcinoma (EIC) is different from atypical hyperplasia and represents the precursor lesion of serous carcinoma. Serous carcinoma, clear cell, and malignant mixed müllerian tumors are found in this category. These histologic types are usually associated with endometrial atrophy or uterine polyps, have a high risk for presence of extrauterine spread at diagnosis, and the tumors have a tendency to relapse outside the pelvis.[13,42]

Histologic grading applies to endometrioid carcinomas, whereas serous and clear cell carcinoma are considered high grade. The grades 1, 2, and 3 correspond with well, moderately, and poorly differentiated carcinoma, respectively. The system is based on the percentage of the tumor mass that is occupied by a solid, other-than-squamous component. The International Federation of Gynecology and Obstetrics (FIGO) classification includes three grades: grade 1, with the percentage of solid growth (other than squamous) in the tumor mass up to 5%; grade 2, with the percentage of solid growth accounting for 6% to 50%; and grade 3, with the percentage of solid growth >50%. In addition, the presence of notable nuclear atypia results in classifying the tumor to a higher grade.[13,43]

Staging

After a series of studies demonstrated that understaging of patients was commonplace, the staging of endometrial cancer was changed in 1988 from clinical to surgical staging (Table 44-1), including pelvic and para-aortic **lymphadenectomy** on the basis of the FIGO criteria.[43,44] The change emphasized the necessity of using a complete surgical assessment of patients to include data for histologic grade, myometrial invasion, lymph node status, and extent and location of extrauterine spread. This provided a significant therapeutic benefit of lymph node dissection (LND) in terms of survival not only in stage II, but in poorly differentiated stage I and IIa disease. This continues to be of controversy in that the recent ASTEC (A Study in the Treatment of Endometrial Cancer) trial did not support the previous findings.[1,41,45,46]

Prognostic Factors

The choice of treatment and prognosis are determined by many factors, including tumor grade, histologic subtype, age, race, endocrine status, depth of

Table 44-1. FIGO Staging of Endometrial Cancer

Stage 0	**No evidence of primary tumor**
Stage I	**Tumor limited to uterus**
	Ia Extent of disease limited to endometrium
	Ib Disease invading less than half myometrium
	Ic Disease invading more than half myometrium
Stage II	**Tumor invading cervix but does not extend beyond uterus**
	IIa Endocervical glandular involvement only
	IIb Cervical stromal invasion
Stage III	**Local and regional extension of tumor**
	IIIa Disease invading serosa and/or adnexa and/or positive peritoneal washings or ascites
	IIIb Tumor extends to vagina (direct extension or metastasis)
	IIIc Tumor invading pelvic and/or para-aortic lymph nodes
Stage IV	**Tumor extending beyond pelvis**
	IVA Diseases invading bladder mucosa and/or bowel mucosa
	IVB Distant metastasis beyond pelvic/local region

endometrial penetration through uterine wall, cervical involvement, presence or absence of positive peritoneal cytology and lymph nodes, and distant metastases. Prognosis is also affected by the presence of adnexal metastases, intraperitoneal spread, and para-aortic involvement.[47]

In addition to the role obesity plays in the genesis of endometrial cancer, obesity also poses a substantial challenge to cancer treatment. Overweight and obese women face increased surgical morbidity. Obesity also offers a challenge to radiation physicists as dosimetry calculation is more difficult. Additionally, there is not a standardized approach to chemotherapy dosing in obese patients. Approaches to dosing in these patients should take into account if the intent of chemotherapy is potentially curative or palliative, and dosages should be adjusted regardless of dosing method based on excessive toxicity. Some healthcare providers may cap dosing at BSA of 2 m^2, whereas others may dose based on total body weight, adjusted body weight, or lean body weight.[16] The combination of capped dosing and increased drug elimination for certain drugs could effectively reduce the chemotherapy dose to tissues and tumors, leading potentially to less effective treatment.[48]

Prevention

Although most cases of endometrial cancer cannot be prevented, some measures offer a protective mechanism and lower the risk of developing this cancer. The use of oral contraceptives lowers risk. The risk is lowest in women who take oral contraceptives for a long time, and this protection continues for at least 10 years after a woman stops taking them.[49,50] Obtaining timely and proper treatment for precursor disorders of the endometrium will decrease the opportunity for the disorder to progress to endometrial cancer. It is postulated that eating a diet high in fruits, vegetables, and whole grain foods is preventative. Participating in regular physical activity and maintaining a healthy weight decreases the risk of endometrial cancer, especially in those women who are obese.[34] A Netherlands cohort study reported a 46% reduction in risk in women who were physically active more than 90 min/day compared with those active less than 30 min/day.[17] There is a significant association between leisure time inactivity and increased risk for endometrial cancer.[22]

Primary Treatment

Most women with endometrial cancer will present with disease limited to the uterus or stage I disease.

If the patient has an acceptable risk for surgery, **peritoneal lavage** for cytology and total abdominal hysterectomy with bilateral salpingo-oophorectomy (TAH/BSO) should be performed. Pelvic and para-aortic nodes should be dissected, and all abdominal organs should be inspected. For patients with stage I disease that is medically inoperable, radiation therapy (RT) alone can be considered, which provides long-term progression-free survival for some women.[3]

For women who have suspected cervical involvement on presentation, a cervical biopsy and MRI should be done to confirm and determine the extent of disease in the cervix. When cervical involvement is determined to be present, the patient should be counseled regarding the need to perform a radical hysterectomy with LND of pelvic and para-aortic lymph nodes if the patient is a surgical candidate. The patient may also be considered for RT before surgery, and for medically inoperable patients, pelvic RT with **brachytherapy** can improve the survival rate.[3]

Women presenting with extrauterine intra-abdominal disease should be managed with a more extensive surgical intervention, including omentectomy and debulking in addition to TAH/BSO, if determined to be a surgical candidate. Patients with extrauterine disease limited to the pelvis are treated with RT and brachytherapy with or without surgery, or chemotherapy. For disease that extends outside of the abdominal cavity, TAH/BSO with or without RT, hormonal therapy, or chemotherapy are available options for these patients.[3]

Nonpharmacologic Treatment

SURGERY

Surgery is the primary treatment for early-stage endometrial cancer. Pathologic assessment of the uterus is critical and should include a ratio of depth of myometrial invasion to the myometrial thickness, tumor size, tumor location within the uterus, histologic subtype with grade, lymphovascular space invasion, and frozen section.

Complete surgical staging will include pelvic washings, bilateral pelvic and para-aortic lymphadenectomy, exploration of nodes to the level of renal vessels, and complete resection of all disease. The incorporation of lymphadenectomy with surgical staging is controversial. Although not standard of practice, LND is critically one of the most precise methods for identifying nodal metastases and is associated with improved survival rates, the most important prognosticator in endometrial cancer.[10,41,45,51] ASTEC preliminary results show lymphadenectomy and surgical staging did not provide a survival benefit but may be used to determine prognosis and tailor treatment.[52,53] The National Comprehensive Cancer Network advocates LND rather than nodal sampling in patients undergoing primary surgical intervention for endometrial cancer.[54] Laparoscopy offers an alternative to conventional open procedure for surgical intervention in the treatment of endometrial cancer. Conversion to laparotomy from laparoscopy is done in case of macroscopic positive pelvic nodes or extrauterine disease. The Gynecologic Oncology Group (GOG) Lap2 phase III study was initiated in 1996. This large randomized study examines the role of pelvic and para-aortic lymph node sampling followed by laparotomy or laparoscopy. Patients with stage I or IIA, any tumor grade, with endometrial or uterine cancer are assigned to both vaginal hysterectomy and BSO by either laparotomy or laparoscopy plus lymph node sampling.[55] Overall risk of intraoperative complications is low, and risk of pulmonary embolism, congestive heart failure, arrhythmia, pneumonia, and small bowel obstruction ranged from 1% to 3%.[56] Conversion to laparotomy is undertaken in 23% of patients. There is a higher rate of arterial injuries but no significant differences in venous, ureteral, bladder, bowel, or nerve injury when compared with open procedure. Length of stay in the hospital is shown to be shorter and operative time longer in the laparoscopy group. Survival results are pending to determine outcomes of the minimally invasive technique vs. open procedure.[55-57] Previous reports demonstrating feasibility and safety of laparoscopy in early-stage endometrial cancer have been confirmed.[58] In patients with a follow-up as long as 51 months, overall survival and disease-free survival were not influenced by the treatment modality (laparoscopic-assisted vaginal hysterectomy or laparotomy) in patients with clinically early stage (stage I) endometrial adenocarcinoma.[57]

RADIATION THERAPY

RT may be used as primary therapy in patients who are deemed medically inoperable and whose operative risk is high. Morbid obesity and severe cardiopulmonary disease are the general reasons a patient with endometrial carcinoma is usually thought to be medically inoperable.

Postoperative uterine brachytherapy can achieve cure rates in excess of 70% and may be combined with external beam radiotherapy (EBRT) in the presence of prognostic factors suggesting a high risk of involved nodes.[43] Patients with increased BMI tend to have more cutaneous complications with external radiation therapy (XRT).[59] Three randomized trials with stage I/II low- and intermediate-risk disease have reached a similar conclusion that adjunctive RT in early-stage intermediate-risk endometrial carcinoma showed significant benefit in local and regional recurrence, but not survival.[60-62]

Additional therapy is warranted in those patients with high tumor grade and increased depth of tumor invasion in the **myometrium,** lymphovascular space invasion, large tumor volume, and involvement of the lower uterine segment or cervix. In a meta-analysis including 1,770 patients with stage I disease—including stage IC, grade 3 pelvic involvement—EBRT added to surgery reduced locoregional relapse. A 72% reduction in the risk of pelvic relapse did not translate into either a reduction in the risk of distant recurrence or death. A subgroup of women with multiple high-risk factors showed a trend toward the reduction in the risk of death from all causes and endometrial cancer death in patients who underwent adjuvant EBRT. In those women with low-risk, surgical stage I endometrial cancer, routine use of EBRT or combination EBRT and brachytherapy is not cost-effective. In women with intermediate risk, adjuvant pelvic radiotherapy reduces the risk of recurrence by 50%, but did not appear to improve survival at a positive net cost to no therapy.[63,64] The decision to treat depends on whether patients have high-risk factors, including the stage of disease, depth of myometrium invasion, grade of tumor, lymphovascular invasion, and the age of the patient.[65] Both pelvic and external beam radiotherapy and vaginal intracavitary brachytherapy carry risks of acute toxicities and long-term complications. Most side effects, including skin reaction and gastrointestinal and genitourinary symptoms, resolve after treatment. Twenty percent of patients have complications of urgency, abdominal cramps, diarrhea, vaginal dryness, and stenosis, which may affect their quality of life. Three percent develop severe long-term complications, mostly of the gastrointestinal tract.[66]

Pharmacologic Therapy

PRIMARY TREATMENT: HORMONAL THERAPY

Some patients may be poor surgical candidates because of comorbidities that put them at an unacceptable mortality risk.[67] For patients with a well-differentiated lesion and contraindications to general anesthesia that are unsuited for radiotherapy, high-dose progestins may be used.[43] In young women with low-grade tumors who wish to retain fertility, hormonal therapy offers an alternative to hysterectomy. Upfront advice should be given that this is not the standard of care and not considered the safest option.[10] In those who undergo conservative therapy with hormonal agents to preserve fertility, 76.5% of those with grade I disease responded to treatment, and 20% were able to become pregnant after completion of treatment; however, definitive surgical treatment should occur on completion of childbearing.[68]

Options for hormonal therapy include progestational agents, tamoxifen, and levonorgestrel-releasing intrauterine device (IUD) (Table 44-2). The levonorgestrel-releasing IUD inhibits the endometrial synthesis of estrogen receptors, making the endometrium insensitive to the circulating estradiol. The local progestogenic effect in the uterine cavity achieves a higher concentration in the uterus instead of plasma. This intervention is useful in the treatment of early-stage disease, particularly in those women medically unfit for surgical therapy.[67] Progestins such as megestrol acetate, hydroxyprogesterone caproate, and medroxyprogesterone acetate have reported response rates as high as 56%; however, on further evaluation and use of more rigorous criteria for response rates, it is likely that these agents have only a 15% to 20% response rate. The response to these agents is limited in duration, averaging about 4 months, with a mean survival of about 8–11 months once these agents are initiated. Tamoxifen also appears to have some efficacy in women, with response rates of 10% to 22%; low-grade endometrial cancers are more likely to respond, with duration of progression-free survival of 1.9 months and an overall survival of 8.8 months.[69,70] Aromatase inhibitors have limited evidence supporting their use in the treatment of endometrial cancer outside of the metastatic or relapsed setting.

CHEMOTHERAPY: ADJUVANT THERAPY AFTER SURGICAL DEBULKING

Adjuvant chemotherapy is sometimes employed for women with unfavorable histology, high histologic grade, lymphovascular involvement, and deep myometrial or cervical invasion. There is currently not much evidence to support that adjuvant chemotherapy results in a better outcome for surgical stage I–II, type I endometrial cancer.[13] However, there are a few small observational studies demonstrating a possible benefit using platinum-based chemotherapy in stage

Table 44-2. Hormonal Agents Used for Treatment of Advanced or Recurrent Endometrial Cancer

Agent	Dosage	Common Adverse Effects
Levonorgestrel-releasing intrauterine device (IUD)	20 mcg release daily continuously (up to 5 yr)	Nausea/vomiting, abdominal pain, fatigue, headache, bleeding, dizziness, breast tenderness
Megestrol acetate	40 mg PO 4 times a day continuously	Thromboembolism, anemia, hypertension, headache, insomnia, malaise, adrenal suppression, weight gain, hyperglycemia, nausea, diarrhea, hepatotoxicity
Medroxyprogesterone	200–400 mg PO in divided doses twice a day continuously	Fluid retention, depression, hyperglycemia, fatigue, dizziness, headache, insomnia, weight gain, nausea, abdominal pain, hepatotoxicity, thromboembolism
Tamoxifen	20 mg PO twice a day continuously	Thromboembolism, thrombocytopenia, anemia, hot flushes, nausea/vomiting, decreased libido, insomnia

PO = by mouth.

I disease. The common single chemotherapy agents used in treatment patients is listed in Table 44-3.

In advanced-stage disease, there is evidence to support the use of combination chemotherapy. A randomized trial comparing the combination of doxorubicin and cisplatin with whole abdominal irradiation following surgery in stage III and IV disease with residual disease <2 cm showed that at

Table 44-3. Summary of Common Single Chemotherapy Agents Used for Treatment of Advanced or Recurrent Endometrial Cancer

Agent	Dosage	Common Adverse Effects
Carboplatin	1) Calvert Formula Dose = AUC (CrCl + 25) 2) Standard dose AUC 4–7.5 IV once every 21–28 days	Nausea/vomiting, myelosuppression (DLT), nephrotoxicity, electrolyte wasting, diarrhea, stomatitis, hypersensitivity reactions
Cisplatin	50 mg/m^2 IV infused over 1 hr once every 21 days **or** With radiation: 40 mg/m^2 IV over 1–4 hr a (cap dose at 70 mg)	Nausea/vomiting, neurotoxicity, ototoxicity, nephrotoxicity, myelosuppression, electrolyte wasting, diarrhea
Doxorubicin	60 mg/m^2 IV over 30 min (maximum lifetime dose = 450 m/m^2) given once every 21 days	Thromboembolism, thrombocytopenia, anemia, hot flushes, nausea/vomiting, decreased libido, insomnia
Gemcitabine	800 mg/m^2–1,200 mg/m^2 IV on day 1, day 8, and day 15 repeated every 28 days	Myelosuppression (DLT), flulike symptoms, headache, somnolence, nausea/vomiting, stomatitis, diarrhea, constipation, rash
Liposomal doxorubicin	40 mg/m^2 IV once every 28 days	Myelosuppression, stomatitis, mucositis, alopecia, flushing, shortness of breath, hypotension, headaches, cardiotoxicity, hand-foot syndrome
Paclitaxel	135–175 mg/m^2 infused over 3 hr once every 21–28 days	Hypersensitivity reactions, peripheral neuropathy (DLT), nausea/vomiting, alopecia
Topotecan	1.5 mg/m^2 IV day 1 to day 5 every 21 days **or** to 4 mg/m^2 IV once a week x 3 followed by 1 week off	Myelosuppression (DLT), nausea/vomiting, diarrhea, stomatitis, abdominal pain, alopecia, SGOT/SGPT elevation

AUC = area under the curve; DLT = dose-limiting toxicity; IV = intravenous; SGOT = serum glutamic oxaloacetic transaminase; SGPT = serum glutamic pyruvic transaminase.

Table 44-4. Summary of Combination Chemotherapy Regimens Used for Treatment of Advanced or Recurrent Endometrial Cancer

Regimen	Dosages	Common Adverse Effects
Doxorubicin/cisplatin	Paclitaxel 60 mg/[2] IV over 30 min followed by cisplatin 50 mg/m^2 IV over 1 hr once every 21–28 days	Myelosuppression, stomatitis, mucositis, cardiotoxicity, alopecia, hypotension, shortness of breath, neurotoxicity, hypomagnesemia
Gemcitabine/cisplatin	Gemcitabine 1,000 mg/m^2 IV over 30 min on day 1 and day 8 with cisplatin 40 mg/m^2 IV over 1 hr on day 8 only repeated every 21 days	Myelosuppression (DLT), flulike symptoms, headache, somnolence, nausea/vomiting, stomatitis, diarrhea, constipation, rash, neurotoxicity, ototoxicity, nephrotoxicity, myelosuppression, electrolyte wasting, diarrhea
Paclitaxel/carboplatin	Paclitaxel 175 mg/m^2 infused over 3 hr with carboplatin AUC 5 to 7.5 IV over 1 hr (Calvert formula [(GFR+25) AUC)] given once every 21 days	Myelosuppression, thrombocytopenia, nausea/vomiting, nephrotoxicity, neurotoxicity, alopecia, hypersensitivity reaction
Paclitaxel/cisplatin	Paclitaxel 135 mg/m^2 over 24 hr followed by cisplatin 75 mg/m^2 over 4 hr given once every 21 days	Neutropenia, nausea/vomiting, hypersensitivity reaction, alopecia, neurotoxicity, nephrotoxicity, ototoxicity, hypomagnesemia

AUC = area under the curve; DLT = dose-limiting toxicity; IV = intravenous.

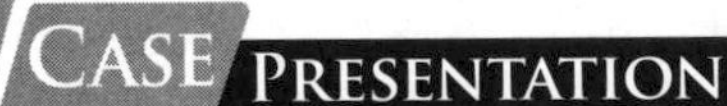

Patient Case: Part 2

Diagnosis: The CXR and CT chest did not indicate any metastatic disease. There was a para-aortic lymph node noted at the level of bifurcation of the aorta on CT of the pelvis. Surgery revealed FIGO stage II, invading 13 mm into a 20-mm-thick myometrium. There was extensive lymph vascular invasion present, including lymphatics in the outer third of the myometrium. The cervix, ovaries, and fallopian tubes showed no evidence of disease.

Treatment plan: After completion of surgery for diagnosis, staging, and primary treatment, H.G. was deemed at risk for recurrence, and a plan was implemented to include whole pelvic RT with 45 Gy in 25 fractions, and three high-dose-rate treatments would follow to the vaginal cuff.

Patient monitoring: At 1 month follow-up, the patient was doing well and dispositioned to serial 3-month follow-up with physical exam and CXR. Surveillance recommendations included CT scans of the chest, abdomen, and pelvis every 3–6 months for the first 2 years, then annually.

Patient education: On completion of therapy, the patient was provided with instructions on diet, skin care, physical activity, and use of a vaginal dilator.

5 years, 55% of the women who received doxorubicin and cisplatin were still alive compared with only 42% of women in the whole abdomen irradiation group.[71] The combination of paclitaxel and carboplatin has also shown overall response rates of 62% to 67% in studies including primary advanced and recurrent endometrial cancer, and complete response rates of 21% to 29%.[72,73] Good efficacy and relatively low toxicity of this regimen make this the standard treatment as employed by many centers in advanced endometrial cancer.[13] A summary of the combination regimens used in the management of advanced/recurrent endometrial cancer are listed in Table 44-4.

Treatment in the Relapsed or Metastatic Disease Setting

SURGERY

Limited local resection may be performed in those patients with recurrence confined to the pelvis. There is likely the need for RT after surgical resection.[3] **Pelvic exenteration** is offered only for potentially curative intent to patients with centrally recurrent endometrial cancer, as there is significant morbidity associated pelvic exenteration. Patients must undergo extensive testing to evaluate for metastatic disease that would exclude them for this massive surgical undertaking. Patients previously treated with XRT at the site of recurrence who are managed with pelvic exenteration with or without intraoperative RT have survival rates of 20%.[74]

RADIATION THERAPY

External beam radiation is the initial choice of treatment for recurrences confined to the vagina with or without lymph node invasion. Pelvic RT is used with vaginal brachytherapy.[3,10] The majority of recurrences are due to vaginal vault recurrences and may be cured with salvage radiotherapy.[13]

CHEMOTHERAPY

A first-line standard chemotherapy regimen has yet to be identified for metastatic or recurrent endometrial cancer. Chemotherapy for recurrent endometrial cancer is palliative in nature, with a median progression-free survival of 9 months and an average median survival of <1 year regardless of the therapy employed.[33,75,76] Chemotherapy may be used as single agent or as a combination of agents with or without RT, with the goal of increasing survival and prolonging time to progression of disease. Active single agents include doxorubicin, cisplatin, carboplatin, and paclitaxel. Ifosfamide, vincristine, and hexamethylmelamine have also demonstrated moderate activity; however, toxicities with these agents are often more significant.[33]

There is some limited evidence to support the use of weekly topotecan in the recurrent setting, as demonstrated by a small case series of eleven patients, with one patient achieving a durable response of 51 weeks and two patients with stable disease for 15 weeks.[77] Pegylated liposomal doxorubicin was evaluated by Muggia et al. in a phase II GOG study in previously treated metastatic endometrial cancer patients. Pegylated liposomal doxorubicin achieved a 9.5% response rate in relapsed disease.[78] Currently, paclitaxel is the only single agent with reproducible response rates >20% in patients who have had prior chemotherapy for their disease.[33]

Combination chemotherapy regimens have been employed for both advanced and recurrent endometrial cancer. These regimens are doxorubicin/cisplatin, gemcitabine/cisplatin, paclitaxel/carboplatin, and paclitaxel/cisplatin (Table 44-4). Although combination chemotherapy has been shown to have a higher response rate and longer progression-free survival, overall survival has not been improved, and there is an increased risk of toxicity with combination therapy. Careful evaluation of risk vs. benefit with more intense therapy must be individualized per patient along with their past medical history and current health status.

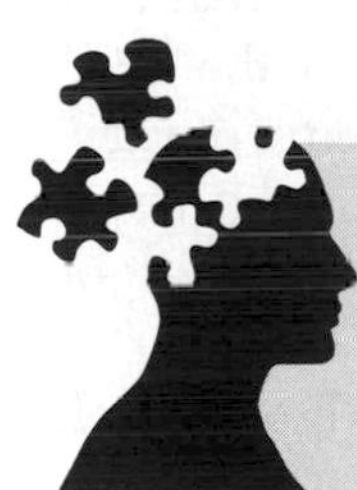

Therapeutic Challenge:

P.N. was recently diagnosed with recurrent stage IIIb endometrial cancer 3 years after completing her primary treatment of TAH/BSO and optimal tumor debulking followed by six cycles of paclitaxel/carboplatin. Her gynecologic oncologist recommended single-agent carboplatin. After three cycles, P.N. had more than 50% reduction in size of her tumor. On cycle four of carboplatin, 4 minutes into the infusion, P.N. had an allergic reaction and coded. P.N.'s tumor is having an excellent response to the carboplatin. How would you proceed with her chemotherapy treatment?

HORMONAL THERAPY

When considering hormonal therapy for metastatic or recurrent endometrial cancer, it is important to determine progesterone receptor positivity of the tumor. The progesterone receptor positivity correlates with the response rates seen when using these agents. The GOG 81 showed a 37% response rate when tumors were progesterone-receptor positive and an 8% response rate when the tumors were negative for progesterone receptors.[70] Progestational agents used in this setting are varied; however, when choosing the dosage, the lowest dose with efficacy for that particular agent should be chosen to limit toxicity.

Tamoxifen is ineffective in women resistant to progestins or chemotherapy, with response rates in the relapsed setting of about 10%, with minimal prolongation of time to disease progression and survival.[79] Aromatase inhibitors have limited use in endometrial cancer. Despite women with endometrial cancer often having significant levels of aromatase, only a moderate response to this therapy has been shown in the metastatic or relapsed patient. Response rates in range from 9% to 14%, with a progression-free interval of 1–6 months.[70] Gonadotropin-releasing hormone receptors are found in endometrial cancer tissue and have the ability to inhibit estrogen. Multiple agents have been tried in the treatment of advanced or recurrent endometrial cancer with conflicting results and response rates.[70]

Treatment-Related Complications

SHORT-TERM COMPLICATIONS

Small bowel obstruction, ileus, and deep venous thromboembolism can occur following surgery. Lymphocysts may occur and require drainage. Small bowel obstruction, not amenable to conservative therapy, may need further surgical exploration.[44] There is also the possibility of wound dehiscence occurring in the postoperative period, with obese patients having a higher risk because of poor healing and moist incisions and tension on tissues. In those patients who undergo surgical intervention, premature menopause is induced, and vasomotor symptoms may begin in the immediate postoperative period.

LONG-TERM COMPLICATIONS

Lymphedema is a possible complication for those patients who have undergone LND. Lymphedema may occur after laparoscopic and laparotomy methods. Lymphedema is most often caused by a disruption of the lymph system as a result of lymphadenectomy or postoperative EBRT. There are significant differences in level of lymphadenectomy and the incidence of developing lymphedema. In those women undergoing more extensive lymphadenectomy (≥10 nodes), 3.4% developed lymphedema compared with 0% of those who underwent less extensive lymphadenectomy (<10 nodes). Treatment of lymphedema includes manual lymphatic drainage, compression wrap, skin care, and exercises to facilitate lymphatic drainage.[80] Patients should be referred to a lymphedema specialist to optimize therapy for this complication.[81]

More than 20% of patients who undergo RT have persistent mild complications, including urgency, abdominal cramps, diarrhea, vaginal dryness, and stenosis. Another 3% develop severe long-term complications related to gastrointestinal disturbances, including obstruction or fistula.[66] Menopausal symptoms are another possible complication for TAH/BSO in surgical candidates who are either pre- or perimenopausal before surgery. Menopause and management of menopausal symptoms will be further discussed in Chapter 45: Ovarian Cancer.

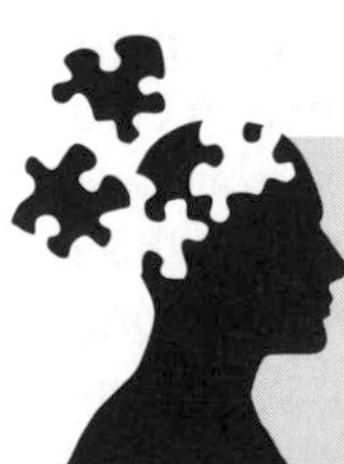

Therapeutic Challenge:

Women with a history of endometrial carcinoma are often denied hormone therapy/estrogen therapy because endometrial cancer is considered an estrogen-dependent cancer. Should hormone therapy be offered to women after achieving a complete response to first-line treatment?

Surveillance Monitoring and Follow-up

The primary goal of surveillance is the early detection of recurrent disease, leading to improved survival and decreased morbidity. All women who have received treatment for endometrial cancer should undergo surveillance.[3,30] Surveillance should include a complete history and physical exam at each visit every 3–6 months for 2 years, then 6-month to 1-year intervals. These visits should also include pelvic and rectal exam. All women should receive a CXR yearly. Vaginal cytology should be monitored every 6 months for 2 years, then monitored yearly. Imaging does not have a well-defined place in the follow-up algorithm, except for those patients with aggressive pathologic subtypes, such as papillary serous and clear cell endometrial cancer. In this group, imaging is mainly performed using CT.[82] Counseling on the symptoms of recurrence is very important in that a great majority of recurrences are symptomatic.

Patient Education

Current guidelines obviate the need for verbal and written instructions about recurrence and the need to seek prompt evaluation for any occurrence of vaginal bleeding, hematuria, and rectal bleeding. Patients with decreased appetite, weight loss, shortness of breath, swelling in the abdomen or legs, and pain—especially pain in the pelvic, abdominal, hip, or back regions—should seek evaluation.[3]

Patients treated with surgery or radiation should be given instruction about the early signs and symptoms of lower-extremity lymphedema and how to access a qualified lymphedema therapist so that early effective interventions can be initiated.

Monitoring of comorbidities present in those patients with endometrial cancer should be ongoing and include monitoring of blood pressure, breast exam, mammogram, and stool guaiac. As obesity is a prime factor contributing to the development of endometrial cancer, women must be counseled on the benefits weight loss, exercise, and change in diet.

Summary

Endometrial cancer is highly curable when discovered as low-grade, early-stage disease. Prompt evaluation of abnormal vaginal bleeding increases the diagnosis of this cancer often before an advanced stage of disease with a much poorer prognosis is reached. There are currently no screening criteria for early detection of endometrial cancer except in those women with genetic predisposition. There are identified risk factors associated with the disease, and women should be counseled about them during preventive provider visits, especially regarding the management of obesity, as it is a significant risk factor for the development and recurrence of endometrial cancer. The primary modality of treatment for endometrial cancer is surgery, and it is often curative in early-stage disease. Some patients with more advanced stage of disease or high-grade features can achieve durable responses with surgery, radiation, and chemotherapy, but responses and duration of response decrease with increasing stage and grade of disease. Treatment for recurrent endometrial cancer beyond a localized solitary recurrence is palliative, and further research is necessary to improve outcomes for these women. Various drug therapies, including both hormonal and chemotherapeutic agents, currently provide little improvement in overall survival. Discovery of endometrial cancer at an early stage and awareness of risk factors ensure the best prognosis for women with endometrial cancer, and any abnormal vaginal bleeding, especially in the postmenopausal period, warrants prompt evaluation.

References

Additional content available at
www.ashp.org/womenshealth

45 Ovarian Cancer

Marisa Navo Mendoza, Pharm.D.; Jubilee Brown, MD

Learning Objectives

1. Identify the possible risk factors associated with the development of epithelial ovarian cancer.
2. Describe the clinical presentations of early-stage, late-stage, and recurrent disease, as well as patterns of metastasis.
3. Assess the pros and cons of preventive strategies based on individual patient risk factors.
4. Construct a treatment plan based on the patient's clinical presentation and previous treatment, if applicable.

Ovarian cancer is the fifth-leading cause of cancer mortality in women and the most common cause of death among gynecologic malignancies in the U.S.[1] It is expected that about 1 in 71 women will be diagnosed during her lifetime; both incidence and mortality rate increase with age.[2] Unfortunately, the majority of patients diagnosed with ovarian cancer often present with disseminated disease because of nonspecific symptoms overlooked by both patients and healthcare providers until widespread, late-stage disease already exists. As a result, ovarian cancer is commonly known as the "silent killer." Moreover, the U.S. Preventive Services Task Force (USPSTF) does not currently recommend the routine screening of asymptomatic patients. A review of the evidence demonstrated that earlier detection of ovarian cancer using current techniques had little effect on mortality and may lead to more potential harm.[3] Currently, screening techniques are difficult to utilize in the general population because of lack of **sensitivity, specificity,** and, consequently, **positive predictive value.** Other barriers include increased cost and patient anxiety.[4-6] Fortunately, a constellation of nonspecific symptoms and signs has recently been identified as crucial in earlier detection of ovarian cancer and is being prospectively studied in a primary care setting to be used as a symptom index.[7,8] Therefore, education with regard to risk factors and symptoms is essential for patients, primary care physicians, and other healthcare professionals to facilitate earlier detection and screening for disease in high-risk patients.

Epidemiology

In the U.S., ovarian cancer incidence and mortality is highest among white women when compared with other races.[2,9] The median age of diagnosis is 63 years, and most women are diagnosed between ages 55 and 64.[2] This is consistent with worldwide data from the International Federation of Gynecology and Obstetrics (FIGO) that show the highest incidence of ovarian cancer occurring in the 50 to 59 year age group.[10] Globally, the incidence of ovarian cancer is highest in more developed countries, such as Europe (specifically Nordic areas and the United Kingdom) and North America. One exception is Japan, which has one of the lowest incidences of ovarian cancer. However, the difference between incidence rates in these countries may be narrowing. Although both the incidence and mortality rates of more developed areas are twice those of less developed countries, the ratio between incidence and mortality does not significantly differ.[11]

Results from the National Cancer Institute's Surveillance and Epidemiology and End Results (SEER) Statistics Review from

2000–2004 demonstrate a 44.9% 5-year survival rate for ovarian cancer patients in the U.S.[2] Internationally, the 5-year survival rate has increased about 20% to 49.7% since changes in treatment started to include debulking surgery and chemotherapy, including platinum and taxane agents.[10] Despite these improvements, most patients with advanced disease relapse within 2 years of treatment, and response rates to available second-line treatment is moderate.

Etiology

Several theories regarding the etiology of ovarian cancer have been studied; however, the exact cause of the disease is still not well understood. The "incessant ovulation" hypothesis was first described in 1971 by Fathalla, who proposed that constant minor trauma to the ovarian epithelium caused by ovulation was a major risk factor for ovarian cancer.[12] Another common theory, the gonadotropin hypothesis, suggests that high levels of gonadotropin and estrogen lead to an increase in proliferation of the ovarian epithelium.[13] In both hypotheses, an increased potential for aberrant repairs and mutations is thought to eventually lead to malignancy. More recently, the idea of chronic inflammatory responses has been under investigation because of observed associations between factors that enhance local inflammation, such as talc and asbestos, with ovarian cancer risk. Unfortunately, inconsistent data from epidemiologic studies do not provide a clear argument for one hypothesis over the other.

Recognizing patient risk factors for ovarian cancer can improve survival by identifying patients who may benefit from prophylactic surgery or close observation. The most significant risk factor for developing ovarian cancer is family history; however, only about 5% to 10% of ovarian cancer cases are thought to be familial or hereditary.[14-16] Hereditary patterns demonstrate the variable penetrance of an autosomal dominant gene.[14] About two thirds of hereditary ovarian cancer cases are associated with *BRCA1* mutations, located on chromosome 17q, with the remaining one third related to *BRCA2* mutations on chromosome 13q.[15] Mutations in these tumor suppressor genes lead to abnormalities in DNA repair mechanisms. Women with a family history of disease have an estimated **lifetime risk** of about 9.4% for developing ovarian cancer, which is increased from 1.4% in the general population.[2,15] The relative risk of ovarian cancer (ROC) for a woman with a first-degree relative diagnosed with the disease is 3.1 and can increase to 7 if two or more relatives are affected.[14] Recently, the Society of Gynecologic Oncologists released a commentary to assist in the identification of patients who may benefit from hereditary cancer risk assessment. The assessment includes evaluation of risk, education, counseling, and possible genetic testing provided by professionals with expertise in cancer genetics.[17] The two common syndromes of familial ovarian cancer are hereditary breast/ovarian cancer (HBOC) syndrome and hereditary nonpolyposis colorectal cancer (HNPCC).

Patient characteristics that may suggest HBOC syndrome include two or more first-degree relatives with breast or ovarian cancer, premenopausal or early onset of disease in the family, multiple cancers in an individual, family history of male breast cancer, *BRCA* mutations, and Ashkenazi Jewish ancestry.[16,18] A small number of families with only an excess of ovarian cancer history are associated mainly with *BRCA1* mutations and called "site-specific" ovarian cancer families.[18] The lifetime risk of developing ovarian cancer for women with *BRCA1* mutations is estimated to be about 40% to 50% and can range from 16% in Ashkenazi Jewish women to 44% in high penetrance families.[15,19] Similarly, the reported risk for women with *BRCA2* mutations is about 27%. Other factors that may contribute to ovarian cancer development in carriers of *BRCA* mutations include the mutation itself, the status of other modifying genes, epigenetic phenomena, and gene-environment interactions (Table 45-1).[15]

Women with HNPCC or Lynch II syndrome are predisposed to hereditary colon cancer and other malignancies such as ovarian, endometrial, gastrointestinal, and genitourinary. This syndrome is associated with mutations in DNA mismatch repair genes, such as *MSH2, MLH1, PMS1,* and *PMS2* and leads to microsatellite instability.[15,19] Mutations in these genes inhibit the ability of cell repair that normally occurs during replication. The lifetime ROC has been reported as 12% in women who are mutation carriers.[20] Ovarian cancer in HNPCC family members may occur at an earlier age when compared with malignancy in the general population. Also, it is more likely to be well or moderately differentiated, and patients are more likely to have a synchronous endometrial cancer (Table 45-1).

Table 45-1. Ovarian Cancer Risk Factors

Family History	
Hereditary Breast/Ovarian Cancer • Genes involved: *BRCA1, BRCA2* • Characteristics ➢ ≥2 first-degree relatives with breast or ovarian cancer ➢ Early onset of cancer in family ➢ Multiple cancers in individual ➢ Family history of male breast cancer ➢ Ashkenazi Jewish ancestry	Hereditary Nonpolyposis Colorectal Cancer (Lynch II syndrome) • Genes involved: DNA mismatch repair genes *(MSH2, MLH1, PMS1, PMS2)* • Characteristics ➢ Predisposed to colorectal cancer ➢ Other possible malignancies include endometrial, gastrointestinal, and genitourinary ➢ Early onset of cancer ➢ More likely to be well or moderately differentiated ➢ More likely to have synchronous endometrial cancer
Reproductive or Hormonal Risk Factors	
• Late menopause • Infertility • Nulliparity	• Early menarche (possible) • Unknown: miscarriages, terminations, ectopic pregnancies, or fertility drug use
Diet or Environmental Risk Factors	
• Resident of high-risk countries • Increased body mass index (BMI)	

In addition to family history, reproductive and hormonal factors may play a role in disease development. Theoretically, any factor that increases the number of ovulatory cycles during a woman's life time may increase ovarian cancer risk through high levels of gonadotropin and estrogen. Therefore, risks may include occurrence of early menarche, late menopause, infertility, nulliparity, and use of fertility drugs. Although possible, studies have not confirmed early menarche as a risk factor. In contrast, a positive association has been demonstrated for patients who have experienced menopause at a later age. Similarly, an established connection has also been shown between ovarian cancer risk and infertility or nulliparity.[14,15] Data from epidemiologic studies demonstrate a 40% to 60% risk reduction for multiparous when compared to nulliparous women. Also, each additional birth can decrease risk by another 10% to 22%.[21,22] However, it is unclear whether miscarriages, terminations, ectopic pregnancies, or fertility drug use have an influence on risk (Table 45-1).

The risks of developing ovarian cancer for women who emigrate from low-risk to high-risk countries increase to those of native-born women.[15] This may signify a potential role for dietary and environmental factors.[14] However, conflicting data have been reported. Observed associations between ovarian cancer and exposure to environmental factors that irritate the ovarian epithelium support the chronic inflammatory response hypothesis. For instance, the proposed mechanism for the association of talcum powder in the perineal region with ovarian cancer risk is by ascending through the lower genital tract and aggravating the ovarian epithelium.[14,16] Also, although the effects of diet are questionable, a connection between body mass index (BMI) and ovarian cancer risk has been reported.[14,23,24] However, this link may be due to the presence of excess adipose tissue and increased conversion of androstenedione to estrone in overweight or obese patients. Nonetheless, the Women's Health Initiative incorporated a randomized control trial of dietary modification intervention to determine whether a low-fat dietary pattern could reduce the risk of cancer, including ovarian cancer, among postmenopausal women. Although not statistically significant, risk reduction was seen among the intervention group during the latter years of the study, suggesting that diet may be relevant (Table 45-1).[25]

CASE PRESENTATION

Patient Case: Part 1

J.J. is a 60-year-old black woman who presents to her primary physician with a 6-month history of dyspepsia, new onset early satiety, and increased abdominal girth.

HPI: She reports ulcerlike symptoms and blames aspirin use. Despite an increase in clothing size, she experienced a 10-lb weight loss in the month before presentation with no change in physical activity. She attributed this to eating less because of the abdominal discomfort.

PMH: Her past medical history is significant for osteoarthritis and hypertension. Medications include hydrochlorothiazide, aspirin, a multivitamin, and glucosamine/chondroitin. Menarche occurred at age 9, and she was diagnosed with infertility at age 30 (gravida 0, para 0).

Social history: She denies tobacco, alcohol, or recreational drug use. She had a family history of hypertension, and both her mother and maternal grandmother were diagnosed with breast cancer before menopause.

Lab values: Complete blood count, electrolytes, liver function tests, and urinalysis are within normal limits. Baseline CA-125 level is 632 units/mL (normal CA-125 <35 units/mL).

Physical exam: Height of 160 cm and a weight of 80 kg. Blood pressure 130/75 and resting pulse of 85 beats/min. Her temperature is 99°F and her respiratory rate is 20. Abdominal examination shows an abdominal distention and a fluid wave consistent with ascites, with fullness in the upper abdomen. On rectovaginal examination, a fixed mass was noted to fill the pelvis and involve the rectovaginal septum.

Diagnostic tests: Abdominal pelvic CT and transvaginal ultrasound revealed bilateral adnexal masses, an omental cake, and ascites. Chest radiograph revealed no lesions.

Patient assessment: J.J. was referred to a gynecologic oncologist for further assessment and treatment.

Clinical Presentation

SIGNS AND SYMPTOMS OF EARLY- VS. LATE-STAGE DISEASE

Ovarian cancer is known as the "silent killer" because patients frequently experience nonspecific symptoms and present with late-stage disease. Early-stage disease is not usually associated with symptoms except for the occasional patient with pelvic pain that may be due to ovarian torsion.[18] Rarely, an incidental diagnosis may occur during evaluation for other symptoms or after routine pelvic examination reveals an **adnexal** mass. In contrast, patients with advanced-stage disease experience nonspecific symptoms that indicate spread of the disease to the upper abdomen. Because there are usually no early warning signs with regard to symptoms or signs when the mass is confined to the ovary, the presence of symptoms typically reflect voluminous spread to the upper abdomen with the presence of ascites produced by the tumor mass. Symptoms may include abdominal or pelvic discomfort or pain, fullness, a change in bowel movements, early satiety, dyspepsia, bloating, change in urinary frequency, and weight changes.[18,26] Unfortunately, these symptoms can indicate other disease states, such as irritable bowel syndrome, and possible delays in diagnosis can occur. The most reported barriers to receiving a prompt diagnosis of ovarian cancer include patients personally ignoring their symptoms and wrong diagnosis. However, Goff and colleagues have recently identified a constellation of symptoms—including pelvic/abdominal pain, increased abdominal size/bloating, and difficulty eating/feeling full quickly—and developed a symptom index that may signal a prompt evaluation for malignancy. Furthermore, these recent findings suggest that symptom severity, duration (<12 months), and frequency (>12 times/month) are all vital in distinguishing patients in need of further diagnostic testing.[7,8]

On examination, physicians may observe a few signs that would indicate the need for further testing. One sign of ovarian cancer that may be identified even with early-stage disease is the presence of an adnexal mass on pelvic examination. Therefore, pelvic and rectovaginal examinations are integral components of a complete physical examination. Any presence of irregularity, solid features, and nodularity can suggest ovarian cancer.[18] In addition, patients with late-stage disease may show signs of abdominal distension that is due to ascites and massive disease, or dyspnea or cough that are due to pleural effusions.

PATTERN OF METASTASIS

Ovarian cancer may spread to other parts of the body through several mechanisms. First, the disease can penetrate through the ovarian serosa and extend to surrounding organs, such as the uterus, fallopian tube, bladder, rectum, or pelvic peritoneum by direct extension.[27] Metastasis may also occur through the lymphatic system, typically involving the pelvic and para-aortic lymph nodes, which may be enlarged on palpitation.[18,27] Although this may occur in 20% of patients with early-stage disease, nodal metastases most often occur in advanced-stage disease. Ovarian cancer can also spread through the peritoneal cavity by dissemination through the peritoneal fluid. Tumor cells then are able to adhere, implant, and invade these abdominopelvic organs, resulting in multifocal disease disseminated throughout the cavity.[27] Other sites may include the surfaces of the diaphragm and liver as well as pulmonary and pleural involvement.[10]

Pathophysiology

The incessant ovulation theory suggests that constant irritation of ovarian epithelium resulting from trauma during ovulation makes it more likely for mutations to occur in the serosa. Women who experience menarche at an early age or those with late menopause are at a higher risk. Also, patients with fewer ovulatory cycles—such as those women with multiple births, history of breast-feeding, and oral contraceptive use—may be protected against the development of ovarian cancer. Several theories exist with regard to subcellular mechanisms involving inflammatory mediators and mutations occurring during repair processes. Also, although the development of malignant disease is unclear, changes in the normal ovulation process through increased gonadotropin and estrogen levels may contribute.

In 1973, a World Health Organization (WHO) committee published a histologic typing of ovarian cancers and categorized tumors into epithelial, sex-cord stromal, and germ cell tumors. More than 90% of ovarian cancer cases arise from the epithelium.[9,15,18] Of these 90%, about 10% to 20% are considered borderline tumors, or low-malignant-potential tumors, of the ovary.[15] Sex-cord stromal and germ cell tumors account for most of the remaining cases.[9,28] These entities are considered separately.

Epithelial ovarian cancer is categorized further with the most common type being serous tumors, which account for 75% to 80% of invasive ovarian cancer.[15,18] This type of cancer is often of high grade and may be associated with *BRCA1* and *−2* mutations.[18] About 10% of invasive cancer is described as endometrioid, resembling the endometrial lining and sometimes associated with endometriosis.[18] Mucinous tumors account for about 10% of invasive cancer.[9,15] These cells have a different natural history, often produce copious mucinous ascites, may lead to the clinical syndrome of pseudomyxoma peritonei, and may have elevated serum CEA levels but not CA-125 levels. Mucinous ovarian cancer appears to be a distinct clinical entity, and research is ongoing to further delineate these differences and optimal treatment strategies. Clear cell carcinoma is also uncommon (4%); however, it is considered to be highly aggressive.[9,18] Unfortunately, both mucinous and clear cell carcinoma have a low response rate to standard chemotherapy regimens used in other types of epithelial ovarian cancer.

Histologic grade is an important prognostic factor for patients with epithelial ovarian cancer. The grade of tumor is associated with prognosis and is based on cell differentiation. A grade designated as “x” (Gx) describes cells that cannot be assessed. Grade 1 (G1) and grade 2 (G2) cells are cells that are well differentiated and moderately differentiated, respectively. Low-grade tumors appear to be a distinct entity and are less aggressive, with an indolent course suggesting a better prognosis. A designation of grade 3 (G3) denotes poorly differentiated cells and a worse prognosis. Grade 2, although commonly found in pathology reports, may have significant interobserver variability and may not be a realistic designation. There is a trend in some centers to reclassify grade 2 tumors into either grade 1 or grade 3, thereby establishing low-grade and high-grade epithelial ovarian cancers. Further research is needed to determine the utility of such approach. Standard nomenclature remains grade 1, 2, and 3.[29]

Screening and Diagnosis

Existing techniques used in the screening of ovarian cancer include routine pelvic and rectovaginal exams, the serum tumor marker CA-125, and ultrasound testing. Unfortunately, currently available tests do not have a high enough positive predictive value when used alone; however, multimodal screening using a combination of available screening tests is being investigated. All women should continue annual rectovaginal pelvic exams as part of routine gynecologic clinical care, but no other screening guidelines or programs are currently recommended for women among the general population. However, the National Institutes of Health (NIH) recommends surveillance consisting of an annual rectovaginal pelvic exam, CA-125 measurements, and transvaginal pelvic ultrasonography for high-risk patients, specifically those with significant family history.[30]

PELVIC EXAMINATIONS

Pelvic exams are important for initial patient assessment and consist of examination of the ovaries and uterus for size, shape, and consistency. Further assessment of patients with an ovarian mass will depend on various factors, such as the patient's history and the mass size. Also, although a definitive diagnosis is not possible, characteristics most often associated with a malignancy are described as a lobulated surface with variable consistency and nontender nodules in the pouch of Douglas. Some limitations that may affect the accuracy of a pelvic exam include obesity, uterine size, abdominal scar, and the experience and technique of the healthcare professional performing the exam.[31]

SERUM TUMOR MARKER CA-125

CA-125 is a nonspecific antigen normally expressed by cells lining various parts of the body such as the fallopian tubes, endometrium, endocervix, peritoneum, pleura, pericardium, and bronchi. Elevated levels of CA-125 can indicate physical changes, including pregnancy, menstruation, benign cysts, endometriosis, and pelvic inflammatory disease.[26,32] In addition, increasing levels of CA-125 are more likely to occur in women with ovarian cancer. Values <35 units/mL are considered normal; however, monitoring the trend of levels may be more useful. Monitoring CA-125 levels is fairly inexpensive, easy, readily available, and relatively noninvasive; therefore despite its lack of sensitivity and specificity for screening, it has become the most commonly used serum tumor marker in ovarian cancer assessment.[4,6]

TRANSVAGINAL ULTRASOUND

Transvaginal ultrasound is considered a safe and time-efficient method for screening ovarian cancer. It provides qualitative information needed for treatment decisions by providing a clearer morphologic assessment.[26] Unfortunately, an estimated specificity of 95% would result in 50 unnecessary surgical procedures for every ovarian cancer detected.[18] Although promising, the low sensitivity and a disappointing positive predictive value would decrease its usefulness in the general population.

MULTIMODALITY SCREENING

A review of 22 prospective studies, 18 cohorts, and 4 randomized controlled trials was conducted to evaluate the numerous screening strategies available. A multimodal approach using CA-125 measurement followed by ultrasound was found to be the superior screening strategy.[33] In one prospective trial conducted between 1986 and 1993, 22,000 postmenopausal women randomized to three annual incidence screens showed the value of using a variety of ultrasound criteria in combination with an elevated CA-125 level to achieve a screening tool with high sensitivity, specificity, and positive predictive value.[34]

From the previous trials, a new screening strategy called the ROC algorithm was developed and is currently being studied in a large randomized controlled trial called the United Kingdom Collaborative Trial of Ovarian Cancer Screening (UKCTOCS).[35] Data from a prospective screening trial support the feasibility of the ROC algorithm for further assessment in the UKCTOCS trial. Investigators report a high specificity of 99.8% and a positive predictive value of 19%.[36] The UKCTOCS study is designed to involve 200,000 postmenopausal women and will randomize women to a multimodal group (annual CA-125 using ROC algorithm), an annual transvaginal ultrasound group, and a control group followed with annual pelvic examinations. The patients will then be followed for 7 years to determine the impact of ovarian cancer screening on ovarian cancer mortality.[6,36]

Although several screening strategies have been explored, none have been found to decrease ovarian cancer mortality.[33] Because of the potential risks involved, such as unnecessary surgeries and patient anxiety, routine screening is not recommended by any medical organization.[3] However, screening in high-risk patients may be warranted. In addition, the American College of Obstetricians and Gynecologists (ACOG) with the Society of Gynecologic Oncologists (SGO) put forth recommended diagnostic criteria based on physical exam, blood tests, and imaging techniques to be considered when contemplating patient referrals to a gynecologic oncologist for further surgical evaluation.[37] However, these guidelines are more useful for predicting advanced-stage disease.[38]

SURGERY

Conventionally, the first method of diagnosis and treatment of ovarian cancer is surgery performed by a gynecologic oncologist. Women with possible ovarian cancer should first undergo a thorough history and physical examination to determine if the patient is a good surgical candidate, the risk of malignancy, and extent of disease. Other possible tests to consider include abdominal and pelvic computerized tomography (CT); chest radiograph or CT; and baseline labs, including complete blood counts and electrolytes. Also, before surgery, the risks and benefits of all treatment options must be discussed with the patient, such as **laparoscopy** vs. **laparotomy** and neoadjuvant vs. adjuvant chemotherapy.[39]

Surgery is performed via a large midline abdominal incision (laparotomy) or an infraumbilical incision (laparoscopy). During surgery, the surgeon first collects ascites for cytologic evaluation or performs peritoneal washings. The next step is exploration of the pelvis and inspection of the adnexal mass to determine the site of origin. The upper abdomen is then examined to determine the extent of disease and resectability to achieve optimal disease status. The first determination is whether the adnexal mass represents malignancy; the mass is removed and sent for intraoperative pathologic evaluation. If cancer is present, the next determination is if optimal disease status can be achieved (any remaining nodule <1 cm remaining at completion of surgery). If this is not possible, appropriate surgery is performed to relieve symptoms (e.g., bowel obstruction), and the patient is closed. If this is possible, a maximal surgical debulking, also called **optimal cytoreduction,** should be undertaken to leave no nodule >1 cm remaining at the completion of surgery; if possible, all macroscopic disease should be removed. If abdominal disease measuring >2 cm is present, the patient is already staged as IIIC, and no further diagnostic staging biopsies are warranted. However, if there is small volume or no visible upper abdominal disease, then a full staging procedure is indicated, including multiple peritoneal biopsies, diaphragmatic cytology, **infracolic omentectomy,** and pelvic and para-aortic lymph node sampling.[27,38] If apparent early-stage disease is present in a reproductive-aged woman, fertility-sparing surgery is an option with **unilateral salpingo-oophorectomy** and a staging procedure, conserving a normal-appearing contralateral ovary and uterus. However, in patients with advanced-stage disease and women who no longer desire fertility preservation, the standard treatment is total abdominal **hysterectomy, bilateral salpingo-oophorectomy,** infracolic omentectomy, and staging or tumor reductive surgery.[27]

Although laparoscopy was initially used as a diagnostic tool, accumulating data have supported the minimally invasive technique demonstrating both safety and efficacy.[40] Although there are currently no data comparing survival between patients managed with laparoscopy vs. laparotomy, there are several advantages of using laparoscopy, such as magnification of pelvic and abdominal anatomy, better visualization of metastases of the upper abdomen, surface of the liver and diaphragm, posterior and anterior cul de sac, quick postoperative recovery, reduction in operative morbidity, and, therefore, avoidance of chemotherapy delays.[41] Moreover, because most adnexal masses are benign, laparoscopy can help avoid overtreatment and unnecessary laparotomy. However, because of the possibility associated with laparoscopy of intraoperative rupture or spillage leading to intraperitoneal dissemination and poorer prognosis, staging should be performed by a gynecologic oncologist.[27] Additionally, the presence of extraovarian disease should warrant laparotomy.

INTERNATIONAL FEDERATION OF GYNECOLOGY AND OBSTETRICS STAGING

According to FIGO, the surgical staging of ovarian cancer consists of laparotomy and biopsy of all suspected sites of involvement with histologic and cytologic data. Staging of ovarian cancer is based on the extent of tumor involvement and divided into four stages (Table 45-2).[10]

PROGNOSTIC FACTORS

The most important prognostic factor of ovarian cancer is stage at diagnosis.[15] According to the SEER data from 1988 to 2003, the 5-year survival rate of patients with localized, regional, distant, and unstaged disease is 92%, 67.6%, 27.7%, and 28.5%, respectively.[2] Increasing grade and histology of clear cell or small cell carcinoma confers a worse prognosis.[15]

Other significant prognostic factors include residual disease after initial cytoreductive surgery and patient age.[15] Patients who undergo optimal cytoreductive surgery with residual disease <1 cm (per nodule) have a better prognosis than those with >1 cm remaining (suboptimal); patients with no visible

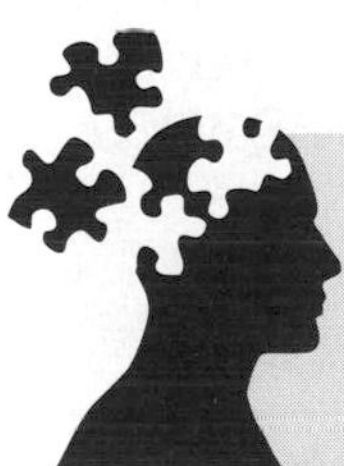

Therapeutic Challenge:

L.K. is a 34-year-old single woman with a family history of both breast and ovarian cancer. Her mother died of ovarian cancer at the age of 48. L.K. has strong desire to have children of her own someday. She presents to clinic to learn about her options for prevention of ovarian cancer. What is her best option to prevent ovarian cancer?

Table 45-2. FIGO Staging System for Ovarian Cancer

Stage		
Stage I	**Tumor Limited to Ovaries**	
	Ia	Tumor present in one ovary (capsule intact) with negative ascites/peritoneal washings and negative tumor on external surfaces
	Ib	Tumor present in both ovaries (capsule intact) with negative ascites/peritoneal washings and negative tumor on external surfaces
	Ic	Tumor present in one or both ovaries (capsule(s) ruptured) with or without ascites/peritoneal washings and/or tumor on external surfaces
Stage II	**Tumor involving one or both ovaries with pelvic extensions**	
	IIa	Tumor extension and/or implants to uterus and/or fallopian tubes with negative peritoneal washings, no ascites
	IIb	Tumor extension and/or implants to other pelvic organs (bladder, rectum, vagina) with negative peritoneal washings, no ascites
	IIc	Tumor extension and/or implants to any pelvic organs (IIa or IIb above) with positive peritoneal washings and/or ascites
Stage III	**Tumor involves one or both ovaries with microscopic confirmed peritoneal metastasis outside pelvis and/or regional lymph node metastasis**	
	IIIa	Microscopic peritoneal metastasis or histologically proven extension to small bowel or mesentery; regional lymph nodes are negative
	IIIb	Macroscopic peritoneal metastasis; implants ≤2 cm in diameter; regional lymph nodes are negative
	IIIc	Microscopic or macroscopic peritoneal metastasis; implants >2 cm in diameter; regional lymph nodes are positive
Stage IV	**Growth involving one or both ovaries with distant metastasis beyond the pelvis (i.e., pleural effusion with positive cytology; parenchymal liver metastasis)**	

FIGO = International Federation of Gynecology and Obstetrics.

residual disease at the completion of surgery represent a subgroup with an improved survival advantage.[42,43] SEER data demonstrate the impact of age on 5-year survival rate. For instance, the 5-year survival rate of women <45 years of age is 73.1% compared with 27.7% in women age 65 and older. Moreover, about 40% of patients ≤49 years are diagnosed with localized disease vs. the 14% of women ≥50 years old.[2]

Prevention

CHEMOPREVENTION

Protective factors found to suppress ovulation and the gonadotropin surge, such as oral contraceptive use, support both the incessant ovulation and gonadotropin hypotheses of disease development.[14,15] A review of data regarding oral contraceptive use reports a reduction of ovarian cancer risk of about 30% for women who have ever used oral contraceptives. Reduction of risk was found to increase about 5% with each year of use, totaling to 50% with 10 or more years of use. Additionally, the protection continued for 20 years after discontinuation of use. This beneficial effect was not dependent on parity, age, histologic type of ovarian cancer, or type of oral contraceptive used.[44] In another case-control study, the maximum protective effect of oral contraceptive use was seen at 3–5 years of use in women with *BRCA* mutations.[45] Other potential agents currently being investigated include cyclo-oxygenase-2 (COX-2) inhibitors and retinoids. A critical review of the current literature evaluating the use of aspirin, ibuprofen, and other nonsteroidal anti-inflammatory drugs in cancer prevention estimated a 47% risk reduction of ovarian cancer.[46] However, these studies have had numerous limitations and have not been confirmed in randomized, controlled study settings. There have also been several in vitro studies demonstrating the benefits of retinoids. More studies are needed to help define the efficacy of these possible chemopreventive strategies.

SURGERY

Surgical procedures that decrease the ROC include bilateral salpingo-oophorectomy (BSO), **tubal ligation,** and hysterectomy. Before surgery, the risks and benefits of each must be fully discussed with the patient. Moreover, patients must be aware that surgical strategies are not absolute with regards to risk reduction. For instance, BSO in high-risk patients with *BRCA* mutations provided an overall reduction in cancer risk of 80%; however, a residual risk for peritoneal cancer remained in these patients, with an estimated cumulative incidence of 4.3% at 20 years after BSO.[47] Moreover, although a maximum gain of 1.7 life expectancy years is projected for a 30-year-old woman who underwent prophylactic oophorectomy, this gain decreases with age at the time of surgery and is minimal in a 60-year-old woman.[48]

Although the mechanism is unclear, both bilateral tubal ligation and hysterectomy have also been found to be beneficial in reducing ovarian cancer risk. This may be due to ovarian function impairment or decreased passage of inflammatory substances and interruption of retrograde transport of carcinogens through the fallopian tube.[16,49] Reductions in ROC have been reported as >30% for tubal ligation and hysterectomy, respectively. Furthermore, the risk reduction persists for 20 to 25 years after the procedure.[50,51]

CASE PRESENTATION

Patient Case: Part 2

Diagnosis: Because of the presence of multiple risk factors and abnormal physical exam, there was a high suspicion of malignancy. The gynecologic oncologist discussed diagnosis and treatment options with J.J. Unfortunately, malignancy can only be truly diagnosed by surgery. J.J. was determined to be a good surgical candidate, and risks/benefits of laparoscopy vs. laparotomy were discussed.

Treatment plan: J.J. underwent exploratory laparotomy. The intraoperative frozen-section analysis of the suspicious sites was performed, and malignancy was confirmed. The gynecologic oncologist continued with staging and optimal debulking surgery, including total hysterectomy, BSO, and partial omentectomy. The surgery confirmed a diagnosis of high-grade stage IIIc papillary serous ovarian cancer. Surgery was followed by chemotherapy with paclitaxel 175 mg/m^2 intravenously (IV) over 3 hours and carboplatin (AUC = 5) IV over 1 hour repeated every 21-day cycle for a total of six cycles.

Patient monitoring: Before each chemotherapy administration, blood counts and electrolyte laboratory tests should be evaluated. Response to therapy can be assessed by the CA-125 level.

Patient education: J.J. should be counseled on the side effects of paclitaxel and carboplatin, including potential for hypersensitivity reactions, infusion-related reactions, myelosuppression, nephrotoxicity, neurotoxicity, alopecia, and acute and delayed nausea and vomiting. She should be given information on neutropenic precautions (i.e., hand washing, monitoring fever, and prevention of infection) and encouraged to drink noncaffeine fluids throughout treatment.

Treatment

PRIMARY TREATMENT

The primary treatment of patients with early disease is surgery alone; however, adjuvant chemotherapy may be considered in patients with unfavorable prognostic factors.[18] The cornerstone of diagnosis and initial therapy for patients with advanced ovarian cancer is maximal cytoreductive surgery, as detailed above, followed by combination chemotherapy with platinum and a taxane.[52] Management of the side effects of chemotherapy used in the treatment of ovarian cancer is detailed extensively in Chapter 47: Management of Treatment Complications.

CHEMOTHERAPY

Historically, the treatment of ovarian cancer has progressed from single-agent alkylating therapy to the current gold standard of combination chemotherapy with platinum and taxane agents. The initial use of the alkylating agents for ovarian cancer showed modest response rates and median survival time in responders vs. nonresponders; unfortunately, prolonged use of alkylating agents was associated with nonlymphocytic leukemia. In the 1970s, superior response rates were reported with the use of combination vs. single agent therapy. However, in the 1980s, studies started to demonstrate significantly better response rates and progression-free and overall survival with the use of platinum-containing agents, specifically cisplatin. Moreover, the taxane agent paclitaxel was identified and reported to be active in **platinum-resistant disease.**[18]

The current gold standard first-line treatment for patients with stage IC disease or above is six to eight

Table 45-3. First-Line Agents Used in Treatment of Ovarian Cancer

Agent	Dosage	Common Adverse Effects
Carboplatin (given with taxane)	1) Calvert Formula Dose = AUC[a] (CrCl +25) 2) Standard dose AUC 5 to 7.5 IV once every 21 days	Nausea/vomiting, myelosuppression (DLT), nephrotoxicity, electrolyte wasting, diarrhea, stomatitis, hypersensitivity reactions
Cisplatin (given with taxane)	75 mg/m² IV infused over 4 hr once every 21 days ***or*** 100 mg/m² IP once every 21 days	Nausea/vomiting, neurotoxicity, ototoxicity, nephrotoxicity, myelosuppression, electrolyte wasting, diarrhea
Cyclophosphamide	750 mg/m² IV once every 21 days	Hemorrhagic cystitis, SIADH, alopecia, myelosuppression (DLT)
Docetaxel	75 mg/m² IV once every 21 days	Hyperlacrimation, fluid retention, nail disorders, myelosuppression
Paclitaxel (Given with platinum analogue)	175 mg/m² infused over 3 hr (with carboplatin)[a] once every 21 days ***or*** 135 mg/m² infused over 24 hr (with cisplatin) once every 21 days	Hypersensitivity reactions, Peripheral Neuropathy (DLT), Nausea/vomiting, Alopecia

AUC = area under the curve; DLT = dose-limiting toxicity; IP = intraperitoneally; IV = intravenously; SIADH = syndrome of inappropriate antidiuretic hormone.

[a]Current gold standard of care.

cycles of carboplatin (AUC = 5 to 7.5) and paclitaxel 175 mg/m² administered every 21 to 28 days (Table 45-3). Carboplatin was approved for palliative treatment of ovarian cancer in 1989; however, it did not immediately replace cisplatin as standard treatment. Subsequently, several studies comparing the combination of paclitaxel-cisplatin vs. paclitaxel-carboplatin were conducted to demonstrate efficacy of the newer combination. In each study, data showed no significant difference in progression-free or overall survival, and the paclitaxel-carboplatin combination had a better toxicity profile.[53-56] Other first-line treatments include paclitaxel and cisplatin, docetaxel and carboplatin, and cyclophosphamide and cisplatin (refer to Table 45-3).

INTRAPERITONEAL CHEMOTHERAPY

Administration of chemotherapy via intraperitoneal (IP) delivery is a not a novel concept; however, recent studies have reported data that may bring its use to the forefront in the first-line setting. The goal of IP administration is to increase drug concentration in the site of disease, specifically the abdominal cavity. A meta-analysis of six randomized controlled trials was designed to quantify the effect of IP cisplatin vs. IV cisplatin in newly diagnosed ovarian cancer. The primary outcomes studied were progression-free survival, overall survival, and toxicity. Review of the trials found statistically significant improvement in both progression-free and overall survival. Furthermore, the few reported toxicities were increased specifically because of IP therapy and variations in toxicities were thought to be due to individual regimens. However, catheter-related complications could not be included in the toxicity assessment because of insufficient data.[57]

Phase III trials investigating IP therapy conducted in the past decade include the Southwest Oncology Group (SWOG) 8501/Gynecologic Oncology Group (GOG) 104 trial, GOG 113/SWOG 9227 trial, and the GOG 172 trial.[58] The goal of the SWOG 8501/GOG 104 trial was to compare the effects of IP and intravenous (IV) cisplatin on survival of women with previously untreated, stage III ovarian cancer. After initial exploratory laparotomy and resection, patients received six courses of IV cyclophosphamide plus either IV of IP cisplatin every 3 weeks. Results showed a longer estimated median survival in patients receiving IP therapy.[59] Similarly, in the GOG 114/SWOG 9227 trial, an increase in progression-free survival was seen in patients who received the experimental arm of IV carboplatin followed by IV paclitaxel and IP cisplatin when compared with patients treated with IV cisplatin and paclitaxel. However, there was only borderline improvement in overall survival, and more toxicity was associated with the experimental IP group.[60] Last, GOG 172 compared IV paclitaxel-cisplatin and IV paclitaxel plus IP cisplatin and paclitaxel in stage III patients. Although the median duration of overall survival was higher in the IP group (65.6 months) vs. the IV group (49.7 months), the quality of life was significantly worse for patients treated with IP therapy.[61] Although the data reported give strong evidence with regard to IP use, there are some limitations that need to be considered. For instance, because of changes in standard therapy during the course of each study, the control arms do not represent the current standard of care. Moreover, many patients in GOG 172 could not complete the planned courses of IP therapy, and quality of life was decreased.[58]

Ideal candidates for IP administration of therapy should be selected carefully. These should include patients with advanced disease (stage III) who have undergone optimal cytoreduction, patients with adequate renal function, and those who can tolerate the toxicities with IP chemotherapy, such as infection, abdominal pain, discomfort, and nausea.[62-64] The presence of extensive intra-abdominal adhesion may be considered a relative contraindication because of decreased distribution of therapy.[62,63]

Placement of an IP port usually occurs at the time of surgery unless otherwise contraindicated. During administration, the optimal volume of infusate to be delivered to the peritoneal space is not known; however, the National Cancer Institute suggests reconstitution of drug in 1 L of normal saline followed by another liter to help distribution if tolerated.[63] Fluids introduced into the peritoneal cavity need to be warmed before infusion to decrease side effects such as cramping, burning, and pain.[64] After infusion, patients may need to change positions or turn to ensure proper distribution.[63,64] Additionally, all patients should receive supportive care therapies, such as routine premedications, hydration, antiemetics, and pain medications.[62-64]

NEOADJUVANT CHEMOTHERAPY

Neoadjuvant chemotherapy has been proposed as an alternative to primary debulking surgery in advanced ovarian cancer. The goal of neoadjuvant chemotherapy is to decrease tumor volume and ultimately increase the chance of maximal tumor resection at time of surgery. A retrospective study of patients with stage IIIC or IV epithelial ovarian cancer demonstrated an increase in progression-free and overall survival in patients with extra-abdominal disease treated with neoadjuvant chemotherapy. Additionally, advantages of neoadjuvant chemotherapy included less preoperative morbidity, less need for aggressive surgery, and a similar survival to patients who underwent primary debulking surgery.[65] Other retrospective analyses do not support the use of neoadjuvant chemotherapy in place of primary cytoreduction as standard of care. However, it is a viable alternative in patients who are unable to tolerate initial cytoreduction.[66-68] Most studies of neoadjuvant chemotherapy are retrospective analyses; therefore, a prospective trial is necessary to determine the use of neoadjuvant chemotherapy.

TREATMENT OF RECURRENT DISEASE

Despite the improved response rates for advanced ovarian cancer, almost 75% of patients eventually relapse and die from their disease.[54,69-71] Recurrence can appear as pelvic masses in the surgical bed, lymphadenopathy, peritoneal carcinomatosis, liver metastasis, and pleura and lung metastasis.[72] Unfortunately, there is no current standard for treatment of recurrent disease, and goals for therapy are improvement in quality and length of life.[73] One major factor in determining treatment for recurrent cancer is the relapse-free period following final dose of first-line platinum treatment. In ovarian cancer, patients with disease recurring ≥6 months after last platinum therapy are considered to have **platinum-sensitive disease** and may respond to a second course of platinum-taxane–based treatment with a response rate ranging from 20% to 70%.[70] For patients with platinum-resistant disease (relapse <6 months postplatinum therapy) or **platinum-refractory disease** (lack of response or progression during platinum therapy), treatment options include taxanes, topoisomerase I inhibitors,

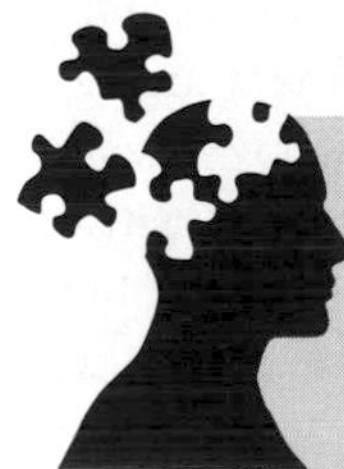

Therapeutic Challenge:

J.J. was considered to have had a complete response to her first-line treatment. After 9 months of follow-up and routine monitoring, J.J.'s CA-125 levels increased to 115 units/mL. A CT scan of the abdomen and pelvis was obtained, and multifocal recurrent disease was detected with multiple peritoneal and perihepatic implants. Should J.J. receive additional taxane/platinum chemotherapy?

Table 45-4. Second-Line Agents Used in Treatment of Ovarian Cancer

Agent	Dosage	Common Adverse Effects
Altretamine	260 mg/m²/d in four divided doses at meals and bedtime in 14- to 28-day cycle	Nausea/vomiting, diarrhea, abdominal cramping, myelosuppression
Carboplatin	1) Calvert Formula Dose = AUC (CrCl +25) 2) Standard dose AUC 5 to 7.5 IV once every 28 days	Nausea/vomiting, myelosuppression (DLT), nephrotoxicity, electrolyte wasting, diarrhea, stomatitis, hypersensitivity reactions
Docetaxel (single agent)	30–40 mg/m² once weekly ***or*** 75 mg/m² IV once every 21 days	Myelosuppression, fluid retention, hyperlacrimation, nail disorders
Etoposide	100 mg daily or 50 mg/m²/d PO for 10–21 days, followed by 1 week rest	Myelosuppression, nausea/vomiting, hypotension, anorexia, alopecia, headache, fever
Gemcitabine	800 mg/m²–1,000 mg/m² IV on day 1, day 8, and day 15 repeated every 28 days	Myelosuppression (DLT), flulike symptoms, headache, somnolence, nausea/vomiting, stomatitis, diarrhea, constipation, rash
Leuprolide acetate	7.5 mg IM once every 30 days	Peripheral edema, gynecomastia, hot flashes, hyperphosphatemia, nausea/vomiting, weight gain
Liposomal doxorubicin	40 mg/m² IV once every 28 days	Myelosuppression, stomatitis, mucositis, alopecia, flushing, shortness of breath, hypotension, headaches, cardiotoxicity, hand-foot syndrome
Paclitaxel (single agent)	135–175 mg/m² infused over 3 hr once every 21–28 days	Hypersensitivity reactions, peripheral neuropathy (DLT), nausea/vomiting, alopecia
Tamoxifen	20 mg PO daily continuously	Thromboembolism, hot flashes, decreased libido, nausea/vomiting thrombocytopenia, anemia
Topotecan	1.5 mg/m² IV day 1 to day 5 every 21 days ***or*** to 4 mg/m² IV once a week x 3 followed by 1 week off	Myelosuppression (DLT), nausea/vomiting, diarrhea, stomatitis, abdominal pain, alopecia, SGOT/SGPT elevation

AUC = area under the curve; IM = intramuscularly; IV = intravenously; DLT = dose-limiting toxicity; PO = by mouth; SGOT = serum glutamic oxaloacetic transaminase; SGPT = serum glutamic pyruvate transaminase.

anthracyclines, cytidine analogues, aromatase inhibitors, antiestrogens, and luteinizing hormone-releasing hormone agonists (Table 45-4). Another option for patients that should be discussed is investigational trials. Because of the lower response rates of second-line agents in recurrent ovarian cancer, there are no guidelines outlining the sequence of therapy. Treatment decisions should be based not only on sensitivity of disease to platinum-containing therapies but also on patient specific factors such as age, comorbidities, and past medical history and treatments. These factors will influence both toxicity profile and ease of administration for the patients.[73]

Summary

Although the prevalence of ovarian cancer is low, it is the fifth-leading cause of cancer mortality in women.[1] Moreover, this mortality rate increases with age.[2] Because of the vague presentation of disease, it is necessary to educate both women and healthcare providers regarding the risk factors, signs, and nonspecific symptoms of ovarian cancer to help recognize patients at higher risk and diagnose patients at an earlier stage. To provide guidance to healthcare providers, investigators are developing a symptom index, which may help to identify patients in need of further diagnostic screening.

Screening is not currently recommended in the general population because of the increase in associated risks with surgery, poor positive predictive value, and patient anxiety. However, in high-risk patients who have not had prophylactic surgery, the NIH recommends monitoring with an annual pelvic exam, CA-125 measurements, and transvaginal pelvic ultrasonography. Clinical studies are being conducted to improve diagnostic techniques through multimodal strategies.

The basis of diagnosis, staging, and treatment of ovarian cancer is surgery via laparotomy or laparoscopy. The goal of surgery in patients positively diagnosed with malignancy is optimal cytoreduction. Additional treatment with adjuvant platinum-taxane based chemotherapy is dependent on disease stage, residual tumor, and other prognostic features. Because of the chronic nature of ovarian cancer, new therapies are necessary for treatment of resistant and recurrent disease. Current research is focusing on intraperitoneal and targeted therapies (Figure 45-1).

References

Additional content available at
www.ashp.org/womenshealth

Figure 45-1. Assessment and treatment algorithm.

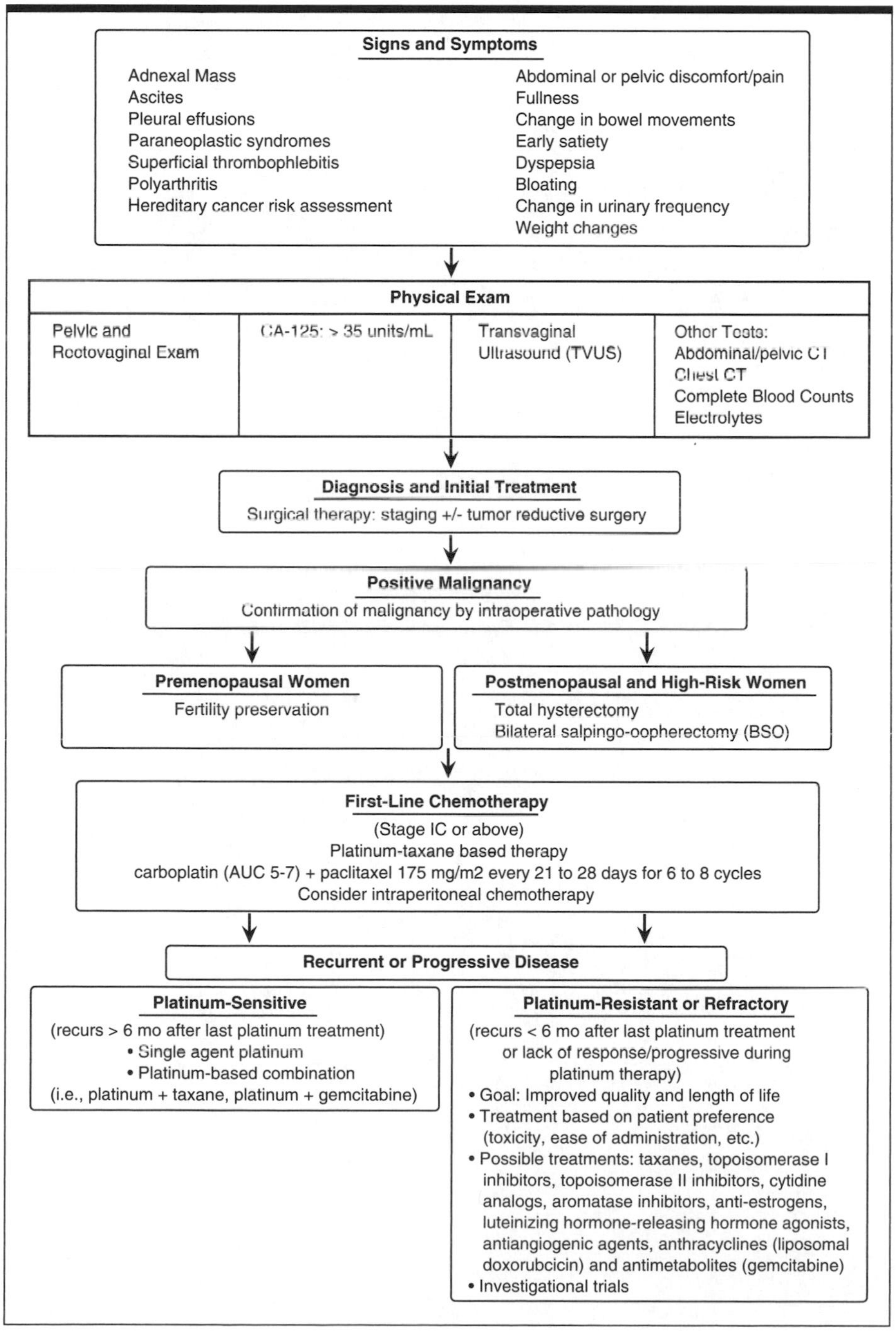

Signs and Symptoms

Adnexal Mass	Abdominal or pelvic discomfort/pain
Ascites	Fullness
Pleural effusions	Change in bowel movements
Paraneoplastic syndromes	Early satiety
Superficial thrombophlebitis	Dyspepsia
Polyarthritis	Bloating
Hereditary cancer risk assessment	Change in urinary frequency
	Weight changes

↓

Physical Exam

Pelvic and Rectovaginal Exam	CA-125: > 35 units/mL	Transvaginal Ultrasound (TVUS)	Other Tests: Abdominal/pelvic CT Chest CT Complete Blood Counts Electrolytes

↓

Diagnosis and Initial Treatment
Surgical therapy: staging +/- tumor reductive surgery

↓

Positive Malignancy
Confirmation of malignancy by intraoperative pathology

↓

Premenopausal Women
Fertility preservation

Postmenopausal and High-Risk Women
Total hysterectomy
Bilateral salpingo-oopherectomy (BSO)

↓

First-Line Chemotherapy
(Stage IC or above)
Platinum-taxane based therapy
carboplatin (AUC 5-7) + paclitaxel 175 mg/m2 every 21 to 28 days for 6 to 8 cycles
Consider intraperitoneal chemotherapy

↓

Recurrent or Progressive Disease

Platinum-Sensitive
(recurs > 6 mo after last platinum treatment)
- Single agent platinum
- Platinum-based combination
(i.e., platinum + taxane, platinum + gemcitabine)

Platinum-Resistant or Refractory
(recurs < 6 mo after last platinum treatment or lack of response/progressive during platinum therapy)
- Goal: Improved quality and length of life
- Treatment based on patient preference (toxicity, ease of administration, etc.)
- Possible treatments: taxanes, topoisomerase I inhibitors, topoisomerase II inhibitors, cytidine analogs, aromatase inhibitors, anti-estrogens, luteinizing hormone-releasing hormone agonists, antiangiogenic agents, anthracyclines (liposomal doxorubcicin) and antimetabolites (gemcitabine)
- Investigational trials

46 Cervical Cancer

Judith Ann Smith, Pharm.D., BCOP, FCCP, FISOPP

Learning Objectives

1. Demonstrate understanding of the etiology and risk factors associated with the development of cervical cancer.
2. Explain the risk and benefits of the human papillomavirus (HPV) vaccine and chemoprevention options available for decreasing the potential risk of developing cervical cancer.
3. Interpret and understand the utility of the **Pap test** and HPV testing screening tests for diagnosing precancerous cervical lesions.
4. Describe the physical signs and symptoms of cervical cancer.
5. Recommend the appropriate surgical, radiation, and chemotherapy treatment options for newly diagnosed and recurrent cervical cancer patients.
6. Compare and contrast chemotherapy options for women with recurrent platinum-resistant cervical cancer.

Cervical cancer is a cancer that can almost exclusively be attributed to high-risk behaviors that increase risk of exposure to the common sexually transmitted disease human papillomavirus (HPV) as well as limited access to healthcare or poor compliance with routine annual screening with Pap test for early detection of cancer cells. Although primary treatment interventions are fairly successful in achieving a cure, if and when cervical cancer recurs, there are limited treatment options associated with poor response rates. Prevention is the critical component for eliminating cervical cancer. The introduction of the HPV vaccine has been a preliminary step on the road to eliminating cervical cancer, but more research on its longevity of immunogenicity—as well as improvement in patient education and overall access to healthcare—will be necessary to succeed in elimination of cervical cancer.

Epidemiology

Cervical cancer is the second most common cancer among women worldwide.[1] Approximately 80% of the cases occur in developing countries, where it is the most common female cancer and the second most common cancer-related cause of death. Although fairly common in developing countries, in the U.S., cervical cancer is only the seventh most common cancer in women.[2]

With the exception of childhood cancers and lymphomas, patients with cervical cancer die younger (average age 60 years) than women with any other cancer. The median age of diagnosis for cervical cancer is 48 years.[2] Approximately 1 of every 145 women in the U.S. will develop invasive cancer of the cervix during her lifetime.[2] In 2009, it is estimated that 11,270 new cases of cervical cancer will be diagnosed, associated with 4,070 deaths in the U.S.[3] There is a slightly higher incidence of cervical cancer in black and Hispanic populations: 25% and 38% higher, respectively, compared with the incidence in white women.[2]

Etiology

The use of tobacco products is considered a risk factor for cervical cancer by the International Agency for Research on Cancer (IARC).[4] Smoking may affect a number of pathways leading to cancer and has been associated with **metaplasia, angiogenesis,** and proliferation in epithelial cells. The formation of chemically stable DNA adducts as a result of smoking may promote genetic instability within the cervical epithelium. Although nicotine and cotinine are not classified as carcinogens, the presence of these compounds in the cervical mucus indicates that some of the approximate 4,000 chemical compounds found in cigarettes (at least 60 of which are known to be toxic or carcinogenic) could also be crossing into the blood and transported to the cervix, where cellular and DNA damage could occur.[4,5] Prokopczyk and colleagues performed a study to evaluate this theory and identified one of the tobacco-specific nitrosamines, 4-(methylnitrosamino)-1-(3-pyridyl)-1-butanone (NNK) in cervical mucus, which is a relatively abundant and the most active tobacco-specific carcinogen in animal models.[5] NNK was identified at higher levels in smokers and a lower level in nonsmokers, indicating that not only is smoking a risk factor, but environmental exposure and secondhand smoke may also be a risk factor.[5]

The sexually transmitted disease HPV is a major risk for cervical cancer and will be discussed in the pathogenesis section of this chapter. The number of sexual partners a woman has is directly correlated with the risk of developing cervical cancer.[6] Risk of developing cervical cancer is also more common in women with lower social status and in women with male partners that engage in high-risk sexual behaviors.

Other high-risk factors include history of cervical cancer, in utero exposure to diethylstilbestrol (DES), immunosuppression (including human immunodeficiency virus [HIV]), three or more lifetime sex partners, first sexual intercourse before the age of 18, contact with partner who has had partners with cervical cancer or HPV infection, smoking, or a previous abnormal Pap test.

CASE PRESENTATION

Patient Case 1: Part 1

C.H. is a 47-year-old black woman who presents to her primary physician with symptoms of intermittent bleeding and pain during intercourse.

HPI: C.H. has noticed increasing pain during intercourse over the past 6 months. She has also noticed breakthrough bleeding/spotting between her menstrual cycles.

PMH: Menarche at age 9. Diagnosed with infertility at age 30.

Family history: Both her mother and maternal grandmother were diagnosed with breast cancer.

Social history: Married, no children, denies any tobacco or alcohol use. She has had four sex partners in her lifetime.

Medications: Aspirin daily.

Allergies: NKDA.

Vitals: 5′4″, 140 lb, BP 126/70, Temp 97.6° F, RR 20.

Lab values: Within normal limits.

Physical exam: Discomfort with exam. Palpable mass approximately 1 cm x 2 cm at vaginal apex.

Patient assessment: C.H. is 47-year-old woman presenting with new pelvic mass that requires additional evaluation.

Clinical Presentation

SIGNS AND SYMPTOMS OF CERVICAL CANCER

Patients with early-stage cervical cancer are typically asymptomatic, and diagnosis is often an incidental finding on cytologic screening tests. However, patients with more advanced tumors may report early signs associated with disruption of the cervical mucosa, such as abnormal vaginal bleeding, postcoital bleeding, or a watery or foul discharge. Patients may report pain during or after intercourse as well.

As tumor grows before reaching the pelvic wall, patients may experience some flank pain that is due to an ureteral obstruction. As tumor continues to grow and reach the pelvic side wall, patients will often report pain in the hip or buttock similar to sciatic pain and may have unilateral leg swelling because of impingement of lymphatic or hematologic circulation. If the tumor invades the bladder, symptoms of urinary frequency or hematuria may occur. Very rarely there is rectal involvement, which could be associated with difficult bowel movements with blood or mucus in the rectum.

PATTERNS OF METASTASIS

Local Invasion

Cervical tumors can directly infiltrate locally along the uterosacral ligaments and parametrium and to the ureters and bladder, resulting in obstruction. Rectal invasion is very uncommon.

Distant Invasion

Both lymphatic and hematologic spread is associated with the progression of cervical cancer. The risk of lymphatic spread corresponds to the depth of invasion of the primary tumor and more often contributes to regional spread to the surrounding organs in the pelvis. Because the cervix is a midline structure, it can spread to both right and left pelvis. Hematologic spread occurs in more advanced disease, most often as **metastasis** to the liver or lung. Neuroendocrine and small cell cervical cancers often spread to the brain and bone. Otherwise, bone and brain metastases are uncommon in cervical cancer.

Pathophysiology

More than 99% of cervical cancers are associated with a persistent HPV infection.[5] HPV is the most common sexually transmitted infection in the U.S., with an estimated 20 million adults currently infected with an additional 6.2 million becoming infected each year.[7] It has been estimated that the lifetime likelihood of exposure to HPV is 75% to 90%, with a 15% to 25% risk associated with each new partner.[5] There is a strong association between HPV and cervical cancer, as 99.7% of more than 1,000 biopsies from a multicenter study of women with cervical cancer tested positive for HPV.[5]

HUMAN PAPILLOMAVIRUS

HPV is a group of small nonenveloped double-stranded DNA viruses with genomes of approximately 8,000 base pairs. These viruses can be characterized into two types: mucosal and cutaneous HPV infections. There are approximately 40 subtypes of mucosal HPV that infect the genital tract. There are nearly 200 characterized subtypes of HPV, among which are 15 that are considered to be high-risk types (HPV 16, 18, 31, 33, 35, 39, 45, 51, 52, 56, 58, 59, 68, 73, and 82), 3 that are most likely high-risk types (HPV 26, 53, and 66), and 12 that appear to be low-risk types (HPV 6, 11, 40, 42, 43, 44, 54, 61, 70, 72, 81, and CP6108).[8]

Cervical dysplasia, premalignant lesions, and cervical cancer are associated with infections with the high-risk HPV subtypes. Infections with the low-risk subtypes, such as HPV 6 or HPV 11, are associated with genital warts and laryngeal papillomas, respectively.

Following the initial exposure and infection, HPV enters a dormant period from 2 to 12 months or longer. More than 90% of subclinical infections will clear spontaneously within 2 years, most likely as the result of a cellular immune response that begins after about 3 months of being infected with HPV. Because of the limitations of the HPV assays methods, it is unclear whether an HPV infection that is clinically cleared has truly been eliminated or if it is below the level of detection. Some HPV infections may remain in a latent state for years, as evidenced in some women with genital warts that appear to spontaneously resolve and then reoccur during pregnancy or if a patient is physiologically stressed, such as immune suppression because of medications or another infection or disease.

As early as 3 months (and sometimes not until years later) after HPV infection, if the immune system cannot clear the virus, the infection can lead to cervical dysplasia and/or low-grade lesions of the cervix. After years of persistent infection with a high-grade HPV, the development of cervical intraepithelial neoplasia (CIN) II or CIN III can occur, and if left untreated can progress to invasive cervical cancer.[9]

The multiple factors that affect progression of HPV infections to cervical cancer are unknown. Unfortunately, some women will have an accelerated progression to advanced disease in a short period despite close monitoring. Some speculate that this may be due to patient-specific factors, such as immune system function or possibly the viral load.

CASE PRESENTATION

Patient Case 2: Part 1

L.R. is a 32-year-old white woman who presents to her gynecologist for a routine well-woman exam with concerns about HPV testing.

HPI: L.R. has recently seen multiple television advertisements promoting HPV testing. She has never been tested but knows she used to practice unsafe sexual behaviors when in college. Now that she is divorced and considering new relationships, she wants to know if she has HPV.

PMH: L.R. is in good health.

Social history: Divorced, three children, history of smoking tobacco but denies alcohol use. She has had 15 different sex partners in her lifetime.

Medications: Oral contraceptives.

Allergies: NKDA.

Vitals: 5′6″, 130 lb, BP 106/72, Temp 98.6° F, RR 22.

Lab values: WNL.

Pelvic exam: Normal.

Patient assessment: L.R. is a 32-year-old woman with past social history that puts her at a high risk for HPV infection.

Screening and Diagnosis

SCREENING

Screening for cervical cancer should begin approximately 3 years after the onset of vaginal intercourse but no later than 21 years of age.[10] Screening should consist of an annual Pap test and pelvic examination. After a 30-year-old woman at low risk for cervical cancer has had three or more consecutive annual exams with a normal finding, the Pap test could be performed less often at the discretion of her gynecologist, Most guidelines recommend that women with one or more high-risk factors to continue cervical cancer screening with an annual Pap test and pelvic examination. In clinical practice, however, most gynecologist continue annual testing because it is difficult to confirm that the patient is really considered low risk; the behaviors of sex partners can only be assumed, not confirmed. The recommendation for annual Pap test and pelvic examination applies to all women regardless of risk factors, including current absence sexual activity or age. After age 30, HPV testing should be repeated whenever abnormal Pap test occurs or periodically if a woman has multiple sex partners.

Table 46-1. Pap Test Terminology

Previous Systems and the Bethesda System		
Pap Classes	**Description**	**Bethesda 2001**
I	Normal	Normal and variants
II	Reactive changes	Reactive changes
	Atypia	ASC, AGC
	Koilocytosis	Low-grade SIL
III CIN I	Mild dysplasia	Low-grade SIL
III CIN II	Moderate dysplasia	High-grade SIL
III CIN III	Severe dysplasia	High-grade SIL
IV	Carcinoma in situ, suspicious	High-grade SIL
V	Invasive	Microinvasion (<3 mm)
		Frankly invasive (>3 mm)

ASC = atypical squamous cells; AGC = atypical glandular cells of uncertain significance; CIN = cervical intraepithelial neoplasia; SIL = squamous intraepithelial lesion.

PAP TEST

Cytologic screening was not accepted into routine gynecologic medical practice until approximately 1941, when Dr. Papanicolaou's study on a cytologic screening tool was published and findings accepted. With the introduction of the Papanicolaou test (more commonly referred to as the Pap test) as a screening tool and the improvement in access and compliance with routine cervical cancer screening, a 74% reduction in the incidence of cervical cancer was observed from 1955 to 2004.[10] The Pap test is a fairly noninvasive cytology sampling test of the surface of the cervix for early detection of cancer cells. It is completed during the pelvic exam and does not cause any pain or side effects. The cells collected with the Pap test are sent for pathology for histologic evaluation.

Table 46-1 summarizes both the old and new systems for classifying cervical cytology. The old system of Pap test classification was updated to the current Bethesda classification system in 2001.[11] The 2001 revised Bethesda system includes reporting adequacy of sample; incidental findings, such as evidence of infection; and evidence of lesions with reporting of low-grade and high-grade squamous intraepithelial lesions, or cancer. The Pap test is read by a pathologist, who is responsible for the diagnosis and recommendations for follow-up cytology sampling.

The new Bethesda System classifies Pap test results into four categories: low-grade squamous intraepithelial lesion (LSIL), high-grade squamous intraepithelial lesion (HSIL), **atypical squamous cells (ASC),** and **atypical glandular cells (AGS).**[11] LSIL is classified as cellular changes associated with HPV or mild (slight) dysplasia/CIN 1. HSIL is defined by moderate dysplasia/CIN II, severe dysplasia/CIN III, or carcinoma in situ/CIN III. ASC can be unspecified (ASC-US) and can favor benign conditions or inflammation, and ASC cannot exclude HSIL (ASC-H). AGC is broken down into favoring endocervical, endometrial, or not otherwise specified origin or endocervical adenocarcinoma in situ (AIS). AGC can be unspecified (AGC-US) or can favor neoplastic cells (AGC-H). The adequacy of a Pap test is determined by the yield of endocervical cells. *Atypia* is a clinical term for atypical cells such as ASC-US and ASG-US, and Pap test results showing atypia should include a recommendation for follow-up.[11]

HUMAN PAPILLOMAVIRUS TESTING

Serologic HPV tests cannot distinguish between past and current infections; therefore, diagnosis of current infections can only be detected through identification of viral DNA in clinical samples.[12] This requires sensitive type-specific HPV DNA tests. There are currently two U.S. Food and Drug Administration (FDA)-approved tests: the Hybrid Capture Tube test (HCT) and the Hybrid Capture® 2 assay (HC2 assay) (Digene Corporation, Gaithersburg, MD). The HCT test was FDA approved in May 1995 and could detect the presence of HPV types 16, 18, 31, 33, 35, 45, 51, 52, and 56. The HC2 assay, which was FDA approved in March 1999, includes a cocktail of full-length HPV type-specific RNA probes for 13 high-risk HPV types (HPV 16, 18, 31, 33, 35, 39, 45, 51, 52, 56, 58, 59, and 68). This technology works by hybridizing HPV-DNA in a sample followed by capture of the DNA/RNA hybrids on a solid phase with signal amplification by conjugate antibodies that recognize the DNA/RNA hybrids. Testing can be done on Pap test samples. The HPV testing cannot distinguish the subtype of HPV but is quantitative for the viral load present. In March 2003, HPV DNA testing was approved by the FDA for women 30 years of age or older combined with the Pap test, with HPV DNA testing recommended to be done not more often than every 3 years.

FOLLOW-UP FOR ABNORMAL RESULTS

If any abnormalities are detected with Pap test, additional follow-up will be recommended. For any atypical cells (mild dysplasia up to CIN I), repeating the Pap test within 6 months is recommended. For CIN II or CIN III, additional evaluation, including **colposcopy** exam with endocervical **curettage,** is recommended, with three to five biopsies of any suspicious sites on the cervix, which are sent to pathologist for histologic evaluation. If follow-up samples are also classified CIN III, any grade, removal of effected cells is recommended. This can be accomplished by a surgical conization or loop electrosurgical excision procedure (LEEP), which will be discussed in the treatment section of this chapter. If cervical cancer is diagnosed in the follow-up samples, patients will undergo additional diagnostic tests, including blood tests and imaging either by computed tomography (CT) scan, magnetic resonance imaging (MRI), or positron-emission tomography (PET) scan to determine the extent of disease.

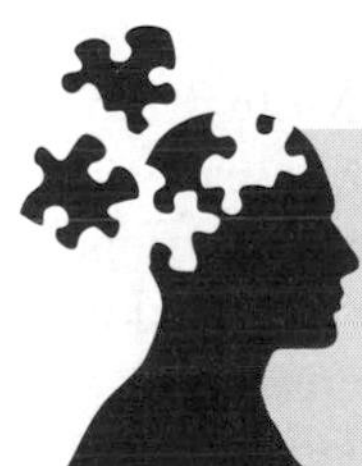

Therapeutic Challenge:

K.B. is a 35-year-old woman who presents to your outpatient clinic concerned about the risk of developing cervical cancer and asks about the HPV vaccine. Her gynecologist has tested her for HPV, which came back negative. K.B. has been married for 9 years and has two daughters. Is K.B. a good candidate for the HPV vaccine?

HISTOLOGIC DIAGNOSIS

The classification of cervical cancer has been developed by the World Health Organization and the International Federation of Gynecology and Obstetrics (FIGO). The majority of cervical cancers can be classified as squamous carcinomas. Adenocarcinomas occur less frequently and tend to be more aggressive and less responsive to treatment interventions such as radiation and chemotherapy. Rare histologies include neuroendocrine and small cell tumors, which tend to be less responsive to radiation. A mixed histology is fairly common in cervical cancer, hence the need for multimodality treatment.

INTERNATIONAL FEDERATION OF GYNECOLOGY AND OBSTETRICS STAGING

Unlike other gynecologic cancers that are surgically diagnosed and then staged using the FIGO staging algorithm, cervical cancer is diagnosed by biopsy and clinically staged by results from imaging tests. Although clinically staged, cervical cancer staging is still defined by the FIGO staging system (Figure 46-1).

PROGNOSTIC FACTORS

The stage of disease at the time of initial diagnosis has the greatest impact on the overall prognosis and survival. The limited or early disease is often curative, with minimal impact on quality of life. In advanced disease, the treatment interventions are associated with complications that often affect the overall quality of life, such fistulas, neuropathies, and permanent damage to bowel associated with bouts of diarrhea and constipation. Histologic subtype is often predictive of response to radiation and chemotherapy, with squamous carcinomas having the best potential to respond to chemotherapy, and radiation and neuroendocrine or small cell carcinomas having the least likelihood of responding to treatment. Achieving a

Figure 46-1. International Federation of Gynecology and Obstetrics (FIGO) staging algorithm.

Stage 0 Carcinoma *in situ* or intraepithelial carcinoma

Stage I

1a: Microscopic invasion: limited invasion of stroma (less than or equal to 5 mm in depth and less than or equal to 7 mm in width

Ia1: Less than or equal to 3 mm depth and less than or equal to 7 mm in width

Ia2: Greater than 3 mm (still less than 5mm) depth and less than or equal to 7 mm in width

Ib: Clinical lesions also limited to cervix but larger than 1a

Stage II

Tumor extends beyond cervix but does not involve the pelvic wall and/or involves upper two thirds of the vagina

IIa: Parametrium not involved; involves up to the upper two thirds of the vagina

IIb: Parametrium involved but does not involve the pelvic wall

Stage III

Tumor involved with pelvic side wall, and/or involve entire vagina

IIIa: No involvement of pelvic sidewall, but entire vagina is involved

IIIb: Tumor involves pelvic sidewall or hydronephrosis or nonfunctioning kidney

Stage IV

Carcinoma is extended beyond pelvic region or involving bladder and/or rectum

IVa: Spread to adjacent pelvic organs

IVb: Spread to distant organs

"complete response" to primary treatment is critical for overall prognosis and survival. In the recurrent setting, the response rates to chemotherapy decrease to <20%, and radiation is often only palliative.

Prevention

The number-one approach for successful prevention is abstinence from sexual encounters, but this is unrealistic over one's entire reproductive life. Abstinence is an effective method of preventing all sexually transmitted diseases; mutual monogamy and condoms are less likely to be effective. Mutual monogamy with someone who has had prior partners harbors the inherent risk that one or more of the prior partners has had HPV exposure; each additional prior partner adds another 25% increase in risk of exposure to HPV. Because HPV exposure is not exclusively genital-to-genital contact but includes all contact with infected epithelial sites, condoms offer only limited protection against HPV infections.[13] In a meta-analysis, Manhart and Koutsky discovered that there is a lack of published studies regarding condom use and HPV infection; that very limited evidence supports that there is no protective effect of condom use on HPV DNA detection; and that some studies actually showed an increased incidence of HPV lesions with condom use.[13]

HUMAN PAPILLOMAVIRUS VACCINE

The HPV quadrivalent (types 6, 11, 16, and 18) vaccine, Gardasil® (Merck & Company, South Granville, NSW), was approved by the FDA in 2006 for the prevention of HPV infections in women ages 9 to 26 years. HPV 6 and 11 are associated with genital warts, and HPV 16 and 18 are associated with up to 70% of all cervical cancer cases. Ideally, the HPV vaccine should be administered before any potential exposure to the virus—that is, before any sexual activity. However, it is effective in those individuals that have been sexually active but currently test HPV negative. The current HPV vaccine (Gardasil®) is not effective for treatment of HPV infections or cervical cancer.

The HPV vaccine is prepared from highly purified viruslike particles (VLPs) of the major capsid protein (L1) of HPV types 6, 11, 16, and 18. The HPV L1 protein, when expressed in yeast, forms noninfectious VLPs that are indistinguishable from native virions but lack viral DNA.[14] These VLPs elicit an immune response and induce a higher geometric mean titer (GMT) of virion-neutralizing antibodies compared with placebo.[15]

LIMITATIONS OF THE HUMAN PAPILLOMAVIRUS VACCINE

The HPV vaccine is effective against HPV 16/18/11/6 specifically and has limited cross-neutralization ability against other HPV genotypes.[16] Hence, there are concerns about increased incidence of infections with other high-risk types not contained in the vaccine, as well as the evolution of another subtype superseding HPV 16/18 that would be resistant to the vaccine. From the preliminary follow-up studies, data suggest that the immunity achieved from the HPV vaccine is not likely to be lifelong, and studies to determine the timing for boosters or repeating series is unknown. However, current studies indicate that the HPV vaccine is effective for 5 years for HPV 16, but additional evaluation to determine effective GMT is needed. The HPV 18 titers decrease similar to placebo by 36 months.[17] The complete three-shot series must be completed within the 6-month time frame for an adequate GMT to be achieved. There are concerns about compliance and the lack of efficacy in those not completing the full three-shot series.[18] In addition, women older than age 26 (and no men) are currently being vaccinated, so the HPV virus will not be eliminated. The total impact of the use of the HPV vaccine will not be apparent for decades, but it has been a significant step forward in the prevention of cervical cancer.

CURRENT HUMAN PAPILLOMAVIRUS VACCINATION RECOMMENDATIONS

At this time, the Centers for Disease Control and Prevention (CDC) Advisory Committee on Immunization Practices (ACIP) recommends the HPV vaccine for girls between the age of 11 and 12, as well for girls as young as 9 to 10 and those between 13 and 26 who have not been vaccinated and may become sexually active. The HPV vaccine should not be given to women with allergy to yeast, who are pregnant, or who have moderate to severe illness (i.e., immunosuppression) until they completely recover. Completion of all three shots at 1, 2, and 6 months is required to achieve immunogenic protection. There are no data on efficacy if HPV vaccine series is not completed. Currently, most major insurance companies will cover the cost of the HPV vaccine for the FDA label indications. In most cases, reimbursement is denied for use outside FDA labeled indications, such in boys or women older than age 26. In the U.S., the Vaccines for Children federal health program for those without health insurance will cover the cost for the HPV vaccine for the FDA indications. Although some states have attempted to mandate HPV vaccination for entry into public school systems, parents/patients can refuse.

CASE PRESENTATION

Patient Case 2: Part 2

Diagnosis: Normal Pap test that is positive for HPV.

Treatment plan: There currently is no available treatment for the eradication of HPV infections. Since L.R. is older than age 30, she likely has a persistent HPV infection and is at a higher risk of developing cervical cancer.

Patient monitoring: She should have annual Pap tests and pelvic exams.

Patient education: L.R. should be counseled on safe sexual behaviors and her risk for spreading HPV to other partners. She needs to be told of her own increased risk of developing cervical cancer and the importance of routine screening for prevention of cervical cancer.

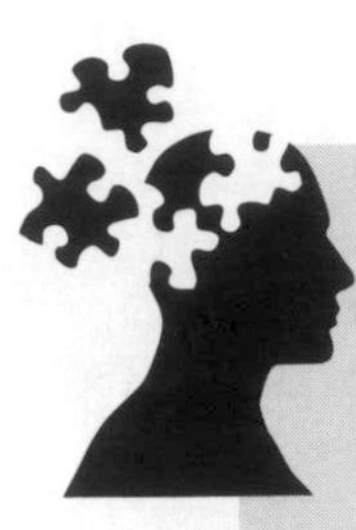

Therapeutic Challenge:

D.G. is a 24-year-old Hispanic woman who presents with stage IA cervical cancer. She is recently married and would like to maintain her fertility. What are her treatment options and associated risks vs. benefits?

Treatment of Cervical Intraepithelial Neoplasia

There is a significant risk of developing cervical cancer in women diagnosed with CIN, which is considered stage 0 cervical cancer. CIN I will often resolve without any treatment interventions, but patients should Pap tests repeated in 6 months. The high grades of dysplasia diagnosis of CIN II or CIN III, however, require treatment to prevent further progression into invasive cervical cancer. Both can be treated with a simple, relatively painless outpatient procedure, such as LEEP or cone biopsy, which removes the surface of the cervix to 1- to 3-mm depth. LEEP and conization of the cervix affect the integrity of the cervix and have been associated with adverse outcomes in later pregnancies, including preterm delivery, low birthweight infants, incompetent cervix, and cervical stenosis.[19,20] Hence, women who have had multiple LEEPs or cone biopsies are often treated as high-risk pregnancies or a least monitored closely for signs of potential complications with delivery.

Treatment of Cervical Cancer

PRIMARY TREATMENT

Surgery

Surgery is typically reserved for stage IA and IB1 disease when it is possible to completely excise the tumor and have negative margins. A **hysterectomy**—vaginal or abdominal—with pelvic lymph node dissection is the standard initial surgical treatment of stage IA1 cervical cancer (Figure 46-2).[21] This is a definitive treatment of cervical cancer but does eliminate possibility for reproduction.

Figure 46-2. Diagram of female reproductive tract (uterus, fallopian tubes, ovaries, vagina). Dash line box outlines what is removed during the total abdominal hysterectomy with bilateral salpingo-oophorectomy (TAH/BSO).

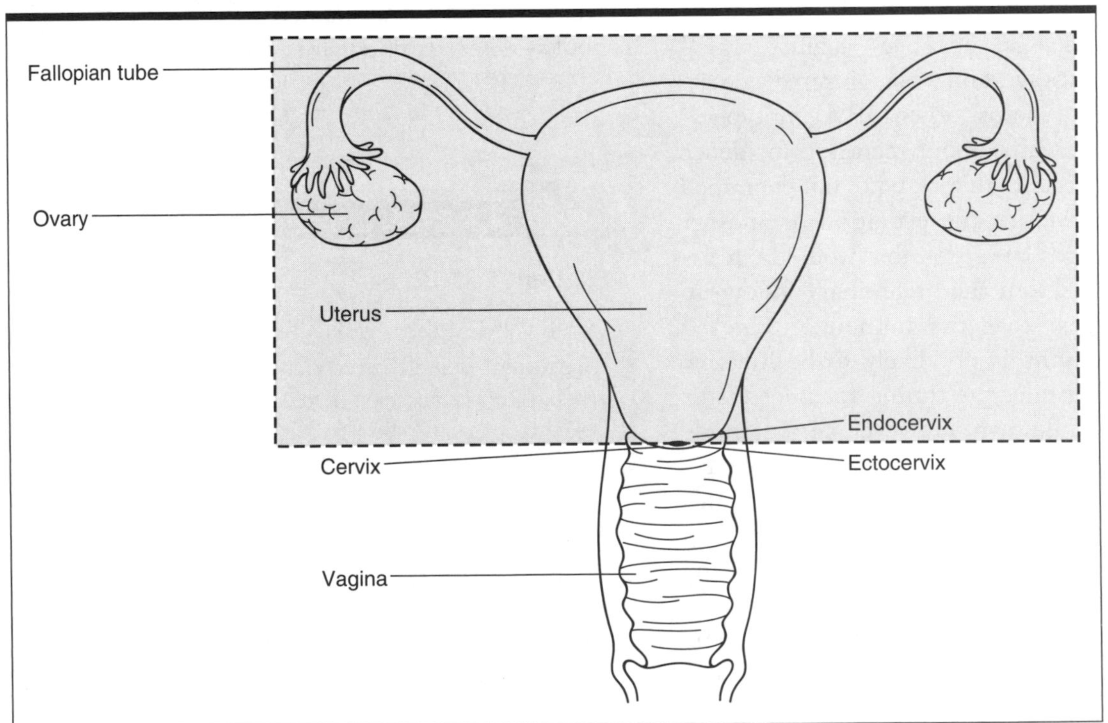

Often patients are seeking fertility sparing surgical interventions. A radical trachelectomy (surgical removal of the cervix and parametrium [Figure 46-2]) and **laparoscopic** lymphadenectomy was first proposed in the early 1990s and continues to gain acceptance.[22] However, compared with a simple hysterectomy, this is a more complicated surgical intervention, and surgeon skill is critical for successful outcome.[23] Overall, there have been more than 236 cases reported in the literature, with an impressive 3.4% recurrence rate; in these patients, there have been more than 50 pregnancies with 30 live births.[23] Conservative, fertility-sparing surgery is typically only considered in patients with stage IA cervical cancer. The risk of recurrence is higher in stage IB and above, so aggressive primary treatment is necessary to achieve a cure. In patients with bulky tumors, stage IB2 and above, surgery is not considered for primary treatment; rather patients are dispositioned for chemoradiation.

Chemoradiation

Chemoradiation is currently considered the standard of care for locally advanced and metastatic cervical cancer. Pelvic radiation and concurrent cisplatin-based chemotherapy is considered the standard of care for stages IIB, IIIA, IIIB, and IVA disease. The chemotherapy regimen most often used includes weekly cisplatin dosed as 40 mg/m²/week (maximum of 6 doses) while receiving 45 Gy of external beam pelvic radiation, followed by internal radiation (brachytherapy) administered via tandem and ovoid insertion (**ALTO**). The tandem is a cylinder that is used to hold the radiation source and is inserted into the vagina, and the ovoids are circular devices to hold radiation sources inserted just below each ovary to deliver radiation to the tumor. The tandem and ovoids are left in place for 72 hours; during this time, patients are required to stay horizontal in bed, with no outside visitors and minimal nursing contact to reduce radiation exposure to others. Two ALTO procedures are recommended, but patients often refuse the second ALTO because of the mental and physical discomfort. In addition, cisplatin is often administered with the first or second ALTO to improve outcomes (Table 46-2). The addition of chemotherapy to the radiation has improved overall survival rates to more than 67%.[24]

Chemotherapy

In patients with advanced cervical cancer, the relief of symptoms through regression of the primary and metastatic tumors is a reasonable goal for treatment for an incurable cancer. Although historically single-agent platinum-based therapy (Table 46-2) has been a standard care in this setting, the emergence of new data has supported the use of combination platinum-based regimens (Table 46-3). Cervical cancer is considered to be a platinum-sensitive disease, with cisplatin achieving better response rates compared with carboplatin; the combination regimens therefore more often include cisplatin. Unlike other gynecologic cancers (ovarian or endometrial), the substitution of carboplatin for cisplatin to decrease toxicity is not well accepted or recommended.

Table 46-2. Platinum Agents for the Treatment of Cervical Cancer

Agent	Dosage	Common Adverse Effects
Cisplatin (+/− XRT) (Gold Standard)	40 mg/m² (maximum total dose 70 mg) infused over 1 hr once a wk for 5 wk and with ALTO	Neurotoxicity (DLT), nausea/vomiting, ototoxicity, nephrotoxicity, myelosuppression, electrolyte wasting, diarrhea
Cisplatin	**Single agent:** 75 mg/m² infused over 4 hr once every 21 days	Neurotoxicity (DLT), nausea/vomiting, ototoxicity, nephrotoxicity, myelosuppression, electrolyte wasting, diarrhea
Carboplatin	AUC 5–6 infused over 1 hr once every 28 days	Myelosuppression (DLT), nephrotoxicity, nausea/vomiting, electrolyte wasting, diarrhea, stomatitis, hypersensitivity reactions

ALTO = internal radiation administered via tandem and ovoid insertion; AUC = area under the curve; DLT = dose-limiting toxicity; XRT = radiation therapy.

Table 46-3. Recommended Combination Platinum-Based Regimens for the Treatment of Advanced and Recurrent Cervical Cancer

Agent	Dosage	Common Adverse Effects
Gemcitabine + cisplatin	Gemcitabine 1,000 mg/m^2 IV infused over 30 min on days 1 and 8 + cisplatin 100 mg/m^2 on day 1 only Regimen is given once every 21 days	Myelosuppression (DLT), flulike symptoms, headache, somnolence, nausea/vomiting, stomatitis, diarrhea, constipation, rash neurotoxicity (DLT), ototoxicity, nephrotoxicity, myelosuppression, electrolyte wasting
Paclitaxel + carboplatin	Paclitaxel 175 mg/m^2 IV infused over 3 hr + carboplatin AUC = 5 IV infused over 1 hr Regimen is given once every 21 days	Peripheral neuropathy (DLT), nausea/vomiting, alopecia, hypersensitivity reactions; myelosuppression (DLT), nephrotoxicity, electrolyte wasting, diarrhea, stomatitis
Paclitaxel + cisplatin	Paclitaxel 135 mg/m^2 IV infused over 24 hr + day 2: cisplatin 75 mg/m^2 IV infused over 4 hr Regimen is given once every 21 days	Peripheral neuropathy (DLT), nausea/vomiting, alopecia, hypersensitivity reactions, neurotoxicity (DLT), ototoxicity, nephrotoxicity, myelosuppression, electrolyte wasting, diarrhea
Topotecan + cisplatin	Cisplatin 50 mg/m^2 infused over 1 hr on day 1 followed by topotecan 1.2 mg/m^2 infused over 30 min on days 1, 2, and 3 Regimen is given once every 21 days	Myelosuppression (DLT), nausea/vomiting, diarrhea, stomatitis, abdominal pain, alopecia, SGOT/SGPT elevation
Vinorelbine + cisplatin	Vinorelbine 25 mg/m^2 on day 1 and day 8 + cisplatin 80 mg/m^2 on day 1 only Regimen is given once every 21 days	Constipation, neutropenia, anemia, thrombocytopenia, neurotoxicity (DLT), nausea/vomiting, ototoxicity, nephrotoxicity, myelosuppression, electrolyte wasting, diarrhea

AUC = area under the curve; DLT = dose-limiting toxicity; IV = intravenously; SGOT = serum glutamic oxaloacetic transaminase; SGPT = serum glutamic pyruvate transaminase.

Post-treatment Surveillance

After LEEP or conization, patients should have routine Pap tests every 3–4 for the first 2 years, then every 6 months for 3 years. If Pap tests remain normal with no detection of abnormal cells for all 5 years, the patient can return to annual screening thereafter.

Patients with cervical cancer who achieve a complete response (CR) to primary treatment with surgery or chemoradiation or chemotherapy (rare) should continue to have a pelvic exam, Pap test, and chest x-ray every 3 months for the first year. In the second year to the fifth year, chest x-rays are only needed every 6 months. After 3 years, the pelvic exam is completed twice a year and a Pap test annually. If Pap tests remain normal with no detection of abnormal cells and there is no detection of disease recurrence for all 5 years, the patient can return to annual screening thereafter.

CASE PRESENTATION

Patient Case 1: Part 2

Diagnosis: PET Ssan reports stage IIB cervical cancer with no para-aortic lymph node involvement.

Treatment plan: C.H. will be dispositioned to initiate chemoradiation with cisplatin.

Patient monitoring: Throughout chemoradiation, C.H. should be monitored for myelosuppression, infection, and electrolyte wasting.

Patient education: C.H. should be counseled on the side effects of cisplatin, including myelosuppression, nephrotoxicity, neurotoxicity, alopecia, and acute and delayed nausea and vomiting. She should be given information on neutropenic precautions (i.e., hand washing, monitoring fever, and prevention of infection) and encouraged to drink noncaffeine fluids throughout treatment. Because she will be receiving pelvic radiation, management of diarrhea and good bathroom habits to prevent infection should also be reviewed.

RECURRENT DISEASE

Chemotherapy

In the recurrent setting, platinum sensitivity of the tumor is assessed first. If it has been <6 months or disease progresses while receiving a platinum-based regimen, the cancer is considered to be platinum resistant. The duration of time since completion of prior treatment influences the goal of treatment in the recurrent setting. If still platinum sensitive, combination regimens are employed as aggressive treatment with a curative intent. Unfortunately, when the recurrence happens at <6 months and is considered platinum resistant, the goal for treatment is palliative care; then, often single therapy is used, with nonplatinum agents such as gemcitabine, paclitaxel, topotecan, irinotecan, vinblastine, vincristine, vinorelbine, liposomal doxorubicin, ifosfamide, or cyclophosphamide (Table 46-4). Overall single-agent activity in the recurrent cervical cancer setting has poor response rates (between 0.1% and 31%).[35] Although an investigational study has just as much likelihood of achieving a response as well or better than the current single agents used, completing clinical trials in this setting is fairly difficult because of the (fortunate) very limited number of patients available to enroll to achieve the number needed to demonstrate statistically significant improvements in response rates.

Radiation

The utility of radiation in the recurrent setting depends on the location of the recurrence. If the recurrence is within the radiation field (i.e., pelvis), additional radiation cannot be used. However, if the tumor is outside the previous radiation field and it is an isolated recurrence, then radiation can be effective in achieving another CR. If there are multiple sites of recurrence, radiation could be used with a palliative intent to relieve symptoms such as pain or persistent vaginal bleeding.

Table 46-4. Examples of Nonplatinum Agents for the Treatment of Recurrent Cervical Cancer

Agent	Dosage	Common Adverse Effects
Capecitabine	1,800–2,500 mg/m² PO as divided dose twice for 14 consecutive days followed by 1 wk of rest	Myelosuppression, hand-foot syndrome, nausea/vomiting, edema, stomatitis, diarrhea, cardiotoxicity, rash
Cyclophosphamide	Cyclophosphamide 750 mg/m² IV over 30 min	Nausea/vomiting, nephrotoxicity, myelosuppression, cardiotoxicity, alopecia, hemorrhagic cystitis
Liposomal Doxorubicin	40 mg/m² IV infused over 3 hr cycle 1 and 2, then infused over 1 hr thereafter; repeat every 28 days	Myelosuppression, stomatitis, mucositis, alopecia, flushing, shortness of breath, hypotension, headaches, cardiotoxicity, hand-foot syndrome
Irinotecan	100 mg/m² infused over 90 min once a wk for 3 consecutive wk, followed by 1 wk of rest given on a 28-day cycle	Neutropenia, diarrhea (acute and/or delayed), thrombocytopenia, anemia, alopecia, nausea/vomiting
Gemcitabine	800 mg/m² IV infused over 30 min once a wk on days 1, 8, and 15 followed by 1 wk of rest	Myelosuppression (DLT), flulike symptoms, headache, somnolence, nausea/vomiting, stomatitis, diarrhea, constipation, rash
Paclitaxel	Peripheral neuropathy (DLT), nausea/vomiting, alopecia, hypersensitivity reactions	Peripheral neuropathy (DLT), nausea/vomiting, alopecia, hypersensitivity reactions, neurotoxicity (DLT), ototoxicity, nephrotoxicity, myelosuppression, electrolyte wasting, diarrhea
Topotecan	1.5 mg/m² infused over 30 min daily on days 1 through day 5 on a 21-day cycle	Myelosuppression (DLT), nausea/vomiting, diarrhea, stomatitis, abdominal pain, alopecia, SGOT/SGPT elevation
Vinorelbine	30 mg/m² IV infused over 15 min on days 1 and 8; repeat every 21 days	Constipation, neutropenia, anemia, thrombocytopenia, neurotoxicity

DLT = dose-limiting toxicity; IV = intravenously; PO = by mouth; SGOT = serum glutamic oxaloacetic transaminase; SGPT = serum glutamic pyruvate transaminase.

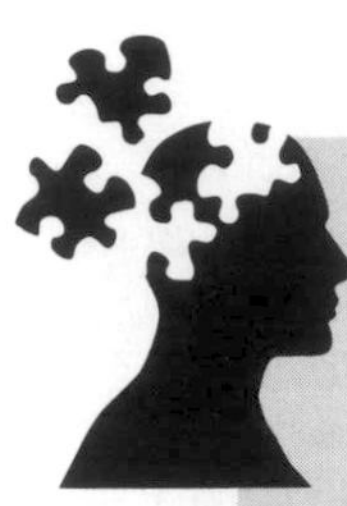

Therapeutic Challenge:

R.K. is a 47-year-old woman of Asian descent with history of stage IIB cervical cancer but has had no evidence of disease for more than 3 years. At her surveillance follow-up visit, one isolated nodule in her pelvis was noted on her PET exam report. Otherwise, she is in excellent health. Is she a candidate for an exenteration surgery?

Surgery

The consideration for surgical interventions in the recurrent setting also depends on the location of the recurrence, as well as the extent of disease. Unless it is an isolated tumor recurrence, it is unlikely that additional surgery would be considered. In those few cases in which the recurrence is isolated tumor in the pelvis region, patients can be considered for a pelvic exenteration.

EXENTERATION

An exenteration involves multiple surgical procedures to completely remove the tumor and any potential adjacent organs that could have microscopic invasion. There are three types of pelvic exenteration: total, anterior, or posterior. A total pelvic exenteration will involve the removal of the bladder, descending colon, rectum, uterus, ovaries, fallopian tubes, and vagina. To maintain bodily elimination functions, two stomas are places for urine and fecal elimination. In an anterior exenteration, the colon and rectum are not removed, so only one stoma is placed for urinary elimination. Conversely, in a posterior pelvic exenteration, the bladder is not removed, so only a colostomy is placed. Some patients will be eligible for the vagina to be rebuilt so that patient can still have sexual intercourse.

Any type of pelvic exenteration has a significant potential to affect quality of life for the rest of the patient's lifetime. Although exenteration can be considered in the primary setting, it is often reserved as an option for recurrent disease only. There are multiple postoperative complications to consider—most often fistulas and gastrointestinal complications.[26] Before embarking on pelvic exenteration, patients undergo extensive diagnostic imaging to verify that there is no evidence of disease elsewhere in the body, head to toe. Intraoperatively, if there are any suspicious sites or doubt, the surgery is aborted.

Summary

Fortunately, cervical cancer is not as common in the U.S. as it once was, which is attributed primarily to the effective Pap test screening tool. However, worldwide cervical cancer is second only to breast cancer in incidence, primarily affecting developing countries, where there is limited access to healthcare with appropriate screening.[27] Almost all—more than 99%—of cervical cancer cases can been attributed to an HPV infection. The introduction of the HPV vaccine effective against two (HPV 16/18) of the fifteen oncogenic subtypes of HPV has been a major advancement in the U.S.; however, additional research is needed to optimize its use for long-term prevention of cervical cancer over a woman's lifespan. Unfortunately, vaccination is developing countries is more of a challenge then Pap test screening because of the cost of the vaccine itself and lack for resources to fund these efforts.

Once cervical cancer is diagnosed, aggressive primary treatment to achieve a CR is a priority, and both surgery for early stage or chemoradiation for advanced stages have been definitive treatment interventions to successfully achieve a CR in most patients. Close surveillance is necessary for 5 years after completion of treatment. In the recurrent setting, there are limited effective treatment interventions with average overall 5-year survival <30%.

References

Additional content available at
www.ashp.org/womenshealth

47 Management of Treatment Complications

Claire Saadeh, Pharm.D., BCOP; Makala Pace, Pharm.D., BCOP;
Sheetal Sheth, Pharm.D., BCOP

Learning Objectives

1. Describe the short- and long-term complications most frequently encountered in women receiving pharmacologic treatment for cancer.
2. Discuss the etiology of chemotherapy-induced nausea and vomiting, and list the risk factors placing women at higher risk.
3. Discuss the pharmacologic agents used for the management of treatment-related menopausal symptoms (i.e., hot flashes, decreased vaginal lubrication, and osteoporosis).
4. Identify the risk factors commonly associated with ovarian dysfunction in women receiving treatment for cancer, and discuss the nonpharmacologic and pharmacologic treatment modalities.

It is estimated that 692,000 new cancer cases will be diagnosed in women in 2008.[1] The five most common cancers to be diagnosed in women include breast cancer, lung cancer, colorectal cancer, ovarian cancer, and non-Hodgkin's lymphoma.[1] These five cancers will account for 56% of all new estimated cancer cases among women (Table 47-1). Approximately 271,500 women will die from cancer in 2008 (Table 47-1).[1] Cancers of the lung and bronchus and breast will account for half of the total cancer deaths in women. In women, when stratified by age, leukemia is the leading cause of cancer death in those younger than age 20, breast cancer is the leading cause of cancer death in those ages 20–59, and lung cancer is the leading cause of cancer death in those age 60 and older.[1] Long-term trends in lung cancer incidence rates seem to be plateauing in women after rising for many decades, whereas the incidence rate in men has been declining. This difference is based on the historical aspect that cigarette smoking in women peaked approximately 20 years later than in men.[1] Colorectal cancer incidence rates continue to decrease in both men and women, and female breast cancer rates have begun to plateau as well, potentially reflecting the decline in use of hormone therapy and the utilization of mammography for earlier detection and diagnosis of breast cancer.[1]

The treatment of cancer involves a multimodality approach, using combinations of surgery, radiation therapy, and pharmacologic therapy. The pharmacologic therapies that may be used in the treatment of cancer in women include chemotherapy (platinum agents, taxanes, alkylating agents, antimetabolites, topoisomerase inhibitors), hormone therapies (selective estrogen receptor modulators, aromatase inhibitors, progesterone and estrogen derivatives), and targeted (biological) therapies (monoclonal antibodies, growth factor inhibitors). These pharmacologic options may be implemented as single-agent pharmacologic therapy, combination chemotherapy, or chemotherapy combined with targeted therapy.

Sex-specific differences are seen in patients undergoing cancer therapy. Women have been noted to have higher survival rates and to tolerate cytotoxic therapy better than men in nearly all tumor types that affect both sexes.[2] Although it is not extensively studied nor well understood, one of the explanations given for these differences is body composition. On average, women have a higher proportion of fat and less lean body mass compared with men.[2] This may affect pharmacokinetic behavior in some cytotoxic drugs correlating to higher toxicity and efficacy in women.[2] Additionally, psychological, cultural, and social factors, although extremely difficult to quantify, do contribute to physiologic diversity and influences cancer treatment and complications.[2]

Table 47-1. Ten Leading Cancer Types for the Estimated New Cancer Cases and Deaths in Women[1]

	Ranking of Estimated Newly Diagnosed Cancer Cases (N cases/%)	Ranking of Estimated Number of Cancer-Related Deaths (N cases/%)
1	Breast [182,460 cases (26%)]	Lung and bronchus [71,030 cases (26%)]
2	Lung and bronchus [100,330 cases (14%)]	Breast [40,480 cases (15%)]
3	Colon and rectum [71,560 cases (10%)]	Colon and rectum [25,700 cases (9%)]
4	Uterine corpus [40,100 cases (6%)]	Pancreas [16,790 cases (6%)]
5	Non-Hodgkin lymphoma [30,670 cases (4%)]	Ovary [15,520 cases (6%)]
6	Thyroid [28,410 cases (4%)]	Non-Hodgkin lymphoma [9,370 cases (3%)]
7	Melanoma of skin [227,530 cases (4%)]	Leukemia [9,250 cases (3%)]
8	Ovary [21,650 cases (3%)]	Uterine corpus [7,470 cases (3%)]
9	Kidney and renal pelvis [21,260 cases (3%)]	Liver and intrahepatic bile duct [5,840 cases (2%)]
10	Leukemia [19,090 cases (3%)]	Brain and other nervous system [5,650 cases (2%)]

CASE PRESENTATION

Patient Case: Part 1

K.J. is a 24-year-old woman who presents to clinic today for routine follow-up during her breast cancer treatment. She reports some fatigue but, most importantly, is bothered by hot flashes, occurring almost every hour throughout the day and night. She also mentions significant discomfort during intercourse because she is "so dry there."

HPI: K.J. was diagnosed with early-stage breast cancer (T2N1M0) at age 23. Estrogen and progesterone receptors were positive, and HER-2-neu protein was negative. She underwent a right radical mastectomy, radiation therapy, and is currently receiving chemotherapy. Menstrual periods are still occurring, however sporadic (approximately every other month).

PMH: Gastroesophageal reflux.

Family history: Mother—hypothyroidism, uterine problems; father—unknown; maternal grandmother—breast cancer at age 37.

Social history: Denies use of alcohol, tobacco, or illicit drugs. K.J is currently in medical school.

Medications: Currently enrolled in a clinical trial consisting of doxorubicin weekly × 15 weeks (completed), cyclophosphamide (oral) weekly × 15 weeks (completed), and paclitaxel every 2 weeks × 6 cycles (completed 2 cycles). Multivitamin daily, calcium and vitamin D supplements.

Allergies: NKDA.

Vitals: 5′8″, 134 lb (BSA 1.7 m^2), BP 109/67, HR 85, T 98.1°F, RR 18, pain score 0.

Physical exam: Normal; status post–right breast mastectomy.

Laboratory values: Significant findings include WBC 2.5 × $10^3/mm^3$ (ANC 1.5 × $10^3/mm^3$), serum creatinine 0.9 mg/dL.

Just as response rates and toleration have sex differences, the treatment complications of each of these pharmacologic therapies and their distinct set of potential adverse effects can differ between men and women. Treatment complications that commonly are encountered by women receiving pharmacologic cancer therapy can be broadly classified into short-term complications (**nausea,** vomiting, and alopecia) and long-term complications (menopause and its associated symptoms and sterility/fertility).

Short-term Toxicities Associated with the Pharmacologic Treatment of Cancer

Cytotoxic therapy generally affects rapidly growing cells, including cells that line the gastrointestinal (GI) tract and hair matrix, and form the immune system defense. Acute toxicity that develops from chemotherapy generally remains short-lived in nature and resolves once the course of chemotherapy is completed or discontinued. Myelosuppression, peripheral neuropathy, mucositis, diarrhea, nausea and vomiting, and alopecia are examples of the acute toxicities induced by chemotherapy. The two short-term adverse effects that will be discussed further are nausea and vomiting and alopecia.

NAUSEA AND VOMITING

Clinical Presentation

Nausea and vomiting is still considered to be one of the most feared adverse effects produced by chemotherapy for patients.[3] Before the introduction of serotonin antagonists, a trial was conducted for patients to rate the most severe adverse effects induced by chemotherapy. Vomiting and nausea were ranked as first and second most severe adverse effects, respectively. A follow-up study (after the introduction of serotonin receptor antagonists) illustrated that nausea was considered to be the most severe adverse effect, but vomiting had fallen to fifth ranking.[3]

Because a variety of chemotherapeutic agents cause nausea and vomiting, patients' initial perceptions about chemotherapy may be negatively affected. As a result, healthcare providers may find it challenging to provide effective therapy. This adverse effect can negatively affect a patient's daily functions and quality of life. Uncontrolled nausea and vomiting can produce further problems, such as electrolyte and nutritional imbalances, weight loss, and anorexia.

Clinical presentation of this condition may include nausea, **retching,** or vomiting. Chemotherapy-induced nausea and vomiting is categorized into three broad classes: acute, delayed, and anticipatory. Additional classes include **breakthrough nausea** and vomiting and refractory nausea and vomiting. Chemotherapy-induced vomiting has been reported in approximately 70% of cancer patients actively receiving treatment; however, the specific impact on women is not yet defined. This condition may be a critical aspect of overall patient satisfaction and willingness to continue and complete cancer treatment.[4]

Pathophysiology

The pathophysiology behind nausea and vomiting induced by chemotherapy is a multifactorial process that involves a variety of neurotransmitters and receptors in the peripheral and central nervous systems. The activation of the dopamine, histamine, opiate, acetylcholine, serotonin, and neurokinin (NK)-1 receptors initiates this multifactorial pathway. Chemotherapy and radiation therapy both provoke vomiting in part by causing the release of serotonin from the enterochromaffin cells lining the GI tract, but nausea may not progress in this same manner. The serotonin adheres to the vagal serotonin type 3 receptors (GI tract) then fires signals to the vomiting center positioned in the lateral reticular formation located in the medulla of the brain.[5] The chemotherapy trigger zone, vestibular apparatus, and brain cortex additionally fire signals to the vomiting center, which in turn activates a vomiting cascade of efferent impulses to the vasomotor, respiratory, salivary centers, and cranial nerves VIII and X.[5] Vomiting finally results after the signals reach the esophagus, resulting in opening of the gastric cardia, dropping of the diaphragm, and tightening of the abdominal muscles.[5,6]

The severity of vomiting or nausea can depend on numerous factors, such as the emetogenicity of chemotherapy agent or regimen, route, administration (bolus vs. continuous infusion), and frequency. Several patient-related factors also play a role in determining the severity of vomiting. These include sex (women are more susceptible than men), age (younger patients more susceptible than older patients), history of motion sickness, history of morning sickness during pregnancy, and history of alcohol abuse (positive risk factor).[5,6]

An important consideration is that uncontrolled nausea and vomiting can affect a patient's quality of life. Patients that experience uncontrolled nausea and vomiting as a consequent of chemotherapy are less likely to continue with daily activities or interactions (e.g., household tasks or spending time with others). Patients suffering from nausea and vomiting can be incapable of caring for themselves, working, or administering prescribed medications. Nausea seems to have a lesser influence on daily activities than vomiting.[5]

Table 47-2. Combinations of Chemotherapeutic Agents[3,5,7-9]

Levels of Emetogenicity	Selected Common Regimens	General Recommended Antiemetic Prophylaxis
Highly emetogenic	AC (doxorubicin + cyclophosphamide) Cisplatin + vinorelbine Cisplatin + docetaxel Cisplatin + pelvic radiation	Serotonin antagonist + corticosteroid +/− neurokin 1 (NK1)-antagonist
Moderately emetogenic	FOLFOX (fluorouracil + leucovorin+ oxaliplatin) Irinotecan + cetuximab Carboplatin + paclitaxel	Serotonin antagonist + corticosteroid
Low emetogenic potential	Weekly paclitaxel Weekly vinorelbine	Corticosteroid

Prevention and Treatment

Nonpharmacologic Treatments

Several factors related to the selection and amount of food, fluid intake, positioning, and physical location can all have an impact on nausea and vomiting. For example, eating smaller, nongreasy meals throughout the day may help keep food in patient's stomach. If a foul taste develops, eating peppermint-flavored candy, brushing teeth/tongue after eating, or using a nonalcoholic mouth rinse may be beneficial. Drinking plenty of noncaffeinated, nonalcoholic beverages several times throughout the day can be advantageous in preventing dehydration. Sitting upright for at least 30 minutes after a meal may also prevent nausea and vomiting. In addition, eating meals in an open, ventilated area may avert the possibility of accumulation of foul odors that could potentially induce nausea or vomiting.[5]

Pharmacologic Treatments

As described previously, chemotherapy induced nausea/vomiting can present as anticipatory, acute, and delayed. For each, the treatment can be very different. For prophylaxis of acute vomiting of a moderately to highly emetogenic regimen, several guidelines recommend use of corticosteroids and a serotonin receptor antagonist with possible addition of a NK-antagonist with platinum-based regimens. Mildly emetogenic regimens do not routinely require preventative measures for acute vomiting. Those receiving a highly emetogenic regimen may additionally receive preventative therapy for delayed nausea with a combination of agents such as corticosteroids and a serotonin receptor antagonist with possible addition of aprepitant. Benzamides (i.e., metoclopramide) may be substituted for the serotonin receptor antagonists in this setting. **Anticipatory vomiting** is generally prevented with the addition of a benzodiazepine (i.e., lorazepam) to the antiemetic regimen. Additional agents such as butyrophenones and phenothiazines may be added on an as-needed basis to the selection of medications previously described if breakthrough nausea and vomiting persists despite the use of scheduled medications. Furthermore, it is important to consider patient- and treatment-related risk factors when choosing antiemetic agents.[4-9] See Table 47-2 for common chemotherapy agents and their respective emetogenicity.

Guidelines and Position Statements

The American Society of Clinical Oncology (ASCO), Multinational Association of Supportive Care in Cancer (MASCC), and National Comprehensive Cancer Network (NCCN) have all published guidelines for the prevention and treatment of chemotherapy-induced vomiting. Each set of guidelines recommends similar antiemetic regimens for the prevention of high-, moderate-, or low-emetogenic combinations of chemotherapeutic agents.[7-9]

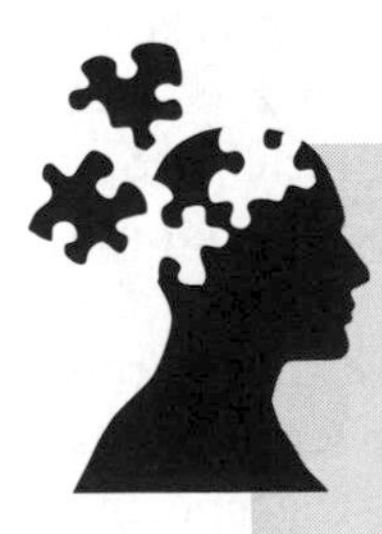

Therapeutic Challenge:

What would be the optimal treatment regimen for delayed nausea and vomiting for a patient who has failed the combination of dexamethasone and metoclopramide?

ALOPECIA

Clinical Presentation and Pathophysiology

Alopecia is a direct effect from cytotoxic therapy and radiation therapy (only if the radiation field encompasses the scalp). The clinical presentation associated with adverse effect includes complete or partial baldness on the scalp. Alopecia may occur within 2 weeks of the initiation of chemotherapy. Alopecia peaks in most patients around 1–2 months after beginning cytotoxic therapy. Although not considered a health risk, it can be an emotional and traumatic experience for women.[10]

Chemotherapeutic agents that possess the cytotoxic characteristic of the ability to kill healthy and cancerous cells (e.g., anthracyclines, etoposide, methotrexate, taxanes, platinum agents, vinca alkaloids) can generate partial or total inhibition of mitoses of the hair matrix (i.e., **anagen hairs**) or impair metabolic processes. This results in thin, weakened hair shafts that are vulnerable to fracture and damage. Repetitive exposure to chemotherapeutic agents results in complete scalp hair loss. Other terminal hair follicles (i.e., eyebrows, eyelashes, axillary hair, and pubic hair) are affected differently based on a number of factors such as rate of hair matrix growth, percent of anagen hairs, and the dose of the cytotoxic drug. This treatment complication is usually reversible as the hair does grow back once treatment ceases. The hair that returns to the scalp may be different in texture and color due to unknown reasons.[10,11]

Prevention and Treatment

Nonpharmacologic Treatments

The key method for prevention or minimization of chemotherapy-induced alopecia is by nonpharmacologic therapies. Scalp tourniquets were once used to decrease blood flow to the scalp, therefore decreasing the amount of cytotoxic therapy delivered to hair matrix. This treatment is no longer recommended because of patient discomfort. Hypothermia of the scalp by employing temperature cooling devices to the scalp may reduce drug uptake in the hair matrix and/or modify the drug metabolism in hair follicle cells.[10,11] This method remains under clinical investigation. Scalp tourniquets and hypothermia of the scalp are currently not recommended and are considered to be impractical means for alopecia prevention when chemotherapy is infused continuously.[10,11] Cranial prostheses (i.e., wigs) are used by many patients as a treatment modality. These are made available with or without prescriptions and are generally reimbursed by many insurance companies. The process of purchasing and using a cranial prosthesis for cosmetic benefit may additionally have significant economic and psychological impact and advantage.

Pharmacologic Treatments

Several pharmacologic therapies have been studied, but at present, there are no approved drug treatments for chemotherapy-induced alopecia. In general, these agents should be applied before administration of cytotoxic therapy. Topical and systemic cyclosporin A has been considered to promote hair growth and prevent hair follicle deterioration in experimental models.[11] The use of cyclosporine A was discovered through its adverse effect profile. It has been known to cause hypertrichosis via direct effect on hair follicles not linked with immunosuppressive actions. Another immunomodulator, AS101, exerts its protection through macrophage-mediated factors and possible relation to prostaglandin E_2 secretion. AS101 was shown to reduce severity of alopecia induced by carboplatin and etoposide.[11]

Minoxidil has been proven to stimulate hair growth by decreasing the telogen stage and shifting the hair follicles into the anagen phase. Several mechanisms of action have been proposed, such as activation of keratinocyte reproduction, prevention of collagen synthesis and development, opening of potassium channels via the sulphated metabolite, prostaglandin development, and activation of vascular endothelial growth factor (VEGF).[11] In one clinical trial conducted by Duvic and colleagues, topical minoxidil (2% solution) was applied to the scalps of breast cancer patients receiving a doxorubicin-based chemotherapy regimen.[12] Minoxidil was applied to the scalp twice daily for the duration of chemotherapy and for up to 4 months after completion of chemotherapy. The results of this trial showed a statistically significant longer time interval to maximal hair loss and a shortened time interval from maximal hair loss to first regrowth.[12]

Several cytokines and growth factor receptors are expressed on hair follicles. The growth and development of hair follicles is affected by one or more of these receptors via possible autocrine or paracrine pathways. Topical or systemic antioxidants have also been evaluated and shown to inhibit chemotherapy-induced alopecia in animal models. In addition, inhibitors of the p53 tumor suppressor gene have also been studied in animal models to prevent apoptosis of hair follicles from exposure to chemotherapy.[11]

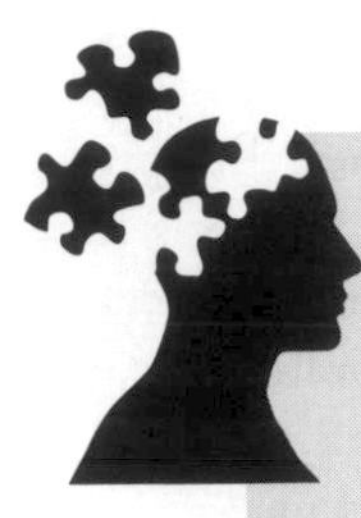

Therapeutic Challenge:

If an advanced ovarian cancer patient scheduled to start receiving a taxane-based regimen is emotionally distressed about the thought of hair loss, would you recommend minoxidil to help prevent it?

Various pathways have been discovered that could potentially prevent or retard the process of chemotherapy-induced alopecia. However, most studies have been conducted in animals in which only one cytotoxic agent was evaluated at a time. Minoxidil has been shown to prolong the interval time to maximal hair loss but has yet to prevent alopecia altogether. Future studies will need to incorporate several agents that possess different mechanisms of prevention but do not compromise efficacy of the anticancer agents.

Long-term Complications Associated with the Pharmacologic Treatment of Cancer

One of the most significant long-term complications associated with cancer treatment includes chemotherapy-induced ovarian failure characterized by **amenorrhea,** the onset of menopause and associated symptoms, and subsequent loss of fertility. Many adult cancer patients are diagnosed with cancer at a younger age and are surviving longer. Approximately 22% of breast cancer cases occur in women younger than the age of 50 years.[13] The majority of these patients will undergo treatment with adjuvant chemotherapy and hormone therapy (HT) (if hormone receptor positive). Menopause may also be induced abruptly secondary to oophorectomy, as in the case of patients with ovarian, uterine, and vaginal cancers. Radiation therapy to the pelvic region may also result in damage to the ovaries, causing premature menopause. The impact of premature ovarian failure or menopause has a significant impact on quality of life for long-term cancer survivors.[14]

MENOPAUSE

Clinical Presentation

According to the NCCN, menopause is defined as the permanent cessation of menses, including a profound and permanent decrease in ovarian estrogen synthesis.[15] Criteria for determining menopause (in breast cancer patients) may include any of the following: 1) prior bilateral oophorectomy; 2) age ≥60 years; 3) age <60 years and amenorrheic for ≥12 months in the absence of chemotherapy, tamoxifen, toremifene, or ovarian suppression, with follicle-stimulating hormone (FSH) and estradiol in the postmenopausal range; or 4) taking tamoxifen or toremifene, age <60 years, with FSH and plasma estradiol level in postmenopausal ranges.[15] For most women undergoing natural menopause, the perimenopausal period may persist for up to 4 years, but in patients experiencing chemotherapy-induced ovarian failure, this transition may be more abrupt and more symptomatic.[14,16]

Treatment of the gynecologic malignancies (e.g., cervical, endometrial, or ovarian cancer) often involve total abdominal hysterectomy and bilateral salpingo-oophorectomy. These procedures will cause "surgical menopause," which can be associated with severe onset of menopausal symptoms/complications.

Complications associated with menopause typically consist of vasomotor symptoms (hot flashes and night sweats), central symptoms (insomnia, changes in memory and mood, depression), vaginal atrophy, urinary atrophy, osteoporosis, and increased risk for cardiovascular complications.[16,17]

Pathophysiology

In healthy menstruating women, FSH produced by the pituitary gland stimulates follicular granulosa cells in the ovary to produce estradiol. Estradiol levels and low FSH levels (<10 milli–International Units/mL) are maintained in premenopausal women by means of negative feedback inhibition on the pituitary gland. In chemotherapy-induced ovarian failure, the ovaries are depleted of follicles and are unable to produce estradiol, resulting in decreased circulating levels of estrogen and progesterone and an increase in FSH levels. Depletion of ovarian follicles in cancer patients may also result from direct damage to the ovaries from radiation treatment to the pelvic region. FSH levels >40 milli–International Units/mL are usually associated with menopause.[14,16]

The timing of cancer treatment and the type of chemotherapy also have an impact on ovarian function and subsequent amenorrhea or menopause. Chemotherapy-induced amenorrhea primarily depends on the age of the patient and chemotherapy agent(s) received. Women older than age 40 are more sensitive to the damaging effects of chemotherapy than those younger than 40.[13] Alkylating agent–based chemotherapy regimens, such as those containing cyclophosphamide, have been highly implicated in producing amenorrhea in breast cancer patients receiving adjuvant therapy.[13] In patients younger than age 40, the incidence of amenorrhea with cyclophosphamide-based therapies ranges between 18% to 61%, compared with 61% to 97% in women older than age 40.[13] Other chemotherapeutic agents have also been studied with regard to their impact on ovarian function but with varying and inconsistent results. These include the anthracyclines (doxorubicin and epirubicin) and taxanes (paclitaxel and docetaxel).[13]

Prevention and Treatment

Although HT has been effectively used to treat menopausal symptoms in healthy women, recent concerns have arisen surrounding the potential for HT to increase the risk of breast cancer in women at high risk or increase the risk of recurrence in cancer survivors. The HABITS (hormonal replacement therapy after breast cancer—is it safe?) study was a prospective randomized trial conducted in women with previously treated breast cancer to determine whether 2 years of HT for menopausal symptoms was safe.[19] The primary outcome was any new breast cancer event. Twenty-six out of 174 women randomized to the HT group developed a new breast cancer event vs. 8 out of 171 women in the best supportive treatment group (non-HT). It was determined that these findings indicated an unacceptable risk for breast cancer survivors, and therefore the trial was terminated. Because of the concerns surrounding the effects of HT (estrogen with or without progesterone) on breast cancer risk and recurrence, these agents are currently not recommended for the treatment of menopausal symptoms in breast cancer survivors.[15,17-19,20] Nonhormonal treatment strategies—such as nonpharmacologic interventions, complimentary therapies, and nonestrogen containing pharmacologic treatments—are therefore needed for the management of symptoms/complications of menopause, such as hot flashes, vaginal atrophy, and prevention of osteoporosis.[21]

HOT FLASHES

Clinical Presentation

Hot flashes are often characterized by the sudden onset of heat in the face, neck, and chest. Other symptoms associated with hot flashes include sweating, red blotching of the skin, palpitations, anxiety, and irritability. The frequency, duration, and intensity will vary and may be severe enough to affect a women's ability to function at work, social life, sleep pattern, and compliance with further cancer treatment.[4] As many as 20% of women who experience hot flashes find them intolerable.[6]

Pathophysiology

The exact mechanism of the occurrence of hot flashes is unknown, but it has been postulated that changes in circulating estrogen levels lead to a heat-loss response of the central thermoregulatory center. Subtle changes in room temperature, hot or cold beverages, alcohol intake, and higher body mass index may contribute to hot flash symptoms and/or be responsible for increased intensity of symptoms.[14,16] Adjuvant treatment with tamoxifen or an aromatase inhibitor (anastrozole, letrozole, or exemestane) may also contribute to the increased frequency and severity of hot flashes experienced in breast cancer patients. Hot flashes are one of the most common adverse events reported with these agents. Hot flashes were reported in 40.9% and 35.7% of patients receiving tamoxifen and anastrozole, respectively.[22]

Prevention and Treatment

Nonpharmacologic Treatment

Simple, nonpharmacologic strategies to help alleviate hot flashes include wearing lightweight and light-colored clothing, dressing in layers, decreasing the room temperature, drinking cold beverages, and avoiding alcohol, spicy foods, hot drinks, and hot foods.[21] Other nonpharmacologic treatment strategies that have been suggested include maintaining an active lifestyle (exercise), acupuncture, and behavioral modification techniques; however, limited data exist on the success of these strategies.

Pharmacologic Treatment

The progestational agents megestrol acetate and medroxyprogesterone have been effective in managing hot flashes. In a double-blind, randomized, placebo study in breast cancer survivors, megestrol 20 mg twice daily for 4 weeks indicated an 85% reduction in hot flashes compared with a 21% reduction in those receiving placebo.[23] Medroxyprogesterone given as a depot intramuscular injection (500 mg every 2 weeks) has also been shown to reduce the incidence of hot flashes by as much as 90%.[24,25] Adverse effects of progestational agents may be significant and include abnormal vaginal bleeding, withdrawal bleeding, weight gain, cramping, and increased appetite.[20] The long-term safety of these agents has not been established in patients who have survived cancer. Because of similar concerns with HT, the use of progestational agents for the management of menopausal symptoms is currently not recommended as first-line therapy. These agents may be considered for women who are refractory to other therapies and who have been appropriately counseled on the potential risks and benefits.[26]

Several complementary therapies have been studied in breast cancer survivors, including vitamin E, soy phytoestrogens, and black cohosh. In a randomized, placebo-controlled, cross-over trial, vitamin E (800 International Units daily) administered to breast cancer patients was associated with minimal effects. The frequency of hot flashes was only reduced by one hot flash per person per day.[27] Side effects were minimal. There is very limited evidence to support the use of vitamin E in cancer patients, and further evidence on the long-term toxicity needs to be established. Vitamin E may be considered for women with mild symptoms that do not interfere with daily function or sleep.[14]

Soy protein, a major source of phytoestrogen, has been investigated for the management of hot flashes. Phytoestrogens exhibit less estrogenic activity than 17-beta-estradiol and some antiestrogenic activity. Phytoestrogens are found in the diet and are classified into two main types: isoflavones (most common) and lignans. Isoflavones are found in soy products, and lignans are typically found in flaxseed.[16] Several studies comparing red clover isoflavones with placebo in breast cancer patients have not shown improvement in hot flash episodes or other menopausal symptoms.[28-32] Standardization of soy content and variability in doses make assessments of these products difficult. Because of the lack of efficacy and lack of long-term safety in patients with a history of cancer, phytoestrogens (from any source) are not recommended for the management of hot flashes or other menopausal symptoms.

Black cohosh (*Cimicifuga racemosa*) is a North American plant that has been used to manage menstrual cramps and menopausal symptoms. Although the mechanism of action is unknown, black cohosh is thought to have an inhibitory effect on the estrogen receptor. It also binds to the following receptors: serotonin (stimulatory effects), dopamine (inhibitory effects), and gamma-aminobutyric acid (GABA; inhibitory effects).[16] Randomized controlled trials conducted in women with a history of breast cancer have compared black cohosh with placebo.[33,34] Doses have ranged between 40 and 80 mg/day. These studies demonstrated a decrease in the number and intensity of hot flash episodes, but there was no significant difference between the treatment and placebo groups. Other reviews have also concluded that black cohosh has no clinical efficacy for the management of hot flashes.[35] Cases of hepatotoxicity in women taking black cohosh have been reported, and there are concerns that this agent may interfere with the antineoplastic effects of cancer therapy.[16] Other side effects include nausea, vomiting, headache, and dizziness.

Clonidine, a centrally acting alpha-adrenergic receptor agonist, has been beneficial in healthy women experiencing hot flashes.[36] Small benefits have also been reported in women experiencing tamoxifen-induced hot flashes. Women receiving transdermal clonidine (equivalent oral dose of 0.1 mg daily) reported a decrease in the frequency of hot flash episodes by 20% and the severity by 10% in one study.[37] Clonidine taken orally (0.1 mg daily) also showed a reduction in hot flashes by 38% (vs. 24% in placebo group) at 8 weeks.[38] Side effects associated with clonidine may be significant and may limit the tolerability of this agent. Side effects most commonly reported in these studies include dry mouth, constipation, itching (transdermal patch site), drowsiness, and difficulty sleeping.

Gabapentin, a GABA analogue, has traditionally been used for the treatment of epilepsy and neuropathic pain. Recent studies have also suggested efficacy for the management of hot flashes. Significant benefit in healthy postmenopausal women taking gabapentin 900 mg/day was reported in a randomized, placebo-controlled trial.[39] A reduction in hot flash frequency of 45% and a reduction in hot flash composite score of 54% was reported. A double-blind, placebo-controlled trial of gabapentin 300 mg/day or 900 mg/day was conducted in breast cancer survivors experiencing greater than or equal to two hot flashes per day.[40] The percentage decreases in hot flash severity score from baseline to 8 weeks were 15% in placebo group, 31% in the gabapentin 300 mg group, and 46% in the gabapentin 900 mg group. Gabapentin 900 mg/day was associated with the greatest decrease in both hot flash frequency and severity. The most common side effects reported in these gabapentin studies include somnolence, fatigue, dizziness, and rash with or without edema.

The selective serotonin reuptake inhibitors (SSRIs) that have been studied in the management of hot flashes in cancer survivors include fluoxetine, paroxetine, sertraline, and venlafaxine (an SSRI and noradrenaline reuptake inhibitor). Interest in these agents developed based on anecdotal observations of improvements in premenopausal symptoms and hot flashes. Results of a randomized, placebo-controlled, 4-week crossover study comparing fluoxetine 20 mg daily with placebo demonstrated a decrease in hot flash scores in both groups (50% decrease in fluoxetine group and 36% decrease in placebo group; $p = 0.02$).[41] Two open-label pilot studies in women either with a history of breast cancer or undergoing active or recent treatment with chemotherapy demonstrated promising results with the SSRI paroxetine.[42,43] Both of these pilot studies reported a reduction in the frequency and severity of hot flashes with improvements also noted for other symptoms, such as depression, sleep, anxiety, and quality of life. A larger randomized, double-blind, crossover, placebo-controlled study in women with a history of breast cancer compared paroxetine 10 mg or 20 mg with placebo.[44] A significant reduction in frequency of hot flashes was reported with both doses of paroxetine. Paroxetine 10 mg vs. placebo demonstrated a reduction of 40.6% and 13.7%, respectively ($p = 0.0006$). Paroxetine 20 mg vs. placebo demonstrated a reduction of 51.7% and 26.6%, respectively ($p = 0.002$). Similar results were also reported for hot flash composite scores. Significant side effects were mainly noted in the paroxetine 20 mg group and consisted of nausea and drowsiness. Paroxetine may not be an optimal choice for women who are receiving tamoxifen concurrently. A significant decline in plasma concentration of endoxifen, a metabolite of tamoxifen, has been reported.[45] The clinical implications of this interaction need further clarification. Sertraline has also been studied in one randomized study in breast cancer patients taking tamoxifen, but there was no significant difference in hot flash frequency between those taking sertraline and placebo.[46]

Venlafaxine has demonstrated significant activity for the management of hot flashes in several studies. Women with a previous history of breast cancer were randomized to receive placebo or venlafaxine extended release at 37.5 mg or 75 mg or 150 mg daily.[47] At 4 weeks, a significant decrease in hot flash score was reported: 27% placebo group vs. 40% venlafaxine 37.5 mg, 61% venlafaxine 75 mg, and 61% venlafaxine 150 mg. Adverse events were dose dependent and most pronounced in those receiving venlafaxine 150 mg. Dry mouth, decreased appetite, nausea, and constipation were most frequently reported. After completion of the previous 4-week study, participants were requested to continue on study for an additional 8 weeks of venlafaxine therapy.[48] At the end of this period, hot flashes were reduced by 26% in the venlafaxine 37.5-mg group and 60% in the venlafaxine 75-mg and 150-mg groups. Similar results have also been reported in healthy postmenopausal women receiving venlafaxine 37.5 mg daily for 1 week, followed by venlafaxine 75 mg daily for 11 weeks.[49] Venlafaxine is the preferred agent compared with other SSRIs based on the clinical data presented. Venlafaxine is a weaker inhibitor of CYP2D6 than paroxetine and has little impact on plasma endoxifen concentrations in those receiving tamoxifen.[21] Venlafaxine is typically initiated at a dose of 37.5 mg daily for 1 week and then titrated to benefit thereafter. It is currently recommended that venlafaxine 75 mg daily is the most effective therapeutic dose for managing hot flashes in this patient population based on published studies, but some patients may be titrated up to 150 mg daily if tolerated. Patients should be counseled that resolution of hot flash symptoms may not be fully appreciated for a minimum of 4 weeks after starting venlafaxine and possibly longer.

VAGINAL ATROPHY

Clinical Presentation and Pathophysiology

Symptoms of vaginal atrophy include vaginal dryness, pruritus, burning/soreness, discharge, and **dyspareunia.** Vaginal dryness has been reported as one of the most important aspects of sexual health in female patients.[50] The onset of symptoms may vary and can occur after the resolution of hot flashes.

Estrogen receptors have been identified in the vulva, vagina, bladder, urethra, pelvic floor musculature, and endopelvic fascia. Loss of estrogen receptors, decreased levels of circulating estradiol, and decreased production of vaginal moisture may result from the direct effects of pelvic irradiation, hormonal therapy, or chemotherapy, resulting in a decrease in the size of the uterus, ovaries, vaginal canal, and vulva. Vaginal atrophy may have a negative impact on sexual desire and activity, and often results in uncomfortable and/or painful intercourse.[16]

Prevention and Treatment

Nonpharmacologic Treatment

Counseling to support the patient and provide appropriate tools for communication with her partner should be discussed with all cancer patients experiencing sexual dysfunction.[14] Patient education regarding potential for drug-induced sexual dysfunction should be provided before treatment. Symptoms associated with vaginal atrophy (dryness) usually require pharmacologic intervention.

Pharmacologic Treatment

Vaginal lubricants, such as polycarbophil, may be helpful in alleviating vaginal dryness and dyspareunia with an indirect improvement of other sexual dysfunction.[14] Intravaginal low-dose estrogen preparations, however, may be more efficacious than vaginal lubricants. Preparations that have been used include conjugated estrogens (vaginal cream, 0.3 mg or 0.625 mg intravaginally daily for 3 weeks, then 0.3 mg twice weekly), estradiol (vaginal tablet, 25 mcg inserted daily for 2 weeks, then twice weekly thereafter), and estradiol-releasing vaginal ring (containing 2 mg of 17-beta-estradiol, which delivers at a constant rate of 7.5 mcg/day).[16] The vaginal ring may be left in place for 90 days. Systemic absorption, although minimal, has been reported with these products and will depend on the dose of the estrogen preparation and thickness of the vaginal mucosa. Patients with estrogen-dependent cancers (breast, ovarian, uterine, or vaginal) should discuss the risks and benefits of using these low-dose estrogen preparations before their use.

OSTEOPOROSIS

Clinical Presentation

Osteoporosis is a skeletal disorder of decreased bone mass and strength that leads to an increased risk of fractures. Premenopausal women who develop surgical, radiation, or chemotherapy-induced ovarian failure after adjuvant therapy for cancer undergo an accelerated and highly significant bone mineral loss.[14,16] Common fracture sites include the femoral neck, radius, vertebral spine, and lumbar spine. Often, these fractures may be associated with loss of mobility and chronic pain.

Cancer survivors are at an increased risk of bone loss and osteoporosis, especially in those who develop premature menopause as a result of treatment. Estrogen deficiency has been suggested as an important etiologic factor in this process. Decreased intestinal calcium reabsorption and increased renal fractional calcium excretion that is due to estrogen deficiency leads to an increase in parathyroid hormone with resulting persistent bone turnover. Estrogen-blocking therapies (tamoxifen, toremifene, and aromatase inhibitors) and gonadotropin-releasing hormone (GnRH) analogs have also been associated with a decline in bone mineral density and enhanced bone loss. Direct tumor effects on osteoclasts may also increase bone turnover. Other factors that may contribute to the osteoporosis risk in cancer patients include poor calcium and vitamin D intake, physical inactivity, and use of corticosteroids.[14,51] Several chemotherapeutic agents have exhibited adverse effects on the skeletal system, independent of hormone status. These agents include methotrexate, ifosfamide, cyclophosphamide, and doxorubicin.[51]

Prevention and Treatment

Nonpharmacologic Treatment

Important lifestyle modifications that may potentially reduce the risk of osteoporosis in all patients include maintenance of physical activity (aerobic and weight-bearing exercise), smoking cessation, healthy diet with sufficient calcium and vitamin D, and decreased intake of caffeine and alcohol.[14,16]

Pharmacologic Treatment

All women who are at risk for chemotherapy-induced ovarian failure (with normal bone mineral density), those meeting the criteria for osteopenia, or those with established osteoporosis should receive basic therapy with calcium (1,000 mg–1,500 mg daily) and vitamin D (800 International Units–1,000 International Units daily) through diet and additional supplementation.[14,16,51]

Bisphosphonates are pyrophosphate analogues that reduce bone turnover by inhibiting osteoclastic bone resorption. Favorable effects on bone health have been well established for the prevention and treatment of osteoporosis in postmenopausal women with no previous history of cancer.[51] Data are limited, however, for the prevention or treatment in patients with chemotherapy-induced bone loss that is due to premature menopause. The following bisphosphonates have been studied in patients with a cancer history: clodronate, risedronate, and etidronate. Although other bisphosphonates are currently available for the management of osteoporosis in patients without a history of cancer, these agents should be used with caution until further efficacy is established in patients with bone loss that is due to cancer treatment.

The effects of clodronate on bone mineral density and bone loss have been evaluated in breast cancer women without metastases. After 2 years of therapy with clodronate and an antiestrogen (either tamoxifen or toremifene), an increase in bone mineral density in both the lumbar spine (2.9%) and femoral neck (3.7%) was reported.[52] Premenopausal women receiving chemotherapy with cyclophosphamide, methotrexate, and fluorouracil (CMF regimen) were randomized to receive clodronate 1,600 mg daily or control.[53] Rapid bone loss was reported for those women who developed amenorrhea. Bone loss was significantly reduced in those who received clodronate. At 2 years, bone loss was 9.5% (lumbar spine) and 4.6% (femoral neck) for the control group vs. 5.9% and 0.4% for the clodronate group (p = 0.005 and 0.017, respectively). Positive findings on bone mineral density were also reported in another study of breast cancer patients who received chemotherapy +/− tamoxifen.[54] Clodronate increased the bone mineral density by 1.72% in lumbar spine, 1.85% in hip, and 2.3% in the trochanter at 2 years. Risedronate also prevented bone loss in women with menopause induced by chemotherapy.[55] Etidronate has been well established in preventing glucocorticoid-induced bone loss and increases the bone mass in patients with established glucocorticoid-induced osteoporosis.[51] A significant reduction (85%) in fracture rate was also reported.

Calcitonin is not as potent as the bisphosphonates and may be used as an alternative in those who cannot tolerate bisphosphonate therapy.[51] The efficacy in reducing fractures has not been well established.

An in-depth discussion on the management of osteoporosis in women without cancer can be found in Chapter 40: Bone and Joint Disorders.

STERILITY AND FERTILITY

Patients who are diagnosed with cancer believe fertility preservation is of great significance, and infertility that can result from anticancer treatment can be related to psychosocial distress. Physicians and patients need to have a discussion that addresses fertility preservation options well before any anticancer treatment is implemented. Fertility preservation options such as embryo cryopreservation and oocyte preservation require time to harvest the eggs or oocytes, respectively. For further discussion on fertility, refer to Chapter 22: Infertility.

Infertility is described as failure to conceive without contraception after intercourse for 1 year.[56] Various cancer treatments and additional factors can result in compromised fertility or rates of infertility. For example, radiation, depending on the field of exposure, duration, dose, and if given concurrently with chemotherapy, may be the likely cause of nausea and vomiting in patients with gynecologic malignancy. Furthermore, fertility can be affected by any treatment that may bring about a reduction in the amount of the primordial follicles, an imbalance hormone equilibrium, or damage to a functioning uterus,

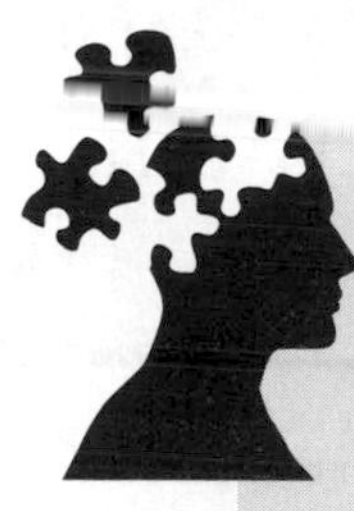

Therapeutic Challenge:

How should fertility issues be addressed in a 25-year-old single woman without a current sex partner who has just been diagnosed with stage I ovarian cancer?

ovaries, fallopian tubes, and cervix. Vascular and anatomic changes to the vagina, cervix, and uterus that are due to cancer treatment can affect natural conception and pregnancy.[56]

Fertility may be altered temporarily or permanently depending on the cancer treatment and can present as premature ovarian failure (cessation of menses before the age of 40). Even though continuation of cyclic menses may return after completion of cancer treatment, this does not correlate with the return of fertility. Additionally, any decline in ovary reserve may lead to a lower possibility of subsequent pregnancy and increased risk of early-onset menopause.[56,57] Patients typically do not present with any specific signs or symptoms with this condition after receiving their cancer treatment (Table 47-3).

Guidelines and Position Statements

The American Society of Oncology and the Practice Committee of the American Society for Reproductive Medicine have both published guidelines and recommendations regarding fertility preservation options for women.[56,58]

Cancer Treatment During Pregnancy

Pregnancy associated with cancer is rare, with a reported incidence of 0.1%.[65] The decision to initiate chemotherapy in this patient population is extremely difficult and must be individualized. The goals of cancer treatment (i.e., cure vs. palliation) must be clearly defined to optimize the risks and benefits to both the mother and fetus. Because there is limited knowledge on the safety of chemotherapy on the fetus, oncologists have difficulty weighing the risks and benefits of particular anticancer agents when recommending a course of therapy for the pregnant patient.

Immediate effects of chemotherapeutic agents on the fetus include spontaneous abortion, teratogenesis leading to fetal chromosomal abnormalities, fetal developmental problems, and inhibited fetal growth. The potential toxicities of chemotherapy that may affect the mother may also adversely affect the fetus, such as myelosuppression, nausea and vomiting,

Table 47-3. Treatment Approaches to Fertility Preservation[55-64]

Nonpharmacologic Procedures	Description	Reported Birth Rates	Comments
Embryo cryopreservation	Stimulation of the ovaries with daily injections of FSH at the onset of menses Follicle growth is followed by serial U/S and laboratory tests An hCG test is given at the initiation of ovulatory cascade, then the oocytes are gathered via U/S transvaginal needle aspiration In vitro oocytes are fertilized and subsequently cryopreserved	Survival rate per thawed embryo: 35% to 90%	Live births depend on the total number of cryopreserved embryos and the patient's age Hormone-sensitive tumors need to find alternative methods for stimulation of the ovaries
Oocyte cryopreservation	Ovarian stimulation and collection of oocytes is similar to those related to embryo cryopreservation	Survival rates per thawed oocyte: 2%	Unfertilized oocytes are more susceptible to harm during cryopreservation; therefore, pregnancy, fertilization, and survival rates are lower with this procedure Executed in centers with expertise (IRB-approved protocols)
Ovarian tissue cryopreservation and ovarian cortical tissue transplantation	Primordial follicles containing immature oocytes can be frozen without need for ovarian stimulation	Two live births	No delay in initiating cancer treatment Primordial follicles are significantly less susceptible to cryo injury due to minute size, decreased metabolic rates, and deficiency of zona pellucida Executed in centers with expertise under the IRB protocol Not recommended in patients older than age 40 years because of the decreased number of primordial follicles
Pharmacologic Procedures	**Description**		**Comments**
Gonadotropin-releasing hormone agonist (GnRH-a)	Mechanism of action exerted is to protect fertility. However, several theories have been presented that further illustrate the mechanism elicited for chemoprotection.		Limited trials evaluating GnRH-a chemoprotective effects have been conducted in humans. Therefore, the optimal dose of these agents has yet to be identified.
Sex steroids (i.e., progesterone, combination of estrogen/ progesterone products)	The mechanism of chemoprotection exerted by the sex steroids includes suppression of the ovaries, which decreases the possibility of chemotherapeutic agents inflicting damage onto them. The mechanism of chemoprotection exerted by antiapoptotic agents is extrapolated to be through protection of the ovaries from chemotherapeutic harm because many chemotherapeutic-induced gonadotoxic effects are mediated by apoptosis.		Antagonizing the effects of cytotoxicity from chemotherapeutic agents on the ovaries has been studied in limited capacity. No dosing recommendations for these agents have been listed to any degree in any of the references.

FSH = follicle stimulating hormone; U/S = ultrasound; hCG = human chorionic gonadotropin; IRB = investigational review board.

diarrhea, or multiorgan toxicity, leading to organ toxicity, premature birth, or low birth weight. However, the risk of not treating the cancer could potentially be fatal to both mother and the fetus.

During the first trimester, congenital malformations and spontaneous abortion may occur after exposure; therefore, it is recommended to avoid treatment if possible during this period. If treatment

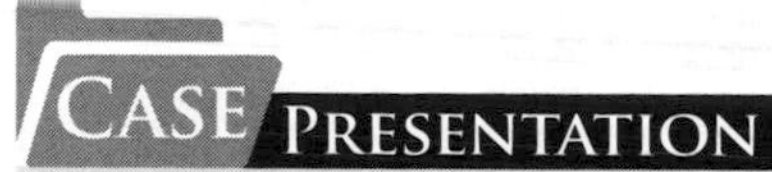

Case Presentation

Patient Case: Part 2

K.J. is currently receiving chemotherapy for her breast cancer and is feeling well, other than bothersome hot flashes that are interfering with her daily activities and sleep. She is not amenorrheic at the present time.

Plan:

1. Venlafaxine extended release: Start 37.5 mg daily, then increase to 75 mg daily after 1 week.
2. Discuss simple strategies to manage hot flash symptoms, including avoidance of triggers.
3. Continue chemotherapy (paclitaxel × 4 more cycles), multivitamin, calcium, and vitamin D.
4. Discuss topical lubricants that can relieve symptoms of vaginal dryness and eliminate discomfort during intercourse.
5. Follow up in clinic in 4–5 weeks

Rationale: The most significant reductions in hot flash symptoms have been reported with venlafaxine. Venlafaxine is preferred because of its clinical benefit, low side-effect profile, and lack of potential interaction in patients receiving concurrent therapy with tamoxifen. Although significant benefit was noted in patients receiving venlafaxine 37.5 mg daily, 75 mg daily appears to provide optimal benefit with similar side-effect profile.[47-49] Venlafaxine at a dose of 150 mg daily does not offer any additional clinical benefit than 75 mg daily and may be associated with more adverse effects.

Monitoring: Number of hot flash episodes per day, reports of excessive sleepiness or somnolence.

Patient education: Reduction in hot flash symptoms may be achieved in 3–7 days after the initiation of venlafaxine. However, in some patients, it may take up to several weeks for clinical benefits to be fully appreciated. Avoid alcohol, spicy foods, hot beverages, hot foods, or any other known triggers. Clothing should be lightweight and layered. K.J. needs to be reminded that use of topical lubricants will help relieve vaginal dryness but have no protective effect against sexually transmitted diseases, and other barrier precautions should be used.

is desired, the option to postpone treatment until the second or third trimester should be discussed. Chemotherapeutic drugs administered during the second or third trimester in general do not cause significant malformations, but fetal growth and development may be impaired.

Some potential long-term complications (delayed effects) of in utero exposure to chemotherapeutic agents include carcinogenesis, sterility, altered physical or mental growth and development, and second-generation teratogenesis.[65] Discussions surrounding the potential early and delayed effects of chemotherapy treatment may involve all family members, physicians (oncologist, obstetrician, pediatrician, neonatologist), and any other ancillary healthcare providers (pharmacist, nurse, social worker, nutritionist) who may be able to provide support for the mother's decision for treatment.

Further information on the safety of specific chemotherapeutic agents used for treatment of cancer in pregnant patients is reviewed in Chapter 26: High-Risk Pregnancies. Discussion of the more complex ethics surrounding management and treatment of cancer during pregnancy is discussed in Chapter 49: Ethical Decision Making.

Summary

A large number of women are diagnosed with cancer each year. Several complications can occur during cancer treatment that significantly affect women. Pharmacologic complications commonly encountered by women during cancer therapy can be generally classified into short-term and long-term complications. Short-term complications include nausea and vomiting and alopecia, and long-term complications include menopause, its associated symptoms, and sterility/infertility. Each one of these individual complications can be managed via pharmacologic and nonpharmacologic interventions as discussed.

References

Additional content available at ***www.ashp.org/womenshealth***

SECTION EIGHT

Ethical Issues in Women's Healthcare

48 Ethics and Ethical Dilemmas

Amy M. Haddad, Ph.D.

Learning Objectives

1. Examine the intersection of law and ethics and gender and ethics.
2. Define the following ethical principles: nonmaleficence, beneficence, respect for autonomy, and justice.
3. Compare and contrast the principlist, care-oriented and feminist approaches to ethics decision making.
4. Apply an ethical decision making model to a complex clinical case in pharmacy practice.

Every area of healthcare practice in the past few decades is changing and broadening its focus to include more patient-centered care and recognition of professional responsibilities. The more health professionals become involved with patients and all of the complexities of their lives, the more aware they are of related ethical issues, which are part of the professional and patient relationship. This chapter and the next one explore ethical issues involved in women's health and pharmacotherapy. The chapters assist readers in the often complicated task of distinguishing ethical from other kinds of issues with medication use and offer insights into the theoretical basis of ethical choice and moral conduct. Additionally, the chapters include the application of principles and alternative approaches of ethical decision making to clinical cases that highlight commonly encountered issues in pharmacy and healthcare.

Law and Ethics

Before focusing primarily on **ethics,** it is important to distinguish ethics from the law. Prescription medication use is highly regulated. So, it is understandable that pharmacists and others involved in medication therapy often turn to the law for clarification about the right thing to do regarding their duties to patients. Although law orders social and institutional relationships, it is too crude a measure of what is right to resolve complex ethical problems. So, rather than ask, "Is it legal?" one should ask, "Is the issue one in which a moral obligation is involved?" If the answer is yes, practitioners look to ethics for preliminary answers and then see if there is also a legal requirement of practice. Table 48-1 helps distinguish between what is ethical and what is legal.

An example of an action that is both ethical and legal is the doctrine of informed consent. The ethical development of informed consent reflects the view that individuals should have the freedom to make decisions about their health and adequate, understandable information to do so. An action that some pharmacists believe is unethical but is presently legal is dispensing emergency contraception or "the morning after pill." If a pharmacist holds that human life begins at conception then any action taken to disrupt the normal course of events that leads to implantation and development is morally wrong. Even though a patient has a legal prescription, a pharmacist could view dispensing a prescription for emergency contraception as unethical because of personal beliefs. An example of an action that is illegal but ethical is dispensing a medication without a prescription. A pharmacist may decide that it is ethical to dispense a partial fill of a prescription drug to a patient without a prescription to get them through a weekend or until a valid refill on the prescription can be obtained from the physician. Exceptions to the law allowing partial

Table 48-1. The Relationship Between Law and Ethics

	Ethical	Unethical
Legal	**Ethical and Legal**	**Unethical and Legal**
	Informed consent	Dispensing emergency contraception[a]
Illegal	**Ethical and Illegal**	**Unethical and Illegal**
	Dispensing medication without a prescription[b]	Insurance fraud

[a]Not all healthcare providers would consider this unethical.
[b]Some states might have partial fill laws, which would make this practice in such states ethical and legal.

filling of a maintenance medication in the absence of a prescription reflect how this particular action can fall into both categories of being ethical and illegal. If the drug is not a maintenance drug, the ethical question of whether one should dispense or not becomes more problematic. Finally, an action that is illegal and unethical is insurance fraud particularly if it is undertaken to benefit the pharmacy because it breaks a law and is deceptive, which breaks the moral rule of **veracity** or truth telling. Thus, for any proposed action one can ask questions about its legal and ethical status keeping in mind that there is disagreement about what is ethical and unethical and what should be legal or illegal.

Gender and Ethics

All of the factors that comprise the complex healthcare system in the U.S. such as fragmentation, barriers to access, cost containment issues, and legal and regulatory concerns also breed complex ethical problems for both genders. In some aspects, ethical concerns regarding women and their healthcare do not significantly differ from other patient populations. All of the standard ethical concerns on the individual level of healthcare delivery can be found in women's health: competency to make choices, **confidentiality,** the rights or **autonomy** of patients, **beneficence** or the duty of health professionals to do good, veracity or truth telling, and distribution of scarce resources to specific patients. However, though some of the issues are the same, other ethical issues related to women's health are not. Pathologies exist that only women experience because of anatomy such as uterine cancer and other diseases that seem to afflict women more than men such as multiple sclerosis. Within pathologies that occur in both sexes, sex disparities in treatment outcomes raise questions about **justice** and fairness in the healthcare system. For example, young women hospitalized for a myocardial infarction have a higher risk of death than young men hospitalized for the same diagnosis.[1]

There are also corollary concerns of ethics that are encountered only or more frequently in the area of women's health. For example, if one were to consider the merits of various treatment approaches to ectopic tubal pregnancy (a health problem unique to women), such as administration of systemic methotrexate vs. laparoscopic salpingostomy (a surgical incision into a fallopian tube by way of a scope inserted into the abdomen), it might seem that the treatment decision is purely a scientific one that has nothing to do with ethics. However, if one looks a little deeper, one can see that decisions like this in reproductive health involve appraisals of the worth of human life, the importance of the ability to bear future children, and distinctions between the worth of the woman who is pregnant vs. the fetus, to name a few ethical concerns.

Besides the physical and physiological differences encountered in women's health that give rise to unique ethical concerns, there are the ethical issues of how disease and illness are experienced by women that may not be as obvious. Patients, in general, must face the challenges of having their everyday routine altered by illness or injury. The patient role includes physical, psychological, and spiritual challenges, whether the condition is short or long term.[2] Patients also suffer from several kinds of isolation—". . . isolation from the healthy, isolation from loved ones, and isolation from the body and self."[3]

Sociologists long ago noted that patients are subjected to a litany of losses that literally strips them of power and identity. Although the following description of the admission of a patient to a hospital uses the masculine pronoun, it applies equally to male and female patients: "Simultaneously, he is expected to check most of his individualized wants and desires and his long-standing habit of making decisions for himself and others. It is assumed that he will place himself implicitly in the hands of medical and hospital staff and cooperate with them in what they are doing for his good. However, as the stripping process continues and its effect on him becomes cumulative, he often feels as if he were losing one layer after another of his self-identification."[4]

The imbalance of power within healthcare that places patients in a dependent position and health professionals in positions of strength still exists today.[5] Unfortunately, there is also an implicit "gendered" stereotype in healthcare that has its origins in the broader society (i.e., the dependent, helpless patient fills the traditional weaker feminine role and health professionals are in the masculine role of authority).[6] Additionally, women's health issues are often reduced to a "... focus on the reproductive functions of women rather than general health and well-being of all females at all times in their lifespan."[7] Women who are patients, therefore, have several barriers to overcome (i.e., the powerless position of patients and gender stereotypes about women in general and women's health), in order to balance the inequities in power within the health professional and patient relationship. It is important to note that the role of patients and what health professionals and others expect of them is socially constructed just as gender and social relationship are in the broader, mainstream society.

Until recently, **normative ethics**—the branch of ethical inquiry that considers ethical questions whose answers have a relatively direct bearing on practice—was not questioned as being anything other than objective and neutral. Major theories such as **utilitarianism** (which is a type of consequentialist theory that balances good and bad consequences in order to bring about the most good for the most people) and **deontological ethics** (upholding specific duties to make an ethical decision; if an act is not in accord with a moral code, it may not be undertaken, no matter the good consequence that it might produce) assume equality among the human beings in question.[8]

Feminist philosophers and others who dealt more directly with patients, such as nurses, began to question this claim of objectivity and the objective stance.[9-11] According to **feminist ethics** (focus on the status of women and the vulnerability of those involved) and **care-oriented ethics** (attention to the impact on relationships), human beings are not all equally situated. Furthermore, relationships between human beings whether they are within families or between a health professional and patient are important and have inherent moral worth. So, traditional approaches to ethics itself appear to have a gendered nature that tends to ignore or discount power differentials, context, and relationships, which are all part of a full view of the moral life. These are only a few examples of places that traditional theories and newer approaches to ethics differ. The traditional theories, feminist, and care-oriented ethics are discussed in more detail later in this chapter.

Key Concepts in Ethics

To have a clearer understanding of ethics in general and its application to clinical pharmacy practice in the area of women's health, it helps to have some basic information about key terms such as the definition of ethics itself, **values** and dilemmas. Ethics is a branch of philosophy that studies human behavior and makes judgments about what is good or bad and right or wrong. Whenever one asks a question such as "What is the right thing to do?" and the question involves the rights or welfare of others and not just matters of personal taste, the question is an ethical one. One is also asking an ethical question when one wonders "What kind of person or professional do I want to be?" Questions like this about actions and character are ethical in nature because the evaluation is ultimate or beyond an appeal to other values, it possesses universality in that they are evaluations (i.e., what is a morally correct action), which all persons ought to be able to make and understand, and they have an "other regarding" focus.[12]

Values also play an important role in ethical questions. Values are deeply held beliefs that should be evident in one's actions. Values are learned as one grows and develops, and they are influenced by many factors including family, friends, religion, ethnicity, socioeconomic status, and geographic location. By the time one reaches adulthood, key values are fixed and it takes a major, life-altering event to change such deeply held attitudes and beliefs. Health professionals, as a group, hold particular virtues or character traits to be of special importance. It has been proposed that the virtues of compassion, faithfulness, and fairness are especially important virtues to the practice of pharmacy.[13] As a member of the healthcare team, pharmacists should take their professional relationships with patients seriously. Therefore, health professionals who hold the virtue of compassion in high regard would behave in a manner that upholds patient relationships such as protecting the patient from harm, treating the patient with kindness and patience, and respecting a patient's right to self-determination.

Finally, an **ethical dilemma** is a conflict between two moral goods or two equally unappealing moral alternatives. Consider the case of a pharmacist who has been asked by a family member to withhold bad news about a diagnosis from a patient. If the pharmacist in this case values honesty, it will be particularly troubling if the patient who is supposed to be kept in the dark asks the pharmacist about her diagnosis. For the time being, set aside the complicated question of whose responsibility it is to tell the patient about her diagnosis or if she is capable of understanding the news if she were told, and focus on the presenting dilemma. The pharmacist is faced with two unappealing choices. One choice involves telling the patient the truth thereby going against the wishes of the family and hurting the patient with the bad news and potentially removing her hope for the future. The second choice would be to keep the patient ignorant of her diagnosis and act against the pharmacist's value of honesty and the patient's basic right to know. No one would want to be in the pharmacist's position. Either way, harms will occur in this situation. Even if the pharmacist doesn't act, that is making a decision of sorts and would result in not telling the patient. It should be emphasized here that even when one arrives at a thoughtful, ethical resolution, one may experience tragedy or loss as that is the nature of dilemmas.

A Process for Resolving Ethical Dilemmas

Pharmacists and other health professionals often go through the process of determining the correct ethical action in a specific case unconsciously rather than following a stepwise process to arrive at a sound decision. Furthermore, if asked, they might find it difficult to trace how they arrived at a decision or provide justification or reasoning for the "soundness" of the decision. There are many normative models for resolving ethical problems in the health professions' literature, but all require critical thinking and should result in a choice that is morally justifiable.[14-17] Here, a general framework is offered in Table 48-2, which includes a step-wise process to systematically resolve ethical problems in particular cases.[18,19] The six steps provide the structure for the decision-making process and should be followed in the order that they are listed so as not to miss important information.

The steps in the model outline a process or a way of making judgments about what should be done in a particular situation (Table 48-2). The basic framework is sufficient to focus moral judgments and simple enough to recall and apply in actual clinical practice. A brief explanation of what each step requires follows as well as examples of the kinds of questions one might ask at each step.

Table 48-2. A Model for Ethical Decision Making

Step 1	Respond to the sense of feeling something is wrong
Step 2	Gather information
Step 3	Identify the ethical problem/moral diagnosis
Step 4	Seek a resolution
Step 5	Work with others to determine a course of action[16]
Step 6	Evaluate/review outcomes of decisions/action[18]

The first step in the decision-making process is not logical and rational but calls on ethical intuition, which indicates something is morally wrong in a situation. When one feels that an action isn't right or something is about to go "wrong" we should attend to this warning. Moral sensitivity is not sufficient to resolve ethical problems but is a starting point to quickly move to the next step of gathering information. In order to make an informed decision, one needs solid information. The most important method of gathering relevant information, whether clinical or situational, is to listen and observe. By reflecting and questioning what is occurring, it will help focus on the initial ethical intuition that triggered the decision process in the first place. The third step deals with the identification of the ethical problem or problems in the situation. Depending on what approach one is using, a problem can be identified according to principles such as **nonmaleficence,** beneficence, respect for autonomy, and justice or other concerns including inequities in power or threats to relationships. The fourth step moves to the level of the application of rules to determine what is or are ethically justifiable course(s) of action. Theories, which are discussed in fuller detail following the case analysis, provide a means to justify decisions by focusing on fair consequences (utilitarianism), specific duties **(deontology),** relationships (care-oriented ethics), and the vulnerability of those involved (feminist ethics). Step five asserts that ethical decisions should not be made alone and that one should seek the perspectives and wisdom of others in arriving at the best resolution. Step six encourages the review of the outcomes of a decision or action that will provide insight into whether an action was the ethically best choice or not for those more directly affected and, in some cases, the larger community.

Approaches to the Ethical Decision-Making Process

As has been noted previously, there are various ways to proscribe ethical decision making, but by far the most popular and predominant approach in healthcare ethics is the principlist approach.[19] The strength of the four principles' approach (respect for autonomy, nonmaleficence, beneficence, and justice) is compatibility with both consequentialist and deontological theories.[20] Additionally, the four principles reflect the basic duties common to all health professionals (i.e., to respect patients, do good for others, avoid harm, and be fair). However, the principlist approach, or at least the abridged way, is often put into practice in healthcare and has been criticized for being too limited in its moral outlook. As one critic notes, the principlist paradigm, ". . . blinds clinicians from seeing a fuller set of moral obligations to the patient and limits the range of options that are available to navigate through such impasses."[21] There are other duties—such as promise keeping, the obligation to make amends, and the ability to appreciate being human and vulnerable to disease and disability—that the four principles wouldn't recognize. Even with these limitations, the principlist approach deserves specific attention because it is so widely used in healthcare ethics. Also, it is often helpful in determining just what the ethical problem is in many situations in healthcare and what should be done.

PRINCIPLIST APPROACH

Four fundamental principles are often cited as the core or major duties of all those working in healthcare. The principles—nonmaleficence, beneficence, respect for autonomy, and justice— provide a framework or guide for action in which to consider ethical obligations, enable clear thinking about the issues involved in specific cases as well as broader implications, and help ensure that important factors aren't overlooked.[20,22]

Nonmaleficence is one of the most basic principles in healthcare, which requires that health professionals avoid doing harm. Some philosophers refer to nonmaleficence as a "perfect duty" in that health professionals owe the duty not to harm to everyone regardless of the relationship they have with others. Doing good for patients or beneficence is often the reason a person decides to enter a health profession in the first place. Beneficence is a pre-eminent moral duty. However, this seemingly simple principle is actually quite complicated. For example, there are questions about the determination of what is considered "good," whose good health professionals are focusing on such as an individual or society, and how much good is obligatory as opposed to supererogatory (i.e., beyond the call of duty) on the part of the health professional.

Respect for autonomy requires that we respect the capacity of persons to make and express choices, which are substantially free from constraints. According to this principle, health professionals are not necessarily required to respect any and all decisions a patient might make, but health professionals should always respect a patient's right to exercise this freedom of choice. For example, patients may choose to reuse insulin syringes to save money even after they have been told about the danger of contamination and possible infection. Although a health professional probably wouldn't agree with this choice or the patient's balancing of harms (possible infection) and goods (saving money, avoiding trips to the pharmacy) involved in such a decision, the health professional could still respect the fact that a competent patient has a right to make such a choice even if it doesn't appear very wise.

Justice is the moral principle that assists in decisions about how resources are distributed. Justice in healthcare requires that health professionals act in fairness and only use morally relevant criteria such as need in deciding when it is morally permissible to treat different patients differently. Of course, people may differ in their views about what "relevant" criteria are, but generally need and prognosis are morally permissible principles to use to determine who gets resources and in what order.

Ethical principles are general guides or criteria that make human actions morally right or wrong. Principles are broad and in order to apply them to specific cases, health professionals must turn to intermediate rules to help make a decision about what principle should take priority or how to react to moral problems of a certain kind. Generally, there are two kinds of rules in ethics: 1) rules of practice, and 2) summary rules.[12] Rules of practice function to specify behavior that is required independent from individual judgment in a specific case. For example, a rule of practice in pharmacy is that it is wrong to participate in the killing of a patient. This particular rule of practice is directly linked to the right-making principles of nonmaleficence and avoidance of killing. So, the rule against killing justifies a practice that is supported more generally by the principles. Even if in a specific case it would seem that more good would come from assisting a patient to die by relieving extreme pain, the rule of practice view would deem it unacceptable. Summary rules, on the other hand, merely summarize the experiences of dealing with similar situations in the past. An example of a summary rule might be based on past experience in dealing with patients; it is generally better to tell the truth.

The final question is what ought to be done in specific cases. In the patient case that follows, the overarching problems of how to relate facts to values, identify the role of ethical principles, and what ought to be done are posed to come to a morally justifiable resolution. The principlist approach and the traditional theories of utilitarianism and deontology are also applied to the case.

APPLICATION TO A COMPLEX CASE—CONFIDENTIALITY AND A MATURE MINOR

C.L. has dealt with the problems and limitations of systemic lupus erythematosus (SLE) for the past 7 years. C.L. was diagnosed with SLE when she was 10 years old. C.L. was fortunate in that early in her illness she was seen by D.M., a pediatric rheumatologist, with whom she shares a good relationship. During a routine office visit, D.M. asked C.L. many of the same questions he usually did about school, friends, etc. C.L. blushed but didn't answer when D.M. asked, "Any new boyfriends?" D.M. waited until C.L.'s mother left the exam room to answer her cell phone and then asked, "Seriously, C.L., are you involved with someone?" CL responded, "I do have a boyfriend and it is serious. My mom would never understand but I really think I love him." D.M. continued, "This may be hard for you to answer, but I have to ask, are you planning to be intimate with this young man or have you already been sexually involved with him? It is important that I know this because of your lupus." C.L. stated that she had not yet had sexual relations, but they had come close. She also stated that she didn't want to get pregnant and knew that this would be a real problem with her lupus. D.M., in consultation with C.L., decided that some form of contraception was in order. C.L. stated that she wanted to be on the pill because most of her friends used that form of contraception. D.M. knew that oral contraceptives (OCs) were the preferred method of contraception in adolescents with SLE and stable disease. C.L. fit this category of patients as she had low antiphospholipid antibodies (aPL) and no history of thrombolytic events in the past 3 years.[12] D.M. wrote a prescription for an OC and encouraged C.L. to have her partner use a condom as well to prevent the transmission of sexually transmitted disease. While her mother went to get the car, C.L. took the prescription to the clinic pharmacy and told the pharmacist that she would pick it up in 2 weeks the next time she had an appointment. "My mom doesn't need to know," C.L. hurriedly told the pharmacist as she left the pharmacy.

When the pharmacist finally had time to really look at the prescription, he was shocked and concerned on several counts. He didn't think it was right for 17-year-old girls to be sexually active. Second, he knew about the diagnosis of SLE and was concerned about the risk of thrombotic events from estrogen exposure that would occur with OCs. Additionally, there were other risks from OCs, which he thought would be difficult for C.L. to assess such as myocardial infarction, stroke, or peripheral artery disease. Of course, he acknowledged the fact that a pregnancy was not risk free either. In a way, he could respect C.L.'s decision to use some kind of contraception if she was going to be sexually active particularly because she had SLE. Given all of this, the pharmacist could not decide if he should talk to D.M. about his concerns, call C.L.'s mother and tell her about the prescription because C.L. is a minor, or fill the prescription and try to talk C.L. out of taking the OCs when she comes in to pick it up explaining his concerns.

This case is complex but reveals potential ethical concerns. The pharmacist involved in the case is poised at the point of making an ethical decision about which action or actions is morally justifiable. The six-step model can help the pharmacist and the other members of the healthcare team involved in C.L.'s care to determine a justifiable resolution.

SIX-STEP MODEL

Respond to the Sense That Something Is Wrong

The first step in the ethical decision-making process is to respond to the intuitive sense that something is wrong in a given situation. Unlike obvious signs and symptoms such as ashen skin color or a drop in hemoglobin, there are no objective signs that one is involved in an ethical problem. Busy ambulatory clinics, like the one where C.L. receives her care, can be fraught with stress and emotion. Additionally, the management of a chronic, possibly life-threatening condition like SLE is also stressful for the patient and her family. It is obvious that C.L.'s case is full of emotion: The pharmacist was described as shocked and concerned. C.L. was anxious and secretive. Do these emotional signs indicate that an ethical problem is in progress? The answer, as is often the case in ethics, is yes and no. Just because people are emotionally upset with each other or under a lot of stress does not necessarily mean that an ethical problem is involved. However, heightened emotional sensitivity along with "... stress and tension intrapersonally or interpersonally; and ineffective communication patterns such as avoidance, nagging, or silence" are often warning signs that one is involved in an ethical problem.[24] In C.L.'s case, the pharmacist believed that something wasn't right when he saw the prescription was for OCs. The pharmacist's response to the prescription is the most obvious emotional reaction in the case but not the only one. C.L. is silent when D.M. asks if she has a boyfriend. He notes her blush at his question and waits for an opportunity to ask her about this in private when her mother leaves the room. All of these emotions and potential conflicts are indications that an ethical problem may be present. One should then move on to the next step.

Gather Information

The two general categories of information that are needed to arrive at an informed decision are clinical and situational.[24] Clinical information deals with relevant clinical data in the case such as diagnosis, prognosis, action, contraindications, side effects of medications, risks and benefits of proposed treatment(s), risks and benefits of alternative treatments, as well as outcomes from doing nothing. In C.L.'s situation, the type of clinical information that is needed to understand the case seems fairly straightforward. Specific clinical information would include general etiology of SLE, specific data on adolescents with SLE, and therapeutic approaches to managing the disease. Furthermore, information about the action and side effects of all methods of contraception, especially OCs, and specific implications for patients with SLE would be essential. The general information then needs to be applied to the specific patient, C.L., with all of her idiosyncrasies and differences, which are part of her history with this chronic illness. The risks of pregnancy and unprotected sexual intercourse would also be appropriate clinical information in this case. As much as possible, the clinical facts of the case should be clarified before moving on to a more in-depth analysis of what these facts mean morally.

Situational information includes data regarding the context and personal information of those involved in a case such as age; gender; cultural issues such as religious and ethnicity/race beliefs; and other values. Additionally, setting and time constraints are important facts as they can influence the conditions under which a decision is made. The values of the people most intimately involved in the case are of particular importance.

The main players in the case are C.L., the physician, the pharmacist, and C.L.'s mother. All of these individuals hold values about many things including privacy, health, freedom, and honesty. We know that C.L. has a mother. Does she also have a father? If so, does he need to be involved and would he be more or less understanding than the mother? Also, we only have C.L.'s opinion on how her mother would react to the news that her daughter is considering being sexually active. Is C.L. right in her estimation of her mother's and potentially father's reaction? It appears D.M. values safe sexual practices for his adolescent patients because he is willing to prescribe OCs to a minor and counsel her on the use of condoms without the involvement of her mother. Does D.M. behave this way with all of his patients or just those who are at high risk? The pharmacist doesn't think it is right for 17-year-old girls to be sexually active. What does this tell us about the pharmacist's values? What isn't right about adolescents being sexually active? The pharmacist may think that this isn't legally right as a 17-year-old is not yet a consenting adult. He may think it isn't right because of religious beliefs about the wrongness of sexual intercourse outside the state of marriage. Or, he might object to adolescents being sexually active because of the risk of unintended pregnancy and its impact on completing high school and the future socioeconomic status of the mother and child and societal impact. These are only some of the reasons that could explain the pharmacist's reaction to the prescription.

The responsibility for C.L.'s care rests with various members of the healthcare team as well as her family. Each member's responsibilities are distinct but also overlap. As part of the information gathering step, it is important to sort out the responsibilities in order to identify moral accountability. For example, the mother has responsibilities for the care of her daughter including her physical and moral health. Thus, she cannot be completely eliminated from decisions about her daughter's welfare unless there is a strong reason to do so (i.e., that she is making a decision that would harm her daughter). These are only some of the situational facts that impact an ethical decision from all of the information provided in the case. Once the facts are outlined and questions are sufficiently answered about unknown facts, one can examine them to see if the case has the characteristics of an ethical problem.

Identify the Ethical Problems/ Moral Diagnosis

As has been noted in the opening of this chapter, ethics deals with the rights or welfare of others and not just matters of personal taste. Clearly, C.L.'s case involves questions about the right of an adolescent to obtain OCs without parental consent and also her welfare and that of others involved in the case. Ethical principles are sources of ethical guidance and can serve as a method to identify the ethical problems in a case. Principles can often be in conflict with one another, which creates the ethical problems. The ethical principles in conflict in the case are respect for autonomy (which implies the patient's right to make an informed decision about her treatment), nonmaleficence, and beneficence (raising the question about the weighing of harms and benefits involved in the treatment decision to prescribe OCs to a minor with SLE). Because the patient's wishes generally take priority over other parties involved, patient's wishes should be considered first. The principle of respect for autonomy requires that health professionals follow the wishes of competent, informed patients. Therefore, it is important to determine if the patient in question is competent. Is C.L. capable of making a competent decision? According to the law, C.L. is not competent because she has not reached the age of majority. She is still considered a minor. However, because of her long-standing illness she might be considered a **mature minor,** that is, an adolescent who can demonstrate that she has a substantial understanding of the choices to be made and sufficient autonomy to make a choice consistent with a life plan. There is controversy over whether clinicians like D.M. have the authority to declare minors mature for consenting to treatment. Over the last 30 years, states have expanded minors' authority to consent to healthcare including care related to sexual activity. This trend reflects the recognition that while parental involvement is desirable, many minors will remain sexually active but not seek healthcare services if they have to tell their parents. Because confidentiality is vital to promoting minors to seek contraceptive services, several states explicitly permit minors to consent to contraceptive services if a physician determines that the minor would face a health hazard if she is not provided with contraceptive services.[25] Although the law might support D.M.'s action, he might want to seek judicial approval before acting on the basis of the consent of a mature minor. This is especially true when a parent might object to the proposed choice of his or her daughter.

Nonmaleficence is the principle underlying D.M.'s decision to prescribe OCs to C.L. to prevent pregnancy. Prevention of pregnancy is particularly important in C.L.'s case because she has SLE. In addition to the normal risks of pregnancy, there are also the potential harms of teratogenicity of medications used to treat SLE and the risk of SLE flares during pregnancy.[23] Nonmaleficence motivates D.M. to strive to protect C.L. from these harms because it appears that she is seriously contemplating sexual activity. The harms from OCs were balanced against the harms of unwanted pregnancy. Included in this calculation is knowledge about the best contraceptive to use in cases like C.L.'s, which would include concerns about adherence to treatment, side effects, and efficacy. Beneficence is closely tied to nonmaleficence in the case as D.M. is trying to maximize good for his patient. OCs are the contraceptive method of choice in adolescents with SLE and stable disease.[23] D.M. also demonstrated a commitment to the welfare of his patient by pressing the discussion of sexual activity with her, a discussion that is often avoided by physicians because it is very often difficult for both parties.

The principles of nonmaleficence and beneficence are also at work in the pharmacist's thinking. He is concerned about whether the risks and harms of OCs have been seriously considered by D.M. and the patient. Perhaps he believes that sexual abstinence is a better choice with far less risks than OCs for a patient with SLE. In any case, he is concerned that C.L.'s mother has not been involved with the decision, which could have a direct impact on C.L.'s welfare in the long run. In other words, would C.L.'s best interests be better served if her mother also knew about the side effects of OCs so that she could observe for them as well? At this point, health professionals can move to the fourth step of the decision-making process by exploring various courses of action that requires determining which principles are involved and what the implications are.

Seek a Resolution

The working phase of a decision-making model is proposing more than one course of action and examining the ethical justification of the various actions. The pharmacist has proposed at least three courses of action: 1) call CL's mother and tell her about the prescription; 2) talk to D.M. about his concerns; or 3) fill the prescription and try and talk C.L. out of taking the OCs when she comes in to pick it up. Of course, there are other actions such as filling the prescription, which the pharmacist hasn't considered.

The three proposed actions fall into the category of overriding C.L.'s autonomy, trying to change D.M.'s mind and indirectly overriding C.L.'s autonomy, and trying to change C.L.'s mind when she comes in to pick up the prescription. Of course, other options could be to fill the prescription and counsel C.L. as he would any other patient receiving an OC prescription, or have another pharmacist who doesn't object to the prescription prepare it and counsel C.L. The fact that the pharmacist didn't see these last two options as possibilities shows us how values shape considerations regarding moral actions. This "blindness" to certain options is another reason why working with others is important in ethical decision-making to ensure that a variety of options are considered.

To determine which options are morally justifiable of those that the pharmacist has proposed, one must project the probable consequences of each action and the underlying intention of the action as well as whether there are moral duties or obligations that hold sway independent of consequences. This process involves the application of the ethical principles described earlier and the ethical theories described below. Choosing the first option would be hard to reconcile with the principle of respect for autonomy, which includes the legal rights of the patient in this area, but could be supported by more consequence-oriented ethics that stress beneficence and nonmaleficence.

One version of utilitarianism holds that health professionals should choose the action that brings about the most good for the greatest number. Informing C.L.'s mother of the prescription without telling D.M. or C.L. clearly overrides the autonomy of both D.M. and C.L., which could result in anger at a minimum or seriously damage the working relationship with D.M. and C.L. If the pharmacist uses the utilitarian theory, he would have to weigh the goods and harms of keeping quiet or informing the mother. If he believes that by informing the mother more good would come to C.L. either because her mother could observe for serious side effects if she agrees to the treatment of OCs or somehow persuade her daughter to refrain from sexual activity until she is legally able to decide for herself, then he must tell her. The harms that will result in addition to overriding autonomy would also need to be considered. The pharmacist may cause a serious rift in the mother/daughter relationship. Another harm involves breaching confidentiality, which is a moral problem and also a legal one because C.L. did not give explicit permission to speak to her mother about her prescription. Confidentiality is somewhat muddied by the fact that C.L. is a minor. Furthermore, C.L. may remain sexually active without the benefit of contraception, which places her at risk for pregnancy. Depending on how one assesses the consequences and whose consequences to include, one could accept or reject the first option.

The second option indirectly ignores the autonomy of C.L. but opens the door to a deeper understanding between the physician and the pharmacist. There are risks and benefits from OCs that are particularly important when the patient has SLE. D.M. appears to have weighed these risks and benefits differently than the pharmacist. The pharmacist has a duty to the patient to fulfill his professional obligations among which are the duties to provide competent patient care and be a patient advocate. In order to fulfill these obligations, the pharmacist must make certain that C.L. is capable of making an autonomous choice. By talking to D.M., the pharmacist could ascertain if C.L. received adequate information to make such a decision. He could also find out how D.M. has determined that this is the best treatment decision given C.L.'s diagnosis of SLE. The weighing of goods and harms might take on different meaning if he had more information. However, it could also be that the pharmacist and physician disagree on the more basic question of whether adolescents, regardless of maturity, have the right to consent to treatment without the involvement of their parents. If that is the case, further discussion might not resolve the issue.

Option three is a variation on option two in that the pharmacist is trying to influence the patient's decision by trying to talk her out of the choice to take OCs when she comes in to get the prescription. If he honors the duty to respect patient autonomy, he would have to measure his comments to C.L. to make certain he doesn't coerce her unnecessarily or force a decision on her that she doesn't want to make. He would have the opportunity to talk to her about her understanding of the risks and benefits, offer any additional information that would be helpful in making her decision, and gain some insights into her ability to make a competent decision. The principle of respect for autonomy would dictate his intention to give her the benefit of the doubt regarding her capacity to make a treatment decision of this nature.

The options are not mutually exclusive in that the pharmacist could first talk to D.M. and then speak to C.L. when she comes in to get the prescription. He could then decide to respect C.L.'s autonomy. However, if he is still troubled about the long-term risks and C.L.'s inability to monitor for these symptoms, he could then inform C.L. about his lingering concerns and his decision to discuss his concerns with her mother. In the end, the pharmacist will have to decide whether he will be guided by a more consequence-oriented ethic or one that holds that in the end the duty to respect patient autonomy must prevail.

Work with Others to Determine a Course of Action

No one makes clinical decisions in a vacuum, or if they do they will certainly learn the limits of their perspective and knowledge when it comes to patient care. The same is true for ethical decisions. Ethical concerns are more likely to be resolved and fair decisions reached if the individuals involved have the chance to share their perspectives, values, and concerns. Group process can enrich decision making by providing insights into the reasoning of others involved in a situation, clarify assumptions, and provide a variety of options that one couldn't supply alone. Also, group discussion about ethical issues such as those involved in this case, help support and validate the ethical norms of the professional group as a whole. For example, the clinic in which the pharmacist and D.M. work will probably see other adolescent patients with rheumatic disease who are contemplating sexual activity. Discussions about how the clinic chooses to handle the question of minors' access to contraceptive services would be a fruitful one for setting policy or guidelines and determining how consent will be handled. Because a decision has not yet been determined in the case, step six of the decision model, which requires evaluation and review of the consequences of a decision or action, cannot be reviewed here.

Although moral issues may begin as a vague sense or feeling that something is wrong, it has been demonstrated through systematic reflection that they can be more clearly articulated.[26] However, the moral life is not just a series of problems to be solved. Rather ethical living is about how to live with ineluctable human difficulties.[27]

At this juncture, the perspective will change to examine alternative approaches to principle-based ethics that do not divide the moral life into discerning the ethically justifiable choice in a given situation but looks at the "ineluctable human difficulties" such as those found in human relationships and power inequities that pervade healthcare interactions.

CARE-ORIENTED AND FEMINIST ETHICS APPROACHES

Although there are numerous approaches to ethics, two different approaches from the principlist perspective will be applied to C.L.'s case. Because the overall focus of the book is on women's health, two approaches that pay particular attention to the experiences of women—care-oriented ethics and feminist ethics—are considered. It should be noted, however, that there are often great differences in fundamental understandings between care-oriented and feminist ethics, which are too complex to elucidate here.

Also, unlike the principlist ethics and theories like utilitarianism, care-oriented ethics and feminist ethics are not decision directed; that is they do not lead to a neat list of possible resolutions nor necessarily to a morally justifiable action in a particular situation. Rather, these two approaches highlight differences in values, family dynamics including connectedness and relationships, power imbalances, and cultural issues. Table 48-3 outlines general differences between traditional ethical theories and care-oriented and feminist ethics.

Care-oriented ethics are briefly defined as an ethic of care concerned with the particularity and partiality of relationships. It considers the impact of the relationship on all those involved, so **reciprocity** is a central focus. Reciprocity is the ability to consider situations from other persons' point of view, to think as others think, and to feel as they feel. Whereas the principlist approach aims for impartiality and universalizability, care-oriented ethics notes the importance of a particular context and those involved. In other words, if an ethical problem occurs in an ED in the context of high stress, life and death decisions, and serious time constraints, these factors

Table 48-3. General Differences Between Traditional Theories and Care-Oriented and Feminist Ethics[28]

Traditional theories	Care-oriented/feminist ethics
Detachment	Attachment
Individual rights	Relationships
Impartiality	Partiality
Universalizability	Particularity
Abstraction	Context

will have an impact on the kind and quality of the ethical decision that is made.

An ethic of care focuses on preservation of relationships and the implications of such relationships on those involved. In pharmacy, the notion of pharmaceutical care describes the relationship between pharmacist and patient as a covenant that is a "mutually beneficial exchange in which a patient promises to grant authority to the provider, and the provider promises competence and commitment (responsibility) to the patient."[29] The traditional scriptural meaning of covenant emphasizes the gifts that each party brings to a relationship, the promises that each makes to the other, and the transformative effect of the covenant on each. Because the term *covenant* is used in the Code of Ethics for Pharmacists to describe the nature of the relationship between the pharmacist and the patient, it is appropriate to explore this particular interpretation of care.[29]

In applying this meaning of care to the relationship between pharmacist and patient, the gifts that each brings to the relationship are noted. Patients begin by giving the gift of themselves by allowing health professionals to care for them. Patients also provide the opportunity for personal and professional growth on the part of health professionals. The actual act of caring changes not only the recipient of care, but also the provider of care in ways that may not be immediately apparent. Pharmacists bring to the relationship gifts such as the gift of competent care, compassion for the predicament of their patients, and ability to protect their patients from harm. Because patients are vulnerable, pharmacists are often in the position of doing good for them but determining *good* depends on knowing the individual patient not just patients in general. Pharmacists need the gift of listening, especially to the particular patient's story. Thus, the promise that pharmacists make to patients is one of listening in order to help the patients in the way they want to be helped. In the case of C.L., it might mean listening more closely to her particular story, her concerns, and values.

Feminist Ethics

Feminist ethics takes many forms. Feminist ethics begins with female experience. Feminist ethics question all societal principles concerning how women's lives ought to be lived. Thus, it is common for feminist ethics to move from the concrete experiences of women's lives to the societal level where personal injustices (e.g., unequal pay for equal work) become part of a larger social structure that sustains injustices. For example, from a feminist ethical perspective, one must ask "For this and every medical decision, how does this affect the recipient as a woman?"[31]

Rather than help with a resolution to a specific problem, feminist ethics address broader concerns and call for resolution or changes on that level. In other words, feminist ethics work at a social analysis level and provide a way of seeing different from the traditional principlist, objective perspective that is dominate in healthcare ethics. One of the most contentious areas in healthcare involves reproductive issues, which places women in the center of these difficult questions. Feminist ethics assert that social structures, which limit a woman's ability to participate in decision making in whatever way she deems appropriate, are unjust and should be changed. Feminist ethics encourage us to examine the ways social institutions shape the experiences of women and the possibilities for new systems and structures that address inequalities. In the case of C.L., a feminist perspective would encourage deeper focus on systems that would empower female mature minors in making informed decisions about their health and healthcare.

Summary

Competence in ethical decision making not only requires familiarity and use of traditional tools of analysis such as principlism but also an understanding and application of other perspectives on the moral life, such as care-oriented ethics and feminist ethics. If the opinions of pharmacists and other health professionals regarding ethical issues in clinical practice are to be taken seriously, they need to be well reasoned. The tools of ethics provide a means to ensure that one's ethical views are expressed in a clear and compelling manner, which incorporates other key decision makers such as patients, other health professionals, and family members. The perspectives of care and feminism assure that these views are informed by an awareness of the lived realities and experiences of all human beings, not just those in power.

References

Additional content available at
www.ashp.org/womenshealth

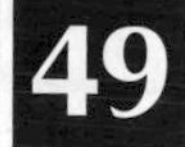

49 Ethical Decision Making

Jean Abbott, MD, MH; Peter V. Tortorice, Pharm.D., BCOP; Jacyln Michelle Graham, Pharm.D.

Learning Objectives

1. Use an ethical framework to identify, analyze, and resolve ethical dilemmas involving pregnancy and contraception issues.
2. Examine the tensions between maternal and fetal interests using an ethical framework.
3. Articulate the process involved in considering and teaching patients about high-risk treatments during pregnancy.
4. Explore the healthcare provider's obligations to the patient and the limits of those obligations when they conflict with personal values.

Ethical dilemmas occur both in personal and professional life. Sometimes it is easier to recognize and practice resolving ethical dilemmas in the daily choices of professionals and persons. Healthcare providers are regularly asked to choose between two or more good choices that have advantages and disadvantages. Do you choose to fire an employee who alters your narcotics log when she has a count discrepancy, or do you warn her when she explains the circumstances and "comes clean," showing compassion by giving her another chance (justice vs. mercy)? How do you balance positive and negative attributes in your letter of reference for a colleague (truth vs. loyalty)? Do you grab a quick lunch that is less healthy so that you have more time to study, or do you spend the extra time to eat something more healthy (short term vs. long term)? How do you balance your desire for a safe and large but fuel-consuming car with your global obligations to reduce energy consumption (individual vs. community)?[1] These choices must be resolved in order to act but have valid arguments to favor each side. Either choice is less than ideal because it involves *not* choosing to emphasize a value that is also important. Persons of good faith may emphasize different values and make different choices, as does the same person in different situations. These ethical dilemmas should not be confused with ethical temptations, in which persons may be tempted to do something that is wrong (choose to skip teaching the patient about his medication because it is hard to access a translator—a "right" vs. "wrong" problem).[1]

Ethical choices in professional life are increasingly complex as medical treatments become more potent and have correspondingly increased risks. In Chapter 48: Ethics and Ethical Dilemmas, the foundational principles of bioethics—autonomy, beneficence, nonmaleficence, and justice were presented as well as newer approaches to ethical reasoning (i.e., **care-oriented ethics** and **feminist ethics.** Cultural diversity around core values and increased focus on patient-centered decision making also contribute to increasing tensions about how to serve the patient best. What should you do when your assessment of a patient's "best interest" diverges from her understanding of her best interest? It is "good" to respect the patient (autonomy) who wants to use an untested herbal remedy, but it is also important to encourage treatments that are worthwhile (beneficence) or avoid recommending a treatment that may cause harm (nonmaleficence). Different professionals will resolve the conflict between core values differently. There may be several valid options for resolving a particular ethical dilemma, as well as some options that are unacceptable. The purpose of ethical analysis is to make the moral dilemma explicit and to provide a structured method for highlighting what values may be in tension, for discerning valid choices or compromises, and for

Table 49-1. Five Steps in Analysis of Ethical Dilemmas

1. Recognize or respond to the existence of an ethical dilemma.
2. Gather information to clarify details of the dilemma in the particular case.
3. Clarify the ethical values that are in tension.
4. Articulate ethical options that could resolve the moral dilemma, as well as those options that are not ethical.
5. Choose a justifiable resolution, working with others through compromise and dialogue to understand and respect the values of the stakeholders involved and act.

making your choice with intention. Resolution of an ethical dilemma involves recognizing other options, but making a valid choice in this particular situation that allows you to move forward to action. This chapter will expand on the foundational principles of bioethics and a method of analysis (Table 49-1) presented in Chapter 48: Ethics and Ethical Dilemmas, via two patient cases related to pharmacy practice are discussed (see Web Resources for Patient Case: Category X Medication in a Woman with Child-Bearing Capacity.)

Additional content available at ***www.ashp.org/womenshealth***

Other Important Influences on Healthcare Professional Ethical Decision Making

While the tension between core ethical principles is the most common source of bioethical dilemmas, there are other sources of **moral distress** and ethical conflict in professional life. These influences on ethical decision making are listed in Table 49-2.

Table 49-2. Sources of Professional Ethical Dilemmas

1. Conflicting medical ethical values
Patient autonomy
Beneficence
Nonmaleficence
Justice or fairness
Resource utilization
Truth telling or honesty (veracity)
Confidentiality
Privacy
Fiduciary commitment
Faithfulness or loyalty
Compassion or kindness
Family relationship
Respect for persons
Integrity
Cultural diversity
2. Personal moral values
3. Legal constraints to practice
4. Employment or contractual commitments
5. Interprofessional relationships

CHARACTERISTICS OF PHARMACY AS A PROFESSION

The primacy of the patient separates professions from business exchanges, in which the consumer must be the one to protect his or her own interests. The term *fiduciary* is sometimes used to refer to the special obligations and commitments required of healthcare professionals (and others like your financial advisor or auto mechanic who have specialized expertise), which protect the patient against the power imbalance intrinsic to the interaction (see Chapter 48: Ethics and Ethical Dilemmas). The fiduciary compact affirms the trust that the patient—in need, often ill, and without expertise—must have in the pharmacist and healthcare professional who commits to being competent and to placing the patient's interest above her/his own. There are limits to the fiduciary commitment (patients cannot ask the professional for help in harming themselves or others), but this compact is central to distinguishing healthcare interactions from business transactions.[2]

Medical professions are also characterized by special benefits and corresponding responsibilities based on the "social contract" under which they practice. The pharmacist possesses specialized information, and s/he works within a closed association, which prevents patient access to pharmaceutical dispensing services from nonauthorized sources in the wider marketplace. Most effective medicines are available only through physicians or pharmacists, making this a "professional monopoly."[3] The protection afforded by the "guild" nature of pharmacy raises the bar of responsibility to respect the patient's values and honor their needs in that professional role.[4]

The codes and position statements from the national organizations representing pharmacists codify the professional duties and boundaries of the **profession.** The Pharmacist Code of Ethics addresses the roles and responsibilities of the pharmacist as a health professional and outlines explicitly the responsibilities of being in a **fiduciary relationship.**[5] It articulates the covenantal relationship to the patient, which makes the patient's well-being central and empowers the patient when possible. The pharmacist pledges to promote the dignity and autonomy of the patient and to encourage the patient to participate in decisions regarding her health. While the pharmacist's primary obligation is to the individual patient, the code acknowledges the importance of respect for colleagues and other healthcare professionals, as well as societal needs and distributive justice in regard to healthcare resources. The more recent Oath of a Pharmacist, revised in 2007, is more vague in committing graduating pharmacists to "service to others" and to the profession, with the goal of assuring "optimal outcomes for my patients." This new oath does not clarify how to balance patient values with the values of the pharmacist but affirms the general commitment to competency and the "highest principles of moral, ethical and legal conduct."[6] A recent position statement by the American College of Clinical Pharmacy (ACCP) has delineated the situations (including capital punishment, euthanasia, termination of pregnancy, or contraception) in which pharmacists may decline to participate in care due to their personal moral, ethical, or religious beliefs.[7]

PERSONAL MORAL BELIEFS

Healthcare providers may face conflicts between professional duties and personal values. Each person has core values deriving from her/his family, cultural, or religious grounding and history. These core values can clash with requests made of them in their professional roles. The pharmacist who doesn't believe in premarital sex may still be asked to dispense birth control pills to unmarried women (or sildenafil to unmarried men). Pharmacists who may decry homosexuality are still asked to fill antiretroviral medication prescriptions. **Conscientious objection** is supported by tradition, and is a longstanding right of citizens, though individuals may expect consequences when they decline to perform duties expected of them in their roles as citizens or professionals. Sometimes, other core personal **moral values** allow the healthcare provider to emphasize her/his values of respect for the patient and the "ethic of responsibility" to the public and to accept dispensing medications s/he may not personally affirm. Resolving differences in deeply held beliefs regarding when life begins or death and dying can be particularly problematic. It is often left to the legal arena to resolve such difficult value conflicts and protect both professional and patient.[3,8]

LEGAL REQUIREMENTS

Legal mandates can require pharmacists to engage in a wider scope of practice than they may individually want, as with the laws requiring dispensing of emergency contraception pills (ECPs). Before 1990, three duties were considered part of common law: "(a) to dispense medication properly; b) to identify obvious errors in prescriptions; and (c) to take appropriate action when alerted to additional facts."[9] In the most recent Omnibus Federal OBRA 1990 bill, these duties were codified and expanded to include the duty to warn about possible interactions, proper use, common side effects, and other relevant information unless the customer declines to receive the information. Justification for the increased responsibilities of pharmacists has been made on the basis of the advanced education by pharmacists regarding prescription drugs, the rapid rate of introduction of new drugs, and the increased specialization and numbers of physicians managing a given patient, requiring increasing need for coordination of medication treatments.[9]

Educational mandates, which are included in the recent laws, can be a source of moral distress in clinical practice. How much should pharmacists educate the patient in the course of dispensing medications? How much information should pharmacists disclose about risks and benefits? How much information must they know about a patient's situation and medical issues to do "informed" dispensing? Obligations may not be limited to prescription medications but also to nonprescription and herbal medications. How active should pharmacists be in encouraging informed decision making for unproven medications? What responsibilities do pharmacists have to advocate for evidence-based decision making by their patients? These ethical dilemmas have grown as the scope of practice has expanded in relation to legal and professional mandates.[10]

Legal constraints on dispensing can also vary among states. Each pharmacist is required to understand his or her legal responsibilities in the state in which he or she practices. For instance, some states have adopted statutes that require a pharmacist to either dispense Plan B contraceptive therapy or assure the patient has timely access, even if the pharmacist has different personal moral values. Other states still restrict access.[11] Laws in many states, however, have conscience clauses that protect pharmacists and their personal values, parallel to the position statements of the ACCP (see above). The Food and Drug Administration (FDA) action to allow over-the-counter distribution of ECPs has served to protect both the woman and the pharmacist by assuring that decisions about pregnancy prevention are private and access to ECPs is more widespread. Direct dispensing by pharmacists or behind-the-counter access may still provide an ethical challenge for some professionals.

OPERATIONAL OR INSTITUTIONAL CONSTRAINTS

Other ethical conflicts occur when operational or institutional constraints limit the healthcare provider's ability to live up to his or her professional responsibilities, as happens when the pharmacist's dispensing workload doesn't allow adequate time for counseling, or when business-associated activities such as sale of nonbeneficial products go against a pharmacist's personal values.

The ethical conflict between being an agent of a company or institution and being the advocate for the patient is becoming more common. In an era of increasing managed care, formularies are commonly restricted, often with input from physicians and pharmacists and evidence-based research, but also driven by business perspectives derived from hospitals, insurance companies, or the government.[12] Indeed, this tension is a major source of what some have called moral distress in medical care: distress that occurs when professionals feel they know what is right for the patient but are blocked from doing what is right by institutional or business-based constraints.[13] Long waits, time pressures, being forced to act against one's conscience, and lack of tolerance for diverse opinions in the workplace are all cited by pharmacists as sources of moral distress.[14]

INTERPROFESSIONAL RELATIONS

The pharmacist also works within a community of medical professionals; those interprofessional relations may precipitate ethical dilemmas. How and when should the pharmacist communicate with other professionals about concerns, potential errors, and disagreements about medical management? Should s/he intervene when an uninsured patient presents an expensive prescription where a cheaper equivalent is available? Should s/he call the practitioner when s/he determines that the patient is not adherent to the prescribed medications? Should s/he dialogue with the physician during an influenza epidemic when nonindicated antibiotics are prescribed? Should s/he recommend that a patient change practitioners if s/he sees that a patient's chronic pain regimen is not allowing the patient to function adequately? These tensions are perceived as ethical issues by many pharmacists but most professionals have not received sufficient training in a process for explicitly resolving difficult scenarios that involve balancing such values as paternalism, provision of information, loyalty to the profession, loyalty to the employer, and obligations under the law.[15]

The role of the pharmacist within the team of healthcare professionals has expanded in the past 50 years as physician domination of patient management has been replaced by inclusion of many healthcare professionals in healthcare delivery.[8] Not only are patients increasingly self-educated, but pharmacist responsibilities have expanded from basic dispensing to patient counseling and education, recognition and resolution of medication related problems such as adverse events, and maintenance of patient profiles. Such books as *Our Bodies, Ourselves* have raised awareness of the uniqueness and importance of women's health since the 1970s and the locus of "authoritative knowledge" is no longer just with physicians, but has grown to include women themselves and other healthcare providers. The interdisciplinary team practice model is growing, and dialogue among professionals caring for a patient has been recognized as enhancing patient care.[16-18]

Special Considerations for Women's Health

Women who are or may become pregnant present a common setting for ethical challenges to healthcare practice. Ethical dilemmas may arise from obligations professionals might have to the fetus, as separate from the patient-mother. They may involve short-range treatment of the woman balanced against potential risk to future conception. In addition, personal values around pregnancy are strongly held and vary among persons (e.g., When does conception occur? When does life begin? Is abortion morally acceptable? What cultural or community beliefs inform provider's and patient's definition of sexual assault?). How are commonly held societal values reconciled with those of citizens (either patients or healthcare providers) who have different moral priorities? How do healthcare providers reconcile conflicts between personal moral values and professional requirements? The case on the web discusses chemotherapy during pregnancy (see Web Resources for Patient Case: Category X Medication in a Woman with Child-Bearing Capacity).

Additional content available at
www.ashp.org/womenshealth

CASE PRESENTATION

Patient Case 1: Part 1—Breast Cancer Treatments in Pregnancy

P.F. is a 32-year-old woman who presents to her medical oncologist with a left breast mass at 22 weeks of pregnancy. Pathology reports from a left breast biopsy 2 weeks prior showed an invasive ductal carcinoma, histologic grade III. P.F. had noticed the mass 1 month prior. The mass had quickly enlarged, was painful, and thought to be related to pregnancy. She experienced extreme morning sickness during weeks 6–12 of pregnancy, resulting in 11-lb weight loss. A left axillary mass was palpated on examination, consistent with a metastatic lymph node. Her family history is negative for breast cancer.

At the present time several treatment options are being considered:

1. Left modified radical mastectomy, possibly with later radiation and/or chemotherapy depending on pathologic staging of tumor.
2. Presurgical or neoadjuvant chemotherapy to be administered now, four cycles over 4 months. After delivery the following treatments may be necessary: (a) breast conservation surgical excision and axillary dissection; (b) radiation therapy of axilla; and (c) other cancer chemotherapies considered too toxic to administer during pregnancy. P.F. is eligible to receive cytotoxic chemotherapy because she is the 2nd trimester of the pregnancy and fetal exposure is less likely to increase chances of stillbirth, spontaneous abortion, or congenital abnormalities.

P.F. chooses to begin chemotherapy with doxorubicin and cyclophosphamide, four cycles at 28-day intervals. Supportive care medications for this regimen include dolasetron, metoclopramide, aprepitant, and ondansetron. The hospital pharmacist is asked to consult with the oncology team not only on the dosing but also on the overall plan for P.F.

Fetal vs. Maternal Rights

Traditional legal and philosophic opinions recognize the mother's right to make autonomous choices regarding her body. There is a strong presumption, as expressed by the most recent American College of Obstetrics and Gynecology (ACOG) Committee Opinion, of a woman's "basic rights to privacy and bodily integrity."[20] This means that women may not be forced to undergo treatments or surgery for the sake of the fetus. Forced treatment would undermine a central principle of respect for persons by requiring one person (the mother) to submit to risk for the sake of another. The pregnant woman's decisions regarding the management of her health take precedence, regardless of fetal consequences.

While some have pitted the rights of the mother against those of the fetus, most ethicists emphasize that the mother is the strongest advocate for an unborn fetus and that their interests are mutual in most instances.[20-22] It is true that respect for the mother may result in a range of outcomes, depending on her values and priorities. Her personal moral choices are rooted in societal, cultural, and or religious traditions. For some mothers, the unborn child may need to be sacrificed for the greater good of the mother. For other women, their child should be saved even at the cost of their own life.[23] Given a societal lack of consensus, P.F. and her husband may make the difficult but valid choice to abort her pregnancy in order to maximize the treatment for her cancer. If the healthcare providers cannot honor that difficult choice, s/he needs to remove self from the treating team based on personal moral beliefs.

In recent legal decisions, there has been an increasing trend to consider the fetus as an independent "patient," with rights that perhaps diverge from those of the mother. This development has been met with alarm by some women's health advocates, as it devalues the interests and rights of women and implies that third parties can advocate for the fetus better than the mother.[22] If the rights of a mother to decide on behalf of herself and her unborn child are constrained by legal "protection," her rights as an autonomous agent become constricted. Recently cases describe criminalization of maternal actions. These have included instances of maternal alcohol or drug abuse, forced Cesarean section, barring women from at-risk workplaces, and excluding women of childbearing age from drug trials that may uncover therapeutic information important to pregnant women. Some have observed that the current status of **fetal rights** is greater than that of the child after birth, citing, for instance, mandated assessment and treatment of fetal pain without a corresponding mandate in the case of painful procedures like circumcision or forceps delivery.[22] Several observers of the maternal-fetal debate have been disturbed by the observation that overriding maternal wishes through court orders and interventions by healthcare providers occurs disproportionately in low income women, and that these are the women who do not have personal relationships with their pharmacists, physicians or other healthcare providers.[22,24]

How is the healthcare provider to approach the responsibility to advocate for beneficence for both patients—mother and fetus? Making therapeutic choices in pregnancy involves balancing estimated benefits and harms for both the mother and the fetus. This medical calculus is not easy to formulate. While it can feel straightforward to present risks and benefits of therapeutic agents, they are only estimates and often not well researched, particularly in pregnancy.[25-27] While treatment of cancer may be perceived as "emergent," there are limited data on relative survival risks of waiting until after birth to initiate toxic treatments. There are likewise scant data on the effect either of the hormonal stimuli of pregnancy or the withdrawal of those stimuli on breast cancers.

In addition, healthcare providers must be aware that unknown social and community-based components of patient decision making exist. Experts have made a plea that pregnancy ethics should be based on relational theories, in which healthcare providers work to understand the situation of the pregnant woman in community. These emphasize that principle-based ethical analyses are difficult to apply to intimate relationships, as that between fetus and mother. Humility and curiosity are more appropriate for healthcare providers tempted to judge their patient. The ACOG and others have recognized the risk of healthcare provider's presumptive knowing "what is best" for medical decision making by a pregnant woman.[20,21] What appears on the surface to be a conflict that pits maternal against fetal interests may represent lack of understanding of complicated circumstances that can play strongly into maternal decision making: How desired is this pregnancy in the context of this woman's life? What other children or maternal demands on this patient exist in the family unit? What resources does this patient's community have to care for either a disabled or a motherless infant? Are the mother's and father's decisions in synchrony? Does the patient have cultural values that may differ from the ones assumed in mainstream society? Is this patient pregnant by her own father or by a man who is not her husband? What external forces may impact the mother's or fetus' situation?

Ultimately, the healthcare provider must recognize that individuals have deeply felt and varied beliefs about the relation of mother and fetus. Some see the fetus as having independent life from the time of fertilization, whereas others believe that the fetus gains independent existence at some time after birth. Some ethicists argue that the previable fetus has a dependent moral status, which exists only in so far as the mother conveys that status on the fetus and affirms her desire to protect its health-related interests. When the woman does not confer moral status on a fetus, it is very risky for healthcare providers to confer personhood and protection on a fetus over the wishes of the mother.[28] Others, particularly from other cultural origins, feel the mother/fetus relationship is one based on interdependence, both in utero and for a period after birth, with essential linkages to family units or communities.

When a pregnant patient is seemingly unwilling to cooperate with medical advice from the healthcare providers, the healthcare team should learn more about circumstances in this patient's life, seek to understand barriers to medical recommendations, and nurture "the development of health-promoting behavior."[20,21] The most problematic ethical dilemmas occur when healthcare providers face a clearly evidence-based fetal risk from dangerous maternal behavior. This is particularly hard when alcoholism, drug addiction, or other behaviors that society sees as harmful or morally ambiguous are involved. Society and healthcare providers will continue to grapple with those true ethical dilemmas in which unhealthy maternal choices truly oppose fetal interests.

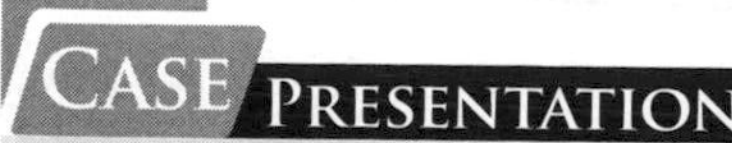

Patient Case 1: Part 2—Ethical Analysis

1. *Recognize the existence of an ethical dilemma*—How should the pharmacist and the rest of the healthcare team balance the risks to health and survival for P.F. with the risks to her unborn child? In the best case scenario, P.F. survives her cancer and her child is born healthy. At the other end of the spectrum, P.F.'s disease progresses and she dies, and her child dies or is born with medical issues arising from treatment for P.F. Many intermediate outcomes can be postulated. Should the team be aggressive with cancer treatment, delay it, or recommend pregnancy termination to be able to maximize aggressive treatment of P.F.'s breast cancer?
2. *Gather information to clarify the details of the dilemma in this particular case*—Significant facts need to be collected regarding the odds of fetal injury for the particular cytotoxic, teratogenic, and carcinogenic agents being proposed. For most of these, use in the first trimester, when organogenesis is occurring, is associated with a higher risk of birth anomalies and spontaneous abortion. However, most clinical series have not indicated a higher rate of developmental delays or cancer in offspring of women who have received chemotherapy during pregnancy (see Chapter 43: Breast Cancer). These agents are less likely to be teratogenic when administered in the 2nd and 3rd trimester, but in many cases data for use in pregnancy are incomplete. Several other questions need to be answered: Does the time period from diagnosis to delivery affect the progression of the disease? How does the risk/benefit change with the use of chemotherapeutic agents before or after delivery? What are the risks of later infertility for P.F. with various treatment options?
3. *Clarify the ethical values that are in tension*—In essence, this ethical dilemma is one of how to best assure beneficence and nonmaleficence in a difficult situation where harm is a risk with all choices. The case is best analyzed by thinking of the values held by each **stakeholder** in the problem.

   For P.F., as a mother, beneficence toward both her and her unborn child are represented by preserving both their lives. P.F. also wants protection from harm, both for her and her baby (nonmaleficence). She wishes to be respected in making an autonomous decision on her and her baby's behalf and to be given the tools (best knowledge available) to make an informed choice. She may have to make the difficult decision of whether to place her child or herself first in her priorities; she may or may not want to risk her own death for the sake of her unborn child. She might have other children to also consider. This is a difficult and complex personal decision for which P.F. deserves and needs the respect of her medical professionals.

   The unborn child's interests are for a right to a good future: healthy survival without injury from potentially hazardous compounds. The father and rest of the family have a desire for beneficence in the form of getting the best treatments possible for P.F. and their unborn baby. The father wants a healthy partner as well as a healthy baby. P.F. and her family need to rely on the expertise of the healthcare team to know what is technically best in this area of complex choices. P.F. and her family need respect for their participation in decision making, because they bring information about their own family's perception of costs (tangible and intangible) and benefits that the healthcare providers may not know.

   The healthcare team, including the pharmacist and the physicians, want to provide the best treatment and do the least harm to P.F. and to her unborn baby. They also are committed to respecting her and encouraging her to pursue the most informed decision. They do this by committing to learn as much as they can about the facts, as listed in step 2. They deserve to have their expertise and recommendations respected. This is best accomplished by dialogue with P.F. and her family, and by educating them as much as possible in making this difficult plan of action. Likewise they need to listen and learn about P.F.'s values and priorities, and to share the information—medical and nonmedical—with the healthcare team.
4. *Articulate ethical options that could resolve the moral dilemma, as well as those options which are not ethical*—The healthcare team could offer P.F. cancer treatment during the 2nd and 3rd trimesters of pregnancy, delay cancer treatment until after delivery of child, or offer to terminate the pregnancy to allow P.F. to get the most potent cancer treatment. P.F. must be made aware of what is known about the risks of her options before making a choice in order to fulfill the healthcare team's obligation to beneficence to administer chemotherapy. The choices involved in treatment decisions for P.F. are so difficult that respect for the patient requires conversation, sharing knowledge, and enhancing P.F.'s autonomous decision making ability as much as is practical. As in the case

(*Continued on next page*)

above, the Pharmacists' Code of Ethics requires recognition and encouragement of the autonomy and dignity of each patient, and compassionate respect for the patient and her ultimate decisions.[5]

5. *Choose a justifiable resolution, working with others through compromise and dialogue to respect the values of the "stakeholders" involved in the ethical dilemma and act*—The details of resolution in this case cannot be derived from this ethical analysis, but the process of decision making is key. Dialogue among the family and the healthcare team can be led by any member of the healthcare team. The goal is to reach a resolution after allowing all the parties involved (P.F., family, friends, healthcare providers) to have their voices, expertise, and values heard. There is no resolution here that does not result in the risk of some harm.

Discussion:

Ultimately P.F. and her husband have nonmedical knowledge and personal values that, along with medical information, will inform their decision. The healthcare team may not be aware of P.F.'s financial situation, personal support available during treatments, beliefs regarding abortion, the impact on other children or plans to have more children, or how other family members would be affected by the various options. In care-oriented ethics, family particularities need to become explicit and respected as key to arriving at a plan of care. The process of sharing values and justification for medical choices is important for all involved (for family and professionals). It helps them all "buy in" to support each other through the difficult times ahead.

Pharmaceutical Research in Pregnancy

A related ethical dilemma facing healthcare providers in a case like this is the lack of research information about the risks and benefits of therapies for pregnant women. But the lack of knowledge about drug effects in pregnancy is concerning because the pharmacokinetics, complications and benefits can be different for the pregnant woman as well as the fetus. Many drug trials exclude pregnant women or those of childbearing age, resulting in a knowledge gap in such important areas of women's health as treating mental illnesses, epilepsy, or cancer.[29,30] Both treatment and nontreatment hold potential risks in pregnancy. Federal regulations rightly insert additional protections for pregnant women and their fetuses in the conduct of research. The researchers evaluating medication effects during pregnancy must understand the fetal-maternal issues discussed above and be ready to accept maternal wishes in such high risk treatment situations. Paradoxically, recognition of the fetus as a person is necessary before responsible pharmacologic research protocols can be developed. For example, the mother needs to be able to decide about the subsequent course of her pregnancy if there are adverse consequences to the fetus, including the right to access a legal abortion. While it is easiest to protect women by excluding them from clinical trials, such decisions are paternalistic and not without ethical risks. Both patients and their healthcare providers must recognize the current uncertainty for many therapeutic agents with regard to pregnancy risk and develop mechanisms for answering safety questions that allow women to avoid, when possible, the kind of difficult therapeutic decisions faced in this case.[28,29]

CASE PRESENTATION

Patient Case 2: Part 1—Emergency Contraception and the Pharmacist

S.B. is a 21-year-old college student who presents to the consultation window at her local community pharmacy at 9 p.m. on a Monday evening. S.B. explains that she wants to purchase the "morning after pill" and wants to know how to take it properly. She explains that she and her boyfriend had celebrated their anniversary on Saturday and during sexual intercourse the condom broke. She is not on the pill because of a history of deep vein thrombosis on oral contraceptive pills (OCPs) at age 18 years. She is very worried about getting pregnant and how mad her parents would be if she had to drop out of school. The pharmacist looks at the clock and is reminded that she is only one hour into her twelve hour shift and is the only pharmacist on duty with two technicians. The pile of prescriptions that needs to be addressed is getting higher. The pharmacist knows that if S.B. is to use Plan B with the greatest chance of success she needs to use it soon. This pharmacy is the only 24-hour pharmacy in a small rural college area; the other local pharmacies are now closed. The pharmacist has been well educated on dispensing Plan B through several continuing education programs sponsored by her employer. The pharmacist objects to dispensing this medication on religious grounds, because she relates the use of Plan B to a medication induced abortion.

(*Continued on next page*)

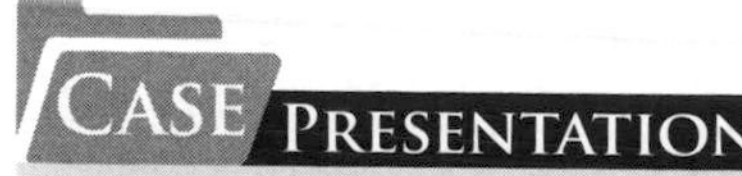

Case Presentation

Patient Case 2: Part 2—Ethical Analysis

1. *Recognize the existence of an ethical dilemma*—The pharmacist feels that Plan B is a form of abortion and she is morally opposed to dispensing this medication and contributing to the possible termination of an unborn child. She is being asked as a professional to do something that she finds morally objectionable. Should she refuse to dispense Plan B? Should she refer S.B. to another pharmacy? Should she fill the prescription over her own moral concerns?
2. *Gather information to clarify the various details of the dilemma in this particular case (much of the situation detail is already in the case presentation)*—Pertinent clinical information includes the particulars noted above, including the fact that S.B. is an adult who has been trying to avoid pregnancy, is unable to use OCPs, and is relatively young and a student. The situational details about alternative access to Plan B are key to balancing patient autonomy with the pharmacist's personal beliefs: What alternative options does S.B. have to access ECPs? Are other pharmacies open? Is there a physician or family planning clinic available to dispense for her in a timely fashion? Does S.B. have transportation allowing her to get Plan B from another source?
   - *Mechanism of action of Plan B*—The exact mechanism of Plan B is unknown. It may work by inhibiting or delaying ovulation, interfering with tubal transport or inhibiting implantation.[31,32] It does not interfere with an established pregnancy, which begins (as currently defined in society) as expressed by federal regulations and ACOG at implantation of the blastocyte on the endometrium.[31] It does not cause the abortion of an implanted or established pregnancy as RU-486 or other abortifacients do. Because Plan B may work in some women to prevent implantation after fertilization, pregnancy prevention after unprotected intercourse may be ethically problematic for persons who consider that life begins with fertilization of the ovum. However, emergency contraception (EC) is comparable to other forms of hormonal contraception, such as OCPs, the transdermal patch, the vaginal ring, and the progestin-containing IUD, which inhibit ovulation but may also prevent implantation (see Chapter 19: Hormonal Contraception).

     Plan B is more efficacious the sooner it is used following unprotected intercourse, although its actual effectiveness continues to be debated in the literature.[32-34] It is effective when used within 120 hours of the unprotected act although FDA approval is for only 72 hours postintercourse. No laboratory tests or physical examination are recommended prior to use, as Plan B has no effect on an established pregnancy.[31] Pharmacists must be well versed in the scientific facts about ECPs in order to avoid perpetuating myths for themselves and their patients; deficits in pharmacists' understanding are not uncommon and have contributed to confusion in the public debate.[35-37]
   - *Legal obligations*—The FDA in 2006 approved over-the-counter availability for Plan B to women over the age of 17 years; however, pharmacist participation is required because ECPs are stocked behind the counter and patient identification must be checked before purchase. If a girl is under 18 years old, she must present a prescription for ECPs. Some states have provisions that allow pharmacist dispensation to minors without physician prescriptions under collaborative practice agreements or state protocols. Several states have developed laws to protect pharmacists' right to refuse to dispense ECPs, while others have laws mandating dispensing.[11,31] The pharmacist must be aware of the laws in her/his particular state or other state-based directives regarding S.B.'s rights to obtain ECPs and the pharmacist's duty to dispense.
   - *Professional codes*—The Pharmacist Code of Ethics states that the pharmacist is obligated to "place concern for the well-being of the patient at the center of professional practice" and to promote "the right of self-determination."[5] If the pharmacist does not dispense Plan B, S.B. will have to wait another 12 hours until another pharmacy opens, theoretically decreasing the efficacy of Plan B. Such a delay may also change the mechanism of action of the EC, increasing the chances that Plan B works postfertilization.[33] If S.B. does not receive Plan B, her chance of becoming pregnant is increased and, from her interaction with the pharmacist, it seems that she does not feel she is ready to mother a child in her current circumstances. Such an outcome might force S.B. to face choices about abortion—a decision she may not have had to make if given Plan B. Both of these "unintended" consequences may be important in the pharmacist's moral system.

(*Continued on next page*)

However, a 2005 position paper from ACCP, *Prerogative of a Pharmacist to Decline to Provide Professional Services Based on Conscience,* affirms the right of pharmacists to "decline to personally participate in situations involving legally sanctioned provision and/or use of medications and related devices or services that conflict with that pharmacist's moral, ethical or religious beliefs."[7] The paper acknowledges the professional responsibility to assure that the patient wanting legally permissible services be referred in such a way that she can receive such services in "an effective, professional, timely, confidential, and nonjudgmental manner."[7]

- *Contractual obligations*—The agreement between the pharmacist and employer or between the employer and the public is unknown. Has the pharmacist agreed to work at a pharmacy that commits to dispensing Plan B? Has the pharmacist committed to working shifts without another pharmacist or when other pharmacies are not open? Does the pharmacist's pharmacy advertise itself as providing all women's health services? Does the pharmacy restrict dispensing for certain pharmacotherapeutics? What does the pharmacy have to say about how to resolve potential conflicts between its pharmacists' values and patient values?

3. *What are the ethical values that are in tension in the dilemma?*—This case provides an example of the central conflict between the patient's right to obtain treatment (i.e., patient autonomy) and the pharmacist's personal values. Likewise, the conflict between professional duties and personal morals is central for the pharmacist. Secondary questions—Who gets to decide what is "beneficent" or "good" for this patient or whether Plan B "harms" the patient? as well as the question of whether denying the patient's request constitutes "obstruction" of her rights, as defined by the law.[36]
4. *What are options for resolving the ethical dilemma?*—1) Tell S.B. to come back when another pharmacist is on duty; 2) refer S.B. to another pharmacy; 3) dispense Plan B as S.B. requests; and 4) call supervisor or colleague who would dispense Plan B. None of these options are win-win resolutions of the ethical dilemma. To choose the first or second course of action and ask S.B. to either return or go to another pharmacy (when it is open) poses several problems. Plan B is less efficacious the more delay there is in taking it after unprotected intercourse. The patient may not have transportation. For some pharmacists, even referring S.B. to an in-house colleague or another pharmacist is considered a breach of personal values. The third course of action that the pharmacist could take is to put aside her own moral/religious convictions and dispense the Plan B. For some professionals, separating and constraining those personal values while in their professional roles is acceptable; they emphasize instead the moral value of respect for their patients, employer and societal standards. For some, however, this compromise of personal moral values could be unacceptable and could put the pharmacist at odds with religious tradition, family, and friends. The fourth course of action is for the pharmacist to call her supervisor and tell her that she can not dispense the medication and request her assistance. This option could have negative consequences for the pharmacist employer relationship, particularly if the pharmacist had not discussed this with the employer previously so that a contingency plan for such circumstances could have been developed. In this rural town it is also possible that the supervisor lives far away and it would take time to respond, also delaying treatment. On the other hand, such a call would assure that S.B. receives the medication in a timely fashion without undue inconvenience or direct compromise of the pharmacist's moral values.

   Unacceptable options would include refusing to dispense without offering a realistic alternative that would assure S.B. timely access to EC. Likewise, it is not acceptable for the pharmacist to impose personal values on S.B. by trying to convince S.B. that ECPs are immoral and she should carry this pregnancy instead. This would fail to respect S.B. or the pharmacist's fiduciary responsibilities to put her patient first. Despite knowing some details of S.B.'s narrative, it is presumptuous and unprofessional for the pharmacist as a pharmacist to assume that personal values can be imposed on others, especially when S.B.'s values are legally protected and access to ECPs are is legally protected in society.
5. *Choosing a reasonable resolution and working with others to move forward*—The pharmacist will have to decide if personal values can be put aside to help S.B. as the patient has requested or not. If the pharmacist cannot, the pharmacist needs to be responsible to see that S.B. is "referred to another pharmacist or other healthcare provider in an effective, professional, timely, confidential, and nonjudgmental manner."[7]

(*Continued on next page*)

Most crucial to solving this ethical dilemma is to prevent it. Resolution should occur at an individual and at a policy level. As the ACCP position statement supporting conscientious refusal to be involved in providing services that conflict with personal moral beliefs states, the pharmacist "is responsible for prospectively informing colleagues and employers" as well as others at the practice setting about situations that would create conflict.[7] The pharmacist should have clarified the professional expectations before starting the position, as well as the state and federal legal policies that govern pharmacy practice. The pharmacist must discern the extent and limits of individual ability to "bracket" personal values in the current employment situation. The pharmacist could negotiate an agreement with the employer to only be on duty with another pharmacist willing to serve this need, or seeking employment where Plan B is not dispensed. The FDA decision to make Plan B over-the-counter has expanded access to ECPs for women 18 years and older but has not eliminated the need for participation by pharmacists. In some states, legal mandates may also constrain the pharmacist's options to either dispense or refuse to dispense.[11]

Discussion:

The debate about how to resolve ethical conflicts between patient needs and personal values of healthcare providers has dominated public healthcare debate recently. When do the patient's autonomy and respect for her perceived medical needs trump the healthcare provider's values? What are the extents or the limits of professional duties if they conflict with personal values? These are questions that professional organizations and society as a whole are grappling with, particularly as society increasingly emphasizes religious or moral values and individual rights. In an essay, a prominent lawyer and a lawyer-physician articulated the most prominent arguments on each side of this debate.[36] Their discussion was subsequently debated widely in the pharmacy literature.[38] The points elucidated by these professionals and others need to be understood to move toward solutions for these difficult ethical dilemmas.

Arguments Supporting a Pharmacist Obligation to Dispense ECPs

The Code of Ethics for pharmacists affirms a "covenantal" obligation that puts the well-being of the patient central. This articulation of the fiduciary duty requires respect for the patient's autonomy even when personal and cultural values vary among patients.[5,36,38] A *New York Times* editorial promoted the argument that entering the profession of pharmacy is a choice, and "any pharmacist who cannot dispense medicines lawfully prescribed by a doctor should find another line of work."[39] The monopoly or guild nature of pharmacy and medical practice also argues for a special duty to patients.[4] The professional's duty to honor autonomous patient wishes is particularly compelling in situations where alternative access is not readily available. The community pharmacist may not be permitted as much freedom when presented with patient requests as colleagues who have practices where they can avoid situations not in alignment with their values. Analogous issues exist for physicians; gynecologists may be able to limit their practice to avoid performing abortions if they wish, but emergency medicine specialists, who cannot select their patients, do not have the same ethical claim to limit prescribing ECPs to women who walk in without choice about who attends them and with an expectation that their needs will be honored. Obligations to the patient increase when patient options are limited.[40]

Arguments which focus on the harm done to women's health as a consequence of refusal to provide ECPs emphasize that it is a time-sensitive medication and that the consequence of an unintended pregnancy may be abortion. Barriers to access differentially affect poor and rural women who may not have alternatives available in a timely fashion.[36] In the case of ECPs, the alternative of safe and timely referral may not be a practical option.[40]

Arguments can also be made from consideration of the pharmacist's professional role in healthcare delivery. Philosophers, physicians, and pharmacists have argued that the pharmacist does not have sufficient information to be making independent judgments about the appropriateness of medications and to override a legitimate prescription by another professional.[41] The ECPs are not abortifacients and some have even suggested that those who oppose ECPs either do not understand its proposed mechanisms or are expressing a desire to punish women for sexual activity.[36,37,40-42] Indeed, because all contraceptives have virtually the same spectrum of mechanisms of actions, arguments based on mechanism are often due to misunderstanding of the science. Writers in a leading medical journal warn of the potential for abuse if pharmacists are allowed to refuse to fill prescriptions (the "slippery slope" of injecting personal judgments on patients' conduct). Exercising personal moral values by professional pharmacists could lead to the option of refusing to dispense OCPs to unmarried women, condoms or erectile dysfunction treatments to unmarried men, or oral hypoglycemics for obese patients who won't lose weight.[4,37]

Arguments Supporting Pharmacist Refusal to Dispense ECPs

Each healthcare provider is a moral agent and should not be required to abandon values in the workplace or as part of professional commitment. Pharmacists are professionals and, as such, function as independent members of the healthcare team. One argument is that pharmacists are moral agents, even if their situation "at the counter" is fraught with uncertainty and a dearth of information with which to judge the propriety of a prescribed drug and the potential for patient abuse. Pharmacists should be held "accountable for their choices and entitled—within limits—to decide in which activities they will participate."[37] Another rallying cry for the right to refuse states, "Healthcare without conscience—unconscionable!"[43]

The right to object or refuse to participate in certain situations for reasons of conscience is a longstanding core value of society. As one editorialist points out, it would be ironic if promotion of personal choice for the patient is offset by denying such choice to the pharmacist.[36] And it is clear that healthcare providers have the right and obligation to say "no" to some requests by patients. The fiduciary duty to put the patient's needs and wishes first is not unlimited. Healthcare providers cannot be asked to perform duties that result in death or serious harm to their patient or to another. Pharmacy duties not required include early refill for opioids that are being dispensed in a pattern suggesting abuse; honoring requests for large amounts of pseudoephedrine suggesting manufacture of amphetamines; dispensing erythropoietin to bicycle racers; or filling a prescription for large doses of sedatives suggesting that the patient may wish to attempt suicide. The justification for these limits is that healthcare providers do not consider dispensing in such circumstances to be in the patient's best interest (beneficence) but instead to risk harm. Pharmacists who do not believe in birth control can rightly say that what is considered of benefit to the patient may not be considered beneficial within their personal value system. Indeed, some pharmacists and physicians argue that ECPs encourage irresponsible sexual behavior (unprotected intercourse), and there is little evidence that ECPs decrease the rate of unintended pregnancies or reduce abortion rates.[33,34]

Toward Resolving the Ethical Dilemma About Emergency Contraception

Virtually the same ethical dilemmas apply to the dispensing of ECPs as to dispensing other contraceptive methods. This essential element in resolving the ethical dilemma is rooted in correct understanding of the physiology of contraception, a professional obligation of each healthcare provider. The use of contraception after intercourse remains, however, more intuitively problematic for some people. Where is the common ground between those who would mandate dispensing of ECPs by pharmacists and those who support refusal? Clearly there is common ground that must be emphasized in any reasoned dialogue:

- Patients deserve respect in responding to their healthcare needs and should be at the center of decision making about their own health.
- U.S. society is diverse where people disagree about fundamental concepts of when life begins and the status of the fetus before it is viable.
- Pharmaceutical practice involves duties to patients that may conflict with duties to self.
- Laws must be obeyed and contracts must be honored in healthcare practice.
- Conscientious objection is a traditional core societal right.
- Prospective planning to avoid situations in which a conflict between patient needs and personal beliefs will occur is part of the professional duty of the healthcare provider whenever possible.
- Refusal to provide professional services based on conscience, while protected, may incur consequences for the healthcare provider in terms of what employment situations are possible and what are not.
- Discrimination, injustice, or abuse of other humans cannot be supported, even in a culturally diverse society, because justice and equality are core values.[44]

Societal values are evolving. As noted by one lawyer observing these trends, "With autonomy and rights as the preeminent social values comes a devaluing of relationships and a diminution of the difference between our personal lives and our professional duties."[45] From common values such as the above, the healthcare professions and society as a whole need to continue to dialogue about how to respect each other and work with integrity to support the community as well as individual and professional integrity.[42] State and federal statutes may be required to affirm common values and to protect the patient, but the autonomous patient's right to receive services is not absolute. Some instances are outside of society's legally protected and ethical understanding of acceptable behavior. Addiction, suicide, and drug abuse are not supported. In such situations, the pharmacist can and should refuse dispensing or should initiate actions to confirm a physician's intent and a patient's diagnosis. In contrast, society at present accepts a wide range of reproductive preferences by women. The state does not intervene in prevention of pregnancy or reproductive options in the first or second trimester. In such a society, can it be tolerable for healthcare providers to be "barriers" to legally and socially acceptable health-seeking behavior by their patients?[36]

Narrative ethics emphasizes the importance of listening empathetically to the patient's story. It reminds healthcare providers that humility is a key to counterbalancing temptation to judge patients. Two prominent ethicists warn that the context for clinical decision making is often complex and beyond the scope of questioning possible at the community pharmacy counter.[41] Is this unprotected intercourse the result of condom failure, sexual assault, abuse by a parent/relative, or an out of control alcohol-fueled party? How do you clarify and judge the validity of such options at the point of interaction? Suspending judgment and acknowledging uncertainty in understanding of the origins of a woman's needs is often required.

Summary

A structured explicit framework allows healthcare providers to recognize ethical dilemmas and proceed to analyze them, recognizing the professional values that may conflict, as well as personal values, laws, contractual commitments, and interprofessional relationships that may impact deliberations. Women's health is an area where ethical dilemmas are not uncommon and it provides a rich arena for practicing the ethical reflection that is required throughout everyone's personal and professional lives. In many cases the process is either as important or more important than the answer. Virtuous healthcare providers grapple with these difficult and humbling problems, even as they come to different solutions in their personal and professional lives. Core values include respecting the patient, honoring the values of all who care for her through empathetic listening, recognizing the value of the community and of relationships in healthcare, balancing risks and benefits in an increasingly complex therapeutic environment, and recognizing the nonmedical values that enter into a patient's decision making. The commitment is to take healthcare provider covenants seriously by being patient-centered in all efforts to promote women's health.[5]

References

Additional content available at
www.ashp.org/womenshealth

Glossary

Abruption of the placenta—Condition in which the placenta separates prematurely from the wall of the uterus.

Acetylcholinesterase—A protein found in the central nervous system that leaks into the amniotic fluid in fetuses with an open neural tube defect.

Acrosome—The part of the head of the sperm, derived from the Golgi complex which produces enzymes that help the sperm penetrate the egg.

Acrosome reaction—Fusion of parts of the acrosomal membrane and the plasma membrane of the egg that liberates the enzymes stored in the acrosome.

Acute coronary syndrome—An umbrella term that includes any group of clinical symptoms consistent with acute myocardial ischemia.

Add-back therapy—Hormone replacement therapy, in which various (steroid) agents are combined with GnRH agonists, in order to maintain a therapeutic response and prevent potential adverse effects of GnRH agonist treatment in patients with endometriosis.

Adenomyosis—Uterine thickening that occurs when endometrial tissue, which normally lines the uterus, moves into the outer muscular walls of the uterus. The presence of ectopic endometrial tissue (tissue that lines the inner lining of the uterus) within the myometrium (outer walls of the uterus muscular layer); causes painful and/or profuse menses.

Adnexa—The region of pelvis including ovaries, fallopian tubes, broad ligament, and structures within the broad ligament.

Ageism—Stereotyping, prejudice or discrimination on the basis of age.

Alcohol use disorders identification test (AUDIT)—12 question screening tool used to obtain more qualitative information about alcohol consumption.

Allele—Any of the alternate forms that one gene can take, such as dominant or recessive.

Allen-Masters syndrome—Pelvic pain resulting from an old laceration of the broad ligament received during delivery.

Allograft—A tissue or organ harvested from one individual and transplanted to another individual of the same species with a different genotype.

Alopecia—Loss of hair from head or body.

ALTO—Internal radiation administered via tandem and ovoid insertion.

Ambulatory reflux monitoring—A test used in a patient to record the frequency, timing and duration of abnormal reflux.

Amenorrhea—Absence or abnormal cessation of the menses.

Amnion—An extra embryonic membrane that that forms a fluid-filled sac.

Anastomosis—Surgical union of parts.

Anencephaly—Congenital neural tube defect that occurs when the cephalic end of the neural tube fails to close resulting in the absence of a major portion of the brain, skull, and scalp.

Aneuploidy—An alteration in the number of chromosomes.

Angiogenesis—Development of blood vessels.

Anorgasmia—Persistent inability to achieve orgasm with adequate sexual arousal or activity.

Anovulation—Failure, absence, or suspension of ovulation frequently noted by an absence of menstrual cycles.

Anterior drawer test—Patient is positioned on her/his back with the knee in 90 degrees of flexion with the foot firmly on the table. The provider puts pressure on the shin with both hands and tries to move the shin forward. A positive test for anterior cruciate ligament injury is abnormal looseness of the knee.

Antinuclear antibodies—Antibodies directed against various nuclear components, including histone proteins, nucleosomes, RNA, and DNA. The staining pattern associated with the antinuclear antibodies, homogeneous, diffuse, nucleolar, or peripheral are associated (though not diagnostic) for different autoimmune diseases.

Apgar scores—A method to assess the health of a newborn immediately after childbirth based on appearance, pulse, grimace, activity, and respiration.

Apolipoprotein A1—A lipoprotein found in high density lipoprotein particles and prevents the accumulation of cholesterol loaded macrophages into the arterial wall as foam cells.

Apoptosis—A form of cell death in which a programmed sequence of events leads to the elimination of unnecessary or abnormal cells.

ASC—Atypical squamous cells.

ASG—Atypical glandular cell of uncertain significance.

Asherman's syndrome—A condition characterized by the presence of scars within the uterine cavity commonly caused by trauma or infection.

Atresia—Congenital absence or closure of normal tubular structure.

Autograft—Transplant tissue from one area in the body to another area in the same individual.

Autonomy—The ethical principle that asserts an individual's right to self-determination

Axis I disorder—Any mental health diagnosis (excluding personality disorders) such as depression, anxiety disorders, schizophrenia, phobias, etc.

Bartholin gland ducts—Glands located on both sides of the vagina at the bottom. They help to lubricate the vagina.

Basal body temperature (BBT)—Temperature measured immediately upon awakening and before any physical activity takes place

Beneficence—The ethical principle that requires that benefits to others be maximized and harms minimized.

Bidis—Flavored, unfiltered cigarettes imported from India. They come in many flavors including chocolate, vanilla, cherry, licorice, menthol, and mango, which appeal to youth. Mistakenly believed to be safe, Bidis are just as likely or more likely to produce the health risks associated with cigarettes.

Bilateral salpingo-oophorectomy—Surgical removal of the fallopian tubes and ovaries.

Bisexual—An identity label used by some people whose emotional and sexual attractions are for both women and men.

Blastocyst—The embryonic stage that follows the morula. It is a spherical mass of cells having a central, fluid filled cavity surrounded by a single layer of cells.

Blastomeres—Cells that make up the blastocyst.

Body mass index (BMI)—An individual's body weight divided by the square of their height; this term frequently is used to describe how an individual's weight varies from the desired range.

Brachytherapy—Radiotherapy in which the source of irradiation is placed close to the surface of the body or within the body cavity.

B-type natriuretic peptide—A 32-amino-acid polypeptide secreted in response to excessive stretching of muscle cells in the ventricles of the heart. Concentrations are increased in patients with left ventricular dysfunction.

CAGE—A four-question tool used to screen for alcohol problems over the lifetime. Two positive answers are considered a positive test requiring additional assessment.

Capacitated sperm—Postejaculation sperm that have been made capable of fertilizing an egg through a process of sperm maturation in the female reproductive tract.

Carcinogenesis—Production or origin of cancer.

Cardiomyopathy—Disease of the heart muscle.

Care-oriented ethics—An approach to ethics that is concerned with the context of moral actions rather than abstractions. Care-based ethics particularly focus on relationships and attachments between healthcare professionals and patients and what these mean for moral life and ethical dilemma resolution.

Carotid endarterectomy—Surgical procedure that removes stenosing plaques from the carotid arteries, reducing stroke risk.

Catamenial epilepsy—Seizures which occur more frequently around the time of menses.

Catamenial—Menstrual.

Cervical cerclage—A suture placed with around the cervix.

Cervical ripening—Biochemical changes in the cervix that gradually take place over the pregnancy.

Cholelithiasis—A solid formation in the gallbladder or bile duct composed of cholesterol and bile salts, also known as gallstone.

Chorioamnionitis—Inflammation of the fetal membranes indicating intrauterine infection.

Chorion—The outermost of the extraembryonic membranes that is the fetal contribution to the placenta.

Chorionic villus sampling—An invasive diagnostic test that may be performed in the first trimester between 10 and 13 completed weeks. Fetal tissue for chromosomal analysis may be obtained by either a transcervical or a transabdominal approach.

Clinical institute withdrawal assessment of alcohol scale (CIWA-AR)—A validated scale used to assess the severity of alcohol withdrawal symptoms. Patients with a score of 8–15 would benefit from pharmacotherapy and a score greater than 15 are at risk for significant complications if not treated with pharmacotherapy.

Coarctation of the aorta—Narrowing of the aorta between the upper-body artery branches and the branches to the lower body.

Cosmesis—Effect of procedure on appearance or external beauty.

Cognitive behavioral therapy—A form of psychotherapy based on cognitions, assumptions, beliefs, and behaviors with the aim of influencing negative emotions that relate to inaccurate appraisal of events.

Colposcopy—Examination of the vagina and cervical tissues by using magnifying lens (colposcope).

Combined hormonal regimen—A form of EC that utilizes a combination of estrogen and progestin containing pills.

Conceptus—The fertilized egg.

Confidentiality—A duty of particular importance in health professional and patient relationships that requires the protection of the patient's private information.

Confounding—A type of bias that occurs when two factors are closely associated and the effects of one confuses or distorts the effects of the other factor on the outcome. The distorting factor is a confounding variable.

Congenital rubella syndrome—A constellation of complications such as small head circumference, low birth weight, mental disabilities, deafness, and seizures that occur in a developing fetus of a pregnant woman who contracts rubella in her first trimester.

Conscientious objection—The right to refuse to participate in acts that conflict with personal ethical, moral, or religious convictions.

Contraception—The prevention of pregnancy.

Co-occurring disorders—Patients with comorbid psychiatric- and substance-use disorders are often known as having co-occurring disorders.

Coronary heart disease—Heart disease due to an impaired perfusion of the arteries that supply blood and oxygen to the heart.

C-reactive protein—An acute phase reactant used as a general screening aid for inflammatory diseases, infections, and neoplastic diseases. Studies have suggested that higher concentrations are associated with increased cardiovascular risk.

Cultural humility—A process that requires an individual to continually engage in self-reflection and self-critique as a life-long learner to bring into check the power imbalances that exist in the dynamics of communication by using patient-focused interviewing and care.

Culture—The learned and shared knowledge that specific groups use to generate behavior and interpret their experience of the world; also a set of beliefs, customs, values, and experiences, as well as manners of communication, concepts of identity, relationships, and roles in society.

Curandera—A lay healer in Hispanic or Latino communities who possesses special wisdom and knowledge about healing with traditional methods.

Curettage—Scraping of tissue.

Decidualization—The procedure of enlargement of endometrial stromal cells into round cells surrounded by a membrane, which forms scaffolding for trophoblast attachment.

Deep vein thrombosis—A condition marked by the formation of a clot within a deep vein.

Deformations—Abnormalities due to an abnormal external (mechanical) force on an

Deontology—The theory of duties based on respect for persons and promise keeping regardless of the consequences. Deontology holds that certain aspects of actions are inherently right or wrong.

Diabetic ketoacidosis—Complication of diabetes in which chemical balance of body is too acidic.

Dilatation and curettage (D&C)—Dilatation of the cervix and scraping of the endometrium for the removal of growths, abnormal tissues, or to obtain material for diagnosis.

Disability—Physical and mental limitations that result from a variety of health problems and make it more difficult to perform normal daily activities.

Disparity—Differences in quality of care not due to clinical need or patient preferences, instead attributable to differences in healthcare operations and potentially discrimination, biases, stereotyping and uncertainty.

Dizygotic—Multiple gestations arising from separate embryos.

DMT—Disease modifying therapy, often used in multiple sclerosis treatment, includes interferon-β, glatiramer acetate, and mitoxantrone.

Douglas pouch—A sac or recess formed by a fold of the pelvic peritoneum; the anterior surface of the uterus and the bladder (anterior Douglas pouch), and the posterior surface of the uterus and the rectum (posterior Douglas pouch).

Dual diagnosis—Another term for co-occurring disorders.

Dumping syndrome—A condition characterized by weakness, dizziness, flushing and warmth, nausea, and palpitation immediately or shortly after eating and produced by abnormally rapid emptying of the stomach, particularly in individuals who have had part of the stomach removed.

Dyschezia—Difficulty in defecation.

Dysmenorrhea—Difficult and painful menstruation.

Dysmorphology—The study of the etiology, prevention, treatment, and prognosis of birth.

Dyspareunia—Pain during sexual intercourse.

Dystocia—A difficult labor and is characterized by an abnormally slow progress of labor.

Dystopia—Malposition or displacement of any organ.

Eclampsia—General tonic clonic seizures without other etiology occurring in women with preeclampsia.

Ectocervix—Is part of the cervix next to the vagina.

Ectopic pregnancy—A pregnancy that occurs outside of the uterus, most commonly in the fallopian tubes.

Effacement—Thinning of the uterine cervix.

Electrocardioversion—An abnormally fast heart rate (cardiac arrhythmia) is corrected by the administration of an electric current to the heart during a specific part of the cardiac cycle.

Embolism—The sudden obstruction of a blood vessel by an embolus.

Embryoblast—The inner cell mass of the blastocyst that will become the embryo itself.

Embryopathy—A developmental abnormality of an embryo or fetus especially when caused by a disease in the mother.

Emergency contraception—(EC) a postcoital form of contraception that may be used within a specified time after intercourse to prevent pregnancy (e.g., when a woman recognizes that her regular contraceptive method has failed or if she has not used any method of contraception).

Emotional work—Efforts made by women to make others (e.g., coworkers, clients, family members) comfortable and happy, oftentimes to the detriment of their own health and wellbeing. Emotional work often begins with a heightened social awareness of others' desires and needs but leads to small and not so small extra efforts to be sure others' comforts are assured.

Empathy—The ability to be emotionally sensitive to or understanding of another, or to see a patient's problems from the patient's perspective. Empathy is contrasted by some with detachment (cognitive without emotional understanding of a patient) or with sympathy, which involves embracing the patient's emotional state and merging the patient's problems with the professional's emotions.

Endocervix—Part of the cervix closet to the body of the uterus.

Endometrial hyperplasia—An increase in the number of normal cells in the mucous membrane comprising the inner layer of the uterine wall.

Endometrial polyps—Abnormal benign growths that can protrude from the lining of the uterus.

Endometrioma—Ovarian cyst with endometriotic content.

Endometriosis—A condition in which the endometrial tissue, which makes up the uterine lining, grows outside the uterus; causes dysmenorrhea and metrorrhagia.

Endometritis—Refers to inflammation of the lining of the uterus, often caused by infection, or the presence of bacteria. Symptoms may include lower abdominal pain and abnormal vaginal bleeding or discharge.

Endomyometritis—Infection which occurs postpartum involving the endometrium, myometrium, and parametrial tissues characterized by maternal temperature elevation, and uterine tenderness.

Erectile dysfunction—A persistent inability to achieve or maintain an erection sufficient to accomplish a desired sexual behavior such as coitus to orgasm. Earlier known as impotence.

Erosive esophagitis—Inflammation of the esophagus due to acid reflux.

ESR—Erythrocyte sedimentation rate, a marker of inflammation that is often used to monitor response to therapy in inflammatory disorders.

Ethical dilemma—A conflict between two moral goods or two equally unappealing moral alternatives.

Ethics—A branch of philosophy that provides insight and justification into what is right or wrong, good or bad, or obligatory in human relationships.

Eye movement desensitization and reprocessing—A comprehensive, integrative psychotherapy approach containing elements of many effective psychotherapies in structured protocols that are designed to maximize treatment effects. These include psychodynamic, cognitive behavioral, interpersonal, experiential, and body-centered therapies. EMDR is an information processing therapy and uses an eight-phase approach to address the experiential contributors of a wide range of pathologies. It addresses the past experiences that have set the foundation for pathology, the current situations that trigger dysfunctional emotions, beliefs and sensations, and the positive experience needed to enhance future adaptive behaviors and mental health.

Factor V Leiden deficiency—The most common hereditary coagulation disorder in the U.S., which is associated with over a threefold risk of venous thrombosis in heterozygotes and an over 30-fold risk among homozygotes.

Facultative parasite—An organism that my live with or without a patient (host) support.

Fecundity—The capacity to conceive in a given period of time (usually one ovulation cycle) and to reproduce.

Feminist ethics—An approach to bioethics that looks at the power inequality in society between those with a special expertise (e.g., healthcare providers) and patients, between men and women, and between the dominant cultural norms and those emphasized in other communities and cultures.

Fenestration—Surgical technique for the removal endometriomas.

Fertility—The ability to reproduce (attain a pregnancy).

Fetal blood sampling (FBS)—An invasive procedure performed under direct ultrasound guidance using a spinal needle, which is placed directly into the umbilical vein or hepatic vein to obtain fetal blood. Fetal blood may be sent for fetal karyotype or other laboratory studies.

Fetal rights—Claims of beneficence and nonmaleficence made on behalf of an unborn baby.

Fibromyalgia—Chronic widespread pain involving all four quadrants of the body and the presence of 11 of 11 tender points on examination.

Fiduciary relationship—A relationship in which a person in a position of trust or responsibility has specific duties to act in the best interest of another, who is often vulnerable or dependent on the integrity of that professional.

Fistula—An abnormal connection between intestinal and adjacent structures as a result of inflammation.

Fitz-Hugh-Curtis syndrome—A rare complication of PID that involves a perihepatitis as a result of inflammation and scarring.

Follicular phase—Phase occurring during the first half of menstrual cycle (days 10–14).

Fourchette—The location where the labia minora meet behind the vestibule.

FTM—Acronym for female-to-male transgender or transsexual person. Also *trans man*. Typically referred to with male pronouns (he, him).

Gametes—The sex cells ovum (i.e., eggs) and sperm.

Gametogenesis—The production of eggs or sperm by the process of meiosis.

Gastroesophageal reflux disease—A highly variable chronic condition that is characterized by periodic episodes of gastroesophageal reflux usually accompanied by heartburn and that may result in histopathologic changes in the esophagus.

Gastroschisis—Congenital fissure of the ventral abdominal wall.

Gastrulation—An early stage in development during which differentiation begins by the formation of three germ layers: ectoderm, endoderm, and mesoderm.

Gelling—Joint stiffness following rest or decreased activity level.

Gender—The nonbiological aspects of being a woman or man, such as ideas, traits, behaviors, dress, actions, and roles. These aspects and expectations can be created by social, cultural, environmental, and personal influences.

Gender expression—An individual's presentation of their gender through clothing, behavior, mannerisms, etc.

Gender identity—A person's sense of being a woman or man, irrespective of biological sex.

Gender norm—A rule or set of rules that instruct women and men about how they should think, act, dress, talk, etc. Because gender norms are widely adopted social rules, they are enforced and people who break the rules are usually punished in some way. For example, it is a gender norm that women are supposed to be mothers or are better caregivers than men. Another gender norm is that women should be thin; thus, beauty norms are gender norms.

Gender presentation—*See* gender expression.

Gendered society—Gender is a backdrop and major organizing principle for how individuals organize their lives. Men and women are expected to think and act differently, fill different roles, and thus are treated differently in this society.

Genetic amniocentesis—Amniocentesis is performed between 15- and 20-weeks' gestation for the purposes to obtain a fetal chromosomal analysis and amniotic fluid AFP.

Gestation—The time from conception to birth when the embryo or fetus is developing in the uterus.

Gravid—Pregnant.

Gummas—Granulomas that are a result of tertiary syphilis. These granulomas may involve multiple organs including the respiratory tract, gastrointestinal tract, and bones but not limited to these areas.

hCG—Human chorionic gonadotropin (hCG) begins to increase in the maternal serum following successful implantation of the embryo into the uterine lining. Increased levels of hCG are associated with Down syndrome while low levels of hCG (along with low MSAFP and low uE_3) are associated with trisomy 18.

Health—Culture or individual beliefs that define state of being well or of being balanced emotionally, physically, mentally, socially, and spiritually.

Health literacy—Degree to which individuals have the capacity to obtain, process, and understand basic health information and services needed to make appropriate health decisions.

Hermaphroditism—An older term for intersex; see intersex definition.

Higher-order multiples—Three (triplet) or more fetuses.

HLA (human leukocyte antigens)— HLA is the designation of the major histocompatibility molecules in humans. These molecules are necessary for antigen presentation to T cells for activation of these cells. Some of these molecules are associated with specific autoimmune diseases.

Homocysteine—An amino acid is derived from methionine and is produced as a byproduct of ingesting meat. Elevated concentrations of homocysteine have been associated with an increased risk of cardiovascular disease in certain patient populations.

Hyperandrogenemia—Laboratory evidence of excessive production of androgens, such as increased testosterone concentrations.

Hyperandrogenism—Clinical signs of excessive production of androgens, including hirsutism, acne, and alopecia.

Hyperemesis gravidarum—Excessive vomiting during pregnancy.

Hyperestrinism—A condition marked by the presence of excess estrins.

Hyperstimulation—More than five contractions in 10 minutes or a contraction that lasts 2 minutes or more in duration, or contractions that are of normal duration but occur within 1 minute of each other and may or may not be accompanied by nonreassuring changes in the fetal heart rate pattern.

Hysterectomy—Surgical removal of the uterus.

ICSI—Intracytoplasmic sperm injection. The procedure involves the injection of a sperm into the cytoplasm of an oocyte. It is used in conjunction with IVF in couples with male factor.

Illness—An individual's experience of signs, symptoms, and disability of disease; the state of not being well or the state of imbalance.

In vitro fertilization (IVF)—The process of retrieving oocytes (eggs) from the female and allow then to become fertilized by the sperms in a Petri dish. IVF is usually followed by embryo transfer, a procedure to transfer embryo to the uterus.

Incontinence—Inability of the body to control the evacuative functions.

Infertility—The inability to achieve conception after persistent attempts over a given period of time, usually 1 year.

Informed consent—The willing acceptance of a medical intervention by a patient after adequate disclosure by a healthcare professional of the nature of the intervention with its risks and benefits and alternatives, along with the risks and benefits of those alternatives.

Infracolic omentectomy—Surgical excision of the omentum beneath the transverse colon.

Inhibin-A—The fourth serum protein used in the quad screen. An elevated value is found with Down syndrome. The level of Inhibin-A in the maternal serum does not contribute to the detection rate of trisomy 18.

Insurance— A contract designed to compensate some or all of future services in exchange for a periodic payment/premium.

Interconception care—Efforts to address health status between pregnancies, birth spacing, and intendedness of subsequent conception.

Intersex—Condition in which a person is born with both male and female genitalia or reproductive organs, or with ambiguous genitalia. Previously referred to as hermaphroditism, intersex is now the preferred term.

Intrapartum—During the course of pregnancy.

Intrauterine device (IUD)—A form of contraception that is inserted into the uterus by a medical provider and provides longer term (i.e., 5–10 years) contraception as compared to other available options.

Justice—The ethical principle that is concerned with the equity or fairness of the patterns of the distribution of benefits and harms.

Kallmann syndrome—A syndrome of hypogonadism caused by a deficiency of gonadotropin-releasing hormone (GnRH) secretion from hypothalamus with a defect in smelling ability (anosmia or hyposmia).

Knee valgus—Knee is twisted abnormally outward away from the midline.

Labia majora—The outer lips; fleshy skin folds, partially covered in pubic hair, that extend from the mons veneris downward on either side of the vulva.

Labia minora—The inner lips; hairless, loose folds of skin located between the labia major and immediately flanking the vestibule.

Labor—The presence of uterine contractions of sufficient intensity, frequency, and duration to bring about demonstrable effacement (*thinning*) and dilatation of the cervix.

Lachman test—The patient is placed in the supine position with the knee flexed 30 degrees. The examiner places one of his/her hands on the femur and the other on the tibia. A gentle anterior force is placed on the tibia. The anterior translation of the tibia is noted. This is compared to the uninjured side. A difference of 3 mm from side to side is considered a positive test.

Lanugo—Fine, unpigmented hair that appears on the fetus.

Laparoscopic—Abdominal exploration or surgery employing a type of endoscope called laparoscope.

Laparoscopy—Visual examination of the inside of the abdomen by means of a laparoscope.

Laparotomy—Surgical incision of the abdominal wall.

Left ventricular ejection fraction—Fraction of blood pumped out of the ventricle with each heart beat.

Leiomyoma—A uterine fibroid that is a benign smooth muscle tumor of the uterus.

Leopold's maneuver—Use of four steps in palpating the uterus in order to determine the position and presentation of the fetus.

Lesbian (gay woman)—An identity label used by some women whose primary emotional and sexual attractions are toward other women.

Life stage—A major social and culturally defined period in life. Different theorists may define life stages differently, but childhood, adolescence and adulthood are three commonly understood life stages. Midlife and late life, or old age, are also life stages discussed in recent times. Usually these life stages are marked by particular events, responsibilities, and either social or biological transitions. For instance, the beginning of adolescence is often marked by age 12 or 13 and the start of puberty.

Lifetime risk—Probability of developing or dying of a disease sometime during a person's lifetime.

Lower esophageal sphincter—A ring of smooth muscle fibers at the junction of the esophagus and stomach.

Lp(a)—A type of cholesterol made by the liver consisting of LDL-cholesterol attached to apolipoprotein a. It is generally not responsive to standard drug therapy such as statins.

Lumpectomy—Surgical removal of tumor of the breast; only tumor removed, no tissue or lymph nodes.

Luteal phase—Phase occurring during the second half of the menstrual cycle; begins with lymph nodes and the accumulation of large amounts of lymph in the affected region.

Lymphadenectomy—Excision of the nodes.

Lymphedema—Swelling as result of obstruction or damage of lymphatic vessels or

Macrosomia—Abnormally large body (i.e., big baby syndrome) defined as a birth weight more than 8 lb, 13 oz.

Malformation—The irregular, anomalous, abnormal, or faulty formation of a structure.

Mammogram—X-ray of the breast.

Mastalgia—Pain in the breast.

Mastectomy—Excision of the breast.

Mastitis—Infection of the mammary glands and surrounding tissue characterized by fever, swelling of the breast tissue, and pain.

Maternal serum alpha-fetoprotein (MSAFP)—This was the first serum protein to be identified and used in prenatal diagnosis. Low levels of MSAFP are associated with Down syndrome and trisomy 18. Elevated levels of MSAFP are associated with ONTD and abdominal wall defects.

Matrix metalloproteinases—Group of enzymes that break down proteins such as collagen and are normally found in the spaces between cells in tissues. Matrix metalloproteinases are involved in angiogenesis and other roles.

Mature minor—A person below the age of majority, usually 18, who possesses internal knowledge and intellectual capacity and is sufficiently free from external constraints to be as autonomous as an adult. Generally the presumption is that minors lack the capacity to make medical decisions on their own.

Meiosis—The process whereby the adult chromosome number is reduced (halved) producing haploid gametes.

Menarche—The first menstrual period in a female's life; the onset of menstruation.

Meningoceles—Protrusion from the vertebral canal that contains the neural membranes (meninges).

Menopause—Permanent cessation of menstruation resulting from the loss of follicular activity.

Menorrhagia—Excessively prolonged or profuse menses.

Metaplasia—Conversion of normal tissue to abnormal (cancerous) tissue.

Metastasis—Movement or spread of disease from one organ or part to new location not directly connected.

Metrorrhagia—Irregular, frequent uterine bleeding of varying amounts but not excessive.

Michigan alcoholism screening test (MAST)—Twenty-two question screening tool that can be useful in identifying alcohol dependence.

Micrognathia—Small size of the lower jaw.

Mindfulness-based stress reduction—Brings together mindfulness-based meditation techniques and yoga as a lifestyle intervention to improve overall mental health and well being.

Mittelschmerz—One-sided lower abdominal pain associated with ovulation (can occur before, during, or after ovulation); occurs in 20% of women.

Molimen—Abnormal strain or tension associated with a normal physiological function, especially menstruation.

Monozygotic—Multiple gestations arising from one embryo.

Moral distress—Stress due to ethical dilemmas in which institutional constraints or legal regulations prevent the pharmacist (or other healthcare provider) from acting according to that they consider morally right.

Moral values—Those beliefs or principles used to make personal decisions, based on upbringing, cultural, religious, and societal standards that the person affirms.

Morula—A solid ball of identical ells that results from repeated division of the zygote.

Mosaicism—A condition where an individual has two or more cell populations that differ in genetic makeup.

MTF—Acronym for male-to-female transgender or trans-sexual person. Also *trans woman*. Typically referred to with female pronouns (she, her).

Multiparity—Condition of having given birth to multiple children.

Multiparous—A woman having borne more than one child.

Mutuality—Recognition of the self in others.

Myometrium—The muscular wall of the uterus.

National Institute on Drug Abuse (NIDA)—A federally funded research institution under the National Institute of Health. NIDA provides research support for drug abuse and addiction. More information can be found at their website (http—//www.nida.nih.gov/nidahome.html).

Navicular—A bone of the foot which articulates with the talus and cuneiform bones.

Neural tube defects—Birth defects of the brain and spinal cord. Two most common neural tube defects are spina bifida and anencephaly.

Nondihydropyridine calcium channel blockers—These calcium channel blockers include verapamil and diltiazem, which may slow the heart rate.

Nonmaleficence—The ethical principle that requires us to refrain from harming others.

Normative ethics—The branch of ethical inquiry that considers ethical questions whose answers have a relatively direct bearing on practice.

Nuchal translucency—A measurement of the thickness of the fluid collection at the back of the fetal neck.

Nulliparity—The condition of not having carried a pregnancy to term.

Nurses' Health Study—A large ongoing cohort study first started in 1976 that has produced data on the major risk factors for many chronic diseases such as diabetes and cardiovascular disease in women.

Oligoovulation—Irregular ovulation frequently noted by irregular menstrual cycles (eight or fewer menstrual cycles per year).

Omentum—Double fold of peritoneum that attaches stomach to abdominal viscera.

Oncotic—Caused or marked by swelling.

Oocyte—One of several stages in the production of a mature ovum. The primary oocyte will undergo the first meiotic division. The secondary oocyte will undergo the second meiotic division.

Oogenesis—The process whereby the female sex cell, the ovum, is formed.

Oogonia—A germ cell that differentiates into an oocyte in the ovary.

Optic neuritis—Inflammation of the optic nerve, which can lead to partial or total loss of vision.

Optimal cytoreduction (debulking)—No residual tumor mass larger than 1–2 cm in diameter.

Orgasm—Rhythmic contractions of the uterus, vagina, and pelvic muscles.

Orthographic language—The aspect of language concerned with the sequence of letters and words.

Osteophytes—A pathological bony enlargement.

Ovarian hyperstimulation syndrome (OHSS)—A condition usually associated with the use of gonadotropin. The ovary becomes massively enlarged because it contains many follicles. Changes in fluid dynamics (caused by vasoactive factors by the ovaries) causes intravascular fluid to move to the third space (such as abdominal cavity, pleural cavity) and results in hemoconcentration. It can be a life-threatening condition.

Palpebral fissures—Opening for the eyes between the eyelids.

Pancolitis—Inflammation involving the majority of the colon in patients with inflammatory bowel disease.

Papanicolaou (Pap) smear—Cytology sampling test of the surface of the cervix for early detection of cancer cells.

PAPP-A and free or total β-hCG—Serum proteins used in conjunction with NT in first trimester screening to calculate the risk of Down syndrome, trisomy 18, trisomy 13, or other chromosomal abnormalities. First trimester screening takes place between 10–13 weeks.

Parametria—The extension of the subserous coat of the supracervical part of the uterus laterally between the layers of the broad ligament. Each of them contains part of the ureter, uterine vessels, nerves, and lymphatic tissue.

Parturition—Giving birth.

PCOS—Polycystic ovary syndrome. It was first described by Stein and Leventhal in the 1940s. The syndrome consists of hyperandrogenism (excess male hormone), irregular periods (or no period), and enlarged ovaries with multiple follicles beneath the ovarian surface. PCOS is usually associated with obesity and infertility; it also has long-term health effects such as heart disease.

Pelvic exenteration—Removal of the urinary bladder, distal ureter, vagina, uterus, adnexa, rectum, anus, and adjacent lymph nodes; renders a colostomy and urinary diversion or substitution necessary.

Pelvic varicocele (pelvic congestion syndrome)—Dilatation of the pampiniform plexus veins (which drains into the ovarian and uterine trunks).

Perfect use failure rate—The rate at which pregnancies occur in 1 year when a contraceptive method is used perfectly; product failure not user failure.

Perimenopause—The time leading up to menopause, usually characterized by irregular menstrual bleeding.

Perinatal mortality—Loss of a fetus after 20 weeks of gestation or loss of neonate up until 28 days of life.

Peritoneal lavage—The washing out of the peritoneal cavity with copious injections and rejections of fluid.

Philtrum—Vertical groove in the upper lip.

Phocomelia—A congenital condition that results in the absence of upper arm(s) and/or upper leg(s). This results in hands and/or feet being attached directly to the trunk by short stump(s). This abnormality is rare, but it is a major side effect noted in the offspring of women who have taken the medication thalidomide during early pregnancy.

Phonologic language—The acoustic transmission and perception of the sound of speech.

Phonophobia—Sensitivity to sounds and loud noises.

Photophobia—Abnormal sensitivity to or intolerance of light.

Placenta previa—Occurs during pregnancy when the placenta implants in the lower part of the uterus and is close to or covering the cervical opening to the vagina.

Placental abruption—Separation of the placenta from the site of uterine implantation before delivery of the fetus.

Platinum-refractory disease—Disease that does not respond or progresses during platinum treatment.

Platinum-resistant disease—Disease recurring <6 months after last platinum therapy.

Pluripotent—Cells that are capable of forming many cell type. After formation of the trophoblast, embryoblast cells become pluripotent, having lost the ability for extraembryonic membrane formation.

Plyometrics—An exercise in which muscles are stretched quickly and repeatedly and then contracted such as when jumping from an elevated platform to the ground.

Polyploidy—Possession of more than two sets of chromosomes per nucleus.

Polyspermy—Fertilization of the egg by more than one sperm.

Positive predictive value—Probability of disease among patients with a positive test.

Postcoital—The time following sexual intercourse.

Posterior cul-de-sac obliteration—Cancellation of the pouch of Douglas due to adhesions.

Postterm pregnancy—Pregnancy that has extended to or beyond 42 weeks of gestation (294 days from the last menstrual period).

Preconception care—A set of interventions that aim to identify and modify biomedical, behavioral, and social risks to a woman's health or pregnancy outcome through prevention and management.

Preeclampsia—A condition occurring after the 20th week pregnancy that is characterized by an abrupt onset of hypertension, albuminuria/proteinuria, and edema.

Prenatal diagnosis—Broad term that involves detecting the presence of a chromosomal or structural abnormality in the fetus prior to birth.

Preterm labor—Regular contractions associated with cervical change before the completion of 37 weeks of gestation.

Primary amenorrhea—Absence of menses in a girl who has reached the age of 16 years

Primary prevention—Efforts to reduce the development of disease such as a first myocardial infarction.

Primigravid—A woman during her first pregnancy.

Primigravida—First time pregnancy.

Privacy—Ability of individuals to protect and control information about themselves.

Proctitis—Inflammation confined to the rectal area in patients with inflammatory bowel disease.

Profession—A discipline or practice that involves a distinct body of knowledge used for the public good, and whose members act with extensive autonomy. In consequence to this freedom and expertise, practitioners have special moral obligations to subordinate their own interests in favor of those of their clients or patients.

Progestin-only EC—A form of postcoital contraception containing levonorgestrel (LNG) but not estrogen (i.e., Plan B™).

Prostaglandins—Naturally occurring hormone-like lipid compounds derived from fatty acids, which participate in a wide range of body functions. They are mediators with a variety of strong physiological effects.

Psychosocial perspective—The psychological and social factors that influence one's health, wellbeing, and healing. A psychosocial perspective is a lens that highlights the things in society that will influence women's health-related behavior positively or negatively that are not a fact of their different physiology or biology. For instance, a psychosocial perspective could help illustrate how gender norms affect women's beliefs about their bodies and their health.

Puerperium—The period between childbirth and the return of the uterus to its normal size.

Pulmonary embolism—Embolism of a pulmonary artery or one of its branches that is produced by foreign matter and most often a blood clot originating in a vein of the leg or pelvis.

Quickening—The conventional term used to denote movement of the fetus when felt by the pregnant woman.

Radiofrequency ablation—A procedure in which electrodes are used to destroy abnormal tissue.

Raynaud's phenomenon—Abnormal spasms in the blood vessels, leading to peripheral vasoconstriction with a diminished blood supply to the local tissues, especially the extremities. Initially, the involved tissue(s) turn white because of the diminished blood supply and then turn blue because of prolonged lack of oxygen. When the blood vessels reopen there is a local flushing causing the tissues to become red.

Reciprocity—The willingness and ability to look at a situation from another's point of view and to take that point of view into account when making your own choices.

Reiter syndrome—Occurs as a result of a number of infectious agents including Chlamydia, which results is an acute or chronic triad of symptoms including postinfectious arthritis, urethritis, and conjunctivitis.

Reproductive health—More than maternal or sexual health. It is also more than just a set of problems or illnesses women might face because of their biological capacities to bear children. The World Health Organization defines reproductive health very broadly as a state of physical, mental, and social well-being in all matters relating to the reproductive system at all stages of life.

Retroverted uterus—A uterus that is tilted toward the back of the pelvis.

Return to Fertility—The amount of time that is takes for the ability to conceive after discontinuing a contraceptive method.

Rheumatoid factors—Autoantibodies directed to the Fc region of the IgG molecule.

Rheumatoid nodules—Firm, nontender nodules that develop subcutaneous in patients with RA. The nodules are generally found at pressure points, such as the elbow, back of the forearm, and metacarpophalangeal joint.

Rose bengal test—A method of evaluating patients for dry eye syndrome. The rose bengal dye, when applied to the surface of the eye, stains damaged epithelial cells. When epithelial cells take up the stain, this is positive for a diagnosis of dry eyes.

Russell's sign—Scarring of the dorsum of the hand or on the knuckles due to self-induced vomiting.

Sandwich generation—Adult persons, usually middle-aged women, who are simultaneously caring for young children and older parents. That is, they are "sandwiched" between two generations that are dependent on them for regular care.

Schirmer's test—A test for dry eyes and involves placing a thin tear strip (paper) inside the lower eyelid for a given interval of time (usually 5 minutes). The tear strip is then removed and the length of the strip that is wet from tears is measured and compared to a standard. Individuals with dry eye syndrome will have less wetting of the tear strip than normal controls.

Scleroderma—An autoimmune disease of connective tissue characterized excessive deposits of collagen and scar tissue formation (fibrosis) in the skin and organs.

Second trimester screening (triple screen or quad screen)—Screening for Down syndrome, trisomy 18, and open neural tube defects that is performed between 15- to 20- weeks' gestation.

Secondary amenorrhea—Cessation of menses in a woman previously menstruating for at least 6 months.

Secondary prevention—Efforts to reduce the risk of developing a second events such as a recurrent myocardial infarction.

Self-management—A rational, cognitive-behavioral approach to change, specifically defined as individual degrees of exercise and fitness, nutrition, coping, health screenings, and lifestyle choices to increase balance in a woman's life.

Semantic language—The meaning of spoken words and speech.

Sensitivity—Probability of a positive test among patients with disease.

Serotonin syndrome—A potentially life-threatening medication reaction that causes the body to have too much serotonin. Symptoms include rapid changes in vital signs (fever, oscillations in blood pressure), sweating, nausea, vomiting, rigid muscles, myoclonus, agitation, delirium, seizures, and coma.

Severe preeclampsia—New onset hypertension and proteinuria in pregnancy that is also associated with signs and symptoms of end organ involvement.

Sex—The biologic classification of a person determined by chromosomes; a woman (female) is XX and a man (male) is XY.

Sex confirmation surgery—Also known as sex reassignment surgery; procedure(s) in which the body is altered to bring it into alignment with a person's gender identity.

Sex discrimination—Inequitable treatment based on gender and includes discriminatory hiring and promotion practices, salary differentials, and sexual harassment.

Sexual attraction—Feelings of sexual desire and/or fantasy, which may or may not relate to sexual behavior.

Sexual behavior—Behavioral aspect of sexuality, distinct from sexual identity and attraction. These dimensions are not always congruent (e.g., some women who have sex with women do not label themselves as lesbian or bisexual).

Sexual harassment—A wide array of offensive behavior of a sexual nature, often in the workplace; including acts of coercion, psychological bullying, and more violent activities such as forced sexual activity.

Sexual identity—How people label themselves with regard to their sexuality (e.g., lesbian, heterosexual, asexual, etc.).

Sexual minority—An umbrella term used to describe those whose sexual identity, behavior, or attraction renders them a minority in a predominantly heterosexual population,

Sexual orientation—One aspect of a person's sexuality, involving sexual attraction, sexual identity, and sexual behavior.

Sheehan's syndrome—A syndrome of panhypopituitarism due to infarction of the pituitary gland mainly caused by severe postpartum bleeding and shock.

Situs inversus—Organs of chest and abdomen are arranged in mirror image reversal of normal positioning.

Sleep apnea—The temporary cessation of breathing during sleep; can be caused by narrowing of the airways resulting from swelling of soft tissue.

Socioeconomic status (SES)—A broad concept referring to the placement of persons, families, households, and census (land) tracts or other aggregates with respect to the capacity to create or consume goods valued in our society. SES encompasses basic elements related to the characteristics of the individual and of the individual's environment such as age, gender, race, ethnicity, marital status, income level, education, insurance coverage, access-to-care, occupation, place of residence, and number of children.

Specificity—Probability of a negative test among patients without disease.

Spermatogenesis—The process whereby the male sex cell, the spermatozoan is formed.

Spina bifida—A neural tube defect due to incomplete closure of the embryonic neural tube resulting in an incompletely formed spinal cord and exposure of the vertebral column.

Stakeholder—A person or entity who can influence or be influenced by a decision, such as a healthcare decision.

Steatorrhea—Excess fat in the stools.

Steatosis—Fatty degeneration of the liver.

Stents—Tiny metal mesh tubes placed in an artery to keep it open; stents may either be bare metal or drug-eluting in which drugs such as sirolimus or paclitaxel are released to maintain patency.

Stricture—A narrowing of the intestinal lumen secondary to build up of scar tissue as a result of longstanding inflammation.

Substance abuse—A diagnostic term defined as maladaptive pattern of substance use, which results in clinically significant impairment as manifested by one (or more) specific criteria within a 12-month period. Examples of criteria include repeated substance use resulting in a failure to fulfill major role obligations at work, school, or home, during physically hazardous situations or despite substance-related legal problems.

Substance dependence—A diagnostic term defined as a maladaptive pattern of substance use, which results in clinically significant impairment as manifested by three (or more) of specific criteria and having occurred at any time in the same 12-month period. Criteria include development of tolerance or withdrawal; consuming larger amounts over a longer period than intended; persistent desire to reduce use; spending excessive amount of time seeking, using, or recovering from substance; reduction in social, occupation, or recreational activities; and continued use despite knowledge of recurrent physical or psychological problems.

Superficial thrombophlebitis—Superficial inflammation of a vein with formation of a clot.

Supraventricular tachyarrhythmia—An arrhythmia consisting of rapid, irregular heart beats where the impulses originate above the ventricles.

Synovitis—Inflammation of the synovial membrane of the joints.

Teratogen—A drug or other substance capable of interfering with the development of a fetus thereby resulting in various congenital anomalies.

Teratology—The study of the etiology and prevention of malformations and abnormal.

Thelarche—The start of breast development in a female at the beginning of puberty.

Thromboembolism—The blocking of a blood vessel by a particle that has broken away from a blood clot at its site of formation.

Torsades de pointes—A form of ventricular tachycardia characterized by a long QT interval.

Total abdominal hysterectomy, salpingo-oophorectomy (TAHBSO)— Surgical removal of the uterus along with the ovaries and oviducts through the abdomen.

Transgender—An umbrella term for persons whose gender identity or gender expression is not congruent with their birth sex, including those who identify with neither (or both) female and male sex.

Transsexual—A transgender person who has transitioned to the other sex or who wishes to. Not all transsexual people access medical services (such as hormones or surgery).

Transverse lie—Lying at right angles to the long axis of the body

Trigeminal neuralgia—A disorder of the trigeminal nerve (the nerve that enervates the face and jaw), which results in episodes of intense pain of the lips, eyes, nose, scalp, and jaw.

Trophoblast—The outer layer of the embryonic blastocyst that will form the fetal contribution to the placenta.

Troponin—A protein with three isotypes (I, T, and C) that is released from dead and injured cells in heart muscle and is increased during a heart attack.

Tubal ligation—Surgical process of tying up the fallopian tubes to prevent passage of ova from the ovaries to the uterus.

Turner's syndrome—A genetic disorder caused by missing of an X-chromosome in female (45, XO) characterized by underdeveloped gonads, primary amenorrhea, infertility, short stature, webbed neck, shield chest, low hairline, low-set ears, heart defects, skeletal abnormalities, and kidney problems. Clinical features vary among affected females.

TWEAK—A five-question tool designed to screen women for risk drinking during pregnancy.

Typical use failure rate—The rate at which pregnancies occur in 1 year when due to the inability of the user to use the contraceptive method properly; user failure in addition to product failure.

Unconjugated estriol—A placentally derived steroid hormone in which low levels are associated with Down syndrome.

Unilateral salpino-oophorectomy—Surgical removal of a single ovary and fallopian tube.

Unintended pregnancy—Pregnancies that are identified by the mother as either unwanted or mistimed at the time of conception.

Universal healthcare— A guarantee of basic healthcare to all in the context of a nation's citizens.

Uterine fibroids (myomata or leiomyomata)—A type of benign growth that can protrude from the lining of the uterus.

Uterine retroversion in fixed position—Congenital or acquired condition in which the uterus is retroverted and loses its normal mobility.

Utilitarianism—The consequentialist ethical theory that asserts the morally correct action in any situation is the one that maximized goods and minimizes harms for all concerned.

Values—Deeply held beliefs that should be evident in one's actions.

Vascular endothelial growth factor (VEGF)—A subfamily of growth factors that are important signaling proteins involved in the formation and growth of blood vessels. The most important member is VEGF-A.

Vasocongestion—Swelling of tissue caused by pooling of blood.

Veracity—The ethical principle that requires honesty in human interactions.

Vermillion border—Red margin of the upper and lower lip.

Vestibule—The space between the left and right labia minora.

Violence against women—The United Nation's Declaration on the Elimination of Violence against Women (1993) defines violence against women as "any act of gender-based violence that results in, or is likely to result in, physical, sexual or mental harm or suffering to women, including threats of such acts, coercion or arbitrary deprivation of liberty, whether occurring in public or in private life."

Vulva—The female external genitalia.

Wellness—Philosophy of life and personal hygiene that views health as not merely absence of disease but the fullest realization of one's physical and mental potential, as achieved through positive attitudes, fitness training, a diet low in fat and high in fiber, and avoidance of unhealthful practices.

Wilson's disease—A genetic disorder in which copper accumulates in body tissues such as the liver initially, as well as the brain, eyes, and kidneys.

Withdrawal bleed—Menstrual bleeding that occurs when hormones are discontinued.

Women of reproductive age—Refers to women between the ages of 15 and 49 years.

Workforce—Number of women and men available for employment in professional, technical, healthcare, clerical, and service jobs.

Zona pellucida—A thick, noncellular membrane that surrounds the maturing oocyte.

Zygote—A single celled, fertilized egg.

LABORATORY REFERENCE VALUES

Lab Test	Reference Range Traditional Units	Conversion Factor	Reference Range SI Units	Comment
A1C	4% to 6%	(A1C%–2.15) × 10.93	20–42 mmol/mol	
Absolute neutrophil count	<1,500 cells/mm^3			ANC
Anticyclic citrullinated peptide antibody	<20 IU/mL	1	<20 kIU/L	Anti-CCP
Antinuclear antibody	<1:80 or negative	Same	<1:80 or negative	ANA
Anti-T4-binding globulin	<20 IU/mL	1	<20 kIU/L	Anti-TBG
Antithyroid peroxidase	<10 IU/mL	1	<10 kIU/L	Anti-TPO
C3 complement	70–160 mg/dL	0.01	0.7–1.6 g/L	C3
C4 complement	20–40 mg/dL	0.01	0.2–0.4 g/L	C4
Cancer antigen 125	<35 IU/mL	1	<35 kIU/L	CA-125
CD4 (T cell subpopulation)	42% to 59% or 580–1,929 mm^3	1	580–1,929 mm^3	CD4
C-peptide	0.5–4.5 ng/mL	0.33	0.17–1.5 nmol/L	
C-reactive protein	<0.9 mg/dL	10	9 mg/L	CRP
Antidouble strand DNA antibody	<1:10 or negative	same	<1:10 or negative	dsDNA
Erythrocyte sedimentation rate (female)	≤30 mm/hr	1	≤30 mm/hr	ESR
Estradiol				E2
Prepubertal	<8 pg/mL	3.671	29.4 pmol/L	
Early follicular phase	10–100 pg/mL	3.671	36.7–367.1 pmol/L	
Pre ovulatory/late follicular phase	100–400 pg/mL	3.671	367.1–1,468.4 pmol/L	
Luteal phase	15–260 pg/mL	3.671	55.1–954.5 pmol/L	
Postmenopausal	<14–35 pg/mL	3.671	51.4–128.5 pmol/L	
Estriol (serum; pregnancy)				E3
28–31 weeks	3–13.6 ng/mL	3.467	10.4–47.2 nmol/L	
32–35 weeks	3.6–15.5 ng/mL	3.467	12.5–53.7 nmol/L	
36–37 weeks	4.6–18 ng/mL	3.467	15.9–62.4 nmol/L	
38–40 weeks	5.4–19.8 ng/mL	3.467	18.7–68.6 nmol/L	
Estrone				E1
1–10 days of cycle	43–180 pg/mL	3.7	160–665 pmol/L	
11–20 days of cycle	75–196 pg/mL	3.7	275–725 pmol/L	
20–39 days of cycle	131–201 pg/mL	3.7	485–745 pmol/L	

(Continued on next page)

Lab Test	Reference Range Traditional Units	Conversion Factor	Reference Range SI Units	Comment
Ferritin	18–300 ng/mL	1	18–300 mcg/L	
Follicle stimulating hormone		1		FSH
Follicular phase	2.5–10.2 mIU/mL		2.5–10.2 IU/L	
Midcycle	3.4–33.2 mIU/mL	1	3.4–33.2 IU/L	
Luteal phase	1.5–9.1 mIU/mL	1	1.5–9.1 IU/L	
Pregnancy	<0.3 mIU/mL	1	<0.3 IU/L	
Postmenopausal	23.0–116.3 mIU/mL	1	23.0–116.3 IU/L	
Hematocrit (female)	36% to 44%	0.01	0.36–0.44	HCT
High density lipoprotein	>45 mg/dL	0.0259	>1.17 mmol/L	HDL
Human chorionic gonadotrophin (urine)				HCG
Nonpregnant	<5 mIU/mL	1	<5 IU/L	
Pregnant 0.2–1 week	5–50 mIU/mL	1	5–50 IU/L	
Pregnant 1–2 weeks	50–500 mIU/mL	1	50–500 IU/L	
Pregnant 2–3 weeks	100–5,000 mIU/mL	1	100–5,000 IU/L	
Pregnant 3–4 weeks	500–10,000 mIU/mL	1	500–10,000 IU/L	
Pregnant 4–5 weeks	10,000–50,000 mIU/mL	1	10,000–50,000 IU/L	
Pregnant 5–6 weeks	10,000–100,000 mIU/mL	1	10,000–100,000 IU/L	
Pregnant 6–8 weeks	15,000–200,000 mIU/mL	1	15,000–200,000 IU/L	
Pregnant 2–3 months	10,000–100,000 mIU/mL	1	10,000–100,000 IU/L	
International Ratio	1	1	1	INR
Luteinizing hormone				LH
Follicular phase	1.9–12.5 mIU/mL	1	1.9–12.5 IU/L	
Midcycle	8.7–76.3 mIU/mL	1	8.7–76.3 IU/L	
Luteal phase	0.5–16.9 mIU/mL	1	0.5–16.9 IU/L	
Pregnancy	<1.5 mIU/mL	1	<1.5 IU/L	
Postmenopausal	5.0–52.3 mIU/mL	1	5.0–52.3 IU/L	
Low density lipoprotein	50–190 mg/dL	0.0259	1.3–4.91 mmol/L	LDL
Mean corpuscular hemoglobin	25–35 pg/cell	1	25–35 pg/cell	MCH
Mean corpuscular hemoglobin concentration	31–37 g/dL	10	310–370 g/L	MCHC
Mean corpuscular volume (female)	78–102 mm^3	1	78–102 fL	MCV
Platelet	130–400 × $10^3/mm^3$	1	130–400 × 10^9/L	
Progesterone				
Follicular phase	ND–0.7 ng/mL	3.18	ND– 2.2 nmol/L	
Midluteal phase	3.5–25 ng/mL	3.18	11.1–79.5 nmol/L	
Luteal phase	2.3–25 ng/mL	3.18	7.3–79.5 nmol/L	
Postmenopausal	ND–0.7 ng/mL	3.18	ND–2.2 nmol/L	
Prolactin (normal menstruation)	<25 ng/mL	1	<20 mcg/L	
Proteinuria	<150 mg/day	1	<150 mg/day	

(*Continued on next page*)

Lab Test	Reference Range Traditional Units	Conversion Factor	Reference Range SI Units	Comment
Reactive rapid plasma reagin	Nonreactive	Same	Nonreactive	RPR
Rheumatoid factor	<1:40 or negative	Same	<1:40 or negative	RF
Sex hormone binding globulin	40–120 nmol/L	1	40–120 nmol/L	SHBG
Testosterone (free; female)				
20–40 yr	0.6–3.1 pg/mL	34.67	20.8–107.5 pmol/L	
41–60 yr	0.4–2.5 pg/mL	34.67	13.9–86.7 pmol/L	
61–80 yr	0.2–2.0 pg/mL	34.67	6.9–69.3 pmol/L	
Testosterone (total; female)	6–86 ng/dL	0.03467	0.21–2.98 nmol/L	
Thyroid antithyroid globulin antibody	<1:400	Same	<1:400	
Thyroid peroxidase antibody	<1:100	Same	<1:100	
Thyroid stimulating hormone	0.25–4.3 μIU/mL	1	0.25–4.3 mIU/L	TSH
Thyroid stimulating immunoglobulin	130% basal activity			
Thyroglobulin antibody	0–2.0 IU/mL	1	0–2.0 kIU/L	
Total cholesterol/high density lipoprotein ratio	<4.0	Same	<4.0	TC/HDL
Triglycerides	40–150 mg/dL	0.0113	0.45–1.69 mmol/L	TG
White blood cell count	4.5–11 × 10^3/mm^3	1	4.5–11 × 10^9/L	WBC

ND = not detected.

INDEX

A

B

C

D

E

F

G

H

I

J

K

L

M

N

O

P

Q

R

S

T

U

W

Z